FREDERIC J. KOTTKE, M.D.

Professor,
Department of Physical Medicine and Rehabilitation,
University of Minnesota Medical School,
Minneapolis, Minnesota

G. KEITH STILLWELL, M.D.

Professor,
Department of Physical Medicine and Rehabilitation,
Mayo Clinic,
Rochester, Minnesota

JUSTUS F. LEHMANN, M.D.

Professor and Chairman,
Rehabilitation Medicine Department,
University of Washington,
Seattle, Washington

Krusen's Handbook of Physical Medicine and Rehabilitation

Third Edition

1982

W. B. SAUNDERS COMPANY

*Philadelphia / London / Toronto
Mexico City / Rio de Janeiro
Sydney / Tokyo*

W. B. Saunders Company: West Washington Square
Philadelphia, PA 19105

1 St. Anne's Road
Eastbourne, East Sussex BN21 3UN, England

1 Goldthorne Avenue
Toronto, Ontario M8Z 5T9, Canada

Apartado 26370 — Cedro 512
Mexico 4, D.F., Mexico

Rua Coronel Cabrita, 8
Sao Cristovao Caixa Postal 21176
Rio de Janeiro, Brazil

9 Waltham Street
Artarmon, N.S.W. 2064, Australia

Ichibancho, Central Bldg., 22-1 Ichibancho
Chiyoda-Ku, Tokyo 102, Japan

Library of Congress Cataloging in Publication Data

Main entry under title:

Krusen's Handbook of physical medicine and rehabilitation

Third ed. of: Handbook of physical medicine and rehabilitation.
2nd ed. 1971.

1. Medicine, Physical.   2. Physically handicapped —
   Rehabilitation.   I. Krusen, Frank Hammond, 1898–
   1973.   II. Kottke, Frederic J.   III. Stillwell,
   G. Keith.   IV. Lehmann, Justus F.   V. Handbook
   of physical medicine and rehabilitation.   [DNLM:
   1. Rehabilitation.   2. Physical medicine.
   WB 460 K942]

RM700.K74 1982   615.8   81-48403

ISBN 0-7216-5501-7   AACR2

Listed here is the latest translated edition of this book together with the language of the translation and
the publisher.

Japanese (2nd Edition) — Ishiyaku Publishers, Inc., Bunkyo-kiu, Tokyo, Japan

Spanish (2nd Edition) — Salvat Editores, S.A., Barcelona, Spain

Krusen's Handbook of Physical Medicine and Rehabilitation   ISBN 0-7216-5501-7

Last digit is the print number: 9   8   7   6   5   4   3   2   1

DEDICATION

The title of the third edition of this Handbook has been changed to *Krusen's Handbook of Physical Medicine and Rehabilitation* in dedication to Frank Hammond Krusen, under whose editorship this textbook was first written. Dr. Krusen was a great teacher and leader, and an inspiration to young physicians entering the field of physical medicine and rehabilitation. He recognized that physical medicine and rehabilitation would become an integral part of medical practice only to the extent that the knowledge and skills of this specialty become incorporated in medical education. As a consequence, he devoted his time and energy mainly to research to increase knowledge of the specialty and to the education of physicians and others in the rehabilitation professions. In 1941 he authored *Physical Medicine* (Philadelphia, W. B. Saunders Co.) as the first general textbook on physical medicine in this country. Over the next six years he worked with John S. Coulter, Walter J. Zeiter, Kristian G. Hansson, Howard A. Rusk, and others to establish the American Board of Physical Medicine and Rehabilitation under the auspices of the American Board of Medical Specialties in 1947. These founders of the medical specialty emphasized that physical medicine and rehabilitation are essential components of comprehensive medicine and that handicapped patients have not had full treatment until they have been rehabilitated to their optimal level of performance.

Under Dr. Krusen's leadership in 1958 a number of academic physiatrists, many of whom had been students of his, began to meet periodically and formed a policy advisory group called the American Rehabilitation Foundation (ARF) Medical Committee. The Handbook first evolved in 1965 from the deliberations of this committee. The ARF Medical Committee has continued to meet each year to consider current issues related to educational needs in rehabilitation medicine.

CONTRIBUTORS

MICHAEL A. ALEXANDER, M.D.

Clinical Assistant Professor of Pediatrics and Orthopedics, University of Pittsburgh, Pittsburgh, Pennsylvania. Clinical Assistant Professor of Physical Medicine, Ohio State University, Columbus, Ohio. Medical Director, D. T. Watson Rehabilitation Hospital for Children, Sewickley, Pennsylvania

Management of Motor Unit Diseases

THOMAS P. ANDERSON, M.D.

Professor of Physical Medicine and Rehabilitation, University of Minnesota Medical School, Minneapolis. Staff Physiatrist, University of Minnesota Hospitals, Minneapolis, Minnesota.

Rehabilitation of Patients with Completed Stroke

GARY T. ATHELSTAN, Ph.D.

Professor, Physical Medicine and Rehabilitation and Psychology, University of Minnesota Medical School, Minneapolis. Director, Counseling Psychology Service, University of Minnesota Hospitals, Minneapolis, Minnesota.

Vocational Assessment and Management

LEONARD F. BENDER, M.D., M.S.

Professor and Chairman, Department of Physical Medicine and Rehabilitation, Wayne State University School of Medicine, Detroit, Michigan. President and Chief Executive Officer, Rehabilitation Institute, Detroit. Chief of Service, Department of Physical Medicine and Rehabilitation, Detroit Receiving Hospital and University Health Center, Detroit. Active Medical Staff, Harper-Grace Hospital, Detroit. Consultant, Sinai Hospital and Children's Hospital of Michigan, Detroit, and Veterans Administration Hospital, Allen Park, Michigan.

Upper Extremity Orthotics; Upper Extremity Prosthetics

DAVID R. BEUKELMAN, Ph.D.

Associate Professor of Rehabilitation Medicine, University of Washington School of Medicine, Seattle. Director of Speech Pathology Services, University of Washington Hospital, Seattle, Washington.

Speech and Language Disorders

RITA BISTEVINS, M.D., Ph.D., F.R.C.P.(C)

Clinical Assistant Professor, Department of Physical Medicine and Rehabilitation, University of Minnesota, Minneapolis, Minnesota.

Footwear and Footwear Modifications

RENE CAILLIET, M.D.

Chairman and Professor, Department of Rehabilitation Medicine, University of Southern California School of Medicine, Los Angeles. Chief, Department of Rehabilitation Medicine, Santa Monica Hospital Medical Center, Santa Monica, California.

Spine: Disorders and Deformities

SANDRA S. COLE

Instructor and Health Educator, Department of Psychiatry and Department of Physical Medicine and Rehabilitation, University of Michigan Medical School, Ann Arbor, Michigan.

Rehabilitation of Problems of Sexuality in Physical Disability

THEODORE M. COLE, M.D.

Professor and Chairman, Department of Physical Medicine and Rehabilitation, University of Michigan Medical School, Ann Arbor. Chairman, Department of Physical Medicine and Rehabilitation, University of Michigan Hospitals, Ann Arbor, Michigan.

Goniometry; Rehabilitation of Problems of Sexuality in Physical Disability

BARBARA J. DE LATEUR, M.D.

Professor, Department of Rehabilitation Medicine, University of Washington, Seattle. Chief of Rehabilitation Medicine, Harborview Medical Center, Seattle, Washington.

Diathermy and Superficial Heat and Cold Therapy; Therapeutic Exercise to Develop Strength and Endurance

PAUL M. ELLWOOD, Jr., M.D.

Clinical Professor in Pediatrics, Neurology, and Physical Medicine and Rehabilitation, University of Minnesota Medical School, Minneapolis. President, Interstudy, Minneapolis, Minnesota.

Bed Positioning; Transfers; Prescription of Wheelchairs

GARY FELL, M.D.

Second Assistant, University of Melbourne, Melbourne, Australia. Consultant Surgeon, Austin Hospital, Melbourne, Australia.

Management of Vascular Disease

STEVEN V. FISHER, M.D., M.S.

Assistant Professor of Physical Medicine and Rehabilitation, University of Minnesota Medical School, Minneapolis. Attending Physician, Department of Physical Medicine and Rehabilitation, St. Paul-Ramsey Medical Center, St. Paul, Minnesota.

Spinal Orthoses

WILBERT E. FORDYCE, Ph.D.

Professor of Psychology, Department of Rehabilitation Medicine, University of Washington School of Medicine, Seattle. Attending Physician, University Hospital and Harborview Medical Center, Seattle, Washington.

Psychological Assessment and Management

MURRAY M. FREED, M.D.

Professor and Chairman, Department of Rehabilitation Medicine, Boston University School of Medicine, Boston. Chief, Department of Rehabilitation Medicine, and Director, New England Regional Cord Injury Center, University Hospital, Boston, Massachusetts.

Traumatic and Congenital Lesions of the Spinal Cord

JEROME W. GERSTEN, M.D.

Professor, Physical Medicine and Rehabilitation, University of Colorado School of Medicine, Denver. Active Staff, University Hospital and Spalding Rehabilitation Hospital, Denver. Consulting Staff, Craig Hospital, Englewood, Colorado.

Rehabilitation for Degenerative Diseases of the Central Nervous System

PROFESSOR FRANJO GRAČANIN, M.D., Dr. Sci.

Head, Clinic for Physical Medicine and Rehabilitation, University Hospital Dr. M. Stojanovič, Zagreb, Yugoslavia. Associate Professor, Medical School of University E. Kardelj, Ljubljana, Yugoslavia.

Functional Electrical Stimulation

CARL V. GRANGER, M.D.

Professor of Community Health and of Family Medicine (Physical Medicine and Rehabilitation), Frederick Henry Prince Distinguished Scholar in Physical Medicine and Rehabilitation, Brown University Program in Medicine, Providence, Rhode Island. Director, Institute for Rehabilitation and Restorative Care, The Memorial Hospital, Pawtucket, Rhode Island.

Health Accounting

DANIEL HALPERN, M.D.

Adjunct Professor, Department of Rehabilitation Medicine, University of Wisconsin, Madison, Wisconsin. Attending Physician, University of Wisconsin Hospital and Clinics; Consultant in Rehabilitation Medicine, Madison General Hospital, St. Mary's Hospital, and Methodist Hospital, Madison, Wisconsin.

Rehabilitation of Children with Brain Damage

DAVID HEIMBACH, M.D.

Professor of Surgery, University of Washington, Seattle. Attending Surgeon, University of Washington Hospital and Harborview Medical Center. Consulting Surgeon, U.S. Public Health Hospital,

Veterans Administration Hospital, and Children's Orthopedic Hospital, Seattle, Washington.

Management and Rehabilitation of Burns

H. FREDERIC HELMHOLZ, Jr., M.D.

Associate Professor Emeritus, Mayo Graduate School of Medicine, Rochester, Minnesota.

Rehabilitation of Respiratory Dysfunction

DAVID L. HOOKS, M.Ed., C.R.C.

Clinical Coordinator, Vocational Rehabilitation Unit, Department of Rehabilitation Medicine, University of Washington, Seattle, Washington.

Prevocational Evaluation

MASAYOSHI ITOH, M.D., M.P.H.

Associate Professor of Clinical Rehabilitation Medicine, New York University School of Medicine. Assistant Director, Department of Rehabilitation Medicine, Goldwater Memorial Hospital, New York University Medical Center, New York, New York.

Epidemiology of Disability

ERNEST W. JOHNSON, M.D.

Professor and Chairman, Department of Physical Medicine, The Ohio State University College of Medicine, Columbus. Chief, Division of Physical Medicine and Rehabilitation, Ohio State University Hospitals, Columbus. Consultant, Children's Hospital, Columbus, and Community Hospital, Springfield, Ohio.

Electrodiagnosis; Management of Motor Unit Diseases

MILAND E. KNAPP, M.A., M.D.

Clinical Professor Emeritus, University of Minnesota Medical School, Minneapolis. Member of Staff, Metropolitan Medical Center and Hennepin County Medical Center, Minneapolis, Minnesota.

Massage; Aftercare of Fractures

MICHAEL KOSIAK, M.D.

Assistant Professor, Department of Physical Medicine and Rehabilitation, University of Minnesota, Minneapolis. Director, Department of Physical Medicine and Rehabilitation, St. Paul–Ramsey Hospital, St. Paul, Minnesota.

Prevention and Rehabilitation of Ischemic Ulcers

FREDERIC J. KOTTKE, M.D.

Professor, Department of Physical Medicine and Rehabilitation, University of Minnesota Medical School, Minneapolis, Minnesota.

Neurophysiology of Motor Function; Therapeutic Exercise to Maintain Mobility; Therapeutic Exercise to Develop Neuromuscular Coordination; Common Cardiovascular Problems in Rehabilitation

MYRON M. LaBAN, M.D., M.M.Sc.

Clinical Associate Professor, Wayne State University Medical School, Detroit. Director, Department of Physical Medicine and Rehabilitation, William Beaumont Hospital, Royal Oak, Michigan.

Rehabilitation of Patients with Cancer

MATHEW H. M. LEE, M.D., M.P.H.

Professor of Clinical Rehabilitation Medicine, Clinical Professor of Oral and Maxillofacial Surgery, and Clinical Professor of Behavioral Sciences and Community Health, Schools of Medicine and Dentistry, New York University. Director, Department of Rehabilitation Medicine, Goldwater Memorial Hospital, New York University Medical Center, New York, New York.

Epidemiology of Disability

JUSTUS F. LEHMANN, M.D.

Professor and Chairman, Department of Rehabilitation Medicine, University of Washington, Seattle. Chief of Rehabilitation Medicine, University Hospital, Seattle, Washington.

Gait Analysis; Diathermy and Superficial Heat and Cold Therapy; Lower Extremity Orthotics

LOREN R. LESLIE, M.D.

Assistant Professor, University of Minnesota Medical School, Minneapolis. Active Medical Staff, Minneapolis Veterans Administration Medical Center, Minneapolis, Minnesota.

Training for Functional Independence; Training in Homemaking Activities

GORDON M. MARTIN, M.D.

Professor Emeritus of Physical Medicine and Rehabilitation, Mayo Medical School, Rochester, Minnesota. Consultant Emeritus, Department of Physical Medicine and Rehabilitation, Mayo Clinic and Mayo Foundation, Rochester, Minnesota.

Prescribing Physical and Occupational Therapy

MAURICE H. MILLER, Ph.D.

Professor of Speech Pathology and Audiology, New York University. Chief of Audiology, Center for Communication Disorders, Lenox Hill Hospital, New York, New York.

Rehabilitation and Management of Auditory Disorders

JOACHIM L. OPITZ, M.D.

Associate Professor in Physical Medicine and Rehabilitation, Mayo Medical School. Consultant, Department of Physical Medicine and Rehabilitation, Mayo Clinic and Mayo Foundation, Rochester, Minnesota.

Reconstructive Surgery of the Extremities

EDWARD J. O'SHAUGHNESSY, M.D.

Associate Professor, Department of Rehabilitation Medicine, University of Washington School of Medicine, Seattle. Staff Physician, University of Washington Hospital, Harborview Medical Center, and Veterans Administration Hospital, Seattle, and Overlake Hospital, Bellevue, Washington.

Management and Rehabilitation of Burns

INDER PERKASH, M.D., M.S., F.R.C.S. (ENG.-EDIN.)

Paralyzed Veterans of America Professor of Spinal Cord Injuries and Associate Professor of Surgery, Stanford University School of Medicine. Chief, Spinal Cord Injury Center, Veterans Administration Medical Center, Stanford, California.

Management of Neurogenic Dysfunction of the Bladder and Bowel

BERNARD SANDLER, M.D.

Acting Chairman, Department of Physical Medicine and Rehabilitation, Rutgers Medical School, Piscataway, New Jersey. Medical Director, Robert Wood Johnson, Jr., Rehabilitation Institute, John F. Kennedy Medical Center, Edison, New Jersey.

Cranial Nerve Palsies and Brain Stem Syndromes

JEROME D. SCHEIN, Ph.D.

Professor of Deafness Rehabilitation, New York University, New York, New York.

Rehabilitation and Management of Auditory Disorders

G. KEITH STILLWELL, M.D.

Professor of Physical Medicine and Rehabilitation, Mayo Medical School, Rochester, Minnesota. Consultant, Department of Physical Medicine and Rehabilitation, Mayo Clinic and Mayo Foundation, Rochester, Minnesota.

Ultraviolet Therapy; Electrotherapy

WALTER C. STOLOV, M.D.

Professor, Department of Rehabilitation Medicine, University of Washington School of Medicine; Director of Training, Rehabilitation Research and Training Center, NIHR, University of Washington, Seattle. Attending Physician, University Hospital, Harborview Medical Center, and Children's Orthopedic Hospital, Seattle, Washington.

Evaluation of the Patient; Prevocational Evaluation

EMERY K. STONER, M.D., M.Med.Sci. (Phys. Med.)

Clinic Professor of Physical Medicine and Rehabilitation, University of Pennsylvania School of Medicine, Philadelphia. Chief of the Regional Rehabilitation Center of South Jersey at Our Lady of Lourdes Hospital, Camden, New Jersey. Consultant in Physical Medicine and Rehabilitation, Hospital of the University of Pennsylvania, Philadelphia; Underwood Memorial Hospital, Woodbury, New Jersey; and Bryn Mawr Hospital, Bryn Mawr, Pennsylvania.

Management of the Lower Extremity Amputee

HENRY H. STONNINGTON, M.B.B.S., M.S., F.R.C.P.

Associate Professor, Mayo Medical School. Consultant, Physical Medicine and Rehabilitation, Mayo Clinic, Rochester, Minnesota.

Rehabilitation for Respiratory Dysfunction

D. E. STRANDNESS, Jr., M.D.

Professor of Surgery, University of Washington School of Medicine, Seattle. Attending Vascular Surgeon, University Hospital, Seattle, Washington.

Management of Vascular Disease

ROBERT L. SWEZEY, M.D.

Clinical Professor of Medicine, UCLA School of Medicine, Los Angeles. Attending Physician, The

Arthritis and Back Pain Center, Inc., Santa Monica; UCLA Center for Health Sciences, Los Angeles; Saint John's Hospital and Santa Monica Hospital, Santa Monica, California.

Rehabilitation in Arthritis and Allied Conditions

JEROME S. TOBIS, M.D.

Professor, Department of Physical Medicine and Rehabilitation, University of California at Irvine College of Medicine. Attending Physician, University of California at Irvine Medical Center, Irvine, California.

Muscle Testing

CARLOS VALLBONA, M.D.

Professor and Chairman, Department of Community Medicine, and Professor of Rehabilitation and Family Medicine, Baylor College of Medicine, Houston. Chief, Community Medicine Service, Harris County Hospital District; Active Staff, General Medicine Service, Texas Children's Hospital, and Family Medicine Service, St. Luke's Episcopal Hospital; Distinguished Medical Staff, The Institute for Rehabilitation and Research, Houston, Texas.

Bodily Responses to Immobilization

DAVID WIECHERS, M.D.

Assistant Professor, Department of Physical Medicine, Ohio State University College of Medicine, Columbus. Attending Physician, Division of Physical Medicine and Rehabilitation, Ohio State University Hospitals, Columbus. Consultant, Grady Memorial Hospital, Delaware, Ohio.

Electrodiagnosis

HELEN J. YESNER

Professor Emeritus, School of Social Work, University of Minnesota, Minneapolis. Member Health Commission, Rancho Bernardo, San Diego, California.

Psychosocial Diagnosis and Social Services

KATHRYN M. YORKSTON, Ph.D.

Assistant Professor, Department of Rehabilitation Medicine, University of Washington, Seattle. Clinical Chief, Speech Pathology Service, University Hospital, Seattle, Washington.

Speech and Language Disorders

PREFACE

When physical medicine and rehabilitation, or physiatry, was recognized formally as a medical specialty in 1947 by the establishment of the American Board of Physical Medicine and Rehabilitation, comprehensive rehabilitation was not being taught in our medical schools and was practiced in very few civilian centers in the United States. At that time only four years had elapsed since Dr. Howard A. Rusk had conclusively demonstrated to the Army that rehabilitation rather than convalescence was essential to restore soldiers to fitness for return to duty. Only three years previously, because of a nationwide demonstration under the auspices of the American Medical Association of the benefits of early ambulation, doctors in civilian hospitals were just beginning to abandon the time-honored custom of keeping patients bedfast for two to three weeks after abdominal surgery. Although the benefits of early ambulation were striking and patients were beginning to be mobilized more rapidly, physicians were still focusing almost exclusively on identification and eradication of acute pathology, after which patients were allowed to convalesce for weeks or months, and all too frequently to stagnate for years. At that time Dr. Rusk began to refer to rehabilitation as "the third phase of medical care" to be instituted following the first phase, preventive medicine, and the second phase, curative medicine and surgery.[1] He emphasized that "in that period when the 'fever is down and the stitches are out,' in the period 'between the bed and the job,'" the patient should be engaged in an active rehabilitation program rather than in passive convalescence.[2] When rehabilitation was applied in this way it represented a great stride forward. However, only a small minority of chronically disabled patients received rehabilitation as a part of the plan of medical management. All too frequently patients experienced further deterioration rather than recovery of neuromusculoskeletal function during a stage of inactive convalescence. Many months and often years would go by with no evidence of improvement of function. In the mid-1950's the Office of Vocational Rehabilitation reported that the average interval from the onset of a stroke to the referral for rehabilitation services was still four years (compared to experience today that the average time for *completion* of the rehabilitation program after the onset of a stroke is approximately two months).

Much progress has been made because of the teaching and advocacy of Drs. Krusen and Rusk and their students. Rehabilitation medicine is recognized today as a necessary and integral part of the management of chronic diseases and disabilities.[3] Rehabilitation services are being paid for increasingly under the various insurance systems for financing health care. Hospitals, extended care facilities, and nursing homes are seeking rehabilitation services for the chronically ill and disabled. The demands for rehabilitation services are growing faster than professional personnel are being trained. As Dr. Rusk has said, "Rehabilitation of the chronically ill and the chronically disabled is not just a series of restorative techniques; it is a philosophy of medical responsibility. Failure to assume this responsibility means to guarantee the continued deterioration of many less-severely disabled persons until they, too, reach the severely disabled and totally dependent category. The neglect of disability in its early stages is far more costly than an early aggressive program of rehabilitation which will restore the individual "to optimal self-sufficiency and functional performance.[4] The American public—that is the relatives and friends of the chronically ill and disabled—has accepted this philosophy and seeks its application as a part of standard medical care.

That demand for rehabilitation services as indicated by the shortage of rehabilitation personnel appears most promising until it is compared with the relative effort devoted to the teaching of rehabilitation by our medical schools at the present time. Although in numbers more persons need rehabilitation services for significant handicaps resulting from chronic diseases and disabilities than are being admitted to hospitals for treatment of acute diseases, chronic diseases receive only a tiny fraction of the emphasis placed on diagnosis, clinical pathology, and treatment of acute diseases by our medical schools (Fig. 1). Rehabilitation still has not achieved sufficient stature to become an essential part of the education of the medical student. It suffers from the "one-down" effect described by Forman and Hetznecker.[5]

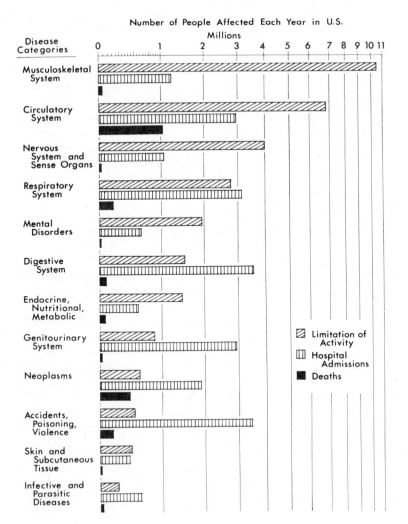

Major Disease Categories
Ranked According to Limitation of Activity

Number of People Affected Each Year in U.S.

FIGURE 1. Two thirds of the persons with limitation of activity, which means significant impairment of self-care, ambulation, or ability to carry on the usual daily activities, have diseases of the musculoskeletal, circulatory, or nervous systems. The incidence of dependency-producing disabilities is not proportional either to annual mortality or to hospital usage by persons in each of the 12 major disease categories.

The medical establishment thrives on short term care and dramatic cures. Sophisticated drug regimens and surgical interventions – the essentials of (acute) medical methodology – are of limited usefulness in the treatment of a handicap. At bottom, the handicapped patient is not particularly attractive in terms of the medical challenge and opportunities he presents. But not only is the handicapped patient "one-down"; so is his physician. . . . The status of the physician is determined, to a major extent, by the status of his patient, and this phenomenon may be described as the "status rub-off effect."

This "one-down" phenomenon pervades the policies of medical education also, so that rehabilitation of the handicapped, although a major problem of our society today, receives only minor attention in the medical curriculum. Only half of the medical schools in the United States have organized departments of physical medicine and rehabilitation. Even those departments are allowed very little time in the curriculum to teach concepts of rehabilitation medicine or procedures and skills. Only 0.5 per cent of medical graduates have been selecting physical medicine and rehabilitation as a specialty for practice. Currently there are only 2200 physiatrists in practice, although 5 to 10 per cent of the total population are estimated to be in need of physical medicine and rehabilitation services at this time. At least three times as many physiatrists would be needed to provide those services. Most other physicians have had little or no training to enable them to use physiatry knowledgeably. Therefore, while the need is great and still increasing, the rate of training of physiatrists and other physicians to practice rehabilitation medicine at present does not indicate that the supply of services will begin to approach the need for services within the next two decades unless a major increase in education in rehabilitation medicine can be achieved.

In the face of this changing pattern of need with the rapid ascendency of chronic diseases and disabilities as major problems, rehabilitation to restore the disabled to optimal levels of performance in society will test the efficiency of medical care in the foreseeable future. However, achievement of efficiency in medical care will require better organization of the resources for provision of health services so that those services are directed toward the return of individuals to the community at optimal functional levels, whether they are disabled by acute illness or by chronic dysfunction. Over the last 50 years medicine and surgery have prevented the deaths of countless persons who were critically ill. Many have been cured. However, there also have been a progressively increasing number left with chronic disabilities. A high proportion of these have not been restored to their optimal levels of functioning in relation to their remaining abilities; multiple sample surveys have estimated that between 5 and 10 per cent of the total population fall into this category of disability. These disabled persons have greatly increased costs for maintenance in addition to the costs of medical care required because of the continuing disability. The costs of dependency resulting from such disabilities have a negative effect on the economy, whether those costs are paid by private or by public funds. In either case dependency consumes resources without enhancing productivity or quality of life for the patient.

The development of rehabilitation as an integral part of comprehensive medical care and its application to restore persons with continuing impairments to the optimal level of performance in their homes and communities will increase the efficiency of our system of health care, as measured by cost-benefit analysis. Just as we do for other modern industries and services, we need to relate the costs involved to the product obtained from medical care. This product is the outcome of medical care as measured by the effect on the life of the patient. There is an economic efficiency to be considered and also a human efficiency.

$$\text{Economic Efficiency} = \frac{\text{Benefits Obtained}}{\text{Investment}}$$

$$= \frac{(P + C_{\bar{s}R} - C_{\bar{\tau}R})\, T - C_R}{C_R}$$

where P = vocational productivity
$C_{\bar{s}R}$ = cost of care and maintenance without rehabilitation
$C_{\bar{\tau}R}$ = cost of care and maintenance after rehabilitation
C_R = cost of rehabilitation
T = time of survival in years

$$\text{Human Efficiency} = \frac{\text{Actual Performance}}{\text{Optimal Performance}}$$

Too often when economic efficiency of rehabilitation is considered, only vocational productivity rather than savings in the cost of maintenance is taken into account. It is nearly impossible to obtain data regarding the full cost of the unrehabilitated handicapped because support must come from so many sources. However, the data that have become available demonstrate the high efficiency of rehabilitation as a newly emerging component of medical care.[6] The reduction of dependency through rehabilitation is cost effective.

The best measure of the value of medical services is the outcome, measured by the degree of improvement of function and the quality of life of the patient. Outcome should be measured by parameters of patient performance throughout the life span rather than by length of survival. Anderson et al.[7] have developed a general scale of functional outcome of rehabilitation modified from Williamson[8] to assess levels of performance across the entire range from normal to death, as shown in Table 1.

TABLE 1. SCALE OF FUNCTIONAL OUTCOME OF REHABILITATION

1. Normal or asymptomatic
2. Symptomatic
3. Partially independent (more than 50 per cent independent)
4. Partially dependent (more than 50 per cent dependent)
5. Totally dependent
6. Death

This scale focuses on the change of functional performance of the patient as increasing illness or disability increases dependency until death supervenes. Conversely, with rehabilitation the patient moves upward through stages of increasing independence to the optimal level of functional performance. Although the assumption often is true in acute episodic diseases that if patients survive they will return to normal activity, the 30 million persons in the United States with disabilities that influence their life styles attest to the fact that commonly cited statistics on mortality and survival do not present an adequate evaluation of healthfulness or of the need for health services. The development of quantitative scales of functional outcome of medical care which define smaller changes in function would make it possible to provide more precise evaluation of patients throughout the entire range of performance. For all patients the assessment of changes in functional performance should be used to define the benefits of therapy. Programs for

health services should be designed to restore patients to the optimal level of function that they can achieve and sustain in relation to the intrinsic and extrinsic resources available to them.

What is the economic cost of dependency? Currently in the United States 10 million people receive disability payments for assistance in maintaining themselves.[9] This represents 7 per cent of the Gross National Product being devoted to disability payments made to approximately 5 per cent of the population. Among the working population, ages 20 to 65, the disability payments amount to $47.6 billion annually. In addition, medical program expenditures for this same group amount to $13 billion annually. Beyond that, the direct services provided to this group cost $2.4 billion annually. Therefore, the total federal disability-related expenditures for the adult working-age population were $63 billion in 1977 and have been increasing about 35 per cent per year—faster than the cost-of-living increases due to inflation. To understand the full cost of disability we must also add the increased costs of care and maintenance of handicapped children and of the disabled among the geriatric population. For disabled persons the costs of maintenance represent approximately 75 per cent of the direct costs of disability (disregarding loss of earned income).

Maintenance of the disabled has been recognized as a major part of the cost of disability for many years. In 1949, in Hennepin County, Minnesota, Stinson studied the distribution of payments by the county welfare program.[10] Forty-nine per cent of the costs were payments to nursing homes for maintenance of the disabled. Twenty-five per cent of the cost was for acute hospital care. Fifteen per cent of the cost was for physician services, and 10 per cent of the cost was for pharmaceutical and other supplies.

In 1980 the Minnesota Department of Public Welfare reported spending $566 million for Medicaid. Fifty-three per cent of the expenditures went for nursing home care, 14 per cent for care in state hospitals, 14 per cent for acute hospital care, and 2 per cent for hospital outpatient services (Fig. 2). Sixty-seven per cent of these costs were spent on institutional maintenance services. If acute hospital care, physicians, dentists, and pharmacy costs are included as a therapeutic group, 28 per cent of the costs went for those therapeutic services. Usually when

Minnesota medicaid expenditures

Fiscal 1980
Total dollars $566,368,921.00

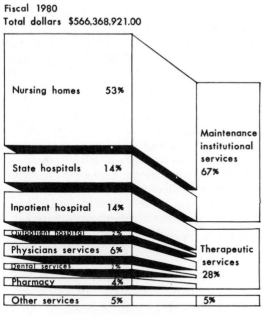

Data:Department of Public Welfare

FIGURE 2. Sixty-seven per cent of expenditures by the state of Minnesota through Medicaid in 1980 were for maintenance of the chronically ill and disabled in nursing homes or chronic care hospitals. (Republished with permission from the Minneapolis Tribune, Dec., 1981.)

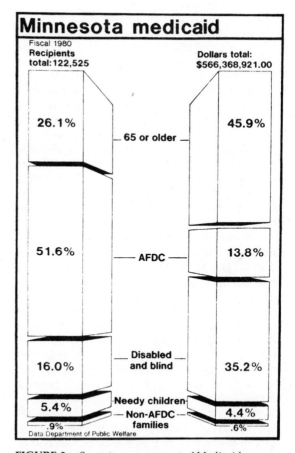

FIGURE 3. Seventy-one per cent of Medicaid expenditures by Minnesota in 1980 provided chronic care for geriatric patients or disabled younger persons. (Republished with permission from the Minneapolis Tribune, Dec., 1981.)

costs of illnesses are calculated, only the costs of therapeutic services are considered and the much higher costs of maintenance services are ignored because, in general, they are paid from other sources. This separation of costs has caused us to fail to recognize the magnitude of potential savings to be obtained through rehabilitation.

Who received these Medicaid services? (Fig. 3). Forty-six per cent of the dollars spent for Medicaid in Minnesota went to the geriatric population. Thirty-five per cent of Medicaid was paid out for services to the disabled and blind of the state. Fourteen per cent of Medicaid was spent for medical services to families with dependent children. In each of these groups there were many individuals who could be made independent or less dependent so that the costs of dependency would be reduced.

The major disease categories leading to dependency have not changed significantly over the last 20 years. Therefore, data from the National Center for Health Statistics in 1972 provide a reasonable representation of our status today. The top 12 major disease

categories presented in Figure 1 are arranged in descending order by (1) prevalence of limitation of activity, and also showing (2) hospital admissions annually and (3) deaths annually. Limitation of activity is defined as significant impairment of ability for self-care, ambulation, or ability to carry on the usual daily activities. Hospital admissions are an approximation of the relative costs of hospital care for these major disease categories. Limitation of activity shows no relationship either to deaths annually or to hospital costs. Note that one third of all disabilities are due to conditions of the musculoskeletal system, especially back problems and disabilities of the joints. Back injury is the most common disability in industry and also the most common of all disabilities in the United States. Limitation of activity due to heart disease, stroke, and peripheral vascular disease is considered under diseases of the circulatory system, which constitute about 21 per cent of all significant disabilities. Disabilities due to diseases of the nervous system and sense organs constitute 12 per cent of all limitation of activity. Disabilities in these three categories of diseases constitute two thirds of all of the disability as measured by limitation of activity in the United States. The physiatrist has been concentrating on and should continue to concentrate on this group of disabilities. However, since physiatrists constitute only 0.5 per cent of physicians in the United States, the impact of rehabilitation services on disabilities is far below the need for services.

Limitation of activity has a highly significant societal impact because it carries with it the major economic costs of dependency maintenance and loss of productivity. However, limitation of activity has not been a major focus of medical education which has concentrated its attention on the major causes of death, the pathologic aspects of disease, and the diagnostic processes by which pathology is identified. Neither has dependency resulting from disability been of major concern for acute medical care services nor for acute hospital care. These resources have been focused on the eradication of pathology that jeopardizes survival or limits the ability to live outside of the hospital, but they have not been committed to carrying the patient through to full restoration.

Why have we not used our health care resources for restoration of patients to optimal functional performance? The reasons are not obvious. In part, it may relate to the historical perspective that less than 100 years ago medical attention was directed almost entirely to survival or relief of pain. Not until

about 60 years ago did we began to develop specific cures for diseases. The development of antibiotics and physiological support systems over the past 40 years has increased the number of disabled persons who survive for many years. Health maintenance has changed from an abstraction to a process for application over the past 15 years. However, we are still groping for parameters to measure the changes that can be achieved in the process of rehabilitating the patient to optimal performance (see Chap. 12). Until we can measure meaningful changes in performance and establish relationships between the health services provided and the improvement of performance achieved, we will not be able to establish systematic service programs. Until such time we will continue to have fractionated, disorganized, and unfocused health services.

Comprehensive rehabilitation needs to become outcome oriented, by developing means to measure outcome and then providing the guidance that is necessary so that the application of the entirety of medical services is oriented toward the optimal outcome for the individual. This goal should be optimal functional performance in the home and community throughout life. A simple illustrative diagram of human performance plotting the Scale of Functional Outcome of Rehabilitation against life span is shown in Figure 4. From birth there is a progressive increase of function through childhood up to a peak performance in early adulthood. If good health is maintained throughout life, function should persist near maximal until far into old age, and death would terminate that high level of function. We might liken that possibility to Oliver Wendell Holmes'

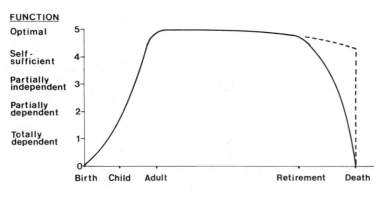

FIGURE 4. The functional performance of the normal, healthy person develops during childhood and is maintained throughout adult life.

Human Performance of Adult Disabled as the Measure of Rehabilitation

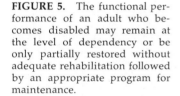

FIGURE 5. The functional performance of an adult who becomes disabled may remain at the level of dependency or be only partially restored without adequate rehabilitation followed by an appropriate program for maintenance.

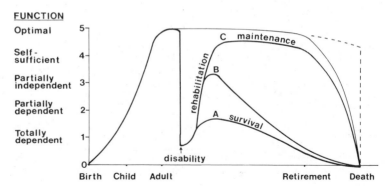

one-hoss shay, which fell apart "all at once and nothing first, just as a bubble when it bursts."

A functional life history when severe disability intervenes in adulthood is illustrated in Figure 5. Illness suddenly decreases functional capacity to total dependency. Medical care alone may ensure survival (curve A) but may leave patients totally or partially dependent throughout the remainder of their lives. Acute medical care plus limited rehabilitation may restore individuals to a higher level of function, but if the rehabilitation is not followed by an adequate maintenance program, there may be progressive loss of function to the level of dependency (curve B). The goal of every rehabilitation program should be to restore patients to a level of in-

dependent living so that at the end of the rehabilitation program they have adequate training and understanding to use available resources to maintain their functional levels throughout life. An optimal outcome of such a program is indicated by curve C.

One indication of the success that may be attained in the maintenance of function is indicated by the maintenance of mobility of a group of 80 stroke patients who underwent rehabilitation[11] (Fig. 6). An assessment of these patients at an average of 6 years (range 3 to 10 years) after rehabilitation showed that while 25 per cent of these patients had become nonambulatory or required supervision during walking, 75 per cent had maintained the functional ability that they had gained through rehabilitation. All of our

Mobility Level

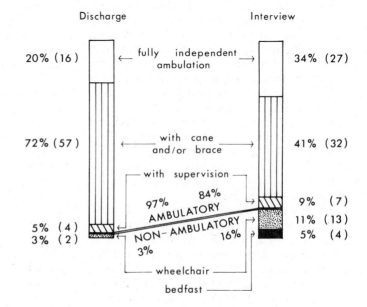

FIGURE 6. Rehabilitation followed by appropriate maintenance can preserve a high level of function for years, as indicated by the maintenance of independent walking in patients for 3 to 10 years following a stroke. (From Anderson, E., Anderson, T. P., and Kottke, F. J.: Stroke rehabilitation: Maintenance of achieved gains. Arch. Phys. Med. Rehabil., 58:345–352, 1977.)

Human Performance of Developmentally Disabled as the Measure of Rehabilitation

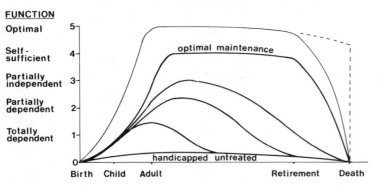

FIGURE 7. Rehabilitation of disabled children is especially important, since without it they do not have an opportunity to develop and may remain severely dependent throughout a survival time of many decades.

services should be assessed by evaluation of outcome similar to this.

The potential functional outcome curves of children with developmental disabilities are illustrated in Figure 7. Children without rehabilitation remain very severely dependent, highly expensive invalids who survive for decades today in complete dependency. Inadequate or incomplete rehabilitation may raise level of performance for a variable period of time but leave the individual with significant dependency needs. In many cases this is the best outcome today. A great deal of research is needed in rehabilitation of developmentally disabled children. Again, the goal for restoration and maintenance for these children should be self-sufficiency, independent living, education, and productivity throughout a normal life span.

This third edition of *Krusen's Handbook* presents the concepts and practices of comprehensive rehabilitation and continuing maintenance of patients with disabilities, consistent with the needs described above. Since comprehensive rehabilitation has not been fully integrated into the medical curriculum, many medical students and practicing physicians lack knowledge of both principles and techniques of physical medicine and rehabilitation. Both aspects are presented here, so that *Krusen's Handbook* is a textbook for medical students, residents, and therapists as well as a ready reference for physicians in practice.

The book is organized into three general sections: evaluation, therapy, and rehabilitation of the major disabling conditions. The 12 chapters of the first section present the components of evaluation that provide the basis for comprehensive rehabilitation. Chapters 1 and 2 explain clinical evaluation of the patient for rehabilitation, and succeeding chapters discuss special techniques of performance evaluation, including electrodiagnosis and electromyography, gait analysis, evaluation of speech and communication, psychological assessment and management, prevocational evaluation, epidemiology of disability, and reflex evaluation to assess neuromuscular function. Chapter 12 presents a system for health accounting in which systematic organization and recording of the ongoing rehabilitation process help to define the patient's status on admission and to evaluate the response to rehabilitation.

The second section, on therapeutics, consists of 17 chapters. Those dealing with standard aspects of therapy which have been of proven value for more than 50 years — thermotherapy, ultraviolet therapy, electrotherapy, massage, and exercise — have been updated to present recent innovations and newly developed techniques in addition to well-established principles and practices. Significant advances of the past decade in techniques of exercise for mobility, coordination, strength, and endurance are presented. A chapter has been devoted to the newly emerging application of functional electrical stimulation for patients with neuromuscular impairments. The following aspects of rehabilitation training have been updated: bed positioning, transfer training, wheelchair use, training for functional independence, and training for homemaking. Three chapters are devoted to the principles of design and application of orthotics for the upper extremities, the neck and trunk, and the lower extremities. One chapter considers specific aspects of the prescription of physical and occupational therapy by the physician.

The third section consists of 23 chapters

dealing with the evaluation and rehabilitation management of disabling conditions that are encountered in physical medicine and rehabilitation. Arthritis and back disorders are most frequently encountered, with 5 per cent of the population significantly limited in daily self-care, ambulation, or vocational activity and many affected individuals home-bound or sequestered in nursing homes. Therefore, knowledge of the rehabilitation management of arthritis and back disorders is important to all physicians in primary care as well as to physiatrists. Another large category of disability for which specific techniques of rehabilitation management are presented includes neurologic problems: stroke, closed head injuries, spinal cord injuries, cranial palsies, and traumatic and degenerative diseases of the nervous system. Rehabilitation management of cerebral palsy and other neurologic diseases of childhood involves consideration of the developmental aspects of childhood, both physical and psychosocial, as well as the specific aspects of therapy for motor and intellectual impairments. The techniques of rehabilitation of the cardiac patient either in the acute phase or in the convalescent phase of recovery are presented. Two chapters deal with the selection of prosthetics for upper extremity amputation and for lower extremity amputation and the fitting and training of the patient in their use. Chapters on specific organ system management discuss neurogenic bowel and bladder, prevention of ischemic ulcers, care of the feet, problems of sexual function and disability, and deafness. Each is presented from the aspect of comprehensive rehabilitation. Finally, new chapters have been included in this third edition of *Krusen's Handbook* on rehabilitation of patients with cancer and on the response of the body to immobility.

The editors wish to express their deep appreciation to each of the authors who made a contribution to *Krusen's Handbook*. The major recompense that the authors receive is their awareness that they are making a significant contribution to the training of young physicians and others in the rehabilitation professions in the principles and application of physical medicine and rehabilitation. The eventual benefits are the improved and extended rehabilitation services that are made available to handicapped persons. However, in addition to that, the wide acceptance and use of this text in its first two editions indicate that many readers have appreciated the contributions of these authors. The contributing authors have been picked because they are authorities on their subjects, who not only select but also interpret and present from the literature the most pertinent information in a manner most meaningful to the reader. This careful preparation of each chapter with selected references provides the basis for entry into the biomedical literature by any reader who wishes to study a subject in greater depth.

We wish to thank Edna Maneval for her extensive editorial assistance, Jean Magney for her excellent illustrations, and, for secretarial help, especially Joan Odegard and Marion Hunter.

Grateful appreciation is expressed to the staff of the W. B. Saunders Company for their willing collaboration and excellent support in the editing and publishing of this book.

FREDERIC J. KOTTKE

JUSTUS F. LEHMANN

G. KEITH STILLWELL

REFERENCES

1. Rusk, H. A.: Rehabilitation. JAMA, 140:286–292, 1949.
2. Rusk, H. A.: Advances in rehabilitation. Practitioner, 183:505–512, 1959.
3. Krusen, F. H.: Concepts in Rehabilitation of the Handicapped. Philadelphia, W. B. Saunders Company, 1964.
4. Rusk, H. A.: Preventive medicine, curative medicine — then rehabilitation. New Phys., 13:165–167, 1964.
5. Forman, M. A., and Hetznecker, W.: The physician and the handicapped child. JAMA, 247:3325–3326, 1982.
6. Kottke, F. J.: Historia, obscura hemiplegiae. Arch. Phys. Med. Rehabil., 55:4–13, 1974.
7. Anderson, T. P., McClure, W. J., Athelstan, G., Anderson, E., Crewe, N., Arndts, L., Ferguson, M. B., Baldridge, M., Gullickson, G., and Kottke, F. J.: Stroke rehabilitation: Evaluation of its quality by assessing patient outcomes. Arch. Phys. Med. Rehabil., 59:170–175, 1978.
8. Williamson, J. W.: Assessing and Improving Health Care Outcomes: The Health Accounting Approach to Quality Assurance. Cambridge, Ballinger, 1978.
9. Joe, T. C.: Professionalism: A new challenge for rehabilitation. Arch. Phys. Med. Rehabil., 62: 245–250, 1981.
10. Stinson, M. B.: Medical care and rehabilitation for the aged. Geriatrics, 8:226–229, 1953.
11. Anderson, E., Anderson, T. P., and Kottke, F. J.: Stroke rehabilitation: Maintenance of achieved gains. Arch. Phys. Med. Rehabil., 58:345–352, 1977.

CONTENTS

1

EVALUATION OF THE PATIENT

WALTER C. STOLOV

The reader might ask why the need for a chapter on patient evaluation in a textbook on physical medicine and rehabilitation. He has, after all, learned and gained experience on how to elicit symptoms and signs from the history and physical examination of a patient. He already knows how to use these data for the establishment of a diagnosis of a patient's disease. Why not get on with the special therapeutics?

The reason is simple. *The symptoms and signs required for the diagnosis of disability are not synonymous with those required for the diagnosis of disease.*

Consider the following example:

A 22-year-old medical student in a skiing accident fractures his left humerus. As the history is being taken, he complains, "I can't raise my hand." "I can't straighten my fingers." "My grip is weak." Examination reveals paralysis of the wrist and finger extensors, and hypesthesia over the dorsum of the first digit.

The diagnosis of the *disease* is clear. The patient has, in addition to a fracture, a radial nerve palsy. The *disability*, however, is not clear and has not yet been diagnosed. One question must yet be asked: "With which hand do you usually write?" If the answer is "The left," one additional examination finding must be elicited. After the fracture is reduced and the arm placed in a cast, the patient's writing skill must be assessed. If he is unable to write, then at least part of his disability diagnosis (there may be other func-

tions interrupted) includes the *inability to write.*

Neither the question, "With which hand do you usually write?" nor the examination of his writing skill after casting was necessary to make the diagnosis of the disease, but both were necessary to diagnose the disability. The history and physical examination required for the two diagnoses were different.

Consider further the possibility that the patient may have answered, "I write with my right hand." The writing disability would therefore not be present, yet the disease is still the same. This illustrates:

There is no one-to-one correlation between a disease and the spectrum of disability problems that may be associated with it. The disability is dependent on the patient's total requirements.

Consider further that our patient with the writing disability is advised that his radial nerve will not regrow successfully. As a result, he enters a deliberate systematic training program to develop writing ability with his normal right arm, and succeeds. He then has removed his disability, although the radial nerve palsy that caused it in the first place is still present. This illustrates:

There is no one-to-one relationship between a disease and the amount of residual disability. Disability problems can be removed even though the disease is unchanged.

This principle further points out a second important reason for a chapter on patient evaluation in a textbook on rehabilitation.

The ability of a patient and his physician to remove disability in the face of chronic disease is dependent on the residual capacity of the patient for physiological and psychological adaptation. His residual strengths must be evaluated and built upon to "work around" impairment in order to remove disability.

Disability means lost function. Our initial example dealt with the loss of a physical function, writing. Other kinds of functional losses can occur:

A 55-year-old male outdoor construction worker complained of "shortness of breath" and "weakness." History and physical examination along with laboratory data confirmed the diagnosis of chronic obstructive pulmonary disease.

What, however, of his disability! Inquiry about employment revealed he was fired from his job because of a gradual reduction in work output. The patient confirmed that he no longer had the energy for the work. His physician indicated that response to treatment of the lung disease would not be sufficient to allow for a return to outdoor construction work. The disability diagnosis will then include the problem of *unemployment.*

Were the same patient engaged in a minimum energy white-collar job, unemployment would not be a problem. On the other hand, a white-collar worker with chronic obstructive pulmonary disease, while not disabled from work, may have the disability problem of loss of his major avocational pursuit (e.g., hunting) because of his disease.

The examples indicate the character of those diseases that produce disability. They are either diseases in which part or all of the pathologic process is irreversible and hence are always present, i.e., chronic diseases, or they are diseases in which a significant period of time must elapse before the pathologic process can be reversed. In either class, they may produce problems of dependency on others in activities of basic *physical* function. They may produce problems that relate to *social* functions in the home and with the family unit. They may produce problems in *vocational* functions and in the ability to engage in *avocational* pursuits. And finally, they may produce chronic emotional stresses that may produce *psychologi-*

cal problems requiring adjustments not only by the patient but by his family unit as well.

A host of conditions exist for which diagnosis of disease alone without also the diagnosis of disability will lead to insufficient treatment. The disabilities must first be identified. The spectrum of disability problems that occur depends upon the interaction of the patient with his environment. This interaction is shown schematically in the diagram below (Fig. 1–1). It indicates that the total disability (i.e., the disability diagnosis — the total list of disability problems) derives from factors specific to the patient and specific to the environment.

Weed's problem-oriented approach[12] to the process of patient care is particularly suited to the evaluation of a patient with chronic illness and disability. The reader will profit by reviewing his monograph. He divides the patient treatment process into four phases. *Phase 1* includes the history, physical examination, and the initial laboratory studies as a data base. *Phase 2* identifies a specific problem list from the data base. *Phase 3* identifies a specific treatment plan for each of the problems. *Phase 4* describes the effectiveness of each of the plans and describes subsequent alterations in each of the plans, depending on progress.

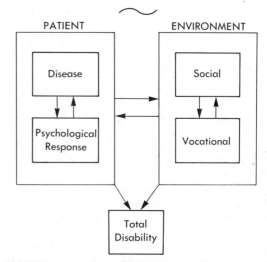

FIGURE 1–1. Schematic representation of the interaction of the patient with his environment. On the left, disease factors are reciprocally influenced by psychological factors. On the right, social factors are mutually influenced by vocational factors. The patient and his environment mutually influence each other. The Total Disability is fed by all areas.

The data base, therefore, goes beyond diagnosis determination. While a problem list will include known diagnoses, it will also include physiological syndromes, symptoms, signs, and laboratory abnormalities for which a disease diagnosis is as yet undetermined. The problem list also includes the specific impairments of function in the basic physical self-care skills, and those specific problems in social, vocational, and psychological function either secondary to or concurrent with the diseases. The individual identification of these functional problems leads to a plan for their solution, and hence for the removal of disability.

In this chapter are discussed specific methods of patient evaluation that will create the appropriate data base necessary to allow the physician to achieve a diagnosis of disability. History and physical examination data pertinent to an evaluation of lost function are described, and problem list formulation is introduced.

HISTORY

Historical data of prime importance in diagnosing disability are obtained from the *Chief Complaint, Present Illness,* and *Social and Vocational History* sections of the usual patient work-up. The nature of the *Chief Complaint* may provide a hint to the existence of disability. The *Present Illness* data can determine the extent of lost function in basic self-care activities. The *Social and Vocational History* evaluates the environment and provides insight into the psychological make-up of the patient. The *Review of Systems* and *Past Medical History* contribute to the assessment of residual capacity.

Chief Complaint

All chief complaints or main reasons a patient may seek the assistance of a physician derive from changes in health or in well-being. These changes create within the patient either (1) fear or anxiety, (2) discomfort, or (3) an inability to function. Chief complaints in which information on inability to function is included are the ones most apt to be associated with chronic illness and are those most likely to indicate that disability is present. The class of diseases most likely to produce complaints of loss of function are those that involve either the *musculoskeletal system,* the *neurologic system,* or the *cardiovascular system.*[6]

The list of chief complaints and final discharge diagnoses presented in Table 1–1 was extracted from a series of charts.* In this list, the statements referring to function are in italics.

While the majority of chief complaints related to loss of function are associated with

---

*The charts from which the statements have been abstracted are those of 50 patients consecutively discharged from a Veterans Administration hospital in 1967 — 10 each from a Medical, Surgical, Neurologic, Psychiatric, and Rehabilitation Medicine Service.

TABLE 1–1. EXAMPLES OF CHIEF COMPLAINTS ASSOCIATED WITH DIAGNOSES IN NEUROLOGICAL, MUSCULOSKELETAL, AND CARDIOVASCULAR SYSTEM DISEASES

Chief Complaint	Discharge Diagnosis
"Pain in calves after *walking* several blocks"	Peripheral vascular disease
"Can't *control* right leg"	Stroke
"Right-sided *clumsiness,* trouble with *balance*"	Multiple sclerosis
"Inability to *use legs* well"	Multiple sclerosis
"Can't *walk* or *talk* well"	Parkinsonism
"Leg weakness, unable to *stand* alone"	Transverse myelitis
"Pain in back and left leg. The more I *do physically,* the more I hurt"	Herniated disc
"*Walking* and *bladder trouble*"	Parkinsonism
"Low back pain increased by *walking* and *sitting*"	Lumbar disc disease
"Difficulty *walking*"	Musculoskeletal trauma
"Unable to *stand* up"	Stroke
"Aching wrist aggravated by *activity*"	Degenerative joint disease
"Difficulty with *ambulation* control"	Brain trauma

TABLE 1–2. EXAMPLES OF CHIEF COMPLAINTS RELATED TO DIAGNOSES OF DISEASES IN OTHER SYSTEMS

Chief Complaint	Discharge Diagnosis
"Severe chest pain while *driving car*"	Chronic lung disease
"Pain after *eating*"	Peptic esophagitis
"Trouble *breathing* after *exercise*"	Obstructive pulmonary disease
"*Weakness*"	Carcinoma of the lung

chronic diseases of the musculoskeletal, neurologic, or cardiovascular system, diseases in other systems also may yield statements related to loss of function (Table 1–2).

In these illustrations, the chronic diseases were in the pulmonary and gastrointestinal systems.

Complaints related to loss of function are presented also by patients with psychiatric disease and without organic pathologic changes, as in the following examples extracted from charts of patients hospitalized on a psychiatric ward:

"Unable to *take care of myself*"

"Fear of going places"

"*Incapable of doing* job"

"Continuous ache in neck made worse by *movement and exercise*"

"I just can't *work, eat, or sleep*"

"I have had a *terrible family life*"

These examples illustrate that psychological responses to the stress of chronic disease may aggravate disability from organic pathologic changes.

When, therefore, chief complaints contain statements related to loss of function, the physician is alerted to pursue carefully a search for disability. He must search for the dependency of the patient on others to carry out his basic self-care skills. He must search for problems in social functions in the home and family unit, problems of employment, and problems secondary to chronic psychological stress. He is further alerted to the need for careful study of the musculoskeletal, neurologic, and cardiovascular systems.

Present Illness

One of the hallmarks of disability is a dependency on others for the performance of basic self-care activities, sometimes termed activities of daily living. Historical information about this dependency is best included under the category of *Present Illness*. Such data are really part of the symptom complex of the disease and are the essence of the disability the disease is producing. For example, it is not so much weakness that a patient is concerned about but the reduced ambulation that results. It is not the tremor that worries a patient, but the lost ability to hold a cup of coffee. Similarly, it is not so much the reduction in shoulder and elbow range of motion that a patient wishes to correct, but rather the lost ability to comb his hair or attend to his perineal hygiene after defecation.

The basic activities for which inquiry should be made as part of the *Present Illness* review can be divided into five categories: (1) ambulation, (2) transfer activities, (3) dressing activities, (4) eating skills, and (5) personal hygiene activities. The quantification of dependency in the performance of any of these activities of daily living is achieved by determining from the patient who in the family unit provides the assistance and the nature of the assistance provided. Assistance is in one of the following categories:

1. *Standby assistance.* As the activity is being performed by the patient, he may not always do it safely or correctly. The assistant then is "standing by" to guard against the occurrence of accidents and to ensure the correctness and completeness of performance by pointing out errors or omissions.

2. *Partial physical assistance.* As the activity is being performed, the patient is able to do a good part but not all of it by himself. The assistant then provides partial physical assistance. For example, the assistant may buckle the patient's belt after the patient himself puts on his pants, or he may hold the wheelchair stationary while the patient is transferring himself into bed.

3. *Total physical assistance.* For the ac-

tivity to be accomplished, the assistant has to do all of it because the patient can contribute little or nothing toward its execution. He is, therefore, totally dependent.

Ambulation History. Ambulation may be defined in the broadest sense as *travel from one place to another over a finite distance.* Ambulation thus includes not only walking but also wheelchair travel, and even crawling. To assess the extent of disability with regard to ambulation, the patient's capacity for ambulation in different environments must be obtained.

The environments of significance are his home, its immediate vicinity, and the community at large. A patient may, for example, be totally independent in walking within and around his house but not in the community. The environments found in theaters, restaurants, subways, or downtown stores may require that he have partial physical assistance in order to negotiate them safely. The disability diagnosis for such a patient will therefore include the problem of *decreased community ambulation.*

If a patient is not walking but uses a wheelchair, the extent of his independence in its use needs to be known. For example, the examiner should determine whether the patient is able to maneuver it independently within the home, whether he is also independent in its use outside his home, and if he can take it successfully into the community at large without assistance.

Sample questions in an exploration of ambulation skill are:
1. Can you walk without assistance?
2. Do you use equipment (canes, crutches, braces)?
3. Do you use a wheelchair?
4. Is there a limit to how far you can walk (or use your wheelchair) outside the home?
5. Can and do you go out visiting friends, or to restaurants, theaters, or stores?
6. Do you have falls?
7. Do you drive a car?
8. Can you climb stairs?

Transfer History. Transfers are movements that involve *changes of position in place.* They include such activities as going from a bed to a wheelchair or regular chair; going from a wheelchair to a toilet, bathtub, shower, or car; and going from a wheelchair, regular chair, or toilet seat to a standing position. These activities are more basic than ambulation. For example, while a patient may be independent in walking, he may be physically dependent on others to get out of his chair into a standing posture. His independent ambulation therefore is not always available to him if the assistance for the transfer into the upright posture is not always present.

Sample questions to begin on assessment of disability in transfer abilities are:
1. Can you get in and out of bed unaided?
2. Can you get on and off a toilet unaided?
3. Can you get in and out of the tub unaided?

Dressing History. A disabled patient's ability to put on and take off his clothes must be carefully assessed. If a patient is not independent in dressing, he is less likely to leave his home and is less likely to receive guests other than his immediate family. Dressing dependency therefore greatly restricts the environments available to the patient.

In obtaining a history of performance in dressing skills, it is not sufficient merely to ask, "Do you dress yourself?" An untrained disabled patient may have for some time abandoned the use of those garments more difficult to put on. Typically abandoned are shoes, socks, pants, clothes with buttons, and close-fitting undergarments. A patient therefore may answer "Yes" to such a question without realizing how few clothes he still wears. A more complete probe is therefore necessary to gain insight into his performance.

Sample questions that may be asked to explore competence in dressing are:
1. Do you dress in street clothes daily?
2. Can you put on without assistance your shirt, pants, dress, undergarments, and so forth?
3. Do you need help with shoes and socks?

Eating History. The loss of independence in a patient's ability to feed himself can be most devastating to his self-image. Unlike the activities already discussed, it is the one activity that *must* still go on even if total physical assistance is necessary. A patient who is dependent on others to feed him is literally reduced to the level of a two- to three-year-old.

Eating skills include the use of a fork, spoon, and knife, and the handling of cups and glasses.

Sample questions in an exploration of this area include:

1. Can you feed yourself unassisted?
2. Can you cut meat?
3. Do you have trouble holding glasses and cups?

Personal Hygiene History. Personal hygiene activities include the spectrum of skills concerned with cleaning and grooming: toothbrushing, hair combing, shaving, the use of tub and shower, perineal care, and the successful handling of bowel and bladder elimination. Loss of independence in the performance of these skills is severely disabling to the patient. This is particularly so when the patient cannot handle bowel and bladder elimination in a socially acceptable manner. If a patient has to concern himself with the possibility that he may soil his trousers or the bed or someone's car with feces or urine, the emotional stresses to him and his family can be quite severe. The adult who requires that his spouse clean him after defecation may soon deal with a strained marriage. Efforts at increasing social functioning and directed toward vocational rehabilitation will be unsuccessful until the patient can develop a system of elimination that is consistently successful.

Socially acceptable elimination does not necessarily require that the systems be physiologically normal. Patients with catheters can develop a successful system if they can handle the emptying of collecting bags and can satisfactorily hide the collecting system under trousers or skirts.

Sample questions to explore the personal hygiene area include:

1. Can you shave (use make-up) and comb your hair unaided?
2. Can you shower or bathe without assistance?
3. Can you use a toilet unaided?
4. Do you need help in cleaning up after a bowel movement?
5. Are bladder and bowel accidents a problem for you?

General Principles in Determining Disability in Basic Functions. In exploring for disability in the five basic functions of ambulation, transfers, dressing, eating, and personal hygiene, several principles should be kept in mind:

1. When the patient reports he is not independent, determine the type of assistance: standby, partial physical, or total physical.
2. Determine who is supplying the assistance.
3. Separately interview the people (usually family members) who are supplying the assistance. The assistant may indicate that the degree of assistance is actually greater than reported by the patient. The two may not interpret in the same way what is actually occurring. A significant difference in the context of their remarks may indicate neither is satisfied with what is going on.
4. When it is expected or anticipated that the patient may be dependent, questions of the "Can you . . ." or "Do you . . ." type should be rephrased to "Who helps you. . . ." Questions asked this way may yield more information. Patients may wish initially to appear more independent than they actually are.
5. When the disability is of acute onset, the inquiry should also include the premorbid level of independence. This is particularly important in the older patient. Earlier disease or trauma may have left some residual dependency. Therapeutics brought to bear on the new problems are not likely to result in a degree of independence greater than pre-morbid levels.
6. If dependency is present and the disease is of a chronic progressive type, determine the time course of the loss of independence. Therapeutics are more likely to remove disability in more recently lost functions rather than in those lost many years previously.
7. For some patients, the answers to certain of the preceding sample questions may be obvious and hence need not be asked. It is best, however, to assume less and inquire more, thereby avoiding omissions of significant data.

When an inquiry into the basic self-care functions of ambulation, transfers, dressing, eating, and personal hygiene is complete, specific disability problems become identified. They need to be identified separately in the patient's list of problems even though they are secondary to a specific disease. Since the pathologic condition may be irreversible in part or in whole, these functional problems will not be eliminated by reversal of the disease process and will have to be attacked individually. Before therapeutics can be applied, however, problems must be identified.

Review of Systems

As already indicated, the ability of a patient and his physician to remove disability is dependent on the patient's residual capacity. Often, specific exercise and training activities are required to remove disability and restore function. The status of four systems in particular must be evaluated to assess the patient's capacity for this training. The *Review of Systems* inquiry, therefore, requires careful study of the cardiovascular, respiratory, neurologic, and musculoskeletal systems. The cardinal symptoms in each of these systems are:

Cardiovascular. Dyspnea, orthopnea, chest pain, limb claudication, palpitation, and cough.

Respiratory. Cough, sputum, hemoptysis, chest pain, and dyspnea.

Neurologic. Numbness, weakness, fainting or loss of consciousness, dizziness, pain, headache, and defective memory or thinking.

Musculoskeletal. Pain, deformity, weakness, limitation of movement, and stiffness.

Past Medical History

Like the *Review of Systems,* the *Past Medical History* provides information on the residual capacity of the patient. Concurrent disease or previous trauma and surgery may have produced residual impairments. Although these impairments no longer produce disability themselves, they may compound the disability of the present illness when added to the new impairments.

A few examples may help clarify this principle:

A patient suffered a severe left brachial plexus injury, which resulted in paralysis of the triceps and the muscles of the wrist and hand. His past medical history revealed an earlier right hip fracture. Although the hip fracture had healed well, residual hip abductor muscle weakness required the use of a cane in his left hand for safe ambulation. Prior to the brachial plexus injury, the patient had not been disabled, since he could then handle all his ambulation needs with his cane.

The profound paralysis of the left arm, as a result of the brachial plexus injury, has now disabled the patient for ambulation.

Loss of ambulation is never a consequence of a brachial plexus injury alone. The past medical problem has compounded the disability.

A patient in an automobile accident suffered a complete paraplegia as a result of injury at the level of the tenth thoracic vertebra. His past medical history revealed a problem of recurrent shoulder dislocation, which was successfully repaired by surgery. The patient, after paraplegia occurred, began a heavy exercise program for his upper extremities in preparation for training in transfer activities. During a bout of exercise, shoulder dislocation occurred. After reduction, immobilization of the arm for six weeks was recommended.

The patient, therefore, became disabled for transfer activities not as a result of his paraplegia but because of the compounding effect of his previously dormant past medical problem.

A careful *Past Medical History* review is therefore an essential component of the evaluation of a patient with disability. A simple recitation of past or concurrent disease or trauma may not be enough. The inquiry requires an understanding of residuals, however slight they may seem.

Social and Vocational History

The social and vocational history of the patient is the source for the necessary data about the environment with which the patient must interact. A careful review will identify environmental problems secondary to or concurrent with the disease. It also provides insight into the personality of the patient. Information on his ability to adjust to the stress of chronic disability can be obtained, and the psychological problems that may need to be dealt with can therefore be identified early.

It is convenient to divide the personal

history data of the patient into three categories: *social, vocational,* and *psychological.*

Social History. When dependency on others for the performance of basic self-care skills occurs, or if a job is lost because of disease, the patient's family unit is compromised. The need to help the disabled person perform his activities of daily living and the loss of income may force some family members to alter their own plans greatly. A major disability of one member of a family unit will create problems of adjustment for all and even threaten the integrity of the unit. Superimposition of a major disability on a family unit already beset with social problems is particularly threatening. Identification of secondary and concurrent social issues as *patient problems* and inclusion of them in the patient's problem list allows the physician to begin to attack the environmental problems at the same time that he attacks problems directly related to organic pathologic processes.

The assessment of social impairment is obtained from inquiries into the stability of the family unit, the history of the unit, the resources within the unit, the responsibilities of the patient within the unit, and the physical environment of the home and the community.

The physical environments are important because independence or dependence in the performance of an activity is directly related to where the activity is being carried out. The following examples illustrate the influence of physical environments on independence:

A patient who is independent in wheelchair travel may require physical assistance to transfer from toilet to wheelchair if the toilet seat is too low. Similarly, a patient may be dependent in bed transfers if the bed is too high. On the other hand, a patient who is independent in wheelchair travel and in transfers, regardless of the toilet seat height, may still be dependent on others for bathroom activities if the door to the bathroom is too narrow to allow for entrance of the wheelchair.

A patient who lives in a large city may be totally confined to his home and be unable to go downtown or to a store because such a trip may require the use of the subway and hence the ability to negotiate three flights of stairs. If he is not independent in such stair-climbing skills, subway travel will be beyond his reach and downtown inaccessible. On the other hand, a patient with identical skills who lives in a smaller city or in a suburban or rural community and who can perform automobile transfers and knows how to drive or has someone who can drive for him will have downtown accessible to him.

Sample questions to begin a search for problems in social functioning can include:

1. Where do you live? (Urban? Suburban? Rural?)
2. Do you rent or own?
3. Are the bedroom, bathroom, kitchen on the same floor?
4. Are there entrance stairs or stairs within the home or apartment?
5. Who else is at home? (Wife, husband, children [ages], and friends?) Do any of them go to work or school? Are they in good health? Are the children having trouble in school?
6. Do your parents, brothers, and sisters live in the area? Do you maintain any contact with them?
7. Are you (how long have you been) married? Is this your first marriage?
8. What activities and functions did you do at home for the family that you no longer can do? (Examples are discipline, financial management, chores, sexual functions, avocational activities.) How are these functions now handled?
9. Where were you born?
10. Where else have you lived?
11. What did (or do) your father and siblings do for a living?
12. When did you leave your parents' home?
13. What was your family life as a child like?

The answers to these questions will provide the social background and current resources, as well as suggest current or potential problems. "Abnormal" responses to these questions should be pursued. For example, if a patient has been married before, inquiry into the number of previous marriages, their lengths, reasons for break-up, other children, and financial obligations will yield further insight.

Vocational History. A patient's disease may also produce the disability of unemployment. Whether there is or will be a problem in this area requires an understanding of the physical, intellectual, and interpersonal requirements of the patient's job.

Sample questions to determine if the disease and the lost function in the activities of daily living will be compatible with employment are:

1. When did you last work?
2. For whom did (do) you work?
3. How long did you (have you) work(ed) for them?
4. Describe what you did (do) on the job. Be specific. Start with what you do when you first arrive.
5. Was (is) your income sufficient to support your family or do you have other sources? Do you have debts?

If job instability is suspected — for example, if the last (current) job was held for less than two years, or if the last (current) job seems to be incompatible with the current illness even after rehabilitation treatment — then further inquire:

1. What kind of work do you plan to do in the future?
2. Obtain chronological history of employment, job requirements, and reasons for change.
3. Inquire about special skills, licenses, union memberships, and ratings received.
4. Inquire about highest attained educational level, age at time left school, and level of school performance.

These additional facts will indicate whether there have been work adjustment problems. The strengths in the patient's vocational background on which one can build will also become clear. If the patient has not been working, inquire into his current sources of financial support and their sufficiency.

For the housewife who is not employed outside the home, inquire:

1. When did you last do the cooking? Shopping? Light housekeeping? Heavy cleaning?
2. Who does these things now?
3. Is this arrangement satisfactory for you and your family?

Avocational activities are also an important aspect of a patient's function. Many patients derive more of their enjoyment of life from their avocational pursuits than from vocational activities. *To seek for problems in this area, the following sample questions are useful:*

1. What do you do with your leisure time after work and on weekends by yourself? With your family?
2. What organizations or religious groups are you active in?
3. When did you last participate in these activities?

Psychological History. Psychological function needs to be assessed in patients with a chronic illness or physical disability for several reasons: (1) Since the organic pathologic changes may be incompletely reversible, the stress of the disease is always present. This stress may be of great magnitude. For example, a patient who loses his leg has to adjust not only to this loss but also perhaps to the secondary stress of loss of his job. The physical requirements of the job may be incompatible with activity limits of an artificial limb. (2) The patient and his family may have to relinquish established goals and old ways of doing things. The patient may have to learn new ways to protect his health that are not at all consistent with his personality. These new modes of behavior are usually not his preferred way of doing things, and often not society's preferred way. (3) The patient's psychological make-up needs to be understood, for if new learning is to be facilitated in treatment, an understanding of what is likely to motivate the patient and reinforce new learning is necessary. (4) For patients with brain damage from trauma or disease, an understanding of intellectual function will be required if they are to be trained successfully in the removal of disability in the basic functions.

Psychological problems should be included in the patient's problem list when the reaction to the stress of the disease is inappropriate or insufficient and when new learning is not occurring during treatment. While the *Mental Status* examination can assess current function, the social and vocational history data will yield a great deal of information about the patient's basic personality.

Interpretation of social and vocational data to yield psychological characteristics is a relatively simple matter when organized into four categories:

1. The patient's previous life style.
2. The patient's past history or response to ordinary life stresses.
3. The patient's current response to the stress of his disease.

4. The activities likely to motivate the patient to "train around" his disability.

Life Style. Characterization of a patient's life style is an attempt to identify a common thread in his social, vocational, and avocational activities. A *symbol-oriented* person is concerned predominantly with the world of ideas, abstract concepts, words, and numbers. A *motor-oriented* person is concerned with the world of objects or physical movement. An *interpersonally oriented* person's life is dominated by activities involving close personal contact with others.

For many people, their usual style is heavily invested in only one of these areas. If such a person suffers a loss of function that interferes in his ability to maintain his mode of living, the psychological burden his disease produces will be great. For example, a professional athlete whose illness produces lower limb paralysis will have a greater psychological burden to adjust to than will a bookkeeper with identical paralysis. If, however, the bookkeeper's major source of enjoyment of life was derived from his hunting, fishing, and camping activities, his burden may be as great as the athlete's. Those whose life style is well balanced among these three areas will be more likely to adjust to disability that affects only one of the areas.

Knowledge of the patient's usual life style and the effect of his disease will yield insight into the psychological response and the problems the patient may have.

The following sample groupings of vocational and avocational data obtained from the history will assist in this determination:

Symbol-Oriented
> *Vocations:* Law, accounting, science, clerical fields.
> *Avocations:* Reading, conversation, theater, museums.

Motor-Oriented
> *Vocations:* Manual labor, tools, machinery, athletics.
> *Avocations:* Active sports, hobby shop, hiking, camping.

Interpersonally Oriented
> *Vocations:* Sales, service, teaching.
> *Avocations:* Church groups, clubs, meetings, parties.

Past Response to "Ordinary" Life Stresses. For some people the simple business of living produces stresses that they are unable to handle successfully. For these it can be anticipated that the superimposition of the stress of disability may be overwhelming. Such patients may actually be more psychologically comfortable with the state of dependency the disability creates. To achieve success in the removal of disability for such patients may be a difficult task.

The physician is alerted to this potential problem when the social and vocational data reveal such things as multiple marriages, multiple vocational and business failures, alcoholism, psychiatric hospitalization, police involvement, delinquent children, and excessive debts.

When, however, the history is devoid of such social and vocational events, the patient may be more likely to be successful in removing his disability and regaining independence.

Current Response to the Disease Stress. If a patient is being evaluated some time after the onset of the disability-producing disease, insight into his ability to handle stress can be obtained from what has transpired. If the social history and present illness data reveal that the patient has been getting his prescriptions filled, taking his medicine, keeping his appointments, altering his habits, monitoring his diet, and avoiding preventable secondary complications, then he is exhibiting a satisfactory adjustment. Such a patient is more likely to be able to remove disability and achieve independence.

Motivational Factors. The same social and vocational data that identify the patient's life style will also identify the type of activities that can be used as goals toward which the patient works as he strives to remove dependency during treatment. The likelihood of success in an activity consistent with his pre-morbid life style will serve as a motivational factor, even if the work the patient must perform to achieve his goals includes activities that are in themselves alien to his usual style.

For example, an interpersonally oriented individual may be motivated to perform certain heavy exercises important for his health if, on achieving a required level of strength, increased visitation with others is permitted. Similarly, a symbol-oriented individual may be motivated to develop transfer skill independence (a motor-oriented task) if, on success, the opportunity to attend a play or concert is made available.

Thus, the social and vocational data provide information that will allow the physician to build on the patient's strengths as he attempts to assist the patient in the removal of disability.

Summary

When the classic approach to the history is elaborated in certain key areas, a patient's total disability can be properly diagnosed.

If the *Present Illness* is studied with regard to the patient's status in ambulation, transfers, eating, dressing, and personal hygiene, the spectrum of problems in self-care functions can be identified.

Study of the *Review of Systems* and the *Past Medical History* provides information on the residual capacity of the patient.

If the *Personal History* is elaborated to include careful study of the *Social and Vocational History*, then the problems within the environment can be identified. When such data are also scrutinized with regard to the psychology of the disabled patient, then problems of his reaction to the stress of the incompletely reversible pathologic condition can also be identified.

Not until these four classes of problems are identified (*physical, social, vocational,* and *psychological*) can the rehabilitation treatment process begin.

THE PHYSICAL EXAMINATION

The information obtained from the physical examination of a patient whose history reveals the presence of disability serves three functions. First of all, the examination searches for the signs that signify deviations from normal structure and function. Correlation of these signs with the patient's history and laboratory data will yield the disease diagnoses. Secondly, in the examination of a disabled patient the physician searches for those signs that signify secondary problems that are not a necessary direct consequence of the disease. Such secondary problems may occur either as a result of treatment of the disease or as a result of lack of institution of appropriate preventive measures. Finally, the third main function of the physical examination is to assess the residual strengths in the systems or parts of systems unaffected

by the disease. It is on these strengths that the patient and his physician build to remove the disability and reestablish the lost functional skills. These residual abilities are what the patient uses to "train around" the impairment induced by his chronic disease.

Some examples of secondary problems that occur as a result of treatment are as follows:

The arm of a patient with a Colles' fracture of the wrist is placed in a cast. To prevent motion of the proximal fragment the elbow is incorporated into the cast in a position of flexion. When the cast is finally removed, elbow flexion contracture is observed. Such a contracture is not a natural consequence of the wrist fracture but is secondary to correct treatment.

An elderly patient receives a severely comminuted hip fracture for which operative reduction and internal immobilization are not feasible. A hip spica cast is applied. As a result of total bed immobilization, the secondary problems of generalized disuse weakness, urinary retention, and postural hypotension develop. These problems are natural direct consequences not of the fracture but of the appropriate treatment.

Examples of secondary problems that result from inappropriate preventive measures are:

A patient develops a partial radial nerve palsy secondary to trauma. The strength of the wrist dorsiflexors is insufficient to produce a full active range of wrist dorsiflexion. The patient is later found to have a wrist flexion contracture with shortening of wrist and finger flexor muscles. These contractures are not natural consequences of radial nerve palsy but are secondary to the omission of the preventive measure of regularly performed passive range of motion exercises of the wrist and fingers.

A patient suffers a fracture-dislocation of the seventh thoracic vertebra with resultant total paraplegia. During his hospitalization, a decubitus ulcer develops over his sacrum. Such an ulcer is not a direct natural consequence of the paraplegia. While the anesthesia over the sacrum is a direct consequence, the ulcer itself is secondary to omission of the preventive measure of periodic relief of pressure over the sacrum.

The major importance of secondary problems, whether treatment-induced or secondary to omission of prevention measures, is that they add to the patient's disability and they lengthen the treatment time necessary to remove the disabilities induced by the primary disease process. For example, the elbow flexion contracture will need to be treated before the patient can get full use of his healed fractured wrist and hand. Disuse weakness and postural hypotension will need to be treated before the patient with the healed hip fracture can achieve meaningful ambulation. The sacral ulcer has to heal before the paraplegic patient can begin to learn dressing skills or begin to sit for long periods.

The particular areas of the physical examination that need close consideration in the search for secondary problems and for the evaluation of residual strengths are *skin, eyes, ears, mouth and throat, cardiovascular, respiratory, genitalia and rectum, neurologic, musculoskeletal, functional neuromuscular,* and *mental status.*

What follows is not an exhaustive description of the examination of these areas. Pertinent highlights only are given.

Skin

Examine the skin over bony prominences in patients with anesthetic areas or those who have been on prolonged bed rest. Look for vasomotor changes in the skin of the hands and the feet in patients with arm and leg weakness, joint contractures, or pain.

Eyes

Carefully assess for near and far visual acuity, for visual field defects, diplopia, and adequacy of glasses. Since the patient may need to relearn new motor acts to eliminate disability in basic self-care skills or may require vocational alterations, visual skills may need to be maximized.

Ears

Assess hearing acuity. Impaired acuity will impair relearning.

Mouth and Throat

In order to ensure adequate nutrition, disabling factors that interfere with mastication and swallowing will need attention. Status of teeth, gums, and dentures should be made optimal.

Cardiovascular System

Retraining to restore basic self-care skills that are lost as a result of musculoskeletal and neurologic disease usually requires specific therapeutic exercise regimens. An adequate cardiovascular reserve and optimized cardiovascular function are therefore essential.

Examination of the blood pressure (supine, sitting, and standing), liver size, peripheral pulses, carotid pulses, venous return systems, peripheral skin temperature, peripheral skin hair, and peripheral edema should therefore be done. Cardiac size, cardiac rhythms, and cardiac sounds will need correct interpretations. All treatable abnormalities will need identification.

Respiratory System

Much like the cardiovascular system, the respiratory reserve needs assessment in the evaluation of exercise tolerance.

Examination of the respiratory rate and rhythm, the chest shape, the fingers for clubbing, the facies for cyanosis, and the lungs for congestion and obstruction is essential. Pulmonary function laboratory tests may also be needed to supplement the physical examination of the respiratory system.

Genitalia and Rectum

Particularly critical for patients with diseases affecting functions of micturition and defecation are examinations for cystocele and rectocele, prostate size, sphincter tone, anal wink reflexes, perineal sensation, the presence of orchitis and epididymitis, and the presence of the bulbocavernosus reflex.

The bulbocavernosus reflex, if present, means that the sacral conus of the spinal cord at the level of S2 to S4 is intact. The afferent sensory stimulus is elicited by pressure on the clitoris or glans. For patients with catheters, a tug on the catheter will stimulate the afferent response. The efferent response is contraction of the external sphincter. A finger in the anus will detect this response.

Neurologic Examination

This examination should be performed with the same care as is exercised by the neurologist searching for signs in a difficult diagnostic problem.[7] All 12 cranial nerves must be reviewed. Sensory examination should include superficial touch and pain, deep pain, position sense (large joints as well as small), vibration sense, stereognosis, two-point discrimination, hot and cold perception, and the presence or absence of extinction to bilateral confrontation. Cerebellar and coordination functions need careful review, as do the deep tendon and pathologic reflexes. Language functions will need to be evaluated with regard to articulation, visual and auditory reception, and verbal and written expression.

Musculoskeletal System

The functional unit of the musculoskeletal system is the joint and its associated structures: synovial membrane, the capsule, ligaments, and muscles that cross it. Examination of this complex anywhere in the body cannot be completed unless the underlying anatomy is known. A screening examination is useful in localizing abnormalities when the disability problems are minor.[9] For conditions that may result in major disability, individual joint examinations are necessary. Such examinations include *Inspection, Palpation, Passive Range of Motion, Stability, Active Range of Motion,* and *Muscle Strength.*

Inspection. The two sides should be observed for symmetry in contour and size and differences measured. Atrophy, masses, swellings, and skin color changes must be noted.

Palpation. The origin of a pain symptom may be localized by palpation of the various anatomic structures about the joint. Palpation of the bones can determine their continuity in fracture assessment. Palpation of masses and swellings for consistency can distinguish between bony masses, edema, and joint effusions. To determine the presence of muscle spasm, muscle palpation when the patient is at rest can detect a sustained involuntary reflex contraction usually secondary to pain.

Passive Range of Motion. These tests are performed by the examiner while the patient is relaxed. When range of motion is limited, the examiner must determine if the limitation is due to joint surface incongruities, joint fluid excess or loose bodies, or capsule, ligament, or muscle contractures. Methods of measurement of passive range of motion and normal values for all of the various joints are described in the next chapter.

Stability. These tests assess whether a pathologic condition of the bone, capsule, or ligament is causing abnormal movement (subluxations or dislocations). The joint should be moved under stress in the direction it is not supposed to move by virtue of its contour, ligaments and capsule, with the patient at rest. Tears in ligaments or laxity of capsule will result in abnormal mobility. During movement, joint stability is also supported by active muscle contraction.

Active Range of Motion. These tests should be performed prior to strength tests in the event pain is a problem. Muscle tension and joint compressions induced by an active movement are less than in a strength test. If pain is minimal in an active range of motion, the examiner can more easily proceed with a strength test. When active range of motion is less than passive range of motion, the examiner must decide between true weakness, hysterical weakness, joint stability, pain, or malingering as possible causes.

Muscle Strength. Muscle strength can be tested if the prime action of a muscle is known. The body part can then be positioned to allow this prime action to occur. Grading systems are based on the ability of the muscle to move, against the force of gravity, the part to which it is attached.

GRADE 5. *Normal strength.* The muscle can move the joint it crosses through a full range of motion against gravity and against "full" resistance applied by the examiner.

GRADE 4. *Good strength.* The muscle can move the joint it crosses through a full range of motion against gravity with only "moderate" resistance applied by the examiner.

GRADE 3. *Fair strength.* The muscle can

move the joint it crosses through a full range of motion against gravity only.

GRADE 2. *Poor strength*. The muscle can move the joint it crosses through a full range of motion only if the part is positioned so that the force of gravity is not acting to resist the motion.

GRADE 1. *Trace strength*. Muscle contraction can be seen or palpated but strength is insufficient to produce motion even with gravity eliminated.

GRADE 0. *Zero strength*. Complete paralysis. No visible or palpable contraction.

The key muscle grade with regard to disability assessment is grade 3. Since any activity a patient may perform is done in a gravity field, if he has at least grade 3 function, then the involved body part can be used. For grades less than 3, external support may be necessary to make the involved part useful to the patient. In addition, joints having muscles across them with less than grade 3 strength are prone to develop contractures.

Different examiners should agree on whether a muscle should be graded 0, 1, 2, or 3. For grades 4 and 5, there may be differences among examiners depending on their expectations of different age groups and the amount of resistance they apply. As an examiner's experience increases, so will his accuracy. For asymmetrical problems, grades 4 and 5 are useful even for inexperienced examiners as the two sides of the body are compared.

For conditions in which weakness is associated with spasticity, the grading system described is not as useful in predicting how much use the patient may get out of the muscle for the performance of his basic skill needs.

The next chapter discusses the major muscles in the body and describes how they are best tested, as well as their innervations.

Functional Neuromuscular Examination

The functional examination is the actual translation of the objective neurologic and musculoskeletal examinations into performance. It defines at a given point in time the skill of the patient in the execution of the activities of daily living. It is the starting point from which improvement can occur through treatment even if the objective neurologic and musculoskeletal signs may not be alterable owing to the nature of the disease.

The functional examination confirms the skill status reported by the patient in the history under *Present Illness* with regard to ambulation, transfers, eating, dressing, and personal hygiene. The functions to be tested are as follows:

Sitting Balance. This is a necessary prerequisite for most transfer skills. Test by placing the patient in the sitting posture, with his feet on the floor, his back unsupported, and his hands in his lap. If he can hold this position, then nudge him in various directions and observe his ability to recover.

Transfers. Abilities to be examined include turning from supine to prone and back, rising to a sitting position, rising from sitting to standing, and moving from a bed or low examining table to a chair.

Standing Balance. This is a necessary prerequisite for safe ambulation. It should be assessed without support and, if balance is present, nudging from side to side should then be done to assess the patient's ability to recover.

Eating Skills. These can be assessed by demonstration of hand-to-mouth abilities utilizing various examining room objects or by means of actual observation at mealtime.

Dressing Skills. These skills are easily assessed in the examining room if the examiner is present at the time the patient removes his clothes prior to the examination and puts them on at the conclusion. If the examiner remains in the examining room while the patient undresses and does not leave before he dresses, much information on patient skill and patient family interaction can be gained.

Personal Hygiene Skills. The motions necessary for face, perineal, and back care can usually be mimicked in the examining room. Direct observation of the specific task when actually performed may be necessary if personal hygiene functions are significant disability problems.

Ambulation. Walking should be observed if the patient has standing balance. The patient should be essentially unclothed. Walking should be inspected with and without street shoes, and from the front and back, as well as from the side. Abnormalities should be described in relation to the phase of the gait at which they occur. If pain is present, it too should be related to the phase of the gait.

Observation and description should be systematically performed and recorded:

Cadence: Symmetrical? Asymmetrical? Consistent?

Trunk: Fixed abnormal posture? Abnormal movements anterior, posterior, or lateral?

Arm Swing: Symmetrical?

Pelvis: Fixed abnormal posture? Abnormal pelvic tilt or drop?

Base: Narrow? Broad?

Stride Length: Short? Asymmetrical?

Heel Strike and Push Off: Present?

Swing Phase: Knee flexion? Circumduction?

Chapter 4 elaborates on gait evaluation, Chapter 28 describes lower extremity braces, and Chapter 49 describes protheses for the lower extremity.

If walking is not present, *wheelchair ambulation* should be evaluated. The patient's ability to produce straight line travel and to negotiate turns should be observed.

Mental Status

The mental status examination, coupled with the psychological history, provides the data base for understanding the patient's basic personality structure and his current emotional reactions to his disease and disability.

In addition, since removal of disability is a retraining and hence a relearning process for the patient, the mental status examination can be used to assess his learning potential. The examination becomes particularly pertinent in patients whose disease or trauma has produced brain damage.

Mental status examinations as they appear in psychiatric textbooks are oriented specifically toward the patient with psychiatric disease. When performed on the patient with physical disability, some of the areas investigated need to be elaborated upon.

For psychiatric patients, the outline described by Storrow[11] includes:

1. Appearance and general behavior
2. Intellectual functions
   a. Orientation
   b. Level of consciousness
   c. Memory
   d. General information
   e. Numerical ability
3. Perception
4. Speech and thinking
5. Affect
6. Insight
7. Judgment

The reader should consult Storrow's textbook[11] for the specific techniques he recommends to evaluate these areas.

For the disabled patient, additional evaluation beyond these usual techniques is necessary in the areas of *Recent Memory, Perception, Affect,* and *Judgment.*

Recent Memory. An understanding of recent memory function in a disabled patient is necessary because his rehabilitation treatment will require him to learn new ways of performing those functions he has lost. He may, for example, need to learn a specific technique to execute a safe transfer or to coordinate crutch and leg movements for ambulation.

Teaching of these skills requires that the patient assimilate, retain, and reproduce new material not previously learned.

Recent memory functions with regard to language information may be assessed by asking the patient to remember, for example, an address that is given him. Retention is then evaluated when he is asked to reproduce the address later and perhaps the next day. With regard to non-language inputs, the patient can be taught a simple new motor task during the examination. Retention of this motor skill can then be assessed by later calling for its performance.

The emphasis should be on memory for totally new information. Asking the patient to recall what he ate for breakfast, although in a sense a recent memory check, is not really new material for him.

When recent memory functions are decreased, the physician is alerted to the fact that much repetition should be used when the patient is in training to remove disability.

Perception. Perception includes the process by which the patient organizes sensory inputs into information about the environment. This term, as used in the context of the psychiatric interview, refers to statements by patients that represent either gross misinterpretations of observable stimuli or hallucinations. Disturbances of this nature are gross departures from reality and are easily detected. Interpretation of wallpaper designs as ants crawling on the wall, the hearing of voices in a quiet room, and the interpretation of radiator noises as special communication codes are examples of disturbed perception associated with psychiatric disease.

There are more subtle disturbances in perception that are not associated with psychiatric disease, and these must be evaluated when retraining of motor skills is to be considered in a brain-damaged disabled patient. These disturbances deal with the interpretation of visual inputs of form, space, and distance. Such visual inputs require correct interpretation for the patient to be able to make a correct motor response based on them. For example, a patient in a wheelchair about to make a transfer onto a bed needs to interpret correctly first that both of his feet are on the floor, that he is close enough to the bed, and that nothing is in his way that will interfere with his performance. Similarly, a patient about to put on his shirt needs first to interpret correctly the inside and outside parts of the shirt and that both sleeves are right side out.

Disturbances in perception of this type are more likely to occur in brain damage that affects the right cerebral hemisphere. They can be tested for by asking the patient to copy figures such as a square, a triangle, and a Maltese cross. He can also be asked to reproduce from memory a clock face. When disturbances in perception of form exist, these reproductions are distorted.[5] Asking a patient to put on a shirt that is presented to him rolled up with one sleeve inside out is also a useful test.

When perception disturbances exist the examiner will recognize that the teaching of basic self-care skills by demonstration will not be as successful as verbal instruction.

Affect. A reactive depression is common following acute onset of a major disability in a previously normal patient, or following a relatively sudden additional functional loss in a patient with long-standing disease. It is a healthy response and indicates that the patient is at least able to recognize his losses. With such a recognition, he is more likely to be successful in removing disability.

A reactive depression requires remedial action if it is associated with disturbances of vegetative function or interferes with the patient's ability to respond to treatment. Judging whether such interference exists comes from observing patient participation during treatment rather than from what he says he is or will be doing.

The absence of a reactive depression may be a disturbing sign. If the patient is unable to face the loss, his ability to overcome the disability created by the loss may be reduced.

Mood swings are another feature of affect to consider. Rapid transitions from laughter to tears and back can represent the lability of an emotionally ill patient. Organic lability secondary to brain damage may show similar mood changes. Organic lability can, however, be more easily interrupted. Vigorously changing the subject matter of the conversation or sometimes a simple snapping of the fingers more easily curtails a flood of tears when such a lability is of organic origin. The presence of pseudobulbar neurologic signs will also suggest that the lability of mood is of organic origin.

Judgment. Judgment factors in brain damage relate to difficulties that the patient may have in monitoring his own behavior. In manner of dress or activities of physical function, he may fail to detect errors and be unaware of mistakes. These problems need to be distinguished from simple apathy, carelessness, or sloppiness. If such behavior is observed in the general assessment of the patient's appearance and the various activities he performs during the course of the examination, judgment problems may exist. Insight into judgment can also be obtained during observation of the patient as he performs the various tasks given him as part of the intellectual function inquiry. Family reports of exposure of genitals and other evidences of embarrassing behavior imply poor judgment. When such behavior represents changes in the patient's personality that are associated in time with the disease or the trauma, an organic origin is possible. When judgment problems are present, standby assistance may have to be provided for the patient as he performs his various basic functional activities.

Summary

The physical examination of the disabled patient, as for any patient, combines with the history and the laboratory data to achieve diagnosis of disease. In the disabled patient it also reveals secondary physical problems that are not direct consequences of the disease and indicates the residual strengths on which the physician and patient must build to remove disability and reestablish function. It also verifies the functional self-care historical data discussed in the *Present Illness* part of the history. This section has emphasized the specific features to be considered when an examination is performed on a patient with disability.

THE PROBLEM LIST

The problem-oriented approach to medical management is a helpful technique in the management of patients with disability, as the following example illustrates.[10]

A 19-year-old woman fractured her cervical spine in a small-plane accident, with resultant quadriplegia. Her male companion, with whom she had been living for the previous year and a half, was killed in the crash. Their relationship had been close and family-oriented, since she served as "stepmother" for her companion's two small children from a prior marriage. Following the accident, responsibility for the children was legally assumed by their natural mother.

The patient was hospitalized for a short period on an acute neurosurgical service and then transferred to a comprehensive rehabilitation center for inpatient care. Her problem list following a complete comprehensive evaluation shortly after admission to the rehabilitation center included:

1. C 7 fracture dislocation
2. C 7 complete quadriplegia
3. Ambulation dependent
4. Transfer skills dependent
5. Eating, dressing, personal hygiene skills dependent
6. Neurogenic bowel dysfunction
7. Neurogenic bladder dysfunction
8. Decreased respiratory function
9. Potential for pressure sore
10. Potential for thrombophlebitis
11. Immature personality
12. Reactive depression
13. Home architecture incompatible with paralysis
14. Financially dependent
15. Estranged from parents
16. Unemployed, no prior work history
17. Homemaking skills deficient
18. Transportation dependent

Eighteen problems make for an impressive list and one might argue that it need not be this long because nearly all are secondary to the first, *C 7 fracture dislocation,* and hence this one alone should be sufficient. Such an approach would be valid if there were a therapeutic technique that could reverse the spinal cord damage and restore full nervous system function. Unfortunately, such a technique does not exist. There does exist, however, a set of techniques for each of the 18 individual problems. These techniques can be used in minimizing the severity of the problems and in fully solving some of them — hence the importance of their identification.

Referring to the scheme in Figure 1–1 reveals problems 1, 2, 6, 7, 8, 9, and 10 to be of the character of "classic" medical problems. Problems 3, 4, 5, and 18, while also a direct result of the trauma, relate to the patient's physical disabilities. Problems 11 and 12 relate to the patient's psychological condition and problems 13, 14, 15, and 17 to the social sphere. Problem 16 succinctly identifies the vocational disability.

The problem-oriented approach to tracing the course of a problem includes:

1. The recording of subjective (S) data (patient symptoms and personal impressions).
2. The recording of objective (O) data (patient physical signs, laboratory and other test data, and quantified progress).
3. The assessment (A) of the problem (the interpretation of subjective and objective data into an impression of the status of the problem).
4. The plan (P) (the necessary additional consultations, diagnostics, therapeutics, or patient education required).

Thus the acronym SOAP serves as a means of organizing continuing management.

The utilization of the problem-oriented approach to patients with significant disability by personnel in rehabilitation wards and centers has led to several suggested modifications and variations. The reader should consult these for additional information.[1-4, 8]

CONCLUSION

It is essential for us to stress those parts of the classic history and physical examination on which special emphasis and elaboration are necessary when evaluating the disabled patient. Application of the techniques described will yield the diagnosis of disability.

Diagnosis of disease alone is insufficient for the planning of a comprehensive rehabilitation treatment program. The symptoms and signs required to diagnose disease are *not* synonymous with the symptoms and signs required to diagnose disability. To diagnose the disability — that is, the specific losses in physical, social, vocational, and psychological functions — requires investigations not ordinarily considered in the treatment of acute short-term disease.

The techniques described also identify those medical problems that are secondary but not natural consequences of a chronic impairment. To achieve a successful treatment program that removes disability, the physician must understand his patient's residual strengths. The methods to achieve this understanding have also been emphasized.

Following an appropriate evaluation, the physician is able then to list all of his patient's problems. Such a problem list will include disease diagnoses and secondary abnormalities. It must also include the specific losses in *physical* basic self-care functions, *social* functions, *vocational* functions, and *psychological* functions.

Once the problem list is established, the rehabilitation treatment process can begin. It begins with a specific plan for each of the problems on the list. It succeeds when each of the problems is solved to the highest degree obtainable by available therapeutic techniques.

Some of the other chapters in this book deal with further elaboration of evaluation methods and the therapeutics that can be brought to bear on the solution of disability problems. The reader will find that the therapeutic techniques described will fall within one of six general areas: (1) methods to prevent or correct secondary problems, (2) methods to enhance the capability of systems unaffected by the disease, (3) methods to enhance the functional capacity of affected systems, (4) methods to promote function through the use of adaptive equipment, (5) methods to modify the social and vocational environment, and (6) methods from psychological theory to enhance patient performance.

REFERENCES

1. Abrams, K. S., Neville, R., and Becker, M. C.: Problem-oriented recording of psychosocial problems. Arch. Phys. Med. Rehabil., 54:316–319, 1973.
2. Dinsdale, S. M., Gent, M., Kline, G., and Milner, R.: Problem-oriented medical records: Their impact on staff communication, attitudes and decision making. Arch. Phys. Med. Rehabil., 56:269–274, 1975.
3. Dinsdale, S. M., Mossman, P. L., Gullickson, G., Jr., and Anderson, T. P.: The problem-oriented medical record in rehabilitation. Arch. Phys. Med. Rehabil., 51:488–492, 1970.
4. Grabois, M.: The problem-oriented medical record: Modification and simplification for rehabilitation medicine. South. Med. J., 70:1383–1385, 1977.
5. Heimburger, R. F., and Reitan, R. M.: Easily administered written test for lateralizing brain lesions. J. Neurosurg., 18:301–312, 1961.
6. Lehmann, J. F.: Patient care needs as a basis for development of objectives of physical medicine and rehabilitation teaching in undergraduate medical schools. J. Chronic Dis., 21:3–12, 1968.
7. Mayo Clinic: Clinical Examinations in Neurology, 4th Ed. Philadelphia, W. B. Saunders Company, 1976.
8. Milhous, R. L.: The problem-oriented medical record in rehabilitation management and training. Arch. Phys. Med. Rehabil., 53:182–185, 1972.
9. Rosse, C., and Clawson, D. K.: The Musculoskeletal System in Health and Disease. New York, Harper and Row, 1980.
10. Stolov, W. C., and Clowers, M. R. (Eds.): Handbook of Severe Disability. Washington, D.C., U.S. Government Printing Office, 1981.
11. Storrow, J. A.: Outline of Clinical Psychiatry. New York, Appleton-Century-Crofts, 1969.
12. Weed, L. L.: Medical Records, Medical Education and Patient Care: The Problem-Oriented Record as a Basic Tool. Cleveland, Ohio, Case Western Reserve University Press, 1969.

2

MEASUREMENT OF MUSCULOSKELETAL FUNCTION

THEODORE M. COLE
JEROME S. TOBIS

GONIOMETRY

THEODORE M. COLE

Goniometry is the measurement of joint motion. It is an essential step in the evaluation of function in a patient with muscular, neurologic, or skeletal disability. The diagnosis of the way in which a patient functions in daily life and how one moves about or manipulates the environment physically may depend heavily upon the degree to which the parts of his body can tolerate passive or active motion. The presence of voluntary muscular contraction, the application of a prosthetic or orthotic device, or the preservation of sensation in a part of the body may be of little value to the patient if the joints of that part are unable to be moved through all or part of their normal range of motion. In other cases — for example, when limitation of joint motion may still permit the patient to walk — endurance may be greatly hampered by the fatiguing effect of muscles exerting their forces at a biomechanical disadvantage.

In addition to helping the physician make a diagnosis of the patient's functional loss, the careful examination of joint motion can reveal the extension of a disease process or provide objective criteria for determining the effectiveness of a treatment program. With-

out such evaluation, not only is the patient's care impaired but legal determination of disability,[12] which in some cases depends upon joint motion, may be muddled and the extent of feasible rehabilitation misjudged.

An accurate medical record is not possible without accurate measurement. Should there be a change in the patient's therapist, should subsequent follow-up of a patient's disease be necessary, or should a dormant disease become reactivated, correct treatment depends upon accurate clinical measurement. If review of data from a patient's record should become necessary for purposes of research, the study will be meaningful only to the extent that procedures such as goniometry were performed and recorded correctly.

The reader setting out to learn the skillful employment of goniometry may have little interest in the accumulated years of controversy over tools and methods to measure the motion of joints. The reader will, however, be interested in readily acquiring the skill and applying it to patients so that they may benefit. One should also want to learn how to communicate findings accurately to colleagues and how to understand their records.

To that end the physician should be acquainted with some of the more commonly used tools and techniques.

TOOLS AND INSTRUMENTS

Although many types of goniometers or arthrometers have been described,[11] the instrument most commonly used in the clinic is the universal goniometer, examples of which are shown in Figure 2–1. The two arms of the goniometer, with a pointer on one and a protractor scale on the other, are joined by a pivot, which provides enough friction so that the instrument remains stable when picked up and held for reading. Some goniometers are made with full-circle scales and others with half-circle scales, but all should be clearly marked in degrees so that the scale may be easily read by the unaided eye at 18 inches. The length of the arms of an easily portable goniometer is usually about 6 inches. However, if more accurate measurements are required for joints of very large[1] or very small members, then longer or shorter arms may be preferred. The tool should also be lightweight, durable, and washable in order to assure that it will be carried in the examiner's pocket or bag often enough to ensure its frequent use.

Only rarely will other joint-measuring tools be useful for the bedside examination. The exception to this generalization is the spine: meaningful measurements of joint motion in the spine are confounded by the multiplicity of participating joints, the paucity of reliable landmarks, and the bulk of soft tissue overlying the joints being measured. Spinal x-rays in extremes of motion offer more useful, readily available, and easily understood information. Bubble goniometers, plumb lines, electronics devices, and certain other tools are used only in special settings and will not be discussed here.[2, 3, 8]

SYSTEMS OF MEASUREMENT

Many of the systems suggested for recording measurements of range of motion were reviewed by Moore,[9, 10] who argues strongly that, whatever method is selected for use, it would be wise for everyone working in the same hospital, department, or clinic to utilize the same system of notation. The method put forth in this chapter is an adaptation of the system used by Knapp and West[6] and is based upon relating the range of motion of a joint to a full circle, or 360°. Since the bones of the body may be considered as levers or systems of levers, they may be thought of as moving in a rotary fashion about an axis of rotation located in the center of their joints. When motion occurs about a joint, every point in the moving bone must describe an arc of a circle, the center of which lies on the axis of rotation.

It is important to locate correctly the axis of rotation of a joint in order to perform

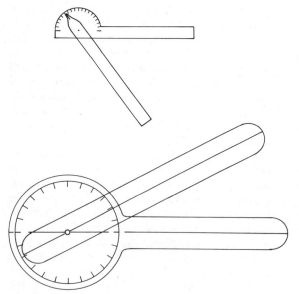

FIGURE 2–1. Two examples of universal goniometers commonly used by the clinician.

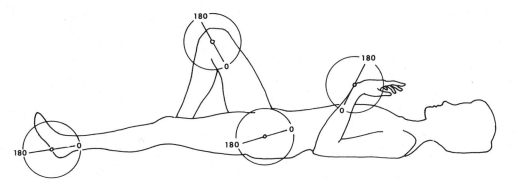

FIGURE 2–2. The full-circle or 360° system of goniometry applied to several joints of the body, illustrating the locations of the zero degree (0°) position.

accurate goniometry. In almost all joints, the axis of a goniometer can be placed so as to coincide with the axis of rotation of the joint. The angle thus formed by the two arms of the goniometer corresponds to the angle formed by the two members of the joint.

The 0° position of a circle superimposed upon the joint has been arbitrarily assigned. With the patient in the anatomical position, 0° is designated as the point directly over the patient's head, with 180° toward the patient's feet. As shown in Figure 2–2, when the proximal member of a joint is moved from the anatomical position, the 0° position moves accordingly and will no longer lie over the patient's head. In the full-circle system, almost all joint motions can be considered as rotating away from or toward the overhead zero point in the frontal or the sagittal planes. Thus, in the sagittal plane flexion is motion that rotates the distal member toward the 0° position on the circle and extension rotates it away from 0°. Abduction is motion toward and adduction motion away from the 0° position in the frontal plane.

The horizontal or transverse plane applies to certain joints that rotate about the longitudinal axis of the body. Neck rotation is an example of such a configuration. The 0° position is designated on the superimposed circle as that point directly in front of the tip of the patient's nose.

Since the 0° position is defined in terms of one of the joint members expressing the position of a joint in degrees signifies a definite relationship between the two members of the joint. Thus, when two arms of the goniometer are laid along the longitudinal axes of two joint members, and a measurement is made at the two extremes of motion, the examiner at once defines the limits of motion, the range of motion, and the many angles that may be formed at that joint.

Other systems of recording joint motion are based upon a different set of numerical figures attached to the zero points or starting points. Some argue for defining the anatomic position as 0° and recording motion as deviation from 0°. Others suggest modifications of this depending upon the joint and the motion being measured. Still other systems require the joining of positive and negative values to compute a range for the entire motion in question. Some workers argue for the use of small numbers, 180° or less for a single motion, believing that smaller numbers can be more easily visualized.

When used consistently, the method of recording joint motion offered here has been found to be readily understood by therapists, nurses, and physicians. Examiners have been able to learn quickly where the zero or starting point is located. The notion that large numbers are difficult to visualize has not been borne out by examiners who use this method of recording in their daily work. Indeed, the 360° system was employed years ago by Knapp to facilitate quick learning by persons without medical or anatomic training.[7]

The 360° system has an added advantage. A flexion contracture, which produces an inability to move the part to its normal position of extension, or a recurvatum deformity, which is present when there is an excessive laxness of a joint permitting motion beyond normal extension, can be easily recorded. There is no need for awkward expressions. Further, there is no need to add or subtract numbers to arrive at the limits of motion.

TERMINOLOGY

As in almost all other areas of medical communication, agreement on goniometric terminology has not been universal. The problem of communication is made worse by the insistence of some persons that the nomenclature should not include such terms as *dorsiflexion* or *radial deviation* but should utilize the "purer" terms of *flexion, extension, abduction, adduction,* and *medial* and *lateral rotation.* However, the choice of words should depend wholly upon whether or not they accurately communicate what the writer intends. The following glossary lists many of the terms commonly used in the language of goniometry.

Glossary of Goniometric Terms

Goniometer: an instrument for measuring angles.

Sagittal plane: the vertical, anterior-posterior plane through the longitudinal axis of the trunk, dividing the body into right and left halves.

Frontal or *coronal plane:* any vertical plane at right angles to the sagittal plane, dividing the body into ventral and dorsal portions.

Horizontal or *transverse plane:* any plane through the body parallel with the horizon.

Flexion: bending of a joint so that the two adjacent segments approach each other and the joint angle is decreased.

Extension: straightening of the joint so that the two adjacent segments are moved apart and the joint angle is increased.

Rotation: turning or moving of a part around its axis.

Supination: rotating the forearm so that the palm is up (anterior in the anatomic position).

Pronation: rotating the forearm so that the palm of the hand is down (posterior in the anatomic position).

Deviation: moving away from a starting position; frequently to denote abduction or adduction relative to the midline, or rotation from a starting point.

Inversion: turning inward; turning the sole of the foot so it tends to face medially.

Eversion: turning outward; turning the sole of the foot so it tends to face laterally.

Abduction: motion at a joint so that segment is moved laterally away from the midline.

Adduction: motion at a joint so that a segment is moved medially toward the midline.

Dorsiflexion: flexing or bending of the foot toward the leg so that the angle between the dorsum of the foot and leg is decreased.

Plantar flexion: flexing or bending the foot in the direction of the sole so that the angle between the dorsum of the foot and the leg is increased.

Opposition: moving the thumb away from the palm in a direction perpendicular to the plane of the hand.

Axis of rotation: a line at right angles to the plane in which adjacent limb segments move and about which all moving parts of the segments describe circular arcs.

Longitudinal axis: a line passing through a bone or segment, around which the parts are symmetrically arranged, and lying in both frontal and sagittal planes.

ACCURACY

Accuracy is an objective of all measurement techniques. However, like other aspects of the clinical examination, accuracy is a relative term implying careful training and attention to technique, thereby keeping the variability of measurements to an acceptable minimum while making observations and compiling data that closely approximate the true state of affairs. The ultimate test of the data that are recorded is in their interpretation and utilization. Interpretation, in turn, depends upon the level of expectation of the interpreter, who must have a realistic understanding as to just how accurate the data really are. Unless goniometry is carried out by a highly trained examiner using specialized equipment in a time-consuming method, measurement of joint motion cannot be expected to yield figures closer to true value than 3° to 5°.

Hellebrandt[4] found that the mean error for an average trained physical therapist was 4.75°. For a thoroughly experienced physical therapist, it was 3.76°. Since the average physician measures joint motion less frequently than the average physical therapist, a 5° error seems reasonable if the equipment is reliable and careful attention is given to technique.

In some cases previous disease or surgical intervention will alter the usual bony landmarks so as to render measurements less reliable. For example, the chronically dislocated hip will make the measurement of hip flexion-extension unreliable, as would the presence of an Austin-Moore prosthesis.

CONDITIONS AFFECTING MEASUREMENT OF JOINT MOTION

The examiner must indicate the conditions under which range of motion was measured. Was it done passively or actively; that is, did the patient move the part himself or did the examiner position the part? Was motion achieved with or without forcing the part through some portion of its total range? Did the patient experience pain during motion? Was motion opposed by voluntary or involuntary resistance? If resistance was detected, did it yield to sustained force exerted by the examiner or was the resistance unyielding? Was the patient able to cooperate with the examiner or was the examination carried out, for example, on a disoriented or confused patient who attempted to oppose the examiner? Was the patient under tension and anxious or was he relaxed? Was the examination encumbered by such things as a restrictive cast, a surgical wound, an appliance, or hypertrophied musculature? In addition to all these aspects, the patient's sex and age are known to influence the variability of normal joint motion.

Thus, many factors can influence the results of the examination, and since one or another of them may be present on one day and absent on the next, including such pertinent information is essential to an accurate interpretation of the data. Interpretation, of course, is the basis for decision making.

GENERAL PRINCIPLES IN MEASUREMENT OF JOINT MOTION

All motions that are commonly measured are carried out in one of three geometric planes. In the sagittal plane the following motions take place: flexion-extension and rotation at the shoulders; flexion-extension at the elbows, wrists, and fingers; and flexion-extension at the hips, knees, and ankles. Motions in the frontal or coronal plane are abduction and adduction at the shoulders and hips. Rotation of the hips and the cervical spine, which occurs in the horizontal plane of the body, radial and ulnar deviation at the fingers and wrists, and pronation-supination of the forearms are exceptions to the full-circle, 360° system.

Not all possible joint motions are measured in the usual clinical examination, because not all of the body's possible joint motions are important to the patient's pathologic or functional diagnoses or to the treatment plan. Also, some joint motions can be only crudely measured and efforts at accurate representation are not warranted. Instead, motions such as toe flexion-extension or back rotation are recorded descriptively in

TABLE 2–1. JOINTS AND MOTIONS THAT CAN BE MEASURED ACCORDING TO FULL-CIRCLE OR 360° GONIOMETRY AND EXCEPTIONS TO THE SYSTEM

Joints and Motions Measured on a Full Circle (360°)		Exceptions to the Full-Circle System
Sagittal Plane	*Frontal Plane*	
Shoulder: flexion-extension, rotation	Shoulder: abduction-adduction	
Elbow: flexion-extension		
Wrist: flexion-extension		Forearm: supination-pronation (abduction-adduction) Wrist: ulnar and radial deviation (abduction-adduction)
Finger: flexion-extension		
Hip: flexion-extension	Hip: abduction-adduction	Hip: rotation
Knee: flexion-extension		
Ankle: dorsiflexion-plantar flexion		Ankle: inversion-eversion

those cases in which their examination is germane to the patient's problem.

The examiner should become familiar with the normal ranges of motion for each joint. In many cases the patient's unaffected, contralateral extremity can be measured to establish a normal value for that patient.

TECHNIQUE OF JOINT MEASUREMENT

Joint — Shoulder

Motion: Flexion-extension (Fig. 2–3)
Plane of Motion: Sagittal
Positioning the Patient: The arm is at the patient's side.
How to Measure: The goniometer is centered on the shoulder just below the acromion. One arm of the goniometer is placed parallel to the midaxillary line of the trunk; the other arm of the goniometer is placed parallel to the longitudinal axis of the humerus along the lateral side of the patient's arm. The patient's arm moves anteriorly in flexion or posteriorly in extension. Readings are taken at the completion of motion.
Normal Limits and Range of Motion: 10° — 240°

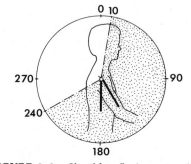

FIGURE 2–3. Shoulder: flexion-extension.

Motion: Abduction-adduction (Fig. 2–4)
Plane of Motion: Frontal
Positioning the Patient: The arm is at the patient's side with the palm toward the body. The arm is raised in the frontal plane to 90°. As it continues upward, the arm is externally rotated so that the palm faces the midline at completion of movement. The greater tuberosity of the humerus is a limiting factor in abduction, and by rotating the arm it is partially removed from the line of action.
How to Measure: The goniometer is centered on the posterior aspect of the shoulder joint (on a level with a line projected posteriorly from below the acromion). One arm of the goniometer is aligned parallel to the midline of the body (vertebral column). The other arm of the goniometer is aligned with the longitudinal axis of the humerus, posteriorly, after the patient's arm is moved.
Normal Limits and Range of Motion: 10° — 180°

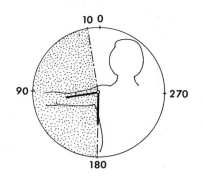

FIGURE 2–4. Shoulder: abduction-adduction.

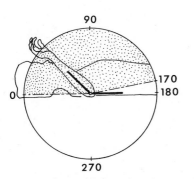

FIGURE 2–5. Shoulder: external and internal rotation.

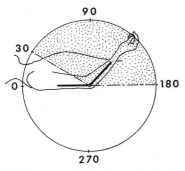

FIGURE 2–6. Elbow: flexion-extension.

Motion: External and internal rotation (Fig. 2–5)

Plane of Motion: Sagittal

Positioning the Patient: The humerus is abducted to 90°; the elbow is flexed to 90°. The forearm is positioned in pronation with the palm facing the feet.

How to Measure: The goniometer is centered on the elbow joint. One arm of the goniometer is held parallel to the midaxillary line of the thorax. The other arm of the goniometer is aligned with the longitudinal axis of the forearm. Measurements are made in extremes of external and internal rotation.

Normal Limits and Range of Motion:
External rotation,   0°
Internal rotation,   170°

Joint — Elbow

Motion: Flexion-extension (Fig. 2–6)

Plane of Motion: Sagittal

Positioning the Patient: The arm is held at the side in the anatomical position. For the convenience of the sitting patient, the shoulder may be flexed.

How to Measure: The goniometer is centered over the elbow joint laterally. The forearm is maintained in supination. One arm of the goniometer is parallel to the longitudinal axis of the humerus and the other arm is parallel to the longitudinal axis of the radius. Measurements are made in extremes of flexion and extension.

Normal Limits and Range of Motion: 30° — 180°

Joint — Radioulnar Joints

Motion: Pronation-supination (Figs. 2–7, 2–8)

Plane of Motion: This motion is an exception to the full-circle or 360° system of measurement. Motion takes place in the frontal plane.

Positioning the Patient: The humerus is adducted to the thorax and the elbow flexed to 90° with the radial aspect of the forearm directed toward the patient's head. This is the 0° position.

How to Measure: To measure pronation (see Fig. 2–7), the forearm is first fully pronated. The goniometer is held against the dorsal surface of the wrist and centered over the ulnar styloid; one arm of the goniometer is placed parallel to the longitudinal axis of the humerus. The other arm of the goniometer remains across the dorsum of the wrist.

To measure supination (see Fig. 2–8), the forearm is first fully supinated. The goniometer is held against the volar surface of the wrist and centered on the ulnar styloid. One arm of the goniometer remains across the volar surface of the wrist while the other is aligned with the longitudinal axis of the humerus.

Normal Limits and Range of Motion: The 0° reading is as described in *Positioning the Patient.* The normal limits of pronation and supination are 90° in each direction, totaling 180° of range.

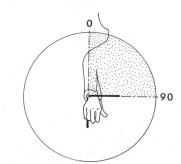

FIGURE 2–7. Radioulnar joint: pronation.

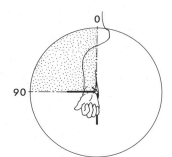

FIGURE 2–8. Radioulnar joint: supination.

Joint — Wrist

Motion: Flexion-extension (Fig. 2–9)
Plane of Motion: Sagittal
Positioning the Patient: The forearm and hand are held in pronation.
How to Measure: The goniometer is centered on the ulnar styloid; one arm of the goniometer is parallel with the longitudinal axis of the forearm along the ulnar border; the other arm is parallel with the longitudinal axis of the fifth metacarpal and is moved with the fifth metacarpal to measure flexion or extension.
Normal Limits and Range of Motion: 90° — 250°

Motion: Radioulnar deviation (abduction-adduction) (Fig. 2–10)
Plane of Motion: This motion is an exception to the full-circle or 360° system of measurement. Motion takes place in the horizontal plane.
Positioning the Patient: With the elbow at 90° of flexion-extension, the forearm is held in pronation and the wrist at 180° of flexion-extension.
How to Measure: The goniometer is placed over the dorsum of the hand and centered over the proximal portion of the third metacarpal bone; one arm of the goniometer is placed along the midline of the forearm, the other is placed

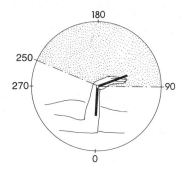

FIGURE 2–9. Wrist: flexion-extension.

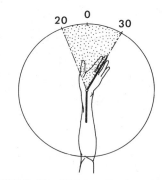

FIGURE 2–10. Wrist: radioulnar deviation.

parallel to the longitudinal axis of the third metacarpal bone. Measurements are made when the hand completes maximum deviation to the radial (abduction) and ulnar (adduction) sides.

Normal Limits and Range of Motion: Since this motion is an exception to the full-circle or 360° system of measurement, the 0° position is as described in *Positioning of Patient* above. Normal motion is 20° of radial deviation and 30° of ulnar deviation, totaling 50°.

Joint — Metacarpophalangeal Joints

Motion: Flexion-extension (including the thumb) (Fig. 2–11)

Plane of Motion: Sagittal

Positioning the Patient: The hand is held in any restful position and the thumb and fingers are extended.

How to Measure: The patient flexes each finger at the metacarpophalangeal joint. The goniometer is centered over the metacarpophalangeal joint being measured. One arm of the goniometer is placed on the dorsum of the hand and the other arm is placed on the dorsum and parallel to the longitudinal axis of the finger being measured. Measurements are made at maximum flexion and extension.

Normal Limits and Range of Motion: 90° — 180°.

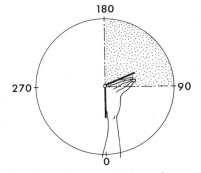

FIGURE 2–11. Metacarpophalangeal joint: flexion-extension.

Joint — Interphalangeal Joints (Including Thumb)

Motion: Flexion-extension (Fig. 2–12)

Plane of Motion: Sagittal

Positioning the Patient: The hand is held in any restful position.

How to Measure: The goniometer is centered over the joint to be measured. One arm of the goniometer is placed on the dorsal surface of the proximal phalanx and the other arm is placed over the dorsal surface of the distal phalanx. Readings are taken at positions of maximum flexion and extension.

Normal Limits and Range of Motion:
Proximal interphalangeal joints, 60° — 180°

Distal interphalangeal joints, 110° — 180°

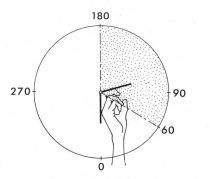

FIGURE 2–12. Interphalangeal joint: flexion-extension.

Joint — First Metacarpophalangeal Joint

Motion: Abduction-adduction of the thumb (Fig. 2–13)

Plane of Motion: This joint is an exception to the full-circle or 360° system. Motion is in a plane parallel to the palm of the hand.

Positioning the Patient: The hand is in any restful position and the fingers are extended.

How to Measure: The goniometer is centered over the volar aspect of the first carpal-metacarpal joint. One arm of the goniometer is placed parallel to the longitudinal axis of the third metacarpal; the other arm is aligned with the longitudinal axis of the first metacarpal. Readings are made in maximum abduction and adduction of the thumb.

Normal Limits and Range of Motion: 20° 50°

Motion: Opposition of the thumb (Fig. 2–14)

Plane of Motion: This motion is an exception to the full-circle or 360° system of measurement. The motion is made in a plane perpendicular to the plane of the palm.

Positioning the Patient: The hand is in any restful position with the fingers extended.

How to Measure: The goniometer is centered over the radial aspect of the first carpal-metacarpal joint. One arm of the goniometer is placed on the radial surface of the hand parallel to the longitudinal axis of the second metacarpal; the other arm is aligned parallel to the longitudinal axis of the first metacarpal. Measurements are made when the thumb is maximally approximated to and opposed from the palm.

Normal Limits and Range of Motion: 0° — 35°

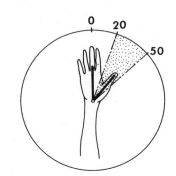

FIGURE 2–13. First metacarpophalangeal joint: abduction-adduction of the thumb.

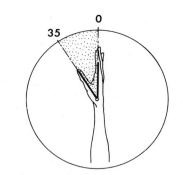

FIGURE 2–14. First metacarpophalangeal joint: opposition of the thumb.

Joint — Hip

Motion: Flexion-extension (Fig. 2–15)

Plane of Motion: Sagittal

Positioning the Patient: The patient may be supine, lying on his side, or standing.

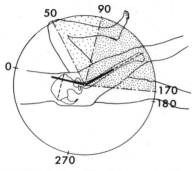

FIGURE 2–15. Hip: flexion-extension.

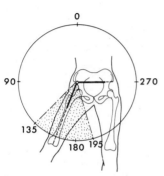

FIGURE 2–16. Hip: abduction-adduction (Method No. 1).

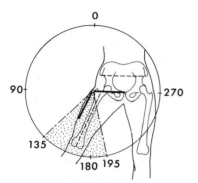

FIGURE 2–17. Hip: abduction-adduction (Method No. 2).

How to Measure: Draw a line on the patient's skin from the anterior-superior iliac spine to the posterior-superior iliac spine. Drop a perpendicular from this line to a point on the skin overlying the anterior-superior aspect of the greater trochanter. One arm of the goniometer is placed on this line with the center of the goniometer placed over the anterior-superior aspect of the greater trochanter. The other arm is placed parallel to the longitudinal axis of the femur on the lateral surface of the thigh. Caution must be taken to ensure that the marks drawn on the skin continue to overlie their bony landmarks as the hip is moved into positions of flexion and extension. If they do not, draw new ones.

Normal Limits and Range of Motion:
With the knee extended, 90° — 170°
With the knee flexed, 50° — 170°

Motion: Abduction-adduction (Figs. 2–16, 2–17)
Plane of Motion: Frontal
Positioning the Patient: Patient supine or standing
How to Measure: Draw a line on the skin connecting the anterior-superior iliac spines (see Fig. 2–16). Place one arm of the goniometer on this line. Align the other arm so that it falls on a line parallel to and overlying the midline of the anterior thigh.

An alternate method (see Fig. 2–17) uses the same reference line between the anterior-superior iliac spines, but one arm of the goniometer is placed parallel to and below the reference line rather than on the line, and the goniometer is centered over the trochanter of the hip being measured. The other arm lies parallel to the long axis of the thigh.

Normal Limits and Range of Motion: 135° — 195°

Motion: External and internal rotation (Figs. 2–18, 2–19)
Plane of Motion: This joint is an exception to the full-circle or 360° system of measurement. Motion takes place on the horizontal or transverse plane and is measured as deviation in the direction of internal or external rotation from the neutral or anatomic position of the lower extremity.

Positioning the Patient: The patient is supine. To measure motion in the hip-flexed position (see Fig. 2–18), the hip and knee are flexed to approximately 90° each. To measure motion in the hip-extended position (see Fig. 2–19), the thigh is flat on the table but the lower leg hangs over the end and the knee is flexed to 90°.

How to Measure: The goniometer is centered on the knee joint. Both arms of the goniometer are placed parallel to the longitudinal axis of the tibia on its anterior surface. One arm is moved to overlie the anterior surface of the tibia after it swings laterally or medially, while the other arm remains held in the position where the tibia had been prior to hip rotation.

Normal Limits and Range of Motion:
  External rotation (hip flexed, 40°)
  External rotation (hip extended, 45°)
  Internal rotation (hip flexed, 45°)
  Internal rotation (hip extended, 40°)

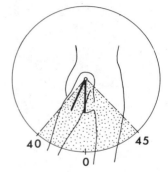

FIGURE 2–18. Hip: external-internal rotation in the hip (flexed position).

Joint — Knee

Motion: Flexion-extension (Fig. 2–20)
Plane of Motion: Sagittal
Positioning the Patient: The patient may be supine or sitting on the edge of a chair or table.
How to Measure: The goniometer is centered over the knee joint laterally; one arm is parallel to the longitudinal axis of the femur on the lateral surface of the thigh; the other arm is parallel to the longitudinal axis of the tibia on the lateral surface of the leg and pointing toward the ankle just anterior to the lateral malleolus.

Normal Limits and Range of Motion:
  45° — 180°

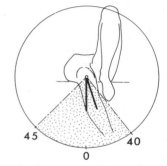

FIGURE 2–19. Hip: external-internal rotation in the hip (extended position).

Joint — Ankle

Motion: Dorsiflexion–plantar flexion (flexion-extension) (Fig. 2–21)
Plane of Motion: Sagittal
Positioning the Patient: The patient may be sitting or supine, but the knee should be flexed to permit maximum dorsiflexion of the ankle.
How to Measure: One arm of the go-

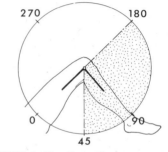

FIGURE 2–20. Knee: flexion-extension.

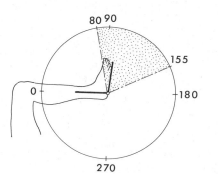

FIGURE 21–21. Ankle: dorsiflexion — plantar flexion.

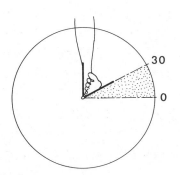

FIGURE 2–22. Ankle: inversion.

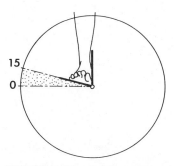

FIGURE 2–23. Ankle: eversion.

niometer is placed on a line parallel to the longitudinal axis of the fibula on the lateral aspect of the leg. The goniometer is centered on the sole of the foot in line with the longitudinal axis of the fibula. The other arm of the goniometer is placed parallel to the longitudinal axis of the fifth metatarsal. Care should be taken to avoid forced dorsiflexion or plantar flexion of the forefoot.

Normal Limits and Range of Motion: 80° — 155°

Motion: Inversion-eversion (Figs. 2–22, 2–23)

Plane of Motion: This motion is an exception to the full-circle or 360° system of measurement. Movement takes place in the frontal plane.

Positioning the Patient: The patient may be sitting or supine. If patient is sitting, the knee should be flexed over the end of the table and the sole parallel to the floor. If patient is supine, the sole of the foot should be perpendicular to the longitudinal axis of the trunk (vertebral column).

How to Measure: The goniometer is set at 90°. This position is considered 0°. One arm is placed parallel to the longitudinal axis of the lower leg. The goniometer is held laterally to measure inversion (Fig. 2–22) and medially to measure eversion (Fig. 2–23). The other arm is held parallel to the plantar surface of the forefoot behind the head of the first metatarsal.

Normal Limits and Range of Motion: Movement is recorded as deviation from the 0° position at which the sole of the foot is either parallel to the floor or perpendicular to the longitudinal axis of the trunk, depending upon whether the patient is sitting or supine.
Inversion, 30° (see Fig. 2–22)
Eversion, 15° (see Fig. 2–23)

Joint — Cervical Spine

The clinical measurement of motion in the cervical spine is probably the least accurate of all common measurements of the joints of the body because of the paucity of available landmarks and the depth of the soft tissues overlying the bony segments. Kottke and Mundale[5] believe that measurement should be made by x-ray of the specific joints involved.[4] However, approximations of cervical flexion, extension, internal and external rotation, and right and left lateral bending can be made by using the universal goniometer. For more precise measurements, however, roentgenographic examination of the cervical spine will be necessary.

Motion: Flexion-extension (Figs. 2–24, 2–25)

Plane of Motion: Sagittal

Positioning the Patient: The patient should sit erect. (Measurements made in the supine position, with the weight of the head removed from its compressive position, show increased range of motion.) The head is vertical, the eyes are forward in a "natural" position, and the shoulder girdle is relaxed. The patient holds the end of a tongue depressor blade firmly between his molars on the same side that the examiner is standing.

How to Measure: The examiner opens the goniometer about 60°. He grasps that corner of the protractor which is at the furthermost end of the goniometer arm. In order to steady the goniometer, the examiner braces his forearm against the patient's shoulder. The goniometer is centered over the angle of the jaw. The protractor arm should be parallel to the long axis of the protruding tongue depressor. The other arm is pointing in the direction of the motion to be measured. During flexion or extension, the pointer arm is adjusted to lie parallel to the new position of the tongue depressor.

Motion: Lateral bending (Fig. 2–26)

Plane of Motion: Frontal

Positioning the Patient: The position is the same as for neck flexion-extension except that a tongue depressor is not used.

How to Measure: The goniometer is centered at the spinous process of the seventh cervical vertebra; one arm of the goniometer is held in a position parallel with the floor; the other, or moving arm, is aligned with the external occipital protuberance. As the neck flexes from right to left, the movable arm records right and left lateral bending.

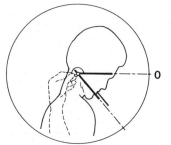

FIGURE 2–24. Cervical spine: flexion.

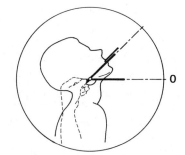

FIGURE 2–25. Cervical spine: extension.

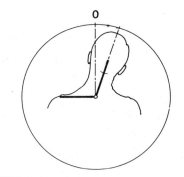

FIGURE 2–26. Cervical spine: lateral bending.

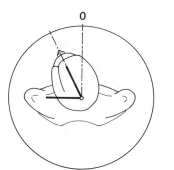

FIGURE 2–27. Cervical spine: rotation.

Motion: Rotation (Fig. 2–27)

Plane of Motion: This motion is an exception to the full-circle or 360° measurement. The motion takes place in the transverse or horizontal plane and is recorded as deviation from the zero position, which is achieved when the head is vertical with the eyes forward in a "natural" position. Rotation is recorded as deviation from zero to the right or left.

Positioning the Patient: The position is the same as for neck bending, above.

How to Measure: The examiner should stand on a low stool directly behind the patient. The goniometer is set at 90° and is centered over the vertex of the head. One arm of the goniometer is held steady in a line with the acromion process on the side being tested. The other, or moving arm, is in line with the tip of the nose. The movable arm follows the tip of the nose as the head is rotated from side to side. Readings are taken at the points of maximum rotation.

MUSCLE TESTING

JEROME S. TOBIS

Manual muscle testing permits one to evaluate the strength of a movement. The strength of an individual muscle cannot be routinely isolated and tested unless it is solely responsible for moving the body part in the performance of a particular movement. For example, the gastrocnemius and soleus are the plantar flexors of the ankle. Since the heads of the gastrocnemius attach to the condyles of the femur, it is possible to reduce the role of the muscle markedly by testing plantar flexion with the knee flexed. In this way the strength of the soleus can be tested. However, the gastrocnemius still makes some contribution in this posture.

It is important that substitution be avoided in evaluating the strength of a muscle responsible for a movement. Thus, in the presence of a paretic muscle or group of muscles, a movement may be performed by a muscle that ordinarily does not serve in that role. For example, the hamstrings flex the knee. In full extension, as in standing, the hamstrings may permit the knee to be fully extended even though the quadriceps — the prime extensor of the knee — is paralyzed.

Manual muscle testing is of value in the peripheral neuropathies and may be helpful in differentiating injury of the peripheral nerves from radicular damage. The peripheral and radicular innervations of skeletal muscles and their actions and tests are shown in Table 2–2 and Figures 2–28 to 2–55 and the following outline, which are from the Mayo Clinic's *Clinical Examinations in Neurology.*

Outline of Anatomic Information Required for Tests of Strength of Specific Muscles. In the following descriptions of the tests, the name of each muscle is followed in parentheses by the peripheral nerve and spinal segmental supply. There is considerable variability in segmental supply, particularly to certain muscles, as given by different authorities. Furthermore, there is some anatomic variation both in the plexus and in the peripheral nerves. The segments listed cannot, therefore, be regarded as absolute. The principal and usual supply is underlined. Under Action are listed only the principal and important secondary or accessory functions — those particularly useful in testing and those that may cause confusion by substituting for the activity of other muscles. In the description of the test itself the position and movement given first refer to the patient

TABLE 2–2. NEUROLOGIC MUSCLE CHART

Fascicul.	Tone	Size	Strength	R MUSCLES L	Strength	Size	Tone	Fascicul.
				CRANIAL NERVES				
				Temporal Cr.N. V				
				Masseter V				
				Pterygoid V				
				Forehead VII				
				Orbicularis oc. VII				
				Mouth VII				
				Platysma VII				
				Soft palate X				
				Pharynx X				
				Sternomastoid XI				
				Trapezius XI				
				Tongue XII				
				Neck, flex. C 1-6				
				Neck, ext. C 1-T1				
				Diaphragm C 345				
				Levator scapulae C 345				
				Rhomboids 45				
				Serratus anterior 567				
				Supraspinatus 456				
				Infraspinatus 456				
				Pect. maj. (clav.) 567				
				Pect. maj. (stern.) 678 T1				
				Subscapularis 567				
				Latissimus dorsi 678				
				Teres major 567				
				Deltoid 56				
				Biceps, Brachialis 56				
				RADIAL N.				
				Triceps C 678				
				Brachioradialis 56				
				Ext. carpi rad. lg. 678				
				Ext. carpi rad. br. 678				
				Supinator 567				
				Ext. digitorum 678				
				Ext. digiti quinti 78				
				Ext. carpi ulnaris 78				
				Abd. pollicis lg. 78				
				Ext. pollicis lg. 78				
				Ext. pollicis br. 78				
				Ext. indicis 78				

Table continued on opposite page

TABLE 2–2. NEUROLOGIC MUSCLE CHART *(Continued)*

Fascicul.	Tone	Size	Strength	R MUSCLES L	Strength	Size	Tone	Fascicul.
				MEDIAN N.				
				Pronator teres C 67				
				Flex. carpi rad. 67				
				Palmaris longus 78 T1				
				Flex. dig. sublimis 78 1				
				Flex. dig. prof. II, III 78 1				
				Flex. pollicis lg. 78 1				
				Pronator quadratus 78 1				
				Abd. pollicis br. 8 1				
				Opponens pollicis 8 1				
				Flex. poll. br. (sup.) 8 1				
				ULNAR N.				
				Flex. carpi ulnaris C 78 T1				
				Flex. dig. prof. IV, V 78 1				
				Hypothenar 8 1				
				Interossei 8 1				
				Flex. poll. br. (deep) 8 1				
				Adductor pollicis 8 1				
				Back				
				Abdomen (upper) T 6-9				
				Abdomen (lower) 10-L1				
				Iliopsoas L 1234				
				Adductors, thigh 234				
				Abductors, thi. (Glut. med.) 45 S1				
				Med. rot., thigh 45 1				
				Lat. rot., thigh 45 12				
				Gluteus maximus 5 12				
				Quadriceps 234				
				Hamstrings, int. 45 12				
				Biceps fem. (ext. hamstr.) 5 12				
				PERONEAL N.				
				Tibialis ant. 45 1				
				Ext. digitorum lg. 45 1				
				Ext. hallucis lg. 45 1				
				Peronei 45 1				
				Ext. digitorum br. 45 1				
				TIBIAL N.				
				Gastroc., Soleus 5 12				
				Tibialis post. 5 1				
				Toes, flexors 5 12				
				Foot, intrinsic 5 12				

unless otherwise clearly stated. In some instances the movement is adequately indicated by the action of the muscle and, hence, is omitted here. The term "resistance," unless otherwise specifically stated, refers to the pressure applied by the examiner, and this is in the direction opposite to that of the movement. For brevity and uniformity in description of the tests, the method of testing in which the patient initiates action against the resistance of the examiner is given except when the other method is distinctly more applicable. However, *this concession to uniformity and brevity of description is not meant to imply a preference for the method of testing in which the patient initiates action.* The location of the belly of the muscle and its tendon is often given in order to stress the importance of observation and palpation in identifying function of that particular muscle. As participating muscles, only those are listed that have a definite action in the movement being tested and that may substitute at least in part for the muscle being discussed.

Trapezius (Figs. 2–28 and 2–29). (Spinal accessory N.)

ACTION: Elevation, retraction (adduction) and rotation (lateral angle upward) of scapula, providing fixation of scapula during many movements of arm.

TEST: Elevation (shrugging) of shoulder against resistance tests upper portion, which is readily visible.

Bracing shoulder (backward movement and adduction of scapula) tests chiefly middle portion.

Abduction of arm against resistance intensifies winging of scapula.

Participating Muscles:

Elevation — Levator scapulae (Cervical N's. 3 and 4 and Dorsal scapular N., C 3 4 5).

Retraction — Rhomboids.

Upward rotation — Serratus anterior.

In isolated trapezius palsy with the shoulder girdle at rest, the scapula is displaced downward and laterally and is rotated so that the superior angle is farther from the spine than the inferior angle. The lateral displacement is due in part to the unopposed action of the serratus anterior. The vertebral border, particularly at the inferior angle, is flared. These changes are accentuated when the arm is abducted from the side against resistance. On flexion (forward elevation) of the arm, however, the flaring of the inferior angle virtually disappears. These features

are important in distinguishing trapezius palsy from serratus anterior palsy, which produces an equally characteristic winging of the scapula but in which movement of the arm in these two planes has the opposite effect. Atrophy of the trapezius is evident chiefly in the upper portion.

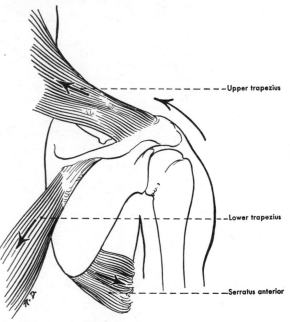

FIGURE 2–28. Upward rotators of the scapula. (Redrawn from Hollinshead, W. H.: Functional Anatomy of the Limbs and Back.)

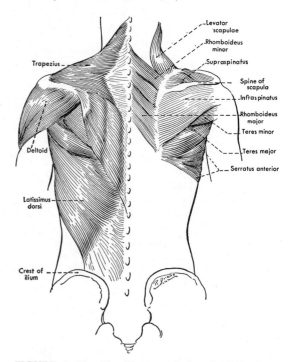

FIGURE 2–29. Musculature of the shoulder from behind. (From Hollinshead, W. H.: Functional Anatomy of the Limbs and Back.)

Rhomboids (Fig. 2–29). (Dorsal scapular N. from anterior ramus C 4 5)

ACTION: Retraction (adduction) of scapula and elevation of its vertebral border.

TEST: Hand on hip, arm held backward and medially. Examiner attempts to force elbow laterally and forward, observing and palpating muscle bellies medial to scapula.

Participating Muscles:
Trapezius; levator scapulae — elevation of medial border of scapula.

Serratus Anterior (Fig. 2–28). (Long thoracic N. from anterior rami C 5 6 7)

ACTION: Protraction (lateral and forward movement) of scapula, keeping it closely applied to thorax.

Assistance in upward rotation of scapula.

TEST: Forward thrust of outstretched arm against wall or against resistance by examiner.

Isolated palsy results in comparatively little change in the appearance of the shoulder girdle at rest. There is, however, slight winging of the inferior angle of the scapula and slight shift medially toward the spine. When the outstretched arm is thrust forward, the entire scapula, particularly its inferior angle, shifts backward away from the thorax, producing the characteristic wing effect. Abduction of the arm laterally, however, produces comparatively little winging, demonstrating again an important difference from the manifestations of paralysis of the trapezius.

Supraspinatus (Fig. 2–30). (Suprascapular N. from upper trunk of brachial plexus, C 4 5 6)

ACTION: Initiation of abduction of arm from side of body.

TEST: Above action against resistance.

Atrophy may be detected just above the spine of the scapula, but the trapezius overlies the supraspinatus and atrophy of either muscle will produce a depression in this area. Scapular fixation is important in this test.

Participating Muscle:
Deltoid.

Infraspinatus (Fig. 2–31). (Suprascapular N. from upper trunk of brachial plexus, C 4 5 6)

ACTION: Lateral (external) rotation of arm at shoulder.

TEST: Elbow at side and flexed 90°. Patient resists examiner's attempt to push

the hand medially toward the abdomen.

The muscle is palpable and atrophy may be visible below the spine of the scapula.

Participating Muscles:
Teres minor (axillary N.); deltoid — posterior fibers.

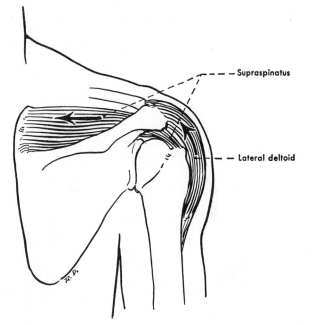

FIGURE 2–30. Abductors of the humerus. (From Hollinshead, W. H.: Functional Anatomy of the Limbs and Back.)

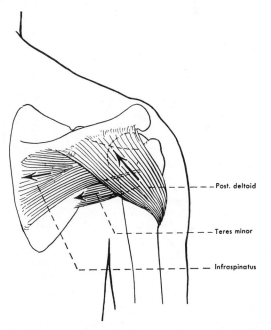

FIGURE 2–31. The chief external rotators of the humerus. (Redrawn from Hollinshead, W. H.: Functional Anatomy of the Limbs and Back.)

Pectoralis Major (Fig. 2–32). Clavicular portion (Lateral pectoral N. from lateral cord of plexus, C 5 6 7)

Sternal portion (Medial pectoral N. from medial cord of plexus, Lateral pectoral N. C 6 7 8 T 1)

ACTION: Adduction and medial rotation of arm.

Clavicular portion — assistance in flexion of arm.

TEST: Arm in front of body. Patient resists attempt by examiner to force it laterally.

The two portions of the muscle are visible and palpable.

Latissimus Dorsi (Fig. 2–33). (Thoracodorsal N. from posterior cord of plexus, C 6 7 8)

ACTION: Adduction, extension, and medial rotation of arm.

TEST: Arm in abduction to horizontal position. Downward and backward movement against resistance applied under elbow.

The muscle should be observed and palpated in and below the posterior axillary fold. When the patient coughs, a brisk contraction of the normal latissimus dorsi can be felt at the inferior angle of the scapula.

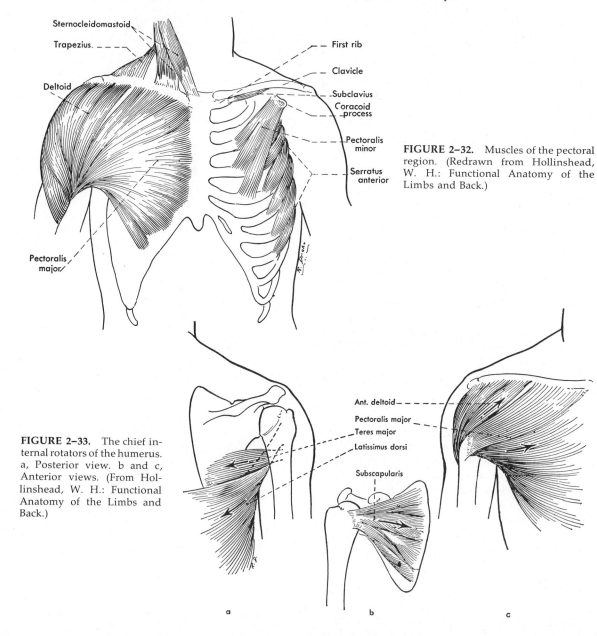

FIGURE 2–32. Muscles of the pectoral region. (Redrawn from Hollinshead, W. H.: Functional Anatomy of the Limbs and Back.)

FIGURE 2–33. The chief internal rotators of the humerus. a, Posterior view. b and c, Anterior views. (From Hollinshead, W. H.: Functional Anatomy of the Limbs and Back.)

Teres Major (Fig. 2–33a). (Lower subscapular N. from posterior cord plexus, C 5 6 7)

ACTION and TEST are the same as for latissimus dorsi.

The muscle is visible and palpable at the lower lateral border of the scapula.

Deltoid (Figs. 2–32 and 2–33b). (Axillary N. from posterior cord of plexus, C 5 6)

ACTION: Abduction of arm.

Flexion (forward movement) and medial rotation of arm — anterior fibers.

Extension (backward movement) and lateral rotation of arm — posterior fibers.

TEST: Arm in abduction almost to horizontal. Patient resists effort of examiner to depress elbow.

Paralysis of the deltoid leads to conspicuous atrophy and serious disability, since the other muscles that participate in abduction of the arm (the supraspinatus, trapezius and serratus anterior — the last two by rotating the scapula) cannot compensate for lack of function of the deltoid.

Flexion and extension of the arm against resistance.

Participating Muscles:

Abduction — given above.

Flexion — Pectoralis major — clavicular portion; biceps.

Extension — Latissimus dorsi; teres major.

Subscapularis (Fig. 2–33b). Upper and lower subscapular N's. from posterior cord of plexus, C 5 6 7)

ACTION: Medial (internal) rotation of arm at shoulder.

TEST: Elbow at side and flexed 90°. Patient resists examiner's attempt to pull the hand laterally.

Since this muscle is not accessible to observation or palpation, it is necessary to gauge the activity of other muscles that produce this movement. The pectoralis major is the most powerful medial rotator of the arm; hence, paralysis of the subscapularis alone results in relatively little weakness of this movement.

Participating Muscles:

Pectoralis major; deltoid — anterior fibers; teres major; latissimus dorsi.

Biceps; Brachialis (Fig. 2–34). (Musculocutaneous N. from lateral cord of plexus, C 5 6)

ACTION: Biceps — Flexion and supination of forearm.

Assistance in flexion of arm at shoulder.

Brachialis — Flexion of forearm at elbow.

TEST: Flexion of forearm against resistance. Forearm should be in supination to decrease participation of brachioradialis.

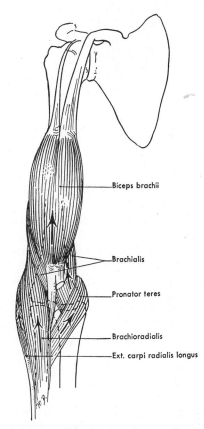

FIGURE 2–34. The flexors of the elbow. (From Hollinshead, W. H.: Functional Anatomy of the Limbs and Back.)

Triceps (Fig. 2–35). (Radial N., which is continuation of posterior cord of plexus, C 6 7 8)

ACTION: Extension of forearm at elbow.

TEST: Forearm in flexion to varying degree. Patient resists effort of examiner to flex forearm further. Slight weakness more easily detected when starting with forearm almost completely flexed.

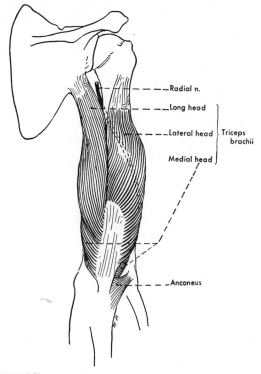

FIGURE 2–35. Muscles of the extensor (posterior) surface of the right arm. (From Hollinshead, W. H.: Functional Anatomy of the Limbs and Back.)

Brachioradialis (Fig. 2–36). (Radial N., C 5 6)

ACTION: Flexion of forearm at elbow.

TEST: Flexion of forearm against resistance with forearm midway between pronation and supination.

The belly of the muscle stands out prominently on the upper surface of the forearm, tending to bridge the angle between the forearm and arm.

Participating Muscles:
Biceps; brachialis.

Supinator (Fig. 2–36). (Posterior interosseous N. from radial N., C 5 6 7)

ACTION: Supination of forearm.

TEST: Forearm in full extension and supination. Patient attempts to maintain supination while examiner attempts to pronate forearm and palpates biceps.

Resistance to pronation by the intact supinator can usually be felt before there is appreciable contraction of the biceps.

Extensor Carpi Radialis Longus (Fig. 2–37). (Radial N., C 6 7 8)

ACTION: Extension (dorsiflexion) and radial abduction of hand at wrist.

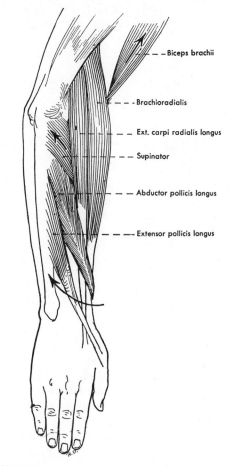

FIGURE 2–36. The chief supinators of the forearm. (From Hollinshead, W. H.: Functional Anatomy of the Limbs and Back.)

TEST: Forearm in almost complete pronation. Dorsiflexion of wrist against resistance applied to dorsum of hand downward and toward ulnar side.

The tendon is palpable just above its insertion into the base of the second metacarpal bone. The fingers and thumb should be relaxed and somewhat flexed to minimize participation of the extensors of the digits.

Extensor Carpi Radialis Brevis (Fig. 2–37). (Posterior interosseous N. from radial N., C 6 7 8)

ACTION: Extension (dorsiflexion) of hand at wrist.

TEST: Forearm in complete pronation. Dorsiflexion of wrist against resistance applied to dorsum of hand straight downward.

The tendon is palpable just proximal to the base of the third metacarpal bone. The

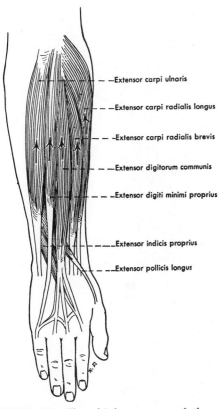

FIGURE 2–37. The chief extensors of the wrist. (From Hollinshead, W. H.: Functional Anatomy of the Limbs and Back.)

Labels in figure:
- Extensor carpi ulnaris
- Extensor carpi radialis longus
- Extensor carpi radialis brevis
- Extensor digitorum communis
- Extensor digiti minimi proprius
- Extensor indicis proprius
- Extensor pollicis longus

fingers and thumb should be relaxed and somewhat flexed to minimize participation of the extensors of the digits.

Extensor Carpi Ulnaris (Fig. 2–37). (Posterior interosseous N. from radial N., C 7 8)

ACTION: Extension (dorsiflexion) and ulnar deviation of hand at wrist.

TEST: Forearm in pronation. Dorsiflexion and ulnar deviation of wrist against resistance applied to dorsum of hand downward and toward radial side.

The tendon is palpable just below or above the distal end of the ulna. The fingers should be relaxed and somewhat flexed in order to minimize participation of the extensors of the digits.

Extensor Digitorum (Fig. 2–37). (Posterior interosseous N. from radial N., C 6 7 8)

ACTION: Extension of fingers, principally at metacarpophalangeal joints. Assistance in extension (dorsiflexion) of wrist.

TEST: Forearm in pronation. Wrist stabilized in straight position. Extension of fingers at metacarpophalangeal joints against resistance applied to proximal phalanges.

The distal portions of the fingers may be somewhat relaxed and in slight flexion. The tendons are visible and palpable over the dorsum of the hand.

Extension at the interphalangeal joints is a function primarily of the interossei (ulnar nerve) and lumbricals (median and ulnar nerves).

The extensor digiti quinti and extensor indicis (posterior interosseous nerve, C 7 8), proper extensors of the little and index fingers, respectively, can be tested individually while the other fingers are in flexion to minimize the action of the common extensor. In a thin person's hand the tendons can usually be identified.

Abductor Pollicis Longus (Fig. 2–36). (Posterior interosseous N. from radial N., C 7 8)

ACTION: Radial abduction of thumb (in same plane as that of palm, in contradistinction to palmar abduction, which is movement perpendicular to plane of palm).

Assistance in radial abduction and flexion of hand at wrist.

TEST: Hand on edge (forearm midway between pronation and supination).

Radial abduction of thumb against resistance applied to metacarpal.

The tendon is palpable just above its insertion into the base of the metacarpal bone and forms the anterior (volar) boundary of the "anatomic snuffbox."

Participating Muscle:

Extensor pollicis brevis.

Extensor Pollicis Brevis. (Posterior interosseous N. from radial N., C 7 8)

ACTION: Extension of proximal phalanx of thumb.

Assistance in radial abduction and extension of metacarpal of thumb.

TEST: Hand on edge. Wrist and particularly metacarpal of thumb stabilized by examiner. Extension of proximal phalanx against resistance applied to that phalanx, while distal phalanx is in flexion to minimize action of extensor pollicis longus.

At the wrist the tendon lies just posterior

(dorsal) to the tendon of the abductor pollicis longus.

Participating Muscle:

Extensor pollicis longus.

Extensor Pollicis Longus (Fig. 2–37).

(Posterior interosseous N. from radial N., C 7 8)

ACTION: Extension of all parts of thumb but specifically extension of distal phalanx.

Assistance in adduction of thumb.

TEST: Hand on edge. Wrist, metacarpal, and proximal phalanx of thumb stabilized by examiner with thumb close to palm at its radial border. Extension of distal phalanx against resistance.

If the patient is permitted to flex his wrist or abduct his thumb away from the palm, some extension of the phalanges results simply from lengthening the path of the extensor tendon. At the wrist the tendon forms the posterior (dorsal) boundary of the "anatomic snuffbox."

The characteristic result of radial nerve palsy is wristdrop. Extension of the fingers at the interphalangeal joints is still possible by virtue of the action of the interossei and lumbricals, but extension of the thumb is lost.

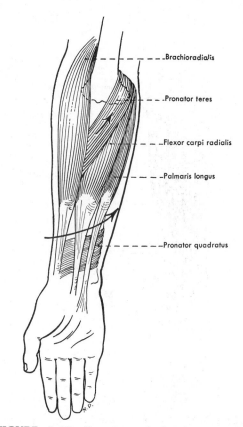

FIGURE 2–38. Pronators of the forearm. (From Hollinshead, W. H.: Functional Anatomy of the Limbs and Back.)

The next group of muscles examined is that supplied by the median nerve, which is formed by the union of its lateral root, from the lateral cord of the brachial plexus, and its medial root, from the medial cord of the plexus. Then the muscles supplied by the ulnar nerve (arising from the medial cord of the brachial plexus) are tested. However, for convenience in order of examination some of the muscles in the ulnar group are tested with the median group.

Pronator Teres (Fig. 2–38). (Median N., C 6 7)

ACTION: Pronation of forearm.

TEST: Elbow at side of trunk, forearm in flexion to right angle, and arm in lateral rotation at shoulder to eliminate effect of gravity, which, in most positions, favors pronation. Pronation of forearm against resistance, starting from a position of moderate supination.

Participating Muscle:

Pronator quadratus (Anterior interosseous branch of median N., C 7 8 T 1)

Flexor Carpi Radialis (Figs. 2–38 and 2–39). (Median N., C 6 7)

ACTION: Flexion (palmar flexion) of hand at wrist.

Assistance in radial abduction of hand.

TEST: Flexion of hand against resistance applied to palm. Fingers should be relaxed to minimize participation of their flexors.

The tendon is the more lateral (radial) one of the two conspicuous tendons on the volar aspect of the wrist.

In complete median nerve palsy, flexion of the wrist is considerably weakened but can still be performed by the flexor carpi ulnaris (ulnar nerve) assisted to some extent by the abductor pollicis longus (radial nerve). In this event, ulnar deviation of the hand usually accompanies flexion.

Palmaris Longus (Figs. 2–38 and 2–39). (Median N., C 7 8 T 1)

ACTION: Flexion of hand at wrist.

TEST: Same as for flexor carpi radialis.

The tendon is palpable at the ulnar side of the tendon of the flexor carpi radialis.

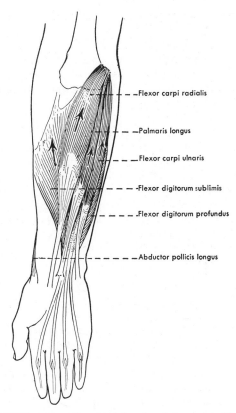

FIGURE 2–39. The chief flexors of the wrist. (From Hollinshead, W. H.: Functional Anatomy of the Limbs and Back.)

Flexor Carpi Ulnaris (Fig. 2–39). (Ulnar N., C 7 8 T 1)

ACTION: Flexion and ulnar deviation of hand at wrist.

Fixation of pisiform bone during contraction of abductor digiti quinti.

TEST: Flexion and ulnar deviation of hand against resistance applied to ulnar side of palm in direction of extension and radial abduction. Fingers should be relaxed.

The tendon is palpable proximal to the pisiform bone.

Flexor Digitorum Sublimis (Fig. 2–39). (Median N., C 7 8 T 1)

ACTION: Flexion of middle phalanges of fingers at first interphalangeal joints primarily; flexion of proximal phalanges at metacarpophalangeal joints secondarily.

Assistance in flexion of hand at wrist.

TEST: Wrist in neutral position, proximal phalanges stabilized. Flexion of middle phalanx of each finger against resistance

applied to that phalanx, with distal phalanx relaxed.

Flexor Digitorum Profundus (Fig. 2–39).

Radial portion — usually to digits II and III (Median N. and its anterior interosseous branch, C 7 8 T 1)

Ulnar portion — usually to digits IV and V (Ulnar N., C 7 8 T 1)

ACTION: Flexion of distal phalanges of fingers specifically; flexion of other phalanges secondarily.

Assistance in flexion of hand at wrist.

TEST: Flexion of distal phalanges against resistance with proximal and middle phalanges stabilized in extension.

With middle and distal phalanges folded over edge of examiner's hand, patient resists attempt by examiner to extend distal phalanges.

Flexor Pollicis Longus (Fig. 2–40). (Anterior interosseous branch of median N., C 7 8 T 1)

ACTION: Flexion of thumb, particularly distal phalanx.

Assistance in ulnar adduction of thumb.

TEST: Flexion of distal phalanx against resistance with thumb in position of palmar adduction and with stabilization of metacarpal and proximal phalanx.

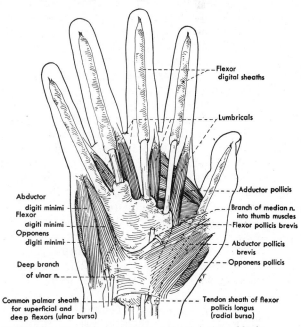

FIGURE 2–40. Short muscles of the thumb and little finger. (Redrawn from Hollinshead, W. H.: Functional Anatomy of the Limbs and Back.)

Abductor Pollicis Brevis (Fig. 2–40).
(Median N., C 8 T 1)
ACTION: Palmar abduction of thumb (perpendicular to plane of palm).

Assistance in opposition and in flexion of proximal phalanx of thumb.

TEST: Palmar abduction of thumb against resistance applied at metacarpophalangeal joint.

The muscle is readily visible and palpable in the thenar eminence.

Participating Muscle:

Flexor pollicis brevis (superficial head).

Opponens Pollicis (Fig. 2–40). (Median N., C 8 T 1)
ACTION: Movement of first metacarpal across palm, rotating it into opposition.
TEST: Thumb in opposition. Examiner attempts to rotate and draw thumb back to its usual position.

Participating Muscles:

Abductor pollicis brevis; flexor pollicis brevis.

Flexor Pollicis Brevis (Fig. 2–40). Superficial head (Median N., C 8 T 1) Deep head (Ulnar N., C 8 T 1)
ACTION: Flexion of proximal phalanx of thumb.

Assistance in opposition, ulnar adduction (entire muscle), and palmar abduction (superficial head) of thumb.

TEST: Thumb in position of palmar adduction with stabilization of metacarpal. Flexion of proximal phalanx against resistance applied to that phalanx while distal phalanx is as relaxed as possible.

Participating Muscles:

Flexor pollicis longus; abductor pollicis brevis; adductor pollicis.

Severe median nerve palsy produces the "simian" hand, wherein the thumb tends to lie in the same plane as the palm with the volar surface facing more anteriorly than normal. Atrophy of the muscles of the thenar eminence is usually conspicuous.

Three muscles supplied, at least in part, by the ulnar nerve have already been described: flexor carpi ulnaris, flexor digitorum profundus, and flexor pollicis brevis. The remaining muscles supplied by this nerve follow.

Hypothenar Muscles. (Ulnar N., C 8 T 1)
ACTION: Abductor digiti quinti

Flexor digiti quinti — abduction and flexion (proximal phalanx) of little finger.

Opponens digiti quinti —opposition of little finger toward thumb.

All three muscles — palmar elevation of head of fifth metacarpal, helping to cup palm.

TEST: Action usually tested is abduction of little finger (against resistance).

The abductor digiti quinti is readily observed and palpated at the ulnar border of the palm. Opposition of the thumb and little finger can be tested together by gauging the force required to separate the tips of the two digits when opposed, or by attemping to withdraw a piece of paper clasped between the tips of the digits.

Interossei (Figs. 2–41 and 2–42). (Ulnar N., C 8 T 1)
ACTION: Dorsal — abduction of index, middle, and ring fingers from middle line of middle finger (double action on middle finger — both radial and ulnar abduction, radial abduction of index finger, ulnar abduction of ring finger).

First dorsal — adduction (especially palmar adduction) of thumb.

Palmar — adduction of index, ring, and little fingers toward middle finger.

Both sets — flexion of metacarpophalangeal joints and simultaneous extension of interphalangeal joints.

TEST: Abduction and adduction of individual fingers against resistance with fingers extended. Adduction can be tested by retention of a slip of paper between fingers, and between thumb and index finger, as examiner attempts to withdraw it.

Ability of patient to flex proximal phalanges and simultaneously extend distal phalanges.

Extension of middle phalanges of fingers against resistance while examiner stabilizes proximal phalanges in hyperextension.

The long extensors of the fingers (radial nerve) and the lumbrical muscles (median and ulnar nerves) assist in extension of the middle and distal phalanges. The first dorsal interosseous is readily observed and palpated in the space between the index finger and the thumb.

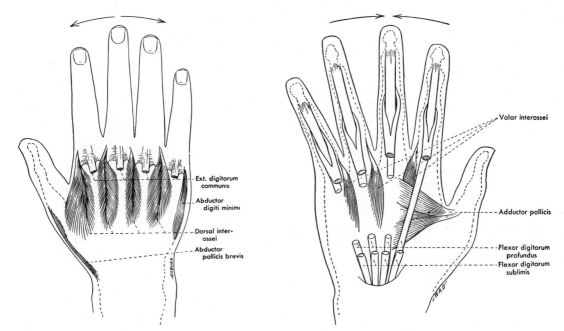

FIGURE 2–41. Dorsal view of the chief abductors of the digits. (Redrawn from Hollinshead, W. H.: Functional Anatomy of the Limbs and Back.)

FIGURE 2–42. The chief adductors of the digits. (From Hollinshead, W. H.: Functional Anatomy of the Limbs and Back.)

Adductor Pollicis. (Ulnar N., C 8 T 1)

ACTION: Adduction of thumb in both ulnar and palmar directions (in plane of palm and perpendicular to palm, respectively).

Assistance in flexion of proximal phalanx.

TEST: Adduction in each plane against resistance.

Retention of slip of paper between thumb and radial border of hand and between thumb and palm, without flexion of distal phalanx.

It is often possible to palpate the edge of the adductor pollicis just volar to the proximal part of the first dorsal interosseous.

Participating Muscles:

Ulnar adduction — First dorsal interosseous, flexor pollicis longus, extensor pollicis longus, flexor pollicis brevis.

Palmar adduction — First dorsal interosseous particularly; extensor pollicis longus.

In severe ulnar nerve palsy, atrophy is evident between the thumb and index finger, between the extensor tendons on the dorsum of the hand, and in the hypothenar eminence. The little finger is separated from the ring finger and cannot be brought into contact with it. The little and ring fingers especially are hyperextended at the metacarpophalangeal joints and flexed at the interphalangeal joints. The index and middle fingers are much less affected because of the intact lumbricals of these fingers (supplied by the median nerve). The true "clawhand" (*main en griffe*) is found only in combined median and ulnar nerve palsy. Attempt at adduction of the thumb is usually accompanied by flexion of the distal phalanx, indicating activity of the flexor pollicis longus (median nerve) in an effort to compensate for paralysis of the adductor. Froment's sign of ulnar palsy is an application of this phenomenon (Fig. 2–43). The patient grasps a piece of cardboard firmly with the thumb and index finger of each hand and pulls vigorously. If flexion of the distal phalanx of the thumb occurs, the test is positive and indicative of ulnar palsy.

Localization of lesions of the brachial plexus (Fig. 2–44) is based on the pattern of muscular weakness (and the distribution of sensory impairment).

Damage to the most proximal elements of the plexus (anterior primary rami) is manifested by weakness or paralysis of one or more of the muscles deriving nerve supply from the rami, such as the rhom-

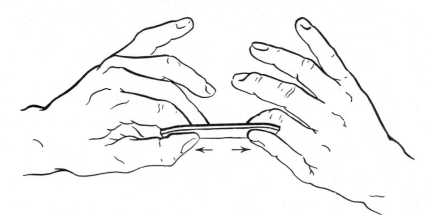

FIGURE 2–43. Froment's sign of ulnar palsy. Positive in the left hand, as indicated by flexion of the terminal phalanx of the thumb. (From Mayo Clinic: Clinical Examinations in Neurology.)

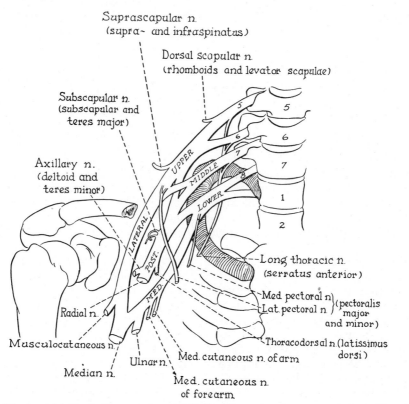

FIGURE 2–44. The brachial plexus. The muscles supplied by the various nerves are in parentheses. (From Mayo Clinic: Clinical Examinations in Neurology.)

boids and the serratus anterior, as well as by segmental distribution of muscular weakness (and sensory deficit) in the more distal portions of the upper extremity. Injury to the anterior ramus T 1 produces Horner's syndrome.

Lesions involving the most distal parts of the plexus spare some of the muscles of the shoulder girdle, and the pattern of muscular weakness (and sensory impairment) is more like that due to peripheral nerve injuries.

Lesions affecting the upper portion of the plexus, such as the upper trunk, impair the function of muscles supplied by segments C 5 and C 6 (syndrome of Duchenne-Erb) such as the supraspinatus, infraspinatus, deltoid, biceps, brachialis, brachioradialis, and supinator. The arm tends to hang limply at the side, medially rotated and pronated.

Injuries of the lower elements of the plexus, such as the lower trunk, C 8 and T 1 (syndrome of Klumpke), produce disability chiefly of the intrinsic muscles of the hand and flexors of the digits.

These examples illustrate the general principles of localization of lesions on the basis of examination of muscular strength.

The muscles of the neck and trunk may be examined in groups in most instances.

Flexors of Neck. (Cervical N's., C 1–6)
TEST: Sitting or supine. Flexion of neck, with chin on chest, against resistance applied to forehead.

Extensors of Neck. (Cervical N's., C 1–T 1)
TEST: Sitting or prone. Extension of neck against resistance applied to occiput.

Diaphragm. (Phrenic N's., C 3 4 5)
ACTION: Abdominal respiration (inspiration), as distinguished from thoracic respiration (inspiration) which is produced principally by the intercostal muscles.
TEST: Observation of patient for protrusion of upper portion of abdomen during deep inspiration when thoracic cage is splinted.
Ability of patient to sniff.
Litten's sign — successive retraction of lower intercostal spaces during inspiration.
Fluoroscopic observation of diaphragmatic movements.
Weakness of the diaphragm should be suspected in diseases of the spinal cord, when the deltoid or biceps is paralyzed, for these muscles are supplied by neurons situated very near those innervating the diaphragm.

Intercostal Muscles. (Intercostal N's., T 1–11)
ACTION: Expansion of thorax anteroposteriorly and transversely, producing thoracic inspiration.
TEST: Observation and palpation of expansion of thoracic cage during deep inspiration while maintaining pressure against thorax.
Observation for asymmetry of movement of thorax, particularly during deep inspiration.
Other more general tests of function of the respiratory muscles are:

Observation of patient for rapid shallow respiration, flaring of alae nasi, and use of accessory muscles of respiration.
Ability of patient to repeat three or four numbers without pausing for breath.
Ability of patient to hold his breath for 15 seconds.

Anterior Abdominal Muscles. Upper (T6–9), Lower (T10–L 1)
TEST: Supine — Flexion of neck against resistance applied to forehead by examiner.
Contraction of the abdominal muscles can be observed and palpated. Upward movement of the umbilicus is associated with weakness of the lower abdominal muscles (Beevor's sign).
Supine — Hands on occiput. Flexion of trunk by anterior abdominal muscles followed by flexion of pelvis on thighs by hip flexors (chiefly iliopsoas) to reach sitting position. Examiner holds legs down.
Completion of this test excludes significant weakness of either the abdominal muscles or the flexors of the hips. Weak abdominal muscles, in the presence of strong hip flexors, result in hyperextension of the lumbar spine during attempts to elevate the legs or rise to a sitting position.

Extensors of Back.
TEST: Prone with hands clasped over buttocks. Elevation of head and shoulders off table while examiner holds legs down.
The gluteal and hamstring muscles fix the pelvis on the thigh.

The movements of the lower extremities are not as complex as those of the upper extremities, hence the examination is somewhat simpler. Since the muscles of the pelvic girdle and thigh do not lend themselves as well to a sequence of examination based on the anatomy of the lumbosacral plexus (Fig. 2–45) as the muscles of the upper extremities, the order is determined largely by clinical convenience with some consideration to segmental innervation.

Many of the muscles are so powerful that when little or no weakness is present they can be tested profitably by certain maneuvers performed by the patient on his feet.

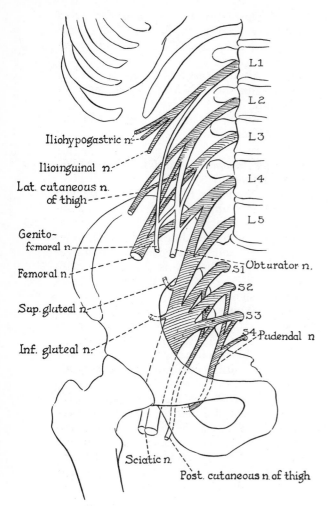

Iliohypogastric n.

Ilioinguinal n.

Lat. cutaneous n. of thigh

Genito-femoral n.

Femoral n.

Sup. gluteal n.

Inf. gluteal n.

L1

L2

L3

L4

L5

S1 Obturator n.

S2

S3

S4 Pudendal n

Sciatic n.

Post. cutaneous n. of thigh

FIGURE 2–45. The lumbosacral plexus. (From Mayo Clinic: Clinical Examinations in Neurology.)

Observation of the patient's gait will reveal weakness of certain muscles, and atrophy may be visible:

Iliopsoas — difficulty in bringing affected leg forward.

Abductors of thigh (chiefly gluteus medius and gluteus minimus) —sagging opposite side of pelvis and lateral displacement of pelvis to affected side when weight is on that leg.

Quadriceps — keeping knee locked when weight is placed on affected leg.

Tibialis anterior and extensors of toes — varying degrees of "steppage gait" and footdrop.

Gastrocnemius and soleus — limp produced by difficulty in raising heel from floor.

Certain maneuvers by the patient will make muscular weakness more apparent. The principal muscles involved are given:

Stepping up on a step.

Raising leg up to step — Iliopsoas.

Raising body — Gluteus maximus and quadriceps.

Squatting and rising — Quadriceps particularly.

Walking on heels — Tibialis anterior and extensors of toes.

Walking on toes — Gastrocnemius and soleus.

When there is little or no weakness, it is feasible to conduct the more detailed examination of the muscles of the lower extremities with the patient in the sitting posture throughout. However, the action of certain muscles is somewhat different in the sitting posture as compared with the supine or prone position. In particular, some of the lateral rotators of the thigh function also as abductors. Furthermore, the sitting posture interferes seriously with observation and palpation of some muscles — particularly the gluteus maximus and to a lesser extent the hamstrings. The muscles mentioned are therefore more accurately tested in the prone position.

In some instances it is convenient and advantageous to test the corresponding muscles of the two sides simultaneously for comparison. Examples are the adductors and abductors of the thighs and the extensors (dorsiflexors) and flexors (plantar flexors) of the feet and toes.

Iliopsoas (Fig. 2–28). Psoas major (Lumbar plexus [Fig. 2–45], L 1 2 3 4); Iliacus (Femoral N., L 2 3 4)

ACTION: Flexion of thigh at hip.

TEST: Sitting — Flexion of thigh, raising knee against resistance by examiner.

Supine — Raising extended leg off table and maintaining it against downward pressure by examiner applied just above knee.

Participating Muscles:

Rectus femoris and sartorius (both — Femoral N., L 2 3 4); Tensor fasciae latae (Superior gluteal N., L 4 5 S 1).

Adductor Magnus, Longus, Brevis (Fig. 2–46). (Obturator N., L 2 3 4. Part of adductor magnus is supplied by sciatic N., L 5, and functions with hamstrings.)

ACTION: Principally adduction of thigh.

TEST: Sitting or supine   Holding knees together while examiner attempts to separate them.

The two legs can also be tested separately and the muscles palpated.

Participating Muscles:

   Gluteus maximus; gracilis (Obturator N., L 2 3 4).

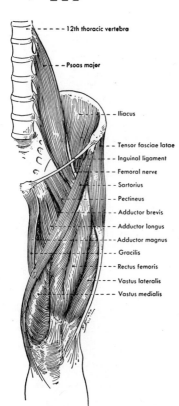

FIGURE 2–46. The more superficial muscles of the anterior aspect of the thigh. (From Hollinshead, W. H.: Functional Anatomy of the Limbs and Back.)

Abductors of Thigh (Fig. 2–47). (Superior gluteal N., L 4 5 S 1)

Gluteus medius and gluteus minimus principally.

Tensor fasciae latae to a lesser extent.

ACTION: Abduction and medial rotation of thigh.

   Tensor fasciae latae assists in flexion of thigh at hip.

TEST: Sitting — Separation of knees against resistance by examiner.

In this position the gluteus maximus and some of the other lateral rotators of the thigh function as abductors, hence diminishing the accuracy of the test.

Supine — Same test as above. More exact.

   Lying on opposite side —Abduction of hip (upward movement) while examiner presses downward on lower leg and stabilizes pelvis.

The tensor fasciae latae and to a lesser extent the gluteus medius can be palpated.

Medial Rotators of Thigh. Same as abductors.

TEST: Sitting or prone — Knee flexed to 90°. Medial rotation of thigh against resistance applied by examiner at knee and ankle in attempt to rotate thigh laterally.

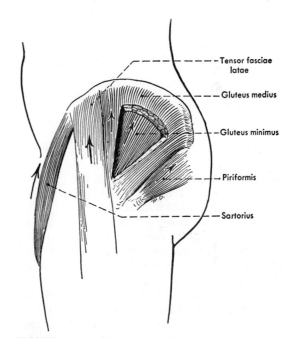

FIGURE 2–47. The abductors of the thigh. (From Hollinshead, W. H.: Functional Anatomy of the Limbs and Back.)

Lateral Rotators of Thigh (Fig. 2–48). (L 4 5 S 1 2)

Gluteus maximus (Inferior gluteal N., L 5 S 1 2) chiefly

Obturator internus and gemellus superior (N. to obturator internus, L 5 S 1 2)

Quadratus femoris and gemellus inferior (N. to quadratus femoris, L 4 5 S 1)

TEST: Sitting or prone — Knee flexed to 90°. Lateral rotation of thigh against attempt by examiner to rotate thigh medially.

The gluteus maximus is the muscle principally tested and can be observed and palpated in the prone position.

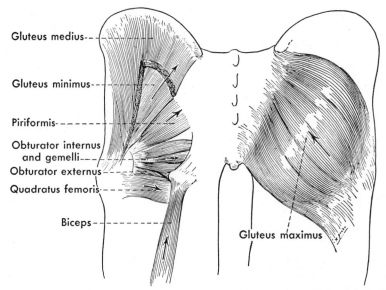

FIGURE 2–48. The posteriorly placed external rotators of the thigh. (From Hollinshead, W. H.: Functional Anatomy of the Limbs and Back.)

Gluteus Maximus (Fig. 2–48). (Inferior gluteal N., L 5 S 1̲ 2̲)
ACTION: Extension of thigh at hip.
  Lateral rotation of thigh.
  Assistance in adduction of thigh.
TEST: Sitting or supine — Starting with thigh slightly raised, extension (downward movement) of thigh against resistance by examiner applied under distal part of thigh.
  This is a rather crude test and the muscle cannot be observed or readily palpated.
      Prone — Knee well flexed to minimize participation of hamstrings. Extension of thigh, raising knee from table against downward pressure by examiner applied to distal part of thigh.
  The muscle is accessible to observation and palpation in this position.

Quadriceps Femoris (Fig. 2–49). (Femoral N., L 2 3̲ 4̲)
ACTION: Extension of leg at knee.
  Rectus femoris assists in flexion of thigh at hip.
TEST: Sitting or supine — Lower leg in moderate extension. Maintenance of extension against effort of examiner to flex leg at knee.
  Atrophy is easily noted.

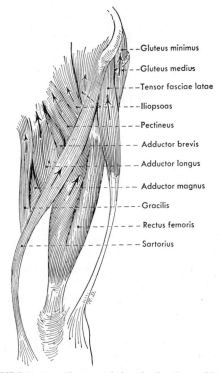

FIGURE 2–49. Flexors of the thigh. (From Hollinshead, W. H.: Functional Anatomy of the Limbs and Back.)

Hamstrings (Fig. 2–50). (Sciatic N., L 4 5̲ S 1̲ 2)
  Biceps femoris — external hamstring (L 5 S 1̲ 2)

Semitendinosus internal hamstrings (L 4 <u>5</u> S <u>1</u> 2)

Semimembranosus (L 4 <u>5</u> S <u>1</u> 2)
ACTION: Flexion of leg at knee.
       All but short head of biceps femoris assist in extension of thigh at hip.
TEST: Sitting — Flexion of lower leg against resistance.
       Prone — Knee partly flexed. Further flexion against resistance.
       Observation and palpation of the muscles and tendons are important for proper interpretation.

Tibialis Anterior (Figs. 2–51, 2–52, and 2–53).   (Deep peroneal N., L <u>4</u> 5 S 1)
ACTION: Dorsiflexion and inversion (particularly in dorsiflexed position) of foot.
TEST: Dorsiflexion of foot against resistance applied to dorsum of foot downward and toward eversion.
The belly of the muscle just lateral to the shin, and the tendon medially on the dorsal

aspect of the ankle, should be observed and palpated. Atrophy is conspicuous.
    Participating Muscles:
       Dorsiflexion — Extensor hallucis longus; extensor digitorum longus.
       Inversion — Tibialis posterior.

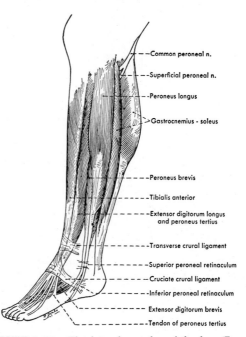

FIGURE 2–51. The lateral muscles of the leg. (From Hollinshead, W. H.: Functional Anatomy of the Limbs and Back.)

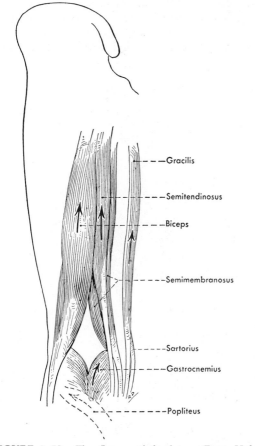

FIGURE 2–50. The flexors of the knee. (From Hollinshead, W. H.: Functional Anatomy of the Limbs and Back.)

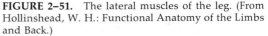
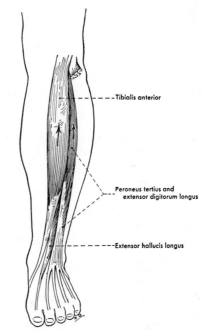

FIGURE 2–52. The dorsiflexors of the foot. (From Hollinshead, W. H.: Functional Anatomy of the Limbs and Back.)

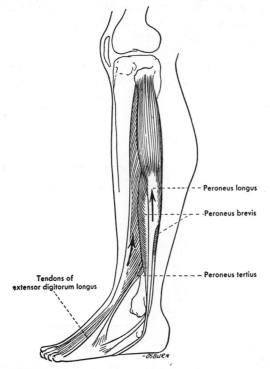

FIGURE 2–53. Evertors of the foot. (From Hollinshead, W. H.: Functional Anatomy of the Limbs and Back.)

Extensor Hallucis Longus (Fig. 2–52).
(Deep peroneal N., L 4 5 S 1)

ACTION: Extension of great toe and dorsiflexion of foot.

TEST: Extension of great toe against resistance while foot is stabilized in neutral position.

The tendon is palpable between those of the tibialis anterior and the extensor digitorum longus.

Extensor Digitorum Longus (Figs. 2–51 and 2–52). (Deep peroneal N., L 4 5 S 1)

ACTION: Extension of lateral four toes and dorsiflexion of foot.

TEST: Similar to above.

The tendons are visible and palpable on the dorsal aspect of the ankle and foot lateral to that of the extensor hallucis longus.

Extensor Digitorum Brevis (Fig. 2–51).
(Deep peroneal N., L 4 5 S 1)

ACTION: Assists in extension of all toes except little toe.

TEST: Observe and palpate belly of muscle on lateral aspect of dorsum of foot.

Peroneus Longus, Brevis (Fig. 2–53).
(Superficial peroneal N., L 4 5 S 1)

ACTION: Eversion of foot.

Assistance in plantar flexion of foot.

TEST: Foot in plantar flexion. Eversion against resistance applied by examiner to lateral border of foot.

The tendons are palpable just above and behind the external malleolus. Atrophy may be visible over the anterolateral aspect of the lower leg.

Gastrocnemius; Soleus (Fig. 2–54). (Tibial N., L 5 S 1 2)

ACTION: Plantar flexion of foot.

The gastrocnemius also flexes the knee and cannot act effectively in plantar flexion of the foot when the knee is well flexed.

TEST: Knee extended to test both muscles. Knee flexed to test principally soleus. Plantar flexion of foot against resistance.

The muscles and tendon should be observed and palpated. Atrophy is readily visible. The gastrocnemius and soleus are very strong muscles, and leverage in testing favors the patient rather than the examiner.

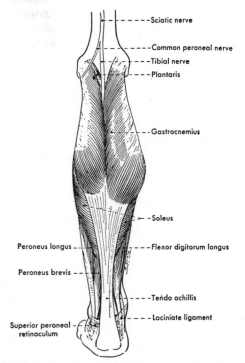

FIGURE 2–54. The musculature of the calf of the leg, first layer. (From Hollinshead, W. H.: Functional Anatomy of the Limbs and Back.)

For this reason slight weakness is difficult to detect by resisting flexion of the ankle or by pressing against the flexed foot in the direction of extension. Consequently, it is advisable to test the strength of these muscles against the weight of the patient's body. Have the patient stand on one foot and flex the foot so as to lift himself directly and fully upward. Sometimes it is necessary for the examiner to hold the patient steady as he performs this test.

Participating Muscles:

Long flexors of toes; tibialis posterior and peroneus longus and brevis (particularly near extreme plantar flexion).

Tibialis Posterior (Fig. 2–55). (Posterior tibial N., L 5 S 1)

ACTION: Inversion of foot.
Assistance in plantar flexion of foot.

TEST: Foot in complete plantar flexion. Inversion against resistance applied to medial border of foot and directed toward eversion and slightly toward dorsiflexion.

This maneuver virtually eliminates participation of the tibialis anterior in inversion. The toes should be relaxed to prevent participation of the long flexors of the toes.

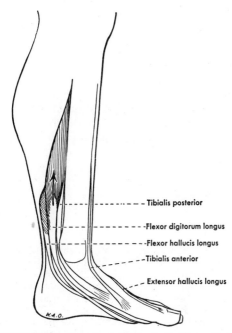

Tibialis posterior

Flexor digitorum longus

Flexor hallucis longus

Tibialis anterior

Extensor hallucis longus

FIGURE 2–55. Invertors of the foot. (From Hollinshead, W. H.: Functional Anatomy of the Limbs and Back.)

Long Flexors of Toes. (Posterior tibial N., L 5 S 1 2)

Flexor digitorum longus
Flexor hallucis longus

ACTION: Plantar flexion of toes, especially at distal interphalangeal joints.
Assistance in plantar flexion and inversion of foot.

TEST: Foot stabilized in neutral position. Plantar flexion of toes against resistance applied particularly to distal phalanges.

Intrinsic Muscles of Foot. Virtually all except extensor digitorum brevis (Medial and lateral plantar N's. from posterior tibial N., L 5 S 1 2)

ACTION: Somewhat comparable to that of intrinsic muscles of hand. Many people have very poor individual function of these muscles.

TEST: Cupping sole of foot is adequate test for most clinical purposes.

If paretic muscles are found that have different peripheral innervations but similar root innervation, such an observation would tend to support the localization of the lesion at either the root or the plexus level. This diagnostic technique can be supplemented by testing for sensory loss and by employing electrical nerve testing, including electromyography and determination of conduction velocity.

In the presence of an upper motor neuron lesion, manual muscle testing has limited value. It may give the examiner a gross estimate of the severity of the motor loss in a hemiplegic patient. However, spasticity does not permit voluntary movements to be performed with ease and may mask the motor power that the patient possesses for a given movement.

Before obtaining a more detailed evaluation of motor skill, a routine neurologic examination should be performed in order to evaluate the total clinical picture. For example, the presence of a sensory deficit will exaggerate a motor disability. Hemianopia may add to the difficulties of a hemiplegic in receiving adequate visual cues. The presence of spasticity or rigidity will impair motor skill. Thus determination of the neurologic deficits is important not only because of their diagnostic implications but in order to develop an effective program of management.

Motor Skill. In evaluating the patient's

Is patient able to meet the following activity requirements? (Write "N" if not necessary.)

Meal preparation, serving and clean-up _____

Work heights_____ Dominance_____

Marketing_____

Washing and hanging clothes_____

Ironing_____

Bedmaking_____

Light housekeeping (dusting, sweeping, etc.)_____

Heavy household activities (washing floors, windows, etc.)_____

Hobbies and special interests_____

Number of stairs_____ Family members_____

Child care: number of children_____ Ages_____

Will patient be alone for long periods of time?_____

Available help in family and outside_____

Limitations for working and contraindications_____

Budget: Supported_____ Self-sustaining_____ Middle_____ High_____

Ambulation status:_____

Assistive devices:_____

Comments:

FIGURE 2–56. Household activities information.

motor performance, one must test not only for range of motion and strength; the patient's capacity to perform various tasks must also be determined. Such testing may consist of an inventory of the activities that are routinely performed in daily life. It may consist of evaluating the transfer activities from bed to wheelchair or chair, the use of a wheelchair, the ability to ambulate and take care of one's personal hygiene and dressing. In Table 12–1, pages 258–262, is shown a method for recording such an inventory of motor skills.

Since so many of the patients who are treated by physiatric techniques suffer from locomotor disturbances, it is incumbent upon the examiner to study the patient's posture and gait (see Chapter 4).

Figure 2–56 provides a rapid means of analyzing the capacity of the disabled patient to be responsible for his own housekeeping.

REFERENCES

Goniometry

1. Clayson, S. J., Mundale, M. O., and Kottke, F. J.: Goniometer adaptation for measuring hip extension. Arch. Phys. Med., 47:255, 1966.
2. Defibaugh, J. J.: Measurement of head motion, Part I: A review of methods of measuring joint motion. J. Am. Phys. Ther. Assoc., 44:157, 1964.
3. Defibaugh, J. J.: Measurement of head motion, Part II: An experimental study of head motion in adult males. J. Am. Phys. Ther. Assoc., 44:163, 1964.

4. Hellebrandt, F. A., Duvall, E. N., and Moore, M. L.: The measurement of joint motion, Part III: Reliability of goniometry. Phys. Ther. Rev., 29:302, 1949.
5. Kottke, F. J., and Mundale, M. O.: Range of mobility of the cervical spine. Arch. Phys. Med., 40:379, 1959.
6. Knapp, M. E.: Measurement of joint motion. Univ. Minn. Med. Bull., 15:405–412, 1944.
7. Knapp, M. E.: Measuring range of motion. Postgrad. Med., 42:123, 1967.
8. Leighton, J. R.: An instrument and technic for the measurement of range of joint motion. Arch. Phys. Med., 36:571, 1955.
9. Moore, M. L.: The measurement of joint motion, Part I: Introductory review of the literature. Phys. Ther. Rev., 29:195, 1949.
10. Moore, M. L.: The measurement of joint motion, Part II: The technic of goniometry, Phys. Ther. Rev., 29:256, 1949
11. Moore, M. L.: Clinical assessment of joint motion. *In* Licht, S.: Therapeutic Exercise (2nd Ed., Re-

vised), New Haven, Elizabeth Licht, Publisher, 1965, p. 128.
12. The Committee on Rating of Medical and of Physical Impairment: A Guide to the Evaluation of Permanent Impairment of the Extremities and Back. JAMA (Special Edition), Feb. 15, 1958, pp. 1–112.

Muscle Testing

1. Chusid, J. G., and McDonald, J. J.: Correlative Neuroanatomy and Functional Neurology. Los Altos, Calif., Lange Medical Publications, 1962.
2. Glathe, J. P., and Achor, R. W. P.: Frequency of cardiac disease in patients with strokes. Proc. Mayo Clin., 33:417–422, 1958.
3. Haymaker, W., and Woodhall, B.: Peripheral Nerve Injuries, 2nd Ed. Philadelphia, W. B. Saunders Company, 1953.
4. Mayo Clinic: Clinical Examinations in Neurology, 4th Ed. Philadelphia, W. B. Saunders Company, 1976.

3

ELECTRODIAGNOSIS

ERNEST W. JOHNSON
DAVID WIECHERS

ELECTROMYOGRAPHY AND NERVE STIMULATION TECHNIQUES

Neurophysiology

Electrodiagnostic techniques are dependent on the activation and display of the electrical activity of the motor unit. This is the physiologic unit of the nervous system consisting of the anterior horn cell, its axon and terminal branchings, and all the muscle fibers it innervates.[24] The number of muscle fibers per motor unit varies from a few in an extrinsic eye muscle to several thousand in a large limb muscle.[7, 12]

The motor unit is activated in an all-or-none manner, the activation consisting of an electrical disturbance passing from the anterior horn cell down the axon and its twigs to the myoneural junctions, where the liberation of a chemical mediator initiates a wave of excitation along each muscle fiber. The muscle fiber contraction occurs approximately 1 millisecond after the action potential. Each muscle fiber depolarizes and is recorded as a biphasic wave with an initial positive deflection. The summated recording of the individual fibers that belong to a motor unit represents the motor unit action potential and is normally displayed as a triphasic wave.

Each motor neuron — that is, the cell body and axon — has a threshold of stimulation; the reciprocal of this threshold is its excitability. The speed with which the wave of excitation passes down the axon is its *impulse propagation rate*, or *conduction velocity*. This velocity varies almost directly with the diameter of the axon and is influenced favorably by the presence of a myelin sheath. The fastest conducting nerve fibers in man are the IA afferent fibers from muscle spindles and the sensory fibers that carry vibration and proprioception.[11, 13] Their conduction velocity varies from 60 to 100 meters per second. The alpha motor neurons that carry impulses to skeletal muscles are also some of the fastest conducting fibers. Their conduction velocities vary from 45 to 75 meters per second.[4, 11, 13, 16, 17] The thresholds of various "A" fibers in a motor nerve vary; therefore, in a clinical application one must ensure a supramaximal stimulus to activate all the axons to a particular muscle.

The action potential of a muscle or nerve fiber is generated because there is a potential difference of approximately -90 millivolts across the semipermeable membrane. An active transport of NA^+ from inside to outside the cell maintains this potential difference. Extremely small quantities (micromoles) of Na^+ allowed to enter the intracellular space are all that is required to reduce the resting membrane potential difference to approximately -55 millivolts, the threshold for depolarization. Once depolarized, the action potential is propagated in an all-or-none fashion down the cell mem-

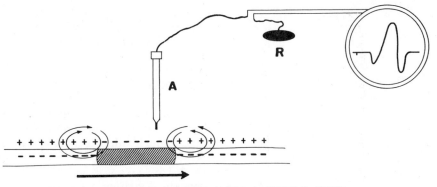

WAVE OF EXCITATION PASSING ALONG A MUSCLE FIBER

FIGURE 3-1. Diagram of the activation of a muscle fiber with the exploring electrode (A) in proximity. Note that tissue is a volume conductor; therefore the shape of the visualized potential will depend on the relationship of the electrode tip to the electrical disturbance.

brane. Recovery to the resting state proceeds immediately following the wave of excitation. The short delay immediately before this recovery is termed the *refractory period*. The first 0.2 millisecond of this delay is termed the *absolute refractory period* because no stimulus, no matter how intense, will excite the cell. A longer period following this is the *relative refractory period,* since a stronger stimulus than normal is necessary to cause excitation.[29]

If an exploring electrode is placed in the vicinity of the cell membrane undergoing change in polarization, the resultant electrical disturbance can be picked up, amplified, and displayed by the electromyograph.

Since living tissue is dispersed in three dimensions, electrical activity is also dispersed in three dimensions. We speak of tissue as a volume conductor; thus, the resultant wave form will depend on the location of the electrode tip with respect to the wave of excitation (Fig. 3-1). It is possible for the action potentials to be monophasic, biphasic, or triphasic, depending on this relationship. The structural distribution of the muscle fibers of one particular motor unit within the muscle as a whole makes more complex the shape of the action potential. Usually the motor unit action potentials are biphasic or triphasic, with fewer than 20 per cent polyphasic in normal individuals.

The excitation disturbance sweeps along the cell membrane of the muscle at 4 to 7 meters per second. Electrical characteristics of the tissue as well as those of the elec-

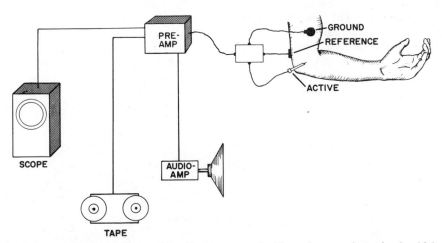

FIGURE 3-2. Schematic representation of an electromyograph. The reference electrode should be placed on the skin near the exploring or active electrode (monopolar).

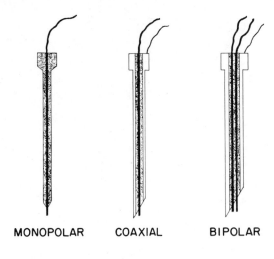

TYPES OF ELECTRODES

FIGURE 3–3. Three types of EMG electrodes.

tromyograph influence the amplitude, duration, and shape of the displayed action potentials.

Instrumentation

The basic components for electromyography and nerve stimulation include a set of electrodes, a preamplifier, an audio-amplifier and loudspeaker, an oscilloscope, and a physiologic stimulator (Fig. 3–2). Provisions for storing the displayed electrical activity include a magnetic tape recorder and a camera.

Electrodes

SURFACE. These vary from 0.5 to several centimeters in diameter. They are useful for kinesiologic studies and also for recording the muscle action potential during nerve stimulation techniques. One, the active electrode, is placed over the middle of the muscle and another, the reference electrode, over the tendon.

MONOPOLAR. These are sharpened pieces of stainless steel wires coated, except for approximately 0.004 to 0.24 sq mm at the tip, with an insulating material such as Teflon. The slippery characteristics of the insulating material make repetitive insertions within the muscle almost painless. A surface electrode or another subcutaneous monopolar electrode is necessary for a reference. Since the insulating material tends to peel off, this electrode is not permanent and should be visually and electrically checked periodically (Figs. 3–3 and 3–4).

COAXIAL. This is a hollow needle with a wire, insulated except at the tip, in the barrel to act as the exploring or active electrode. The barrel serves as the reference electrode. Exposure of the tip surface of the usually platinum inner wire of the coaxial electrode is 0.01 sq m, making this an electrode of high impedance.

There is reduction in the amplitude of the motor unit action potentials of approximately 50 per cent when compared to some monopolar electrodes. The beveled edge of the coaxial electrode results in a directional component toward the action potential recording (see Fig. 3–3).

All of the aforementioned electrodes require a ground electrode placed centrally to the muscle examined. Contact between skin and surface electrodes is enhanced by electrolytic paste, sparingly used.

BIPOLAR. Two insulated wires are inserted in a hypodermic needle to serve as active and reference electrodes, and the barrel serves as a ground (see Fig. 3–3). Bipolar electrodes permit very restricted areas to be investigated.

SINGLE FIBER. This is used to record depolarization of individual muscle fibers and is therefore very selective. It is usually a 25-micron diameter wire lead off the cutting side of a hollow needle. It has a high impedance of approximately 10 megohms. This is a coaxial electrode, and the barrel of the nee-

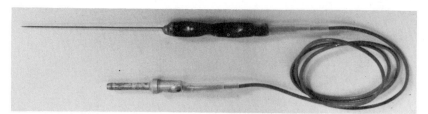

FIGURE 3–4. Close-up view of a monopolar EMG electrode, coated with Teflon.

dle serves as the reference electrode (Fig. 3–5).

Preamplifier. The preamplifier should have a uniform response for frequencies from 16 to 16,000 cycles per second with an input impedance of at least 50 megohms. It should be a differential or "push-pull" amplifier so that the "common mode" signal will be rejected. The rejection ratio of the common mode signal should be at least 100,000:1 for use in general hospital surroundings. Provision should be made for stepwise adjustment of the gain and for the optional insertion of high- and low-frequency filters. These filters may appreciably distort the displayed electrical activity.

Some commercially available electromyographs have features that eliminate or minimize certain interference, for example, a narrow-band elimination filter for 60 cycles, and a filter at the input to remove radio frequency interference. The input impedance of the preamplifier should be at least 10 times the impedance of the active electrode.

For single fiber electromyography the input impedance should be 100 megohms, and the frequency response from 500 to 20,000 Hz (so that distant potentials do not interrupt the base line).

Oscilloscope. The oscilloscope provides a visual display of the electrical signal so that the amplitude, duration, and shape of the potentials can be observed. Sweep speeds used for electromyography vary from 2 to 10 milliseconds per centimeter. For determination of motor and sensory nerve conduction velocities, sweep speeds should range from 2 to 30 milliseconds per centimeter. Single fiber electromyography requires sweep speeds as fast as 200 microseconds per centimeter.

Stimulator. The physiologic stimulator should have sufficient output to ensure a supramaximal stimulus under all clinical conditions. Stepwise and vernier adjustments for intensity and duration of stimulating voltage, as well as step adjustments for frequency and delay of the stimulus, are necessary. The stimulating electrodes are usually bipolar, with the cathode placed distally; however, a monopolar electrode, with either a needle or surface electrode placed over the nerve and with the large indifferent plate electrode placed over another part of the body, may be used. The stimulator must be isolated from ground with an isolation transformer. The stimulator triggers the sweep for nerve conduction velocity measurements and may be coupled to a one- or two-kilocycle oscillator so that the time base is "locked" to the start of the sweep.

Time Base. Crosshatching on the oscilloscope face that corresponds to the known sweep speed will usually give a satisfactory time·base for clinical nerve conduction velocities. It may be desirable to make the time base independent of the sweep speed by introducing a one- or two-kilocycle signal on a second oscillographic channel or superimposing the oscillatory signal on the tracing.

Intramuscular Thermometer. Since changes in temperature may alter the con-

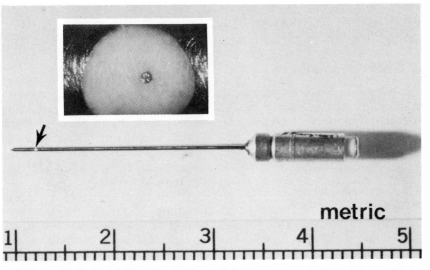

FIGURE 3–5. Photomicrograph of a single fiber electrode. Note the small 25 micron diameter lead-off surface of the single fiber electrode in the center of the insulation material.

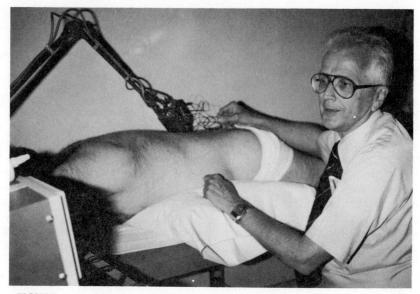

FIGURE 3–6. Electromyographic examination of the lumbosacral paraspinals.

duction velocity, it is helpful to have a needle thermistor to indicate the temperature of the tissue. The thermistor is inserted in the muscle near the middle third of the peripheral nerve being investigated. Several studies suggest that a drop in temperature of 1° C may reduce the conduction velocity by 5 per cent.[16]

Precautions. It is important to take the following precautions: Clean the skin thoroughly. Place electrodes securely. Use electrode jelly sparingly. Use firm pressure on stimulating electrodes. To ensure supramaximal stimulus, increase the stimulus intensity by at least 30 per cent after the "M" response amplitude no longer increases. If peak stimulation voltage has been reached, double the duration of the stimulus.

The Normal Electromyogram[3, 29]

Figure 3–6 shows an electromyographic examination in progress. The patient should be recumbent and comfortable, and the procedure should be thoroughly explained before starting. A brief history and a short but systematic neurologic examination is absolutely necessary in planning the electromyogram.

First, the needle electrode is inserted and the patient is asked to contract the desired muscle to ensure that the electrode is in the correct muscle. Adequate exploration of each muscle examined may require 5 to 10 needle advancements at several locations in the muscle.

There are five steps to the electromyographic examination. Sweep speeds vary from 5 to 10 milliseconds per centimeter, the faster sweeps for detailed examination of the individual action potentials. The gain is usually 50 microvolts per centimeter, except during maximal contraction, when it is 200 to 500 microvolts per centimeter. In chronic neuropathic conditions the gain may be adjusted to 1 to 2 millivolts per centimeter.

Muscle at Rest. When normal muscle at rest is examined, there is electrical silence (Fig. 3–7).

Insertional Activity. When the needle is moved briskly, a burst of electrical activity occurs that stops abruptly when the movement stops. The duration of this burst is dependent on the type of needle and the character of the needle movement but is usually 50 to 250 milliseconds in duration. This results from the activation of muscle fibers with the mechanical stimulus of electrode movement. The absence of insertional activity indicates that there are no functioning muscle fibers or that the electrode is not in muscle tissue.

If the tip of the exploring electrode is in the vicinity of motor end plates, a sputtering burst of electrical activity (diphasic spikes) occurs on a background of high-frequency noise, which has been likened to a sea shell murmur. The "sea shell murmur" comprises

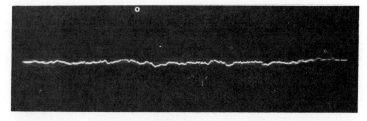

FIGURE 3–7. Normal muscle at rest. Note that there is no electrical activity.

high-frequency (1000 Hz), low-amplitude (8 to 10 microvolts), negative monophasic potentials that are nonpropagated, appearing on the postsynaptic membrane. These are called *miniature end plate potentials* (MEPP). The sputtering diphasic spikes (Fig. 3–8) are single muscle fiber discharges provoked by the unloading of pockets of acetylcholine by the tip of the needle. They have an initial negative phase with duration of 1 to 2 milliseconds, amplitude of 50 to 200 microvolts, and firing with irregular rhythm.

The patient usually complains of pain as end plate potentials are elicited (Fig. 3–8). These potentials are more likely to be encountered in the middle third of the muscle and particularly in the small muscles of the hands and feet. If the needle is advanced slightly farther, these single muscle fiber diphasic spikes may be recorded as positive sharp waves by the tip of the needle now in an injured area of the fiber.

Minimal Muscle Contraction. A single motor unit action potential is elicited by asking the patient just to think of contracting the desired muscle and then carefully moving the needle electrode as close to the firing unit as possible. The sound becomes louder and amplitude increases as the tip of the exploring electrode nears the activated motor unit (Fig. 3–9).

It is important to observe the amplitude measured peak to peak, the duration measured from the take-off to the return to the isoelectric line, and the shape, usually triphasic, of the first recruited and low-threshold motor units. Motor unit characteristics vary with electrode type, the muscle being examined, the strength of contraction, and the age of the patient. The recruitment interval, or the time between firing of the same potential at the point when the next higher threshold motor action potential is recruited, should be noted. The steady recruitment of higher threshold motor units of increasing amplitude should be observed and related to strength of contraction.

Maximal Muscle Contraction. To demonstrate maximal muscle contraction the patient is asked to contract the muscle against maximal resistance by the examiner. Placing the needle electrode superficially will reduce the discomfort.

The interference pattern is normal when the face of the oscilloscope is blotted out with motor unit action potentials. It is es-

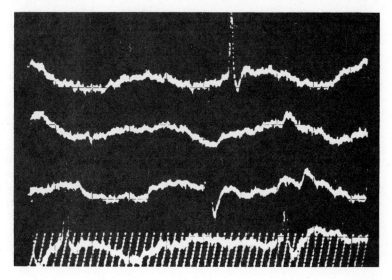

FIGURE 3–8. End plate activity. Calibration signal: 50 microvolts in amplitude; duration of one vertical line is 1 msec.

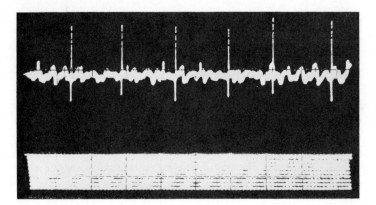

FIGURE 3–9. Minimal contraction. First recruited motor unit. Calibration line, 1 sec total duration; height is 500 microvolts.

timated that there are five to six motor units in the vicinity of the exploring electrode contributing to the interference pattern. Normal motor units begin activating at 5 per second and increase their rate of firing with increasing force of contraction effort. Simultaneously, additional motor units are recruited. Maximal rates of firing are from 30 to 50 per second. The patient's contraction effort is estimated from the rate of firing.

The amplitude is 200 to 2000 microvolts. Sound is more important in determining the duration. Fine crackling sounds indicate shorter duration; thuds suggest increased duration. The number of action potentials should be compared to strength of contraction.

Distribution of Abnormality. If abnormal potentials are observed, it is necessary to identify the anatomic distribution of the abnormalities. Is it a branch of a nerve, a peripheral nerve, a portion of a plexus, or a root or cord segment, or is it diffuse?

Children and Electromyograms. Always separate children from their parents. Explain the procedure to all above the age of four. Often a few words such as, ''You're going to see your muscles on television,'' will put the youngster at ease. Always refer to the electrode as a pin or mosquito bite. Avoid showing the needle electrode if possible, and use the smallest possible diameters (½ to ¾ inch in length). The needle electrode (pin) should be inserted concomitantly with a slap or pinch on the thigh or arm, particularly if the room is semidarkened.

Careful physical examination and planning are necessary to ensure that the minimal number of muscles are examined to make a proper diagnosis. Anesthesia is rarely necessary, but for children under the age of four,

the electromyographer will need assistance to restrain the child.

Obtaining muscle relaxation is the difficult part of the examination, but it may be done by forcibly positioning the muscle at its shortest length. For example, to investigate the anterior tibial muscle in an uncooperative child, the foot should be dorsiflexed as much as possible.

Caution. It is imperative that the electromyogram be performed by a physician for three reasons. First, a neurologic history and examination are necessary to plan the electromyogram; the plan must usually be modified as the electromyographic findings unfold. Second, the displayed electrical activity depends on the actions of the electromyographer at a particular moment as well as on the location of the electrode, and therefore taping of the electromyogram by a technician for later interpretation by the physician is inappropriate. Third, with the physician present, the electromyography findings can be interpreted immediately in conjunction with the history and neurologic examination.

Normal Motor Nerve Stimulation

Almost any nerve that has motor fibers and is placed superficially along a portion of its course can be stimulated with recording from a surface electrode on, or a needle electrode in, a distal muscle. A reference electrode is placed over the tendon and the ground electrode is placed between the active and stimulating electrodes (Fig. 3–10).[5, 6, 18-20, 27, 28]

The conduction velocity is determined by stimulating a motor nerve supramaximally at two points along its course and photograph-

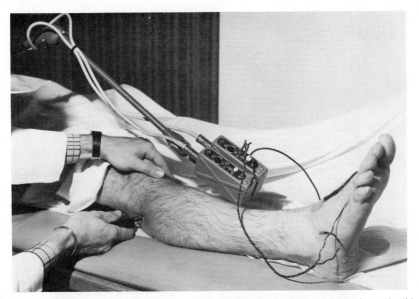

FIGURE 3–10. Peroneal motor nerve conduction study. Bipolar stimulating electrode at the fibular head, the active electrode over the extensor digitorum brevis, the reference electrode on the tendon, and the ground electrode on the dorsum of the ankle.

ing or observing the delay between the stimulation artifact and the muscle action potential. The distance between the points of stimulation is measured on the skin and divided by the conduction latency between the points of stimulation. Results are expressed as meters per second (Fig. 3–11). Figures 3–12 through 3–18 show sample records of conduction velocities.

If a peripheral motor nerve is stimulated at its most distal point — that is, where it enters the muscle — there is a conduction delay of several milliseconds. This latency represents the delay at the myoneural junc-

tion (0.2 to 0.5 millisecond) and the prolonged conductivity along the terminal axon twigs, which are small in diameter and unmyelinated at their endings. This delay is referred to as the *terminal conduction delay*. The difference between this delay and the expected delay (i.e., calculated from the observed velocity along the more proximal nerve trunk) is referred to as *residual latency*.

There is faster (5 to 10 meters/sec.) conduction velocity in more proximal nerve segments.[4] However, measurement errors are more likely in the proximal segments of the

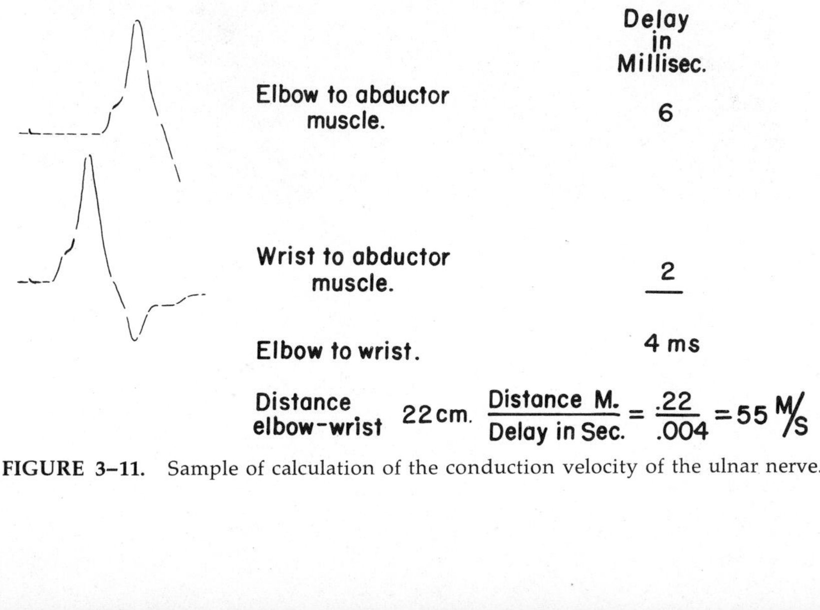

	Delay in Millisec.
Elbow to abductor muscle.	6
Wrist to abductor muscle.	2
Elbow to wrist.	4 ms

$$\text{Distance elbow-wrist} \quad 22\,\text{cm.} \quad \frac{\text{Distance M.}}{\text{Delay in Sec.}} = \frac{.22}{.004} = 55\,\text{M/s}$$

FIGURE 3–11. Sample of calculation of the conduction velocity of the ulnar nerve.

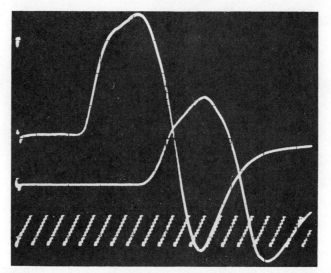

FIGURE 3–12. Recording the conduction velocity of the median motor division (54 m/s). Calibration signal is 2 mvolts in amplitude, and the duration of one vertical line is 1 msec. Note the normal delay in the median nerve at the wrist (less than 5 msec.).

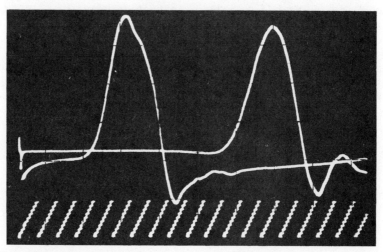

FIGURE 3–13. Recording of peroneal motor nerve conduction velocity (49 m/s). Calibration signal 1 mvolt amplitude, duration of one vertical line is 1 msec.

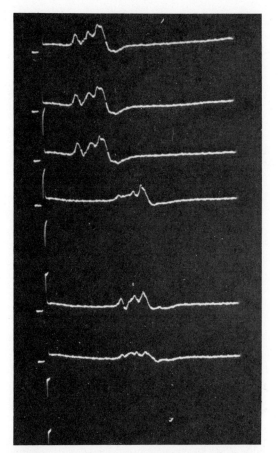

FIGURE 3–14. Actual photograph of peroneal nerve conduction velocity in patient with muscular dystrophy (58 m/s). Note the ragged and low amplitude "M" response, although the velocity is normal.

limbs.[19] A measurement error of 1 centimeter will result in errors of 1 part in 25, or 4 per cent, in an adult arm. Inspection of photographs or determination of the conduction latency permits an accuracy of at best 1 part in 20 if one uses 0.5 millisecond as the time base and a latency of 10 milliseconds (Table 3–1).

Surface electrodes permit comparisons of the amplitude of the "M" response to be made between different locations of stimulations along the nerve and repetitive stimulations at one site. The hand or foot should be firmly immobilized when attempting repetitive stimulations. However, surface electrodes may not isolate the proper muscle response.

Needle electrodes move when the muscle contracts and thus cannot be used to compare amplitudes. They do, however, isolate the response more precisely.

"M" response varies from 5 to 20 milli-

volts in normal subjects when recorded with surface electrodes.

Normal Sensory Nerve Stimulation. Sensory conduction studies can be performed in a similar manner on almost any pure sensory peripheral nerve or on the sensory fibers of mixed nerves.[8, 14, 15] Surface electrodes are placed over the distal sensory branches of the nerve and used for stimulation (orthodromic), with recording electrodes placed proximally over the nerve trunk. Antidromic techniques can also be employed with stimulation over the proximal nerve trunk and recording over the sensory distal branches. The recording electrodes are placed approximately 4 cm apart, with the active electrode proximal. This 4-cm separation of recording electrodes ensures maximal amplitude of the nerve action potential (Fig. 3–19).

The negative spike of the evoked sensory response is approximately 5 to 60 microvolts in amplitude, and under 2 milliseconds in duration, using either orthodromic or antidromic techniques. By convention, latencies in sensory studies are measured to the peak of the negative spike.

Conduction velocities may be determined by stimulating the nerve at two sites and dividing the distance between the sites by the

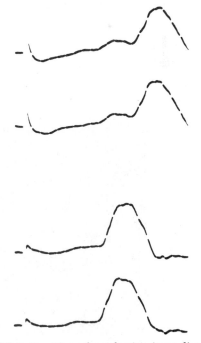

FIGURE 3–15. Normal conduction in median nerve (57 m/s) but prolonged (9 msec) delay at the wrist in a patient with carpal tunnel syndrome.

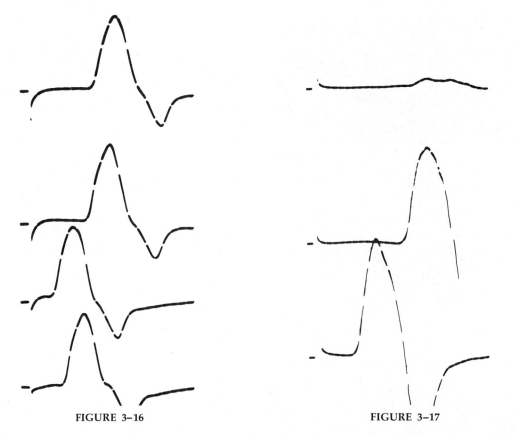

FIGURE 3–16   **FIGURE 3–17**

FIGURE 3–16. Neuroma of the ulnar nerve in the proximal wrist. The top trace is stimulation above the elbow; the next is stimulation below the elbow; the next is stimulation distal to the neuroma at the wrist; the bottom trace is stimulation at the wrist proximal to the neuroma. Note the 4 msec (prolonged) delay proximal to the neuroma. The conduction velocity calculated to the distal wrist is 42 m/s. The conduction velocity calculated to the proximal wrist is 60 m/s.

FIGURE 3–17. Block of the peroneal nerve at the fibular head in a patient with "crossed leg palsy." The top trace is stimulation above the fibular head; the middle trace is stimulation below the fibular head; the bottom trace is stimulation at the ankle. Note the temporal dispersion and reduced amplitude of the "M" response when the peroneal nerve is stimulated above the fibular head. The time base is 1 msec intervals. The stimulus artifact is to the left, the "M" response is to the right.

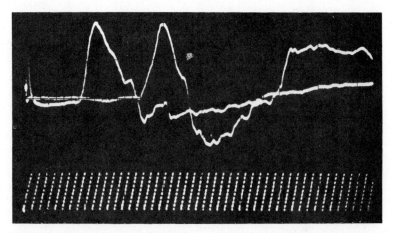

FIGURE 3–18. Marked slowing of the median motor nerve (29 m/sec) in a patient with Charcot-Marie-Tooth syndrome. Calibration signal 100 microvolts in amplitude; duration of one vertical line is 1 msec. Note the ragged and temporarily dispersed (negative spike duration 8 msec) "M" response.

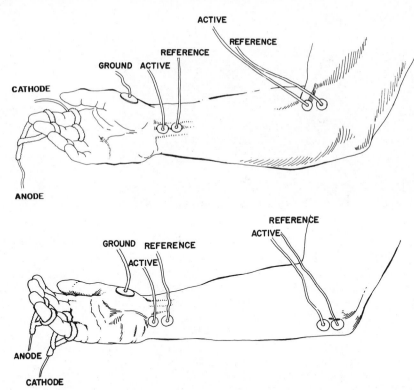

FIGURE 3–19. Placement of electrodes for sensory conduction studies of median nerve (upper) and ulnar nerve (lower). Clinically only the delay from fingers to wrist is obtained. Antidromic technique is done by recording on the fingers and stimulating at the wrist.

TABLE 3–1. PLACEMENT OF ELECTRODE FOR NERVE CONDUCTION STUDIES

Nerve	Sites of Stimulation		Pick-Up	Conduction Velocity M/Sec.	Terminal Conduction Delay (msec.)
	Proximal	*Distal*			
Ulnar	Posterior elbow or axilla	Wrist (Lateral to flexor carpi ulnaris tendon)	Abductor digiti quinti	45–70	2–4
Median	Antecubital area or axilla	Between tendons of palmaris long-us and flexor carpi radialis	Opponens	45–70	3–5
Deep Peroneal	Knee Fibular head or sciatic notch	Ankle (Anterior lateral aspect)	Extensor* Digitorum brevis	40–65	3–5
Tibial	Lateral popliteal area or sciatic notch	Posterior to medial malleolus	Abductor digiti quinti pedis	40–65	4–6
Facial		Under ear lobe	Frontalis	—	4
Radial	Spiral groove	Lateral antecubital space	Extensor indicis proprius	50–70	—
Femoral	Proximal and distal to inguinal ligament	Vastus medialis		—	6–8

*In 20 per cent of individuals an anomalous branch separates from the peroneal nerve and courses below the lateral malleolus to the extensor digitorum brevis.

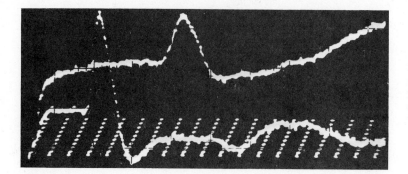

FIGURE 3–20. Normal median sensory conduction study (59 msec) antidromic. Latency is 3.4 msec. Calibration signal is 20 microvolts in amplitude; duration of one vertical line is 1 msec.

difference in latencies. This value also can be determined by dividing the latency into the distance of a single stimulation. To be more accurate, especially for short distances, 0.1 millisecond should be subtracted before calculation to correct for latency of activation (Fig. 3–20).

"H" Reflex. If the tibial nerve is stimulated with a low voltage (10 to 20 volts) and active reference electrodes are placed over the gastrocnemius, a muscle action potential may be observed after a latency of 30 to 40 milliseconds, a delay presumably necessary for the afferent and then the efferent limbs of the two-neuron muscle stretch reflex arcs to conduct the impulse.[25] The "H" reflex is facilitated by placing the cathode of the stimulating electrodes proximally rather than distally and stimulating at a rate of 1 per 2 to 3 seconds. It may also be demonstrated in the femoral nerve and in any peripheral nerve of infants under one year of age.

If found in relaxed muscles of human adults by stimulating the median, ulnar, or peroneal nerves, the "H" wave may indicate upper motor neuron disease due to injury below the midbrain. However, it has been demonstrated in apparently normal adults by having the individual contract the muscle slightly, a maneuver that results in facilitation of the muscle stretch reflex. The "H" reflex was named after Hoffmann, who first described it (Fig. 3–21).

"F" Wave. The "F" wave is a late compound action potential that is evoked inconsistently by supramaximally stimulating a motor nerve and recording from its distal muscle. It has a variable latency with repetitive stimulations in the 20- to 40-millisecond range. It is believed to be the result of antidromic motor conduction, backfiring of the alpha motor neuron, and recording of a second response from a portion of the motor units that responded to this antidromic stimulation. It is evoked by placing the stimulating cathode proximal on the peripheral nerve. The shortest latency of from 20 to 100 supramaximal stimulations is usually record-

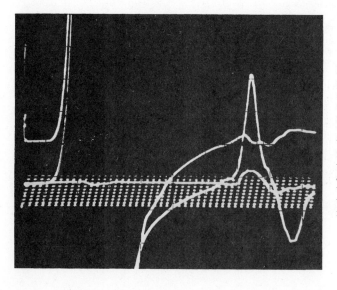

FIGURE 3–21. "H" wave recorded in a normal subject from the medial gastrocnemius stimulating the tibial nerve at the popliteal space. First or lowest "H" wave (on the right) is present before the appearance of the "M" wave (on the left). The second "H" wave is of normal amplitude. As the stimulus intensity increases, the amplitude of the "H" wave decreases until on the top tracing it is almost obliterated and probably contains "F" wave components. Calibration signal 1 millivolt in amplitude; duration of one vertical line is 1 msec.

ed as the "F" wave latency. This "F" wave is identified by a variable shape with each stimulation and an amplitude that is always less than the "M" wave. It is differentiated from the "H" response by its presence on supramaximal stimulation (Fig. 3–22).

Root Stimulation. Stimulation of the C 8 nerve root can be performed with the antidromic technique by insertion of a stimulating electrode (cathode) one finger breadth lateral from the spinous process of the C 7 vertebra, and in contact with the transverse process of C 8. The evoked response may be an "M" wave from a distal C 8 innervated muscle or a nerve action potential recorded over a measured distance along a nerve trunk, e.g., ulnar nerve, along the course of the peripheral nerve. Comparing side to side in normals should reveal a latency difference of less than 1.5 milliseconds. The latency is usually half of the "F" wave from the abductor digiti quinti.

Effect of Age on Motor Nerve Conduction Velocity. At birth, the conduction velocity in the motor fibers of the ulnar nerve averages 28 meters per second. By age two to three it reaches low adult values and by age four or five it averages adult values. In premature infants the conduction velocity correlates well with the degree of prematurity. In a group of premature infants of approximately eight months' gestation, the conduction velocity in the peroneal nerve averaged 19 meters per second.[6]

The conduction velocity of motor nerves in adults beyond the fifth decade is gradually reduced up to 10 per cent per decade, perhaps as a result of metabolic or circulatory disturbances.

Effect of Changes in Temperature. Reduced temperature in an extremity may result in lowered conduction velocities.[16] Estimates for this in the conduction velocity, varying from 1.8 to 4 meters per second per degree Centigrade, should precede clinical interpretation of a reduced velocity. Increase in the temperature of the body can raise the conduction velocity in motor nerves in a similar manner.

Pathophysiology

The lower motor neuron (anterior horn cell and its axon) responds in three ways to an insult: wallerian degeneration, neurapraxia, and axonostenosis or axonocachexia.

Wallerian Degeneration. If it is injured or diseased severely, the entire neuron (if it is an anterior horn cell) or the axon distal to the injury undergoes wallerian degeneration. This is first a dissolution of the myelin sheath and then a disintegration of the axis cylinder. The process ordinarily takes 18 to 21 days in human axons. When the degeneration is complete, the electromyogram shows fibrillation potentials. Injured axons that will undergo wallerian degeneration are excitable and will conduct distal to the injury for about 72 hours, after which time they are no longer excitable.

Neurapraxia. A segment of an axon or an anterior horn cell may temporarily lose its excitability and yet not undergo wallerian degeneration. In this situation, stimulation

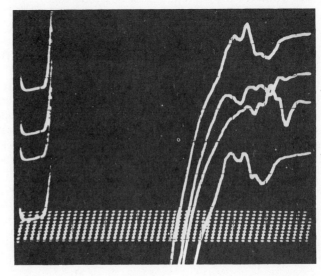

FIGURE 3–22. Normal "F" waves (on the right), "M" waves (on the left) off the screen to demonstrate amplitude difference. Calibration signal is 200 microvolts in amplitude; duration of one vertical line is 1 msec.

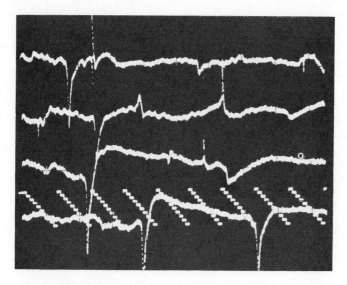

FIGURE 3–23. Positive sharp waves and fibrillation potentials. Calibration signal is 100 microvolts in amplitude; duration of one vertical line is 1 msec.

proximal to the site of compromise will not result in muscle contraction (assuming that all fibers are neurapraxic), but stimulation distal to the compromise will cause contraction (Erb's paradoxical palsy). This is called *neurapraxia*. If not all of the axons in a motor nerve are neurapraxic, then stimulation proximal to the injury will result in a smaller "M" response than distal stimulation (Figs. 3–16 and 3–17).[2]

Axonostenosis or Axonocachexia. If a localized compromise is prolonged or more severe, the axon may retain its excitability, but at a reduced level. This may necessitate an increased intensity of stimulus for excitation, and it also results in reduced conductivity across the involved segment. This is termed *axonostenosis*. Altered excitability and conductivity extending throughout the entire distal axon is called *axonocachexia*. If some of the axons are normal, the amplitude of the "M" response will be roughly proportional to those when stimulating proximal to a segment of axonostenosis. Axonocachexia will result in temporal dispersion of the "M" response as the axons conduct at different velocities proportional to their altered physiology.[2] Combinations of all three may be present with coexistent electromyographic and nerve stimulation abnormalities.

Abnormal Potentials in Electromyography

Fibrillation Potentials. The amplitude of fibrillation potentials is 50 to 300 microvolts;

the duration 0.5 to 2 milliseconds with a regular rhythm and a frequency of 2 to 10 per second (Fig. 3–23). They are usually diphasic or triphasic, with the initial phase positive. Their sound resembles that of eggs frying or cellophane paper being crumpled. This is the electrical activity associated with the spontaneous discharge of a single muscle fiber. This is the result of abnormal muscle membrane irritability produced in a variety of circumstances, such as denervation, inflammation, degeneration, electrolyte disturbances, trauma, and upper motor neuron disease. Single muscle fiber contractions are not visible grossly through intact skin or mucous membrane. Their appearance is enhanced by heat, cholinergic drugs, and mechanical stimulation.[9, 10]

Fasciculation Potentials. The amplitude and duration of fasciculation potentials vary. They may be simple or polyphasic. Fasciculation potentials are identified by the irregular rhythm and a rate of firing less than 3 or 4 per second. These may be visible through intact mucous membrane or skin. They represent spontaneous discharges of part or all of a motor unit, many probably originating at the myoneural junction (Fig. 3–24). These discharges may be simple or complex in shape. Complex fasciculation potentials include the polyphasic type as well as grouped or iterative discharges.[9]

Iterative or grouped discharge fasciculation potentials result when the excitability of the motor unit is heightened so that the relative refractory period is shortened, permitting repetitive activation. Thus the motor

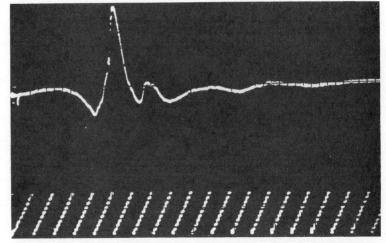

FIGURE 3–24. Benign fasciculation recorded from the biceps of an anxious medical student. Calibration signal is one millivolt in amplitude; duration of one vertical line is 1 msec.

unit may fire two or three or more times (Fig. 3–25). Fasciculation potentials may be pathologic or benign.

Polyphasic Potentials. Polyphasic potentials are usually motor unit action potentials having more than four phases (i.e., crossing the isoelectric line more than four times) (Fig. 3–26). Fewer than 25 per cent of motor unit action potentials in most muscles of normal individuals are polyphasic. Motor units with heightened excitability may fire repetitively and result in a polyphasic potential. Possible origins of these potentials are (1) differences in conduction times over the terminal axon branches; (2) synchronous but not simultaneous firing of multiple motor units; (3) repetitive discharge of part or all of a motor unit; or (4) loss of some muscle fibers in a motor unit so that the anatomic dispersion of the remaining fibers does not permit smooth summation. A special type of polyphasic potential is the previously mentioned repetitive discharge or iterative potential.

Positive Sharp Waves. Positive sharp waves are potentials having a sharp positive deflection associated with a long-duration negative phase. They occur when one or a group of "sick" muscle fibers is activated by the tip of the exploring electrode, when the tip is in the injured or diseased area of the muscle fiber with the depolarization wave moving away from the electrode tip. These are induced by mechanical stimulation, either by tapping the muscle in the vicinity of the needle or by advancing the needle abruptly. They are abnormal only if they persist after electrode movement stops, since the potentials provoked with electrode movement in muscle are also usually of an

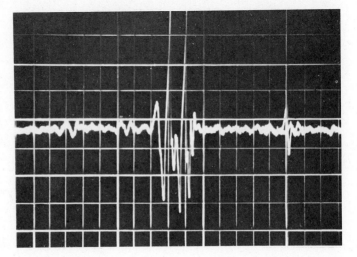

FIGURE 3–25. Repetitive or iterative potential. Calibration: 6 msec per horizontal division, 100 microvolts per vertical division.

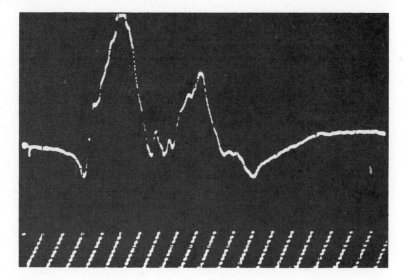

FIGURE 3–26. Polyphasic, long-duration motor unit recorded from a patient with ALS. Calibration signal is 1 millivolt in amplitude; duration of one vertical line is 1 msec.

initial positive deflection. The amplitude and duration vary considerably, as does the frequency. These potentials may appear as trains of discharges at the rate of 50 to 100 per second (see Fig. 3–23).

Bizarre Repetitive Discharges (Bizarre High-Frequency Discharges). High- or low-frequency polyphasic grouped discharges, up to 200 per second, are seen in a variety of motor neuron diseases. Their origin is thought to be reinnervating motor units (Fig. 3–27).

Myotonic Discharges. Myotonic discharges are trains of positive sharp waves or biphasic spikes, which vary in frequency and amplitude. Audibly they have been likened to a diving airplane that pulls out only to dive again, as they wax and wane in frequency and amplitude. They are not specific for myotonic dystrophy or myotonia congenita, since they have been recorded in myotubular myopathy and other conditions (Fig. 3–28).

Cramp. In cramp there is a synchronous, high-frequency discharge of a group of motor units.

Motor Units in Pathologic Conditions. Motor units in disorders of the terminal axon or individual muscle fibers are recorded as a dropout of individual biphasic single fiber depolarization potentials that no longer summate to form the usual triphasic potential. The result is a potential whose amplitude and duration are reduced and whose shape may

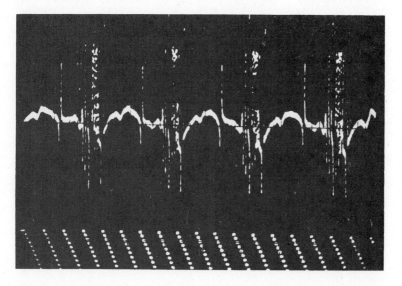

FIGURE 3–27. *Bizarre repetitive discharge* recorded from a patient with Duchenne muscular dystrophy. Calibration signal is 100 millivolts in amplitude; duration of one vertical line is 10 msec.

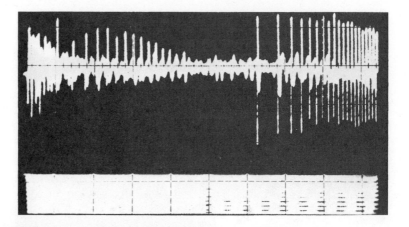

FIGURE 3–28. Myotonic discharge recorded from a patient with myotonia congenita, elicited by needle electrode movement. Calibration signal is one millivolt in amplitude; duration of the entire sweep is 2 sec.

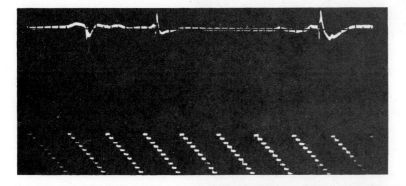

FIGURE 3–29. Low threshold motor units recorded in a patient with Becker muscular dystrophy. Calibration signal is 100 microvolts in amplitude; duration of one vertical line is 10 msec.

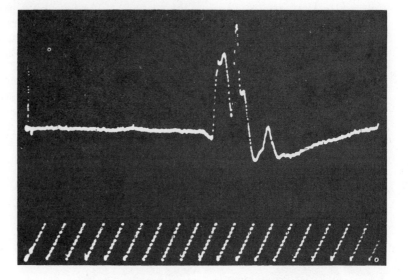

FIGURE 3–30. Motor unit recorded in the anterior tibialis 2 months after onset of Guillain-Barré syndrome. Calibration signal, 200 microvolts in amplitude; duration of one vertical line is 1 msec.

be polyphasic (Fig. 3–29). In disorders of the neuron or axon there is a dropout of motor units.

With reinnervation seen in most neuropathic disorders the number of muscle fibers now belonging to a single motor unit is increased. Early these reinnervation potentials are of low amplitude and highly polyphasic with a long duration (Fig. 3–30). With maturation of the reinnervating axon sprouts and newly formed myoneural junctions, the potentials become large in amplitude and duration and may remain somewhat polyphasic (Fig. 3–31).[23]

Single Fiber Electromyography. Single fiber electromyography permits the record-

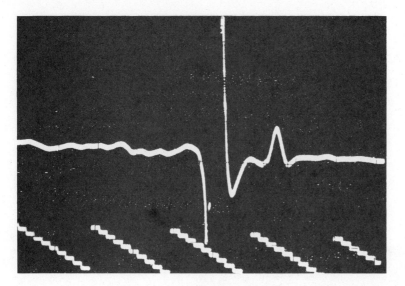

FIGURE 3–31. Giant motor unit recorded from the flexor hallucis longus in a slowly progressive neuropathy. Calibration signal is 5 millivolts in amplitude; duration of one vertical line is 10 msec.

ing of the depolarization of a single muscle fiber or a group of muscle fibers that are within the recording area (200 micron diameter hemisphere) of a single fiber electrode.[26] If a single motor unit is activated voluntarily, then single muscle fibers that belong to one motor unit can be recorded.

Voluntary single fiber depolarizations have the same configuration as fibrillation potentials. They are usually less than 1 to 2 milliseconds in duration. They are biphasic with an initial positive deflection. The amplitude is variable with the distance that exists between the recording surface and the surface of the depolarizing fiber. For quantitative determinations a single fiber depolarization must be greater than 200 microvolts in amplitude and have a rise time of the positive to negative spike of less than 300 microseconds.

If the single fiber electrode is inserted randomly into a voluntarily contracting muscle, in 70 per cent of insertions only one single muscle fiber depolarization is recorded. In 25 per cent of the insertions two fibers that belong to the same motor unit are recorded. Five per cent of the time three or even four fibers are recorded.

If we systematically insert the electrode 20 times, maximizing the amplitude of the first fiber recorded and counting the number of fibers that also belong to the same motor unit that are within the pick-up area of the single fiber electrode, we can calculate a mean

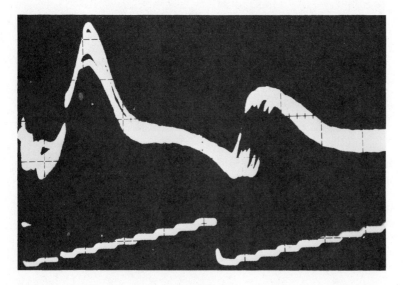

FIGURE 3–32. Normal jitter between two single fiber discharges. Calibration signal is 1 millivolt in amplitude; duration of one vertical slanted line is 200 microsec.

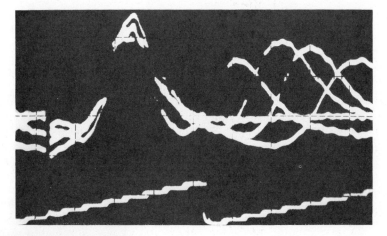

FIGURE 3–33. Blocking of the second single fiber discharge. First fiber has discharged five times and only four depolarizations of the second fiber are recorded. Calibration signal is 1 millivolt in amplitude; duration of one vertical slanted line is 200 microsec.

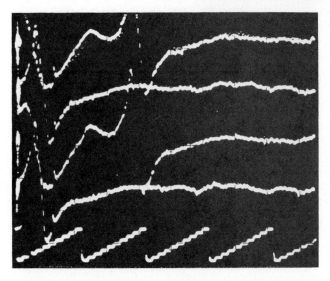

FIGURE 3–34. Neurogenic blocking. Single fiber discharge of fibers 2 and 3 block together in the second and fourth discharge. Calibration signal amplitude is 1 millivolt; duration of one vertical line is 1 msec.

number of fibers per insertion, or a *fiber density*. An increase in fiber density may be the first definite sign of reinnervation.

When recording from two single fibers that belong to the same motor unit, if we hold the first fiber still in time by using an electronic triggering device, we see that the appearance of the second fiber varies in time (Fig. 3–32). This variation in time is due to variation in conduction down terminal axon branches, delays across myoneural junctions, or delays in impulse propagation down muscle fibers.

If we determine the mean of the differences between the time of appearance of these two single fibers for 50 to 200 consecutive discharges of the motor unit, we have a statistical time referred to as the *mean consecutive difference* (MCD). This is the statistical expression of jitter.

Jitter, then, is the statistical variation in microseconds of 50 to 200 consecutive depolarizations of two fibers that belong to the same motor unit. Since the first fiber is held constant in time, the jitter reflects variation in both fibers: conduction times down terminal axons, across myoneural junctions, and down muscle fibers.

If with repetitive firing of a motor unit we note that the second fiber does not appear at times because of failed conduction, this is referred to as "blocking" (Fig. 3–33). Blocking commonly occurs in disorders of neuromuscular transmission. Blocking may also be due to failed conduction at terminal branching sites in reinnervated motor units. In this condition, referred to as "neurogenic blocking," groups of fibers will drop out in an all-or-none fashion (Fig. 3–34).

Clinical Application

Anterior Horn Cell Disease. Examples of anterior horn cell disease include acute paralytic poliomyelitis, amyotrophic lateral sclerosis, progressive spinomuscular atrophy, myelopathies (such as syringomyelia), and intramedullary spinal cord tumors.

Fibrillation potentials appear 18 to 21 days following the death of the anterior horn cell. Voluntary low-threshold potentials are increased in amplitude (up to 8 to 10 millivolts) and in duration (showing a mean of 13 milliseconds) and are so-called *reinnervation potentials*. The number of motor unit action potentials is reduced, and they fire rapidly. Unless the motor units are firing rapidly, it is not possible to evaluate the number of units present.

A myelopathic electromyogram shows a reduced number of motor unit action potentials with an increase in amplitude and duration and fibrillation potentials.

Fasciculation potentials are very frequently seen in anterior horn cell disease, probably as a result of the "sick" neuron. They may be simple or polyphasic. In amyotrophic lateral sclerosis they are quite common and generally are of low amplitude and short duration early in the course of the disease.

Synchronous discharge of motor units in different locations in the muscle frequently occurs early in acute paralytic poliomyelitis.

The motor nerve conduction velocity is normal or low normal in anterior horn cell disease. If it is reduced, the temperature of the extremity should be checked.

Single fiber electromyography demonstrates an increase in fiber density and an increase in jitter with neurogenic blocking. The more acute the process, the greater the abnormality in jitter. The more chronic or long-standing the reinnervation, the more stable the motor unit complexes.

Axonal Disease. Conditions affecting the axon as a whole or in segments include idiopathic polyneuritis (Guillain-Barré syndrome), diabetic neuropathy, Charcot-Marie-Tooth disease, and toxic neuropathy. Examples of localized problems are tardy ulnar nerve palsy and median nerve neuritis (or carpal tunnel syndrome).[10, 16, 17]

If the segment of axon has undergone wallerian degeneration distal to the injury, the electromyogram will show a neuropathic picture. This type of electromyogram exhibits a reduced number of motor unit action potentials and perhaps an increased proportion of polyphasic potentials and fasciculation potentials.

Axonal disease is differentiated from anterior horn cell disease by the reduced motor nerve conduction velocity. In acute disease the reduction may appear after one to two weeks, and after three to four weeks conduction velocity may be markedly reduced. The reduced conductivity is probably the result of the myelin sheath alteration. In chronic polyneuropathies the reduced caliber of the axis cylinder may be a factor. The conduction velocity reduction is heralded at 7 to 10 days by a raggedness and temporal dispersion of the stimulated muscle action potential. The amplitude of the muscle action potential may be lower when the nerve is stimulated proximally than when it is stimulated distally, and the duration may be increased.

Velocities may be reduced 50 to 75 per cent in idiopathic polyneuritis, and in chronic polyneuropathies, such as Charcot-Marie-Tooth disease, they may be even lower. In chronic peripheral neuropathies, fibrillation potentials are rare and insertional activity is reduced.

Localized areas of compromise may be identified by stimulating proximally and distally to the site of compromise and noting prolonged latency across the diseased segment or reduced amplitude of the muscle action potential when stimulation is proximal to the compromise[21] (Figs. 3–15 and 3–17). In chronic compressive (ischemic) compromise of motor nerve, a single stimulation frequently results in a repetitive discharge polyphasic motor unit action potential as recorded by a needle electrode.

Peripheral nerve injury and motor root compression produce neuropathic electromyograms. The distribution of abnormalities permits the localization of the compromise. For example, fibrillation or fasciculation potentials or an increased proportion of polyphasic potentials in the anterior tibial, peroneal, and gastrocnemius muscles, as well as in the sacrospinalis muscle at L5 level, indicates a compromise at or proximal to the root level. The motor and sensory roots join and leave the spinal canal via the intervertebral foramen as a mixed nerve, then split into the posterior primary ramus, which goes to the muscles and skin of the back and the anterior primary ramus. This ramus is distributed to the plexus and then to the extremity. Thus an electromyographic abnormality in the muscles of the extremity, as well as in the paraspinal muscles at the appropriate level, indicates a compromise of the spinal nerve before it divides into the anterior and posterior primary rami.

Myoneural Junction Disease. Myasthenia gravis is a disease affecting the receptor sites on the postsynaptic membrane. Electromyographically, the motor unit action potentials are reduced, or vary, in amplitude and duration as the muscle contraction is sustained. This occurs at more and more of the myoneural junctions, and thus muscle fibers drop out of the firing effort. There is a normal number of motor units, but each unit grows progressively smaller. The electromyogram may show an increase in the number of motor unit action potentials as compared with the strength of contraction.[22]

To obviate the necessity for cooperation by the patient, repetitive nerve stimulation can demonstrate the myasthenic reaction objectively. With surface recording electrodes the motor nerve is stimulated at the distal site two or three times per second for one series. The muscle action potential will show a reduction as the fatigued myoneural junctions fail to contribute when the second or third shock comes along. To make this test more sensitive, the myoneural junction can be sensitized with exercise or curare. If the defect of transmission appears, it may be repaired with Tensilon.

Single fiber electromyography in myasthenia gravis is a more sensitive test and demonstrates an increase in jitter with blocking, especially as the rate of depolarization is increased. This is seen in muscles that are normal by clinical examination and routine electrodiagnostic techniques.[26]

In certain malignancies — particularly small cell carcinoma of the lung — a myasthenia-like syndrome may be present. Here, repetitive stimulation will increase the amplitude of the muscle action potential corresponding to the clinical finding of initial weakness, and then subsequent muscle contractions will increase the muscle strength. With single fiber electromyography in the myasthenic syndrome, slow rates of depolarization demonstrate marked increase in jitter and blocking that is improved somewhat by increasing the rate of depolarization.

Muscle Disease. Examples are muscular dystrophy, polymyositis, thyrotoxic myopathy, and potassium alteration. Here the motor unit is functioning with the exception that it loses the muscle fibers involved in the myopathic disease. Thus the motor unit action potentials are reduced in amplitude and duration (50 to 200 microvolts and 4 to 6 milliseconds). Each contraction results in an increase in the number of motor unit action potentials activated with respect to the strength of contraction. Polyphasic potentials are common and are usually of short duration and low amplitude, as one would expect with the fewer and anatomically dispersed muscle fibers and resultant ragged summation.

Generally the first recruited potentials are affected early in the disease. In this early stage the only electromyographic abnormality may be action potentials of short duration. As muscle fibers degenerate, spontaneous single muscle fiber action potentials appear, so that fibrillation potentials are commonly seen in muscular dystrophy. There are showers of fibrillation potentials in polymyositis, as well as provoked positive sharp waves. Fibrillation potentials indicate active degeneration of muscle fibers. Positive sharp waves are found often in both muscular dystrophy and polymyositis, as well as in other types of myopathies. Again, these represent hyperirritable muscle cell membranes depolarizing away from the electrode tip. Motor nerve conduction velocity is normal in myopathic disease.

Myotonic dystrophy is characterized by a unique electromyographic pattern (see Fig. 3–28). When the needle electrode is inserted or moved, prolonged trains of positive waves that vary in frequency and amplitude appear. The sound is similar to that of a diving airplane. The myotonic potentials are prominent and necessary for diagnosis but not specific for myotonic dystrophy (Steinert's disease) or myotonia congenita (Thomsen's disease). Also, following volitional contraction, an afterdischarge persists as the voluntary effort triggers cycling depolarization and repolarization.

Single fiber electromyography in muscle disease demonstrates an overall increase in fiber density with some long duration complex potentials. Jitter is increased in some, but blocking is not a prominent feature.

Specific Applications

Diabetic Neuropathy. Distal sensory nerve conduction velocity is usually slowed first. Typically the motor nerve conduction velocity is reduced earliest in the peroneal nerve, then in the facial nerve, and finally in the ulnar and median nerves. Usually when onset of diabetic neuropathy is insidious, electromyographic abnormalities are found only in the most distal foot muscles, while the velocity may be reduced 20 to 30 per cent. In a few severe neuropathies, a classic neuropathic electromyogram, with progressively reduced conduction velocities, may be demonstrated.[14]

Diabetes mellitus apparently alters the metabolism of the peripheral nerve so that the nerve becomes more susceptible to local trauma. Tardy ulnar nerve palsy, carpal tunnel syndrome, and other mononeuritides may be frequent manifestations of diabetic neuropathy. The so-called femoral neuralgia seen in diabetic patients has been shown electromyographically to be multiple lumbar radiculopathies rather than a peripheral mononeuropathy, as was suggested clinically.

Carpal Tunnel Syndrome. The median nerve is located within the rigid tunnel at the wrist. Any disease or injury that increases the volume of the tunnel's contents or distorts its structure may thus compromise the median nerve with resultant axonostenosis. The conduction delay from proximal wrist crease to thenar eminence is less than 4.3 milliseconds normally; in carpal tunnel syndrome the delay is greater than 4.3 milliseconds and averaged 8.5 milliseconds in a published series. If compromise is severe, the electromyogram will be neuropathic, but fibrillation potentials are rare. The sensory delay is usually prolonged before the motor delay, and after operation it returns to normal later[21] (see Fig. 3–15).

Tardy Ulnar Nerve Palsy. Stimulation of the ulnar nerve above the elbow will show prolonged delay and reduced amplitude of the muscle action potential of the abductor digiti quinti; stimulation below the elbow may show normal conduction velocity and increase "M" response. The electromyogram will usually demonstrate a reduced number of motor units per strength of contraction with a paucity of fibrillation potentials and reduced insertional activity.

Amyotrophic Lateral Sclerosis. Normal or minimal reduction in conduction velocity is found, but the electromyogram is neuropathic. Fasciculation potentials are numerous and may be polyphasic or simple short-duration potentials. Voluntary motor unit action potentials are increased in amplitude (to 10 or more millivolts) and duration (9 to 18 milliseconds). Fibrillation potentials are present but may be difficult to demonstrate. Positive sharp waves are invariably present. The abnormalities shown with the electromyograph are generalized even though in the clinical findings the weakness is apparently localized.

Acute Idiopathic Polyneuritis. Reduced motor nerve conduction velocity is present together with a neuropathic electromyogram. The motor unit action potentials are usually of normal amplitude. There are fasciculation potentials, fibrillation potentials, and a reduced number of voluntary potentials, of which there is an increased proportion of polyphasic potentials (see Fig. 3–30). The reduction in conductivity may appear as early as 10 to 14 days and may drop 75 to 80 per cent of normal. The earliest abnormality may be a prolongation of the "F" wave or the distal latency. Early in the disease (during the first two weeks) there is usually a temporal dispersion of the "M" response when the nerve is stimulated proximally and an increase in the amplitude in the "M" response when the nerve is stimulated distally or near the muscle. The rise in the conduction velocity follows but lags behind the clinical recovery.

Root Compression Syndrome. Early compromise of the motor root may result in an increased proportion of polyphasic potentials, fasciculation potentials, or only positive sharp waves in the muscle innervated by the root. These would include muscles innervated by the anterior primary ramus (extremity) and the posterior primary ramus (paraspinal). More severe compromise causes reduction in the number of voluntary motor units recruited per strength of contraction with fibrillation potentials (after 18 days). Ordinarily, fibrillation potentials appear earlier, often after 14 days, in the paraspinal muscle (Table 3–2).

When the diagnostic problem includes differentiating an intraspinal tumor from the root compression syndrome, it is helpful to attempt to elicit the sensory fiber action potential in a peripheral nerve having sensory fibers chiefly from that level. If the root is compromised severely, sensory axons will of course have undergone wallerian degeneration and will not conduct. Conversely, if the compromise is within the cord, sparing the

TABLE 3–2. TIME OF PRESENTATION OF ELECTROMYOGRAPHIC ABNORMALITIES IN RADICULOPATHY

Day 1
A. Reduced number of voluntarily recruited motor unit action potentials in the affected nerve root distribution.
B. Abnormal "H" reflex in the S1 nerve root.

Day 4
A. The above abnormalities plus
B. Reduced amplitudes of the evoked compound motor unit action potential in a muscle supplied by the affected nerve root.

Days 7–10
A. The above abnormalities plus
B. Provokable (by needle electrode insertion) positive sharp waves and fibrillation potentials in the paraspinal musculature at the affected level.

Days 18–21
A. The above abnormalities plus
B. Provokable positive sharp waves and fibrillation potentials in limb muscles.

Days 22–25
A. The above electromyographical abnormalities plus
B. Spontaneous fibrillation potentials recorded in the affected muscles.

---

dorsal ganglion, then the intact afferent (sensory) axon will conduct. In these conditions the electromyographic findings would probably be quite similar.

Peripheral Nerve Injury. The distal segment of the injured nerve will conduct for about 72 hours; then, if wallerian degeneration is taking place, no conduction will occur. After 72 hours the amplitude of the "M" response will be proportional to the number of motor fibers that were not injured severely enough to undergo wallerian degeneration. From the time of injury to 18 to 21 days, there will be a reduced number of motor unit action potentials or none at all, depending on the degree of injury (Fig. 3–35). At about 12 to 16 days, positive sharp waves may appear during insertional activity and at 18 to 21 days, fibrillation potentials will appear. These abnormal findings in wallerian degeneration will occur earlier in the proximal muscle — that is, those with shorter motor nerves.

The earliest indications of reinnervation are (1) the disappearance of fibrillation potentials; (2) the appearance of low-amplitude highly polyphasic "reinnervation potentials" (see Fig. 3–30), which in the early period are not under voluntary control but appear when the needle is moved or the muscle is tapped; (3) a supramaximal stimulus proximal to the injured site resulting in a temporally dispersed muscle action potential with the surface electrode or a complex motor unit action potential with the needle electrode. (The conduction velocity of the motor nerve fibers that are regenerating is markedly slowed, by 50 per cent or more, since the diameter of regrowing fibers is considerably reduced.)

After prolonged periods of denervation, muscle fibers may be replaced by fibrous tissue, a condition that reduces the number of fibrillation potentials as well as the amount of insertional activity.

Myasthenia Gravis. With surface electrodes over the abductor digiti quinti and bipolar stimulating electrodes over the ulnar nerve at the wrist, repetitive stimulation at two or three stimulations per second is done. The hand is held securely to avoid movement. Reduction in "M" response of the abductor digiti quinti during supramaximal repetitive stimulation indicates a "myasthenic reaction." This may be confirmed by the repair of the transmission defect with Tensilon. Other tests using curare-like agents or

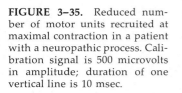

FIGURE 3–35. Reduced number of motor units recruited at maximal contraction in a patient with a neuropathic process. Calibration signal is 500 microvolts in amplitude; duration of one vertical line is 10 msec.

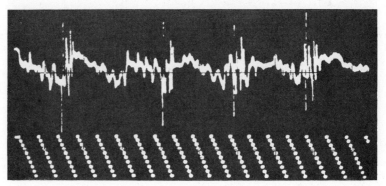

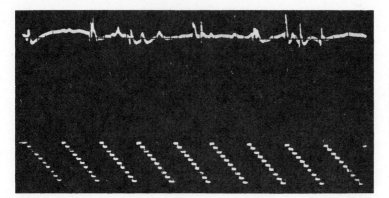

FIGURE 3–36. Low threshold motor units from biceps of a patient with Duchenne muscular dystrophy. Calibration signal is 100 microvolts in amplitude; duration of one vertical line is 10 msec.

depolarizing drugs may be even more sensitive in detection of a myasthenic reaction. Single fiber electromyography is the most sensitive electrodiagnostic test for this disorder.

Muscular Dystrophy

PROGRESSIVE MUSCULAR DYSTROPHY OF LITTLE BOYS (DUCHENNE, X-LINKED RECESSIVE). The electromyogram shows fibrillation potentials (because of disintegrating muscle fibers) and positive sharp waves. There is an increased proportion of polyphasic potentials low in amplitude and of normal or short duration; some are disintegrated potentials (Fig. 3–36). Insertional activity is reduced and there is increased resistance to needle advancement later in the disease as fibrosis and fat infiltration occur.

LIMB GIRDLE (AUTOSOMAL RECESSIVE) AND FACIOSCAPULOHUMERAL (AUTOSOMAL DOMINANT). Insertional activity may be normal, although an occasional positive sharp wave or fibrillation potential may be seen. Motor units in weakened muscles are of reduced amplitude and short duration and of increased polyphasicity. Recruitment demonstrates an increased number per strength of contraction (Fig. 3–37).

MYOTONIC DYSTROPHY (AUTOSOMAL DOMINANT). Myotonic discharges, or trains of positive sharp waves or biphasic spikes that vary in frequency and amplitude, are produced by tapping the muscle, stimulating its nerve, or moving the needle electrode (see Fig. 3–28). Motor units of distal muscles show a reduction in amplitude and duration, and an increase in polyphasicity and number recruited per strength of contraction. Conduction velocity is normal.

INFLAMMATORY MYOPATHY (POLYMYOSITIS, DERMATOMYOSITIS). The electromyogram demonstrates profuse positive sharp waves and fibrillation potentials. Fibrillation potentials parallel the activity of the disease and may be suppressed with steroids. Bizarre repetitive (low- or high-frequency) discharges, are found (see Fig. 3–27). Motor units are of reduced amplitude and duration. An increase in polyphasic potentials and an

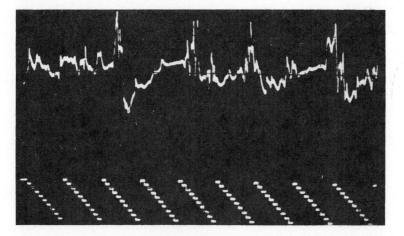

FIGURE 3–37. Moderate strength contraction in a patient with limb-girdle muscular dystrophy, demonstrating an increased number of voluntary recruited motor units per strength of contraction. Calibration signal is 100 microvolts in amplitude; duration of one vertical line is 10 msec.

increase in the number of motor units recruited per strength of contraction are recorded.

Tetany. Incipient tetany may be manifested first by volitional repetitive discharge polyphasic potentials (iterative discharges) as the heightened irritability shortens the relative refractory period. Progressively increased motor unit hyperirritability results in spontaneous appearance of these repetitive discharges, which are grouped fasciculations. Hyperventilation may also produce these abnormal potentials.

Facial Paralysis. It is helpful in prognosticating the outcome of facial paralysis to stimulate the facial nerve under the tip of the ear lobe and record over the frontalis above the center of the brow. In the first 72 hours the excitability should be normal; after this time, if the distal axons are undergoing wallerian degeneration, excitability will disappear. With the use of surface electrodes, the amplitude of the "M" response should be proportional to the number of conducting fibers, those which presumably are neurapraxic in a segment of compromise. If the facial delay is greatly prolonged, the prognosis is less favorable. The contralateral facial nerve should be stimulated for comparison.

Sprouting may occur from the normal side of the face across the midline so that inter-pretation of active potentials under voluntary control as recorded near the midline after prolonged time may lead to a mistaken report that reinnervation is occurring. Here, stimulation of both facial nerves can give the answer.

Anomalous Innervation. Interpretation of a variety of clinical conditions depends on a knowledge of innervation patterns. Since anomalous patterns occur frequently, it is necessary to identify these variations in order to avoid erroneous conclusions regarding electrodiagnostic findings. Isolation of the muscle response, with a needle electrode if necessary, then stimulation of the motor fibers of the involved nerve proximally and distally will indicate the correct pathway. Examples include median nerve fibers communicating with the ulnar nerve in the forearm so that the ulnar nerve of the wrist contains median nerve fibers going to the thenar eminence. Martin-Gruber anastomosis may become apparent during testing for carpal tunnel syndrome. This is the anomalous crossing of motor axons from median to ulnar nerve in the forearm. It is recognized by an initial positive deflection of the "M" response on stimulation at the elbow and calculation of a false, very fast conduction velocity (Fig. 3–38). Similar anomalous connections may occur between the peroneal

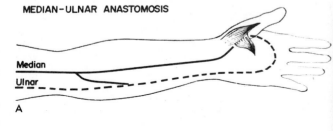

MEDIAN–ULNAR ANASTOMOSIS

Median

Ulnar

A

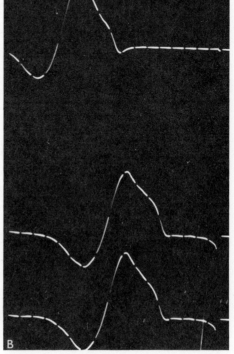

FIGURE 3–38. Martin-Gruber anastomosis (median-ulnar crossover) in a patient with carpal tunnel syndrome. Initial positive deflection in proximal stimulation response represents depolarization of ulnar thenar muscles by median crossing branches. (Top recording reading right to left. Each slashed line is one millisecond.)

and tibial nerves in the leg. In 20 per cent of individuals an anomalous branch separates from the peroneal nerve to innervate a portion of the extensor digitorum brevis muscle. It runs beneath the lateral malleolus, so it will not be stimulated by the usual distal placement of stimulating electrodes on the anterior ankle.

Reporting the Electromyogram

Many types of forms are used to report the electromyographic findings (Fig. 3–39). They are based on the necessity of recording the muscles examined, the electrical activity observed, and the interpretation of the findings.

Muscles Examined. In addition to listing the muscles examined, it is often helpful to record locations of needle insertions (proximal, central, or distal within the muscle). The peripheral nerve and the cord level of innervation should be noted routinely. If differential diagnosis involves a branch of a plexus or a peripheral nerve, more specific identification of the nerve supply is indicated.

Insertional Activity. This report should include the presence or absence of positive sharp waves and fibrillation potentials: Were there few, many, or trains? The presence of bizarre repetitive (high- or low-frequency) discharges or myotonic discharges and their frequency should be noted. The frequency and locations at which one encounters end plate potentials may be helpful and should be reported. A reduction in the amount of insertional activity, provoked activity, or the mechanical resistance to insertion (as seen in fibrosis or myositis) should be included.

Spontaneous Activity

FIBRILLATION POTENTIALS. These are graded according to the number present, on a scale from 1 to 4. Grade 1 usually indicates that fibrillation is difficult to find and is present only when the muscle is stimulated mechanically. Grade 2 represents the presence of a few fibrillation potentials without mechanical stimulation of the muscle. Grade 4 indicates that the oscilloscope screen is filled horizontally with fibrillation potentials. Grade 3 is between 2 and 4. Some electromyographers use simply minimal, moderate, and considerable number of fibrillation potentials.

FASCICULATION POTENTIALS. These should be reported as simple or polyphasic. Their wave form should be followed over

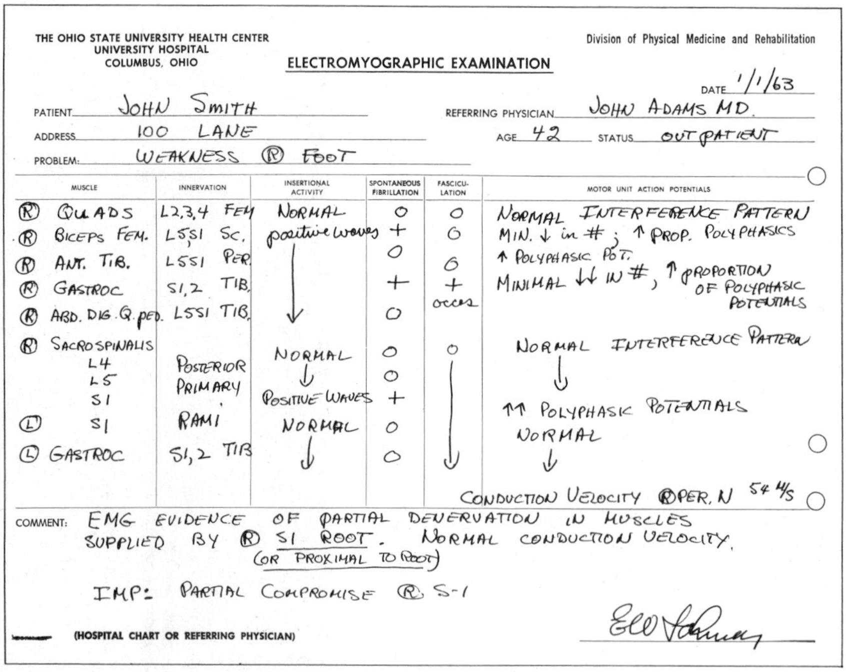
THE OHIO STATE UNIVERSITY HEALTH CENTER
UNIVERSITY HOSPITAL
COLUMBUS, OHIO

Division of Physical Medicine and Rehabilitation

ELECTROMYOGRAPHIC EXAMINATION

DATE 1/1/63

PATIENT JOHN SMITH — REFERRING PHYSICIAN JOHN ADAMS MD.

ADDRESS 100 LANE — AGE 42 — STATUS OUT PATIENT

PROBLEM: WEAKNESS Ⓡ FOOT

MUSCLE	INNERVATION	INSERTIONAL ACTIVITY	SPONTANEOUS FIBRILLATION	FASCICULATION	MOTOR UNIT ACTION POTENTIALS
Ⓡ QUADS	L2,3,4 FEM	NORMAL	O	O	NORMAL INTERFERENCE PATTERN
Ⓡ BICEPS FEM.	L5S1 SC.	positive waves	+	O	MIN. ↓ in #; ↑ PROP. POLYPHASICS
Ⓡ ANT. TIB.	L5S1 PER.		O	O	↑ POLYPHASIC POT.
Ⓡ GASTROC	S1,2 TIB.		+	+ occas	MINIMAL ↓↓ IN #, ↑ PROPORTION OF POLYPHASIC POTENTIALS
Ⓡ ABD. DIG. Q. PED.	L5S1 TIB.	↓	O		
Ⓡ SACROSPINALIS				O	NORMAL INTERFERENCE PATTERN
L4	POSTERIOR	NORMAL	O		
L5	PRIMARY	↓	O		↓
S1		POSITIVE WAVES	+		↑↑ POLYPHASIC POTENTIALS
Ⓛ S1	RAMI	NORMAL	O		NORMAL
Ⓛ GASTROC	S1,2 TIB	↓	O	↓	↓

CONDUCTION VELOCITY Ⓡ PER. N 54 M/S

COMMENT: EMG EVIDENCE OF PARTIAL DENERVATION IN MUSCLES SUPPLIED BY Ⓡ S1 ROOT. (OR PROXIMAL TO ROOT) NORMAL CONDUCTION VELOCITY.

IMP: PARTIAL COMPROMISE Ⓡ S-1

(HOSPITAL CHART OR REFERRING PHYSICIAN)

FIGURE 3–39. Sample EMG report.

multiple discharges to note the stability of the complex. Quiet muscle should be observed for at least one minute. The number of fasciculation potentials present is usually recorded as rare, occasional, few, or many.

MOTOR UNIT ACTION POTENTIALS. The amplitude, duration, shape, rate, and rhythm of firing and the number activated with respect to the strength of contraction should be described.

Nerve Stimulation Studies. The motor or sensory conduction velocity of the stimulated nerves should be indicated, as well as the terminal latency. Normal values should be included for comparison. Any variation in "M" response at the proximal and distal stimulation sites and during repetitive stimulations should be reported. Presence or absence of "H" reflex should be noted.

Comment. The electromyographic findings should be summarized and then translated into a clinical diagnosis. An electromyogram without a clinical impression is of little value to the practicing physician.

TRADITIONAL ELECTRODIAGNOSTIC TECHNIQUES

Rheobase. When a current is allowed to flow for an infinite period, the minimal amount of intensity of current that will stimulate the muscle is termed the *rheobase.* For practical purposes, infinite time is 300 milliseconds of current.

Chronaxie. The duration of flow of a current twice the intensity of the rheobase required to stimulate a muscle is termed the *chronaxie.*

Strength-Duration Curve. It is apparent that the intensity of current and its duration of flow are nerve-exciting parameters that are inversely related. Plotting the duration of current flow against the intensity of current applied results in the strength-duration curve. Instruments are available that give a constant current or a constant voltage so that either the voltage or the current may be plotted as the intensity of stimulus. The chronaxie is one point of the strength-duration curve.

Reaction of Degeneration. When an electrical stimulus is applied to a muscle that has an intact nerve supply, the muscle is activated by impulses arriving from the motor nerve, since nerve tissue is inherently more excitable (has a lower threshold of stimulation) than muscle tissue. Thus if a current that is two times the rheobase is applied to an innervated muscle, the duration of flow needed to produce a contraction could be very short. One current that has an extremely short duration is induced or faradic current.

Conversely, if the muscle has lost its nerve supply, then the muscle fibers must be stimulated directly, and since they are less excitable (have a higher threshold of stimulation) than the nerve tissue, the flow of current must be longer at similar intensities to produce a contraction of muscle. A galvanic or direct current permits current flow of prolonged duration.

Reaction of degeneration (RD) is the reaction of a muscle responding to galvanic but not faradic stimulation (i.e., current flow of less than one millisecond). Innervated muscle also responds best when stimulated at its middle third or at the *motor point,* the point at which the nerve enters the muscle. Conversely, denervated muscle responds equally to the stimulus applied anywhere over the muscle. The muscle twitch is quite brisk in intact muscle, since the stimulus is conducted throughout the muscle by fast-conducting nerve fibers, while in denervated muscle the twitch is quite slow and "worm-like" because the non-nervous tissue is the conducting medium. The cathode closing current is the most effective in exciting nerve tissue, while for denervated muscle it has no such property. This has led to Erb's law for the effectiveness of stimulation of normal muscle CCC>ACC>AOC>COC (cathode, anode, opening, closing, and current).

When alternating current is used, the quarter cycles of the sinusoidal wave compare to CC, COC, ACC, and AOC. Thus one fourth of the wave corresponds to the exciting stimulus, and an alternating current with a frequency of 1000 cycles per second would compare to an induced current having a duration of 0.25 millisecond, a duration too short to activate denervated muscle. However, an alternating current of 100 cycles per second would have a quarter cycle of 2.5 milliseconds, a duration of flow sufficient to excite denervated muscle.

Partial Reaction of Degeneration. When the muscle is only partially denervated, the muscle twitch in response to faradic or other current flowing for short duration would be diminished in proportion to the number of denervated muscle fibers, since they would be unable to respond.

Tetanus Twitch Ratio. Excitation of denervated muscle requires a high intensity of current. A very slight further increase of intensity will tetanize the muscle (ratio almost 1:1). However, very little current is required to excite normal nerve, but considerably more to tetanize it, so that the tetanus twitch ratio is 5:1 (i.e., five times the current intensity is needed to tetanize rather than to cause a twitch).

Summary

These traditional electrodiagnostic techniques require interpretation through several variables: the location of the underlying muscle, the resistance of the skin, the thickness of the subcutaneous layer, and then the visible recognition of a minimal twitch. All these factors compound the variability of the tests and cloud their significance.

Electromyography and efferent and afferent fiber stimulation techniques are considerably more sensitive and objective than obsolescent and less reliable techniques, and thus should supplant them.

REFERENCES

1. Adrian, E. D., and Bronk, D. W.: The discharge of impulses in motor nerve fibers. II. The frequency of discharge in reflex and voluntary contractions. J. Physiol. (Lond.), 67:119–151, 1929.
2. Bauwens, P.: Electrodiagnostic definition of the site and nature of peripheral lesions. Ann. Phys. Med., 5:149–152, 1960.
3. Buchthal, F., Pinelli, P., and Rosenfalch, P.: Action potential parameters in normal human muscle and their physiologic determinants. Acta Physiol., 32:219–229, 1954.
4. Carpendale, M. T. F.: Conduction time in terminal portion of motor fibers of ulnar, median, and peroneal nerves in healthy subjects and patients with neuropathy. Thesis, University of Minnesota, 1956.
5. Cerra, D., and Johnson, E. W.: Motor nerve conduction velocity in "idiopathic" polyneuritis. Arch. Phys. Med. Rehabil., 42:159–163, 1961.
6. Cerra, D., and Johnson, E. W.: Motor nerve conduction velocity in premature infants. Arch. Phys. Med. Rehabil., 43:160–164, 1962.
7. Christensen, E.: Topography of terminal motor innervation in striated muscles from stillborn infants. Am. J. Phys. Med., 38:65–78, 1959.
8. Dawson, G. D., and Scott, J. W.: The recording of nerve action potentials through the skin in man. J. Neurol. Neurosurg. Psychiatry, 12:259–268, 1949.
9. Denny-Brown, D., and Pennybacker, J. B.: Fibrillation and fasciculation in voluntary muscle. Brain, 61:311–332, 1938.
10. Eaton, L. M., and Lambert, E. H.: Electromyography and electrical stimulation of nerves in diseases of the motor unit. JAMA, 163:1117–1124, 1957.
11. Erlanger, J.: Interpretation of action potential in cutaneous and muscle nerves. Am. J. Physiol., 82:644–655, 1927.
12. Feinstein, B., Lindegard, B., Nyman, E., and Wohlfart, G.: Morphologic studies of motor units in normal human muscles. Acta Anat. (Basel), 23:127–142, 1955.
13. Gasser, H. S., and Grundfest, H.: Axon diameters in relation to spike dimensions and conduction velocity in mammalian fibers. Am. J. Physiol., 127:393–414, 1939.
14. Gilliatt, R. W., and Sears, T. A.: Sensory nerve action potentials in patients with peripheral nerve lesions. J. Neurol. Neurosurg. Psychiatry, 21:109, 1958.
15. Gilliatt, R. W., et al.: The recording of lateral popliteal nerve action potentials in man. J. Neurol. Neurosurg. Psychiatry, 24:305–318, 1961.
16. Hendriksen, J. D.: Conduction velocity of motor nerves in normal subjects and patients with neuromuscular disorders. Thesis, University of Minnesota, 1956.
17. Hodes, R., Larrabee, M. G., and German, W. U.: Human electromyogram in response to nerve stimulation and conduction velocity of motor axons: Studies on normal and on injured peripheral nerves. Arch. Neurol. Psychiatry, 60:340–365, 1948.
18. Hursh, J. B.: Conduction velocity and diameter of nerve fibers. Am. J. Physiol., 127:131–139, 1939.
19. Johnson, E. W., and Olsen, K. J.: Clinical value of motor nerve conduction velocity determination. JAMA, 172:2030–2035, 1960.
20. Johnson, E. W., and Waylonis, G. W.: Facial nerve conduction latency in diabetes. Arch. Phys. Med. Rehabil., 45:131–139, 1964.
21. Johnson, E. W., Wells, R. M., and Duran, R. J.: Diagnosis of carpal tunnel syndrome. Arch. Phys. Med. Rehabil., 43:414–419, 1962.
22. Kugelberg, E.: Electromyogram in muscle disorders. J. Neurol. Neurosurg. Psychiatry, 10:122–129, 1947.
23. Lambert, E., and McMorris, R.: Size of motor unit action potential in neuromuscular diseases. Fed. Proc., 12:263, 1953.
24. Liddell, F. G. T., and Sherrington, C. S.: Recruitment and some other features of reflex inhibition. Proc. R. Soc. Lond. (Biol.), 97:488, 1925.
25. Magladery, J., Ward, D., McDougal, B., Jr.: Electrophysiologic studies of nerve and reflex activity in normal man. I. Identification of certain reflexes

in the electromyogram and the conduction velocity of peripheral nerve fibres. Bull. Johns Hopkins Hosp., 86:265–290, 1950.

26. Stalberg, E., and Trontelj, J. V.: Single Fiber Electromyography. U.K., Mirvalle Press, Ltd., 1979.

27. Thomas, J. E., and Lambert, E. H.: Ulnar nerve conduction velocity and H-reflex in infants and children. J. Appl. Physiol., 15:1–9, 1960.

28. Wagman, I. H., and Lesse, H.: Maximum conduction velocities of motor fibers of ulnar nerve in human subjects of various ages and sizes. J. Neurophysiol., 15:235–244, 1952.

29. Weddell, G., Feinstein, B., and Pattle, R. E.: The electrical activity of voluntary muscle in man under normal and pathological conditions. Brain, 67:178–257, 1944.

4

GAIT ANALYSIS: DIAGNOSIS AND MANAGEMENT

JUSTUS F. LEHMANN

GAIT PATTERN

In order to analyze a gait pattern, to diagnose pathology, and to understand therapeutic interventions such as braces and prostheses, it is essential to understand the biomechanics and physiology of normal gait.[8, 16, 23]

Points of the Gait Cycle

The cycle from heel strike on one leg to the next heel strike on the same leg equals 100 per cent of a total gait cycle. One can identify specific points in time during this gait cycle. At 0 per cent, the heel strikes at the beginning of the stance phase. At 15 per cent the forefoot is also in contact with the floor; therefore, it is called "foot flat." At 30 per cent the heel leaves the ground, called "heel off"; at 45 per cent the knee and hip bend to accelerate the leg forward in anticipation of the swing phase, and this is called "knee bend." At 60 per cent the toe leaves the ground, which also signals the end of the stance phase and the beginning of the swing phase. This is called "toe off."

At mid-swing, foot dorsiflexion provides toe clearance. No accurate percentile can be attributed to this event. At 100 per cent, heel strike again occurs with the same leg. Thus,

by definition, the duration of the stance is 60 per cent of the total gait cycle and the swing phase is 40 per cent of the total.

Phases of the Gait Cycle

The terms for the phases from point to point of the gait cycle are as follows: The period from 0 to 15 per cent is called the *heel strike phase*. From 15 to 30 per cent is called *mid-stance;* from 30 to 45 per cent is called *push off;* from 45 to 60 per cent is called *acceleration of the swing leg*. The swing phase is subdivided into the swing-through portion and deceleration of the swinging leg at the end of the period.

At the end of the stance phase of one leg and the beginning of the stance phase of the other, there is a time of double support of the body by both legs. This phase of double support extends over approximately 11 per cent of the gait cycle.

Energy is consumed in two ways. For example, when the leg is decelerated during the end of the swing phase, a swinging mass is decelerated and a forward movement is transmitted to the body so that it is actually accelerated. Energy is also consumed during the shock absorption of heel strike. The body's center of gravity tends to continue forward owing to inertia and downward

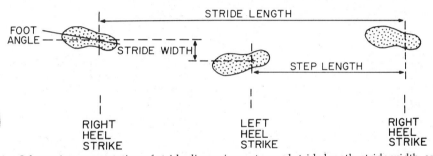

FIGURE 4–1. Schematic representation of stride dimensions: step and stride length, stride width, and foot angle. (Used with permission from Murray, H. P., et al.: Walking patterns of normal men. J. Bone Joint Surg., 46A:2:341, 1964.)

owing to gravity. The restraint exerted by muscles is called *shock absorption*. Energy is also required for propulsion during push off when the center of gravity is actually propelled up and forward. The relative relationship of energy consumption of the two activities is 5:8 between propulsion on the one hand and shock absorption/deceleration on the other.[12] Thus, biologically, more energy is actually consumed in controlling forward movement than in moving forward.[14]

To further clarify terminology, Figure 4–1 shows stride length, defined as the length extending from heel strike to heel strike of the same foot; step length is from heel strike of one foot to heel strike of the other foot. Stride width is determined by the distance between the midline of one foot and the midline of the other foot. On the average, these values are approximately 156 cm for stride length and half that value, for step length. Stride width is 8 cm ± 3.5, and the angle at which we normally toe out from the line of progression is about 6.7° to 6.8°. The mean duration of the total gait cycle is slightly over one second (1.03 ± 0.10). Cadence, the number of steps per minute, is approximately 117, or not quite 60 strides per minute.[15] However, for all these measures there is a considerable amount of variation.

The most important variable influencing energy consumption is the character of the movements of the center of gravity. The center of gravity moves up and down and right and left, and the amplitude of these excursions essentially determines the amount of energy consumption during walking activity. The center of gravity pathway requiring the least energy consumption would be a straight line parallel to the ground. Such a line is possible only with wheels, and our translatory motion during

ambulation occurs as a result of angular changes at the two ends of stick levers. Since a straight line is not feasible, the next best trajectory would be a sinusoidal curve of the least possible amplitude.

Determinants of Gait

Translatory movement of the body such as walking is brought about by alternating angular changes at the upper and lower end of the stick levers that constitute the lower limbs.[19] If the leg consisted of a single lever with mobility only at foot and hip, a "compass" gait would result. If the pivot point were the contact area with the ground, the arc described by the center of gravity would have a vertical excursion of approximately 3 inches. At the low end of the center of gravity curve an abrupt change of direction as well as a deceleration and subsequent acceleration would occur, both energy-consuming processes. This center of gravity pathway curve is modified in reality by six determinants.[18]

The first modification of this inefficient compass gait is *pelvic rotation* of 4° in either direction, a total of 8° (Fig. 4–2). The rotation occurs maximally to one side at the phase of double support, that is, when both legs are on the ground and the center of gravity is at the low end of the pathway curve. Thus the length of the supporting leg is effectively increased and the lowest point of the center of gravity pathway curve is elevated. As the other leg swings forward the pelvis rotates 4° in the opposite direction, with the same effect on the center of gravity pathway curve. This elevation of the low end of the center of gravity pathway curve reduces the total amplitude by 3/8 inch.

The second determinant is that of *pelvic*

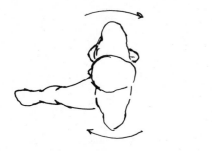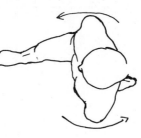

FIGURE 4–2. Pelvic rotation, 4 degrees in either direction.

tilt. As one walks, the pelvis drops on the side of the swinging leg. This drop is controlled by the hip abductors (gluteus medius and minimus) of the stance leg. Since the center of gravity is midway between the hips, the pathway curve also drops. This reduces its greatest elevation from the floor during mid-stance. At about the same time, the swing leg must be foreshortened by hip and knee flexion and ankle dorsiflexion to provide toe clearance. This pelvic drop is about 5° and saves 3/16 inch of vertical excursion at the top of the center of gravity pathway curve.

The third determinant is *knee flexion,* which occurs during the mid-stance. The knee is extended during heel strike, flexed to 15° toward mid-stance, and then extended toward push off. This effectively reduces leg length during mid-stance, when the center of gravity reaches its highest point. The reduction in leg length lowers the center of gravity at its highest point by 7/16 inch; thus, the sum of reductions in vertical excursion caused by the first, second, and third determinants is 1 inch, reducing total amplitude to less than 2 inches (1.7 inches), with considerable energy saving.

However, the abrupt change in direction and the deceleration and subsequent acceleration around the lower point of the center of gravity pathway has not yet been eliminated by these determinants. The fourth and fifth determinants are responsible for smoothing out this part of the curve. This is *knee and ankle motion.* The ankle motion (Fig. 4–3), in combination with the already described knee motion, produces a smooth sinusoidal pathway of the center of gravity. The ankle pivots on the posterior heel with a relatively short radius of motion to the foot flat position. The ankle position then remains the same until the heel leaves the ground at the toe off position; during this phase, the ankle pivots over the ball of the foot with a much

larger radius of the arc. The fourth and fifth determinants convert the vertical center of gravity pathway curve into a smooth sinusoidal curve of less than 2 inches amplitude.

The last determinant concerns the *motion of the center of gravity* in the horizontal plane. To be stable the center of gravity must be brought over the supporting limb. A plumb line should fall over the supporting foot; thus, for one to stand on the left leg, one's center of gravity must shift toward the left side and then sway to the right side when one steps onto the right foot, a total excursion of 6 inches. This is an inefficient use of energy. The normal anatomic valgus at the knee brings the feet closer to the midline; therefore, less lateral sway is necessary. The excursion is again less than 2 inches, an average of about 1.7 inches for an adult. The center of gravity pathway describes a smooth sinusoidal pathway curve, not only up and down but also from side to side.

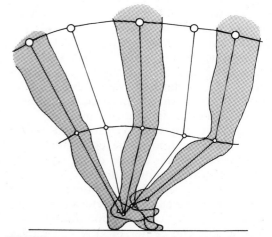

FIGURE 4–3. Knee and foot rotation smoothing the center of gravity pathway. (Redrawn from Saunders, J. B., Inman, V. T., and Eberhart, H. D.: The major determinants in normal and pathological gait. J. Bone Joint Surg., 35A:543, 1953.)

Thus, the center of gravity is found in the midline and at its lowest point during the phase of double support. As weight is put on the right foot, it shifts to its highest and most lateral position toward the right during mid-stance. As the other heel strikes, the center of gravity is back at its lowest point in midline to move up and left laterally toward mid-stance on the left.

The limb also undergoes a considerable amount of rotation during the gait cycle; the pelvis rotates 8°, the femur 8°, and the tibia 9°, a total of 25°. Figure 4–4 shows the direction of rotation. From the beginning, at toe off, all the rotation moves in the direction of internal rotation until a peak is reached at mid-stance (15 to 20 per cent of the gait cycle). Then the rotation begins to reverse toward external rotation until push off. During push off, especially during the very last part of the stance, there is a more rapid change into external rotation, particularly of the tibia. If one walks on the wet sand at the beach, a cake of sand is thrown out at this point, indicating this rotation. This rotation is difficult to imitate in prosthetic replacement of the limb.

Muscle Activity in the Gait Cycle

If we examine the motor power that produces the motion of the limb segments in Figures 4–5 and 4–6, the pre-tibial group shown in the graph is most active during the heel strike phase, where a lengthening contraction of the foot dorsiflexors lets the foot down from heel strike to the foot flat position slowly, in a controlled manner. The small activity during the rest of the stance phase is due to the fact that these same dorsiflexors are also invertors and evertors, a bridle to keep the foot stable in the mediolateral direction, together with the corresponding inver-

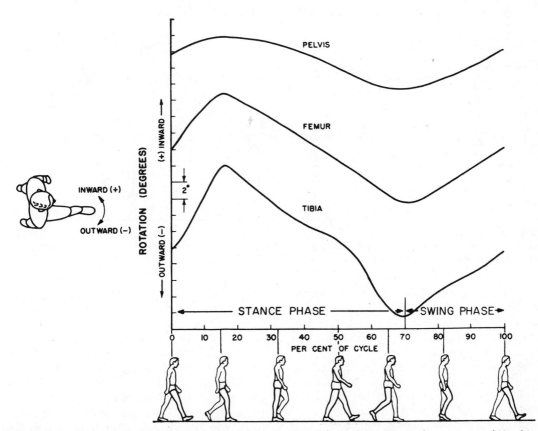

FIGURE 4–4. Relative rotations at knee and hip joints as viewed from above. Pin studies, average of 12 subjects. There is considerable variability in the stride length, step length, stride width, gait cycle duration, and cadence. (From Human Limbs and Their Substitutes by Klopsteg and Wilson. © 1954 by McGraw-Hill Book Company, Inc. Used with permission from the McGraw-Hill Book Co.)

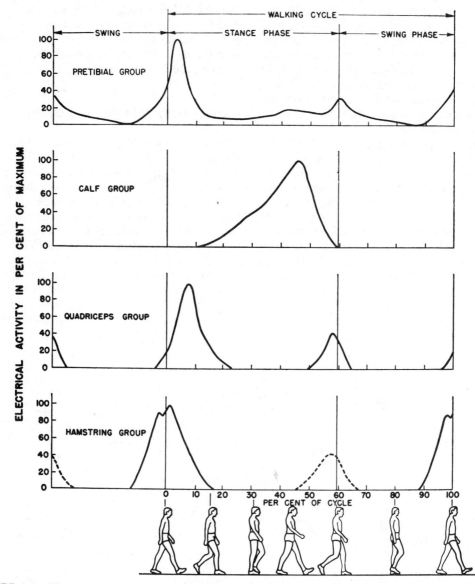

FIGURE 4–5. Phasic action of major muscle groups during level walking. Electromyograph studies, 10 adult males. (From Human Limbs and Their Substitutes by Klopsteg and Wilson. © 1954 by McGraw-Hill Book Company, Inc. Used with permission from the McGraw-Hill Book Co.)

tors and evertors in the calf. This is important for the stability of walking on rough ground or on a hillside. The small activity during the swing phase results from picking up the toe for toe clearance.

The calf group, primarily the gastrocnemius and soleus, shows maximal peak activity during push off to propel the center of gravity up and forward. The quadriceps group is maximally active just after heel strike, acting as a shock absorber to control knee flexion to the allowed 15°. It prevents the center of gravity from being driven down

and forward by gravity and inertia. The rectus femoris again is active during the latter part of the stance phase when the hip is flexed and the leg is accelerated forward. The quadriceps is also active in producing adequate forward swing of the leg below the knee while the hip is flexed. This is an extension action to make the leg follow the thigh segment. The hamstrings have a double peak just before and after heel strike. The first peak occurs during the swing when there is an open kinetic chain — that is, when the leg is not firmly planted on the ground — and this peak decelerates the forward swing of the leg by its extension action across the hip and its flexion action across the knee. The moment the foot is planted firmly on the ground, the open kinetic chain is converted to a closed kinetic chain, and the hamstrings now keep the knee from buckling, that is, from going into further flexion. They act as shock absorbers and also keep the hip from buckling. With the quadriceps they act as knee extensors to limit knee flexion at 15°. The hamstrings may show a second peak of activity at the termination of the stance phase, probably working toward hip and knee extension for push off.

The abductor group, gluteus medius and minimus, is primarily active during heel strike and the early stance phase to stabilize the pelvis tilt to 5°.

The adductor group's first peak of activity occurs right after heel strike. In part this peak may be explained by the hamstring portion of the adductor magnus controlling hip flexion as do the other hamstrings. This is also the time when the femur moves toward internal rotation. The adductor group may assist in this motion. While the adductors are external rotators when the limb is free (open kinetic chain) they allegedly reverse their function and act as internal rotators with the

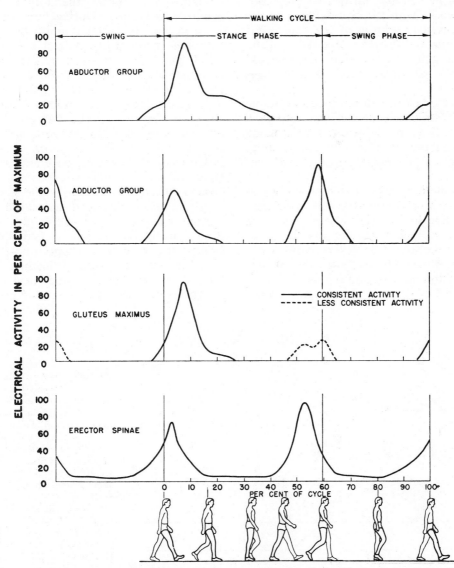

FIGURE 4–6. Phasic action of major muscle groups during level walking. Electromyograph studies, 10 adult males. (From Human Limbs and Their Substitutes by Klopsteg and Wilson. © 1954 by McGraw-Hill Book Company, Inc. Used with permission from the McGraw-Hill Book Co.)

foot planted on the ground (closed kinetic chain).[3, 10] Klopsteg states that they "stabilize the pelvis."[14] The second peak occurs at the end of the stance phase. The explanation may be that they work together with other hip flexors to accelerate the limb forward in preparation for the swing. It is also noted that at this time the limb segments move toward maximal external rotation.

The gluteus maximus is most active during the heel strike phase when the maximus acts as a shock absorber. Its extension function across the hip and knee keeps both joints from buckling and keeps the person from folding down during heel strike. Again there is a peak of activity during the push off, when it works with the hamstrings and the adductor magnus portion of the hamstrings to extend hip and knee for propulsion of the center of gravity. Its function may also add to the external rotation of the limb segments.

The erector of the spine becomes active during heel strike of each leg. This activity is necessary to keep the trunk from folding forward from the forces of inertia and gravity at heel strike. It also stabilizes the trunk mediolaterally.

These functions taken together show that the muscles work during the gait cycle only for short and limited periods of time. For instance, the shock absorbers, like the quadriceps and the foot dorsiflexors, work early during the stance phase, and the plantar flexors, gastrocnemius, and soleus work during the push off phase. The muscles cannot sustain a strong isometric contraction for long periods of time. There must be relaxation between contractions to allow the blood flow to restore itself fully for the resupply of oxygen and nutrients and the removal of waste and carbon dioxide. In an activity like walking, which we can maintain for long if not indefinite periods of time, it is essential that muscles work "on" and "off."

Force Transmission Through the Limb

Figure 4–7 shows the forces exerted against the ground. During heel strike the force vector slants down and forward. This vector is the sum of a vector shearing forward, parallel to the ground, and another perpendicular. During push off the resultant force is down and backward. It is the sum of a posterior shear vector and vertical force, shown in Figure 4–7. The horizontal, dotted line indicates body weight (vertical force): it is exceeded during the shock absorption phase when the dynamic deceleration of the center of gravity produces a force against the ground. Then inertia carries the body forward; therefore, the force against the ground vertically is less than body weight. Finally, during push off when we actually push against the ground to propel ourselves up and forward, the vertical loading on the ground may go up to 120 per cent of body weight as a result of acceleration (Force =

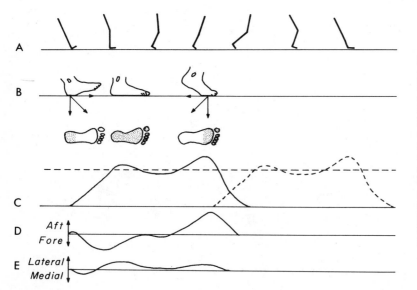

FIGURE 4–7. Forces during phases of the gait cycle. *A,* Points: heel strike, foot flat, heel off, toe off, knee bend, foot dorsiflexion, heel strike. *B,* Force vectors at heel strike and push off. *C,* Vertical ground reactive force. Horizontal dotted line indicates body weight; dotted curve indicates same phases on opposite leg. *D,* Fore and aft shear. *E,* Mediolateral shear. (Redrawn from Klopsteg, P. E., and Wilson, P. D. (Eds.): Human Limbs and Their Substitutes. New York, McGraw-Hill Book Co., Inc., 1954.)

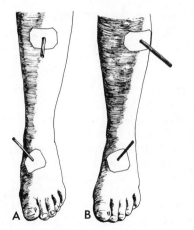

FIGURE 4–8. Pins fixed to the tibia and first metatarsal show the following: *A,* With foot planted on the ground, the tibial pin points straight ahead. *B,* When the tibia rotates externally, the foot is inverted, stiffening the arch. (Redrawn from Inman, V. T.: The Joints of the Ankle. Baltimore, Williams and Wilkins, 1976.)

Mass × Acceleration). The ground reactive force declines, and the dotted line indicates when the other leg takes up the force during the phase of double support.

The fore and aft shear is shown in Figure 4–7. At heel strike there is a small kick backward as the curve indicates.[6, 7, 14] Then through the heel strike phase there is a primarily forward shear. If we step on a banana peel at that time, the leg slides out in front. Then during push off, shear is reversed to the posterior direction; if we then step on the banana peel, the foot slips out from under us backward.

While the leg lands with a medial shear throughout most of the stance, it is followed by a lateral shear. The gluteus medius and minimus act to stabilize the pelvis and limit pelvic tilt. This produces lateral shear against the ground.

Inman[13] found that the subtalar joint complex functions essentially as a mitered hinge to allow force transmission through the foot during push off. When the tibia rotates externally, the arch is increased and the foot is inverted, stiffening the foot for better force transmission (Fig. 4–8*A, B*). Push off occurs just when the maximal rate and degree of external rotation are reached in the tibia (see Fig. 4–4).

Energy Consumption of Ambulation

Efficiency is best illustrated by the number of calories consumed to propel the body over a given distance (e.g., one meter), prorated per kilogram of body weight. This figure has been found by many authors to be very close to 0.8 calorie/m/kg for normal ambulation at a comfortable speed[9] (Table 4–1). Whenever pathology disturbs normal ambulation, this figure is markedly elevated. In Figure 4–9, for normal persons energy consumption is minimal at a certain comfortable walking speed.[2] This speed is approximately 60 to 75 meters per minute; at slower speeds relatively more energy is consumed for stabilization without increase in propulsion. As one walks faster than the comfortable walking speed,

TABLE 4–1. ENERGY REQUIREMENTS IN NORMAL AMBULATION*

Researcher, Date	N	Type of Disability	Speed (meters/min)	Energy Expenditure kcal/min/kg	kcal × 10⁻³/m/kg
McDonald, 1961	583	Normals (F)	80	0.067[b]	0.83
		Normals (M)	80	0.061[b]	0.76
Ralston, 1958	19	Normals (M&F)	74[c]	0.058[b]	0.78
Corcoran, 1970	32	Normals (M&F)	83[c, d]	0.063[b]	0.76
Waters, 1976	25	Normals (M&F)	82[d]	0.063[b]	0.77
Ganguli, 1973	16	Normals (M)	50[c]	0.044	0.088[a]
Bobbert, 1960	2	Normals (M)	81[c]	0.063[f]	0.079[a]
Peizer, 1969	?	Normals (?)	80[g]	0.043[g]	0.57

*From Fisher, S. D., and Gullickson, G.: Energy cost of ambulation in health and disability, a literature review. Arch. Phys. Med. Rehabil., 59(3):124–133, 1978. Used with permission.
[a]Calculated knowing kcal/min and m/min.
[b]Calculated knowing kcal/meter and m/min.
[c]Most efficient speed of ambulation.
[d]Speed chosen by the subjects.
[e]Speed chosen by researcher (the only speed or a representative speed).
[f]Calculation from author's equation and/or percentage figure.
[g]Approximated from a graph.

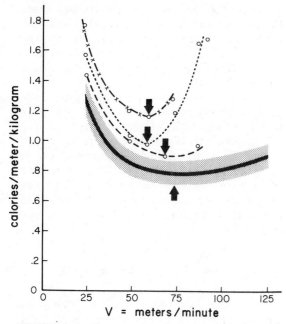

FIGURE 4–9. Energy expenditure in calories/meter/kilogram of normal subjects (heavy curve). Stippled area, one standard deviation. Broken line, amputee walking with suction-socket prosthesis. Dotted line, same, using pylon. x–x–x, same using forearm crutches. (Used with permission from Bard, G., and Ralston, H. J.: Measurement of energy expenditure during ambulation, with special reference to evaluation of assistive devices. Arch. Phys. Med. Rehabil., 40:417, 1959.)

the curve of energy consumption increases at a more rapid rate. When the phase of double support is lost, walking turns to running. As Figure 4–9 shows, when pathology such as amputation produces a gait abnormality, there is an upward shift of the total curve; at any given speed, energy consumption will be greater. The comfortable walking speed — i.e., that speed at which the patient moves over a given distance with a minimal amount of energy consumption — will shift to slower walking speeds. The increase in oxygen consumption at speeds faster than comfortable

speed occurs at a much more rapid rate; the curve rises more steeply. It also ends abruptly at higher speeds, representing the maximum speeds these people can walk safely. Maximal walking speed is reduced; in practical terms, patients with significant limps are usually unable to run.

The efficiency of the total gait mechanism can be measured by determining the ratio of metabolic expenditure in calories per minute over mechanical work, as shown in Table 4–2. This efficiency ratio, according to Ralston,[17] is between 0.21 and 0.24 at the speed of 73.2 meters per minute. Engineers tell us that this is approximately the maximum efficiency that can be achieved by moving a stick-lever system through angular changes to produce the translatory motion of our anatomic system.

In designing devices such as orthoses and prostheses, it is important to realize that adding weight to the body increases metabolic demand, but the amount of increase depends on where the weight is added.[5] If we add a load equal to 17 per cent of body weight to the trunk, metabolic demand increases only three per cent. If we add the same load to the foot, there is a 31 per cent increase in metabolic expenditure.[17] Thus, the weight of lower extremity orthoses can make a significant difference. However, one must keep in mind the influence of design of the orthosis or prosthesis on the center of gravity pathway. It has an even greater role in influencing energy expenditure, because anything that alters the center of gravity pathway means that the total body weight has to be lifted and lowered by that much, therefore changing metabolic demand.

GAIT ANALYSIS

In analyzing a patient with a limp, it is most important to do a thorough, step-by-

TABLE 4–2. METABOLIC EXPENDITURE AND EXTERNAL POSITIVE WORK: GROSS EFFICIENCY OF TWO FEMALES AND ONE MALE WALKING AT 73.2 METERS/MIN*

Subject	Metabolic Expenditure (cal/min)	Positive Work (cal/min)	Ratio
PK	3010	713	0.24
JR	3450	716	0.21
JC	3780	863	0.23

*From Ralston, H. J., and Lukin, L.: Energy levels of human body segments during level walking. Ergonomics, 12:45, 1969. Used with permission.

step appraisal. First one should look at symmetry and smoothness of movement. Stride length and width of the gait base should be observed. One should observe separately and deliberately each component part of the body: head, shoulders, arms, pelvis, hip, knees, ankles, and feet. Shoulders should be observed for dipping, elevation, depression, protraction, retraction, and ease of rotation. Listing of the trunk, asymmetric armswings, abnormal tilting, hiking, dropping, or fixedness should be noted. Circumducting the hip is another sign to watch. The stability of the knee and excessive inversion or eversion of the foot are only some of the other indicators of gait abnormality.

Pathologic Gaits

There may be several general causes of pathologic gait: *structural*, including abnormal bone length or shape; *joint and soft tissue pathology,* such as contractures; and *neuromuscular disorders*, which include the involvement of the central and peripheral nervous system and the musculature itself.

Common Abnormalities

Inequality of leg length is a common structural abnormality. If the difference is moderate, less than 1½ inches, there is an apparent elevation of the shoulder on the opposite swing side and dipping of the shoulder on the affected side. Compensation is sought by dropping the pelvis on the affected side. One observes exaggerated flexion at the hip, knee, and ankle on the opposite side during swing. If, on the other hand, the differential is more than 1½ inches, usually the patient switches to a different mode of compensation — that is, walking on tiptoe on the short leg to lengthen the limb.

If there is an *ankylosis* or *limitation of the joint range* — of the hip, for example — compensatory motion is usually present in the lumbar spine. Since the pelvis and trunk are tilted as a rigid unit to substitute for motion at the hip, excessive motion will be seen in the lumbar spine and in the unaffected hip joint.

If the knee is limited by contracture, the limb is shortened and all the hallmarks of a short leg limp will be present. Usually the problem is apparent only at higher walking speeds if the contracture is less than 30°. If it is greater, it will also be apparent at slower speeds. If the contracture is in extension the leg becomes too long. Circumduction, hip hiking, or tiptoeing on the unaffected side becomes necessary to swing the leg through. During the stance phase the pelvis and center of gravity rise too far because the 15° of knee flexion cannot occur. Heel strike is jarring because shock absorption requires knee flexion.

Equinus deformity of the foot produces a steppage gait, i.e., excessive flexion of hip and knee because the leg segment is too long for the swing phase. *Calcaneal* deformity prevents an effective push off, and its absence is visible.

Joint instability shows up in excessive range of motion, abnormal motion, inability to support body weight, and sudden buckling.

Painful or antalgic gait is characterized by avoidance of weight-bearing on the involved side, shortening of the stance, and an attempt to unload the limb as much as possible. If there is a midline lesion in the spinal column, the gait is slow and symmetrical; the jarring of active heel strike is avoided on both sides. Short steps are taken to limit the weight-bearing period. In lumbar lesions one can see rigid guarding of the back musculature. The lumbar lordosis is often decreased or abolished. Unilateral lesions (for example, the impingement of nerve roots by the disc in the intervertebral foramen) are often relieved by bending the trunk forward to the unaffected side so as to open the foramen. Muscle guarding, small steps, and avoidance of heel strike are observed. The patient with hip pain reduces mechanical stress on the hip joint by shifting the center of gravity over the affected hip joint. Therefore, during the stance one sees a dipped shoulder on the affected side, a relative elevation of the shoulder on the unaffected side, and a sliding of the trunk over the stance leg. In the swing phase, especially if there is an effusion present, the leg is carried in a slightly flexed, externally rotated position that relaxes the capsule and ligaments. Heel strike is avoided because of the jarring. A painful knee is usually carried in slight flexion, especially when effused, to relieve the tension. The patient in this situation may walk on his toes. At the least, heel strike is avoided.

Gaits from Neurologic Deficits

Gaits resulting from neurologic deficits in the central control mechanism may vary greatly depending on the type and localization of the lesion. Only a few common patterns can be mentioned.

One of the most common problems is encountered in patients whose strokes result in hemiplegia. Most patients with *extensor synergies* will ambulate. The extensor synergy includes extension and internal rotation at the hip, extension at the knee, plantar flexion of the foot and toes, and inversion of the foot. The patient is more likely to ambulate if this is not associated with severe sensory loss, especially of joint position sense; unilateral neglect; or equilibrium difficulties. In this gait pattern, heel strike is often missing and the patient strikes with the forefoot. The limb is kept extended during the entire gait cycle; consequently the patient has difficulties advancing the center of gravity during the latter part of the stance because the foot remains in plantar flexion. In severe cases the patient appears to walk up to that foot but not through the next step. For this reason push off is also missing. During the swing phase on the affected side, the limb is too long. Circumduction is used for toe clearance, sometimes in combination with hip hiking. In addition, the leg remains stiff, without knee flexion during the stance. As a result there is an excessive rise of the hip and center of gravity. The arm is held in adduction at the shoulder and in internal rotation and flexion at the elbow, wrist, and fingers. In cases of more flaccid paralysis, knee instability is pronounced. Because of the absence of abductor musculature, exaggerated drop of the pelvis on the opposite side may be noted.

Other lesions, such as those in cerebral palsy, may lead to adductor spasms with scissoring.

The *ataxic gait* that occurs in cerebellar lesions shows a typical dysmetria and incoordination. Staggering and lack of smooth motion are compensated for by a wide-based gait.

Lack of sensory feedback — for example, in posterior column disease (e.g., tabes dorsalis) — produces an uncontrolled motion. Commonly, innervation of the hamstrings and other muscles is not timed appropriately because of lack of sensory feedback. The knee is forcefully extended against the ligaments, which may ultimately be damaged, producing a Charcot joint with genu recurvatum and additional mediolateral instability. Jerky movements during the end of the swing phase and improper placement of the feet on the ground are observed. The gait abnormalities are increased if visual feedback is removed.

Basal ganglia disease such as Parkinson's disease produces a *festinating or propulsive gait*. Noticeable are the lack of armswing and the short quick steps with increasing speed, as if the patient were trying to race after his center of gravity. Ultimately the patient may fall. He cannot stop abruptly or change direction without danger of falling.

Gaits from Lower Motor Neuron Lesions

The gaits produced by lower motor neuron lesions are very characteristic in their effect on specific muscle groups. An understanding of these limps and compensatory mechanisms is essential for remediation.

If the physician suspects weakness in the accelerator group of muscles used in push off, he should direct the patient to walk up an incline; this activity will demonstrate a pronounced deficit in these accelerator muscles. The functioning of the shock absorbers that work during heel strike are more distinct when the patient walks down an incline. Almost all limps, with the exception of the gluteus medius limp, are more exaggerated on fast walking than on slow walking. The gluteus medius limp is obscured because inertia carries the body through, making the gluteus medius limp less visible.

Hip extensor gait, or weakness of the gluteus maximus, is striking because the trunk and pelvis are suddenly thrown backward after heel strike on the affected side, and the affected hip seems to protrude owing to the trunk motion. The knee is tightly extended in mid-stance, which slightly elevates the hip on that side. At heel strike the shock absorption function of the gluteus maximus is missing; hip flexion cannot be controlled unless the trunk is thrown farther back so that the center of gravity force line to the supporting foot falls well behind the hip joint. This action creates a rotatory moment rotating the hip in extension and locking it against tight extensor check ligaments, thus making it stable. The knee must be kept tightly extended because if the knee is flexed when the foot is on the ground the hip is unavoidably flexed as well. This gait cannot be corrected by braces, and a pelvic band is awkward. The best intervention is probably two crutches or canes with a three-point gait if the lesion is unilateral; if the lesion is bilateral, using crutches with an alternating two-point or four-point gait is best.

The uncompensated gluteus medius limp occurs in moderate weakness of the gluteus medius when it can only partly control the pelvic drop on the opposite swing side. In this case one sees a greater dropping of the pelvis on the unaffected swing side and an apparent lateral protrusion of the stance hip; if necessary, the patient may use a steppage gait to clear the swing leg. The best remedy for this limp is a cane in the opposite hand. If the gluteus medius is still weaker or entirely absent, the patient uses another gait pattern, the *compensated gluteus medius* limp. To prevent the pelvis from dropping too far on the opposite swing leg, the patient shifts his trunk so that the center of gravity is balanced over the stance hip joint. This maneuver produces less drop of the pelvis on the affected side than does the uncompensated gluteus medius limp. There is a medial deviation (rather than a lateral protrusion) of the affected hip because of the shift of the trunk. There is lateral bending of the trunk and dipping of the shoulder toward the affected side. The steppage gait on the unaffected swing leg is usually absent or less pronounced, since the hip does not drop as much.

Hip flexor paralysis is demonstrated by a limp that starts at push off, lasts throughout the entire stance, and also persists during the swing phase. The limb is swung forward solely by the musculature of the opposite hip throwing the trunk backward. The affected hip on the swing side becomes tightly extended against the check ligaments. Trunk rotation is transmitted via the ligaments to the swing leg, accelerating the leg forward. When the trunk stops moving, the leg continues forward by inertia into hip flexion.

The *quadriceps gait* pattern appears most obvious during the heel strike phase, the shock absorption phase, but it also shows during the swing phase. The knee is forcibly thrown into extension at or preceding heel strike and is associated with a smooth lurch of the trunk forward immediately following the heel strike. This is done in order to manipulate the center of gravity force line to the ground in front of the tightly extended knee joint, safely maintained in extension against the posterior capsule and ligaments. During rapid walking, the quadriceps is needed to accelerate the lower limb forward, motion that does not occur in the absence of the quadriceps. The leg lags behind by inertia, and an excessive heel rise results.

Weakness of the gastrocnemius-soleus is shown best when the patient walks up an incline. At push off, the heel does not come off and the pelvis-hip center of gravity area is not properly propelled up and forward. The affected side lags compared to the other side.

Moderate weakness of the foot dorsiflexors implies a less-than-effective lengthening contraction during the heel strike phase. The patient comes down to foot flat too fast, producing an audible slapping of the foot against the ground. During the swing phase these muscles may be still strong enough to pick up the patient's foot for toe clearance. However, if the muscles are very weak or absent, there will be a "drop foot" during swing and no slap will be heard after heel strike because the patient no longer strikes the ground with his heel. Rather, he lands on the ball of his foot. During the swing phase the toe hangs down, requiring a steppage gait for ground clearance.

WALKING AIDS

Stability when walking and standing depends on the location of the center of gravity. The center of gravity plumb line or force line to the ground must fall into the area of support to make the stance stable. The area of support can be increased if the patient has difficulties maintaining the center of gravity safely over the support area. The patient automatically assumes a wide-base gait if he cannot control the sway of the center of gravity.

The base of support can be increased by appliances such as a cane (Fig. 4–10) or crutches (Fig. 4–11). The triangular area between the crutches and the feet is the base of support that makes the patient stable. A four-legged cane increases the base of sup-

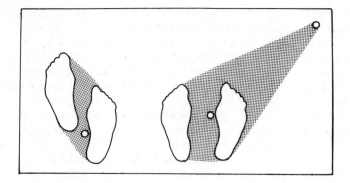

FIGURE 4–10. Foot position showing supporting area and location of center of gravity forceline, and its enlargement with the use of a cane. (Redrawn from Williams, M., and Lissner, H. R.: Biomechanics of Human Motion. Philadelphia, W. B. Saunders Company, 1962.)

port beyond that of a simple cane. A walkerette not only maximally enlarges the area of support but also increases stability beyond that provided by crutches.

The cane is always used in the hand opposite to the leg with muscular weakness or joint pathology in order to provide a normal pathway for the center of gravity. If the cane is carried on the same side it produces an unnecessary and exaggerated trunk sway. In bilateral pathology two canes may be used, usually with an alternating two-point gait. In an alternating two-point gait pattern, cane and opposite leg are advanced at the same time. The cane is commonly used in patients with lesions such as gluteus medius weakness or joint pathology at knee or ankle. The maximum weight that can be put on the cane is approximately 25 per cent of body weight.[21] Forearm crutches may be used in the same fashion as a cane. Maximal loading of the forearm crutches can be up to 45 per

cent of body weight if a single forearm crutch is used.[21]

The following gait patterns are commonly in use: (1) A forearm crutch instead of a cane is used on the side opposite to the affected limb, alternating two-point gait only partially relieving weight-bearing of the legs. (2) A three-point gait can completely eliminate weight-bearing on one extremity. In this case, when the affected leg is on the ground, the patient puts all his weight on the two forearm crutches. This gait pattern can be used in amputees. The intact limb is fully weighted without the support of the crutches. During the stance phase of this leg, the crutches are swung forward together with the affected limb. (3) The other gait pattern used with forearm crutches is the four-point gait. In this case there are always three points of support, either two crutches plus one leg or two legs plus one crutch; that is, the right crutch is moved while both legs

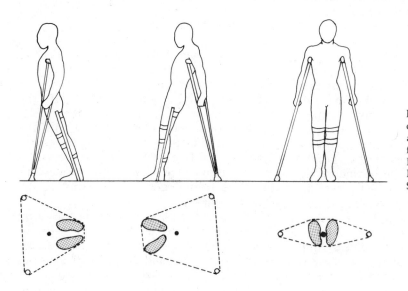

FIGURE 4–11. Different bases of support offering varying amounts of stability. (Redrawn from Williams, M., and Lissner, H. R.: Biomechanics of Human Motion. Philadelphia, W. B. Saunders Company, 1962.)

and the left crutch are on the ground. Subsequently the left leg is moved forward while the two crutches and the right leg are on the ground. Then the left crutch moves while two legs and the right crutch are on the ground. Then the right leg moves while the two crutches and the left leg are on the ground, and so forth. First a crutch, then the opposite limb, is always moved. While this gait pattern is slower than the other patterns described, it distributes weight over three points of support at all times, either through the upper extremities to the crutches and one leg or to two legs and one crutch and upper extremity. This pattern is commonly indicated to reduce weight-bearing by any one extremity to a minimum, for instance, in rheumatoid arthritis involving both upper and lower extremities.

Axillary crutches are used more commonly in such conditions as paraplegia. However, in some lower levels of the lesion, forearm crutches may be used. Axillary crutches can be used with an alternating two-point gait, or three-point or four-point gaits. In paraplegia, a swing-to or swing-through pattern may be used. The swing-to pattern reduces the triangle of support represented by the two crutches and the feet by lifting the body with the arms and sliding the feet forward closer to but never to the same level as the crutches, because anterior-posterior instability would result (Fig. 4–11). The crutches are then moved forward to enlarge the triangle of support and this maneuver is repeated. The patient must be braced at knee and ankle for either swing-to or swing-through patterns.

In the swing-through pattern, at the start the patient leans forward on the crutches and lifts and swings the legs through to a heel strike in front of the crutches. Since the ankle and knee are braced, arching the back makes this position stable. The hip is extended against ligaments which lock in extension because the center of gravity force line to the ground falls behind the hip joint, creating an extension moment. Subsequently the patient swings the crutches forward and again is stable because the center of gravity force line falls in the triangle of support. Gravity acting on the trunk will extend the hip. With this gait pattern the patient is stable twice: once with the crutches in front and once with the crutches behind. This is a mechanically ef-

fective gait pattern that produces a brisk speed of walking. Because the center of gravity pathway amplitude is large and not smooth, this pattern is very energy-consuming. Depending on the level of the lesion, energy expenditure may be between three and four times as much as that in normal ambulation, and in higher lesion levels it may even exceed 10 times normal energy requirements.[9]

In the injured or diseased hip joint, a three-point gait pattern can be used with partial or complete weight-bearing relief. However, a special consideration should be given to the effectiveness of a single cane or crutch in the opposite hand, or an alternating two-point gait in the case of bilateral disease. The loading on the hip of a patient standing on both legs is 50 per cent of body weight on each side. As the patient walks or stands on one leg, pelvic drop is controlled by the force of the gluteus medius on the stance side (Fig. 4–12). This counteracts the gravitational force on the center of gravity. The fulcrum is the hip. The approximate length of the levers is 1 inch for gluteus medius force (F) and 3 inches for the gravitational force (W) on the center of gravity of the body. The rotatory moment created by the gravitational force is 3 times 165 inch-pounds if the body weight is 165 pounds. Thus it must be counterbalanced

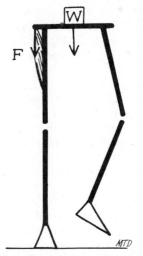

FIGURE 4–12. The abductors of the hip on one side balance the pelvis when the opposite leg is lifted. F is the force exerted by these muscles and operates at the hip in addition to W. (Used by permission from Harper & Row for Rosse, C., and Clawson, D. K.: Introduction to the Musculoskeletal System. New York, Harper & Row, Publ., 1970.)

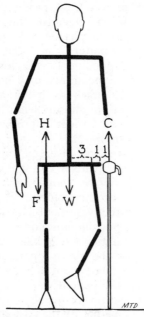

FIGURE 4–13. Schematic representation of forces acting on the hip with the use of a cane. F = gluteus medius force; C = force on cane; W = gravitational force acting on center of gravity; H = reactive force on hip fulcrum. (Used with permission from Harper & Row for Rosse, C., and Clawson, D. K.: Introduction to the Musculoskeletal System. New York, Harper & Row, Publ., 1970.)

by the rotatory moment of the gluteus medius contraction (F). The moment arm is 1 inch; therefore, the gluteus medius force must be equal to 3×165 pounds or 495 inch-pounds. Therefore, the reactive force on the fulcrum of the hip (H) must be gluteus medius force (F) plus gravitation force (W), or 4 times body weight.

If a cane is used (Fig. 4–13) the force put on the cane (C) is multiplied by a moment arm of a total of 8 inches, creating an elevation of the pelvis on the swing side. In addition, the gluteus medius force (F) creates a rotatory moment in the same direction. Thus the sum of the counterclockwise rotatory moment is (F × 1 inch) + (C × 8 inches). The clockwise rotatory moment is created by the gravitational force acting on center of gravity (W) multiplied by 3 inches (W × 3). Clockwise and counterclockwise moments must therefore be in equilibrium:

$$W \times 3 = (F \times 1) + (C \times 8)$$
$$165 \times 3 = F + (60 \times 8)$$
$$F = 15 \text{ lbs,}$$

assuming 60 pounds force is put on the cane.

The force on the hip is therefore the sum of the vertical forces down (F + W) minus the vertical force up on the cane (H = W + F − C) or H = 165 + 15 − 60 = 120 pounds. Thus, because of its leverage the cane eliminates necessary gluteus medius force and reduces the compressional force on the hip. A more accurate and detailed account has been given by Blount.[4]

In summary, understanding normal and abnormal gait is an essential basis for corrective action.

REFERENCES

1. Anderson, M. H., Bray, J. J., and Hennessy, C. A.: Prosthetic Principles — Above Knee Amputations. Springfield, Ill., Charles C Thomas, Publisher, 1960.
2. Bard, G., and Ralston, H. J.: Measurement of energy expenditure during ambulation, with special reference to evaluation of assistive devices. Arch. Phys. Med. Rehabil., 40:415–418, 1958.
3. Basmajian, J. V.: Muscles Alive. Baltimore, Williams and Wilkins, 1962.
4. Blount, W. P.: Don't throw away the cane. J. Bone Joint Surg., 38A:695–708, 1956.
5. Braun, W., and Fischer, O.: Uber den Schwerpunkt des menschlicken, Korpers unt Rucksicht auf die Ausrustung des deutschen infanteristen. Abhandl. Konig. Sachs. Ges. Wiss (Leipzig), 15:559–672, 1889.
6. Bresler, B., and Frankel, J. P.: The forces and moments in the leg during normal level walking. University of California (Berkeley) Prosthetic Research Project Report, Series 11, Issue 6, June, 1948.
7. Bresler, B., and Berry, F. R.: Energy and power in the leg during normal level walking. University of California (Berkeley) Prosthetic Research Project Report, Series 11, Issue 15, May, 1951.
8. Eberhart, H. D., Inman, V. T., and Bresler, B.: The principal element in human locomotion. *In* Klopsteg, P. E., and Wilson, P. D. (Eds.): Human Limbs and Their Substitutes. New York, McGraw-Hill Book Co., Inc., 1954.
9. Fisher, S. D., and Gullickson, G.: Energy cost of ambulation in health and disability, a literature review. Arch. Phys. Med. Rehabil., 59:124–133, 1978.
10. Hollinshead, W. H., and Jenkins, D. B.: Functional Anatomy of the Limbs and Back, 5th Ed. Philadelphia, W. B. Saunders Company, 1981.
11. Inman, V. T., and Mann, R. A.: Biomechanics of foot and ankle. *In* Inman, V. T. (Ed.): DuVries Surgery of the Foot, 3rd Ed. St. Louis, C. V. Mosby Co., 1973.
12. Inman, V. T.: Conservation of energy in ambulation. Arch. Phys. Med. Rehabil., 47:484–488, 1967.
13. Inman, V. T.: The Joints of the Ankle. Baltimore, Williams and Wilkins, 1976.

14. Klopsteg, P. E., and Wilson, P. D. (Eds.): Human Limbs and Their Substitutes. New York, McGraw-Hill Book Co., Inc., 1954.

15. Murray, H. P., et al.: Walking patterns of normal men. J. Bone Joint Surg., 46A:341, 1964.

16. Perry, J.: The mechanics of walking. *In* Perry, J., and Hislop, H. (Eds.): Principles of Lower Extremity Bracing. New York American Physical Therapy Association, 1967.

17. Ralston, H. J., and Lukin, L.: Energy levels of human body segments during level walking. Ergonomics, 12:45, 1969.

18. Saunders, J. B., Inman, V. T., and Eberhart, H. D.: The major determinants in normal and pathological gait. J. Bone Joint Surg., 35A:543, 1953.

19. Steindler, A.: Kinesiology of the Human Body. Springfield, Ill., Charles C Thomas, Publisher, 1955.

20. Stolov, W. C.: The lower extremity. *In* Rosse, C., and Clawson, D. K. (Eds.): Introduction to the Musculoskeletal System. New York, Harper and Row, 1970.

21. Warren, C. G.: Personal communication, 1979.

22. Williams, M., and Lissner, H. R.: Biomechanics of Human Motion. Philadelphia, W. B. Saunders Company, 1962.

23. Normal human locomotion. *In* Lower Limb Orthotics, 1974 Revision. New York University, Post Graduate Medical School, Prosthetics and Orthotics, pp. 19–52.

5

SPEECH AND LANGUAGE DISORDERS

DAVID R. BEUKELMAN
KATHRYN M. YORKSTON

The primary goal of human communication is accurate and rapid transfer of information through the spoken, written, or gestural modes. The ability to share daily experiences, draw up legal agreements, and record history is dependent upon an extensively developed communication system. Since most of us acquire our native verbal language with little voluntary effort, we are unaware of the complexities of human communication until we attempt to learn a second language or to write clear, concise term papers, or until we experience a communication impairment.

Communication impairment may involve any aspect of the hearing, language, or speech processes. Discussion of all possible communication disorders in this chapter would lead to superficial descriptions of each. Therefore, only those speech and language disorders clearly having a physical basis will be discussed. Because of the number of patients with neurogenic speech and language problems served by physical medicine and rehabilitation teams, additional emphasis will be placed on these disorders. In preparation for the discussion of communication disorders, a brief review of normal language and speech processes will be presented.

NORMAL LANGUAGE AND SPEECH PROCESSES

Language

Verbal language is an arbitrary code that symbolically associates sound and meaning in patterns that are produced and understood by members of a linguistic community. The notion of a "code" implies that verbal language involves numerous symbols and rules that are unique to a specific language (e.g., English, Japanese, and Spanish). Although reading and writing heavily involve language processes, the written form of a language is usually derived from its spoken form.

Verbal language may be divided into four subdivisions — phonology, semantics, syntax, and pragmatics.

Phonology refers to the area of linguistic study dealing with the relationships between sounds. Humans are able to produce many different sounds, but only a few of them are used as speech sounds. For example, the

Preparation of this chapter was supported in part by Research Grant No. 16-P-568 18/0-18 from the National Institute of Handicapped Research. Department of Education, Washington, D.C. 20202.

English language system makes use of only about 45 different sound elements (phonemes), which can be differentiated from each other because they change the meaning of a sound sequence. For example, the words "bat" and "cat" have different meanings in English. The "b" and "c" are distinct sound elements because they signal these differences in meaning.

Semantics refers to the study of linguistic units of meaning. As children, we learn that certain sound sequences consistently symbolize specific meanings. As children's language systems mature, the quantity and specificity of their vocabularies increase. For example, a child initially may label all animals "dogs." However, in time, the label "dog" is attached to a specific animal and the words "cat," "horse," "cow," "mouse," and "elephant" are added to the vocabulary. As normal adults speak, appropriate words are selected and produced rapidly (approximately 160 to 180 words per minute).

Syntax refers to the study of word relationships in forming phrases and sentences. The rules that govern these relationships are complex and numerous. For example, if words are combined in one order a certain meaning is communicated; however, if the same words are produced, but the order is changed, a different message is conveyed (The dog bit the boy. *vs* The boy bit the dog.). As children, we learn to generate sentences using nearly all syntactic rules accurately. However, only later do we learn to verbalize the specific grammatical rules of our language. Eventually, we eliminate errors of usage by learning exceptions to these grammatical rules. Language development has been studied extensively.[14] A detailed review is beyond the scope of this chapter. However, Cohen and Cross[11] have edited a resource book describing many aspects of child development, including language development.

Pragmatics refers to the study of the function or use of language in social contexts. For example, language can be used to demand, command, request, protest, threaten, impress, placate, or regulate others. The study of pragmatics also explores dialogue strategies and rules of discourse that occur in human communication. This relatively new field of study is receiving increasing attention in both adult and child language research.[3, 14]

Speech

Speech is the motor activity by which the oral, laryngeal, and respiratory structures produce the sound patterns of a language. Speech production involves the dynamic interaction of various components of the speaking mechanism. Despite the complex interactions between the various components of the speech mechanism, each will be discussed separately. Selected speech mechanism muscles and their motor innervations are listed in Table 5–1.

Respiration. Respiration is the energy source for the speaking process. The respiratory system is responsible for generating subglottal air pressure below the vocal folds. This pressure is maintained or varied depending upon the loudness level the speaker wishes to achieve. Normal speech is produced during the exhalation phase of respiration. Speech loudness (intensity) increases in proportion to the increase in subglottal air pressure. Since the average utterance varies minimally in loudness, the respiratory mechanism must ensure that a relatively constant level of subglottal air pressure is maintained throughout the utterance even though the lung volume level changes and the relative contributions of the elastic recoil forces of the structures of the lungs and thorax and the inspiratory and expiratory muscles change. This interaction between muscle activity and lung volume level during speech is summarized by Hixon[33] as follows: "The amount of muscular pressure required at a given instant during speech depends upon the alveolar pressure (subglottal air pressure) needed and the relaxation pressure available at the prevailing lung volume." During "high" lung volumes, the pressure bias of the muscles of the respiratory system is inspiratory in nature, thus checking the combined recoil forces of the lungs and thorax. During "low" lung volume levels the combined recoil forces of the lungs and thorax are supplemented increasingly by the net expiratory muscular pressure.

Phonation. Phonation refers to laryngeal sound production in speech. Two types of phonation occur during speech — voicing and whispering. Generally voiced phonation occurs during the normal production of all vowels and voiced consonant sounds. Voicing is achieved by adducting the vocal folds to constrict the glottis, thereby momentarily

TABLE 5–1.   SELECTED MUSCLES OF SPEECH MECHANISM WITH MOTOR INNERVATION*

Muscles	Motor Innervation
Respiration	
Diaphragm	Phrenic
Sternomastoid	Accessory (XI)
External intercostals	Intercostals T-2 through T-12
Internal intercostals	Intercostals T-2 through T-12
External and internal oblique	Intercostals T-6 through T-12
Transversus abdominis	Intercostals T-7 through T-12
Phonation	
Interarytenoid	Vagus (X), Inferior
Lateral cricoarytenoid	Vagus (X), Recurrent Branch
Posterior cricoarytenoid	Vagus (X), Recurrent Branch
Thyroarytenoid	Vagus (X), Recurrent Branch
Cricothyroid	Vagus (X), Recurrent Branch
Articulation	
Tongue	
Superior longitudinal	Hypoglossal (XII)
Inferior longitudinal	Hypoglossal (XII)
Transversus	Hypoglossal (XII)
Styloglossus	Hypoglossal (XII)
Palatoglossus	Accessory (XI)
Hypoglossus	Hypoglossal (XII)
Genioglossus	Hypoglossal (XII)
Mandible	
Masseter	Trigeminal (V), Anterior
Temporalis	Trunk of Mandibular Branch
Internal, external, and pterygoid	Trunk of Mandibular Branch
Velopharyngeal Mechanism	
Levator palatini	Vagus (X)
Tensor palatini	Trigeminal (V)
Palatoglossus	Accessory (XI)
Pharyngeal constrictor	Vagus (X)

*After Zemlin, W.: Speech and Hearing Sciences: Anatomy and Physiology. Englewood Cliffs, N.J., Prentice-Hall, Inc., 1968.

interrupting the flow of air from the trachea through the larynx. The build-up of subglottal air pressure below the adducted folds causes the folds to be "blown apart," and a puff of air escapes into the upper vocal tract. A combination of the elastic recoil and muscle force of the laryngeal structures and the Bernoulli effect draw the vocal folds once again into the adducted position. This pattern is repeated many times per second, with an average fundamental frequency being around 125 Hz for men and around 200 Hz for women.[9]

Fundamental frequency (pitch) and intensity (loudness) are two speech parameters controlled primarily by the interaction of the laryngeal and respiratory systems. Fundamental frequency is controlled by changes in vocal fold thickness, mass, length, and tension.[37, 38] Generally, an increasing fundamental frequency contour is associated with an increase of (1) vocal fold length, and with it the longitudinal tension of the folds (stretching the folds), or (2) medial compression (adductory squeeze), or a decrease in vocal fold thickness and mass. With other factors constant, an increase in subglottal air pressure will result in an increase in fundamental frequency.

Intensity adjustments are controlled by subtle interaction between the respiratory and laryngeal systems. There appears to be a close relationship between subglottal air pressure and voice intensity. A doubling of subglottal air pressure is associated with a 9 to 12 decibel increase in voice intensity.[10] Usually, the pattern of vocal fold movement changes as intensity is increased. The duration of the closed phase (time that the vocal folds are approximated) is increased, and the duration of the open phase of each vibratory cycle of the folds is decreased. This change probably occurs because of an increase in medial compression of the folds associated with increases in intensity.

Articulation. The vocal tract is a dynamic tubelike series of cavities beginning at the vocal folds and ending at the lips. The soft palate and pharynx, tongue, lips, cheeks, and mandible are the primary structures of articulation whose movements influence the shape and configuration of the vocal tract. Individual speech sounds are a mixture of acoustic vibration and/or silence which occurs when the air within the vocal tract is set into vibration. The major source of energy for speech sound production is the flow of air from the lungs. When specific speech sounds are produced in isolation, the speaker produces an ideal configuration of the vocal tract.

Speech sounds have been divided into two categories — vowels and consonants. Vowels include a family of sounds that are produced with a relatively open vocal tract. The sound source is at the level of the larynx, and the distinct identity of each vowel depends upon the shape and size of various cavities in the vocal tract. The critical factors in vowel production are the height of the dorsum of the tongue, the front-to-back position of the high point of the tongue in the oral cavity, and the degree of lip opening. The consonant category includes a group of sounds in which the vocal tract is completely or closely constricted during sound production. The sound source for these consonants may be a turbulent source in the oral cavity, e.g., s and f, with no laryngeal sound source (voiceless consonant); a combination of a turbulent sound source in the oral cavity and a laryngeal sound source, e.g., z and v (voiced consonants); or sounds with only a laryngeal sound source, e.g., l.

The articulatory targets of most vowel and consonant sounds include a complete or nearly complete closure of the velopharyngeal port (the passage from the oral into the nasal cavity). The nasal consonants (m, n, and ng) are exceptions to this pattern, as these sounds involve the radiation of acoustic energy through the nasal cavity. The degree of velopharyngeal closure that a speaker achieves during the production of a vowel may vary to some extent depending on the adjacent sounds. If the adjacent sounds require complete velopharyngeal closure, this port will probably be closed during the production of the intervening vowel. If one or both of the adjacent sounds is a nasal consonant, the velopharyngeal port may not be completely closed during the production of the intervening vowel.

Prosody. Prosody encompasses the rate, rhythm, loudness, and pitch contours that signal stress and therefore carry additional meaning beyond individual speech sounds, words, or sequences of words. It is an overall dimension of verbal communication that cannot be ascribed to any of the speech mechanism components described earlier. Overall prosodic patterns are produced by a complex interaction of all of the speech components. A normal speaker will produce the sentence, "Show Sam some snow," differently depending upon whether it is in response to the question, "To whom should I show the snow?" or to "What should I show Sam?" Normal stressing patterns are achieved by subtle changes in fundamental frequency, loudness, and duration.[48]

NEUROGENIC SPEECH AND LANGUAGE DISORDERS

Aphasia

Aphasia is defined as an impairment in the ability to interpret and formulate language symbols as a result of brain damage. Darley[15] describes aphasia as a disorder of the "central language process" that underlies the various language modalities, such as comprehension of verbal material, reading, speaking, and writing. The most common etiology of aphasia (85 per cent) is left cerebral vascular accident.[39] Although specific prevalence figures for aphasia are not available, it has been estimated that two million Americans are handicapped to some degree by stroke.[83] Other common etiologies of aphasia are arteriovenous malformation, tumor, and head injury. Although reports of frequency of aphasia with traumatic head injury vary, incidence of aphasia following head injury in a series of 3500 individuals was reported by Hillbom to be 14.6 per cent.[32]

Terminology

Aphasia is not restricted to one language process; rather, an aphasic individual has reduced ability in all language modalities, including speaking, auditory comprehension, reading, writing, and expression through pantomime. Patients exhibit a variety of different patterns of deficits. For example, some patients exhibit auditory comprehension problems that are disproportionately severe when compared with problems exhibited in naming or other verbal tasks. Other patients may have relatively severe word-finding problems yet perform fairly well on auditory comprehension tasks. These differences in patterns of deficits seen in behavioral examination form the basis for classifying aphasic patients.

One widely used descriptive system to classify aphasic speakers is based on the patients' verbal output.[24] *Fluent aphasia* is characterized by effortless, well-articulated speech with normal speech rhythm and melody. Failure to use the correct word is common. Words devoid of content, nonspecific words, and circumlocutions frequently occur. The verbal output of a severely involved, fluent speaker may contain jargon or nonsense words as well as meaningful ones. Fluent aphasics often do not recognize their errors. *Nonfluent aphasia*, on the other hand, is characterized by limited speech that is uttered slowly, with great effort, and often with poor articulation. The patient's speech may be telegraphic in nature, containing only the information-bearing words and excluding the words necessary for complete grammatical structure, such as prepositions and conjunctions.

More specific subtypes of aphasia can be identified by including other language processes such as auditory comprehension, naming ability, and ability to repeat. The following subtypes of aphasia were described by Goodglass and Kaplan.[26]

Broca's Aphasia. Speech is effortful and halting, with impaired articulation and reduced grammar. Comprehension is relatively good and reading is superior to writing.

Wernicke's Aphasia. Speech is fluent with paraphasic errors (sounds in words may be substituted for one another; order may be reversed). Auditory comprehension, reading, and writing are also impaired.

Anomic Aphasia. Speech is well-articulated, grammatical, and fluent but marked by severe word-finding difficulty and circumlocutory attempts. Auditory comprehension is good, and reading and writing are variable.

Conduction Aphasia. Spontaneous speech is relatively fluent with good comprehension, but there is selective loss of the ability to repeat.

Global Aphasia. Severe deficits are found in all language processes, including speech production, auditory comprehension, reading, and writing.

Transcortical Motor Aphasia. Speech is nonfluent, but auditory comprehension and the ability to repeat are good.

Isolation Aphasia. All language processes are poor, except for the ability to repeat.

Thalamic Aphasia. Recently, an aphasia syndrome resulting from thalamic damage has been described.[4, 62] Spontaneous speech is minimal. Verbal output is characterized by word-finding problems, perseveration, neologisms, and fading volume. Auditory comprehension and word repetition are intact.

Neurologic Correlates

For most people the language centers are in the left cerebral hemisphere. The reported incidence of aphasia with right cerebral insult varied up to 10 per cent in right-handed individuals and from 10 to 20 per cent in left-handed individuals.[54] Within the left hemisphere, fluent aphasia is usually associated with damage in the posterior parietal and temporal lobes and nonfluent aphasia is associated with more anterior lesions in the left hemisphere. Studies of localization of language function have a long history. For 100 years, attempts have been made to specify areas of cortical function via autopsy findings of aphasic individuals who exhibited typical behavioral patterns.[75] This type of investigation has several obvious disadvantages, not the least of which is the fact that long periods of time often elapsed between onset of the disorder and the postmortem examination. With the onset of computerized tomography of the brain, a noninvasive procedure that allows for neurologic localization at any time after onset, various research projects have been reported.[1, 42] Kertesz et al.,[45] in a "blind" research design, compared localization results obtained from CT scans with classifications derived from clinical testing. Results indicate that there are

. . . distinct areas of Broca's, conduction and Wernicke's aphasia along the parasylvian axis of the lateral templates. Lesions of global aphasics covered all of these areas, while transcorticals were outside of them. Lesion size and severity of aphasia showed significant correlations.

Mohr et al.[55] used autopsy reports, arteriograms, and CT scans to compare anatomic and clinical findings of Broca's aphasia. They found that when damage was limited to Broca's area, the clinical symptoms were not those of Broca's aphasia but rather were characterized by mutism replaced by a rapidly improving dyspraxia and effortful articulation. Further, the speech disorder clinically labeled "Broca's aphasia" results from damage extending outside the Broca area.

Localization of language function in the left hemisphere has also been explored via cortical mapping of neurosurgical patients undergoing resection for medically intractable focal epilepsy.[59] During these experiments, weak electric currents were applied to the cortex during a naming task. In a study of 11 patients, results indicated that the extent of the language cortex in an individual can be wider than that traditionally proposed. Only a narrow band of posterior inferior frontal lobe, immediately anterior to the motor strip, showed involvement in all patients. Within the larger language areas, language is discretely localized, with different sites variably committed to the naming function.

In addition to the study of left hemisphere and its language functions, there is a growing interest in the roles played by both the right hemisphere and the thalamic system. Searleman,[72] in his 1977 review of the linguistic functions of the right hemisphere, cited evidence from patients with (1) aphasia secondary to unilateral left hemisphere damage, (2) hemispherectomy, and (3) commissurotomy. Review of this literature leads to the conclusion that the right hemisphere possesses a far greater capacity to comprehend than to produce speech and language. However, Levine and Mohr[49] concluded from a study of the language of individuals with bilateral cerebral infarctions that the right hemisphere may also have some role in normal articulation.

The role of the thalamic system in language has been investigated by the study of spontaneous and stereotaxic lesions and with stimulation of the thalamus and adjacent structures.[58] Results of this work indicate that the dominant lateral thalamus plays a role in naming activities, and disruption in this area results in anomia and perseveration but intact comprehension.

Assessment

Extensive and systematic language assessment can serve a variety of purposes. One of the primary goals of assessment is to arrive at a differential diagnosis of the type of aphasia. In order to do this, systematic samples of a variety of language tasks, including speaking, listening, reading, and writing, must be obtained. This allows the clinician to identify the pattern of deficits in order to differentiate aphasia from other neurogenic communication disorders or to classify subtypes of aphasia.

A second major purpose for assessment of aphasia is to measure the severity of the disorder. The broad classification of aphasia is not sufficient to describe fully the language capabilities of an aphasic individual. Because a wide range of severity levels are possible, some measure of the degree of processing deficits is also necessary. In the area of auditory comprehension, the most severe deficits may be characterized by an inability to understand any verbal message. With less severe deficits, the patient may be able to comprehend single words or single-stage directions and to respond to brief yes/no questions. In the mild range of impairment, an aphasic patient may be able to understand ordinary conversations with only occasional repetition. In the area of verbal output, a patient with severe deficits may not speak or may produce only jargon. With less severe deficits, the patient may produce automatic phrases or name simple objects and actions. In the mild range of impairment, the patient may convey information slowly with some word-finding, grammatical, or articulatory problems. Reading and writing disorders range in severity from inability to read or write single words to slowness in handling adult level material.

The third major function of assessment is to establish a prognosis for recovery of language skills. Both severity and type of aphasia have important prognostic implications. Kertesz et al.,[44] in a long-term follow-up study, found that global aphasic patients frequently exhibited good recovery. Severity of the overall impairment at one, three, and six months after onset can also be used to predict performance at points later in the recovery.[61] For those patients with severe language deficits, recovery is not expected to be as great as for those with moderate or mild deficits. For the severely aphasic patient, changes that occur in communication performance, as measured by standardized tests, may not be reflected in increasing ability to perform functionally in other communication situations. This point can be illustrated with the example of a severely aphasic speaker who may show improvement in test performance on the easier tasks, such as matching identical objects or matching a picture of an object with the actual object. The recovery, however, will probably not make a significant change in the patient's ability to handle ordinary communication situations.

The fourth major function served by the assessment process is the identification of realistic treatment goals and appropriate treatment tasks. Selection of appropriate treatment tasks involves identification of tasks that have functional relevance and are at an appropriate level of difficulty. The difficulty level varies from patient to patient and is defined by that individual's unique skills and needs. Generally, a level is selected at which the patient is able to achieve a high success rate. With a success rate of approximately 80 per cent, the patient does not experience excessive frustration, yet errors are frequent enough that the patient is continually forced to actively process the stimulus and monitor the response for possible errors. Because standardized aphasia tests typically sample many tasks, they allow the clinician to select tasks at the appropriate difficulty levels for each of the language areas. Routine administration of standardized tests allows for the monitoring of performance. Decisions to continue or terminate treatment often are based on this information.

The standardized tests commonly used by speech/language pathologists to evaluate language disturbances in adult brain-injured individuals are listed below with a brief description of each.

Minnesota Test for Differential Diagnosis of Aphasia.[70] This test includes 47 different subtests that focus on five disorder areas, including (1) auditory disturbances, (2) visual and reading disturbances, (3) speech and language disturbances, (4) visual, motor, and writing disturbances, and (5) disturbances of numerical relationships and arithmetic processes. The responses are scored as either correct or incorrect.

Boston Diagnostic Aphasia Examination.[27] This test evaluates auditory comprehension, oral expression, understanding of written language, and writing. Responses are scored either in a plus-minus fashion, on a rating scale, or with longhand notation, depending on the subtest. Test results are arranged on a profile of speech characteristics according to subtest scores. These profiles are particularly useful in classifying patients into the various subtypes of aphasia.

Porch Index of Communicative Ability.[60] This test contains 18 10-item subtests measuring communicative behavior in the gestural, verbal, and graphic output modalities. Responses are scored according to a 16-point multidimensional system based on accuracy, responsiveness, completeness, and promptness. Because of the multidimensional scoring and standardized administration techniques, special training is required in administering and interpreting this test. Results are reported in percentiles comparing the patient's performance with a large group of left hemisphere–damaged individuals. This test can be readministered on a monthly basis and can be used to establish a prognosis and to assess therapeutic progress.

Western Aphasia Battery.[46, 74] This test is sensitive to fluency, information content, comprehension, repetition, and naming ability. Responses are scored on a 1 to 10 or 1 to 100 point scale depending on the subtest. Patterns of performance among the subtests categorize the patient according to the type of aphasia.

Token Test.[21] This is not a comprehensive test but focuses on auditory comprehension skills. The test contains 20 unique tokens of various sizes, shapes, and colors. The patient is asked to follow 36 orally presented commands at various difficulty levels. This test is particularly sensitive to mild auditory comprehension deficits. Cut-off scores separate "normal" from "aphasic" performance. Scores can be adjusted for educational level.

The Functional Communication Profile.[67] This profile consists of 45 communication behaviors that are rated on a nine-point scale. Behaviors are divided into five major groups: movement (gesture), speaking, understanding, reading, and other (handling money, etc.). Data are collected in an interview format.

Communicative Abilities in Daily Living.[36] This test consists of 68 items incorporating everyday language activities presented in a natural style to approximate normal communication. Responses are scored on a 3-point scoring system — wrong, adequate, or correct. Results yield information about the functional communications skills of aphasic patients.

Treatment Goals

The speech/language pathologist's major goal is to establish the most effective means of communication by which aphasic individuals relate meaningfully to those around them. Treatment goals for aphasic patients depend on the nature and severity of the language disorder. For example, goals for a patient with aphasia characterized by severe comprehension deficits and speech consisting largely of jargon are quite different from goals for a patient with fair comprehension and limited but appropriate speech. The following treatment approaches reflect a variety of techniques utilized by speech/language pathologists in dealing with aphasic individuals at different severity levels.

For severely involved patients, direct speech treatment involving drill and repetitive practice is usually not appropriate for several reasons. Tasks easy enough to insure some success may not be functionally relevant. For example, a person's ability to match identical objects does not translate into "real-life" communication skills. For this reason tasks at the appropriate difficulty level for the severely aphasic patient are often not tolerated by the patient. Little direct treatment is employed. However, a good deal of time is devoted to managing the patient's communication environment by counseling his family and training them in techniques to optimize communication potential. The direct treatment of the severely involved aphasic patient may be limited to construction of an individualized "communication book" that includes photographs of the patient's family along with those who are currently providing care for him. Photographs illustrating needs, activities, and locations may also be incorporated. Experience has shown that severely involved aphasic patients tend to respond better to photographs, which are more concrete than symbolic line drawings. The aphasic patient can point to the communication book to indicate specific needs or a general topic. If necessary, the communication partner can obtain more specific information by asking a series of questions. Often patients and their communication partners need training in order to use such a system.

With aphasic individuals in the moderately severe to mild range, more direct speech treatment can be carried out and a variety of approaches can be taken. The *stimulation approach*[71] stresses the repetitive presentation of stimuli designed to increase the patient's ability to organize, store, and retrieve language patterns formerly used. The speech/language pathologist functions not as a teacher but as a stimulator. This approach is based on the notion that the aphasic patient has not lost words but has lost the ability to retrieve, select, and sequence them. Stimuli of sufficient intensity are used so that responses are elicited, not forced. For example, rather than using a difficult confrontation naming task ("Tell me the name of the object.") with a patient who is experiencing word-finding difficulties, a sentence completion task ("You drink coffee out of a _____.") may be more appropriate.

Another widely used approach to direct treatment of moderately aphasic individuals is the *programmed approach*.[35] This approach centers on the application of learning principles, particularly those of shaping and differential reinforcement, to prompt reacquisition of language behavior. This approach is based on principles of programmed learning in which stimuli are controlled as the patient works at a high success rate. As the patient improves, tasks are gradually made more difficult.

With mildly aphasic patients, the speech/language pathologist must consider a new set of treatment strategies. The *context-cen-*

tered approach,[85] although not restricted exclusively to mild aphasia, is particularly useful with this group of patients. This approach de-emphasizes direct language treatment and moves away from the search for specific words into the realm of ideas and thoughts. This technique is often used with high-level aphasics, who are encouraged to embellish and enrich content and move from concrete to more abstract and complete communication.

With the mildly aphasic patient, emphasis is placed on identification and remediation of specific vocational problems that might arise as a result of the communication disorder. Often mildly aphasic individuals are taught compensatory strategies to handle difficult communication tasks. For example, a mildly aphasic patient may be taught to create a detailed outline of business correspondence before actually writing a letter. The outline may contain not only a series of points that the writer wishes to make but also a system for logically organizing and sequencing them. The mildly aphasic speaker is often taught to make his communication partners aware of potential communication breakdowns. Mild language deficits may not be readily apparent yet may cause the speaker a good deal of frustration.

Efficacy of Treatment

With any ongoing treatment program, regardless of severity or type of aphasia, the speech/language pathologist must be able to document the effectiveness of therapeutic intervention. Progress can be measured by re-administering standardized tests and comparing current results with those of earlier testing sessions. The *Porch Index of Communicative Ability*[60] is particularly sensitive to small changes in performance. This test not only gives an overall indication of change but also allows the clinician to identify changes in specific language areas such as verbal output, auditory comprehension, and graphic skills. Another way of monitoring progress is by maintaining careful records of scores on treatment tasks. In this way, the speech/language pathologist can identify trends in performance and document changing skills. Regardless of how it is obtained, a measure of progress is needed to justify continued speech treatment.

In addition to documenting changes in individual aphasic patients as treatment progresses and as recovery occurs, the question of efficacy of treatment has also been studied by examining changes in groups of treated and untreated patients. In this way, the issue of the contribution of spontaneous recovery to changing performance can be addressed. Darley[16] discussed a variety of research design problems, including the need to match groups in terms of age, etiology, site of lesion, initial severity, etc. Despite these methodological problems, the literature contains several examples of group design efficacy studies. Basso et al.[2] studied the influence of language rehabilitation on 281 aphasic patients (162 treated and 119 untreated). They wrote that "... rehabilitation had a significant positive effect on improvement in all language skills" (p. 195). Hagen[29] studied a group of 20 men with aphasia and found that several parameters changed more in treated than in untreated groups, including functional reading comprehension, language formulation, speech production, spelling, and arithmetic abilities. Vignolo[82] found that consistent improvement was noted if treatment was started between two and six months after onset and lasted longer than six months. Sarno et al.[68] found that several different methods of treatment of global aphasics did not result in functional speech. Although this study has been widely quoted as evidence that aphasia treatment is not efficacious, the authors are careful to state that this study relates only to severely aphasic speakers and that their auditory comprehension improved but functional speech did not.

APRAXIA OF SPEECH

Apraxia of speech is a sensorimotor disorder of articulation and prosody that frequently accompanies nonfluent aphasia and may also co-exist with dysarthria.[63] Some writers disagree with the use of the term *apraxia*, feeling that the disorder is too closely associated to aphasia to be considered a separate entity.[51] However, because apraxia of speech includes some characteristics that distinguish it from other neurogenic language and speech disorders and because the treatment strategies typically employed are unique, apraxia of speech will be considered as a separate disorder. Apraxia of speech occurs in the absence of significant weakness or incoordination when performing reflexive or automatic movements.[20] It is characterized by impaired ability to program the positioning of the speech musculature and to sequence the movements for volitional production of speech.

Assessment. Because apraxia almost always appears concomitantly with aphasia, the speech/language pathologist will routinely administer standardized aphasia tests. With the apraxic speaker, these test results will usually indicate relatively intact auditory and reading comprehension skills. Writing skills are better than speaking skills. In addition to these findings, the pattern of articulatory breakdown in apraxia is characteristic.[41] Articulatory errors include omissions, substitutions, distortions, additions, and repetition of speech sounds. Many of these errors appear to be off-target approximations made in an effortful manner. Apraxic speakers often appear to be groping for the proper articulatory position or sequence of positions. Errors are highly inconsistent, varying with the complexity of the sound patterns and length of the target words. There is a discrepancy between the accuracy of automatic-reactive speech and inaccuracy of volitional-purposeful speech. The speaker is often aware of errors but is usually unable to anticipate or correct them. If the patient attempts to monitor his speech, anticipation of errors often leads to a slowed rate and even stress and pacing.

Treatment. Treatment of apraxia of speech typically involves highly structured, controlled, and intensive practice of sound patterns and speech. Rosenbek et al.[65] suggest the use of an eight-step task continuum ranging from maximum cueing (simultaneous production with the clinician after having heard and seen the phrase being produced) to eliciting responses in a role-playing situation.

Another approach often used with nonfluent aphasics who exhibit apraxia is *melodic intonation therapy.*[77] This is a four-level program in which natural melody patterns are used to facilitate speech. Phrases are accompanied by exaggerated natural melody and rhythm patterns. As the patient progresses through the program, the melody and rhythm cues are gradually faded. Candidates for this treatment procedure have good auditory comprehension and good error recognition in the presence of severe articulatory deficits and poor ability to repeat.

DYSARTHRIA

Dysarthria is a term that refers to a group of speech disorders resulting from a disturbance of motor control—weakness, slowness, or incoordination — of the speech mechanism due to damage to the central or peripheral nervous system.[19] Dysarthric speakers usually have normal auditory comprehension and can select words correctly and order them in grammatical strings without difficulty. However, they experience difficulty saying words and sounds precisely with appropriate stress, loudness, and pitch control.

The pattern of speech characteristics produced by a specific dysarthric individual depends upon the site of neurologic lesion and the severity of speech impairment.[19]

Flaccid Dysarthria. Damage to the nerves (or their nuclei) will result in speech characterized by breathy voice, hypernasality, imprecisely produced consonants, reduced speech loudness, and air escape through the nose (nasal emission). Flaccid dysarthria occurs in patients with a low brain stem stroke, polio, or myesthenia gravis.

Spastic Dysarthria. If the site of neurologic lesion involves the upper motor neurons, a spastic condition may result in a speech pattern characterized by imprecise consonant production, monopitch, a strained-strangled voice quality, hypernasality, and occasional pitch breaks. Spastic dysarthric patterns are observed with spastic cerebral palsy and pseudobulbar palsy. Patients with amyotrophic lateral sclerosis will often exhibit a combination of flaccid and spastic dysarthria.

Ataxic Dysarthria. Patients with cerebellar disorders produce a characteristic speech pattern that includes irregular breakdowns and distortions of speech articulation. Prosodic patterns are unusual, in that some patients stress nearly all syllables equally, while others stress words and syllables inappropriately. These dysarthric speakers usually exhibit irregular, imprecise consonant production, distorted vowel production, excessive loudness variation, and occasional harsh voice. Ataxic dysarthria is found in patients with Friedreich's ataxia, some patients with multiple sclerosis, and some patients with severe head injury.

Hypokinetic Dysarthria. Patients with movement disorders also demonstrate unique dysarthric patterns. Parkinsonism is a neurologic disorder of the basal ganglia, and the movements of these speakers are often reduced in rate. Hypokinetic dysarthric individuals usually speak with monopitch, reduced speech stress, short rushes of speech, inappropriate silences, and reduced speech loudness.

Hyperkinetic Dysarthria. Patients with movement disorders resulting in excessive motor activity, such as dystonia and chorea, exhibit hyperkinetic dysarthria. In dystonia the dyskinesia is characterized by muscle contractions building slowly, distorting posture, and subsiding gradually. The dysarthric pattern includes imprecise consonant production, prolonged and distorted vowels, harsh voice, irregular articulation breakdowns, excessive loudness variations, and voice stoppages. Chorea, on the other hand, results in quick hyperkinesis with irregular, random, and unpatterned movements. Speech symptoms include imprecise speech articulation, speech sounds that are abnormally prolonged, variable speaking rate, and harsh voice.

Mixed Dysarthria. While dysarthric speech patterns associated with various lesion sites are distinctive, patients with extensive neurologic involvement due to multiple sclerosis, amyotrophic lateral sclerosis, or brain trauma exhibit a mixed dysarthria with components of different dysarthric types.

Assessment

Assessment of dysarthric speech has taken a variety of forms, including perceptual, component, and overall assessment of speech performance. Each of these approaches provides unique information.

In *perceptual assessment,* Darley et al.[17, 18] rated dysarthric speech along 38 dimensions. Many of these perceptual dimensions were specific to one aspect of speech; for example, imprecise consonants, irregular articulatory breakdowns, and distorted vowels are all closely related to articulation. Other dimensions were more general — for example, intelligibility, bizarreness, and reduced stress. Results of this research revealed that clusters of deviant speech dimensions were associated with specific neurologic disorders. This descriptive, perceptually based tool allows the speech/language pathologist to distinguish the various dysarthrias on the basis of a series of speech dimensions.

In *component assessment,* Rosenbek and LaPointe[64] took a somewhat different approach in their discussion of evaluation. They suggested a model based on the speech physiology work of Netsell.[57] The components of the patients' speech mechanism are systematically evaluated by determining the type of locus of breakdowns at points along the vocal tract where speech activities occur. For example, some speakers demonstrate their neuromotor deficits by failing to shorten the inhalation phase and lengthen the exhalation phase of respiration during speech. Others are unable to maintain relatively stable subglottal air pressure, and the loudness of their speech is abnormally variable or tends to decay toward the end of an utterance. Still others are unable to generate levels of subglottal air pressure (5 to 10 cm H_2O) needed to speak with appropriate loudness. Impairment of phonation may result in aphonia (absence of sound), dysphonia (distortions of sound quality), or disorders of pitch and loudness control. Neurogenic articulatory disorders may result in the inability to accurately achieve the movement patterns associated with target postures of various sounds. Imprecise sound production, substitution of one sound for another, or complete omission of sounds may result. If velopharyngeal mechanism control is deficient, hypernasality and nasal emission (air escape through the nose) will be present. Rosenbek and LaPointe[64] use the evaluation process to focus treatment. Abnormal function of speech mechanism components is identified so that treatment can be organized into a hierarchy based on the contribution of various symptoms to reduced intelligibility.

In *overall assessment,* a third approach to dysarthric speech evaluation focuses on overall indicators of dysarthric speech performance. Reduced intelligibility provides an overall index of the speech disorder that takes into account many different neuromuscular factors along with whatever compensatory strategies the dysarthric speaker may have adapted.[88, 89] Intelligibility also is closely associated with other functional measures of communication, such as the amount of information transferred.[7]

Treatment

The treatment hierarchy for dysarthric speakers who are recovering from a neurologic impairment secondary to stroke, trauma, or surgery includes the following goals and procedures depending upon severity level. Initially, an early communication system is developed for the patient who is unable to speak functionally. Communication augmentation systems for these severely dysarthric individuals will be discussed later in this chapter.

If a severely dysarthric speaker shows the potential for verbal communication, it is necessary to develop the motor skills involved in functional speech. This phase of treatment includes muscle strengthening and control exercises necessary for the production of single sounds. Next, the transition of speech mechanism movement from the target position for one sound to another sound is developed. All through this phase of the dysarthria treatment program, it is important that the speaker produce sounds that can be distinguished from one another by the listener. The next goal in treatment is to have the dysarthric speaker make the transition from producing single words and phrases in the treatment session to functional use of speech for communication for his daily needs. The authors commonly have their patients achieve this transition by teaching the dysarthric individuals to point to the first letter of each word on an alphabet board as they speak.[6] In this way listeners are provided with additional information about the word that the dysarthric speaker is attempting to say. The use of this technique has allowed many dysarthric persons to begin to communicate verbally long before their speech intelligibility level without assistance would have permitted.

After the dysarthric person develops functional verbal communication supplemented by the alphabet board, the focus of treatment shifts to maximizing the intelligibility of speech. This involves training in specific skills and/or prosthetic management. In an attempt to improve speech intelligibility, patients are taught to modify speaking rate, emphasize consonant sounds in important words, control the number of words per breath, and stress important words. Some patients need to be fitted with palatal lifts to reduce hypernasality and nasal emission.[25] The palatal lift consists of a dental retainer that is secured to the teeth (Fig. 5–1). A shelf attached to the retainer elevates the soft palate to the height necessary to reduce abnormal speech characteristics.

Once the recovering dysarthric speaker is intelligible, the last step in the treatment program is to reduce the bizarreness of speech. This is accomplished by teaching appropriate stress, loudness, and pitch patterns with consistently accurate articulation at a rate that allows intelligible speech.

The treatment hierarchy for dysarthria secondary to progressive diseases and conditions such as Parkinson's disease, multiple sclerosis, and amyotrophic lateral sclerosis is obviously different from that for the recovering dysarthric individual. Initially, the pa-

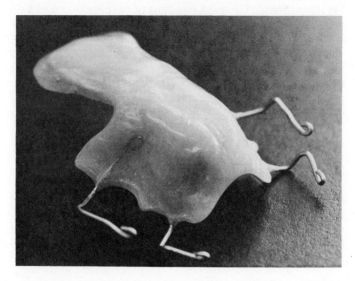

FIGURE 5–1. Photograph of a palatal lift.

tients are encouraged to maximize the functional communication level by paying special attention to the clarity and precision of their speech. At some point, the patients will need to modify their speaking patterns by controlling rate, consonant emphasis, and number of words per breath. Some patients with progressive dysarthria make the adjustments in their speech pattern without specific treatment; others may need to practice these modifications with a speech/language pathologist or trained family member before the changes become habitual. In severe cases communication augmentation systems may need to be considered. These systems are usually chosen or designed to accommodate most easily to the life style of the patient while serving his communicative needs over the longest period of time.

Cerebral Palsy

The neuromotor speech disorder of cerebral palsy places these individuals under the general "dysarthria" label. Owing to the early childhood onset of the defect and depending upon the extent and type of neuromuscular involvement and associated disorders, the communication problems of cerebral palsied individuals may involve language and hearing as well as speech. McDonald and Chance,[52] in a summary description of cerebral palsied children, reported that 25 per cent are normal and above normal in intelligence, 30 per cent are slightly retarded, and 45 per cent are moderately or severely retarded. He also reports that between 10 and 30 per cent of these children have hearing impairment. Up to 35 per cent of cerebral palsied children are reported to have visual disorders other than refractive errors.[40] These factors, combined with reduced ability to move about physically and experience the environment, contribute to language development delays in many cerebral palsied children.

The management of the communication and related disorders of cerebral palsied individuals is a multidisciplinary activity. Usually communication development occurs concurrently with programs to develop swallowing, motor control, and socialization. The description of a complex, coordinated, integrated treatment program is clearly beyond the scope of this chapter and is presented elsewhere.[52, 56, 86]

READING DISORDERS IN NEUROLOGICALLY IMPAIRED ADULTS

The following discussion focuses on adult-onset neurogenic reading deficits, which will be discussed in three broad categories.

The first category includes reading disorders associated with aphasia. Since aphasia is defined as a language deficit that crosses all communication modalities, aphasic individuals will typically experience difficulty with both oral and silent reading. These deficits are usually associated with left hemisphere lesions and are more prominent with posterior than with anterior lesions. Severity can range from the inability to recognize simple words to mild reduction in speech clarity and in the efficiency with which adult-level material is read.

The second category includes reading disorders associated with perceptual problems. These reading deficits are typically associated with right hemisphere lesions and may be accompanied by left-sided neglect and/or visual field cuts. Individuals with perceptual problems will (1) experience difficulty scanning the line of print, (2) fail to return to the left margin of the page, and (3) skip lines of print. Reading rate is often significantly reduced, at times to the point where the individual is unable to understand the material. Difficulties are exaggerated when print size is reduced.

The third category includes reading disorders associated with confused language. Confused language has been characterized by Halpern et al.[30] as the reduced recognition and understanding of and responsiveness to the environment faulty short-term memory, mistaken reasoning, and disorientation in time and place. Reading deficits are often characterized by severely reduced comprehension in the face of relatively intact oral reading.

Assessment. When specific reading deficits are suspected, such as language-based (aphasias) or perceptually based problems, a variety of standardized and/or informal assessment techniques are available. Many standard aphasia test batteries sample reading performance with a variety of tasks that are graded in difficulty. For example, the *Minnesota Test for Differential Diagnosis of Aphasia*[70] contains a series of reading tasks ranging from matching shapes to the reading of paragraph-length passages. LaPointe and Horner[47] have developed a reading battery entitled *Reading Comprehension Battery for Aphasia,* specifically designed to assess and monitor recovery of reading abilities in aphasic individuals. Perceptual deficits may be assessed using a series of written passages graded in perceptual difficulty. This series may range from large print and color-cued margins to standard newspaper print with multiple columns. Performance can be assessed by noting the number of tracking or scanning errors and reading rate as the patient reads the passage orally.

When the clinician is concerned with the extent to which reading deficits interfere with ordinary activities of living, a variety of functional tasks can be tested. A list of functional reading activities might include medicine bottle labels and bus and television schedules. These tasks are typically selected for patients on an individual basis depending on their communication needs. When considering the potential for return to educational or vocational settings, one should compare the reading performance of individuals with relatively mild reading deficits with that of the normal population. Standardized tests that have been normalized on high-school and/or college students can be used for this purpose.

Treatment. With neurogenic reading disorders, treatment varies with the type of disorder. Reading deficits seen in aphasic patients are typically addressed as part of the normal course of treatment. Reading tasks can be ordered into a hierarchy of difficulty based on language-related variables, including word frequency and grammatical complexity. As the patient improves, treatment progressively focuses on more difficult tasks.

Like the treatment of language-based reading deficits, the treatment of perceptually based deficits progresses through the hierarchy of tasks. Tasks can be ordered in terms of perceptual difficulty from easy tasks (large print, colored margins, markers to underscore lines of print) to more difficult tasks (small print, multiple columns, hyphenated words). The research of Weinberg et al.[84] indicates that this approach to remediating visual scanning difficulties is effective.

Reading treatment for severely confused patients is not typically undertaken for a variety of reasons. First, the combination of decreased error recognition and memory makes these patients poor treatment candidates. Second, traumatically caused confusion often clears during the initial phases of recovery. At the point in recovery when the confusion seems to have cleared, treatment of specific language or perceptually based reading deficits can be completed.

CONFUSED LANGUAGE

Confused language is an impairment associated with the neurologic condition of confusion and characterized by reduced recognition, understanding of, and responsiveness to the environment.[30] Other sequelae of the disorder include disorientation to time and place, short-term memory loss, difficulty "tuning in" to novel tasks, impaired comprehension, rambling and incoherent speech, and inability to function on an abstract level. Confused language is often associated with the acute stages of a disease process or the period of time immediately following head trauma. When traumatically induced, lesions are usually either multifocal or mixed focal and diffuse. Confused language may also be a chronic condition secondary to arteriosclerosis or organic brain syndrome.

Assessment. In their initial evaluation, speech/language pathologists are often called upon to distinguish between aphasia and confused language. This distinction is particularly important, since the treatment approaches and management strategies are quite different for these disorders. Chief among these differences is the fact that confused language is part of a generalized disorder, whereas aphasia is specifically a language disorder. Typically the person with confused language will also exhibit confusion in nonlanguage areas. The aphasic patient, on the other hand, will have difficulty only with tasks that require him to use language processes or symbol systems.

In addition to disorders in non–language-related activities, the confused patient will typically exhibit a unique pattern of language deficits that can be identified by administering one of the standard aphasia assessment tests. The pattern of language deficits seen in confusion is different from any of the deficit patterns found in the subclassifications of aphasia. Halpern et al.,[30] in their comparison of aphasic patients with those who exhibit confused language, identified several characteristics. One of the most predominant characteristics was the lack of relevancy in the responses of confused patients. Verbal responses of the confused patient are often rambling, bizarre, and not related to the task. For example, one former seamstress, when asked to name a toothbrush, called it a "pastel material clipper." Her responses were not only irrelevant but also tended to follow a theme centered on her former occupation. She also exhibited an almost total lack of awareness of her errors. The reading deficits exhibited by confused patients are also quite different from those exhibited by aphasic patients. Patients with confused language are often able to orally read single words or even paragraphs. Although they may confabulate and add occasional irrelevant words, their oral reading is not typically marked by articulatory or word recognition errors. However, comprehension of material read is severely limited, often to the point where the confused patient will not be able to match single words with the appropriate picture. Reading comprehension of the aphasic patient, on the other hand, is typically not more impaired than oral reading. Confused patients often tend to have writing deficits that mirror the irrelevant and rambling characteristics of their verbal output.

Wertz[86] suggested that the most useful tasks in diagnosing confused language are those that give the patient enough "room" to show his disorientation and tendency to confabulate, for example, questions that elicit biographical information. Darley[15] reports that if the answers to all of the following questions are "no," then the diagnosis of confused language is highly probable. Is the patient oriented in terms of space and time? Does the patient stay in contact with the examiner? Is the patient aware of his inappropriate responses? Does the patient demonstrate vocabulary and syntax problems?

Treatment. The speech/language pathologist's role in the management of patients with confused language typically does not involve direct treatment of the language disorder. Rather, the speech/language pathologist will offer suggestions to assist in communication management of these patients. Such suggestions may include structuring the environment to be as relaxed and calm as possible. A routine of daily activities should be structured so that the same activity is carried out at the same time and, if possible, by the same people each day. Correct orientation may be encouraged by often reminding the patient of name, date, and location.[23] Rehabilitation staff, family, and friends should be encouraged always to have the patient's attention before initiating communication. They should ask simple and direct questions, allowing the patient time to process the information. Often the patient will be unable to stop talking and will ramble from the original subject. When this occurs, staff should be encouraged to interrupt the behavior and ask a question that will bring the patient back to the original subject. When reading comprehension skills are sufficient, memory aids may be used to improve orientation. These notebooks may contain a schedule of daily events, a calendar, names of the people involved in the patient's care, and a record of special events that have happened or are anticipated in the near future. Confused patients should also be routinely supplied with large wall calendars and clocks to facilitate orientation.[8] The role of the speech pathologist in the management of traumatically head-injured patients may include some direct training. The goal of this training is reorganization of cognitive function, including increasing the patient's attention span and sequencing ability and training him in the use of memory aids.

OTHER PHYSICALLY BASED SPEECH DISORDERS

Voice Disorders

Phonation is a complex neuromotor activity; therefore, disorders of phonation may take several forms. *Aphonia* refers to an absence of phonation due either to hysterical problems or to central or peripheral neurologic problems interfering with the approximation of the vocal folds. *Dysphonia* refers to a number of phonatory disorders of sound quality that have a variety of etiologies. *Vocal nodules* are a callous formation at the anterior to middle third of the vocal folds. *Laryngitis* is an inflammation of the vocal folds, while *vocal polyps* are enlarged structures around a small blood vessel. *Contact ulcers* are an ulceration of the vocal folds on the free approximating margins of the vocal processes. Dysphonia may also result from forms of vocal fold paralysis or cancer of the larynx. In addition to dysfunction of the true vocal folds, adduction of the ventricular or false vocal folds during speech may occur as part of a disordered phonatory pattern. *Spasmodic dysphonia* refers to an intermittent strained, harsh voice with voice stoppage.

The primary objectives of the voice evaluation are (1) a detailed history of the phonatory problem, (2) a physical evaluation of the laryngeal structures by a laryngologist, (3) a description of current phonatory function, (4) identification of use and abuse patterns that are contributing to the disorder, and (5) determination of the patient's potential ability to modify phonatory patterns.

If the phonatory problem does not require medical treatment, a careful description of phonatory function includes an evaluation of pitch, quality, and loudness control. At times there is an interaction among these three parameters. For example, phonatory quality of some patients is dependent upon the pitch range at which they are speaking. If the pitch is too low, the phonatory quality may be excessively harsh. The interaction between the phonatory and respiratory systems is also important. Although no particular pattern of breathing has been shown to be the best, clavicular respiratory patterns with excessive movement of the thorax and reduced diaphragmatic/abdominal activity during breathing are not conducive to clear, flexible, strong phonation.

The speech treatment of noncancerous, nonparalytic voice problems usually involves several steps. First, an active program to minimize vocal abuse and at least temporarily decrease vocal use is initiated. Vocal abuse patterns of concern are smoking, excessive coughing and throat clearing, and talking or shouting over crowd or machine noise. Second, optimal pitch and loudness ranges for efficient phonatory production are selected. Third, the focus of sound resonance is shifted anteriorly from the pharyngeal to the oral and nasal areas through the alteration of tongue position during speech and ear training so that the speaker recognizes the more appropriate pattern. Fourth, hard vocal fold approximations are replaced with easy, gentle approximations. Fifth, if present, abnormal respiratory patterns are modified.

Motor paralysis of the vocal folds can be unilateral or bilateral and may leave the folds in the adducted position or in several stages of abduction. A complete discussion of the etiologies of the various patterns of paralysis can be found in Hart[31] and in Luchsinger and Arnold.[50] In case of complete abductor paralysis (folds in adducted position), the patient usually requires a tracheostomy initially to maintain a functional airway. Phonation may be achieved by plugging the tracheostomy tube with a finger and exhaling for speech. Eventually one of the folds may be surgically repositioned laterally in a somewhat abducted position to establish an airway. However, this surgery results in phonatory quality that is breathy and reduced in intensity. Recently, attempts to reinnervate the abductor muscle with a muscle pedicle transplant have shown some promise in restoring an airway and maintaining quality phonation in patients with abductor paralysis.[78] In the case of adductor paralysis (folds in abducted positions), several surgical procedures may be employed, including surgically repositioning of a fold medially or implanting or injecting material into the fold to displace it toward the midline. Speech treatment for patients with motor paralysis of the vocal folds usually occurs in conjunction with the medical management program. The goal is to assist these patients to develop the most functional voice possible given the physical condition of the laryngeal mechanism.

Laryngeal cancer may initially be reflected in a phonatory disorder. The term *laryngectomy* refers to the partial or total removal of the larynx. An incomplete laryngectomy may or may not influence voice quality, depending upon whether or not vocal fold tissue has been removed. The total laryngectomy results in complete loss of voice and most audible aspects of whisper. Depending upon the type and extent of total laryngectomy surgery, three different speaking options may be available to the laryngectomee. First, a pseudoglottis or shunt constructed of human tissue or prosthetic material allows air to pass from the trachea into the esophagus, and sound is produced by vibrating esophageal tissue. Second, in laryngectomees without a shunt, esophageal voice is produced by vibration of the upper narrow portion of the esophagus when air is injected into the esophagus and released. Third, a neck type or intraoral type of electrolarynx serves as a sound source and the laryngectomee "mouths" his messages. Nearly all laryngectomees can learn to use some form of electrolarynx. For a detailed discussion of management of laryngeal cancer and related communication issues, the interested reader is referred to Diedrich and Youngstrom[22] and Keith and Darley.[43]

Cleft Palate

The congenital orofacial deformity of cleft palate with or without cleft lip occurs in approximately 1 of 600 to 900 Caucasian births and 1 of 1500 to 2000 black births in the United States.[53] Cleft patterns for the individual children may involve the primary palate (lip and premaxillary or alveolar process anterior to the incisive foramen), the secondary palate, or both the primary and secondary palates.[5] Clefts may be unilateral or bilateral, as well as incomplete or complete.

Surgical repair of cleft lip and palate is usually staged as follows. Labial clefts are typically closed first, often within the first month of life. Primary surgical repair of the palate is completed later, with the timing dependent on the philosophy of the cleft palate management team. Prior to surgical repair of the palate, orthodontic appliances often are fitted to maintain or restore the contour of the maxillary arch and to occlude, at least partially, the cleft of the hard palate.

Some individuals with cleft palate remain velopharyngeally incompetent, unable to occlude the port between the oral and nasal cavity. Velopharyngeal incompetence following palatal surgery might be managed in one of several ways. An obturator may be fitted to occlude the velopharyngeal port. Secondary surgery might involve a "pushback" procedure with or without a pharyngeal flap attached to the soft palate. Detailed discussions of primary and secondary procedures can be found in Cooper et al.[13] and Grabb et al.[28]

Speech disorders may result from several factors related to orofacial deformity. Velopharyngeal incompetence results in the escape of air through the nasal cavity (nasal emission) during the production of sounds requiring the impounding of intraoral air pressure (e.g., s, p, b, f, v). Hypernasality during consonant sound production also results from velopharyngeal incompetence.

Dental and occlusal abnormalities may hinder the development of normal articulation by the child with cleft palate. Children with cleft palate have demonstrated a more frequent than average occurrence of mild to moderate conductive hearing impairment. This hearing impairment may contribute to delays in language and speech development in some children.

The communication management of the child with cleft palate focuses on the areas of hearing, language, and speech. Owing to increased occurrence of hearing loss in children with cleft palate as compared to normal children, regular hearing assessments are scheduled. Depending upon the outcome of the dental, orthodontic, and surgical management to achieve velopharyngeal competence and maxillary/mandibular arch alignment, the speech problems vary from child to child. Thorough speech evaluations are required to determine the error patterns and plan instruction programs appropriate to the individual. Because language development delays might occur in children with cleft palate, their language skills regularly should be assessed and additional instruction provided when delays are found.

COMMUNICATION AUGMENTATION SYSTEMS

The term *communication augmentation system* refers to any device or system designed to support, enhance, or augment the communication of individuals who are not independent verbal communicators in all situations. As the result of cerebral palsy, brain trauma, cerebral circulation disorders, degenerative neurologic diseases, severe hearing loss, or severe learning or developmental disorders, some individuals are speechless while others can be understood only by persons very familiar with them. In the past 10 years an increasing number of systems for augmenting communication have been developed. Some systems include electronic or mechanical aids, while others such as hand signing or gesturing do not.

Communication aids usually are composed of three basic components — system control, system process, and system output. As communication options are presented to the user on a display module (a keyboard, screen, etc.), communication aids are con-

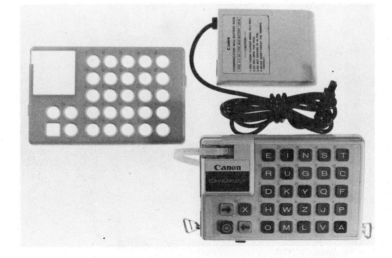

FIGURE 5–2. A photograph of a Canon Communicator. This device is distributed in the United States by Telesensory Systems, Incorporated, 3408 Hillview Ave., P.O. Box 10099, Palo Alto, California 94304.

trolled by physical displacement, touch, electromyography, or light sensor control of single or multiple switches. Single-switch control usually involves a system in which the display is a scanning light or image of some type, while multiple-switch control may control a scanning system or a system in which the specific symbol is directly selected. System processes incorporated into a specific aid vary greatly. Some systems transmit messages without enhancing, storing, or decoding. Such a system would be a typewriter, since the depression of a key corresponding to a letter of the alphabet results in the printing of that letter only. Other aids allow for the retrieval of coded messages, the storage of messages and phrases, or the repeated output of messages. Output choices available in communication augmentation systems can be divided into two broad categories — visual and auditory. The visual output may occur on a screen or a permanent printed display, while the auditory output is usually an audio taped message or a speech-synthesized message.

It is beyond the scope of this chapter to review and describe all of the communication augmentation systems that are currently available. For a more complete description of commercially available systems, the interested reader is referred to the *Non-Vocal Communication Resource Book.*[79] A yearly update of this handbook can be ordered to obtain information about recent advances in system modifications. The following examples are presented to illustrate various types of aids. The Canon Communicator (Fig. 5–2) is a small portable tape typewriter. The con-

trol display consists of a keyboard with numbers, letters, and punctuation displayed beside or on the control keys. The control interface consists of 29 displacement keys that are directly selected by the user. Permanent visual output is produced by a strip printer.

The Zygo Model 100 Scanner is pictured in Figure 5–3. The control display includes 100 squares with a small light centered in each square. There are several interface control options. The light can be controlled in a row-column scanning pattern by a single switch or in the horizontal and vertical directions by multiple switches. Messages can be formulated and stored in memory, to be retrieved as a sequential pattern of light movement. The output of this aid is a transient visual display of lights in selected squares. However, a printer can be added to the basic model when permanent output is required.

The Phonic Mirror Handi-Voice 120 is presented in Figure 5–4. There are three control options available for this aid. The first consists of a keyboard display containing number and control keys. The user retrieves a pre-programmed message by depressing a three-digit code. The second control option involves a sequential visual display of numbers 1 through 9. The interface for this mode involves the activation of a single switch to select the desired number. The third control option consists of the auditory presentation (synthesized speech) of the numbers 1 through 9. The interface control for this option involves the activation of a single switch to indicate the desired number.

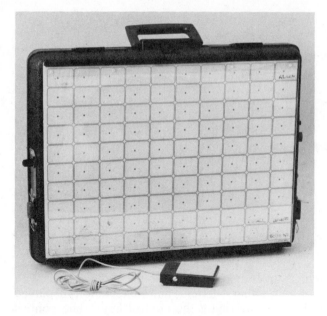

FIGURE 5–3. A photograph of a Zygo model 100 Scanner. This device is distributed in the United States by Zygo Industries, Box 1008, Portland, Oregon 97207.

This device has several system process options. The unit will retrieve a message — word, phrase, or sentence. The vocabulary, which includes 45 phonemes, is factory programmed. With this device new messages can be formulated and placed in one of two memories to be received at a later time. Synthesized speech is the only output option of this aid.

The Prentke-Romich Express I is presented in Figure 5–5. The control display consists of an 8 by 16 LED matrix display behind a front panel. Letters, words, or pictures can

be mounted on the panel square corresponding to a single LED. The control interface options are extensive. With the display and the scan mode, a single switch or multiple switches can be used to indicate the message or system control choice. In the direct selection mode, a light sensory can be held in a hand or mounted on the headband to detect an LED lamp. Thus, message and system control choice can be selected. The system process options of the Express I allow for the retrieval of messages, some of which can be programmed by the user. Messages can

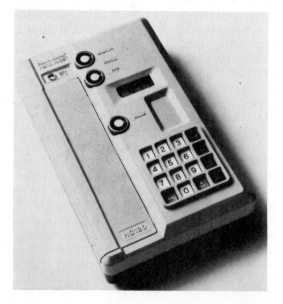

FIGURE 5–4. A photograph of the Handivoice 120. This device is distributed in the United States by HC Electronics, 250 Camino Alto, Mill Valley, California 94941.

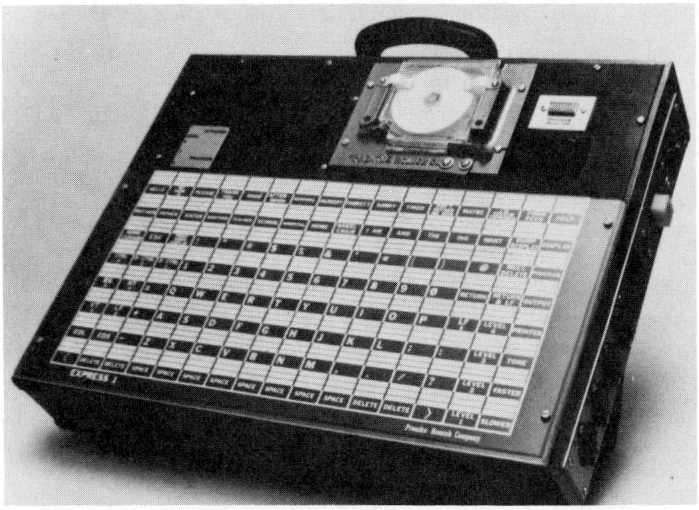

FIGURE 5-5. A photograph of a Prentke-Romich Express I. This device is distributed in the United States by the Prentke Romich Company, R.D. 2, Box 191, Shreve, Ohio 44676.

also be prepared and stored for retrieval at a later time. Output options include a strip printer and a visual transient display (marquee type). Messages from the system can also be displayed on peripheral modules such as a TV screen or computer-controlled line printer.

Guidelines for choosing individuals who would potentially benefit from communication augmentation assistance have been reported by Shane and Bashir.[73] Included is a consideration of cognitive, oral reflective motor control, speech intelligibility, emotional status, chronological age, previous therapy, imitative ability, and environmental factors. The selection of a specific communication aid for a communicatively impaired individual is usually made by a multidisciplinary team that includes experts in communication, motor control, education, device adaptation, and engineering and consultations from medical, psychological, and seating experts. Of course the nonspeaking individual and his family members are involved in the selection process. System selection requires extensive information about the linguistics, motor control, cognitive, and visual abilities of the communicatively impaired individual along with a detailed analysis of current and future communication needs. Training programs to prepare individuals to use communication augmentation systems are rapidly being developed. Several of these approaches are presented in the book entitled *Non-Speech Language Intervention.*[69] The communication augmentation field is changing rapidly; therefore, additional references are provided for interested readers.[12, 66, 76, 80, 81]

REFERENCES

1. Alexander, M. P., and Schmitt, M. A.: The aphasia syndrome of stroke in the left anterior cerebral artery territory. Arch. Neurol., 37:97–100, 1980.
2. Basso, A., et al.: Influence of rehabilitation of language skills in aphasic patients. Arch. Neurol., 36:190, 1979.
3. Bates, E.: Language and Context. New York, Academic Press, Inc., 1976.
4. Bell, D. S.: Speech functions of the thalamus inferred from the effects of thalamotomy. Brain, 91:619–638, 1968.
5. Berlin, A.: Classification of cleft lip and palate. *In* Zoch, K. B. (Ed.): Communicative Disorders Related to Cleft Lip and Palate. Boston, Little, Brown and Company, 1971.
6. Beukelman, D. R., and Yorkston, K. M.: A communication system for the severely dysarthric speaker with an intact language system. J. Speech Hear. Disord., 42:265–270, 1977.
7. Beukelman, D. R., and Yorkston, K. M.: The relationship between information transfer and speech intelligibility of dysarthric speakers. J. Commun. Disord., 12:189–196, 1979.
8. Bollinger, R. L., et al.: Communication Management of the Geriatric Patient. Danville, Ill., The Interstate Printers and Publishers, Inc., 1977, p. 45.
9. Boone, D.: The Voice and Voice Therapy. Englewood Cliffs, N. J., Prentice-Hall, Inc., 1971.
10. Broad, D. J.: Phonation. *In* Minifie, F., et al. (Eds.): Normal Aspects of Speech, Hearing and Language. Englewood Cliffs, N. J., 1973, pp. 127–168.
11. Cohen, M., and Cross, P.: The Development Resource: Behavioral Sequences for Assessment and Program Planning. New York, Grune and Stratton, 1979.
12. Communication Outlook: Focusing on Communi-

cation Aids and Techniques, International Action Group for Communication Enhancement. East Lansing, Michigan State University.

13. Cooper, H., et al.: Cleft Palate and Cleft Lip: A Team Approach to Clinical Management and Rehabilitation of the Patient. Philadelphia, W. B. Saunders Company, 1979.

14. Dale, P. S.: Language Development: Structure and Function, 2nd Ed. New York, Holt, Rinehart and Winston, 1976.

15. Darley, F. L.: Diagnosis and Appraisal of Communication Disorders. Englewood Cliffs, N. J., Prentice-Hall, Inc., 1964.

16. Darley, F. L.: The efficiency of language rehabilitation in aphasia. J. Speech Hear. Disord., 37:3–21, 1972.

17. Darley, F. L., et al.: Clusters of deviant speech dimensions in the dysarthrias. J. Speech Hear. Res., 12:462–496, 1969.

18. Darley, F. L., et al.: Differential diagnostic patterns of dysarthria. J. Speech Hear. Res., 12:246–269, 1969.

19. Darley, F. L., et al.: Motor Speech Disorders. Philadelphia, W. B. Saunders Company, 1975.

20. Deal, J.: Consistency and adaptation in apraxia of speech. J. Commun. Disord., 7:135–140, 1974.

21. DeRenzi, E., and Faglioni, P.: Normative data and screening power of a shortened version of the Token Test. Cortex, 14:41–49, 1978.

22. Diedrick, W., and Youngstrom, K.: Alaryngeal Speech. Springfield, Ill., Charles C Thomas, Publisher, 1966.

23. Folsom, J. C.: Reality orientation for the elderly mental patient. J. Geriatr. Psychiatry, 1:291, 1968.

24. Geschwind, N.: Current concepts, aphasia. N. Engl. J. Med., 12:284, 1971.

25. Gonzalez, J. B., and Aronson, A. E.: Palatal lift prosthesis for treatment of anatomic and neurologic palatopharyngeal insufficiency. Cleft Palate J., 7:91–104, 1969.

26. Goodglass, H., and Kaplan, E.: The Assessment of Aphasia and Related Disorders. Philadelphia, Lea and Febiger, 1972.

27. Goodglass, H., and Kaplan, E.: Boston Diagnostic Aphasia Examination. Philadelphia, Lea and Febiger, 1972.

28. Grabb, W., et al.: Cleft Lip and Palate. Boston, Little, Brown and Company, 1971.

29. Hagen, C.: Communication abilities in hemiplegia. Effect of speech therapy. Arch. Phys. Med. Rehabil., 35:377, 1970.

30. Halpern, H., et al.: Differential language and neurologic characteristics in cerebral involvement. J. Speech Hear. Disord., 38:162–173, 1973.

31. Hart, C. W.: Functional and neurological problems of the larynx. In Sisson, C. (Ed.): Problems of the Larynx. Otolaryngol. Clin. North Am., 3(3):609–623, 1970.

32. Hillbom, E.: After effects of brain injury: Research on symptoms causing invalidism of persons in Finland having sustained brain injuries during the Wars of 1939–40 and 1941–44. Acta Psychiatr. Scand., 35:142, 1960.

33. Hixon, T.: Respiratory function in speech. In Minifie, F., Hixon, T., and Williams, F. (Eds.): Normal Aspects of Speech, Hearing, and Language. Englewood Cliffs. N. J., Prentice-Hall, Inc., 1973, pp. 73–122.

34. Hixon, T., et al.: Dynamics of the chest wall during speech production: Function of the thorax, rib cage, diaphragm, and abdomen. J. Speech Hear. Res., 19:297–356, 1976.

35. Holland, A. L.: Case studies in aphasia using programmed instruction. J. Speech Hear. Disord., 35:377–390, 1970.

36. Holland, A.: Communicative Abilities in Daily Living. Baltimore, University Park Press, 1980.

37. Hollien, H.: Vocal pitch variation related to changes in vocal fold length. J. Speech Hear. Res., 3:150–156, 1960.

38. Hollien, H.: Vocal fold thickness and fundamental frequency of phonation. J. Speech Hear. Res., 5:237–243, 1962.

39. Hook, O.: Aphasia and related communication disorders after brain damage. Lecture presented at the Second Annual Conference: Head Trauma Rehabilitation — Coma to Community. San Jose. Cal., 1979.

40. Ingram, T. T.: Pediatric Aspects of Cerebral Palsy. London, E. S. Livingston, Ltd., 1964.

41. Johns, D., and Darley, F.: Phonemic variability in apraxia of speech. J. Speech Hear. Res., 13:556–583, 1970.

42. Karis, R., and Hornstein, S.: Localization of speech parameters by brain scan. Neurology. 26:226–230, 1976.

43. Keith, R. L., and Darley, F. L.: Laryngectomee Rehabilitation. Houston, Texas, College Hill Press, 1979.

44. Kertesz, A., et al.: Computer tomographic localization, lesion size, and prognosis in aphasia and non verbal impairment. Brain Lang., 8:34–50, 1979.

45. Kertesz, A., et al.: Isotope localization of infarcts in aphasia. Arch. Neurol. 34:590–601, 1977.

46. Kertesz, A., and Poole, E.: The aphasia quotient: The taxonomic approach to measurement of aphasia disability. Can. J. Neurol. Sci. 1:7–16, 1974.

47. LaPointe, L., and Horner, J.: Reading Comprehension Battery for Aphasia. Tigard, Oregon, C. C. Publications, 1979.

48. Lehiste, I.: Suprasegmentals. Cambridge, Mass., MIT Press, 1970.

49. Levine, D. N., and Mohr, J. P.: Language after bilateral cerebral infarctions: Role of the minor hemisphere in speech. Neurology, 29:927–938, 1979.

50. Luchsinger, R., and Arnold, G.: Voice-Speech Language. Belmont, Cal., Wadsworth Publishing Company, 1965.

51. Martin, A. D.: Some objections to the term "apraxia of speech." J. Speech Hear. Disord., 39:53, 1974.

52. McDonald, E., and Chance, B.: Cerebral Palsy. Englewood Cliffs, N. J., Prentice-Hall, Inc., 1964.

53. Millard, D. R.: Cleft Craft: The Evaluation of Its Surgery #1. The Unilateral Deformity. Boston, Little, Brown and Company, 1976.

54. Milner, B., et al.: Observation of cerebral dominance. In DeReuk, A., and O'Connor, M. (Eds.): Disorders of Language. London, Churchill, 1964, pp. 200–222.

55. Mohr, J. P., et al.: Broca aphasia: Pathologic and clinical. Neurology, 28:311–324, 1978.

56. Morris, S. E.: Program Guidelines for Children with

Feeding Problems. Edison, N. J., Childcraft Education Corporation, 1977.

57. Netsell, R.: Speech physiology. *In* Minifie, F. D., Hixon, T. S., and Williams, F. (Eds.): Normal Aspects of Speech, Hearing and Language. Englewood Cliffs, N. J., Prentice-Hall, Inc., 1973.

58. Ojemann, G. A.: Subcortical language mechanism. *In* Whitaker, H., and Whitaker, H. A.: Studies in Neurolinguistics 1. New York, Academic Press, Inc., 1976, pp. 103–138.

59. Ojemann, G. A., and Whitaker, H. A.: Language localization and variability. Brain Lang., 6:239–260, 1978.

60. Porch, B. E.: Porch Index of Communicative Ability. Palo Alto, Cal., Consulting Psychologists, 1967.

61. Porch, B., et al.: Statistical prediction of change in aphasia. J. Speech Hear. Res., 23:312–321, 1980.

62. Reynolds, A. F., et al.: Left thalamic hemorrhage with dysphonia: A report of five cases. Brain Lang., 7:7, 1979.

63. Rosenbek, J. C.: Treating Apraxia of Speech. *In* Johns, D. F. (Ed.): Clinical Management of Neurogenic Communicative Disorders. Boston, Little, Brown and Company, 1978, pp. 191–241.

64. Rosenbek, J. C., and LaPointe, L.: The dysarthrias: Description, diagnosis and treatment. *In* Johns, D. F. (Ed.): Clinical Management of Neurogenic Communication Disorders. Boston, Little, Brown and Company, 1978.

65. Rosenbek, J. C., et al.: A treatment for apraxia of speech in adults. J. Speech Hear. Disord., 38:462–472, 1973.

66. Ross, A., and Flanagan, K.: An Innovative Communication System for the Disabled Using Morse Code to Printed English Translation. Proceedings of the Fourth Annual Conference on Systems and Devices for the Disabled, 1977, pp. 83–85. Seattle, WA., Dept. of Rehabilitation Medicine, University of Washington School of Medicine.

67. Sarno, M. T.: The functional communication profile manual of directions. Rehabilitation Monograph 42, New York Institute of Rehabilitation Medicine, New York University Center, 1969.

68. Sarno, M. T., et al.: Speech therapy and language recovery in severe aphasia. J. Speech Hear. Res., 13:607, 1970.

69. Schiefebusch, R. L. (Ed.): Non Speech Language Intervention. Baltimore, University Park Press, 1980.

70. Schuell, H. M.: Minnesota Test for Differential Diagnosis of Aphasia. Minneapolis, University of Minnesota Press, 1955.

71. Schuell, H., et al.: Aphasia in Adults. New York, Harper and Row, Publishers, 1964.

72. Searleman, A.: A review of right hemisphere linguistic capabilities. Psychol. Bull., 84:503–528, 1977.

73. Shane, H. C., and Bashir, A. S.: Electron criteria for the adoption of an augmentative communication system: Preliminary considerations. J. Speech Hear. Disord., 45:408, 1980.

74. Shewan, C. M., and Kertesz, A.: Reliability and validity characteristics of the Western Aphasia Battery. J. Speech Hear. Disord., 45:308, 1980.

75. Sies, L. F. (Ed.): Aphasia Theory and Therapy: Selected Lectures and Papers of Hildred Schuell. Baltimore, University Park Press, 1974.

76. Silverman, F. H.: Communication for the Speechless. Englewood Cliffs, N. J., Prentice-Hall, Inc., 1980.

77. Sparks, R., and Holland, A.: Melodic intonation therapy for aphasia. J. Speech Hear. Disord., 41:287–297, 1976.

78. Tucker, H.: Human larngeal reinnervation. Laryngoscope, 86:769–778, 1976.

79. Vanderheiden, G.: Non-vocal Communication Resource Book. Baltimore, University Park Press, 1978.

80. Vanderheiden, G., and Grilley, K.: Non-vocal Communication Techniques and Aids for the Severely Physically Handicapped. Baltimore, University Park Press, 1977.

81. Vicker, B.: Non-oral Communication System Project 1964/1973: Iowa City, University of Iowa, 1974.

82. Vignolo, L. A.: Evaluation of aphasia and language rehabilitation: A retrospective exploratory study. Cortex, 1:344, 1964.

83. The Vocational Rehabilitation Problems of the Patient with Aphasia. A workshop sponsored by Western Michigan University. Washington, D.C., U.S. Department of Health, Education and Welfare, Social and Rehabilitation Services, 1967.

84. Weinberg, J., et al.: Visual scanning training effect on reading-related tasks in acquired right brain damage. Arch. Phys. Med. Rehabil., 58:479, 1977.

85. Wepman, J. M.: Aphasia therapy: A new look. J. Speech Hear. Disord., 37:203–214, 1972.

86. Wertz, R. T.: Neuropathologies of speech and language: An introduction to patient management. *In* John, D. F. (Ed.): Clinical Management of Neurogenic Communication Disorders. Boston, Little, Brown and Company, 1978, pp. 1–101.

87. Westlake, H., and Rutherford, D.: Speech Therapy for the Cerebral Palsied. Chicago, National Easter Seal Society for Crippled Children and Adults, 1961.

88. Yorkston, K. M., and Beukelman, D. R.: A clinician-judged technique for quantifying dysarthric speech based on single-word intelligibility. J. Commun. Disord., 13:15–31, 1980.

89. Yorkston, K. M., and Beukelman, D. R.: A comparison of techniques for measuring intelligibility of dysarthric speech. J. Commun. Disord., 11:499–512, 1978.

90. Zemlin, W.: Speech and Hearing Sciences: Anatomy and Physiology. Englewood Cliffs, N. J., Prentice-Hall, Inc., 1968.

6

PSYCHOLOGICAL ASSESSMENT AND MANAGEMENT

WILBERT E. FORDYCE

The purpose of this chapter is to analyze the medical rehabilitation process in behavioral terms in order to provide a basis for developing appropriate courses of action when so-called psychological or motivational problems occur in patient management. Major objectives are to provide the physician and other health care professionals with an appreciation of the implications for intervention strategies and to examine and analyze the rehabilitation processes from a learning point of view.

The clientele of medical rehabilitation are primarily people who, as a consequence of physical disability, are at a functional disadvantage in the performance of life tasks. Medical rehabilitation is concerned with containing or limiting this functional impairment; with slowing its progression; or with reducing or eliminating the functional impairment, as may be indicated by the nature of the medical problem. Whatever the ultimate course of the medical aspects of the disability, rehabilitation is concerned with optimizing functional performance in the face of impairment. Finally, rehabilitation is concerned with assisting the individual with the impairment to become re-engaged in the affairs of society and daily living at an optimal level commensurate with the state of his disability. In a sense it might be said that rehabilitation is trying to do something about

the patient's medical or physical status, whatever that status may be, and also trying to do something about how effectively the patient performs. The former of those two areas of concern focuses primarily on medical problems, broadly defined. The latter area clearly involves problems of learning and performance. This chapter will be primarily concerned with this sector.

There are several reasons why rehabilitation properly emphasizes learning. In the first place, learning is behavior change. When a person incurs a physical disability, there is some immediate change in behavior potential or response repertoire. The patient, for example, who sustains injury to the spinal cord undergoes significant change in a host of behaviors, e.g., ambulation. The disability will change what needs doing as well as what can be done. But the new behaviors that need to be carried out will not occur until the patient has learned them. Effective learning consists both of acquiring the skill or ability to do something and of developing the probability that the necessary actions will occur as often as needed. Using again the example of a paraplegic patient, such a patient needs to acquire skill at transferring from bed to wheelchair, but he also needs to perform those transfers at appropriate times and in appropriate places. Both skill acquisition and increasing probability of perform-

124

1. Observe sign or symptom of illness. ("Illness Behavior")

2. Pursue, identify (or infer) underlying pathology "causing" symptom.

3. Treat by attacking underlying pathology.

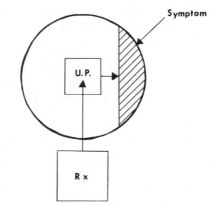

FIGURE 6–1. The disease-medical model.

ance are behavior change processes and therefore learning problems.

Another way in which learning concepts become important in rehabilitation is in the assimilation of disability or adjustment to disability. Traditionally, problems of adjustment have been viewed from a disease-oriented conceptual model. That is, those behaviors the individual engages in that cause others to identify him as either adjusted or maladjusted are seen as under the control of intrapsychic factors within the organism. This approach has evolved from traditional disease concepts in which symptoms are identified as under the control of underlying pathologic conditions. The disease model frame of reference (Fig. 6–1) has been applied by analogy to problems of adjustment. Unfortunately, it has often been the case that people fail to recognize it as an analogy and not a statement of facts. There are alternative descriptive systems one may

use to organize phenomena associated with questions about adjustment to disability. The descriptive system or conceptual model used here (Fig. 6–2) views those behaviors defined as indicative of adjustment or maladjustment as subject to the influence of learning processes. Use of a learning model leads one's effort toward applying appropriate learning principles directly to the behavior to be changed rather than trying to change inferred underlying attitude or feeling states in order that an ensuing behavior change may occur.

When a person incurs a disability, certain behaviors engaged in prior to the onset of disability are no longer appropriate. Those behaviors need to be reduced or eliminated. In addition, the patient needs to acquire new disability-appropriate behaviors. The identification of behaviors to be changed (decreased, eliminated, increased) and efforts to develop conditions favorable for these behavior changes need not await changes in

1. Observe sign or symptom of illness. ("Illness Behavior")

2. Sign or symptom ("Illness Behavior") may be learned behavior.

3. Treat by applying learning principles.

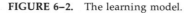

FIGURE 6–2. The learning model.

underlying attitudes or feeling states. In essence, the major distinction between the disease model and the learning model, in the context of assimilation of disability, is that the disease model approach emphasizes changing underlying attitudes and feeling states so that new behaviors may occur. In contrast, the learning model aims directly at changing these behaviors, with the expectation that adjustments in underlying feelings and attitudes, insofar as they are crucial or relevant, will follow.

There is yet another way in which learning concepts are important in medical rehabilitation. One of the major differences between rehabilitation medicine and most other medical fields is the emphasis in rehabilitation medicine on medical problems of a chronic nature. Disabilities usually cannot be totally eliminated or resolved. Residual impairments persist. Medical problems relating to disability are chronic and recurring. This difference has a number of implications for the patient, the family unit, the patient's environment, and for professionals dealing with the patient. Acute, time-limited medical problems ordinarily do not require the patient to make a lasting behavior change. Chronic disease problems, as with physical disability, usually require major and permanent behavior changes. Moreover, as will be developed further in a discussion of motivation, many of the behavior changes dictated by the disability are low-frequency, low-strength, low-value behaviors having little attractiveness to the patient or his family, thereby complicating the learning process. Finally, it is generally the case in rehabilitation that rate of progress is relatively slow in comparison to the patient's prior experiences with acute illness. As a consequence, the learning process may be further burdened by a dearth of the rewards of rapid progress.

Psychological interventions have for the most part been derived from various personality theories, though claiming some allegiance to learning theory. Only in approximately the last two decades, however, has there emerged meaningful and practical remedial technology derived from learning principles. These new, learning-based therapies may be applied directly to a number of facets of the rehabilitation process. Gendlin and Rychlak[22] (p. 156), in reviewing the current state of psychotherapy and problems of maladjustment, say:

The new therapies written about tend to reject the older conception of maladjustment as a long-term illness needing long-term treatment and substitute instead a much briefer intervention . . . instead of deep dynamics, the therapies now tend to make the difficulty a mode of interaction, game, or behavior pattern which is to be knocked out not by years of treatment but simply by taking up some other mode of interaction 'game' or 'behavior' pattern.

It is important to establish a proper perspective with regard to use of behavioral methods. At one extreme, more traditional so-called psychodynamic (e.g., Freudian, neo-Freudian) approaches to an understanding of human behavior have tended to postulate the emergence of a basic personality or a set of attitudes, or a configuration of traits that direct or guide behavior. The emphasis is on alleged or inferred inner or underlying mechanisms within the person. That view has tended to attach little importance either to discriminated stimuli or to contingent consequences in the here and now or the anticipated environment. At the other extreme, some doctrinaire behavioral approaches have seemed to proceed as if behavior is controlled strictly by discriminated stimuli or contingent consequences, thereby underemphasizing the contribution of prior experience or learning. Both are oversimplifications. The position taken here is an "interactionist" one. Behavior is seen as a response to a complex interaction of prior experience and present stimuli. Previous learning will have helped determine which stimuli in the environment will be discriminated and responded to, and which contingencies are likely to prevail as consequences to alternative behaviors. At the same time, the here and now environment will indeed provide cues or indicators of probable consequences to alternative behaviors.

There is another important but often overlooked reason for viewing rehabilitation in behavioral terms. This concerns the behavior of members of the rehabilitation team and what keeps them going. In acute illness, treatment usually provides rapid changes toward improvement. To the extent that this is true, two things follow. One is that treatment methods are exposed to a short feedback loop regarding progress. Since progress is expected, if it does not occur, changes in treatment are likely to be imposed quickly. Outcome tends to have a rapid and strong effect on process or methods. A second consequence is that the health care professional tends to get rapid reinforcement for effort: "What I did made a difference: my patient got better." That performance reinforcement is, in addition to monetary, status, and peer approval reinforcers, somewhat indigenous to health care delivery.

The situation is different in chronic illness and disability. Progress is often slow when compared to the time frame of acute illness. Progress may be minimal. In the case of progressive diseases there may be no improvement, only worsening. It follows that an outcome in the form of improvement has necessarily limited capacity as an effective reinforcer by which to maintain the professional's behavior: How can progress be a reinforcer if it is delayed or missing? Either of these circumstances minimize or negate reinforcer effectiveness. It takes us too far afield to explore this issue in detail here. The point is that in chronic illness or disability settings, one cannot assign to effective outcome a heavy part of the burden of reinforcement from which to expect maintenance of staff performance. There will of course be monetary rewards for effort. Principally, however, a large part of the burden of reinforcement for maintaining professional performance in rehabilitation is likely to reside with peer concensus or approval. That in turn means that it will be especially important to maintain militant self-performance and team performance analysis to be sure that optimal methods and procedures are being used and are being updated. Professional behavior, like that of patients, is sensitive to consequences. If those consequences are not favorably arranged, performance will suffer accordingly. In chronic illness it may require more effort at special arrangement of the consequences to the professional's performance.

The learning principles underlying the behavioral perspective can be described rather briefly. It will not be possible to develop mastery over their application by study of the summary statements and illustrations provided here. It should be possible, however, to develop an understanding of the principles involved, an appreciation of the basic methods sufficient to participate with others in their application, and a grasp of what the adequately trained behavioral engineer is up to when working out detailed applications.

The principles underlying operant conditioning or contingency management methods derive from the work of B. F. Skinner.[48, 49] Concise treatment of operant principles and illustrations of applications are found, for example, in Berni and Fordyce,[10] Marr and Means,[36] Ince,[29] Krasner and Ullman,[33] Michael,[38] Patterson and Guillion,[40] and Reese.[42] The brief statement of the principles given here draws heavily on the work of Michael[39] and of Lindsley and Skinner.[35]

LEARNING PRINCIPLES

A distinction is drawn between respondent and operant behavior. Respondents are responses of the organism involving glandular, smooth-muscle, or reflex phenomena. They are under the control of antecedent stimuli — that is to say, upon occurrence of an adequate stimulus, the respondent follows automatically. Operants are behaviors involving striated muscles or voluntary actions. Operants may be elicited by an antecedent stimulus. However, the strength of an operant response (i.e., the probability that it will occur in a given situation) is subject to influence by consequences. Manipulation of consequences is the critical operation in operant conditioning. When an operant is followed by a positive consequence (reinforcer), its frequency tends to increase. When an operant is followed by a negative or aversive reinforcer (punisher), its rate tends to decrease. When positive reinforcers are withdrawn from an operant, its rate will diminish and ultimately disappear, a process termed *extinction*.

The effectiveness of a reinforcer on an operant is related to the stimulus situation in which the operant has occurred in the past contiguous to that reinforcer. A reinforcer will have more effect on an operant when it is delivered or withheld in the same stimulus setting as has occurred previously. The more the stimulus setting has changed, the less the effect of the reinforcer. As behavior occurs and is reinforced or punished in changing stimulus situations, the new stimuli will tend to act as reinforcers; i.e., they become conditioned reinforcers or conditioned punishers.

A given consequence can be identified as a

reinforcer or punisher only by observation of its effects on the behavior it follows. One cannot assume a given consequence is a positive reinforcer. One may hypothesize that it is and try it out. Having done so, if the behavior it follows in fact increases in rate, it may be inferred that that consequence is a positive reinforcer for that person.

In order to be effective, reinforcers must be delivered as soon as possible following the behavior they are designed to influence. The longer the delay, the less likely the reinforcer will be effective.

Schedules of reinforcement play an important role. When starting a new behavior or increasing the rate of a behavior that previously rarely occurred, it is advantageous to reinforce as many occurrences of the behavior as possible (continuous reinforcement); i.e., one approaches a 1:1 response-reinforcement ratio. When a behavior becomes established, it will become more durable if the reinforcement schedule is reduced (intermittent reinforcement); i.e., a decreasing proportion of occurrences of the response receives reinforcement.

The most important principle to remember in regard to selection and programming of reinforcers is the Premack principle.[41] It states that ". . . high-frequency behavior can be used to strengthen low-frequency behavior. . . ." That can be paraphrased as, "What a person does repeatedly can, when appropriately programmed, be a powerful means of increasing actions that the person does too little of — the behavior to be strengthened."

It would be difficult to overstate the practical importance of the Premack principle in helping people by behavioral methods. One implication is that there is always a potentially effective reinforcer available in any situation because the person is sure to be doing a lot of *something,* even if it is insisting on remaining in bed instead of getting up for treatment.

New and complex responses are acquired by shaping. In shaping, successive approximations of the desired response are reinforced. Systematically varying the stimulus situations for an established response (stimulus fading) helps bring the response under control of increasingly complex or remote stimuli, thereby making it more durable.

Certain rules should be kept in mind in applying these principles.

1. Never simply try to eliminate a behavior. There must be an alternative response available; if there is not, help the person to acquire an alternative.

2. It is easier to accelerate then to decelerate a response. This means that when trying to help a person eliminate or reduce some behavior, it is usually easier to focus on increasing a response incompatible with the one to be reduced, rather than to try only to extinguish the undesired behavior.

3. Reinforcers or consequences naturally occurring in the treatment environment are usually more effective and easier to program than some exogenous consequence. Rest or time out from arduous activity and praise, attention, or social reinforcement are the more common examples.

The sequence for setting up operant-based behavior change projects is as follows: (1) Pinpoint the behavior to be increased or decreased. (2) Define measurable units of that behavior, i.e., the beginning and end of the cycle of movements constituting the behavior. A movement cycle may be said to have occurred when the organism is in a position to repeat. (3) Record the rate at which the behavior is occurring. Rate is always defined as the number of movement cycles over a unit of time. (4) Identify reinforcers anticipated to be effective. Reinforcers should not be used unless they can be made contingent upon the behavior to be influenced. If there is incomplete control over a reinforcer's availability to a patient, it should not be used. (5) Specify a schedule of reinforcement. (6) Try out the program. If the rate of the behavior in question does not change following a reasonable number of trials, each of the preceding steps needs to be reexamined. As progress occurs, it is usually desirable to decrease the rate of reinforcement, i.e., to expect increasing amounts of performance for each unit of reinforcement. In later portions of this chapter, examples will be given of applications of these methods to specific problems in patient management.

The behavioral analysis and contingency management systems described here for modifying behavior represent a departure from more traditional approaches. These new methods can be very effective in bringing about behavior change, but their use requires appropriate training and experience. Their use also raises a number of ethical questions that deserve at least brief consideration here. Further discussion of ethical issues can be found in Berni and Fordyce[10] and in Ulrich et al.[52]

Contingency management methods involve the manipulation of behavior-consequence relationships. When these manipulations are handled with technical correctness, behavior change probably will ensue. The question rightfully should be raised as to whether one is arbitrarily manipulating a patient when these techniques are being applied. Concern about manipulation of patients should be directed toward any treatment approach that fails to specify methods and goals and that fails to provide opportunity for the patient to decide if he will participate.

There is every reason to explain to the patient in detail the design and objectives of a contingency management program. It is sometimes mistakenly inferred that telling the patient about a contingency management program will somehow compromise its effectiveness. Quite to the contrary, a well-planned program involves the patient to a much greater degree than frequently is true of more traditional approaches. Behaviors that are expected by the end of the program, i.e., the program's goals, should be specified. Those goals should be formulated with the patient. The patient should also participate, when possible, in selection of reinforcers. Exceptions to this are only those situations in which the patient is not able to participate because he is too young (preschool) or because he suffers intellectual impairment from cortical deficit.

ADJUSTMENT TO DISABILITY

This section will deal with the process of assimilation of disability and some of the more common patient management problems relating to it. These problems will be grouped arbitrarily into three subheadings: crisis management, assimilation of disability, and participation in rehabilitation. Figure 6–3 portrays graphically the conceptualization used here.

Efforts to identify a personality pattern or style of response specific to a given kind of disability have not proved fruitful. The subsequent behavior of a person who has in-

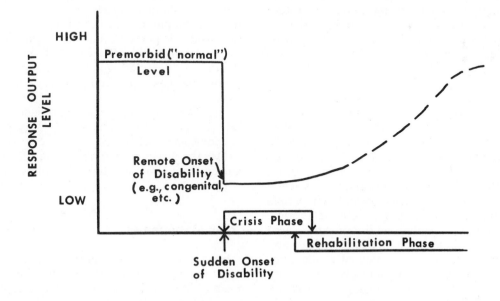

FIGURE 6–3. Assimilation of disability — a behavioral approach.

curred a particular disability will be some function of the behavioral repertoire he had prior to onset, the behaviors left to him by the disability, the meaning or value of the disability to him (i.e., the anticipated loss of reinforcers), and the way those around him behave in relationship to his disability.

For an historic and in many ways definitive analysis of this subject and its critical parameters, one should consult Dembo et al.[13] Extensive reviews of the literature bearing an adjustment to disability and the other major parameters of psychological issues in medical rehabilitation can be found in Trieschmann.[51] Additional helpful reviews include Athelstan,[3] Fordyce,[21] and Woodbury.[56]

Most of the efforts to develop a typology of personality according to type of disability are but another example of the disease model conceptual system applied by analogy to human behavior. That is, since some diseases have fairly fixed patterns of symptoms or manifestations, some people expect that fixed sequences or patterns of physical disability and emotional state or behavioral expressions will also occur. Such a position assumes that the emotional states and behavioral manifestations are under the control of underlying pathologic conditions. When the evidence is clear that behavior is under the control of an underlying pathologic condition (e.g., aphasic signs in a right hemiplegic), there is every reason to expect that behavior will accompany the disability at an appropriate base rate. It should be evident, however, that feelings, attitudes, and general styles of behavior are learned and are not ordinarily under the control of pathologic conditions.

There appear to be only three conditions under which one might expect a systematic relationship between behavior, on the one hand, and a particular kind of disability, on the other. One such condition occurs when the disability itself appears only in people who have certain behavioral characteristics. For example, people who consume large amounts of liquor are more likely to develop cirrhosis of the liver. Perhaps also, diabetics who take poor care of themselves are more likely to sustain loss of vision. In both instances, however, there has been very little specification as to exactly which kinds of behavior the individual will display other than consumption of alcohol in the first ex-ample and careless diet control or insulin management in the second. Little has been said about a wide range of other behaviors of interest in the rehabilitation process.

A second condition in which behavior and disability may have a significant relationship is that in which the disability has a direct causal relationship to certain behavior changes. The example cited earlier of the signs of aphasia in a right hemiplegic is an illustration, as is the increase in physically sedentary behavior in an advanced case of chronic obstructive pulmonary emphysema. Another example of such a relationship is seen in the changes in recreational patterns of a person with significantly limited ambulation resulting from disability. In each of these examples, it is easy to identify a causal relationship between functional impairment and the ensuing behavior.

A third condition in which behavior-disability relationships might occur is that in which the disability has a consistent effect on the behavior of others toward the person with the disability. Facial disfigurement, athetoid movement in a cerebral palsy patient, and obvious blindness in a retrolental fibroplasia patient are illustrations. When the disability has a consistent effect on the behavior of others, their responses in turn are likely to influence the behavior of the person with the disability. The causal relationships in this example are between the behavior of the disabled person and the behavior of others toward him. There is no need for recourse to postulating an underlying mechanism that has produced the behavior observed.

Once it is recognized that there is no need for recourse to a personality typology when considering problems of adjustment to disability, the direct path of observing behavior-consequence relationships becomes more evident.

Crisis Management

Most rehabilitation facilities admit patients a few weeks or even a few months following onset of illness. As a consequence, the process of assimilation by the patient of what has happened will have already begun, whether purposefully or simply in the natural course of events. Sometimes rehabilitation will begin soon after onset. In such cases, crisis management issues are important in early work with the recently disabled patient.

The radical change in body state that accompanies significant disability of sudden onset (e.g., spinal cord injury, stroke, amputation) inherently provides a situation analogous to the work of Hebb[26] of many years ago. Hebb noted that subjecting a person to radical alteration in sensory input nearly always leads to disorganized behavior. Having the lower half of one's body suddenly deprived of sensation is prototypic of that, because that person's central nervous system suddenly receives a quite different configuration of kinesthetic, tactile, and proprioceptive input.

In addition to the neurophysiological sensory changes occasioned by severe injury, the move to a hospital bed and changes in mobility and environment provide sudden and dramatic changes in sensory input.

For the first several days or weeks following onset, confusion and disorganization are to be expected. Familiar faces may be unrecognized. Temper outbursts may occur with little or no provocation. Intellectual confusion and misunderstanding of even simple communications may occur. This does not in itself imply disintegration of coping mechanisms or personality functioning. For some people, the stress of assimilating the fact of serious injury is more than they can readily handle and indeed they become disorganized. However, virtually everyone with serious disability will, initially, show periods of confusion that do not presage lingering disorganization.

The theory of crisis management can be divided into two parts. The first is to recognize that the patient's difficulty will tend to improve if those responsible for his care use reasonable skill.

As Hanford[25] has noted, people in crisis tend to be more suggestible. It follows that stability and calmness in the immediate environment will make a greater difference. Therefore, the first rule of thumb in crisis management is to establish and maintain as much as possible a calm environment. This does not mean that sensory deprivation should be increased by keeping the patient isolated. To do that would likely aggravate the problem. It means to ensure that those working with the patient go about their business in a calm, deliberate, supportive way.

Immediate family should also be helped to recognize that the patient will benefit if they remain calm.

The second part of the theory of crisis management takes us back to one of the basic principles of behavioral management; namely, that if one wishes a person to reduce some behavior (in this case, crisis-related behaviors) it is important to ensure that alternative behaviors are available. One of the more helpful crisis management tactics is to identify a "life-on-the ward" issue in which one can enhance the patient's skill for coping and then pursue this goal. An example would be to note that many people are not effective in asking for help in ways that make the giving of it easier for the helper. Particularly if the patient is disorganized, calls by a recently injured quadriplegic to a nurse to supply water or provide other services may come out in ways not well designed to enhance nurse support. If, however, some person such as the ward psychologist were to begin working with that patient on the very circumscribed task of improving social skills at variations of assertiveness (e.g., ways of asking for help), two goals might be accomplished. One is improving the patient's skill at developing optimal working relationships with treatment staff and the more general ability to foster and maintain needed assistance. The other is building the patient's sense of mastery of an immediately relevant issue and helping him to develop behavior alternatives to ruminating or daydreaming, or random and scattered mentation.

Assimilation of Disability

Rehabilitation as Punishment. The conditions defining punishment also describe the typical situation for a person who has recently incurred a significant disability. Punishment, according to Ferster,[16] Michael,[38] and Reese,[42] can be defined as any consequence that either weakens the behavior that follows or strengthens behavior designed to avoid or escape the punishing stimulus. Another way of stating it is that punishment may be thought of either as the loss of positive reinforcers or the onset of aversive stimuli. When positive reinforcers are no longer accessible following a behavior, the subsequent rate of that behavior diminishes. Similarly, when an aversive stimulus is applied following some behavior, that behavior's rate diminishes and behavior designed to enable escape from the aversive stimulus increases.

Those conditions characterize what happens with sudden onset of disability. The patient immediately loses access to the positive reinforcers previously sustaining his work and leisure behavior. The patient also immediately begins to experience aversive stimuli. There is likely to be pain and physical distress. As discussed previously, there is likely to be relative sensory deprivation and some disorganization. It is probable the patient will perceive his disability and related functional impairments as very aversive. Finally, those around the patient are likely to attribute negative value to the disability and to communicate that to the patient in one way or another.[46, 47, 57]

Punishment, whether in the form of aversive stimuli or loss of positive reinforcers, tends to increase behavior designed to avoid the punishment of escape from it. Moreover, stimuli contiguous to aversive stimuli will tend to take on aversive properties; i.e., they become conditioned aversive stimuli. It follows that the patient is likely to identify disability and the rehabilitation procedures associated with it as stimuli leading to punishment. The patient may avoid what he perceives as punishment by engaging in behavior that keeps him out of the rehabilitation process. Similarly, when he is actively engaged in some rehabilitation activity, escape behavior on his part may serve to terminate the aversive stimuli of disability and rehabilitation. There are many ways in which the patient may engage in avoidance or escape behaviors in the medical rehabilitation setting. He may refuse treatment appointments or be consistently late for them. He may lose himself in a passive withdrawal into fantasy. He may provoke arguments or encourage rejection by angry and rebellious behavior. He may depart precipitously by signing out of the hospital against medical advice. Remedial action for these problems will be discussed later in this section.

Ferster[16] has observed that "... it is problematical whether a repertoire consisting entirely of escape and avoidance behavior can be maintained." The disabled patient who engages in escape or avoidance behavior gains "time out" from a noxious situation, but what he escapes to is not likely to

be effectively reinforcing for long. There are several reasons why that is the case. The act of withdrawing or escaping from rehabilitation does not reestablish access to reinforcers that maintained functioning prior to onset of disability. Similarly, daydreaming about what one used to be able to do does not provide access to the reinforcers to those behaviors. Fantasy provides only temporary relief. Finally, avoidance or escape from rehabilitation limits access to certain other reinforcers. Specifically, the attention and regard of professionals working with the patient will no longer be available. Reinforcers that become accessible only upon completion of an effective rehabilitation program will also be lost.

In the natural course of events, then, the chances of the patient engaging in escape or withdrawal behavior when confronted with significant disability will tend to diminish across time. Exceptions may result if the rehabilitation program has failed to handle the escape or avoidance behavior in effective fashion or the nontreatment environment of the patient reinforces avoidance behavior excessively.

To this point in considering onset of disability relative to the concept of punishment, the focus has been on people with recent and sudden onset. Under certain conditions persons who have had a disability for a long period of time and who then enter a rehabilitation program may present similar problems. The person with remote onset who enters rehabilitation probably does so because of some medical complication or because some change in his functional performance is contemplated. The home environment of such a patient likely will have evolved relationships between his disability and his family's behavior toward it that serve to maintain or reinforce the ways in which he has been doing things. When he enters the rehabilitation program, he will be cut off from those reinforcers. If rehabilitation plans for such a patient involve major changes in how the patient performs, he may perceive the program as the functional equivalent of punishment.

The work of Azrin, Hake, and Hutchinson,[4] Ulrich, Wolfe, and Dulaney.[53] and others has shown that punishment may produce aggressive behavior in animals. The studies cited show that aggressive behavior in response to punishment is more likely to occur when there is an available target to attack.

Experience in medical settings with persons who have suddenly become disabled indicates that man, too, may respond to punishing circumstances with aggressive behavior. When viewed in the context of the concept of punishment, some of the arbitrary and rebellious behavior of recently disabled patients may become more understandable. The patient who lashes out, verbally or otherwise, at therapists working with him may interrupt activities that remind him of his disability or that directly produce pain or discomfort. Temper outbursts and rebellious recalcitrance about engaging in treatment procedures sometimes are viewed as loss of emotional control in an impulse-dominated or emotionally labile personality. Sometimes these behaviors are identifed as self-destructive. Such behaviors may be responses to what is perceived as a punishing situation.

Psychological interventions for problems of withdrawal or aggression should be directed toward decreasing the aversive qualities of rehabilitation and decreasing the positive consequences to avoidance or escape behavior. A critical first step in this process is to establish an effective therapeutic relationship. Conceptually, during the initial phases of rehabilitation, the emphasis should be on substituting the interim reinforcer of positive interaction with an interested and attentive therapist for the natural reinforcers to effective behavior that become accessible to the client when he gains more mobility and functional capacity and re-engages in home and work activities. If those working with the patient are not effective social reinforcers, the reinforcers left to sustain rehabilitation efforts are mainly relief from pain, relief from sensory deprivation, interruption of disturbing ruminative fantasies about disability, and awareness by the patient that he is progressing toward those reinforcers that will become available upon completion of the program. How effective those reinforcers are will vary from patient to patient, depending upon the patient's prior experiences. It is well to remember, however, that reinforcers are more effective if they are delivered immediately following the behavior they are designed to influence. Some of the reinforcers just cited are delayed. The rehabilitation program that fails to establish an effec-

tive treatment relationship with the patient will be proceeding under what may well be seriously compromised circumstances.

At the outset of rehabilitation the attention and positive regard of the therapist should be directed to each increment of engagement in the rehabilitation process. This may be seen as a process of shaping participation in rehabilitation.[29, 37–39] Tactically, the objectives are to delineate graded increments of the treatment task scaled to maximize chances of success; to identify and deliver positive reinforcers, initially on an almost continuous (1:1) schedule; and, as progress occurs, to increase performance expectations by adding components to the task while maintaining or lowering the amount of reinforcement. The goal of this approach is to make involvement in rehabilitation as reinforcing as possible rather than aversive. If it is effective, the patient's positive experiences in treatment are accompanied by reduction of isolation and sensory deprivation, thereby adding a further reinforcement.

The steps just described may decrease the aversive qualities of rehabilitation or increase its positive value. At the same time, when withdrawal or aggressive behavior is encountered, efforts should be made to decrease its reinforcement. In the hospital setting a number of steps can be taken to influence responses of hospital personnel to withdrawal or aggressive behavior.[20, 21]

It is easy for hospital personnel to fall into the trap of paying attention to the patient only when something is going wrong. The patient's long-range objectives are better served if professional attention is contingent upon productive activity. For example, upon observing a disabled patient in what appears to be a withdrawal reverie, a nurse might encourage him to work on a previously prescribed bedside occupational therapy task. If he begins to work at the task, the nurse may then remain to interact with him. If he works for a time and then stops, she may then prepare to leave and say to him something like, "That's fine. Let me know when you feel like doing some more and I'll come join you." If a nurse socializes with a patient on a noncontingent basis, she thereby dissipates her effectiveness as a therapeutic agent. If she socializes only when the patient is not working, she may encourage the very behavior the program is trying to reduce. If her attention is contingent upon his engaging in rehabilitation-appropriate behavior, she contributes directly to treatment objectives.

Family members should be helped to perceive how their interactions with the patient can make a direct contribution to progress. Families are at particular risk in socially reinforcing withdrawal behavior. Two relatively simple steps can be taken to help with this problem. One is to establish contact and communication with the family to help them understand how they can contribute to progress in his rehabilitation program. The second step is to make visible indications of treatment accomplishments. One way of doing this is to draw graphs showing performance in each aspect of the program and affix them to the wall at the patient's bedside. The graphs provide visible evidence of increments in performance, remind the family about the importance of selective responsiveness, and give them a subject that they can discuss appropriately. Care should be exercised in the construction of graphs to ensure that increments in performance are scaled appropriately to the patient's rate of progress in each activity recorded.

Management of Grieving

In most important respects, both conceptually and tactically, the management of grieving parallels closely that of punishment. The conceptualization of grieving used here draws heavily on the work of Ferster.[16] Grieving or depression is seen as a state of deprivation of reinforcers. The sudden shift in life style brought about by onset of disability results in the loss of previously sustaining reinforcers. The result is grieving and depression. This is true of the newly disabled patient. It is true of the person whose spouse has suddenly died. It is true of the patient who, having been in the hospital so long that previously established relationships have faded and a new set of intrahospital relationships have been developed, is suddenly confronted with discharge from the hospital.

The objective of intervention (for problems of grieving) is to help the patient gain access to reinforcers as expeditiously as possible. An analysis should be made of those activities the patient engaged in previously that can be made available readily in the hospital setting. Effort should also be made immediately to provide tasks related to treatment that elicit reinforceable responses from the patient. One way of describing this approach is to note that one does not treat grieving or depression so that the patient can do things; one helps the patient to start doing things as a way of treating the grieving or depression. The essential features of the tactical approaches by which this may be accomplished have already been described in the sections dealing with crisis management and punishment. The steps to follow are to pinpoint units of performance at the highest level of difficulty consistent with guaranteed patient performance, to define movement cycles and their current rate, to identify reinforcers, to schedule reinforcement initially at a near continuous rate, and to monitor carefully the program as it is applied.

Chemotherapeutic intervention with mood-elevating drugs is sometimes indicated. Some depressive patterns are so severe as to leave the patient virtually incapable of producing reinforceable responses. Psychiatric consultation is certainly indicated in that kind of situation. Chemotherapuetic intervention should not be seen as in any way incompatible with the behavioral approaches just described. Quite to the contrary, when chemotherapy is used, it should be coupled with graded introduction of treatment-related tasks and application of the appropriate reinforcing contingencies.

Extinction of Premorbid, Disability-Inappropriate Behavior

As noted in the introductory section, extinction occurs when a behavior is no longer reinforced. Certain behaviors the patient engaged in prior to onset of disability are incompatible with his disability. That is true of specific performance skills in daily activities, in larger complexes of behavior such as vocational or leisure time activities, and in many behaviors subsumed under the terms *self-concept, attitudes about one's self,* and so forth. For a recently disabled patient the concern here is with leisure and vocational behaviors engaged in previously that are no longer feasible. Those behaviors cannot again occur in fact. The patient may, however, daydream about those activities. As noted previously, that kind of withdrawal behavior is intrinsically reinforcing for only a limited time.

A problem arises when people around the patient reinforce fantasy behavior by unrealistic statements implying that the disability is only temporary. Remedial action to this kind of problem is based on the same principles as in dealing with punishment and grieving. The optimal conditions for extinction are that the response occurs, it is not reinforced, an alternative response is available, and that alternative is effectively reinforced. The rehabilitation program should seek to minimize the direct reinforcement of unrealistic fantasies, i.e., minimize reinforcement of withdrawal. The rehabilitation program should also move as rapidly as possible to shape in alternative, disability-appropriate behaviors under optimal conditions of reinforcement. At all costs, one should *avoid punishing for withdrawal or denial* of disability behaviors. To punish for them is to make it more likely that the punisher will become a conditioned aversive stimulus, thereby losing effectiveness as a source of support and reinforcement. At the same time, the punishing of denial behaviors risks suppressing the behavior to be extinguished. That in turn will inhibit extinction.

The patient's family also needs help with problems relating to extinction of disability-inappropriate behavior. One reason families engage in unrealistic denial and reassuring behavior with the patient is because they lack viable alternatives. Providing families with information about what the patient is going to be able to do at the end of the program and about his progress helps give them alternatives about which they can communicate with the patient. The use of performance graphs at the patient's bedside, as discussed earlier, is one illustration of how this may be accomplished.

Family members, like everyone else, need positive reinforcement for their behavior. Often it is not sufficient to provide them with relevant information. The social worker and others on the rehabilitation team can make important contributions to patient progress by systematic contact with family members. These contacts should be designed to help the family anticipate the reinforcers that will become available to the patient and to themselves as the rehabilitation program progresses. Once communication and working relationships are established, less effort should be spent on feelings and more on working out details of what the patient and family will be doing upon completion of the rehabilitation program.

Most recently disabled patients have not yet learned ineffectual behaviors relative to their disabilities, and their families have not evolved a pattern of reinforcing such behaviors. If the recently disabled patient were to leave the rehabilitation program, in most instances he would not likely long receive effective reinforcement for his withdrawal. The outlook for change in both the patient and the family unit under those conditions is favorable. In contrast, the patient who has long had his difficulty may come from an environment that has evolved effective reinforcement patterns for ineffectual or disability-inappropriate behavior. If ineffectual behavior has been going on at a substantial rate, it must have been receiving reinforcement. If such a patient were to leave the rehabilitation program precipitously, he would return to an environment that would sustain his existing behavioral repertoire. If the patient successfully completes the rehabilitation program, he returns to an environment that may fail to reinforce the new behaviors and may resume reinforcing the previously ineffectual behaviors reduced by rehabilitation. It should be evident that those planning rehabilitation programs for patients who have had their disabilities for long periods of time need to be particularly concerned with analyzing the home situation. If a program concerns itself only with the patient's behavioral repertoire and ignores that of the family, behavioral changes brought about in rehabilitation may not persist.

The tactical steps for helping family members to change their behavior are the same as those for helping patients to change behavior. Family members need aid to pinpoint their own and the patient's behavior, to be aware of the rate of these behaviors, and to establish patterns of desired behaviors by the use of contingent rewards.

PARTICIPATION IN REHABILITATION

This section will deal with problems relating to motivation, with techniques for enhancing patient acquisition of disability-appropriate behaviors, and with helping the patient to maintain new behavioral repertoires upon completion of rehabilitation.

Motivation

There can be little doubt that the most frequently mentioned psychological problem in the context of disability and rehabilitation concerns patient motivation. Fishman[17] states, "Empirical evidence substantiates the theoretical consideration that the single most important problem facing the rehabilitation worker concerns the ways and means of implementing marginal motivation."

The conceptualization of motivation implicit in the learning model approach and the management techniques derived from that model are quite different from the more traditional view based on a disease model system.[19, 51] Motivation is not an attribute of behavior but an inference about an inner state of the organism derived from observations of behavior. Typically, a patient is held to be "motivated" if he engages in the behaviors of interest at an acceptable rate. If those behaviors do not occur at an acceptable rate, the patient is considered to be "unmotivated" or to be "motivated" for some less desirable goal. Used in that way, the concept of motivation adds nothing to information about the patient or to the clarification of courses of remedial action. All that has happened is that the observer has noted the extent to which the patient has done what the program hoped he would do and has labeled him "motivated" or "unmotivated," as the case may be. Statements about the patient's motivation, although used characteristically as if they described some inner state of the organism, are in fact based on a relationship between what the patient has done and what observers thought he should do.

Approaching the concept of motivation from a learning model point of view leads to a different formulation. Behavior is sensitive to consequences. If a behavior is occurring at an inadequate rate (i.e., the "unmotivated" patient), some adjustment is needed in the contingencies to that behavior. If a patient is doing too much of something that interferes with performance of rehabilitation-appropriate behaviors at a desired rate (i.e., the "unmotivated" patient or the patient "motivated" for the wrong things), the reinforcers to those undesired behaviors need to be withdrawn. To quote Michael,[39]

From a behavioral point of view, however . . . marginal motivation seems merely to be a case of insufficient or poorly arranged reinforcement. The basic question that should be asked is 'What does the patient get out of his activity?' The problem of motivation is a simple one. One must merely arrange the environment so that its desirable features are only available contingent upon participation and accomplishment in the rehabilitation training activity.

There are several reasons why motivation problems are so prominent in rehabilitation. The earlier discussion of punishment has shown how becoming disabled and entering into rehabilitation may initially be aversive. It is not surprising, therefore, that many patients fail to produce disability-appropriate behaviors at the desired rate. There is another reason for the prominence of motivational problems. Staats[50] points out,

Discussions with therapists in rehabilitation suggest that much of their work, especially with children, involves training new behaviors under circumstances in which the reinforcers are weak. For example, prior to developing skill with the prosthesis the child secures reinforcement more easily for various already learned substitution movements. Thus, some way must be found at first to supply 'prosthetic responses,' in a competitive sense, since these responses are not in themselves 'naturally' reinforcing.

It may be said that disability-appropriate behaviors, particularly in the case of physical disability, initially are low-frequency, low-strength, low-value behaviors to the rehabilitation client without experience with those behaviors.

The essential features in the psychological management of motivation problems in rehabilitation consist of establishing treatment relationships that enhance the reinforcing value of interactions with rehabilitation professionals, of enhancing the value of long-term reinforcers for disability-appropriate behavior, and of carrying out the behavioral analysis and contingency management steps that promote acquisition of the new behaviors provided by effective rehabilitation.

Evaluation

The objectives of psychological evaluation in rehabilitation are to predict what the patient is likely to do in rehabilitation and in relevant situations in the future and to identify stimulus situations and reinforcers likely to influence patient behavior. In addition, in the case of head injury or some suspected or observed form of cortical insult, psychological evaluation via psychometric assessment can shed considerable light on the precise configuration of intellectual, cognitive, and emotional changes produced by the disability. That in turn can provide an important part of the basis for planning rehabilitation. This will be discussed in a later section of this chapter. As the picture of the patient's potential functional capabilities emerges from the diagnostic process, it becomes important to specify the behavioral changes that the patient will need to make and the way in which these changes can more readily be brought about. As noted in the discussion of motivation, disability is likely to require the patient to engage in some low-frequency, low-strength, low-value behaviors.

The more similar what the patient has done in the past is to what he is functionally capable of doing in the future, the less likely the disability behaviors will be low-frequency, low-strength, and low-value. It is important, therefore, to identify what he had done in the past in order to assess whether special reinforcement is going to be needed to establish new, disability-appropriate behaviors. Identifying reinforcers is itself a procedure specifically related to what the person has done in the past. The best estimate of the activities that are reinforcing to a person is derived from the knowledge of the activities that he has pursued frequently in the past.

Evaluation can be carried out in part by obtaining current behavior samples from the patient in the form of direct observations or from psychological testing, as will be discussed later. Evaluation also may be carried out by indirect observation of behavior in the form of history taking about the patient and family members.

The kinds of activities the patient has engaged in in the past that are reinforcing to him are mainly to be found in his recreation and leisure-time pursuits. Those data, supplemented by a detailed job history, should tell much about what is likely to be reinforcing to him in the future. There are many reasons why the patient's past may not be an adequate prologue of the future. Youthfulness of the patient, a vague or incomplete picture of what he has done, or radical changes in what is possible in the future all may make additional information essential.

An additional and frequently very rich source of information for providing estimates of future activities likely to be reinforcing is the activities the patient's early models — usually parents or older siblings — have engaged in. Personality and modes of self-expression are learned. They are learned by a combination of the influence of consequences in the environment in which behaviors have been practiced and of modeling or social imitation learning.[7-9] The most significant models usually will have been parents and older siblings. Many of their behaviors will have been emulated. In addition, these same models will themselves have been exercising some selectivity as to which behaviors of the patient they will have reinforced, ignored, or punished. Their choices in that regard will reflect, in part, what they find reinforcing to themselves. Thus, so long as there has been reasonably effective communication between patient and models, patient behavior will reflect much of the behavior style of the models. It frequently proves fruitful, therefore, to obtain a detailed picture of both the leisure and vocational activities of those in the patient's background who have served as significant models for him.

Psychological testing in patient evaluation needs some consideration. Which tests are used and how frequently they are used varies markedly from psychologist to psychologist. That variability and the sometimes seemingly inexplicable relationship between the stimulus materials in a test and the inferential comments made about test responses make it difficult to maintain a clear perspective as to what psychological testing is all about. Psychological tests are one kind of behavior sample designed to provide a basis for predicting how the tested person will behave in nontest situations.

Sometimes tests, like x-rays, are seen as revealing underlying characteristics that, when understood, permit rather precise predictions of future behavior. That view, however, is of questionable validity. It implies that personality steers the individual into actions somewhat independently of the context in which he functions. It is more accurate to recognize that human behavior is governed by a combination of the repertoire of the individual and influences from the immediate environment. Psychological test responses are one kind of behavior. What the person will do in some other situation is another kind of behavior. The degree to which these two behaviors are in fact correlated cannot exceed the degree of comparability of test stimuli and future situation. As future situations depart more and more from stimuli surrounding testing and the test itself, the predictive efficiency of the test data will be correspondingly diminished.

The accuracy of predictions that a psychologist may make on the basis of test data will depend in part upon the extent to which the test has been standardized in stimulus situations comparable to those about which the predictions are made. This point is illustrated by the obvious fallacy of trying to predict subsequent academic performance of an English-speaking native of upper Sudan based on scores derived from intelligence tests standardized on middle-class American normative groups. Some tests have normative data based on reference populations about which much is known. When the rehabilitation clients being tested are from comparable reference populations, the normative data are directly relevant and few interpretative problems exist. When standardization is carried out on a quite different population or when very limited standardization is carried out, as frequently is the case in many psychological tests, there must be increasing reliance on the extrapolating acumen of the psychologist.

Rehabilitation programs are confronted with many evaluation problems for which few, if any, standardization data are available. The compromise imposed by necessity is to ask the psychologist to make his estimates or predictions according to his best judgment and experience, based on the test data he accumulates. He must therefore have some latitude in selecting the tests to be used so that he can draw upon the instruments with which he is most experienced. Under these conditions, the utility of the psychological test report will be correspondingly greater as the psychologist becomes better acquainted with the stimulus situations in which the behavior he is trying to predict will occur. The psychologist's contribution will be enhanced if he is helped to become better acquainted with the rehabilitation process and the specific styles of the rehabilitation team. The rehabilitation physician can enhance the contribution of the psychologist by encouraging continuing functional exposure to the rehabilitation team and continuing feedback to the psychologist about the accuracy of his predictions. Further discussions of specific tests pertinent to rehabilitation may be found in Fordyce.[18]

Evaluation should lead to a specification of the behaviors required in the environment toward which the client is headed and an understanding of the behaviors likely to be reinforced or punished by that environment. The rehabilitation team sometimes conceptualizes its goals in broad generalities, e.g., greater independence, more mobility. Eventually, a concept like independence must be translated into terms specifying the operations or behaviors that the patient and those about him are to engage in. Failure of the rehabilitation team to arrive at those specifications leads to two kinds of problems. One is that individual therapists may be unclear as to what it is they are to do. What they do may even contradict other aspects of the program. Failure to specify the target behaviors of the program also makes it difficult realistically to identify the extent to which the program has succeeded or failed. The failure to specify goals in operational terms risks fostering the continuation of procedures that are ineffectual or inefficient.

One final point should be made about use of psychological testing in evaluation. This concerns the cost effectiveness of testing compared with other methods the psychologist might use instead. Direct observation of performance is often a better method to obtain a basis for prediction than are giving and analyzing tests. Similarly, for each hour spent in test evaluation, the evaluator might instead have spent time conferring with therapists about structuring an optimal learning and performance environment or in social skill training sessions with a patient. There is ample basis for believing that the latter activities might have made greater contributions to program objectives.

Contingency Management Methods

This section will illustrate the use of consequence manipulation or contingency management systems to bring about behavior change. Evaluation should have yielded specification of the behaviors to be reduced, maintained, and shaped or increased. Evaluation should also have indicated at least a general picture of the behaviors likely to be reinforcing to the patient and the behaviors that are likely to be reinforced or punished by the environment toward which he is headed. There are some additional steps that can be taken to identify reinforcers immediately available to help the patient entering the rehabilitation process.

A useful guide to identification of reinforcers is the previously mentioned Premack principle.[41] To restate, of any two activities, the more probable one will function as a reinforcer for the less probable one. Stated another way, activities that previously have been attractive to a patient are likely, when made available contingent upon completion of specified units of rehabilitation-related efforts, to prove effective positive reinforcers to the rate of those efforts. Reinforcers naturally occurring in the rehabilitation environment offer considerable advantage over more remote reinforcers. History data will tell a lot about what is likely to be reinforcing. In addition, direct observations of what the patient now does should prove helpful.

Two important characteristics of reinforcers are that they be available and that they be contingent upon performance. Rest or periods of time-out from treatment and attention are naturally occurring and readily available reinforcers in rehabilitation. These and other reinforcers will be of little value, however, if they are available to the patient whether or not he performs, i.e., if they are not contingent upon performance. If a reinforcer is not subject to control, it should not be used.

A third functional characteristic of an effective reinforcer is that delivery of the reinforcer should not interfere with the performance one is trying to improve. To illustrate that point, consider a program designed to increase standing in long-leg braces in a paraplegic patient. If rest is the reinforcer and it is programmed so that one minute of standing earns 30 minutes of rest delivered immediately following performance, training sessions would be protracted unduly by reinforcement.

The number of reinforcers that can be used effectively in rehabilitation can be enhanced considerably by the use of token or point systems. When a token economy is used, upon completion of a designated number of movement cycles, the patient receives a token (e.g., poker chip or point) that can be traded in subsequently on some previously designated reinforcer. Token economies make available a range of reinforcers that can be delivered immediately following performance without disrupting the behavior one is trying to strengthen. The use of tokens makes it possible to relate a series of reinforcers to one behavior and, conversely, to make more than one behavior relate to one or more reinforcers.

More detailed discussions of the use of token economies can be found in Berni and Fordyce,[10] Michael,[38] and Krasner.[31] An annotated bibliography on token economies is found in Krasner and Atthowe.[32]

The following example* illustrates an application of contingency management systems to a problem of patient participation in medical rehabilitation. Figure 6–4 illustrates the results.

Case Example 1

The patient was a 62-year-old woman who had had a resection of the left femoral head and neck because of infection. Postoperatively she had hyponatremia, a myocardial infarction, acute tubular necrosis, and anemia. Three weeks after the myocardial infarction, she began rehabilitation for ambulation. She was emaciated and weak and had a painful left hip. She rapidly learned transfers and gained strength. However, routinely she requested a bedpan rather than transfer to a commode. *Target behavior:* Increased use of commode. *Movement cycle:* Transfer to commode and return to bed or wheelchair.

REINFORCERS. It was observed that the patient engaged the staff in conversation at any opportunity and that she seemed to get a great deal of pleasure from these conversations. Therefore, chatting and interacting with the staff were chosen as the reinforcers.

PROCEDURE. (1) *Baseline:* Requests for bedpan or commode were honored without comment and the nursing staff continued to chat with the patient at those times. In general, the patient used the commode once daily and the bedpan the rest of the time. (2) *Selective Reinforcement:* As before, the bedpan or commode was supplied upon request. The nurse would stay to chat only when the commode was used. The patient was not informed of this. Nonetheless, within three days use of the bedpan had fallen essentially to zero. (3) On the 16th day the selective reinforcement program was terminated in order to assess how well the new behavior

---

*The projects in Case Examples 1 and 2 were carried out under the direction of John Kirby, M.D., a resident in Physical Medicine and Rehabilitation.

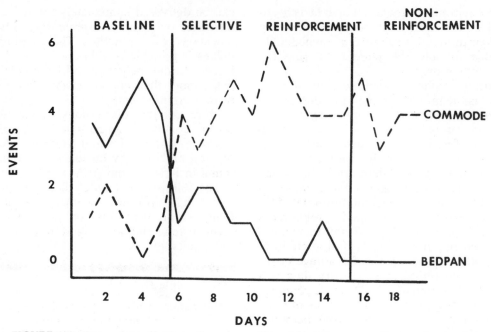

FIGURE 6–4. Improving self-care performance with social reinforcement. (See text for details.)

was established. Use of the bedpan remained at zero, as shown in Figure 6–4.

The second example illustrates use of a simple point or token system with a commonly encountered problem in medical rehabilitation. Results are shown in Figure 6–5.

Case Example 2

The patient was a 28-year-old male who had sustained an L5-S1 fracture-dislocation, with resultant incomplete paraplegia. Owing to the seriousness of the injury, many additional procedures were necessary, including diversionary colostomy, multiple graft and skin flap rotations to repair massive soft tissue injury, multiple surgeries for recurrent renal stone formation associated with primary renal failure at the time of injury, immobilization hypercalcemia, and recurrent urinary tract infections. In addition to these many setbacks, the patient had been under psychiatric care for four years prior to injury and was described as having a schizoid personality. The result in the patient was apprehension, mistrust, and the conviction he was being punished by his injury.

The immediate treatment task considered here was to increase ambulation with a walker and with use of short leg braces with the goal of independence in mobility. The target behavior

was ambulation, and the movement cycle was number of laps walked, expressed in number of feet traversed. In addition, speed of walking was also recorded.

After full discussions by the psychologist with the patient and in collaboration with the physical therapist, a contingency management plan was set up. The reinforcers were praise by the therapist, rest (two minutes following achievement of a quota), and a cup of ice chips, which the patient had been observed to enjoy. For three days, from twice daily sessions and two trials per session, baseline values were obtained without reinforcement. Thereafter the contingency arrangements went into effect. One additional trial was added each session. Thus, additional trials and additional distance constitute a fading of reinforcement, because attainment of the rewards of praise, rest, and ice chips required increasingly greater amounts of performance.

Case Example 3

This case involved a 56-year-old obese woman with adult diabetes mellitus and peripheral neuropathy. She had received a gastric stapling procedure. Shortly thereafter she had sudden onset of "whole body" weakness and severe pain.

After full discussions with the patient and with her agreement, treatment objectives were developed, two of which are reported here, along with the contingency management plan.

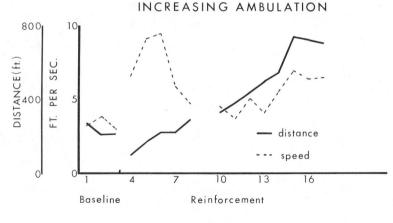

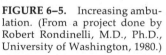

FIGURE 6–5. Increasing ambulation. (From a project done by Robert Rondinelli, M.D., Ph.D., University of Washington, 1980.)

Pain complaints tend to be self-defeating in many instances in chronic illness, because they tend to promote dwelling on the distress, thereby heightening intensity of the pain experience and tending to disrupt other treatment activities. The reduction or extinction of pain complaints was undertaken solely by withdrawing social reinforcers to their concurrence. That is, instead of questions, solicitous comments, reassuring statements, or suggestions by therapists to guard against worsening the pain, pain complaints were simply ignored. The results are shown in Figure 6–6.

The problem of increasing ambulation presents another set of contingency management issues. It was necessary first to restore the patient's ability to ambulate and then to increase it. The contingencies programmed to assist in this effort were praise, rest, and performance feedback through the use of graphs portraying successive performance. In the case of rest, as in

Case No. 2, a simple contingency arrangement was used — one that is typically quite powerful in helping people to increase performance. Instead of working to tolerance (variations on the theme of doing "as much as you can"), specific quotas of performance are worked out, e.g., two laps or round trips in the parallel bars. A rate of incrementing quotas is also set — one additional lap each trial. This arrangement of working to quota lets rest or time out from the arduous task, which is usually a powerful consequence or reinforcer, become contingent on the behavior to be increased — in this case, ambulation. Working to tolerance does not do that.

The patient first was placed on the tilt table for increasing intervals and with decreasing physical support. When sufficient standing and weight-bearing tolerance had been achieved, ambulation in the parallel bars was begun. Results are shown in Figure 6–7.

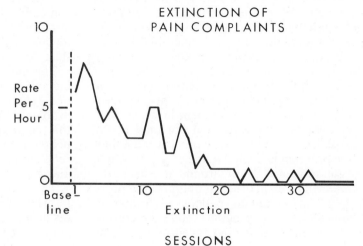

FIGURE 6–6. Extinction of pain complaints. (From a project done by Kenneth Jaffe, M.D., University of Washington, 1980.)

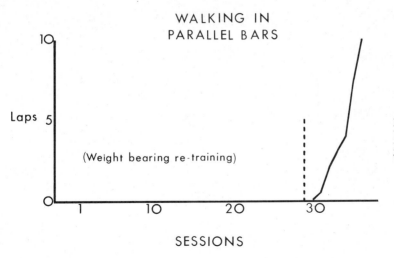

FIGURE 6–7. Walking in parallel bars. (From a project done by Kenneth Jaffe, M.D., University of Washington, 1980.)

These examples illustrate the influence on patient performance of naturally occurring reinforcers in the rehabilitation setting when they are made contingent upon performance. The examples also illustrate pinpointing target behaviors, identifying movement cycles, and recording rate of performance. Further illustrations in the application of these methods to a variety of problems in rehabilitation may be found in Berni and Fordyce[10] and Ince.[29]

MAINTENANCE OF PATIENT PERFORMANCE

It is important to distinguish between the ability to do something and the probability that it will be done.[54] It is easy to lose sight of the fact that these concepts are not the same. That someone has the ability to do something by no means ensures that he will in fact do it. If a rehabilitation program has given a patient the ability to do something but he subsequently does not do it, the program can hardly be considered a success. The objectives of a rehabilitation program ought to be that the target behaviors occur at an appropriate rate in the environment in which they are supposed to occur and not only in the rehabilitation center. Obviously a rehabilitation program is limited in the extent to which it can influence the environment outside the treatment area in order to optimize the probability of adequate patient performance. Nonetheless, the program should be considered incomplete if it has failed to assess the influence of the target environment on the behaviors being developed within rehabilitation and actions have not been taken to influence the environment toward the end of optimizing patient performance.

As noted earlier here and by Staats,[50] rehabilitation may require the patient to perform tasks that are not intrinsically reinforcing and may in fact initially be noxious, cumbersome, or unrewarding. The environment outside the rehabilitation program is not likely to reinforce many disability-appropriate behaviors (e.g., ambulating by wheelchair, drinking large amounts of fluids, wearing an upper extremity prosthesis) at the same rate that it does for corresponding nondisability behaviors. That, in turn, means that special effort must be made to provide contingencies in the environment that will maintain disability-appropriate behaviors. If that effort is not made and the natural environment fails to reinforce disability-appropriate behaviors acceptably, those behaviors will fade or be carried out at a lower than desirable rate.

The maintenance of disability-appropriate behaviors following departure from the formal rehabilitation program is essentially a problem of generalization. Generalization in this context refers to the extent to which behavior that occurs in one time or place (in rehabilitation) will also occur in another time and place (in the natural environment).

There are two major strategies to consider in promoting generalization. One is to bring disability-appropriate behaviors under the control of reinforcers naturally occurring in the target environment. Failing that, the alternative strategy is to make a special effort to reprogram the natural environment so that it will deliver appropriate reinforcement contingent upon performance of the disability-appropriate behaviors.

The first of these strategies, that is, relating the disability behaviors to naturally occurring reinforcers, provides the major conceptual basis for the importance of social and vocational programs to physical or medical rehabilitation. When a patient is effectively employed, for example, the reinforcers available in the work situation are likely to maintain behaviors immediately elicited by the job and such work-related behaviors as effective self-care, mobility, and fluid intake. The reinforcers provided by work may be money, status and prestige, socialization, sense of accomplishment, or others. One or more of those reinforcers may effectively maintain work behavior. For some people they will not maintain work behavior at an adequate rate. For yet other rehabilitation patients, employment may not be a feasible objective. In either case, there may be alternative reinforcers available in the home environment to maintain essential disability-related behaviors. Stimulating recreational and leisure-time activities, for example, may provide sufficient reinforcement to maintain both the behaviors immediately elicited by those kinds of activities and related self-care behaviors.

When it appears likely that the natural environment will fail to provide sufficient reinforcement for essential disability-appropriate behaviors or that it will reinforce disability-inappropriate behaviors, special effort should be made to modify the existing contingency relationships. Earlier discussions about punishment and about family involvement in the rehabilitation process described methods for dealing with these problems.

A rehabilitation program can enhance generalization also by providing for gradual and systematic rehearsal of disability-appropriate behaviors in environments more closely approximating the natural environments in which they are to be carried out following rehabilitation. When a patient is provided the opportunity to exercise his new disability-related skills outside the treatment setting, it is more likely that those behaviors will come under the influence of reinforcers available in the nontreatment environment.

Excellent discussions of the principles of generalization and some illustrative applications are found in Baer, Wolf, and Risley.[6]

PSYCHOLOGICAL FACTORS IN BRAIN DAMAGE

Brain damage presents an important problem for medical rehabilitation. Significant numbers of patients with various forms of cortical or subcortical deficits come for help. Developments in the newly emerging field of cognitive remediation promise an expanding capacity for providing this help. It is essential, therefore, to gain some familiarity with brain-behavior relationships, with typical configurations of cortical deficits and their behavioral consequences, with methods for assessment of these problems, and with principles underlying therapeutic interventions.

The topics of brain-behavior relationships and of cognitive remediation are vastly complex — far too complex to deal with adequately within the confines of a single chapter. In this section, a brief overview is presented of the topography of brain-behavior relationship, with particular attention to the behavioral or functional consequences of the cortical insult problems more commonly encountered in medical rehabilitation. Assessment methods are reviewed. Finally, an overview of cognitive remediation is presented. For more detailed treatment of these complex subjects, additional references should be studied. Comprehensive review and analysis of assessment techniques and relevant aspects of brain-behavior relationships can be found in Boll,[11] Diller,[14] Diller et al.,[15] Hecaen and Albert,[27] Lezak,[34] Reitan,[43] Reitan and Davison,[44] and Walsh.[55]

Excellent discussions and debates concerning laterality and as-yet-unsettled issues may be found in Corballis[12] and Schlesinger.[45]

Brain-Behavior Relationships

Lateralization or hemisphericity can easily be either underestimated or oversimplified. There are clearly differences in left and right brain function, but the exact nature and functional boundaries of these differences are yet to be fully understood. Information available at present permits a number of generalizations having workable validity. One is that handedness or dominance has limited relevance. Virtually all right-handed people are found to have language functions in the left brain; however, on the order of 85 per cent of left-handed people are the same. The balance of 15 per cent or so of left-handed people present a mixed picture. Some have language functions bilaterally, others have them virtually solely in the right brain.

A second generalization is that cognitive tasks involving the appreciation of form, distance, and position and of such nonlanguage perceptual tasks as tone and rhythm discrimination appear to lateralize to the right brain. These functions we shall label here as spatial tasks. Conversely, aside from the aforementioned infrequent differences relating to handedness, language and symbol manipulation tasks lateralize to the left brain. Considerable as-yet-unresolved controversy exists as to whether these differences between left and right brain are simply a function of cognitive styles. It is held by some that one hemisphere, the left, processes propositional or analytic cognitive tasks, whereas the right hemisphere processes matters lending themselves to a synthesizing or gestalt approach. One alternative to that view is that it is more a problem of localization by content. One hemisphere, the left, for some reason, processes language or symbol tasks (i.e., something to which names or words are readily attached) and the other, the right, for some reason processes nonlanguage tasks such as appreciation of tone or music, of form or distance, of position, and of size.

Whatever the outcome of this controversy, and presumably future empirical data will show the way, for the purposes here we can work with the linkage of the two generalizations offered. That is, language and symbol manipulation function is pretty much an affair of the left brain, and movement, form, distance, and position functions relate principally to the right brain. The matter of handedness has limited influence.

In addition to the distinctions between spatial and language-related tasks and their lateralization, some cognitive functions seem better described as general attributes of brain function that play a role in virtually any and all cognitive acts. Memory function is the prime example. It will have a part in all stimulus discrimination, association, and response selection tasks. Memory, therefore, does not localize except in the sense that if language and symbol of spatial tasks are impaired, memory function within either will be correspondingly impaired. With spatial deficit we may have memory deficit for spatial tasks, with little or no memory deficit for language tasks. The more pervasive the damage, the more pervasive the effects in terms of memory difficulties.

Reasoning and judgment may also be seen as general attributes of cognitive function rather than as discrete tasks. Conceptually, they can be seen as analogous to memory. They are discussed later in another context.

Memory is so basic to cognitive functioning that it is of paramount importance to rehabilitation. However, the topic is complex and much remains to be learned. Some generalizations appear to have workable validity. It is useful to think about "memory" as learning efficiency. For "memory" to exist, there must be the assimilation of some stimulus material, its retention, and its retrieval for use at appropriate moments. The first generalization is that deficits in memory function appear to be the single most likely adverse consequence of brain damage, so far as cognitive functions are concerned. Virtually all brain-damaged patients, whatever the etiology or localization of damage, are likely to show some impairment in memory function.

The second generalization concerns the distinction between "recent" and "remote" memory. Recent memory can be taken to refer to recall of information or experience taken in since onset of the cortical insult. Remote memory refers to things learned and retained prior to brain damage. Functionally, the difference is that the rate or efficiency of acquisition and retention after the onset of injury is usually impaired. It is not so much a matter of the length of the interval from presentation of information to recall, although that may have some effect, but of whether the information was learned before injury or is presented for learning after injury. Remote memory function is less frequently impaired and, when it is, severe and pervasive cortical damage is usually present. Clinically, one observes repeatedly that brain-injured patients may have exquisitely precise recall of things they knew before injury but be quite unable to remember a therapy instruction from morning to afternoon.

There are a number of implications to the matter of memory deficit. First, identification of the nature and extent of memory deficit must emphasize assessment of recent memory, not remote memory. Secondly, since recent memory is another term for learning efficiency, and it is so common for recent memory deficit to accompany even minor head injury or brain damage, its assessment is critical to planning a rehabilitation program. Finally, since so much of rehabilitation is made up of the acquisition (learning) of skills and new methods, the design of the treatment program must carefully take into account the extent and nature of the memory deficit.

There is some basis for inferring that the presence of recent memory deficit or learning efficiency deficit does not mean that the person cannot learn, it means that the rate at which learning occurs is compromised. It is not yet possible to predict how far the person may be able to go in relearning, although it seems clear that at least some residual limitations will exist. It has been established that the presence of memory deficit does not permit one to infer that relearning is not feasible. The matter then often becomes one of a mix of logistic opportunity and therapeutic persistence to determine how much can be accomplished.

There appears to be a slight tendency for memory deficit to lateralize. That is, left brain injury tends to result in more impairment of memory for language and symbol material. Right brain damage seems to lead to slightly more memory impairment for spatial (nonlanguage) material.

In addition to language and symbol functions, nonlanguage perceptual tasks, and memory, a fourth dimension of brain behavior relationships bearing on intellectual or cognitive deficit is the matter of affective control, or disinhibition. The behavior referred to here concerns the ability to modulate or control emotional expression and impulse.

It involves the previously mentioned general cognitive functions of judgment and reasoning, as well as the modulation of emotional expression. One often observes in brain-damaged patients an ease of emotional expression. They cry for little or no apparent reason, laugh with sometimes inappropriate vigor, or explode into angry temper outbursts with perhaps minimal provocation. In addition to their unabashed vigor, these emotional outbursts, whatever the particular affect expressed, have the further characteristic of being short-lived. They often may be terminated simply by capturing the patient's attention momentarily by a diverting stimulus. The phenomena are sometimes misunderstood as indicating that the person is overwhelmed with some affect and feels intensely. It would appear more appropriate to consider the difficulty as one of reduced ability to modulate the intensity of emotional expression once it is begun. The emotional expression usually is in response to some stimulus of considerably less intensity than the ensuing response would suggest. Descriptively, it is as if the person starts down the sadness or happiness "road," and once started, cannot moderate the emotional expression. Instead of being expressed as a frown or a sob, or a smile or chuckle, the emotion comes out as vigorous crying or laughter.

There are two more common errors in coping with these problems of affective lability. First, sometimes it is assumed that they reflect accurately the feeling state of the person. It is not, for example, that the crying patient is not sad, but the intensity and pervasiveness of the sadness may be considerably less than crying outbursts suggest. The second error is to assume that the remedy to the sadness that is inferred to lie beneath a crying episode is to "let the person ventilate or get it off his chest." That will not often be therapeutic. It may be counterproductive to permit "ventilation," both because it consumes energy and because it interferes with responding to other stimuli and tasks extant in the treatment environment.

Usually an attention-demanding stimulus is sufficient to interrupt these emotional "jags." Clap the hands once smartly, snap fingers, or ask a brief question in tones loud and firm enough to elicit attention. The question can be about anything, so long as the patient must think about something else besides crying or laughing in order to respond.

The second part of the domain of affective control is more complex, more difficult, and more impairing. Many brain-damaged patients demonstrate defective impulse control as well as defective affective control. These are defects in judgment or reasoning. The behavior shown might be characterized as diminished ability to discriminate effectively relative importance from among diverse incoming stimuli and diminished ability to weigh the consequences to various possible alternative responses. For example, the disinhibited male, on encountering an attractive woman, rather than perhaps subjectively or internally "appreciating" her attractiveness, may make immediate and overt sexual approach responses. He may stare, or touch, or initiate a sexually aggressive conversation. As another example, a disinhibited patient may, when provoked to anger by some environmental stimulus situation, respond by physical assaultive behavior with little or no restraint. A normally prudent and restrained woman, when the target of sexual advances, may respond with little prudence or inhibition. The list of possible examples is long. The essence of the problem should be evident.

Disinhibited behavior may also reflect diminished ability to appreciate and respond to the immediate social feedback that we all receive and that ordinarily exercises elements of control over our actions.

Problems of affective lability and disinhibition may be associated with stroke, particularly of the right brain, and cortical insults involving subcortical structures, as in brain stem contusions associated with closed head injuries. In cases of the latter it is difficult at this point to assess the extent to which the phenomena indeed involve subcortical structures or whether it is just that any injury so severe as to lead to involvement of subcortical elements somewhat inevitably will also involve cortical damage so extensive as to lead to the behavior in question. Whatever the case, affective lability and disinhibition, particularly the latter, pose major problems in rehabilitation.

Defects in reasoning and judgment also are

likely to be observed in another way. Individually, we develop problem-solving techniques. These too are somewhat general functions in that we tend to approach a diversity of problems with at least roughly comparable problem-solving methods. These methods will necessarily emphasize association functions, a scanning of prior experience deemed relevant to the problem. That brings us back to memory deficit. As would be expected, problem-solving skills and methods often are impaired and perhaps seriously disrupted by brain damage.

ASSESSMENT

Innumerable psychometric tests have been developed to assess cognitive parameters. It is quite beyond the scope of a single chapter to review these. Comprehensive reviews or detailed descriptions are found in such references as Boll,[11] Reitan,[43] Heilman and Valenstein,[28] Lezak.[34]

There are two major test batteries having much current use in cognitive assessment, the Halstead-Reitan and the Luria-Nebraska. The former is described in detail in, for example, Reitan and Davison,[44] and the latter in Golden et al.[24] In regard to the Luria-Nebraska, the reader is referred to Adams,[1, 2] and Golden.[23]

The Halstead-Reitan battery is a very comprehensive, empirically based set of behavior samples touching on a full range of cognitive functions. It takes from five to eight hours to complete. As a diagnostic tool, it makes its greatest contribution in sampling a wide range of functions, in identifying whether there is cognitive deficit in not otherwise apparent situations, and in helping to localize those not-so-apparent lesions. It is expensive and time-consuming but effective. It is by far the soundest empirically based device of its kind. Thus far, analyses of test protocols based on the Halstead-Reitan have much to say about what the problems are but little to say about what to do about them.

The Luria-Nebraska is somewhat less extensively grounded in empirical data. It represents an effort to translate Luria's highly subjective assessment methods into more objective and quantified form. It seeks to capture more the flavors of cognitive style of the person — of how problems are dealt with. The pool of experience with Luria-Nebraska is, by a quantum amount, less than that of the Halstead-Reitan. However, if the data from the Luria-Nebraska hold up empirically, they may address better one of the gaps remaining from the work thus far with the Halstead-Reitan — namely, implications and guidelines for remediation.

There are alternative assessment batteries to the Halstead-Reitan or to the Luria-Nebraska. Individually selected intellectual and cognitive tests or behavior samples can be used to address specific questions. For example, the Wechsler Adult Intelligence Scale, also a part of the Halstead-Reitan battery, samples a spectrum of languages and spatial tasks. The Wechsler Memory Scale samples fairly extensively verbal or language and symbol memory, both recent and remote. Similarly, the Benton Memory for Designs or the Bender-Gestalt sample the ability to appreciate and synthesize form, distance, and position, as well as memory for such stimuli. There are other possibilities too numerous to list. Lezak[34] provides a very useful review of this subject.

In the hands of a skilled examiner, virtually all of the tests mentioned, and many others, permit inferences about the matter of disinhibition. These kinds of difficulties tend to show up in the style or type of errors made in the various tests presented. In addition, if there is sufficient language to permit handling the test, the Minnesota Multiphasic Personality Inventory (MMPI) also can be useful in assessing the presence and extent of disinhibition.

When there are major limitations in the ability to emit various forms of response, special tests may be needed. For example, the severely aphasic patient cannot emit verbal responses or can do so only on a seriously compromised basis. How then is one to sample left brain functions of such a person? A number of tests may be used in such cases. The Raven Progressive Matrices, for example, present a blending of reasoning, conceptualizing, counting, and form discrimination problems to which a patient may respond only by pointing a finger, thereby bypassing the inability to write or speak. It is enough for our purposes to be aware that alternatives exist.

REMEDIATION

There are too few data and no comprehensive text from which to permit any kind of definitive description or review of cognitive remediation and too little space to describe fully the piecemeal state of the art. Certain generalizations will be offered and additional references will be cited.

First, the task of cognitive remediation involves new learning, a cognitive function that, as noted, is almost inevitably compromised to some extent by the cortical insult. That in turns means that the learning environment must be structured with care and precision. It is not simply a matter of providing ample rehearsal and demonstration. The teaching environment must be organized to maximize consistency and simplicity. It must also be organized in such a fashion as to organize appropriately the hazards of expecting a person to persist with a learning task when early failures are likely. Here we are referring to the "motivational" problem. There must be an optimization of successes. That means tasks must be broken down into bits and pieces to ensure some early successes.

A second statement is that there must be a precise analysis of the behaviors to be changed. To say, for example, that a relearning objective is to enhance perceptual discriminations is far too general. The point is illustrated by the work of Diller et al.[15] on visual scanning. Right brain-damaged patients often are observed, for example, to become lost or to bump into door frames when moving through doorways. Close inspection of their behavior often reveals that they no longer visually scan to the left. This may occur irrespective of visual field cuts associated with the brain damage. One remediation task, therefore, may be to retrain them to visually scan to the left. Only when that is established can one begin to move beyond to additional perceptual discrimination tasks.

The need for precise analysis of behaviors also means there will be a need for considerable effort at staff preparation and supervision. Cognitive remediation is expensive. That is so because it is time-consuming, but it is also because it requires intensive effort by treatment staff. The need for precision observation and recording is much greater than in virtually any other set of rehabilitation problems.

A third statement is that the learning process inevitably involves not only the acquisition and retention of a task but the ability to express it in different stimulus environments, a problem of generalization. The brain-damaged patient, with his learning impairments, can be expected to display difficulty in generalizing acquired responses. Learning to scan to the left in physical therapy does not automatically mean that the patient will scan to the left outside the hospital, or even on the ward. Special attention and rehearsal regarding generalization and practice in a variety of relevant environments is needed.

A fourth generalization is more of a systems approach issue. In task analysis in preparation for a cognitive remediation approach, there needs to be a clear articulation of the objectives. To illustrate, in the case of a patient displaying marked memory deficits, the objective need not and often should not be understood as improvement of memory functioning. In the final analysis, operationally, the objective is to optimize the proportion of times the person is where he is supposed to be and does what is supposed to be done. One way of optimizing attainment of those objectives is to enhance memory functioning so the person will "remember" where to be and what to do. If one could accomplish that, it would be conceptually the more efficient way to go, but this is not always attainable. There is an alternative. The patient might be equipped with a prosthetic memory in the form of an appointment book carried in a pocket, setting forth the schedule of activities and their content. The remediation task then might become one of training the person to remember to use the appointment book. This often is a far more simple training task.

Use of a prosthetic memory device or strategy illustrates two important points in cognitive remediation. To reiterate the first, because of the often-encountered difficulties in restoring to an adequate level some cognitive skill (e.g., memory), an operational analysis of the essential tasks performed often can lead to discovery of alternative ways of getting the task performed. In the present state of the art, this requires ingenuity, creativity, and thought. It may also require considerable trial and error.

The second point is the proposition that if the response repertoire of the person cannot be changed sufficiently, perhaps the environment can be modified to help make up the deficit. This is of course analogous to building entry ramps into a home to enhance access by a wheelchair-bound patient. In the case of brain damage and associated functional impairments, often the environment can be modified to provide additional and more readily discriminable cues from which the patient can find guidance.

Perhaps the most important consideration in the domain of cognitive remediation is to recognize that the essence of the matter is learning. Learning or relearning in the presence of compromised ability to do so requires special precision and expertise in devising the learning environment.

REFERENCES

1. Adams, K.: In search of Luria's battery: A false start. J. Consult. Clin. Psychol., 48:511–516, 1980.
2. Adams, K.: An end of innocence for behavioral neurology? Adams replies. J. Consult. Clin. Psychol., 48:522–524, 1980.
3. Athelstan, G.: Psychological, sexual, social, and vocational aspects of spinal cord injury: A selected bibliography. Rehabil. Psychol., 25:1, 1978.
4. Azrin, N., Hake, D., and Hutchinson, R.: Elicitation of aggression by a physical blow. J. Exp. Anal. Behav., 8:55–57, 1965.
5. Baer, D., and Wolf, M.: The entry into natural communities of reinforcement. In Achieving Generality of Behavioral Change. Symposium presented at the Meeting of the American Psychological Association. Washington, D.C., September, 1967.
6. Baer, D., Wolf, M., and Risley, T.: Some current dimensions of applied behavior analysis. J. Appl. Behav. Anal., 1:91–97, 1968.
7. Bandura, A.: Behavioral modification through modeling procedures. In Krasner, L., and Ullmann, L. (Eds.): Research in Behavior Modification. New York, Holt, Rinehart and Winston, 1966, pp. 310–340.
8. Bandura, A.: Psychotherapy Conceptualized as a Social-Learning Process. Unpublished manuscript, Stanford University, 1964.
9. Bandura, A., and Walters, R.: Social Learning and Personality Development. New York, Holt, Rinehart and Winston, 1963.
10. Berni, R., and Fordyce, W.: Behavior Modification and the Nursing Process, 2nd Ed. St. Louis, C. V. Mosby Co., 1977.
11. Boll, T.: Diagnosing brain impairment. In Wolman, B. (Ed.): Clinical Diagnosis of Mental Disorders. New York, Plenum Press, 1975.
12. Corballis, M.: Laterality and myth. Am. Psychol., 35:284–295, 1980.

13. Dembo, T., Leviton, G., and Wright, B.: Adjustment to misfortune — a problem of social-psychological rehabilitation (1948). Reprinted in Rehabilitation Psychology, special monograph issue, Vol. 22, No. 1, 1975.

14. Diller, L.: A model for cognitive retraining in rehabilitation. J. Consult. Psychol., 29:13–15, 1976.

15. Diller, L., Ben Yishay, Y., Gerstman, L., Goodkin, R., Gordon, W., and Weinberg, J.: Studies on Cognition and Rehabilitation in Hemiplegia. Behavioral Science Institute of Rehabilitation Medicine, New York University Medical Center, Monograph 50, 1974.

16. Ferster, C.: Classification of behavioral pathology. In Krasner, L., and Ullmann, L. (Eds.): Research in Behavior Modification. New York, Holt, Rinehart and Winston, 1966, pp. 6–26.

17. Fishman, S.: Amputation. In Garrett, J., and Levine, E. (Eds.): Psychological Practices with the Physically Disabled. New York, Columbia University Press, 1962, pp. 1–50.

18. Fordyce, W.: Psychology and rehabilitation. In Licht, S. (Ed.): Rehabilitation and Medicine. New Haven, Elizabeth Licht, 1968, pp. 129–151.

19. Fordyce, W.: Research on influencing level of patient participation in the rehabilitation process. In Fuhrer, M. (Ed.): Selected Research Topics in Spinal Cord Injury Rehabilitation. Rehab. Serv. Admin. Washington, D.C., Department of Health, Education and Welfare, 1975, pp. 55–69.

20. Fordyce, W.: A behavioral perspective on rehabilitation. In Albrecht, G.: The Sociology of Physical Disability and Rehabilitation. University of Pittsburgh Press, 1976, pp. 73–97.

21. Fordyce, W.: Behavioral methods in the rehabilitation process. In Eisenberg, M., and Falconer, J. A. (Eds.): Treatment of the Spinal Cord Injured: An Interdisciplinary Perspective. Springfield, Ill., Charles C Thomas, Publisher, 1979, pp. 82–100.

22. Gendlin, E., and Rychlak, J.: Psychotherapeutic processes. Ann. Rev. Psychol., 21:155–190, 1970.

23. Golden, C.: In reply to Adams' "In search of Luria's battery: A false start." J. Consult. Clin. Psychol., 48:517–521, 1980.

24. Golden, C., Purisch, A., and Hammeke, T.: The Luria-Nebraska Neuropsychological Battery: A manual for clinical and experimental uses. Lincoln, University of Nebraska Press, 1979.

25. Hanford, D.: Life crisis viewed as opportunity. The Bulletin. Division of Mental Health, State of Washington, 9(2):87, 1965.

26. Hebb, D.: The Organization of Behavior. New York, John Wiley and Sons, 1949.

27. Hecaen, H., and Albert, M.: Human Neuropsychology. New York, John Wiley and Sons, 1978.

28. Heilman, K., and Valenstein, E. (Eds.): Clinical Neuropsychology. New York, Oxford University Press, 1979.

29. Ince, L.: Behavior Modification in Rehabilitation Medicine. Springfield, Ill., Charles C Thomas, Publisher, 1976.

30. Kerr, N., and Meyerson, L. (Eds.): Psychological intervention in a spinal cord injury center. Rehabil. Psychol., 22:165–211, 1975.

31. Krasner, L.: Applications of token economy in chronic populations. In Token Economies: Current Status — Future Directions. Symposium presented at the Meeting of the American Psychological Association, San Francisco, September, 1968.

32. Krasner, L., and Atthowe, J.: Token economy bibliography. In Token Economies: Current Status — Future Directions. Symposium presented at the Meeting of the American Psychological Association, San Francisco, September, 1968.

33. Krasner, L., and Ullmann, L. (Eds.): Research in Behavior Modification, New York, Holt, Rinehart and Winston, 1966.

34. Lezak, M.: Neuropsychological Assessment. New York, Oxford University Press, 1976.

35. Lindsley, O., and Skinner, B.: A method for the experimental analysis of the behavior of psychotic patients. Am. Psychol., 9:419–420, 1954.

36. Marr, J., and Means, B.: Behavior Management Manual: Procedures for Psychosocial Problems in Rehabilitation. Arkansas Rehabilitation Research Training Center, Hot Springs, Ark., 1981.

37. Meyerson, L., Kerr, N., and Michael, J.: Behavior modification in rehabilitation. In Bijou, S., and Baer, E. (Eds.): Child Development: Readings in Experimental Analysis. New York, Appleton-Century-Crofts, 1967, pp. 214–239.

38. Michael, J.: Management of Behavioral Consequences in Education. Inglewood, Cal., Southwest Regional Laboratory for Educational Research and Development, 1967.

39. Michael, J.: Rehabilitation. In Neuringer, C., and Michael, J. (Eds.): Behavior Modification in Clinical Psychology. New York, Appleton-Century-Crofts, 1970.

40. Patterson, G., and Guillion, M.: Living with Children. Champaign, Ill., Research Press, 1968.

41. Premack, D.: Toward empirical behavior laws: I. Positive reinforcement. Psychol. Rev., 66:219–233, 1959.

42. Reese, E.: The Analysis of Human Operant Behavior. Dubuque, Iowa, William C. Brown, 1966.

43. Reitan, R.: A research program on the psychological effects of brain lesions in human beings. In Ellis, N. (Ed.): International Review of Research in Mental Retardation. New York, Academic Press, Inc., 1966.

44. Reitan, R., and Davison, L. (Eds.): Clinical Neuropsychology: Current Status and Applications. Washington, D.C., Winston, 1974.

45. Schlesinger, J.: Laterality and myth continued. Am. Psychol., 35:1147–1149, 1980.

46. Siller, J., and Chipman, A.: Attitudes of the Nondisabled Toward the Physically Disabled. New York University School of Education, 1967.

47. Siller, J., Ferguson, L., Vann, D., and Holland, B.: Studies in reactions to disability. Vol. XII. Structure of Attitudes Toward the Physically Disabled. New York, New York University School of Education, 1967.

48. Skinner, B.: The Technology of Teaching. New York, Appleton-Century-Crofts, 1968.

49. Skinner, B.: Verbal Behavior. New York, Appleton-Century-Crofts, 1957.

50. Staats, A.: A case in and a strategy for the extension

of learning principles to problems of human behavior. *In* Krasner, L., and Ullmann, L. (Eds.): Research in Behavior Modification. New York, Holt, Rinehart and Winston, 1966, pp. 27–55.

51. Trieschmann, R.: The psychological, social, and vocational adjustment in spinal cord injury: A strategy for future research. Final Report, RSA, 13-P-59011/9-01, April, 1978.

52. Ulrich, R., Stachnick, T., Mabry, J.: Control of Human Behavior. Glenview, Ill., Scott, Foresman and Company, 1966.

53. Ulrich, R., Wolfe, M., and Dulaney, S.: Punishment of shock-induced aggression. J. Exp. Anal. Behav., 12:1009–1015, 1969.

54. Wallace, J.: An abilities conception of personality: Some implications for personality measurement. Am. Psychol., 21:132–138, 1966.

55. Walsh, K.: Neuropsychology: A Clinical Approach. New York, Churchill, Livingstone, 1978.

56. Woodbury, B.: Psychological adjustment to spinal cord injury: A literature review. Rehabil. Psychol., Monograph Issue, 25:115–174, 1978.

57. Wright, B.: Disabling Myths About Disability. Paper presented at the meeting of the National Society for Crippled Children and Adults, Denver, September, 1963.

7

PSYCHOSOCIAL DIAGNOSIS AND SOCIAL SERVICES — ONE ASPECT OF THE REHABILITATION PROCESS

HELEN J. YESNER

RATIONALE FOR PSYCHOSOCIAL CONCERNS IN REHABILITATION

In order to understand the importance of the psychosocial aspects of diagnosis and treatment in rehabilitation, it might be helpful to restate the definition of rehabilitation. For the purposes of this chapter rehabilitation is defined as a treatment process designed to help physically handicapped individuals make maximal use of residual capacities and to enable them to obtain optimal satisfaction and usefulness in terms of themselves, their families, and their community. Rehabilitation may result in restoring the patient to complete independence and functioning, or it may mean only partial restoration. In some cases rehabilitation goals may include as the best adjustment for the patient only a life of dependence upon others. In a situation of this kind, helping the patient develop as much self-dependence and self-help as possible would be desirable along with helping the patient make a con-structive adjustment to these extreme limitations.

One of the values of our society is that all persons should be able to lead satisfying lives. We know that the well-being of a society is related to the well-being of its individual members. A satisfying life is achieved when basic needs are met and when the individual has opportunity for self-realization in a socially constructive way. Needs are universal in all people but are expressed and gratified in various and individual ways depending upon the culture in which the individual lives out his or her life. Illness and disability interfere with gratification of needs and with self-realization and, therefore, prevent to some extent a satisfying life. Rehabilitation is a means for helping the disabled individual make the most of his or her capacities for wholesome gratification of needs and self-realization. This means maximal physical restoration, more comfortable acknowledgement of the disability, alteration in goals, a substitution of new satis-

151

factions for old, and development of new or unused resources.

Successful rehabilitation demands a highly individualized treatment process based on a full and complete diagnosis of the physical disability and physical functioning of the patient as well as prognosis regarding ultimate physical outcome. The psychological and social functioning of a patient along with the environment and life situation cannot be disregarded. The diagnosis and problem identification, which must go beyond the mere gathering of facts, requires an assessment of facts in order to clarify the interrelationships of the various aspects of the patient's personality, situation, and condition. The potential resources of the patient must not be ignored. Indeed, at times, untapped resources must be explored and exploited. Ultimately, it is the patient, the family, and the community that must be considered, involved, and utilized.

Therefore, the rehabilitation process must use the knowledge and skills of many professional disciplines working together, and it must include the use of community services and resources.

The social worker is the professional who is most competent to perform this type of psychosocial assessment. Social work is a profession whose major concern and arena of work are the interactions of individuals, families, and small groups with the other physical and social systems common to all humanity. The functioning of the microsystems are affected by and have impact on the macrosystems.

In considering psychosocial diagnoses and social services in rehabilitation, it is important to keep in the forefront two major factors. Rehabilitation is a process concerned with all sexes and all ages and encompasses work with individuals who have suffered many and varied illnesses, traumas, and congenital defects that have resulted in impaired physical functioning. In all instances the process has a psychosocial component that must be considered and frequently dealt with to achieve the goals of rehabilitation.

PSYCHOSOCIAL ASPECTS OF DISABILITY

Approach to the Patient. In keeping with the current comprehensive nature of medical care and of rehabilitation, it is essential to view the patient in terms of his or her social functioning, past and present. We all recognize the interrelatedness of the physical, psychological, and social aspects of people. Trouble, disease, or malfunctioning in one area will have their effects in other areas. Thus it becomes imperative to consider the patient's physical functioning, the patient's feelings about it and about self, the patient's relationships to others, and the milieu in which he or she lives and functions. In other words, the physical illness or disability must be viewed not only in terms of its effect upon physical functioning, but also in terms of how it has affected the overall life of the patient. Conversely, it is important to consider how social and psychologic functioning affect adjustment to physical illness and disability. There is a direct relationship between the severity of the disability and the degree to which social functioning is impaired. If the disability is such that extensive residuals remain, one can anticipate an increase in social problems. Further, if the patient has had previous difficulty in social functioning, if social functioning has been at a rather low level, one can expect the patient to have greater difficulty in coping with a severe physical disability and in making use of rehabilitation services.

If the central physical problem is congenital or genetic in origin or occurred during any one of the early life stages that all individuals must pass through and master in order to develop normally to maturity, the patient has most likely had to cope with unusual stress. This intense stress has compounded the normal stress generated at critical life periods in any individual's development and may have interrupted or distorted the normal social and psychological growth processes.

It is also important to consider in the case of ill or disabled children how the increased demands of providing care for, adjusting to, and accepting a disabled or different child may have placed unusual demands upon family members. Experience and research indicate that premature babies and children born with birth defects or suffering critical and chronic illnesses are often most vulnerable to neglect and abuse by parents unless immediate social and psychological support have been made available and utilized.

In working with patients who are adults, life stages continue to be important. Each stage has its normative tasks. For example, in evaluating and treating a young adult early in marriage with a spouse and very young children, one must understand that a recent severe disability has quite different impact and implications than it does in an older person. In the case of the younger person, there is greater demand for participation in family life, often fewer financial resources but also greater resilience, often a more intact support system, and in general a more optimistic outlook. This is not always true, of course, for each situation is different, with its own potential for hope and growth and its own burdens and barriers to be worked on and overcome. So much depends upon the individual's internal strengths and external supports.

In the case of the older person, disability occurs in a life stage in which many individuals are facing stresses of aging, fewer natural support systems, less energy and hope, and thus diminishing capacity for coping.[24]

One aspect of family interaction that must be considered is the impact on children of a disabled parent. This is a crisis for the entire family system, may involve separation, and will have critical impact on children's growth and development. Work must focus on needs of children in the family as well as on the patient.[6]

It is important in the process of a social assessment to consider the history and development of a disability. For example, if the patient has recently experienced severe trauma resulting in quadriplegia, one needs to question how the patient and family were treated during the crisis situation and during the acute phases of the condition and treatment. What was the patient's response in this early phase, and to what extent were the family members supportive? What support system was utilized? One must question and seek to understand the patient's stage in the process of grasping, denying, and accepting the actual condition and possible outcome. This is the essential base for starting the assessment and social treatment process.[9]

Organizing and Assessing Materials. Probably one of the most useful ways of organizing and assessing the complex materials involved in determining any individual's well-being is to attempt to assess the patient's functioning as a social being. Social functioning refers to the effectiveness with which the individual fulfills the many life roles. These roles may include that of marital partner, parent, child, worker, community member, and, in the case of illness, patient. Werner Boehm states, "Social functioning, then, is the sum of the roles performed by a person. . . . One value in the role concept is that it permits identification of affected areas of social functioning."* In applying this concept to rehabilitation, it is necessary to formulate the psychosocial diagnosis in terms of the social roles the patient has ordinarily carried. Further, it is essential to assess the effectiveness with which the patient has carried these roles and to clarify the effect of the disability on the usual role-carrying responsibilities. In turn, it is vital to consider the probable impact of the role-carrying responsibilities on the disability and on treatment.[15]

Probably a more inclusive approach to psychosocial assessment is the problem-solving model. The many steps in this model include problem identification and problem assessment, including identification of major systems involved in and related to the problem. Assessment can include role theory and role dysfunction cited above. The problem-solving model involves active involvement of all systems pertinent to problem identification and solution, e.g., patient, family, caretaking team, and treatment team, as well as actual and potential resources. The problem-solving model involves establishment of goals within a therapeutic relationship with the patient and leads to a contract between the patient, significant others, and members of the team in working toward problem solution. This model not only enhances the assessment process and enables greater focusing, but also allows for use of a goal-attainment scale in evaluating outcome.[25]

It is the social worker's responsibility to determine the model to be utilized, to gather the kind of information needed, and to make the social assessment so that the rest of the rehabilitation team can be helped to bring into focus the effect of the disability on the patient and his or her situation, and the effect of the patient and his or her situation on his or her disability. This assessment is also the

---

*Boehm, Werner: The Social Casework Method in Social Work Education. Vol. X in Social Work Curriculum Study. New York, Council on Social Work Education, 1959. Quoted on p. 374 in Perlman.[15]

basis for social treatment. The role concept concentrates on areas of difficulty in social functioning and provides direction for the gathering of additional pertinent information.[15] The problem-solving approach is more comprehensive and can encompass not only role dysfunction but all significant aspects of other areas of social functioning or dysfunctioning.[25]

As was stated previously, health is a basic need. Illness or disability interferes with the gratification of this need. In addition, illness and disability usually produce increased dependence upon others and arouse fear and uncertainty. These internal reactions, these emotions, immediately affect the individual's equilibrium and, in turn, affect social functioning.[1]

Attitude of the Patient. Many patients are able to use medical treatment effectively. They are well motivated and eager to achieve as much restoration as possible. Other patients find secondary satisfaction in illness and disability because of neurotic and immature attitudes. The first patient will need facilitating help primarily; the second will need help in growing up and finding more appropriate kinds of satisfactions. The amount of help and kind of help needed will in part depend upon how radical the effect of the illness or disability is upon the patient and the situation.[20]

For example, take the case of a patient who has suffered quadriplegia as the result of an accident. The patient soon discovers that he is unable to use any of his limbs. He is unable to control elimination. He is almost totally dependent upon others. In some respects he is like an infant. He is frightened, he may be angry, and very likely he is depressed. He is at least subjectively aware that he has lost a large measure of control over his own life. Internally he begins to wonder whether people care enough about him to give him the very intimate and personalized attention he now needs. To a large extent his present insecurities will be either magnified or diminished by his previous life experiences. Knowledge of these previous life experiences can be helpful in understanding his current reactions. Regardless of his past experiences, it can be anticipated that he will not be able to cope immediately with the catastrophic change in his physical functioning. However, his level of maturation,

his particular personality organization, and his overall situation will in large measure determine the ultimate outcome.

In our contemporary world we have gone beyond the obvious and externally observable impact of disability upon the patient. We have finally acknowledged that all aspects of life functioning must be considered, assessed, and treated. One area long neglected has been that of sexual functioning. In many disabilities sexual functioning may not be affected other than for those psychological and social barriers that may be encountered. In some disabilities there are physical barriers to normal sexual functioning. This area of functioning is an essential consideration in the psychosocial assessment process and social treatment.[26-28]

We do know that this patient will not immediately respond to his family as he did formerly, nor will he respond positively, in all cases, to treatment personnel. Because of his fear of death, his fear of almost total dependency, his fear of loss of family role and of possible repudiation by the family, he may withdraw and become extremely passive or extremely hostile.

Attitude of the Patient's Family. As a result, the family, wishing to cooperate, may feel threatened, confused, and even antagonistic. They may be tangibly threatened by income loss, particularly if the patient has been the main source of income. In those cases in which the patient is either married or emotionally and sexually involved with another person, concern about sexual function is often of paramount importance — particularly as the patient and his partner contemplate their future.

This aspect of functioning should be dealt with in adolescent and younger patients with the goal of preparing the individual for honest, open consideration of sexuality and adaptations that will be required. These factors could increase family tension. Such an antagonistic dialectic could produce an increase of the difficulties. It takes no leap of the imagination to see, from this oversimplified example, that the patient's response to treatment could be affected. Further, with this patient, it is essential to take into account the fact that he will be dependent in some measure upon others the rest of his life. Thus it becomes essential to consider not only the current psychosocial aspects of the patient and his situation but also the long-range psychosocial prognosis.

The Social Worker's Approach to the Patient's Problems. To help this patient involve himself and respond positively to treatment, intervention on several levels must take place. In addition to the medical diagnosis and treatment, both psychosocial assessment and social treatment must now be considered by the social worker. In addition to casework treatment, the social worker may need to use other modes of treatment or involve other social workers with these competencies. These interventive modes include group work treatment and community organization. In other words, treatment must be focused on interrelated medical and psychosocial problems. The social worker will attempt (1) to gather a social history; (2) to compile and assess data about the family situation; (3) to study the patient's current responses and functioning; and (4) to assess and analyze all this material, including information derived from other professional sources, so that a psychosocial diagnosis can be made. Further, the social worker, while engaged in the diagnostic process, will try to help the patient and family resolve their conflicts and their environmental difficulties (provide support and, wherever indicated, develop a working contract toward future goals).

Summary. In summation, the psychosocial aspects of disability must be considered in terms of the patient, the family, and the total life situation. Disability can mean temporary or permanent dependence upon others. It may mean dependence upon others for physical care as well as for economic and social support. It may mean temporary or permanent change in role responsibilites for the patient and for family members. These effects, inasmuch as they are crucial and stressful, must be seriously considered in the treatment of any disabled patient. Finally, any disability has its impact on the psychosocial aspects of the patient and total life situation. The impact may be relatively benign, one that the patient and family can handle with little outside help, or the disability could cause considerable dislocation. Then more extensive help will be required, particularly in the area of psychosocial functioning.

SOCIAL WORK AND REHABILITATION

The social worker is the professional whose central concern is with the social functioning of people in relation to their life problems. Through training and experience the social worker has developed knowledge and skills in working with people in the solution of their social problems. Social work concepts take into account the interrelatedness of physical, social, and emotional factors in the precipitation of social breakdown. Illness and disability come within the purview of physical causes of social breakdown. Since the social worker is committed to helping people lead socially satisfying, useful lives, he or she fits very logically into the physical rehabilitation effort. As a profession, social work has developed methods for working with individuals, groups, and communities in the solution of their social problems. Even though some rehabilitation agencies offer social group work services as well as casework services, for the purposes of this book, we will consider primarily the social casework method and the role and function of the social caseworker in rehabilitation. Social group work, community organization, social policy, and administration are all important methods that have been developed by social work professionals for helping people solve their problems and bring about change in their personal and communal lives. All these methods play a part in the rehabilitation process and all should be considered in greater depth than is possible here.

Social group work should be utilized as extensively as possible in rehabilitation facilities. We do know that many individuals move faster and more effectively in treatment when helped through the group process. Groups can be problem-oriented or can be focused on self growth and development. The group process can enhance milieu therapy, can improve the quality of institutional life, and can help the patient move more quickly toward return to life in the community, to his or her family, or to a more permanent life situation.

Self-help groups have become a major instrument for problem solving and coping with major disabilities. Group experience in the rehabilitation setting should help the patient prepare for this type of participation and should at a minimum help the patient to consider whether or not this is a viable resource.[29]

THE FUNCTION OF THE SOCIAL CASEWORKER IN REHABILITATION

The social caseworker has six major functions in rehabilitation: (1) to participate in the psychosocial diagnostic effort; (2) to give social casework and other social services; (3) to offer consultation to the treatment staff concerning the psychosocial functioning of the patient; (4) to influence the team as a group regarding their attitudes, feelings, and objectives toward and concerning the patient and his or her family; (5) to influence social policy development and social policy changes within the institution and the community toward a more satisfying quality of life for all; and (6) to function in developing effective liaison between the rehabilitation agency and the larger social welfare community.

Psychosocial Diagnosis

The psychosocial diagnosis serves two purposes. First, it contributes to an overall team diagnosis that becomes the basis for rehabilitation goals and treatment. Second, it serves as the basis for determining psychosocial problems and social treatment so that the social worker can fulfill his or her part in the total rehabilitation service in the achievement of rehabilitation goals.

The psychosocial diagnosis and assessment in a rehabilitation setting is threefold. It comprises study, assessment, and evaluation. First, a study must be made of the social functioning of the patient, of the family functioning and relationships, and of the pertinent cultural, social, and environmental factors that are immediately related to the patient's rehabilitation problem. Then an assessment must be made of the patient's strengths, capacities, motivations, and difficulties in functioning. Finally, the diagnostic process demands an evaluation of the interaction of all these factors (cause and effect must be considered) for the purposes of determining the central problem or problems and to establish goals with the patient. Skill-

ful utilization on the part of the social worker of this threefold process — study, assessment, and evaluation — can facilitate physical rehabilitation.[30]

Sources of Information. The social worker draws upon many sources of information to arrive at a psychosocial diagnosis. These sources include social agencies familiar with the patient and his or her family, records of previous contacts with the rehabilitation agency, medical and other treatment personnel currently working with the patient, the patient, and the patient's family. In addition, the social worker's own experience with the patient is a valuable source of information. The patient in almost every case is the best source of information about self and the situation and can provide information that will be most effective in furthering the rehabilitation process. For the most part, diagnosis and evaluation of treatment in social work are based on clinical observations, information collected from others, and case-by-case analytical judgments. This method continues to dominate practice.

Currently client-worker evaluation of outcome based on original goals remains the most frequently used means of evaluation. Professional judgment of worker's and client's views of outcomes are significant and important in the evaluation process. Goal attainment scaling and single case research are other means of attempting to measure outcomes.

Evaluation on a single case basis remains at a somewhat primitive level. In social treatment there are so many forces and variables at play that it is difficult to arrive at conclusive outcomes related to specific interventions. Program evaluation is at a more sophisticated stage but can only speak to groups or classes of cases, services, etc., and not to the individual case.[31]

Clarification of the Social Situation. By utilizing as many of these sources and techniques as possible, the social worker can attempt to clarify the patient's immediate social situation, such as living arrangements, family relationships, financial situation, the effect of the disability on the patient, employment history, educational background and achievement, and in general the patient's level of social functioning. The social worker very specifically attempts to comprehend the patient's feelings about the disability and the nature of the patient's motivations in seeking rehabilitation services. It is essential to determine how the patient has coped with physical limitations, how he or she has adapted to previous stress situations, and what the present condition means to him or her. It is important to clarify family interaction, including family reaction to the patient and the patient's disability. It is also important to know the resources within the family and the impact of the patient's disability on the family functioning and situation. The diagnostic effort must be geared to understanding the meaning of all the significant details of the patient's situation. This diagnostic effort is a continuous one that begins with the admission of the patient and ends only when the patient is considered rehabilitated.

Diagnosis on the part of the social worker carries with it the responsibility for interpreting and sharing this diagnostic material with the rest of the rehabilitation team and for participating with the team in the establishment of rehabilitation goals and treatment. As a member of the team, it is very important that the social worker draw on his or her knowledge of the small group process to help promote teamwork and to meet his or her responsibilities for contributing to and influencing the team's work with the patient.

Social Treatment Services

In rehabilitation, social treatment involves primarily work with individuals, families, and small groups, as was stated earlier. The author will focus primarily on work with individuals and families, recognizing that work with small groups is and can be an important part of social treatment in the rehabilitation process. For purposes of this presentation, work with individuals and families will be referred to as social casework.

Social casework is a problem-solving process. It is the professional method that the caseworker uses in helping an individual in some area of social functioning. Helen Perlman, in her book, *Social Casework,* has described social casework as "a process used by certain human welfare agencies to help individuals to cope more effectively with their problems in social functioning." She described the social casework process as "a progressive transaction between the professional helper and the client (patient). It consists of a series of problem-solving opera-

tions carried on within a meaningful relationship. The end of the process is contained in its means: to so influence the client-person that he develops effectiveness in coping with his problem and/or to so influence the problem as to resolve it or vitiate its effect."[14] In addition, the social worker may influence not only the problem but also the situation so that, for all practical purposes, the effects of the problem are reduced or made more manageable. Furthermore, help with a particular situation may free the person so that he or she can cope more effectively with the problem. For example, the placement of a homemaker may relieve the anxiety of a disabled mother to such an extent that she is freer to contemplate what is expected and required of her in the rehabilitation program. Before the placement of the homemaker she may have been extremely anxious about what was happening to her children because of lack of care and supervision. Preoccupation with this concern could reduce her capacity to participate in treatment. Thus, change in situation, or manipulation of environment, may reduce stress and free the patient to cope more effectively with a central problem.

Another example of environmental assistance is arranging for a caretaker through medical assistance, enabling a severely disabled person to undertake independent living, vocational and educational training, and eventually engagement in a remunerative occupation.

Helping the Patient. The social worker is frequently called upon to help encourage the patient to understand his or her condition. Sometimes internal stress interferes with this. The caseworker, by supportive measures, may reduce the sense of threat, and this can facilitate the patient's participation in treatment and, therefore, facilitate restoration. If stress arises primarily from external difficulties, the social worker can help deal with these difficulties. For example, if the patient is concerned about the financial status of the family, he or she may find it too threatening to consider the permanent nature of his or her disability. The social worker can help the patient and the family consider ways of meeting their financial problem. One of the ways might be to make application for public assistance or total and permanent disability if covered by Social Security. The combination of support and tangible help quite often is enough to enable the patient to begin to take appropriate action to improve his or her condition and, as a result, the situation. Frequently casework help may involve working not only with the patient but also with the family, and often the major help is given to the family. In fact, in every situation in which the patient is a part of a family, the patient and the family should be viewed and worked with as a unit. Much has been written about the value and methods of working with families as units, and, whenever possible, this should be attempted as a part of the rehabilitation process.

Social work help is social in its very process. The help emerges as a result of a professional relationship that is focused on meeting the needs of the patient and on eliciting maximal participation and involvement of the patient in the solution of problems identified.

Social casework is the means for providing the social services offered by the rehabilitation agency. These services include direct help to the patient in utilizing the therapeutic services of the agency, help in coping with the immediate situation during rehabilitation, and help in planning for the future after discharge. At any point in treatment the caseworker may refer the patient or family to other agencies in the community for help with problems that cannot be dealt with in the rehabilitation setting.

The Interview. Basic to all social casework treatment is the relationship between worker and client (patient). The major tool in treatment is the interview, which presupposes the establishment and development of this relationship. Social casework treatment usually involves a series of interviews that are both diagnostic and therapeutic in their focus. Once the initial diagnosis has been achieved, the social caseworker establishes certain mutual and relevant goals with the patient and proceeds with the treatment according to a plan they have agreed upon.

Casework Treatment Methods. Casework treatment usually involves one or both of the following methods: (1) *providing support* and (2) *encouraging change.* The supportive method helps the patient through times of stress so that he or she can function at maximum while engaged in solving crucial life problems. This type of treatment does not envision basic changes in personality

functioning but merely seeks improvements in it. Of course, indirectly, this type of treatment could foster maturation and, as a result, could bring about a change in personality functioning. In the supportive method, the caseworker always employs supportive techniques such as *reassurance, logical discussion, advice and guidance,* and *intervention.* The supportive method would always be concerned with the patient's troubled feelings about self, about the disability, about the situation, and about anything else that interferes with his or her use of treatment and the solution of current problems.

The second type of treatment envisions modification in certain areas of personality functioning that interfere with the solution of problems. This type of treatment combines the use of supportive measures with an attempt to clarify with the patient inappropriate patterns of behavior. By clarification of these inappropriate patterns of behavior, the patient may develop enough insight so that a change in functioning can occur. This type of treatment is employed only when personality function seriously impairs problem-solving and when ego strength seems adequate to tolerate insight.[8]

Crisis theory is a useful theory in the early stages of work with the patient and family, and also at any time additional crises occur during rehabilitation. Social workers have developed effective ways of working and intervening at times of crisis.[12]

Consultation

The social worker shares with all members of the rehabilitation team the responsibility for providing consultation to members of other disciplines. Consultation involves the giving of expert advice, information, or insights related to the treatment of the patient. The social worker's advice is sought on the basis of competence and knowledge about psychosocial aspects of the disability that affect the patient and his or her situation, or vice versa.

Liaison Between Rehabilitation Agency and Larger Social Welfare Community

The social worker is the professional who probably has the most complete knowledge of community social welfare resources. As such, he or she should be the team member responsible for referring the patient and family to the appropriate community resources. In helping a patient and family consider community resources it is important for the caseworker to give enough information about these resources so that they can decide which ones they can best use. At this point the caseworker may have to help the patient and family overcome their feelings of discomfort in making application to a new and different resource.

The caseworker may also have to facilitate the referral by taking appropriate actions. The caseworker's activity depends in part upon the adequacy of the client and the family. In some instances they are able to take a great share of the responsibility in making application to a new resource; in other instances, they may need a great deal of help. This may include such specific aids as a telephone call to the agency, an appointment, a letter of referral, and sometimes a conference with the new agency. In general, people have considerable anxiety about asking for assistance. This must always be taken into consideration in helping the patient consider community resources. The patient must be helped at all times to maintain a sense of worth and of adequacy.

WHEN SHOULD A PATIENT BE REFERRED TO SOCIAL SERVICE?

This question is related in part to the administrative structure and organization of a hospital or rehabilitation facility. In many rehabilitation settings each patient is seen by a member of the social service department at the time of admission. This policy reinforces the current concept of the interrelatedness of the physical, psychologic, and social functioning of a person in the rehabilitation process. As a result the social worker, even though he or she is not working intensively with all patients, is usually familiar with all the patients' situations and can become involved whenever a patient seems to need assistance. In this kind of setting it is helpful if the non-social work staff will alert the social worker to any current problems of a psychosocial nature that the patient seems to manifest so that the social worker can determine whether active involvement is necessary.

In most hospitals for the acutely ill the social service department sees patients only upon referral by other staff or upon request of the patient or family members. In this kind of organization the medical and treatment staff must be unusually sensitive to the psychosocial impact of disability and illness and, in turn, the impact of psychosocial problems or illness and disability and on the treatment of these conditions. A referral to social service should be made in any case in which (1) the patient seems to be reacting inappropriately to the illness or disability, (2) the patient seems unable to cope with the illness, disability, or treatment, (3) family relationships or family problems impinge upon the patient's use of medical care, or (4) the patient's illness and disability create overpowering problems for the family. In general, the social worker can be helpful to the patient in those situations in which the patient's attitude interferes with the use of treatment and in which the actual treatment situation seems to have created conflict for the patient and is, therefore, obstructing treatment. All cases in which there are tangible environmental problems such as a financial need or the need for homemaker service, foster home care, or nursing home care should be referred to the social worker. In fact, all illness or disability has a social and psychologic aspect.

HOW TO REFER PATIENTS TO SOCIAL SERVICE

When a patient is to be referred to social service for help, it is advisable to discuss the referral with the patient. It is important that the referring person clarify with the patient the reason for referral so that the patient has some understanding of why the social service worker has been called in. There may be a few exceptions to this. For instance, it may be impossible to explain the need for referral to a person who is psychotic or mentally incompetent. In the case of children, especially when the social worker will be working more directly with the family, no explanation may be necessary.

Needless to say, the social worker has a responsibility through actions and interpretation to help patient and family understand what can be expected of this service.

COMMUNITY RESOURCES COMMONLY USED IN THE REHABILITATION PROCESS

The community resources can be divided into public and private agencies. Public agencies are supported through tax funds and are under the sanction and auspices of some branch of the government. Private agencies are voluntary in their organization and financing and usually have the sanction of certain groups in the community. The public welfare agencies offer a wide range of services, including aid to dependent children whose fathers are disabled, dead, absent from the home, or, in some states, unemployed. The Social Security Administration administers help to the disabled, aged, and blind through Supplemental Security Income and provides Social Security and Medicare for those covered. Medical assistance administered by the county welfare boards in most states covers those unable to provide for medical care and supplements Medicare when this is insufficient. Most communities provide some form of general assistance that serves to meet the economic needs of all residual problem situations not included in these categorical groups. General assistance could include help to single, unattached individuals under the age of 65, help to families when the head of household is unemployed, or help to any persons or families not covered by categorical aid programs or SSI, or may supplement SSI when the need exists.

Most communities provide additional funds for medical care through state or local hospitals and, in some instances, through private facilities, depending upon eligibility.

Public Welfare Agencies. Departments of *public welfare* offer services to dependent and neglected children in the form of family treatment, guardianship, protection, foster home, and adoption programs. Departments of public welfare also provide for care and supervision of the mentally retarded and the mentally ill. Public welfare agencies provide protective services for adults, counseling, and family services. In some instances they may contract for services with a third party such as a specialized private agency. *State boards of education* provide special services to children who suffer some type of handicap. Public resources include *vocational rehabilitation programs* that are sponsored jointly by federal and state governments. Also under public agencies are *court services* and *probation offices*. The *Veterans Administration* provides many services for veterans, including medical, psychiatric, and rehabilitation care, and also administers disability compensation programs and pension programs. In addition, state and local groups may provide for subsistence needs of veterans and their families. Community mental health centers should also be considered as resources of help to the patient and family.

Mainstreaming in most public schools is mandated and provides for inclusion of disabled and/or handicapped children in classrooms with normally functioning children.

Private Agencies. In most medium-sized or larger urban areas a wide range of social services are available through private agencies, including *social casework counseling* to families who are experiencing parent-child problems, marital difficulty, or problems in normal functioning because of either mental or physical illness of one of the parents. Services in this instance might include *homemaker service* or *foster home care,* as well as *counseling services.* In addition, many communities offer mental hygiene and child guidance services. They may offer institutional care or residential group home treatment for disturbed and delinquent children. Many rehabilitation agencies are sponsored by private groups; we see examples of this in the *curative workshops* and *out-patient physical rehabilitation services.* Privately sponsored resources include a wide range of health agencies such as the *Cerebral Palsy Association,* the *National Society for Crippled Children and Adults,* and the *American Heart Association.* Some communities have developed day care and treatment programs for homebound disabled and in some instances, provide community support systems for persons able to undertake an independent living program. Group homes and community-based care centers have emerged as resources for many types of living in or treatment care.

Long-term care facilities have increasingly focused and specialized in the provision of total care for severely disabled, often grouping them by ages or type of care needed.

The Rehabilitation Act of 1973, Public Law 93–112, mandated environmental requirements, services, and freedom from prejudiced treatment and did much to improve life for the disabled.

WHAT IS THE TRAINING FOR THE SOCIAL WORKER?

Professional social work training involves a two-year graduate course in an accredited school of social work. Satisfactory completion of this course leads to a Master of Arts or Master of Social Work degree.

Professional training for social work involves theoretical courses in human growth and behavior, community organization, administration, research, social policies and programs, social group work, and social casework. The training program provides for heavy concentration in the following areas: dynamics of normal and pathological growth and behavior, social policies and programs, and primary methods courses, such as social casework or basic generalist practice courses. Throughout the two-year training period the student is enrolled in field training for instruction in one of the following concentrations: work with individuals, families, small groups and grass root community group or administration, policy analysis and development, planning, and community development. The field training instruction is provided for in a social agency or in an allied host agency such as a hospital or rehabilitation setting. Each student has experience in two different types of settings during the two-year period. At this point, social work training curricula are undergoing great changes, as are all the helping professions. Instead of being organized around primary methods, the curriculum is frequently organized around concentrations and target populations. Many schools of social work are moving to a strong core with specializations such as work in health settings, etc. Schools are also developing joint degree programs such as Social Work and Public Health.

REFERENCES

1. Bartlett, H. M.: Social Work Practice in the Health Field. New York, National Association of Social Workers, 1961.
2. Bartlett, H. M.: The widening scope of hospital social work. Social Casework J., 44:3–10, 1963.
3. Cooper, R.: Social work in vocational rehabilitation. Social Work, National Association of Social Workers, 8:92–98, 1963.
4. Family Service Association of America: Methods and Process in Social Casework. New York, Report of a Staff Committee, Community Service Society of New York, 1958.
5. De Wolfe, A. S., Barrell, R. P., and Spaner, F. E.: Staff attitudes toward patient care and treatment-disposition behavior. J. Abnorm. Psychol., 74(1):90–94, 1969.
6. Romano, M. D.: Preparing children for parental disability. Social Work in Health Care, 1(3):309–315, 1976.
7. Grosser, C. F.: Changing theory and changing practice. Social Work, 5:16–21, 1969.
8. Hollis, F.: Analysis of casework treatment methods and their relationship to change. Smith College Studies in Social Work, 32:97–117, 1962.
9. Weller, D. J., and Miller, P. M.: Emotional reaction of patient, family and staff in acute-care period of spinal cord injury. Social Work in Health Care, 2(4):369–377, 1977.
10. Ludwig, E. G., and Adams, S. D.: Patient cooperation in a rehabilitation center: Assumption of the client role. J. Health Soc. Behav., 9:322–336, 1968.
11. National Association of Social Workers, Medical Social Work Section: Report of Subcommittee on the Medical Social Worker in Rehabilitation. New York, Committee on Medical Social Work Practice, 1957.
12. Parad, H. J.: Crisis Intervention: Selected Readings. New York, Family Service Association of America, 1965.
13. Parks, A. H.: Short term casework in a medical setting. Social Work, National Association of Social Workers, 8:89–94, 1963.
14. Perlman, H. H.: Social Casework: A Problem Solving Process. Chicago, University of Chicago Press, 1957.
15. Perlman, H. H.: The role concept and social casework: Some explorations. 1. The "social" in social casework. Social Service Review, 35:370–381, 1961.
16. Rapaport, L.: The state of crisis: Some theoretical considerations. Social Service Review, 36:211–217, 1962.
17. Simon, B. K.: Relationship theory and practice in social casework. Monograph IV in series. Social Work Practice in Medical Care and Rehabilitation Settings. New York, Medical Social Work Section, National Association of Social Workers, 1960.
18. Specht, H.: Casework practice and social policy formulation. Social Work, 13:42–52, 1968.
19. Thomas, E. J.: Behavioral Science for Social Workers. New York, Free Press, 1967.
20. Thomas, E. J.: Selected sociobehavioral technologies and principles: An approach to interpersonal helping. Social Work, 13:12–26, 1968.
21. Upham, F.: A Dynamic Approach to Illness. New York, Family Service Association of America, 1960 (reprinting).
22. Vernick, J.: The use of the life space interview on a medical ward. Social Casework J., 44:465–469, 1963.

23. Wright, B. A.: Physical Disability — A Psychological Approach. New York, Harper and Brothers, 1960.
24. McDowell, F. H.: Rehabilitating patients with stroke. Postgrad. Med. 59:145–149, 1976.
25. Compton, B. R., and Galaway, B.: Social Work Processes. Homewood, Ill., Dorsey Press, 1975, pp. 5–50, 223–274, 446–471.
26. Comarr, A. E., and Gunderson, B. B.: Sexual function in traumatic paraplegia and quadriplegia. Am. J. Nursing, 75:250–255, 1975.
27. Eisenberg, M. G., and Rustad, L. C.: Sex education and counseling program on a spinal cord injury service. Arch. Phys. Med. Rehabil., 57:135–140, 1976.
28. Hanson, R. N., and Franklin, M. R.: Sexual loss in relation to other functional losses for spinal cord injured males. Arch. Phys. Med. Rehabil., 57:291–293, 1976.
29. Singler, J. R.: Group work with hospitalized stroke patients. Social Casework, 56:348–354, 1975.
30. Berkman, B.: Innovations for social services in health care. In Sobey, F. (Ed.): Changing Roles in Social Work Practice. Philadelphia, Temple University Press, 1977, pp. 92–125.
31. Wood, K. M.: Casework effectiveness: A new look at the research evidence. Social Work, 23:437–458, 1978.
32. Bracht, N. F.: Social Work in Health Care: A Guide to Professional Practice. New York, Haworth Press, 1978. Part I — "Scope of Social Work and Its Contribution to Health Care," pp. 3–36; Part III — "The Interprofessional Team as a Small Group," pp. 85–108; Part IV — "Assessing the Psychosocial Effects of Illness," pp. 111–136.
33. White, R. B. (Ed.): Approaches to Health Care, Proceedings of the 1976 Medical Social Consultants Annual Meeting, Johns Hopkins University, School of Hygiene and Public Health, Department of Maternal and Child Health, Baltimore, Maryland, 1976.

8

VOCATIONAL ASSESSMENT AND MANAGEMENT

GARY T. ATHELSTAN

DEFINITION AND SCOPE OF VOCATIONAL REHABILITATION

Since rehabilitation services were first established in America by an Act of Congress in 1920, employment has been their primary goal. The Act defined rehabilitation as "the rendering of a person disabled fit to engage in a remunerative occupation."[1] Consequently, governmental support for rehabilitation services has been justified by a financial equation: rehabilitation saves more than it costs, since service recipients become taxpayers instead of tax consumers.

The vocational emphasis of rehabilitation programs was reaffirmed when the medical rehabilitation research and training centers were established in 1961 and placed under the direction of the Office of Vocational Rehabilitation.

Over the years, both the definition of disability and the goals of rehabilitation have broadened. The original act was concerned with disability "by reason of a physical defect or infirmity." Now disabilities due to mental illness, mental retardation, and certain social disadvantages are included. In the 1960s, the goals of rehabilitation were expanded to encompass "(restoration of) . . . the handicapped individual to the fullest physical, mental, social, vocational and eco-nomic usefulness of which he is capable."[2] Even within that broadened framework, however, the disabled person was required to show potential for work in order to be eligible for services.

The Comprehensive Rehabilitation Services Act of 1978 added independent living as a goal. Employment continued to be the desired outcome of rehabilitation services, but did not need to be an immediate objective. Thus, persons who appeared initially to be too severely disabled to work were nevertheless eligible for government-supported rehabilitation services to help them live and function independently in their family or community. The growing concern with the quality of life of disabled persons[3] appears likely to eliminate eventually the "vocational feasibility test" as a criterion of eligibility for services.

The Importance of Work

The importance of work is stressed in the economic goals of the state-federal vocational rehabilitation system. It is also reflected in the value our society attaches to productivity and the negative social and psychological consequences that unemployment has for the individual. Thus the welfare of the pa-

163

tient dictates that the physician consider employment as a possible goal of rehabilitation. Sir Ludwig Guttman, a British pioneer in the rehabilitation of patients after spinal cord injury, wrote:

> The most gratifying result of the return of a paraplegic to useful life, apart from the beneficial effect upon both physical condition and mental outlook, is the realization that employment is essential to human happiness. In this connection it may be noted that many paraplegics with military or industrial pensions, to whom employment may not be essential from a financial point of view, recognize that it is essential for their well being.[4]

Much has been said in the years since that statement about the declining importance of work in our modern "leisure society." Nevertheless, in our society a person's identity, social status, and feelings of self-worth are still often based upon occupation. Prolonged unemployment can be psychologically and socially devastating, even when disability provides a socially acceptable excuse. For these reasons, the physician must always ask at the outset, "What is the effect of disability on this person's ability to work, and how can that effect be ameliorated?"

The Structure of Vocational Rehabilitation Services

State vocational rehabilitation agencies, variously called departments, divisions, or bureaus of vocational rehabilitation, are the primary sources of vocational services for handicapped people. Governed by federal legislation and state administrative plans, and funded mainly by federal money, the agencies in every state conduct rather similar programs of services under the direction of the Rehabilitation Services Administration.

The principal service provider in the state agency is the vocational rehabilitation counselor, who usually has a master's degree or some graduate level training in that specialty. The counselor's functions include vocational evaluation, counseling, coordination of restorative and training services, and job placement. In many agencies, these functions may be divided among a number of specialists.

When a disabled person is referred to the state agency for services, the counselor must make a series of judgments about whether the disability constitutes a vocational handicap, the likelihood of benefit from services, and what can be done to help the individual to achieve independent living or employment. These judgments require medical information, and the formulation of a vocational plan may depend upon medical consultation and further restorative or medical rehabilitation services.

To prevent delay in obtaining consultations and services, many hospitals and medical rehabilitation centers maintain an office for the state agency counselor. This can expedite referrals and permit early initiation of vocational planning. Medical and vocational rehabilitation services can also be closely coordinated. To further facilitate continuity of services, some treatment centers employ their own rehabilitation counselors.

While the state-federal program is the main element in the rehabilitation system, there are also numerous voluntary agencies. The private sector has grown rapidly in recent years, as the carriers of worker's compensation and disability insurance have sought to reduce their costs by employing their own rehabilitation personnel or by contracting directly for services from private providers. Also, a number of large, self-insured business and manufacturing firms have developed their own in-house rehabilitation programs.

Most private rehabilitation agencies provide specialized vocationally oriented services, such as work evaluation, work adjustment training, long-term sheltered employment, and job placement. Many are subsidized by the state agencies and provide most of their services under contract to state agency counselors and insurance companies.

VOCATIONAL ASSESSMENT

Rehabilitation goals must be as specific as possible. If the patient is of working age, the goals should usually include employment. Consequently, accurate assessment of vocational capabilities and potential will frequently be an essential component of the medical rehabilitation process.

As soon as possible after onset of disability, judgments must be made about whether the patient will be able to work and, if so, at what kind of job. Such judgments have implications for compensatory training, use of adaptive equipment, surgery, and other treatment procedures. Planning for employment will also influence the expectations of both the patient and the rehabilitation team. Patients who assume that they will work after completing rehabilitation and are reinforced in that assumption have the best prospects for success.

For the disabled worker who had been employed previously, it may be of critical importance to give the employer an early estimate of vocational potential. Such information can facilitate a return to the previous job or to a different job with the same employer.

The primary responsibility for determination of vocational disability and assessment of vocational potential belongs to a specialist such as the vocational rehabilitation counselor or counseling psychologist. However, it is clear that the physician and every other member of the rehabilitation team contribute to an accurate assessment. Moreover, the physician often plays a central role in deciding when a vocational expert is needed and how that person should be involved in the rehabilitation process.

Assessing the Whole Person

In general, the best predictor of future behavior is past behavior. Thus, vocational potential can be estimated best on the basis of past vocational achievement. However, a disability may impose so many limitations on the individual as to prevent or greatly change the application of skills and abilities that were previously vocationally useful. Moreover, the young rehabilitation patient may have very little history that relates to vocational questions.

For these reasons, assessment must include a thorough review of the patient's past nonvocational performance — in school, hobbies, sports, social groups, or any other activities involving behaviors that may relate to employment. Assessment must also include analysis of the person's abilities, skills, interests, and social and physical environment, and of the disability and the limitations it imposes. Attention must be given to the

ways in which the limitations of a disability interact with all of the other characteristics of the individual and his environment.

In this connection, the physician must keep in mind the distinctions among impairment, disability, and handicap. An impairment is a residual limitation resulting from a congenital defect, a disease, or an injury. Evaluation of an impairment is the function primarily of the physician.

A disability exists when an impairment causes an inability to perform some major life function, such as self-care, mobility, communication, or employment. The judgment as to whether an impairment constitutes a disability is not exclusively a medical one, since that judgment requires consideration of the whole person, including such factors as abilities, skills, and the possibilities of adaptation. Unfortunately, the distinction between impairment and disability is not always recognized, and the existence of an impairment is sometimes taken as *prima facie* evidence of disability. This confusion leads to problems in the medical-legal system in connection with disability determination and compensation proceedings, and in the self-definitions of people with impairments who may be motivated to be considered disabled.

A handicap results when a disability interacts with the environment to impede the individual's functioning in some area of life, such as work, travel, or fulfilling family or other social roles. The importance of the environment in defining a handicap can be illustrated by considering the paraplegic who is confined to a wheelchair. Such a person has a disability, but would not be handicapped at all with regard to mobility in an architecturally accessible environment.

INFORMATION NEEDED FOR ASSESSMENT

As indicated previously, an adequate vocational assessment requires information about all aspects of the individual and his circumstances. However, some personal characteristics, such as abilities, skills, interests, and physical capacities, have special vocational relevance. In what follows, these factors and the principal means of measuring them will be more fully discussed.

Abilities

Abilities are the presumably innate capacities for performance that relate to proficiency in a wide range of activities. They should be distinguished from skills, which are the demonstrated proficiencies in performance resulting from training or practice. Abilities represent a potential for performance in the future and may set limits on ultimate achievement in an activity; however, they relate mainly to the speed of acquisition of a new skill. Thus, the person with high ability in a particular area will generally learn a new skill more quickly than the person with low ability, as well as possibly attain a higher level of proficiency.

Abilities are measured in order to make predictions about the likelihood of success in training or in a job that requires the development of new skills. The relationship of ability to success in school or work is not a simple one in which more ability ensures more success; rather, it appears that most complex activities have an ability threshold. Success may demand that a person possess the relevant abilities beyond a certain minimum level, but once the minimum is surpassed, other factors, such as motivation, perseverance, or personality, are more important.

Two kinds of ability are considered to have vocational relevance. One is general ability, often referred to as general intelligence; the other is special ability, which is synonymous with aptitude. In common usage, the terms ability, aptitude, and skill are often used interchangeably to denote any indication of proficiency in an activity. However, the correct definitions are different and it is both meaningful and important in rehabilitation practice to maintain a clear distinction between skill on the one hand and ability or aptitude on the other.

Research on the structure of ability has not produced a consensus on the number and composition of different aptitudes. Vocational counselors are concerned mainly with those that have been demonstrated by empirical research to be relevant to job performance. Only about a dozen aptitudes meet this criterion.

One of the most widely accepted systems for classifying and measuring abilities has been developed by the United States Department of Labor. The Department's studies have found nine basic aptitudes to be important in training and job performance. These are measured by the General Aptitude Test Battery (GATB) in a testing program carried out by the Employment Service.

The Department of Labor has also analyzed a very large number of jobs with regard to their ability requirements. Continuing studies produce regularly updated information about the ability characteristics of workers in relation to their performance on the job. Thus, norms are available that enable the vocational counselor to evaluate a person's abilities in relation to a wide variety of different jobs.

The aptitudes measured by the GATB comprise the principal components of ability considered important in work.

Intelligence, or general learning ability, is the ability to "catch on" or understand instructions and underlying principles. It includes the ability to reason, to solve problems, and to make judgments, and is closely related to doing well in school.

Verbal aptitude is the ability to understand the meaning of words and to use them effectively. It includes the ability to comprehend language, to understand relationships between words, and to understand the meanings of whole sentences and paragraphs. Verbal aptitude is generally the most conspicuous or easily recognized ability and is frequently the basis for casual judgments about intelligence. However, its significance as a predictor of success is largely limited to performance in school and in highly verbal occupations.

Numerical aptitude is the ability to perform arithmetic operations quickly and accurately. Numerical and verbal aptitude together are the primary components of general intelligence as measured by the GATB.

Spatial aptitude is the ability to think visually of geometric forms and to comprehend the two-dimensional representation of three-dimensional objects. It includes the ability to recognize the relationships resulting from the movement of objects in space. Spatial aptitude is an important component of mechanical ability, which is not in itself considered a basic aptitude, but has elements of several different basic abilities.

Form perception is the ability to perceive pertinent detail in objects or in pictorial or graphic material. It includes the ability to make visual comparisons and discriminations and to see slight differences in shapes and shadings of figures and widths and lengths of lines. Together with spatial aptitude, form perception is important in the skilled trades and many other occupations involving fabrication or assembly. This aptitude is probably also a component of mechanical ability.

Clerical perception is the ability to perceive pertinent detail in verbal or tabular material. It includes the ability to observe differences in copy, to proofread words and numbers, and to avoid perceptual errors in arithmetic computation.

Motor coordination is the ability to coordinate eyes and hands or fingers rapidly and accurately in making precise movements. It is also the capacity to make a movement response accurately and swiftly.

Finger dexterity is the ability to move the fingers and manipulate small objects rapidly and accurately.

Manual dexterity is the ability to move the hands easily and skillfully. It includes the ability to work with the hands in placing and turning motions that also involve the wrist.

There are other dimensions of ability, such as artistic, mechanical, and musical aptitude, which the counselor might assess for specific purposes. Many cognitive abilities, such as judgment, abstract reasoning, and several kinds of memory, may be important in job performance, but occupational norms have not been developed for them. Extensive research shows that the nine GATB aptitudes account for much of the variance in abilities for which vocational relevance has been established.

Whenever there are questions about a patient's capacity for vocational planning, the assessment of abilities must be thorough. Considerable variation is common in brain-damaged persons, and even the normal individual may possess widely varying levels of different abilities. Therefore, it is not safe to assume that either a very high or a very low level of functioning in one area, such as verbal ability, will be accompanied by similar levels in other areas.

Brain injury producing severe impairment of some aspect of ability that is critical in vocational functioning or in everyday life, but that leaves verbal ability intact, is especially frequent. Such cases are often difficult for the physician to detect, because the patient may communicate well and appear normal in a brief encounter, but have memory,

judgment, or other cognitive deficits that rule out competitive employment.

Skills

Skills are the learned proficiencies that comprise the major part of every person's repertoire of vocational behaviors. Abilities underlie and influence the development of skills, but skills represent an achieved level of performance.

The skills a person possesses at the time of assessment are among the most important factors in determining immediate employment prospects. However, disability often impairs skills or prevents the application of those that are still intact. For example, an auto mechanic who has become paraplegic may possess highly developed manual and mechanical problem-solving skills but be unable to employ them in his usual occupation because of the climbing, reaching, kneeling, and other gross bodily movement the work involves. In such cases, identification of transferable skills becomes crucial in vocational rehabilitation.

Whenever a disability requires a change of occupation or limits an initial occupational choice, retraining or special training is often considered. However, vocational assessment should look first at skills that can be transferred from a prior job to a new one. After all, the goal of vocational rehabilitation is to return the person to productive activity as soon as possible. Even when retraining is feasible, the expense in time and money may not be justifiable if the patient already has skills that can be applied in a new combination or under different environmental circumstances in a new occupation.

Every job involves some skills that potentially can be transferred, even if they are as basic as the capacity to understand and follow instructions. With higher level intellectual skills, such as reading, writing, and oral communication, it is usually possible for a person with almost any physical disability to engage in some kind of remunerative employment.

Skills are assessed mainly by history of an individual's accomplishments in school, in the labor market, and in other areas of life. Information about skills is thus usually obtained by interview or through review of written records. If useful information cannot be obtained by interview or from records, job tryouts in work evaluation may be necessary to accurately assess skills.

Most persons possess a wide variety of skills that they have acquired throughout life, not only in work, but in school, avocational activities, and everyday living. This fact has gained wide recognition in recent years as large numbers of homemakers have sought to re-enter the labor market after many years of not being employed outside the home. Such persons were long believed to be handicapped by lack of vocational qualifications, but economic necessity and improved vocational assessment have led to a greater appreciation of the value of the organizational and managerial skills acquired in homemaking. Equally sensitive assessment is needed with disabled persons.

Interests

Interests should be given as much attention as other factors in vocational assessment. However, many rehabilitation professionals appear to implicitly discount interests when a person's options are restricted by disability, since limited alternatives reduce one's chances of obtaining satisfying employment. However, such assumptions should not limit the planning process. Disabled people should have just as much opportunity as the able-bodied to seek realization of their interests. Rehabilitation professionals should provide whatever resources will help make that possible.

The vocational significance of interests appears to reside primarily in their relationship to occupational choice and tenure. People tend to move toward, and to stay longest, in occupations that are consistent with their vocational interests.[5] They tend to move out of occupations that do not fit, presumably because of the part that satisfaction plays in long-term vocational behaviors. Consequently, vocational planning that is guided by accurate assessment of interests can help the disabled make choices that will contribute to both occupational stability and self-fulfillment.

Interests must be measured in the same careful, professional manner as any of the other vocationally relevant qualities of the individual. Most people are able to describe their interests specifically, and it is common practice to take such self-descriptions at face value. However, there is good evidence that stated interests are strongly influenced by limited or inaccurate information and by social and occupational stereotypes. As such, they are not necessarily accurate predictors of occupational satisfaction nor a valid basis for career choice. The vocational counselor tends to place more weight upon standardized measures of interests that correct for such influences and have had their validity established by empirical research.

Physical Capacities

Physical capacities should be assessed in functional terms, rather than in medical or diagnostic terms. This serves several purposes. First, a functional analysis provides the kind of information the vocational counselor needs to determine whether the patient can meet the physical demands of particular jobs. For example, some counselors will have a general idea of what a person with complete C6-7 quadriplegia can and cannot do, but it is necessary to know the extent of the person's independence in transfers and wheelchair use, sitting tolerance, nature and strength of grip, and other such details of physical functioning.[6]

Secondly, the lack of functional precision in even those diagnoses that have an air of exactness argues for a functional approach. A vocational counselor may be very familiar with C6-7 spinal cord injuries but still needs to know precisely where the patient falls in the widely varying distributions of specific physical capacities possessed by such quadriplegics.

Finally, a functionally oriented evaluation of the patient is likely to be less negative or restrictive in its implications than any other approach. A thorough functional assessment will indicate what the patient *can* do, as well as what limitations are present. Specification of remaining abilities is not merely an affirmation of a positive rehabilitation philosophy; it is absolutely essential to the provision of adequate vocational rehabilitation services.

Several systems have been devised to facilitate the physician's evaluation of physical capacities, but most yield information that is of limited value in vocational planning.

Therefore, it is probably most helpful if the physician remembers to be thorough and to describe capacities and limitations in everyday language as they relate to common physical activities.

The physical functions that are important in many jobs include mobility, ambulation, upper extremity and hand function, coordination, motor speed, strength and endurance, and the ability to bend, lift, reach, handle, and feel. In quantifying these capacities, vocational relevance is more important than precision or the type of measure used. Thus, for example, it is more helpful for the vocational counselor to know how many yards or blocks the person can walk or propel a wheelchair without resting, and how long that takes, than to know walking speed in meters per minute. Strength might best be expressed as the ability to repetitively lift weights of 5, 25, or 50 pounds, endurance as the ability to be up and active in a job for two hours, a half day, or a full day, and so on. Similarly, it is less useful for the counselor to learn the degrees of limitation of motion in a person's knee joint than to know that the particular limitation makes it impossible for the person to kneel or climb a ladder. The experienced counselor will often put questions to the physician in exactly these terms, but it is helpful for the physician to be oriented to these aspects of physical function at the time of evaluation.

Other Factors Affecting Vocational Potential

Motivation for Work

The patient's interest in employment is probably the most important single determinant of a return to work. In this connection, rehabilitation professionals often place great importance on the concept of "motivation." Patients are usually categorized as either "motivated" or "unmotivated," and the "unmotivated" patient may be subject to urgent exhortations aimed at increasing motivation. In fact, no patient is ever devoid of motivation. The problem arises when the patient's motivation is different from what the rehabilitation professionals believe it should be.

Most rehabilitation patients are motivated primarily to regain whatever physical function they have lost because of their disability. Patients may be concerned about the impact of disability on their earning capacity, social relationships, and many other areas of their life. However, usually their first wish is simply to recover. This is especially true during the early stages of rehabilitation, while the patient is still in the hospital and focusing all attention on medical treatment. In fact, at this stage of rehabilitation, the patient may not have grasped yet the permanence of the disability and its implications for psychosocial and vocational functioning. Although this can be a critical time for vocational intervention, the vocational counselor is often at a serious disadvantage in attempting to initiate vocational rehabilitation procedures.

Some patients remain uninterested in employment throughout the rehabilitation process. Indeed, it is not unusual to find that the person disabled by a work-related injury was in vocational trouble before the onset of disability. In such cases, it may appear that the disability provided a socially acceptable escape from an intolerable work situation, and it is possible that psychological factors contributed to the onset of the disability. This is sometimes especially evident in instances where unusual accident proneness appeared in the work setting or where psychological components are obvious in "functional overlay," which influences the type and extent of the disability.

Finally, despite the importance of employment to the identity and morale of most people, it is clear that many people simply do not much enjoy working. For some people, work is a major source of satisfaction; for others, it is a necessary unpleasantness. In general, people will work if they have to; but, in the absence of financial necessity, some people would prefer not to. In this connection, Social Security Disability Income, Worker's Compensation payment, and other sources of compensation or support for disabled persons often act as disincentives for employment.

Financial and Psychological Disincentives

Much attention has been given in recent years to the various financial disincentives that work against effective rehabilitation. One of the major problems is that most of the compensation or support systems work with rigid definitions and criteria, and according to inflexible rules. For example, until recently, a person had to be judged "totally and permanently disabled" for any remunerative employment in order to be eligible for Social Security payments. The concepts of permanence and totality seem unreasonable when both individual potential and the environmental circumstances that create a vocational handicap may change. Moreover, the psychological impact on the disabled individual of being labeled "totally and permanently disabled" may contribute to a self-fulfilling prophecy.

Most of the services or financial benefits for disabled people place the burden of proof for eligibility on the applicant. Thus the individual is required to "prove" not only the existence of a disability, but the extent of its handicapping effects, in order to obtain assistance. In behavioral terms, this creates a contingency in which a certain degree of helplessness is the most likely route to reward. Ongoing litigation concerning a personal injury or other cause of disability creates a similar contingency. The anticipated or real size of the settlement of the lawsuit may be directly related to the degree of handicap demonstrated.

Another major problem with the sources of financial support for handicapped persons is that they are treated either as compensation or as a substitute for an earned income. It is very difficult to use such support flexibly in conjunction with a positive program aimed at helping the individual get back to work. For example, benefits may be terminated very soon after return to work, thus creating a major financial risk if the job does not last. Another problem is that some sources of financial support are provided on an all-or-nothing basis and cannot be used to supplement a person's income or to help meet some of the expenses that may be part of the cost of employment for a severely disabled person.

Age and prior work experience are factors influencing future vocational prospects. Up to a point, increasing age is an advantage, since the older person is considered more mature and, therefore, a better employment risk. However, both the very young and the older disabled person are likely to encounter employer prejudice, despite the existence of laws forbidding age discrimination in employment.

Both the quantity and quality of prior work experience affect job prospects. The person who has a "spotty" job history, including frequent job changes and significant gaps between jobs, may be correctly regarded as a poor risk by the potential employer. Similarly, the person who has very little or no prior work experience, and is further disadvantaged by a disability, will have a much harder time finding an accepting employer than will the person with an ample work history.

Family attitudes and beliefs are important. For example, family members may profess to support rehabilitation goals but place subtle obstacles in the way of a return to work if their own needs are met better by having the disabled person remain at home. It is not unusual for family members to believe that the disabled person is too fragile or too disabled to work, or that working entails unreasonable risks to health. Such fears can sabotage the most carefully crafted vocational rehabilitation plan. On the other hand, if the family is psychologically supportive of employment and willing to contribute the time and assistance that may be necessary to facilitate work, most of the tasks of vocational rehabilitation will be much simpler.

The environment of the neighborhood and community must be considered in its relationship to vocational rehabilitation. Very few communities permit easy access by people in wheelchairs or with other mobility impairments. Problems in transportation discourage the kind of mobility needed in many jobs. If the home is not architecturally accessible, it may be easier to stay in it than to leave for work and return each day. In this connection, it may be necessary to evaluate the suitability of the home for home employment.

Small towns and rural areas lack the vocational rehabilitation facilities and services that can be of help to the disabled. They also are less likely to have a range of jobs in different settings, involving a variety of tasks, that might be suitable for handicapped workers.

Of perhaps even greater importance is the lack of social amenities in small towns. Very few offer much opportunity for contact with other handicapped people; social support systems, such as clubs or organizations for the handicapped, are rare. Because of the limited resources for disabled persons in rural areas, relocation may be necessary to permit realization of the individual's full potential.

Timing of vocational rehabilitation intervention is important in several respects. It can be difficult to engage the patient in effective vocational planning or other constructive steps toward re-employment when his energies are focused on medical treatment. Furthermore, the patient must have achieved a reasonably accurate understanding of the nature of the disability and the limitations it imposes, in order to formulate a sensible plan. It is unusual for such an understanding to be reached while the patient is still in the hospital. Some people, especially those with severe disabilities, require months of living at home, "getting used to being disabled," before they are ready to undertake vocational rehabilitation.

Because unemployment itself can constitute a vocational handicap, the need to await patient readiness for vocational rehabilitation must always be balanced against the advantage of an early return to work. Conventional wisdom among vocational counselors maintains that prospects for re-employment diminish steadily over time, to a virtual zero point after five years. However, research on people with spinal cord injuries[7] has not supported this opinion, suggesting, in fact, that employment may never be a completely dead issue. Some persons studied re-entered the labor market after absences as long as 15 to 25 years. Nevertheless, it is clear that considerations of both employer acceptance and patient readiness dictate that re-employment be effected as soon as possible after the onset of disability.

ASSESSMENT TECHNIQUES

The Interview

A correct diagnosis and complete medical evaluation of any disabling condition requires an understanding of its effects on every aspect of the patient's life. Therefore, vocational assessment begins in the first meeting between the physician and a new patient. The routine history and physical examination should give attention to the patient's educational and vocational background, socioeconomic status, lifestyle, and leisure time activities. The individual's behavior in these areas may be related to the onset or to the nature of the medical problem and will certainly have implications for treatment. Moreover, the patient's vocational functioning can be indirectly affected by the impact of disability on other aspects of the patient's life.

Research shows that a work history obtained by interview cannot always be assumed to be accurate.[8] People tend to upgrade their job title, level of responsibility, and income when reporting work history data. In addition, patients tend to tell professionals what they believe professionals want to hear.

Information is more likely to be accurate and significant if it is obtained by narration and asking the patient to "tell his own story." If answers to specific questions are needed, they can always be obtained by following up later, after the patient has made a narrative response to an open-ended question.

The physician should also recognize that work history information will not be very useful unless it includes some behavioral detail, not just a job title. Job titles are unreliable indicators of work activities, since the duties associated with a given job title may vary from one setting to another. For example, the physician might assume that a paraplegic could return to work as a shipping clerk unless it was known that the particular job included lifting and transporting large boxes of merchandise, climbing ladders while stocking and retrieving inventory, and loading and unloading trucks. After learning a patient's job title, the physician should always ask, "Just what do you do in that job? What is your work area like? How does your work come to you?" and other such questions.

Psychological Tests

The vocational rehabilitation counselor or counseling psychologist uses many different tests to evaluate patients' vocationally relevant characteristics as an adjunct to other assessment procedures. Psychological tests provide a basis for making inferences about patients' attributes or predictions about their future behaviors. Although tests measure directly only the behavior involved in taking the test, they substitute for more direct measures of the behavior in which the counselor is interested. At times, heavy reliance upon test data may be necessitated by the limited availability of direct information or by significant change in the patient's attributes due to disability.

The range of tests used includes measures of abilities, skills, interests, and emotional state or personality.

The physician is unlikely to become involved directly in the choice of particular tests or in decisions concerning the timing of testing. However, it is important for the physician to know the purposes, values, and limitations of tests, in order to help create appropriate patient expectations and to encourage cooperation with testing. The physician should also be familiar with the kind of information produced by tests and with the ways in which tests are related to the real world.

A psychological test can be defined as a sample of behavior obtained under standardized conditions, in which the individual's responses to standardized stimuli are recorded for subsequent evaluation. A person's performance is usually quantified in a numerical score, and the significance of an individual's score is determined by comparing it to the scores of other, similar people. This is known as the "normative" approach to evaluation of test performance, and it requires careful adherence to standardized procedures.

One of the best methods of normatively evaluating a test score is to determine its percentile rank in relation to a specific norm group. If a test measures an ability that is significantly related to performance in a training program or an occupation, the percentile rank immediately clarifies the meaning of a score. For example, a clerical aptitude score that stands at the 85th percentile in comparison to employed clerical workers has implications for success in clerical work that are very different from a score at the 10th percentile. A score at the 10th percentile does not necessarily predict failure in clerical work, but would certainly place a person at a competitive disadvantage, since that score is surpassed by 90 per cent of clerical workers. Such a score would suggest careful examination of the specific tasks involved in any clerical job under consider-

ation, followed by selective placement or possibly by special training in clerical skills.

Another advantage of the percentile rank is its uniform interpretation. A given percentile always denotes the same relative standing in a group, regardless of the attribute or the test used to assess it. This is not true of other measures of test performance, such as the IQ, whose interpretation may vary depending on the test and sometimes on the age of the individual tested. For these reasons test reports should usually include the percentile rank of any scores and specify the norms used.

The importance of using norms that are both specific and appropriate can be illustrated by referring to mechanical reasoning ability, for which some occupations are highly selective. For example, a mechanical reasoning score at the 50th percentile against general population norms (i.e., an "average" score) would fall below the 10th percentile on norms for mechanical engineers. Moreover, the difference would not result from the higher educational level or general intelligence of engineers in relation to the general population. In comparison to trade school students in auto mechanics or tool and die making, the percentile rank of such a score would be even lower.

Exactly appropriate norms are not always available, so it is sometimes necessary to approximate from the most relevant ones. For example, a patient's performance may be compared to the norms for students in an architectural drafting training program when norms for employed draftspersons cannot be obtained. However, it is important to remember that the levels of different norm groups may vary greatly, making such substitutions possibly misleading.

In addition to the available norms, the most important qualities of a psychological test are its reliability and validity. Reliability is the ability of a test to measure a patient's attributes consistently. Most psychological tests will show some variation in their measure of a supposedly stable trait from one testing to another. However, if the psychologist is careful to adhere to standard conditions of administration, the extent of variability or unreliability in a test's scores can be rather precisely estimated. It is inappropriate to discuss test scores in terms that imply greater precision than they possess. For example, it is technically incorrect to describe an IQ of 113 as higher than one of 110, since both scores are in the "high average range." On the other hand, it is not reasonable to discount differences that are large enough to be significant, nor to disregard test scores because of their modest reliability.

The validity of a psychological test is determined by the extent to which it measures what it is supposed to measure. Validity is usually expressed in terms of a coefficient of correlation between a test score and some external criterion, such as performance in school or on the job. The most important kind of validity for tests used in rehabilitation is predictive validity.

The validity of most psychological tests is even more modest than their reliability. However, limited validity should not cause test results to be ignored. Test results should not be used to prescribe what a patient *should* do, but they can help suggest alternatives and assist the patient in making decisions about the future.

Most vocational tests are designed for administration to groups in educational settings and personnel selection programs. Consequently, administration procedures make little provision for individual attention, nor for adaptation to the limitations or special requirements of the disabled person. In addition, many vocational tests are timed, so that speed of performance may significantly influence a person's score. Both of these common characteristics of vocational tests limit their use in rehabilitation, especially in the medical setting.

The counselor can sometimes deal with these limitations of vocational tests by finding alternative measures. For example, it may be possible to substitute an untimed test for one with time limits. However, such options are generally limited, because the purposes of vocational testing usually require very specific norms that are seldom available for more than one test. As a rule, a test that lacks relevant norms is not very useful in vocational counseling, even if it accurately measures the attribute of interest to the counselor.

As alternatives, the counselor may delay testing until the patient's condition permits standardized administration, use a test with somewhat inappropriate norms, or rely on other assessment methods. Occasionally, testing may have to be foregone altogether.

This need not block rehabilitation progress, but it can result in delays by forcing the patient to directly explore avenues that could be more quickly evaluated by tests.

Standardization of testing procedures is important because of the effect that conditions of administration can have on performance. If a test is administered under widely varying environmental conditions, or with different time limits or instructions, the performance of individuals will obviously vary. The problem arises in attempting to determine how much of the variation is due to conditions of administration and how much to real differences among the people tested. Also, predictions based on test performance may be invalidated by failure to adhere to standard procedures. This is a frequent problem in rehabilitation, because a patient's physical, sensory, or intellectual limitations may interfere with standardized administration. For example, a test that is ordinarily self-administered may produce different results when the items must be read aloud by the examiner and the responses marked for the patient. Also, the patient's performance may vary from day to day owing to the effects of stress, pain, drugs, and other temporary factors.

These problems do not mean that valid vocational testing is impossible in a medical rehabilitation setting. However, they do impose some constraints on the choice of tests and on the timing of assessment. In addition, the psychologist is sometimes required to exercise special ingenuity to identify and assess the impact of factors that can cause inaccuracy in test results.

Tests Frequently Used in Vocational Assessment

The psychological test library in a comprehensive medical rehabilitation center may contain up to 80 different tests. In practice, however, the counselor will make frequent use of only a few. Many of the tests used in vocational assessment are designed as omnibus instruments that measure simultaneously a number of traits. For example, the GATB covers nine aptitudes; the Strong-Campbell Interest Inventory measures 23 "basic" interest dimensions and has scales for 124 different occupations; the Minnesota Multi-phasic Personality Inventory evaluates

10 major traits and has over 500 special scales for specific aspects of personality or behavior.

Because the patients in a comprehensive medical rehabilitation center usually present a limited range of vocational assessment questions, perhaps 90 per cent of vocational testing will make use of 15 or so different tests, comprising six distinct types: (1) general ability or intelligence; (2) special ability or aptitude; (3) achievement or skill; (4) interests; (5) values or attitudes; and (6) personality. Brief descriptions of each type and examples of some specific tests follow.

General Ability or Intelligence Tests

The Wechsler Adult Intelligence Scale (WAIS) is the most widely used individually administered test of intelligence. It is designed for use throughout the adult age range above 16 years and is available in a similar version for children, the Wechsler Intelligence Scale for Children (WISC). Administration resembles a structured interview in which the subject answers questions, solves problems, and is given tasks to perform. The test must be given by a trained examiner and takes about one and one-half hours to complete, making it expensive to use. However, careful observation of the patient during this test may permit valuable inferences to be drawn about behavior and personality.

The WAIS consists of 11 scales or subtests containing different kinds of tasks. Six of the subtests yield a verbal IQ, based on such tasks as information, comprehension, and vocabulary, while the remaining five, including block design, picture arrangement, and object assembly, produce a performance IQ. Overall ability is represented by the Full Scale IQ. Since educational deprivation, brain damage, or other impairments may affect verbal and performance abilities differently, it is often useful in rehabilitation to be able to evaluate them separately.

Scores can also be obtained on several basic factors that underlie intelligence, such as verbal comprehension, memory, freedom from distractibility, and perceptual organization. Variations among these factors and among the subtest scores are sometimes taken as diagnostic clues to central nervous system problems.

The unit of measurement for the WAIS is the IQ, which, on this test, is statistically designed to have a mean of 100 and a standard deviation of 15. Thus, IQ scores are easily translated into percentile ranks: an IQ of 115 stands near the 85th percentile; 130, at about the 98th; and an IQ of 85 ranks near the 15th percentile.

Because of frequent misunderstanding of the IQ among the general public, it is usually best to describe WAIS performance in terms of percentiles or broad zones, such as "average," "below average," or "above average." It is also desirable to avoid terms that have a value connotation, such as "subnormal," "borderline retarded," "superior," and "genius." The percentile rank is the clearest and most neutral indicator of performance on any ability test, and it should usually be used when discussing performance with a patient or family member.

Since there are no occupational norms for the WAIS, its application in vocational assessment is rather limited. However, WAIS scores are highly related to school performance and to speed of learning in the clinical setting. The test can also contribute to an understanding of the patient's personality, problem-solving style, and specific intellectual strengths and weaknesses. These uses of the test often outweigh its limitations for specific vocational purposes.

Several tests of intelligence have been designed for people with specific limitations, such as the Hayes adaptation of the Stanford-Binet for the blind, the Revised Beta Examination for people with hearing impairment or non-native language background, and the Peabody Picture Vocabulary Test for aphasic and deaf people. There are also a number of nonverbal and other special tests of intelligence. Most of these instruments are rarely used in general rehabilitation practice, but the physician who expects frequent contact with patients having such problems should become familiar with the special tests.

Special Ability or Aptitude Tests

Aptitudes may be tested either by selected single-aptitude tests or by a multi-aptitude test *battery*. The abilities that can be measured range from such complex ones as computer programming, musical aptitude, and sales aptitude, to the more "basic," such as clerical, arithmetic, and spatial aptitude.

Single-aptitude tests are used to answer specific questions concerning a person's chances of success in a particular occupation or training program. General occupational exploration has been completed and counseling is focusing on just one or two options. This allows the counselor to select a single-aptitude test having specific norms and validity that relate directly to the question at hand. Some aptitude tests, devised by large companies to help select workers for particular jobs, may be used before initiating job placement effort.

The principal application of the multi-aptitude test battery is in comprehensive vocational evaluation or initial vocational exploration, when information is needed about the range of the patient's alternatives. A major advantage of the multi-aptitude battery is the opportunity it affords of making intra-individual comparisons. Because all of the tests in a battery have been standardized with the same basic norm group, scores on the different aptitudes can be used to identify a patient's particular strengths and weaknesses.

The General Aptitude Test Battery (GATB) is not only the most widely used multi-aptitude battery; it is one of the most frequently used vocational tests of any kind. It measures intelligence; verbal, numerical, and spatial ability; form and clerical perception; motor coordination; and finger and manual dexterity, the nine basic aptitudes that are described on page 166. The GATB has norms for people employed in more than 400 different specific occupations. The GATB tests are all timed, an important disadvantage in rehabilitation use, since patients are often slowed by pain, medications, or inactivity. However, careful attention to the patient's condition, with some flexibility in the scheduling of testing, can usually avoid any problems with slowness. If a better measure of "power" is needed, a substitute can generally be found, usually in a single-aptitude test.

GATB scores can be evaluated in two different ways. First, the scores on each of the nine aptitudes can be examined and compared. The scores are standardized on the general working population, with a mean of 100 and a standard deviation of 20. Inspection of the "aptitude profile" or list of scores will quickly reveal the individual's strongest and weakest abilities and his standing on each ability in relation to the general population. A second means of evaluating an individual's scores is to compare them to the Occupational Aptitude Patterns (OAPs). OAPs are clusters of aptitudes that correlate with performance in occupations that have similar ability requirements. There are at present 66 different OAPs encompassing approximately 11,000 occupations to which GATB scores have been related. Each OAP has cutting scores for its aptitudes representing the minimum level of ability that is believed to be necessary for success in the occupations within that OAP group. The individual's aptitude profile can be compared to all OAP cutting scores, thus determining the families of jobs for which the person qualifies. Since the cutting scores for occupations within an OAP will usually vary slightly, the suitability of a particular job can be checked by consulting the Specific Aptitude Test Battery (SATB) for that occupation.

The GATB does not assess factors other than ability, such as interests or skills, which may be important to success in an occupation. However, it can be very helpful in opening up possibilities not previously considered.

The Differential Aptitude Test (DAT) is another widely used multi-aptitude test. It has measures of verbal, abstract, and mechanical reasoning, numerical ability, clerical speed and accuracy, space relations, and language usage. However, the DAT is designed primarily for educational evaluation and planning in high schools. It emphasizes abilities that are important mainly in academic activities and it has few norms for adults or for occupational groups. The principal applications of the DAT in rehabilitation would be in educational planning with high school–age patients or in evaluating adults who are considering trade school.

There are other multi-aptitude batteries, such as the Flanagan Aptitude Classification Test and the SRA Primary Mental Abilities, which are sometimes used in vocationally oriented agencies. Also, some agencies and individual vocational counselors have "favorite" tests that they use extensively because of the advantages of familiarity with one test, or because of the needs or characteristics of a particular clientele. However, none of the other tests approaches the GATB in its extensive norms and validation research, nor in its wide applicability.

Achievement or Skill Tests

Large numbers of achievement tests have been developed, mainly for use in schools. Because their different purposes and specific applications are so numerous, no attempt will be made here to describe particular examples. Rather, this section will present the characteristics and uses of achievement tests in general.

Most achievement tests measure academic skills, such as reading comprehension, vocabulary, and arithmetic, or knowledge of specific content areas, such as science, history, and social studies. Some achievement tests have been designed to measure specific vocational skills, but in recent years such tests have been largely supplanted in rehabilitation by work samples or job tryouts in work evaluation.

The most frequent use of achievement tests in rehabilitation is to determine a patient's readiness for vocational training or further general education. Vocational training, even in semiskilled occupations, usually requires the ability to read at a tenth or eleventh grade level. Mastery of eighth grade mathematics is also generally necessary. Training in a skilled trade is likely to demand high school graduate–level achievement in both of these areas.

Even if further training or education is not part of the rehabilitation plan, it may be important to assess a patient's academic skills, since many jobs require eighth to tenth grade literacy. Some jobs with no literacy requirements have application blanks that demand twelfth grade reading ability. Surprisingly large numbers of rehabilitation patients do not possess educational skills at this level.

Academic or educational achievement tests are generally designed to measure skills at specific levels, for example, mathematical achievement among students in grades seven through nine. Because the normal range of achievement varies considerably in different grades, it is important to select the appropriate instrument for the specific testing purpose at hand. This is especially true when the patient is an adult, because adult achievement levels often do not correspond very closely to years of education completed.

Achievement test scores are usually reported in grade level equivalents. For example, a reading comprehension score of 11.2 denotes comprehension at a level that is average for students two months into the eleventh grade in school. Sometimes a percentile rank within a specified grade level is given.

The physician should always ask for thorough interpretation of achievement test data, because the implications may not be obvious, even when the specific meaning is clear. For example, the practical importance of reading skill level is clarified by the fact that most newspapers, including the employment advertisements, are written at about an eleventh grade level of difficulty.

Vocational Interest Tests

Interest tests can contribute greatly to the quality of rehabilitation outcomes by objectively evaluating a patient's likes and dislikes. The information produced by tests can be helpful in exploring avocational possibilities, as well as in selecting an occupational goal.

Among the best known interest tests are the Strong-Campbell Interest Inventory (SCII), the Career Assessment Inventory (CAI), and the Kuder Occupational Interest Survey. Each of these has occupational scales, which compare the individual's likes and dislikes with those of people in selected occupations. The SCII and CAI also have basic interest scales, which measure an individual's *likes* in such general areas as science, nature, art, and athletics.

The Strong-Campbell Interest Inventory is the most extensively used and thoroughly researched of all interest tests. Description of this instrument will illustrate some of the principal features and uses of interest tests. The SCII has 325 items dealing with such things as occupations, school subjects, activities, amusements, and types of people. The individual responds "like," "indifferent," or "dislike" to each of the items, and the responses are scored on both occupational and basic interest scales. There is only one form of the test for both sexes, but the norms for men and women differ. The 124 occupations represented on the SCII are strongly skewed in a professional direction, with many requiring college preparation. The instrument has been criticized for this limitation. However, the Career Assessment Inventory, which is newer, uses the same measurement approach to provide better coverage of occupations with lower educational requirements.

The occuptional scales of the SCII empirically score an individual's responses compared to the responses of various occupational groups. The more similar the individual's likes and dislikes are to those of people in an occupation, the higher will be his score on the scale for that occupation. The average score of an occupational group on its own scale is 50; the average score on that scale of people not in the occupation is about 25.

The SCII does not directly measure interest in an occupation. However, the relationship of interests measured in this way to long-term vocational behavior has been amply demonstrated by research. People tend to enter occupations for which they have high scores (45 and above), and to avoid fields in which they score low (25 or below). People who stay in an occupation that does not fit their interests tend to be engaged in atypical activities. For example, the physician with a low score on the physician's scale will probably be working as a medical administrator, researcher, or medical writer, or engaged in other nonmedical activities.

The SCII also measures a person's interests within broad categories or types, called occupational interest themes. Examples are the artistic, social, and enterprising themes, represented by such occupations as photographer, social worker, and life insurance agent, respectively. A person's occupational theme scores and basic interests provide a basis for extrapolating the test results to occupations that are not represented on the SCII profile. Thus, the SCII and similar instruments can be used very flexibly by the counselor to suggest directions for both vocational and leisure time planning.

Value or Attitude Tests

Most tests of values or attitudes are used by counselors to provide a focus for discussion of personal matters and to assist their clients in gaining better self-understanding. These uses can enhance communication in counseling and facilitate progress in vocational planning. However, the vocational relevance of such tests is generally quite limited. The information they yield relates more to personality and lifestyle than to vocational choice or to questions of vocational success. However, since values and attitudes may influence decisions and behaviors, they can have an indirect effect on the results of rehabilitation.

The Study of Values, developed by Allport, Vernon, and Lindzey and often referred to as the AVL, is one of the oldest and most widely used instruments in this category. It measures the relative strength in the individual of six basic motives or evaluative attitudes: *theoretical,* characterized by interest in discovery of truth and by an empirical, critical, rational, "intellectual" approach; *economic,* emphasizing useful and practical values typical of the businessman; *aesthetic, social, political,* and *religious.* The norms for this instrument are somewhat limited, but include high school and college students and several occupational groups. The value profiles of various samples show differences in the expected directions. For example, medical students score highest on the theoretical scale, theology students in the religious area. Studies also show some relationship between value profiles and academic achievement in areas that correspond to the high value scores, and between values and vocational interests.

The Internal-External Locus of Control (I-E scale) by Rotter is not clearly a value or attitude scale. However, it measures some aspects of an individual's beliefs that are clearly relevant to rehabilitation. The concept of locus of control reflects the perceptions that people have of the relationship between their behavior and subsequent reinforcers. At one end of the continuum are people who believe that chance, luck, or fate are more important than their own behavior in determining what happens to them. At the other end of the continuum are those who perceive reinforcers as contingent mainly on their own behavior or personal characteristics. They believe in internal control.

The scale consists of a series of paired statements dealing with beliefs about locus of control. For example: (a) In the long run, people get the respect they deserve in this world; (b) Unfortunately, an individual's worth often passes unrecognized no matter how hard he tries. The individual selects the one statement from each pair that more closely corresponds to his own view. The inventory contains 29 similar items and the score it yields will place the individual somewhere on the continuum of beliefs. Internal scorers are usually described as more active, independent, effective, and achieving than external scorers. Research on this inventory in rehabilitation settings suggests that internal scorers take more personal responsibility for their treatment and are likely to achieve better outcomes.

The Minnesota Importance Questionnaire (MIQ) is one of a small number of devices designed to measure values specifically related to work. It has 21 scales that measure such vocational needs as achievement, independence, recognition, security, and variety. The MIQ presents a series of statements describing what a person's "ideal job" would be like. The individual ranks the statements within each group to indicate which aspects of a job are most important to him. Examples of the statements are, "On my ideal job . . . the job could give me a feeling of accomplishment" (achievement), ". . . I could work alone on the job" (independence), ". . . I could do things for other people" (social service).

Scores on the MIQ indicate the relative strengths of the different values within the individual. Also, an individual's entire "need profile" can be compared to the profiles of various occupational groups. Similarity between an individual's profile and that of a particular occupational group is believed to predict "probable satisfaction" in that occupation. Extensive occupational norms are available for the MIQ, as well as norms for different groups of students and vocational rehabilitation clients.

Personality Tests

The role of personality measures in vocational assessment is similar to that of most value and attitude measures. There are no vocational norms for personality tests, and the importance of personality in rehabilitation has more to do with overall personal effectiveness, coping skills, and behavior patterns than with questions of vocational choice or specific vocational performance. However, evaluation of coping skills and behaviors is frequently helpful in rehabilitation, and understanding a patient's personality can often facilitate progress in treatment.

There are two schools of thought in psychology concerning personality assessment. One view, held by those with a psychoanalytic or similar "psychodynamic" orientation, advocates the use of projective tests, such as the Rorschach. The other view, sometimes characterized as "empirical," favors objective tests, such as the Minnesota Multiphasic Personality Inventory. The two approaches to assessment are quite different and reflect different concepts of the origins and structure of personality. The language employed by practitioners of these approaches to describe personality also differs. However, research shows that the inferences and predictions of behavior based on the different approaches are of similar accuracy and practical utility.

Because of their lower cost, objective tests are much more widely used in rehabilitation practice, although this varies in different regions of the United States. Most projective tests are individually administered, scored, and evaluated by a licensed psychologist, requiring several hours of professional time. Objective tests, on the other hand, may be administered to groups and can be given by a psychometrician or specially trained clerk. Scoring is entirely a clerical process and is often done by computer. Only evaluation requires the expertise of the psychologist.

Regardless of approach, there is an important caution to observe concerning the use of personality tests in rehabilitation. Most tests have been designed for use in psychiatric settings, to facilitate diagnosis or evaluation of abnormal behaviors. The resulting emphasis on pathology in personality testing is due to habit rather than necessity. With a focus on assets, tests can help to identify the patient's strengths of personality, as well as possible problems.

Rehabilitation patients often experience emotional difficulties because of the stress of disability. However, their rate of mental illness and truly pathological behavior is the same as that of the normal population; they do not need the stigma of a personality description in psychiatric terms added to the burden of disability.

Because of this traditional bias in personality testing, a special effort may be required to balance its potentially negative effects. Therefore, when personality assessment is to be done by a consultant unfamiliar with rehabilitation, the physician should make a point of requesting an evaluation in nonpathological language that includes attention to assets, as well as to problems.

The Minnesota Multiphasic Personality Inventory (MMPI) is not only the most widely used objective test of personality; it is the most frequently used and extensively researched psychological test of any kind. Originally designed as an aid to psychiatric diagnosis, it has nine basic scales that measure such psychiatrically defined traits as hypochondriasis, depression, hysteria, psychopathic deviation, and paranoia. The standard personality profile of the MMPI also includes the trait of introversion-extroversion. Many hundreds of special scales have been developed to assess various aspects of normal, as well as abnormal, behavior. For example, a scale for intellectual efficiency has been devised as a personality-based measure of intelligence.

The MMPI has 550 affirmative statements about one's physical and mental health, attitudes, behaviors, interests, beliefs, self-concept, and relationships with other people. The person being tested responds "true" or "false" to each item to indicate whether it is usually or mostly true or false as applied to himself. Examples of some items are, "I do not tire quickly," "I liked school," "I am happy most of the time," "I believe I am being plotted against," and "My sex life is satisfactory."

Items are grouped into scales on the basis of their ability to distinguish between a "criterion group" having certain defined characteristics or displaying certain distinctive behaviors and the general population. Thus, the hypochondriasis scale includes items to which hypochondriacs respond in a certain way more often than do normals. The original diagnostic or clinical scales, as they are called, were all based on the responses of patients with established psychiatric diagnoses.

Scores on the scales of the MMPI are determined by totaling the number of items to which the individual responds in the same way as people in a selected criterion group. Scores are standardized on the general population, yielding a mean of 50 and a standard deviation of 10. A standard score of 70, at the 98th percentile on general population norms, is usually the level where scores are considered significant in identifying a characteristic of personality, or "abnormal" in psychiatric evaluation.

Although some of the items have frankly abnormal or socially undesirable content and rather obvious intent, MMPI results are not easily distorted. The inventory includes several "validity" scales that measure openness, honesty, and other aspects of test-taking attitude. These scales are quite effective in identifying deliberate attempts at faking and they even provide a sensitive indicator of unconscious or other subtle distortions of responses. As a result, the MMPI can be successfully used in a wide variety of settings and circumstances, even when examinees have little motivation to provide accurate self-reports.

In the years since its original publication, the MMPI has been extensively used in schools, in health care and social service agencies, and in personnel selection efforts. Whenever people are being evaluated or selected for some purpose in which personality is relevant the MMPI has been widely applied. At present, its use in assessment of normal personality characteristics is probably more frequent than its psychiatric or mental health applications.

Many of the special scales of the MMPI have been developed for use in some aspect of medical care: tendencies toward alcoholism or allergies, headache proneness, the "ulcer personality," and rehabilitation motivation. The ready availability of normative data and the established techniques of scale construction make it easy to create new scales for specific applications. In addition, there are extensive MMPI data on specific disability groups, such as patients with spinal cord injury and multiple sclerosis. These data indicate some of the personality characteristics associated with severe physical disability and have contributed greatly to an understanding of psychological reactions to disability.

The California Psychological Inventory (CPI) was derived from the MMPI. Many of the 480 items on the CPI came directly from the MMPI and are still used in their original form, calling for a "true" or "false" response. However, the CPI was designed from the outset to evaluate the normal personality. This is accomplished through the use of 15 scales measuring such traits as dominance, sociability, self-acceptance, and responsibility.

The scales of the CPI were empirically validated; the criterion groups were selected on the basis of displaying certain normal personality traits to an outstanding degree. Thus, the scale for sociability is composed of items that distinguish between students rated "most sociable" and students who lack that trait as rated by the students' peers and teachers. The basic validation of most of the scales proceeded in this fashion, contrasting the responses of people identified on the basis of conspicuous presence or absence of the traits evaluated.

In comparison with the MMPI, the CPI has the advantages of language and topics that are less "sensitive" to most people, and a focus on normal personality. It also has norms for people as young as 13, while the MMPI is of marginal suitability below age 18. The CPI has less research behind it and less information on its use in rehabilitation. However, it is potentially at least as flexible as the MMPI and it deserves to be included in any rehabilitation center's test library.

Referring the Patient for Testing

In preparing the patient for testing, the physician should keep in mind both the strengths and the limitations of tests. Too often, referrals for counseling are made with a statement like, "I am going to send you to the vocational counselor to take some tests and see what you can do." This places an inappropriate emphasis on one procedure when, in fact, tests are usually a small part of the assessment and counseling process. It also tends to subtly reinforce the expectation of many patients that the "magic" of tests will provide all the answers. This can lead to disillusionment with the entire counseling process when hard and fast answers are not forthcoming. Finally, submitting passively to testing and awaiting its "verdict" can diminish the patient's active involvement in other aspects of assessment and planning and contribute to a reduced sense of responsibility for both the process and outcome of rehabilitation counseling.

In keeping with the traditional rehabilitation emphasis on strengths rather than weaknesses, tests should be used in a positive vein, to expand possibilities rather than limit them. However, by specifying a deficit that may virtually rule out certain plans, tests can sometimes prevent frustration and loss of valuable time. For example, I was once asked to evaluate a 40-year-old physician with left-sided hemiplegia due to stroke. Evaluation at another center had seemed to confirm the suitability of his plan to leave his previous practice, which he was physically unable to continue, and enter therapeutic radiology. His memory, verbal ability, and other obvious intellectual capacities appeared intact. However, testing revealed impairment of his mathematical ability, to the extent that he was completely unable to perform the operations involved in calculating radiation dosages. This proved to be irremediable. Unfortunately, he did not fully appreciate the significance of his deficit but was able to conceal it well enough to gain admittance to a residency program. His problem was discovered in time to avert disaster for his patients, but not soon enough to avoid a great deal of anguish for him and others concerned.

When test scores are evaluated by an experienced psychologist or vocational counselor and considered along with information from other sources, they can be highly accurate and meaningful. Their contribution to the planning process can be crucial.

Work Evaluation and Other Observational Techniques

Observation of the patient during participation in a rehabilitation treatment program will yield information regarding qualities such as cooperativeness, the ability to follow instructions, reliability in following schedules or keeping appointments, and ability to get along with others. Qualitative assessments of behavior as related to judgment, memory, impulsivity, and other possible problems can be made. Research on spinal cord–injured patients, for example, has shown that measures of independence, mobility, and diversity of behavior in the hospital are related to community involvement after discharge and to the incidence of medical complications requiring rehospitalization.[9]

Work evaluation is the main observational approach to assessment of rehabilitation patients. It usually consists of a series of situational tests designed to evaluate behaviors of the individual that are not measured effectively by psychological tests or casual observation. The principal uses of work evaluation are to assess work habits, readiness for employment, and tolerance for work. Occasionally, work evaluation is used to determine a patient's interests or skills in certain tasks when psychometrics are not satisfactory.

As indicated earlier, work evaluation is usually carried out in sheltered workshops or other specially designed facilities that can accommodate simulated work settings with a variety of business and manufacturing equipment. However, large, comprehensive medical rehabilitation centers often have work evaluation facilities, sometimes called prevocational evaluation units.

The work samples or tasks used in work evaluation are available in systems or "packages" that can be purchased commercially, such as the TOWER (Testing, Orientation and Work Evaluation in Rehabilitation) and the JEVS (Philadelphia Jewish Employment and Vocational Service Work Sample Battery). Such systems are usually "standardized," which means that there is a prescribed method of administration and "scoring," just as with traditional psychological tests. Also, there are usually norms that permit comparison of the patient's speed and quality of output with those of competitively employed workers, sheltered workers, and hospitalized patients.

The norms provided with commercial work evaluation systems are usually national or otherwise broadly based. However, most work evaluators eventually develop their own norms, which can be related to the standards of local industries that hire handicapped workers.

Work evaluation is often necessary as a supplement to, or substitute for, traditional psychological testing, especially when the patient's motor, intellectual, or behavioral limitations prevent adherence to standardized conditions. Since work evaluation requires individualized observation, it is usually possible to be flexible in changing time limits, physical arrangements, or other conditions of administration.

Work evaluation is not solely an assessment technique. It can also serve as a valuable tool in the management of the vocational rehabilitation process.

MANAGEMENT: THE PROCESS OF VOCATIONAL REHABILITATION

If vocational assessment has been thorough and accurate, most patients will have a vocational objective before discharge from the inpatient rehabilitation service. Ideally, the objective should be clear enough and identified early enough to permit some progress toward it while the patient is still in the hospital. Vocational planning seems most likely to succeed if it starts early and sustains some momentum throughout the rehabilitation process. Such movement is facilitated if the initial steps are taken while the entire rehabilitation team is working with the patient.

Developing a Vocational Plan

The vocational plans made early in rehabilitation need not be firm. Indeed, many factors may preclude definite plans, such as an uncertain medical prognosis or the possibility of major change in financial status, family arrangements, or other aspects of the patient's life. Also, some patients resist planning as a way of denying the reality of their disability. However, plans are needed to guide the treatment program and to establish some landmarks for measuring progress aside from physical restoration.

One way to deal with an uncertain future or a patient's reluctance to plan is to sketch several "what if — — —?" scenarios with the patient. These can provide the frameworks for a series of alternative plans, with the choice of plan depending upon how the contingencies unfold. For example, a paraplegic with an incomplete spinal cord injury may wish to wait for maximum return of function before making plans to change his occupation, even when it is clear that the greatest possible degree of recovery will still necessitate change. Refusing to plan allows him to maintain hope of recovery. The physician could confront such a patient with questions like, "What if you will need a wheelchair to get around after you leave the hospital? What will you do then about your job?" This approach can sometimes ease the implicit threat involved in planning and secure the patient's cooperation "just in case" plans for change are needed.

It is vital to success that the rehabilitation plan be the patient's, rather than the treatment team's. Inevitably, there are differences, especially early in rehabilitation when the patient may be unwilling to work toward anything less than full recovery. However, these differences must and usually can be resolved through a combination of education, counseling, and negotiation.

Success in carrying out a rehabilitation plan is most likely if both the patient and family understand, accept, and actively support the plan. Serious problems can arise when the rehabilitation professionals have imposed their own judgments, values, and beliefs too strongly in planning. This is easy to do despite the best of intentions, since the balance of power and authority is so heavily on the side of the professionals. The danger is that the patient and family may accept the professionals' goals too readily because of unrecognized feelings of intimidation. When this happens, the plan that is launched with ease and enthusiasm by the treatment team may become a nightmare for everyone as it gradually breaks down without meeting anyone's expectations.

Identifying a suitable vocational goal and developing a plan to achieve it may be difficult and time consuming, but it usually requires the direct involvement of only the counselor and the patient. However, implementing the plan may involve the active participation of several members of the treatment team.

Implementing the Vocational Plan

A rehabilitation goal for the patient identifies the steps to be taken to reach the goal. The relationships among assessment, goal setting, and progress in treatment are often complementary, in that goals are identified and refined through a series of successive approximations as limitations become clear and as the patient's hopes and expectations evolve.

The key to successful implementation of a plan is to break it down into small steps, each of which can be easily achieved. This allows the patient to experience frequent success, thus helping to sustain momentum, and it simplifies the measurement of progress as successive steps are accomplished. This approach is especially important if the ultimate goal is unlikely to be reached within a few months of discharge from the inpatient reha-

bilitation program. Employment, in particular, is likely to be a long-term goal, often taking several years for severely disabled patients to achieve.

Psychological and Social Adjustment

Delays in vocational rehabilitation result from the time needed for physical restoration and also from the slowness of psychological and social adaptation and relearning. In a study of paraplegics, Cogswell[10] found that their behavior during the first few months after discharge from initial hospitalization was characterized by a marked reduction in social contacts, in the frequency of entering community settings, and in the number of roles played.

This early post-hospital period seems to the patient like an uneventful time in which the only change is an apparent decline in social functioning as the critically important process of resocialization is taking place. Pre-disability roles and relationships are being discarded, new relationships are gradually being formed, and experimentation with new roles is beginning. The individual gradually ventures out into the community again, first visiting relatively nonthreatening, anonymous public places that are easy to leave. Subsequent outings generally involve increasing risk due to greater intimacy of the settings and the increased difficulty of leaving abruptly. Usually, the last steps in the resocialization process involve private parties, certain kinds of public places such as bars, and places of employment.

This period of resocialization and psychological adaptation entails a high risk of failure for the rehabilitation plan. Both the patient and the rehabilitation professionals are likely to see this as a time of no progress or even regression, failing to recognize the gains that are being made. The danger is that the seeming lack of progress may be taken as a sign of poor potential or insufficient motivation, and as grounds for terminating services. Many severely disabled people may be lost to the system in this manner when their cases are closed due to apparent lack of interest in rehabilitation.

Several things can be done to minimize this kind of failure. The first is to avoid premature termination of services. The responsibility for corrective action belongs mainly to the rehabilitation counselor, because the counselor is usually the professional most involved with the patient during this critical time. However, the physician and other members of the treatment team may see the patient during this period for follow-up care. They, too, should be familiar with the phenomenon of resocialization. The physician, especially, can play an important part in keeping a vocational plan alive by encouraging the patient to maintain or renew contacts with the counselor, even when little seems to be happening.

Steps can also be taken early in rehabilitation, while the patient is still in the hospital, to incorporate a plan for resocialization into the treatment program. Even if no deliberate intervention is planned to facilitate resocialization, giving recognition to it as a necessary and active process can reduce the risk that it will set the occasion for ending the program. If nothing else, everyone involved can be advised of the time that resocialization may take and of the need to remain available but patient during that time. However, it may not be necessary for the treatment team to stand by passively while resocialization proceeds. There is growing evidence[11, 12] that such measures as counseling and social skills training may shorten the duration and improve the results of resocialization.

Preparing the Patient for Employment

For the severely disabled patient, several intermediate steps may have to be taken on the route back to work. These steps include social skills training or other procedures to facilitate resocialization. Enrollment in school can serve this purpose, as well as provide further general education or specific vocational training. In addition, readiness for employment may be enhanced through work adjustment training or sheltered employment.

Work adjustment training is a means of preparing for employment handicapped persons with significant intellectual limitations or behavior problems. Its purpose is to develop an orientation to the world of work and general work-related skills in persons with little or no work experience, or whose capacities have been so changed by disability as to

make their previous work history essentially irrelevant. For example, work adjustment training may aim to develop work habits such as neatness, punctuality, and persistence, to teach the social skills necessary for relating to co-workers and employers, or simply to develop the physical or psychological stamina necessary to tolerate a full day of work. It can be considered a form of treatment for persons who are not initially employable but have the potential to work if their behavior problems or skill limitations can be ameliorated in a work-oriented setting.

Sheltered employment takes place in a controlled environment that is adapted to the special needs and limitations of the workers, under the supervision of staff trained in rehabilitation. The work in sheltered workshops usually consists of manufacturing, assembly, sorting, or packaging jobs obtained through contracts with industry. Some workshops manufacture their own products and have their own retail outlets or distribution channels.

Sheltered workshops provide three essential rehabilitation services: (1) work evaluation, consisting of actual jobs or simulated job tasks to assess work habits and basic work skills; (2) work adjustment training, which usually involves actual work for pay, but with the objectives mentioned above; and (3) sheltered employment, usually intended as preparation for the competitive labor market, but sometimes to provide long-term employment for those whose limitations militate against success in a competitive job.

The Physician's Role

The most important contribution the physician can make to vocational rehabilitation is to ensure that it receives sufficient emphasis in the treatment program. The problem list should consider employment or vocational planning for every appropriate patient. This will include all patients of working age (roughly 16 to 65) whose vocational options or performance might be limited in some way by disability, and any others who express a concern about work. A thorough functional evaluation of the patient provides the counselor with information about functional capacities and limitations as they relate to vocational potential. In consultation with the counselor and perhaps with the occupational therapist and work evaluator, the physician is responsible for decisions about physical restoration that may have implications for a patient's employment potential.

The physician should be careful not to make negative assumptions about the appropriateness of vocational services for some patients, since such assumptions can have a profound influence on the expectations of the patient and the treatment team. For example, severity of disability or age is seldom sufficient, by itself, to rule out employment, and the physician's encouragement of vocational exploration may be of enormous psychological significance.

The physician should avoid assuming that vocational counseling is not needed by the patient who seems to know his interests and states an apparently feasible vocational goal. As indicated earlier, most people's knowledge of occupations is based on stereotypes, and stated interests are not necessarily accurate predictors of vocational satisfaction or success. Incomplete or incorrect ideas about occupational demands could lead the physician to inadvertently reinforce an unrealistic plan, thus seriously impeding vocational rehabilitation efforts. An accurate evaluation of the suitability of a patient's vocational plans requires the same thoughtful application of specialized knowledge and skill on the part of the vocational counselor as does the diagnosis and treatment of a medical condition by a physician.

The physician can play an important part in arousing the patient's interest in vocational rehabilitation by asking directly about the patient's status and plans. Questions such as, "What are you going to do about a job?" or "Have you made any vocational plans?" may raise the patient's anxiety, but can also motivate the patient to face a problem he might prefer to put off. Simply asking about a patient's vocational future also conveys the message that there is one. Such a message may provide valuable reassurance to the patient who has had serious doubts.

Preparing the Patient for Counseling

When referring the patient for vocational counseling, the physician should pay careful attention to the expectations created. It is important for the patient to understand that developing a vocational plan and carrying it out is an active process which demands a substantial commitment of time and energy and for which the patient must take considerable personal responsibility. Such expectations are difficult to establish because they are contrary to much of the patient's experience in treatment. Most of what happens to people in the hospital or other health care setting is "done to" them. Vocational rehabilitation is very different, in that the counselor provides the guidance, the instruction, the technical resources, and some of the psychological support needed for movement to occur, but virtually all of the motivating force must come from the patient. Furthermore, most of the responsibility for the outcome rests with the patient.

Appropriate expectations for counseling can be facilitated by directing the patient's attention to the *process* rather than the outcome. It is best to suggest that "the counselor will talk with you about your vocational possibilities and perhaps help you make some plans," or "the counselor can help you determine what you might be able to do and like to do." Suggesting instead that the counselor will help the patient arrange for school, get a job, or produce any other specific result fails to convey the idea that the process of achieving the desired result may be long and arduous, and that the patient must make a substantial investment of himself in the process. Also, the suggested outcome may not be realistic, owing to limitations of available resources, in the labor market, or in the patient's potential for work. The selection of a realistic goal must be based on a thorough assessment of all these factors. Suggesting specific outcomes for counseling narrows its focus unreasonably. Counseling could lead to other, even better, outcomes, but the patient with specific expectations may be unwilling to consider them. Inaccurate expectations for counseling create a likelihood of disappointment and failure. The physician can avoid such problems by simply encouraging participation in counseling. The patient's questions about possible outcomes should be referred to the counselor.

Unless good communication is established, working with a vocational counselor is often a frustrating experience for the physician because of the differing perspectives of the two professionals. The physician usually expects the counselor to secure employment for the disabled patient. The physician and counselor agree that this expectation is reasonable only for certain patients, but they often disagree on which ones. The patient who responds well to medical treatment is not necessarily a good candidate for employment. The hemiplegic, for example, may be a model patient for the physician, but a source of exasperation for the counselor. Even when the patient has good potential for employment, the physician may be unaware of the obstacles that have to be overcome, and of the time that takes, before the patient can work. The physician may also think of employment as part of treatment, through which many of the patient's problems will be resolved.

Another source of difficulty is the tendency of physicians to measure employment in all-or-none terms; anything less than complete success is viewed as failure. On the other hand, the counselor may regard some degree of productive activity to be a highly successful outcome for certain patients and for others an intermediate step on the way to eventual full employment. Problems that stem from differences in the perspectives of the counselor and physician may be avoided if the counselor specifies an expected outcome of vocational rehabilitation and the steps and timetable needed to achieve that outcome. This defines vocational reality for the physician. The importance of effective communication to the smooth functioning of the treatment team makes it worth considerable effort.

The Counselor's Role

In general, the vocational counselor is responsible for initiating and directing the evaluation, planning, and treatment procedures that relate to the patient's vocational functioning. The details of what the counselor does may vary somewhat depending upon the training of the individual. The vocational rehabilitation counselor is usually trained as a specialist whose expertise is in assessment of disability, vocational evaluation and planning, and coordination of rehabilitation services.

The counselor with a degree in psychology, although he or she may have some specialized training in rehabilitation, is primarily a psychologist. The practice of the counseling psychologist encompasses normal human development, including education, growth of the self, psychological adjustment, and career development. The psychologist may be expected to emphasize psychological assessment and the use of counseling or other psychological techniques to facilitate behavior change in patients. The psychologist will also generally be more interested in the patient's total psychological adjustment, rather than more narrowly concerned with vocational adjustment. When a psychological obstacle to rehabilitation arises, the rehabilitation counselor is likely to refer the patient, while the counseling psychologist is more likely to assume direct responsibility for working with the problem.

It is common practice to refer to the person who is filling the vocational rehabilitation role as the "vocational counselor," or simply the "counselor," regardless of the individual's academic background. Although some counseling psychologists, especially those with the doctorate, may prefer to be identified as psychologists, the term *counselor* is practical and has been used throughout this chapter to denote both professionals. Outside the medical setting, the vocational rehabilitation counselor is usually considered "captain of the rehabilitation team." This is not merely an affirmation of the vocational emphasis of rehabilitation programs; it accurately reflects the central role played by the counselor in planning, directing, and coordinating all of the services included in vocational rehabilitation.

The counselor's interest in medical rehabilitation is usually limited to obtaining accurate medical information and ensuring that the patient will achieve maximum medical benefit before the vocational program is concluded. In addition, the counselor needs a medical evaluation to establish a patient's eligibility for services and to precisely determine physical capacities and limitations.

The counselor treats the patient's disability as only one of the several variables among the skills, abilities, and interests that need to be considered in vocational planning. The counselor's job is simplified if the patient's medical condition is as stable as any of these other variables. If the patient's physical functioning can be stabilized or improved by medical treatment, the counselor may contract with a physician for "physical restoration," which is the general term used by the vocational agencies to denote any medical rehabilitation treatment. Physical restoration may be just one of several specialized services that the counselor will seek from independent professionals, community agencies, and other "service vendors" to help achieve a vocational plan.

Because of the leading role played by counselors in vocational agencies, the counselor who takes a job in a medical rehabilitation setting may have difficulty adjusting to the change in emphasis. Being displaced by a new "captain" of the rehabilitation team and finding that vocational considerations are secondary in the hospital can be distressing to the counselor.

The responsibilities of the vocational counselor often overlap with those of other rehabilitation professionals. In particular, the social worker will share some of the counselor's interest in the patient's family relationships and functioning in the community. Similarly, the clinical psychologist may share the counselor's concern for the patient's psychological adjustment and an interest in the use of counseling and other psychological techniques to induce behavior change. When these other specialists are part of the treatment team, as they often are in a medical rehabilitation setting, frequent communication and careful coordination is needed to ensure that the overlap of professional domains is a source of strength, rather than a hindrance, to the rehabilitation plan.

The counselor is responsible for knowing what vocational services are available in the community, for referring patients to appropriate vocational agencies after discharge from the hospital, and for maintaining liaison with these agencies. The counselor is also usually the only member of the rehabilitation team who has any responsibility for job placement. Since placement involves securing employment that the patient can perform satisfactorily, it entails more than simply "finding a job" for the patient. Placement requires that the counselor know both the jobs and the patients well enough to make good matches between them. A placement must last long enough to give the patient a firm foothold in the labor market. The counselor must also maintain good working relationships with employers who can provide a range of jobs in different settings, suitable for people with a variety of abilities and limitations.

Placement often requires "selling" to the employer the handicapped applicant who is unable to make a convincing presentation of his or her qualifications for work. Few counselors have much taste or ability for sales work. Consequently, in the community vocational rehabilitation agencies, placement is usually handled by a specialist who works directly with employers. Only the largest medical rehabilitation centers can justify having their own placement specialist. However, it is reasonable to expect that the staff counselor will maintain effective liaison with placement services and handle the referral of patients who are ready for placement.

Including a vocational counselor on the inpatient medical rehabilitation team requires attention to effective communication for both the counselor and other team members. Nevertheless, significant benefits can result from early and continuous attention to vocational concerns throughout rehabilitation, and from having the counselor's advice and consultation readily available when treatment decisions are made that relate to a patient's prospects for employment. These benefits are worth the extra efforts required in communication and coordination among the professionals involved.

The Work Evaluator's Role

The work evaluator or prevocational therapist is another important figure in the vocational rehabilitation of some patients. In consultation with the counselor and the physician, the work evaluator takes direct responsibility for carrying out most work evaluation and work adjustment training. The work evaluator can be expected to contribute significant information, not only about the patient's work habits, skills, and readiness for employment, but also about the possibilities of modifying job duties or a job site to adapt to a patient's limitations. The work evaluator also shares with the counselor responsibility for having current knowledge of job opportunities and job performance standards in both competitive and sheltered employment that may be available to patients.

Work evaluators are trained in job analysis, human engineering, and performance analysis techniques. Their expertise includes observation, time sampling and other assessment techniques, and measurement and norming procedures. They must also have knowledge of the worker trait requirements of many different jobs. Traditionally, the background of the work evaluator has been in occupational therapy or industrial arts education. In recent years, however, many people have received special training in this field and it is now possible to earn a graduate degree in work evaluation.

One of the special techniques the work evaluator may use to enhance readiness for employment is to arrange for trial work periods. Sometimes these involve tryouts on simulated jobs in the work evaluation unit, but the work evaluator may also set up work stations in various departments of the hospital or institution where he or she works. Setting up such work stations may be difficult, because of work rules, insurance complications, and the uncertain supply of patients capable of filling a job opening reserved for this purpose. This is especially true when work stations are established outside of the hospital. Nevertheless, such work stations can be of great value by providing a realistic setting and conditions to help bridge the gap between intensive rehabilitation care and actual employment.

SPECIAL PROBLEMS IN VOCATIONAL REHABILITATION

The Progressive or Unstable Disability

Several problems arise in working with people whose disabilities fluctuate or tend to worsen. One of the most important is the difficulty of predicting functional limitations. Vocational plans that are predicated on specific functional capacities may be upset when those capacities diminish. Training to develop vocational skills may be entirely negated if any of the critical underlying abilities change. For example, a journeyman bricklayer was forced to change occupations after becoming paraplegic due to a spinal cord tumor. Because he had the interest and ability, he took training in architectural drafting. However, he had worked in his new job less than a year when progression of the tumor impaired the use of his hands and prevented him from continuing as a draftsman. A progressive disability of this sort may force several major, successive changes in a person's life.

The psychological impact of an unstable disability is another source of difficulty. For example, it is common for the patient with a condition such as multiple sclerosis to insist that planning of any kind is futile, because "I don't know what I will be like tomorrow." Such patients often demonstrate an interplay between their psychological defense mechanisms and the nature of their disability which is very resistant to intervention. On the one hand, their avoidance of planning makes it easier for them to deny the reality or seriousness of their condition. On the other hand, the very uncertainty of the disease provides a "reason" or socially acceptable excuse for not planning which psychologically legitimizes their strategy for coping with it.

Dealing with both the practical and the psychological implications of an unstable disability often requires highly skilled counseling. The denial and avoidance behavior that many patients exhibit is usually based on anxiety about the future, and the patient may need considerable assistance to cope with this anxiety.

Usually, direct confrontation of the possibilities is the most effective way of inducing constructive participation in planning. The patient must be informed, fully and clearly, but in a supportive manner, how the condition may progress and what limitations will result. The patient can then be encouraged to work with the counselor on a series of alternative plans, each of which would seek, despite increasing limitations, to preserve something of importance to the patient. At one end of the continuum of disability, the plans may specify alternative job possibilities; at the other, counseling may focus on how to maintain satisfying social and family relationships. In between, options for various avocational activities may be considered.

From a practical viewpoint, it makes sense to take a somewhat conservative approach to planning, so that the patient does not make too large an investment in alternatives that may later be impossible. Regardless of its focus, the very process of detailed planning can do much to promote a sense of mastery in the patient over his or her destiny. In addition, making the possibilities known and helping the patient to understand how they may be dealt with can contribute greatly to alleviating anxiety about the future.

Vocational Planning for Young People

Vocational rehabilitation of the developmentally disabled or children with severe disabilities of early onset presents some special challenges. The main problem is that the need for special vocational plans may have implications for much of the child's educational program. Valuable time can be saved and consistent educational and vocational progress may be facilitated by making the right decisions about a child's education, sometimes as early as age ten or twelve. For example, if a child has the intellectual potential for a professional level career, many vocational possibilities are open that would be unavailable to the child with lesser ability. However, the need to gain access to such opportunities may dictate the choice of a college preparatory program in high school. In some instances, a college education may be possible, but only if certain deficits in educational skills can be corrected. Then, decisions about remedial education may have to be made early as part of a long-range educational-vocational plan.

Children who do not have the potential for primarily intellectual work may benefit from special attention to their social skills and general work-related skills. This can sometimes be facilitated through enrollment in a work-study program or a vocationally oriented high school curriculum.

The difficulty in making long-range plans for young people stems from the frequent unreliability of early judgments about potential. In the first place, tests of intelligence and special aptitudes are usually less reliable for children than for adults. The greater the distance in time spanned by a prediction based on test results, the less accurate the prediction is likely to be. Repeated measures of multiple predictors may be needed to compensate for the unreliability of tests in long-range predictions.

The unreliability of tests and other measures over time is sometimes compounded by the difficulty of accurate assessment on a single occasion. Because of the skewed social experience of many handicapped children, it is notoriously easy to either over- or underestimate their ability. Habitual avoidance of competitive or stressful situations, or a history of being catered to by overly solicitous parents, may prevent a child from making an optimum effort in testing. On the other hand, social and verbal skills may be overdeveloped in relation to other skills in children who have had extensive experience interacting with rehabilitation professionals. Moreover, sensory, perceptual, and motor impairments, as well as widely varying rates of development of different abilities, may also interfere with accurate assessment.

The resources available for dealing with the vocational needs of handicapped children are rather limited. For example, persons under age 16 are usually not eligible for services from the state vocational rehabilitation agency. Moreover, even when a vocational counselor is available, he or she has usually had little experience with children. On the other hand, a child psychologist may be able to handle the assessment needed, but know little about how to use the results for vocational purposes. Nevertheless, the comprehensive rehabilitation program does afford some possibilities. Frequently, the state agency counselor will provide consultation, even when the child cannot be accepted for direct services. Special education consultants and teachers can also be of help, as can the educational or child psychologist. Many large medical centers either employ such specialists or have reasonable access to them.

A team composed of the vocational counselor, the child psychologist, the teacher, the school counselor, and the physician is needed to develop a suitable long-range educational-vocational plan.

Alternatives to Employment

Some disabled people need an extended period of recuperation or adjustment following onset of a disability before they are ready to attempt work. For others, employment may never be feasible.

Some of the nonworking disabled welcome an opportunity to spend more time with their family. They are sometimes able, in new roles and relationships, to contribute significantly to the well-being of family members. However, others have difficulty adopting new roles or changing their relationships, because of rigid views about the definition of roles. Also, value conflicts may arise from a sense of guilt over not working. All such people can benefit from rehabilitation services to increase their independence, improve their psychological and social adjustment, and help them constructively occupy their time. The physician should be alert to the need for such services and aware of what can be done to help achieve such goals.

If a disability not only prevents employment, but also interferes with the pursuit of previous interests, counseling or occupational therapy may help the individual develop new avocations. In some cases, avocational rehabilitation may involve major changes in lifestyle. For example, a person may be forced by disability to give up former avocations of a largely solitary nature and to depend more on interaction with others for recreation. Occasionally, substitute activities can be found that entail fewer physical demands but are psychologically similar to previous avocations or offer similar satisfactions. For example, the former recreational athlete may be restricted to sedentary activities but may learn to enjoy the contest of scrabble, chess, cards, or other intellectually competitive games. Accomplishing such changes, however, may require extensive assistance in the form of counseling, training, or guided recreation.

Alternative approaches to increasing constructive use of time among the nonworking disabled include participation in organized programs of day activities, work activities, independent living programs, or sheltered employment. Most metropolitan areas, and many smaller communities as well, offer some opportunities of this kind. The programs are usually operated by private rehabilitation agencies, such as the Easter Seal Society, Jewish Vocational Service, or United Cerebral Palsy, with subsidies from the state vocational rehabilitation agency. The activities programs usually have primarily social and recreational purposes, but they are often intended also to improve a person's ultimate prospects for employment through teaching of skills for social interaction and independent living. Sheltered workshops usually have a more explicit vocational orientation, in that their services are intended to lead to competitive employment for those who have the potential, or to provide long-term sheltered work for those who do not.

Whether a disabled person has immediate prospects for employment or no apparent prospects at all, the physician must recognize the importance of constructive activity. Unemployment and inactivity inevitably carry some stigma for the individual, even if there is ostensibly a socially acceptable reason for it, such as severe disability. Also, the person who has activities and interests to fill time and provide a stimulating environment is likely to maintain better mental and physical health and be less of a burden to others.

REFERENCES

1. United States Statutes at Large, Vol. 41, Sixty-sixth Congress, 1920, p. 735.
2. McGowan, J. F., and Porter, T. L.: An Introduction to the Vocational Rehabilitation Process. Washington, D.C., United States Department of Health, Education and Welfare (Rehabilitation Services Administration), 1967, p. 4.
3. Crewe, N. M.: Quality of life: The ultimate goal in rehabilitation. Minnesota Med., 63:586–589, 1980.
4. Guttman, L.: Our paralyzed fellowmen at work. Rehabilitation, 43:9–17, 1962.
5. Strong, E. K., Jr.: Vocational Interests 18 Years After College. Minneapolis, University of Minnesota Press, 1955.
6. Crewe, N. M., and Athelstan, G. T.: Functional assessment in vocational rehabilitation: A systematic approach to diagnosis and goal setting. Arch. Phys. Med. Rehabil., 62:299–305, 1981.
7. Crewe, N. M., and Athelstan, G. T.: Employment after spinal cord injury: A handbook for counselors. Minneapolis, University of Minnesota Medical Rehabilitation Research and Training Center No. 2, 1978.
8. Keating, E., Paterson, D. G., and Stone, C. H.: Validity of work histories obtained by interview. J. Applied Psychol., 34:6–11, 1950.
9. Norris-Baker, C., et al.: Patient behavior as a predictor of outcomes in spinal cord injury. Arch. Phys. Med. Rehabil., 62:602–608, 1981.
10. Cogswell, B. E.: Rehabilitation of the paraplegic: Processes of socialization. Sociological Inquiry, 37:11–26, 1967.
11. Dunn, M. E.: Social discomfort in the patient with spinal cord injury. Arch. Phys. Med. Rehabil., 58:257–260, 1977.
12. Mishel, M. H.: Assertion training with handicapped persons. J. Counseling Psychol., 25:238–241, 1978.

9

PREVOCATIONAL EVALUATION

WALTER C. STOLOV
DAVID L. HOOKS

A physician's commitment to comprehensive rehabilitation includes a determination to develop the maximum vocational potential of every patient. This commitment carries with it specific responsibilities. It is not sufficient for the physician simply to say, "I have diagnosed and provided the best of medical treatment, I have assisted my patient in achieving maximum ambulatory and self-care skills, and I have assisted the patient and his family in developing a safe and satisfactory social interaction and psychological adjustment. I have therefore already maximized his vocational potential and all he need now do is look for a job as might any able-bodied person." Successful employment does not naturally follow the maximum achievement of physical, social, and psychological function. Specific therapeutic processes must be put into play to achieve the vocational goal.

A physician, and in particular a specialist in physical medicine and rehabilitation, has the obligation to include in his patient problem list the problem of *unemployment* when his patient is over 18 years of age (perhaps even as young as 16) and is unemployed, is not in school or in a training program, and has no direction toward achieving an employment goal. There exists a host of various professionals skilled specifically in vocational rehabilitation to whom the physician should refer, or better yet with whom the

physician should become involved, to develop the therapeutic processes necessary to achieve the goal. For the patient who indicates a desire to move into employment, the initial steps may be easy ones. For the patient who makes no such request, the process is a little more difficult. The physician's obligation includes the initiation of a dialogue with his patient to raise the patient's level of awareness of the possibility of employment. Such an educational function by the physician is as important as standard educational efforts in good health habits and in preventive medicine techniques.

Age Relationships

Patients who come under medical rehabilitation care with an unemployment problem and who are in the traditional vocational age range of 18 to 65 years usually fall into one of five categories:

1. There are those *disabled from birth* or essentially within the first five to ten years of life, who by virtue of their disability did not receive the breadth of experiences that normal growth produces and who therefore come to adulthood ill equipped to move smoothly into the labor market.

2. There are those who are *disabled in their teens*, at a most critical stage in their development, who not only also reach adulthood ill equipped because of an impoverish-

ment of experiences but are somewhat further handicapped by a keener awareness of their deficiencies when comparing themselves to their able-bodied friends.

3. There are those *disabled as young adults* who have yet a different set of problems with regard to vocational matters. Maturation for entry into the vocational world usually has already been achieved. They may already have been on a training path or perhaps in the work force. They usually, however, have not yet achieved an enduring, successful vocational history. They have accumulated some knowledge about the world of work, which may keenly point out to them the difficulties presented by their disability. When disability develops in the young adult, from a single traumatic insult, the burden of the shock of acute onset is tempered by the relatively reduced stress of a stable disability not likely to further progress. A heavier burden of stress is borne by the young adult who acquires a chronic disease process, which by its nature has a progressive component. Whether such progression is continuous or is unpredictably intermittent, there is the stress of uncertainty. The set of vocational problems acquired by the latter subgroup within the young adult population is greater generally than those with the acute stable lesion.

4. There are those *disabled as mature adults,* perhaps within the working age of 35 to 55, who have a vocational history that, perhaps more than anything else, describes them. They have a much greater sophistication and understanding of what the world of work is about and, if they have been successful, are perhaps in a better position than the young adult. They carry, however, by virtue of a more advanced age, the added burdens of greater financial responsibility and less adaptability.

5. Finally, there are those *disabled in late life* in the age range between 55 and 65, who may well have the severest burden in readapting to the world of work, particularly if they had not been, during most of their prior life, in self-employed or professional fields.

All of the above categories of patients present the same "unemployment" problem. These simple descriptions suggest that the therapeutic techniques and solutions are likely to be different for each group.[1] For each, nevertheless, the ultimate goal is the achievement of a stable, enduring vocational placement consistent with maximum potential and with opportunities for maximum growth.

The Process

Physicians in the past and unfortunately still in the present have treated the employment problem rather naively. The physician who tells his patient to "Get a different job" or "Learn a new skill" or "Get lighter work" simply is insufficiently sophisticated about the world of work. This type of "advice" has often been directed at the vocational rehabilitation counselor under relatively similar headings, namely, "Get my patient a different job" or "Teach him a new skill" or "Get my patient lighter work." All too often the physician wonders after a week or ten days have elapsed why the rehabilitation counselor has not yet been successful. Primarily focused on acute medical care, the physician often finds it difficult to appreciate that some therapeutics take a little more time.

The vocational rehabilitation process can be divided into four stages:

1. The initial evaluation phase
2. The prevocational (i.e., pre-employment) exploration
3. The job-seeking and placement period
4. The follow-up after placement

Before discussing the prevocational component, it is useful to indicate the required information that the vocational professional needs from a patient's physician in order to establish an effective plan with his client, the physician's patient.

MEDICAL INFORMATION

Simply passing on to the vocational counselor or prevocational professional a copy of the history and physical and the diagnostic impressions or even, if recently hospitalized, a discharge summary, does not provide the information essential for proper planning.

1. The Disease.   The name of the disease is helpful for coding, categorizing, or classifying, but it does not tell the counselor very much. The physician must also include the *location of the pathology* and the systems involved. The physician must make clear the *necessary medications* and *health measures* the patient should be taking to sustain maximal function. The vocational professional must know from the physician whether the injury or the disease produces disability that is *stable* or has a *progressive component* and, if so, what additional systems may become involved. The physician must also communicate *complications* likely to develop if preventive health measures are not undertaken. This permits the counselor to plan in a way that will not contribute to the development of such complications. The physician must communicate to the counselor the patient's need for *continuing medical attention* to maintain health. Such information enlists the aid of the vocational professional in health maintenance. And finally, with regard to the disease, if impending death is a factor to be considered, the counselor should be permitted the physician's best guess (not some number derived from an average of such patients) whether the client being referred will survive two years, five years, or ten or more years. The counselor's approach may appropriately be different for the two-, five-, and ten-year categories.

2. The Function. The knowledgeable physician also transmits to the experienced counselor specific information on the breadth of *ambulatory skills*. Such data includes needs for canes, crutches, braces, and wheelchairs, and whether ambulation skills include the community at large or are restricted. The physician communicates *stair climbing abilities, transportation possibilities* within the community (be it public or automobile), special needs the patient may have with regard to *bowel and bladder function*, and the extent of independence in *transfer skills* and *activities of daily living*. All are useful to the counselor in understanding what it takes for his client to get up in the morning and prepare to go to employment and what needs he may have during the working day.

3. Special Problems. The knowledgeable physician communicates to the experienced counselor information that he has with regard to the strength and weaknesses of the patient in the areas of basic *intellect, personality, vision, hearing acuity,* written and oral *communication ability,* sense of *smell, memory* function, *learning skills,* and overall *cardiac* and *respiratory* function.

4. The Environment. The counselor must know and the physician must communicate his best guesses with regard to whether the patient can sustain *outdoor* as well as *indoor* employment, *temperature* and *humidity* extremes, *mobility* on rough terrain, and variations in *air quality*. Further, requirements with regard to *bathroom accessibility, quality of illumination* in a work environment, and *noise level* limitations, if any, must also be made known.

5. Physical Work Categories. Finally, physician communications to the vocational professional must include an assessment of the physical capacity of his patient. These should be expressed in terms most often used by the vocational community in categorizing the physical demands of an employment activity. The category indicated may well be only the physician's best guess and might well be modified up or down as the prevocational process evolves. Nevertheless, the guidance is still helpful as a starting point. These categories include the following:[2]

a. SEDENTARY WORK. In this activity, the lifting requirements are of a magnitude of 10 pounds (4.5 kg) maximum and usually involve small objects. The work is usually done sitting, although some walking or standing may be required.

b. LIGHT WORK. This activity implies a lifting capacity of up to 20 pounds (9.0 kg), with significant walking or standing requirements. A heavy requirement for pushing, pulling, or leg control is also consistent with most sitting work in this category.

c. MEDIUM WORK. At this level, a lifting maximum of 50 pounds (22.7 kg) with a usual lifting requirement of about 25 pounds (11.4 kg) exists. This type of work and the two types that follow usually require walking and standing capacities.

d. HEAVY WORK. At this level, lifting maximums of up to 100 pounds (45.5 kg) exists, with the usual requirement at the 50 pound (22.7 kg) level.

e. VERY HEAVY WORK. At this highest level of physical exertion, a lifting maximum of greater than 100 pounds (45.5 kg) exists, with a usual carrying capacity of 50 pounds (22.7 kg).

In addition to these categories, additional comments are useful which discuss any potential interferences in lower extremity functions such as *climbing, balancing, stooping,* and *kneeling,* and in upper extremity functions such as *reaching, handling, grasping,* and *feeling.*

INITIAL EVALUATION

Successful employment, both for placement and for maintenance, requires the job candidate or employee to have proficiency in four primary skill sets: (1) interpersonal relationships, (2) work performance, (3) intellectual function, and (4) work behaviors. These four sets are not mutually exclusive, but for ease and clarity of analysis they are considered individually.

Interpersonal Skills

The ability to "get along with" others and good skills in interpersonal communication are often considered to be elements of personality. Concepts such as attitude, friendliness, cooperation, determination, and awareness are components of this set. These are the standards against which an employee is measured when his interaction with the public, peers, and supervisors is assessed and evaluated. An employee must have mastery of these concepts simply to maintain the *status quo* and to avoid negative relationships. To advance and be considered for jobs of increasing responsibility, an employee must have a high level of competence in interpersonal skills. At an initial interview for employment these skills have, with the exception of physical appearance, the highest initial impact on a prospective employer.

Performance Skills

These skills are those that affect the work product. They are measured by quantity and quality. Quantity is simply the total output of a worker (e.g., units). Quality is a measure of the acceptability of the units and is often expressed as a ratio of acceptable units completed to the total number of units attempted. This measurement system, while being "production line" oriented, can be generalized to human services and other work settings as well. There is always a balance between quantity and quality. Rarely are the two expected to be equal (e.g., the perfect worker). The employer sets the balance that is minimally acceptable.

An employee's physical capabilities impinge heavily in the area of work performance. Clearly, the ability to stoop, bend, stand, lift, or push, for example, may well affect performance. Depending on the product, interpersonal skills, intellectual skills, and work behaviors can affect performance. The ultimate measure in work evaluation still remains, "How much and how fast?"

Intellectual Function

These skills include, for example, problem solving, innovation, and rate of knowledge communication. The degree of intellectual skills required varies greatly from job to job. While an employer seldom looks for people who function at low levels, the ability of a person to persevere at routine and repetitious tasks is generally inversely related to intelligence. Some employers are likely to screen out highly educated highly intelligent candidates for repetitive tasks, especially if the job is to be permanent or long term.

Work Behaviors

This fourth category includes a large number of activities that also must be acceptable. Even those with superior interpersonal, performance, and intellectual skills will find little success in their vocational pursuits within our modern society if their work behaviors are not sufficiently acceptable. These are activities common to any job. The following lists examples of work behaviors critical to job success:

1. One's personal hygiene, grooming, and dressing habits must be appropriate to the work setting. Thus, while body odor is not a negative factor for a professional football player during competition, it is indeed a significant factor in a crowded office or where public interaction is required.

2. Personal habits must not be offensive to others. While also highly variable to the setting, such things as nose picking, groin scratching, lack of handkerchief use, floor spitting, and constant humming or whistling are obvious examples of potential deterrents

to successful employment. Even these, however, may be acceptable in some settings.

3. Punctuality and attendance records are obvious in their influence in determining work acceptability.

4. Communication skills directly related to work needs must also meet certain minimums. They are equal to performance skills in order of importance. Employees who cannot effectively communicate with their supervisors or coworkers with regard to their work needs or the work needs of others cannot succeed. Communication skills are a different entity than interpersonal skills (e.g., "He is really a very nice guy and tells great stories, but for the life of me, I can't understand his reports.") Most work-related communication is either written or oral. At least one must be mastered and the two should not conflict.

5. Coping ability refers to how well, when faced with a problem, the employee handles it until it is solved. "Frustration tolerance" is another way of indicating this work behavior. If frustration reaches a level that causes work performance to deteriorate, employability diminishes. Clearly, coping skills rank high in importance.

6. Endurance and vitality, while in a sense performance measures, refer to the ability to perform continually with expected quantity and quality, hour in and hour out, day in and day out, and week in and week out. Particularly for the disabled, the ability to sustain a four- or eight-hour day, day in and day out, is an important behavior to assess. Vitality is a measure that refers to whether performance levels sustain or deteriorate over time. Vitality deterioration usually occurs before the endurance level, the point at which the work quality becomes unacceptable, is reached and the worker must actually stop the activity.

7. Production consistency, while in part related to vitality and endurance, differs in that one must assess, even before the vitality and endurance endpoints are reached, whether the worker's output is predictable or varies from unit to unit, even in the early part of the day when endurance and vitality are not factors.

8. Distractibility, while in part related to consistency, differs in that one may have great vitality and consistency of output but be relatively less productive should neighboring extraneous factors not related to one's work, such as background noise, conversation, and visitors, cause relaxation of concentration and a decline in production.

9. Conformity to safety rules and practices is increasingly important. The high costs incurred by employers for injured workers and the high standards imposed by regulatory agencies may cause the unsafe and careless worker to lose his job in spite of high performance skills.

10. Adverse reactions to changes in work assignments and/or to the occasional or frequent monotonous task can also defeat successful employment. The worker who reacts with anger, hostility, or frustration to a less pleasant job assignment is not likely to endear himself to a supervisor or to his coworker.

11. Work methods refer to how well one organizes his tools and materials. This behavior may relate to personal habits and may, if deficient, affect quantity of output.

12. Supervision requirements, which in part relate to performance and intellectual skills, specifically measure how closely and how often a supervisor must monitor an employee after what may be deemed a sufficient initial period of instruction. Related behaviors in connection with supervision include one's ability to accept the authority of the supervisor, to avoid becoming tense when close supervision is deemed necessary, and to be able to respond favorably to constructive criticism.

Initial Evaluation Phase

The client and counselor have as their ultimate goal a successful and enduring vocational placement with sufficient underpinnings for equally successful future advancement. The Dictionary of Occupational Titles lists 40,000 specific job titles.[2] Obviously, much work is necessary to reduce these options to an appropriate and manageable number and to maximize the four sets of skills previously described.

Armed, it is hoped, with appropriate medical information equally well understood by client and counselor, the two "go to work." This initial phase is an intense intellectual and personal exercise often stressful to both. Its function is to narrow down and select from the world of work those areas or directions in which it may appear that the client may have his best success. This exercise must be pursued with great skill. One must not be too broad and end with too many options that would take too long to pursue successfully. At the same time, one must not be too narrow and hence run the risk of no success. The assessment draws upon all that precedes. Included is prior education and training, prior employment (unsuccessful as well as successful), verbalized personal preferences, clear understanding of physical limits, clear understanding of physical strengths, and an assessment of the four sets of skills required for successful employment. Standard psychometric testing is often administered to supplement this assessment. The counselor has available, in addition, specific tests to evaluate, for example, eye-hand coordination, manual dexterity, spatial perceptual function, fine and gross motor skills, and reaction time.

Development of areas within the world of work that initially look promising for the client are further tempered with what may be available in the job market within the available geographic area. The geographical area open to the client is not only governed by the client's physical skill, but by social requirements and life style as well as the logistic constraints of housing and transportation.

PREVOCATIONAL EXPLORATION

The client and counselor are, after the initial evaluation phase, now ready to test out the initial assessment of potentially suitable work. In this prevocational exploration, the client is directly engaged in the performance of job units. Having the client engage in actual work samples or in a work performance setting allows for an assessment of the best of alternate directions and also provides answers to questions not obtained by the initial phase. Depending on the work setting selected, prevocational exploration can also be therapeutic, in that solutions of work behavior problems that may have been present in the past can be found.

The amount and extent of the prevocational period is highly correlated with the client categories defined on page 190. Thus, what might be necessary for the client who is disabled from birth and has carried his disability throughout his formative years is en-

tirely different than what might be required by the 55-year-old who has developed leukemia or perhaps lost his limb through peripheral vascular disease. Prevocational evaluation can be diagnostic as well as therapeutic. Some of the goals that can be achieved include the following:

1. Interests can be developed, particularly when no useful interests were generated by the initial vocational phase. Interest development may also be required even if interests do exist, for one may not be able to build upon them by virtue of the physical disability present.

2. Skill exploration is another goal of a prevocational program. Psychometric testing and even some of the more specific manual skill instruments may not be sufficient to assess if a client has potential skill in an area. Vocational samples can help assess whether there is inherent skill with certain tools, for example, sufficient to meet employment standards or to warrant specific training.

3. Confidence building is obtainable through a prevocational "on the job" performance without the consequences of failure. Within the protected confines of a prevocational sample, confidence can be created without much stress.

4. For the physically disabled who have achieved maximum levels of independence through rehabilitation in self-care and ambulation skills, the prevocational setting allows for the generalization of achieved skills into the work setting.

5. Endurance is another important factor to be assessed, particularly for the physically disabled. It may not be possible to predict whether the patient can maintain a daily work schedule of four or six or eight hours without a prevocational evaluation that approaches the same levels of stress and duration.

6. Growth in output, sometimes referred to as "work hardening," is another therapeutic goal achievable through prevocational activities. This is particularly useful for the younger age group who have not had much prior work experience. Prevocational activities can simply, through repetition and daily attention to work, increase work productivity.

7. A prevocational work period may be part of skill exploration in that it may help solidify a preliminary decision that specific training, be it at a school or through an apprenticeship, is a worthwhile possibility.

Prevocational explorations occur in quite variable settings. The mode selected is determined by the questions being asked or the goals that must be achieved. They extend from execution of standardized work samples performed in an artificial environment to placements in actual work settings alongside the able-bodied.

Work Samples

Various approaches to work sampling are used by work evaluators and counselors in rehabilitation facilities. The samples are often described as being standardized but may not always be statistically sound. Of the many work samples available, approximately 10 to 12 are consistently used. The most well known include The Philadelphia Jewish Employment and Vocational Service Work Sample System (JEVS), Singer Vocational Evaluation System (Singer), Testing, Orientation and Work Evaluation in Rehabilitation System (TOWER), and the Valpar Component Work Sample Series (Valpar). A brief description of these work sample systems will indicate the differences in their approaches.

The JEVS system, developed under sponsorship of the U.S. Department of Labor, was designed around various work traits that collectively constitute performance skills. There are 26 work samples that are formally administered to a client, and the work traits sampled include such characteristics as handling, sorting, manipulating, inspecting, and drafting. The system uses a realistic work atmosphere and requires six to seven days to complete. The JEVS is highly standardized. Essential to its use is a high level of accuracy of the observations made and the data collected. It is comprehensive and thorough in assessing client potential.

The Singer system, developed by the Singer Educational Division, Rochester, New York, utilizes over 20 different work samples drawn from the skilled trades and assesses potential for specific jobs. The client performs work typical of the job as opposed to the more abstract samples used in the JEVS. Each sample has its own work station, as opposed to some of the other systems in which the tasks are brought to a central work station. The Singer has a strong emphasis on career exploration from an information point of view but is weak in determining client potential.

The TOWER was developed by the Institute for the Crippled and Disabled, New York, and is one of the oldest systems. It consists of 93 work samples that are combined to assess 14 job training areas such as clerical, drafting, jewelry making, mail clerk, sewing machine operator, and assembly. The TOWER is a complete work evaluation system and provides a realistic setting in which to evaluate and analyze job potential. While comprehensive, it is somewhat narrow in focus and does not generalize well to other job areas. Both the dependence on written instructions and the relative complexity of the tasks may eliminate its use by the comparatively illiterate, mentally retarded, and severely disabled. The TOWER has been the "work horse" of work evaluators, and components are often found in occupational therapy settings. Depending on the number of tests used, the TOWER can require up to three weeks to complete. Seldom are all tasks given.

The Valpar was developed by the Valpar Corporation in Phoenix and is one of the newer samples available. It was developed to assess performance of industrially injured workers. The Valpar is a trait and factor system and is based on task analysis. As each sample is self contained, an evaluator might use any one or more of the 12 samples, such as small tools, problem solving, and soldering, to assess a client. This ease of use also contributes to its major criticism, namely, that it lacks a unified analysis and reporting system. The behavioral observations are somewhat subjective, and therefore interrater reliability is low. On the positive side, it is rapidly administered (1 hr/sample) and appeals to clients.

The choice of the work sample evaluation system to be used is based on the patient's medical picture, the job market, and the objectives to be achieved. For further information on work evaluation systems, the comprehensive summaries prepared by the Stout Vocational Rehabilitation Institute at the University of Wisconsin should be consulted.[3]

Most work samples do not evaluate interpersonal skills, nor many of the varied work behaviors adequately, but they are useful for specific performance evaluation and also provide some measure of intellectual skills. Evaluation and assessment of interpersonal skills and work behaviors require other techniques, such as sheltered workshops and job stations.

Sheltered Workshops

Workshop settings are geared for "long-term" prevocational evaluations. They are "sheltered" by appropriate certification by the Federal or State Departments of Labor to be outside general employment rules such as minimum wage regulations. They are further viewed as sheltered in that the quantity of acceptable units of production by its workers is generally below that considered minimum for industrially competitive employment. They are not, however, to be viewed as places for recreation or play. Sheltered workshops typically have specific contracts to produce specific outputs by a specific time for a specific customer. In many instances, the actual work one sees performed in a sheltered workshop is quite similar to what one might see in an ordinary industrially competitive setting. Many industries do not "tool up" for all their production needs and subcontract some of their work. Sheltered workshops often compete with traditional industrial companies for the same subcontract.

For certain clients, sheltered workshops end up as the final placement. For others, they serve as a transitional place of employment prior to entrance into the regular job market. For many, workshops are used for prevocational evaluation toward the goals enumerated earlier.

Job Stations

Perhaps more advanced than the sheltered workshop is the job station in an industrial setting. In this example, a vocational rehabilitation service program develops relationships with specific public or private industrial settings that permit clients to be placed for short periods in work positions alongside the able-bodied. Any one such individual placement is likely to be about one month in duration, although, depending upon the setting and the disability, it may be longer. Appropriate relationships must first be established, both for the protection of the client and for the protection of the company that allows such placements to occur. Essential is the need for the supervisor at the job station to interact with the vocational counselor or work evaluator so that they, as well as the client, get the necessary feedback from the supervisors. This feedback helps to identify problems that the client and counselor must solve together. Direct behavioral observation by the counselor of his client is often utilized in the setting for detection of strengths on which to build or weaknesses in need of solution.

While job stations of this type are obviously longer than job samples, they may not be as suitable as sheltered workshops when the prevocational phase needs to extend into two, three, or four months or more. In the latter instance, the sheltered workshop may well be the more suitable placement. Volunteer work in public or private industrial settings, when well evaluated, is akin to the formal job station. In addition, current federal legislation allows industrially competitive settings to engage in *job tryout*. The employer is able to apply for a special fund and to utilize these funds to pay salaries for a person to participate in a trial work period. If the worker proves to be successful, the trial period may lead to regular employment. If the trial period proves unsuccessful, the client and counselor have gained important information, and, at the same time, the employer has not sustained a financial loss.

Finally, one additional form of prevocational "job station" evaluation needs to be mentioned, although actually there is nothing prevocational about it. This method is suitable for people who were employed at the onset of illness or time of injury and for whom there is a probability of returning to their job following rehabilitation. Assuming that the client has achieved, in the past, a record of reliability and good performance, the employer is often willing to give it a try. In such a situation, the first few weeks or month in a job becomes the prevocational phase, when the person is actually already employed. Care must be used in this approach, because a poor performance may tarnish an otherwise good record. It should be used, perhaps, only when there is at least a 75 per cent probability of success.

RELATIONSHIP OF PREVOCATION PHASE TO DISABILITY ONSET

The discussion now allows for some general statements with regard to what a prevocational exploration must accomplish for each of the categories enumerated on page 190.

Clearly, for those disabled from birth or in the first five to ten years of life, the prevocational phase may well be as much as 6 to 18 months long. Much must be accomplished. Such clients reach working age with very little in the way of experiences that normal growth produces to prepare them for the labor market. All aspects, performance skills, intellectual skills, interpersonal skills, and work behaviors must be developed.

The same applies, but less so, to those disabled in the teens. While maturation is only in part slowed, endurance testing, confidence building, and training might be the more important issues. The prevocational phase for this group is likely to be less than three months.

For those disabled in the young adult years, prevocational exploration needs are further reduced. Interest generation might be important, depending upon the degree of disability, and a certain measure of endurance training and assessment may be necessary.

For those in the age range of 35 to 55 years, the prevocational phase, assuming a good prior work record, has, perhaps as its main function, assessment of performance skills. This again does not require much time in a prevocational setting.

Finally, the adult in a late stage of his vocational life, 55 to 65 years, either moves directly into a job tryout setting or more likely back to his prior job setting, if indeed possibilities for employment exist. If neither of these can be achieved, the likelihood of a return to employment is quite low.

REFERENCES

1. Stolov, W. C., and Clowers, M. R. (Eds.): Handbook of Severe Disability. Rehabilitation Services Administration. Washington, D.C., U.S. Government Printing Office, 1981.
2. Dictionary of Occupational Titles, Vol. 2, 3rd Edition. Washington, D.C., U.S. Government Printing Office, 1965.
3. A Comparison of Vocational Evaluation Systems. Materials Development Center, Stout Vocational Rehabilitation Institute, Menomonie, WI, 1981.

10

THE EPIDEMIOLOGY OF DISABILITY AS RELATED TO REHABILITATION MEDICINE

MASAYOSHI ITOH
MATHEW H. M. LEE

The word epidemiology is derived from the Greek *epidēmios*, meaning "among the people." Thus, it is no coincidence that in the early twentieth century C. O. Stallybrass defined epidemiology as "the science which considers infectious diseases — their course, propagation, and prevention."[89] This rather narrow and restricted definition, although obsolete, has an historic value, since it characterized epidemiology as a science.

Hippocrates stressed meteorological variations and seasonal characteristics as the fundamental elements that determine cyclic variations in epidemic diseases.[82] Until the seventeenth century this theory was widely accepted as the dominant concept for explaining the causes of transmissible disease. Few supported Fracastoro[28] in the sixteenth century when he theorized that infection was a cause and epidemics were a consequence. He further recognized three modes of contagion: (1) by direct contact from person to person; (2) by an intermediate agent; and (3) through the air. Sydenham in the seventeenth century suggested that there were intercurrent diseases that were dependent on the susceptibility of the human body.[82]

Beginning with ancient civilizations, the practitioners of medicine, the church, and governments struggled against epidemics by using theory, superstition, authority, and religion to compensate for lack of scientific knowledge. Throughout the medieval period, it was generally assumed that sorrow and suffering create a particularly favorable environment for the rise and spread of disease. The panic that erupted during epidemics was regarded as furthering the spread of the disease. Thus, municipal authorities in many European cities felt it advisable to forbid tolling the customary death knell, as it would be ringing continuously night and day. Since epidemics were attributed to the sins of man, elders of the church went from house to house hounding those suspected of religious irregularities and immoral conduct. Numerous men and women were expelled from the community in disgrace for minor offenses, since it was believed that eradication of sin and the sinful would halt an epidemic.[33]

As outrageous and primitive as it may sound, these and similar preventive measures were guided by contemporary medical beliefs and prevailed until the twentieth century. Yet, we are not too far away from the day when tuberculosis and epilepsy were considered shameful afflictions. Even today, many still view venereal diseases as a sign of immorality; and superstition and fear doom patients with leprosy to life as social outcasts in many communities of the world. Because of such stigmatization, early discovery in these diseases remains extremely difficult. This is not meant to belittle or negate the tremendous amount of epidemiologic knowledge that has been accumulated in this century. It does, however, suggest that in centuries to come, our present-day knowledge on causation and prevention of diseases and morbid conditions may be considered as primitive as the witch hunt or voodoo rite.

W. H. Welch defined epidemiology as a study of the natural history of disease.[104] Lilienfeld described it as the study of the distribution of a disease or condition in a population, and of the factors that influence this distribution.[60] In these definitions, epidemiology is not restricted solely to the study of transmissible diseases but can embrace all types of diseases as well as disabilities, whether physical or mental.

This chapter on epidemiology discusses conceptual aspects, the classic theory of the natural history of disease, and practical application of an epidemiologic approach to the daily practice of rehabilitation medicine in the office, hospital, extended care facility, or home.

SPECTRUM OF HEALTH

The noted English biographer Izaak Walton stated in his famed *Compleat Angler,* "Look to your health; and if you have it, praise God, and value it next to a good conscience; for health is the second blessing that we mortals are capable of; a blessing that money cannot buy." Benjamin Disraeli, the great English statesman, said in 1877, "The health of people is really the foundation upon which all their happiness and all their powers as a state depend." "Health is an essential preliminary to the best success in the best work, and to the highest attainment in the widest usefulness. Without it there is sadness at the hearthstone, silence and sorrow, instead of cheerful words and happy heart."[27] Whether considered as personal treasure or national strength, health has long been regarded as the prime factor of human welfare. Therefore, prior to a discussion of disease and disabilities, some thought should be given to the concept of health.

One of the most frequently quoted and dynamic definitions of health was issued by the World Health Organization: "a state of complete physical, mental and social well-being and not merely the absence of disease or infirmity."[106]

This rather simply phrased definition contains two distinct thoughts. The words "complete physical, mental and social well-being" imply an infinite number of variables relative to the present and to the ever-changing future. Rogers, in his Health Status Scale,[81] terms this state "Optimum Health" and notes that it is seldom maintained for a prolonged period. The second important aspect of the W.H.O. definition is the phrase "absence of disease or infirmity." This recognizes the existence of a state of health which is neither Optimum Health nor actual illness and which may be called Suboptimum Health. Suboptimum Health can best be illustrated by the patient undergoing the incubation period of bacterial or viral disease or the person with latent diabetes mellitus.

Usually it is not too difficult to recognize the state of Overt Illness or Disability. However, in those diseases with insidious onset, such as multiple sclerosis or arteriosclerosis, it is often difficult to detect this state. When the process of disease threatens life, man reaches the state of Approaching Death. Today, however, this state does not necessarily mean that a man is going to die. A cardiac pacemaker, organ transplantation, or exchange transfusion may bring a man back to Suboptimum Health.

In spite of advancements in scientific knowledge and technology, man reaches a state of Death, which is absolute and irreversible, when all vital organs cease to function. The fundamental goal of medical science is not to produce an immortal man but to maintain man in Optimum Health as long as possible, ideally until death.

The most important aspect of Rogers' Health Status Scale (Fig. 10–1) is that no man can stay in one particular spot on this scale for an indefinite period. If we assume that the sum of the word "health" is constant as is the word "weather," then ill health is discord, while health is concord. Thus, as a

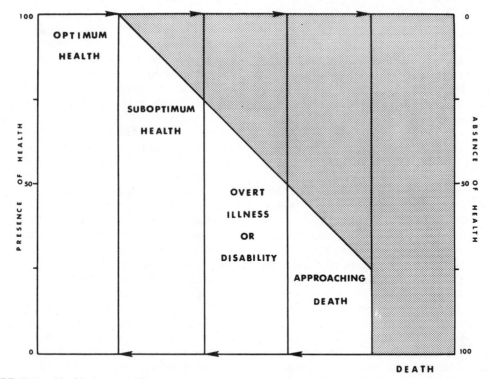

FIGURE 10–1. Health Status Scale. Arrows on the top and bottom of this diagram indicate declining and improving health, respectively. (Modified from Rogers, E. S.: Human Ecology and Health. New York, The Macmillan Company, 1960.)

man's health status declines, a portion of health decreases and that of ill health increases. As a train on a funicular railway, a man's health status constantly goes up and down from the peak of health to the edge of the valley of death.

This concept of health can easily be applied to the diseases or conditions that are observed in a rehabilitation service. Let us take as an example the case of a 60-year-old female who fell and sustained a subcapital fracture of the femur. Prior to the accident, this woman most likely had postmenopausal osteoporosis and possibly impairment of reflexes, of body balance, and of musculoskeletal coordination. Although the patient might have thought she was in perfect health, the presence of these conditions indicates that her health status classification at the time of the fall was, at best, Suboptimum.

Now she is obviously in a state of Overt Disability. If this case is mismanaged, i.e., with prolonged bed rest subsequent to traction, then hypostatic pneumonia and possibly decubiti may develop. Thus, this woman's health enters the Approaching Death stage and may decline until it reaches

Death. Not too long ago, this was the most commonly expected course after this type of accident.

The prognosis for subcapital fracture is poor if the fracture is treated with the Smith-Peterson nail, because the head of the femur will inevitably develop aseptic necrosis within a few months. In order to avoid this disaster and to bring the patient back to Suboptimum Health as rapidly as possible, replacement of the femoral head is the logical treatment.

Such surgical treatment, with proper restorative care, will return the patient to her normal state, Suboptimum Health, in a period of a few weeks. This model of the health status scale is applicable to every disabling condition, including loss of limbs or body organs.[41]

In the case just discussed, even the loss of the femoral head can be analyzed by the use of the health status scale. The femoral head initially was in Suboptimum Health. Trauma from the fall resulted in Approaching Death of the femoral head. Its removal by surgery, since it could no longer function, is tantamount to Death of the femoral head. Insertion of the prosthesis, though it does not restore any portion of health to the femoral head, does restore a portion of health to the patient. In fact, it restores the patient to the level of health she enjoyed prior to the accident. Thus, Death of the femoral head prevented the patient from sliding to a lower level on the Health Status Scale.

NATURAL HISTORY OF DISEASE

In this concept of health it is obvious that there is a specific mechanism by which health changes from one direction to the other. The history of medicine clearly indicates that our predecessors made a great effort to identify the causation of illness. In early times, strange reasons were advanced as the causes of disease. Virtually anything that was beyond human control was, at one time or another, considered as the cause of some · disease or affliction. Astrology and religions held that evil spirits and sins were responsible for the rise and fall of plagues. Evil spirits rising with the stench from sewage or stagnant water were thought to be the cause of epidemics. The initial use of smelling salts by European ladies may well have been an early but vague recognition of environment as a causative factor of disease.

It was not until the seventeenth century that the idea of human susceptibility emerged. During the onslaught of epidemics in the medieval period, the "sinful" people who fell victim to epidemics were obviously highly susceptible to the disease. Those who survived were naturally less susceptible but not necessarily any less sinful.

As early as the mid-seventeenth century, existence of the microorganism as a causative agent of illness was suspected. It was not until the nineteenth century, however, that this obscure theory was proved. Identification and isolation of a specific microorganism as a responsible agent of a particular disease enforced the concept of a single cause of disease, and less attention was focused on causes related to the host and environment.[53]

In the early twentieth century, various epidemiologic investigations on outbreaks of transmissible diseases were conducted. These studies revealed that mere exposure of the human host to a specific agent did not inevitably produce the state of Overt Illness. Thus, the modern epidemiologic concept that illness is caused by simultaneous interaction of host, agent, and environment was established.

In order to comprehend this triad theory, which is highly relevant to later discussions in this chapter, it is essential to analyze each causative factor. The host, being human, has various characteristics: age, sex, race, chromosomal variety, body constitution, immunity, marital status, education, occupation, habit and custom, psychological state, and so forth. The significance of host characteristics may be illustrated by the fact that certain diseases or conditions are more prevalent in persons with similar characteristics than in others lacking those characteristics.

Biological, chemical, mechanical, genetic, nutrient, and physical elements are often cited as qualitative agent factors that may vary in their virulence. It is also important to note the value of the quantitative aspect of agent factors. Quantity may be understood in two categories: *dosage* and *frequency*. Frequent exposure to a low dosage of the agent could develop either of two opposing results: increased resistance or a cumulative effect.

Increased resistance is exemplified by tuberculosis in the New World. White settlers had been exposed to *M. tuberculosis* for centuries in Europe and thus had developed resistance. Despite many hardships in America, there was no marked increase of tuberculosis among the white settlers. At the same time, American Indians and the imported black slaves in Argentina suffered greatly and some tribes and groups were virtually wiped out. Similarly some childhood diseases may afflict adults, who have had little exposure to them and thus offer low resistance.

The cumulative effect of frequent and/or prolonged exposure to a low dosage of agents is often associated with environmental pollution. "Black lung," which is produced only after years of silica dust inhalation, is commonly found among mining workers.[67] However, one visit to a coal mine cannot result in pulmonary silicosis. Similarly, inhalation of asbestos dust seems to be responsible for a high incidence of lung cancer among asbestos workers and ship pipefitters.[5, 36] Byssinosis results from chronic inhalation of fibers in a cotton mill.

The ill effects of pollutant agents are not

limited to occupational exposure to toxic substances. A classic example is the tragic Minamata disease, which was caused by frequent consumption of fish contaminated by mercury compound.[29] While the ecological effect of DDT, fictionalized in *Silent Spring*,[15] is now a historical reality, contamination of drinking water with polychlorinated biphenyls (PCB) and other industrial chemical substances is a major problem today. Soil pollution, which necessitated evacuation of residents in the Love Canal section of Niagara County, New York, was traced back to industrial waste used for sanitary landfill in the area.[9]

It is important to differentiate between the epidemiological concept of environment as the third causative factor of a disease and environmental pollution in epidemiology. The environment is the vessel in which pollutant agents are contained.

Environment may be viewed in terms of physical, biological, socioeconomic, political, and other aspects. Physical environment may refer to the physical characteristics of the immediate surroundings or to atmospheric conditions such as climate, atmospheric pressure, gaseous composition, and quality of air. Such characteristics of socioeconomic environment as education, customs, and nutritional habits may greatly influence host susceptibility.

Paul[73] recognized two types of epidemiologic climate: micro-climate, described as the social climate and representing intimate living conditions within the home or place of work; and macro-climate, which represents climate in the ordinary meteorological sense of temperature, humidity, and rainfall. The concept of micro-climate is more individualized in its interpretation of environment and includes some host characteristics that are related to socioeconomic conditions. For example, certain political climates could make one group of hosts more or less deprived in a socioeconomic sense.

When a disease or condition is analyzed, the factors of host, agent, and environment must be carefully considered. An acceptable and perhaps innocent clinical statement such as "Fracture of the neck of femur is commonly seen in elderly people, mostly women"[42] is far short of satisfactory in an epidemiologic sense. Mere age and sex cannot accurately represent the host characteristics. Such characteristics in an aging female may involve body constitution — for example, postmenopausal osteoporosis, diminished vision, and a propensity for falling — in other words, an impaired sense of body balance. This could be caused by cerebral arteriosclerosis or by medications being administered for hypertension. But this is still a limited analysis. Custom and habit can also contribute to this injury and disability. Many women at home customarily wear house slippers, which cause a shuffling gait and make the wearer more susceptible to falling accidents. Some investigators[7, 100] claimed hip fracture is common among whites but another[80] disputed this by citing a large number of cases among blacks. Thus even the racial factor must be considered when discussing the prevalence of this condition.

Since most hip fractures occur inside the home, the peculiarities of the environment must be studied. Highly waxed or wet floors, slippery throw rugs, or a dangling telephone cord may become menacing obstacles. Cluttered floors, poor lighting, sagging floors or steps, defective hand rails on staircases, or crowded housing indicating a hazardous physical environment may be host characteristics related to the socioeconomic and education factors.

The agent in the accident discussed as an example is mechanical force, which exerted extreme stress to body structure.[18] Unsuccessful attempts to regain body balance resulted in the fall, and stress produced the fracture. However, one can easily ascertain that various host characteristics and environmental factors had existed for some time prior to this accident. Most likely, there had been episodes of loss of balance or near accidents before this incident. The fact that injury did occur at this particular time indicates that the three causative factors — host, agent, and environment — sufficiently and simultaneously interacted and resulted in fracture.

The period when these three causative factors exist independently and have not completed interaction is called the Prepathogenesis Period (Fig. 10–2). Upon completion of simultaneous interaction, a disease stimulus is produced. At this stage, Early Pathogenesis, a man's health status changes from Optimum to Suboptimum Health. However, until the disease process reaches above the Clinical Horizon, the presence of illness is

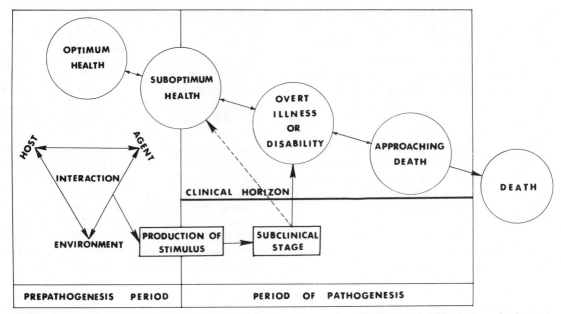

FIGURE 10–2. Natural history of a disease in man, as constructed on the Rogers' health status scale shown in Figure 10–1. Not every disease appears above the clinical horizon. Man may recover from the subclinical stages directly to suboptimum health.

not recognizable. Once reaching the state of Overt Illness, man may recover to Suboptimum and, hopefully, Optimum Health, at which time he returns to the Prepathogenesis Period and commences another cycle. for other disease. This model of the natural history of disease is applicable to virtually all diseases and conditions and is the basis for the epidemiology of disability. A survey done by the Environmental Protection Agency after the Love Canal disaster found 32,254 sites in this country that may cause health hazards, and many may already be affecting the health of people in those areas.[4] The residents in these sites could be considered to be in their period of Prepathogenesis.

LEVELS OF PREVENTION

Health care includes preventive and clinical medicine. Any health care that attempts to halt man's slide down the slope of the health status scale is termed preventive and any attempt to push it up toward the peak, Optimum Health, is called therapeutic. This definition is essential to conceptualization of the Levels of Prevention. While activities in preventive medicine have no direct therapeutic value, every measure administered in

therapeutic or clinical medicine has its preventive aspects. Vaccination or fluoridation of drinking water protects populations from disease but does not cure any disease. On the other hand, antibiotics are therapeutic agents that can also prevent septicemia and death. Similarly, internal fixation of hip fracture is a therapeutic surgical treatment but also prevents pulmonary and peripheral vascular complications.

Within this frame of reference, the total spectrum of health care is classified into three levels of prevention: Primary, Secondary, and Tertiary. Primary prevention is applicable during the Prepathogenesis or Optimum Health periods. The other two levels cover the period of pathogenesis or, let us say, all gradations of the health scale from Suboptimum Health to Approaching Death.

Each level of prevention consists of various representative activities. Table 10–1 shows a comparison of the activities at each level, as interpreted by the authors of this chapter and by others. All the listed authors agree wholly on activities basic to Primary prevention and agree in part with our interpretation of Secondary prevention. Our interpretation of rehabilitation and limitation of disability activities differs from that of the other authors, and they also differ from each other in interpretation of these measures.

TABLE 10–1. LEVELS OF PREVENTION

Authors	Primary	Secondary	Tertiary
Leavell and Clark[18]	Health promotion Specific protection	Early diagnosis Proper treatment Disability limitation	Rehabilitation
Columbia University[25]	Health promotion Specific protection	Early diagnosis Proper treatment	Disability limitation Rehabilitation
Itoh and Lee[41]	Health promotion Specific protection	Early diagnosis Proper treatment Rehabilitation	Disability limitation Custodial care

Rehabilitation is defined as "the ultimate restoration of a disabled person to his maximum capacity — physical, emotional, and vocational."[84] It is widely believed that rehabilitation must be started at the earliest possible time in order to ensure the best results. Thus, the diagnosis must be established in the earliest possible phase of disease and all necessary treatment, including rehabilitation, must be initiated at that time. The belief that rehabilitation should commence after termination of specific treatment of a disease or condition that results in disability is the basis for classifying rehabilitation at the Tertiary prevention level. The writers admit that this idea is regrettably widespread, and such procedure is common practice. But this is obviously a misconception. Inasmuch as rehabilitation should be administered in conjunction with specific medical or surgical treatment of diseases or conditions which can result in disablement, rehabilitation should be considered an integral part of Secondary prevention.

Disability limitation (Table 10–1) refers to preventing an increase in the intensity or scope of an existing disability. This measure, therefore, becomes necessary after termination of active medical or surgical treatment and rehabilitation. Disability limitation is generally known as maintenance treatment. It is particularly indispensable for those who are chronically ill or disabled and absolutely mandatory for geriatric patients. Another example of disability limitation is recreation therapy. Eventually, lack of stimuli, regimented daily life, and hopelessness can mold the population of a chronic disease institution into a depressed, docile, apathetic mass. Recreation therapy, through programs designed to stimulate both groups and individuals, can prevent this kind of psychological crippling.

One of the most important aspects of disability prevention is pain control. Regardless of its origin, intractable pain is an extremely debilitating symptom, emotionally as well as physically. Although the tolerance to pain may vary from one individual to another, no person is immune to pain. Often patients with chronic pain may state that they "have gotten used to pain" or "have learned to live with it." Such statements should not be taken literally as a sign of increased pain tolerance but should be considered a possible sign of resignation, which in itself can be destructive. While there is no ideal analgesic, the discovery of enkephalins and endorphins[90, 91] may revolutionize the concept of and approach to pain management. Relationships between these opiate-like peptides and some old and new pain control techniques such as acupuncture, transcutaneous nerve stimulation, and behavior modification are currently under investigation.[14]

We have included custodial care in our table of health care. The purpose of custodial care is to make man as comfortable as possible for the last few years or days of his life. When custodial care is indicated there is usually no hope for reversal or cure. This does not mean disability limitation is not indicated. It is warranted because it prolongs activity and comfort and it should be listed as an independent entity in Tertiary prevention.

Management of the terminal cancer patient has always been a problem for health care systems and an agonizing experience for patients and their families. Recently, great attention has been focused on pain control and tertiary care for terminal cancer patients. This management of pain is not limited to somatic pain but encompasses social, emotional, and spiritual pain. Following the pioneer work by Saunders at St. Christopher's Hospice in London, the importance and need for hospice type care has been recognized and is gaining worldwide acceptance.[40, 58, 62, 75, 98] The basic concept of hospice care is to alleviate all kinds of pain for patients and their families so that they are able to maintain rewarding relationships and live as fully as possible during the final stages of the patient's illness.

The model of Levels of Prevention that is described here can be applied to each individual disease or condition. Thus, in reality, a man may be subjected to various levels of prevention simultaneously. For example, a 65-year-old man has had a cerebrovascular accident secondary to arteriosclerotic heart disease. He complains of fatigue and shortness of breath after exercise and experiences pitting edema. He was recently discharged to his home from a rehabilitation service and is able to ambulate with a short leg brace but his upper extremity is spastic and nonfunctional. The time is late November and the city health department predicts influenza epidemics during the coming winter.

The cardiac condition receives priority attention; early diagnosis and prompt treatment for cardiac decompensation is in order. This is Secondary prevention. The patient is advised to wear the short leg brace daily and is given a static splint for his upper extremity. Further, ambulation commensurate with his tolerance is encouraged and a visiting physical therapist gives passive exercise to his upper extremity to prevent contracture of fingers. These are disability limitation measures. The attending physician would probably give influenza vaccine to prevent any danger to the patient from the threatened epidemic. This is Primary prevention.

Another example is cardiac surveillance of elderly disabled who are undergoing a rehabilitation program. Solomon and associates[94] found that over 25 per cent of geriatric lower extremity amputees who had no previous history of ischemic heart disease showed changes indicative of myocardial ischemia on telemetric dynamic electrocardiograms taken during ambulation exercise. This finding provides information necessary for regulating the patients' physical activity within the limits of cardiac tolerance so that ische-

mic heart disease might be prevented. While these patients are obviously receiving rehabilitation, the Secondary preventive care, the surveillance program promotes the "specific protection" of Primary prevention.

The purpose of this epidemiologic approach to patient care is to provide the tools that seek and analyze all factors contributing to disease and disability. It demonstrates a rational and individualized approach that assures that no factor is overlooked and no question remains unanswered.

FUNCTIONAL DIAGNOSIS

Prevention consists of two interrelated processes: the anticipation of future events and the action to thwart occurrence. Anticipation is possible only if there is some recall from past experience. When experience is documented in detail and carefully analyzed, prognostication can be reasonable and accurate. Epidemiology systematically studies the process of a disease or condition and demonstrates a chain of events that is known as the natural history. Once the natural history of a disease is established, the weakest link in the chain of events is the point where the attack to prevent the disease should start.

In the early part of this century epidemics of an unknown malady became prevalent in the southern part of the United States. An epidemiologic investigation was launched and certain characteristics regarding the prevalence of the disease were uncovered. Thus, the disease caused by a deficiency of niacin and now known as pellagra was identified.[30, 34] The methods used to discover the identity of pellagra were identical to the approach that previously had been applied only to transmissible diseases. The most important aspect of the pellagra investigation is that the whole epidemiologic study was based solely upon accurate clinical documentation of the condition of each patient so afflicted.

Rehabilitation, one of the secondary levels of prevention, focuses its attention on disability. Other specialties in therapeutic medicine require early and precise diagnosis in order to institute the most effective treatment. The same logic applies to rehabilitation, and the disabled should be given early evaluation and intensive treatment to prevent permanent disability.[51] Dynamic rehabilitation care can be administered only when an explicit early diagnosis of the disability has been established.[95] The longer explicit diagnosis is delayed, the less effective the consequent restorative care becomes.

For example, right hemiplegia due to cerebral artery thrombosis is not sufficiently accurate as a diagnosis to be utilized in making an effective rehabilitation care plan. Because the ultimate goal of rehabilitation is total restoration, the total person, physically, emotionally, vocationally, and socially, must be considered in the diagnosis. Most medical records and case histories do not indicate the physical, mental, or socioeconomic ability of a man.[97] There are no two identical hemiplegics. The aforementioned diagnosis, although medicolegally acceptable, does not indicate the extent of brain damage or note cultural background, which will directly influence the patient's ability to comprehend, retain instruction, or respond to the rehabilitation process. Thus, the conventional non-illuminating diagnostic nomenclature for statistical purposes[107] is insufficient for dynamic rehabilitation care.

Diagnosis of disability may be expressed either in terms of the amount of disability or in terms of the amount of remaining function. The former category is commonly called the disability evaluation or rating. In the latter category, functional diagnosis is the preferred terminology. Regardless of choice, the sum of the results from either system remains constant. It is universally agreed that disability evaluation is, in reality, a quantitative diagnosis as contrasted with the more familiar qualitative diagnosis.[23, 49, 50, 108] Evaluation of disability has long been important in the legal field.[1, 49, 64, 102] Since no single standard wholly fulfills the specific needs of all programs concerned with disability,[77] various rating systems according to diagnostic groups have been reported.[2, 35, 74, 108] One of the most widely used is the cardiac classification ratings of the American Heart Association. A variety of disability scales to evaluate the injured in liability or workmen's compensation cases were developed in the first half of this century.[13, 16, 31, 66, 111]

Countless methods to assess the extent of disability pursuant to a treatment plan and to evaluate the progress of a patient in a rehabilitation program are in the literature. Some are more ingenious or sophisticated than others. Moskowitz and McCann[68] developed a physical profile called PULSES which utilizes a set of ordinal scales. PULSES expresses general physical condition, the function of upper and lower extremities, sensory status, continency, and emotional status by six representative digits. The Sokolow method[92] rates physical, social, emotional, and vocational capacity, but a national field trial[93] revealed that this method contributes little of significant value to vocational counseling. For the past two decades numerous Activities of Daily Living (ADL) scales have been reported.[8, 12, 17, 21, 32, 37, 38, 48, 52, 59, 63, 86, 109] While ADL scales are mainly in the domain of the occupational therapist, Pool and Brown[76] selected certain activities which a physical therapist could evaluate.

A large volume of data must be collected in order to produce one comprehensive functional diagnosis. The accumulation of voluminous information inadvertently necessitates involvement with the problem of effective format and storage that will permit easy retrieval of all the data. In this regard, electronic data processing techniques have been found to be most advantageous.[92, 95]

The expression of disability evaluation or functional diagnosis varies according to the method. The most common method is a numerical presentation in either percentage or digit based upon a specific scale. The other common method is a graphic presentation. Unlike Lawton's method[52] for ADL, Huddleston and colleagues[39] produced a graph called the Patient Profile Chart, on which the value of muscle power and comparative functional capacities were arranged. In reviewing all these methods, there are more numerical presentations than descriptive ones. This tendency is perhaps due to the fact that the use of digits gives simplicity and provides mathematical advantages such as weighting.

The ordinal scale is becoming more popular than the nominal scale. However, one must recognize that a well-conceived nominal scale is superior to a haphazard ordinal scale despite the use of digits. One pitfall in the nominal scale is that innovators sometimes become trapped in their own jargon. There is a need to eliminate or replace vague stereotyped expression with more realistic and accurate terminology.[10] A good example of this type of ambiguous phraseology is "partial independent" or "minimum assistance." The ideal functional diagnosis should be:

1. Simple enough so that rapid evaluation is possible;

2. Reproducible so that constancy may be maintained;

3. Objective and using measurable factors so that the results are statistically more reliable;

4. Descriptive so that the actual situation is accurately reflected;

5. Comprehensive so that the diagnosis is completely and specifically utilizable in the direct care of patients and is practicable for epidemiologic investigation.

To date there is no single standard that measures disability with precision nor is there any set of precise biological units, free of subjective influences, that uniformly conveys universally acceptable measuring criteria.[49]

In relation to functional diagnosis, Wylie and White[110] stated:

In each field of knowledge, such as medicine or public health, a new measuring instrument commonly results in new studies and observation: from these we evolve new hypotheses, and further instruments are invented to test these ideas. . . . When the field knowledge is still in a rudimentary stage, often a scarcity of measuring instruments delays this cycle.

Thus, the use of epidemiology in rehabilitation can aid in defining the natural history of physical disabilities in mankind and it is well recognized that there is a gap in our knowledge of human incapacitation. Better "instrument" or better functional diagnosis means that new studies, new observation, and new hypotheses will emerge.

SECONDARY DISABILITY

In the daily practice of rehabilitation medicine in a hospital-based service or private office, there is a tendency to view disability in a simplistic or superficial way. Excluding iatrogenic disability and physical disability due to psychiatric illness,[56] two types of disabilities exist. Disabilities that are direct consequences of a disease or condition are called primary disability. Paraplegia, quadriplegia following spinal cord injury, hemiplegia, hemianopia, aphasia due to cerebral vascular accident, or traumatic fracture are examples of primary disability. On the other hand, disabilities that did not exist at the onset of the primary disability but subsequently developed are called secondary disabilities.[85] The secondary disability is indirectly related to the disease or condition that is responsible for the primary disability. Examples are joint contracture, subluxation of shoulder joint in hemiplegia, disuse muscle atrophy, and decubiti.

The epidemiology of primary disability, a subject outside the province of conventional rehabilitation medicine, will be discussed later in this chapter, under Preventive Rehabilitation. Since the secondary disability develops while the patient is under the physiatrist's care, it is important to discuss it in depth. However, literature related to the epidemiology of secondary disability is minimal. Abramson et al.[1] claimed that among injured workers there is a correlation between the degree of disability, the circumstances of injury, and the sex, age, employment status, economic status, and place of residence of the injured. This finding should not be interpreted as proof of the existence of malingering among workers covered by workmen's compensation but rather as proof that many complex factors are responsible for disablement. The group of secondary disabilities commonly found in cases of Hansen's disease has received intensive epidemiologic study,[70, 96] perhaps because the nature of the illness requires that a large number of epidemiologists be engaged in control of the disease.

An epidemiologic analysis of secondary disability reveals certain characteristics in the causative factors. Elderly people and those who have had a primary disability for an extended period are more susceptible to a secondary disability. Further, when the disease or condition causing the primary disability is accompanied by pain or spasticity, the prevalence of secondary disability increases. The frequency of flexion contracture in the hip joint of above-knee amputees or the multiple contractures in rheumatoid arthritis or multiple sclerosis are examples of these. On the other hand, if the original disease diminishes skin sensation, particularly pain or temperature, the patient is also predisposed to the secondary disability. Decubiti in paraplegics, plantar ulcers in patients with diabetes, and plantar ulcers and absorbtion of fingers in patients with Hansen's disease are representative. When nutrition is poor, certain disabilities such as decubiti are more easily developed. Socioeconomic and vocational factors may have indirect relationship to the causation of secondary disability. The level of intelligence, often related to cultural and educational background, and individual motivation are other indirect causative factors.

The environmental factor involved in the development of secondary disability is simply the position of the body itself. The idea of considering body position as an environmental factor may be unorthodox. However, positioning of either hemiplegic extremities or the stump after an amputation is external to the host and thus constitutes a contrived man-made environment. Negligence or ignorance on the part of paramedical personnel or family members results in placing the disabled in positions that foster secondary disability. Certain body positions that involve maintaining a particular position for a prolonged period may well prevent one disability but inadvertently cause another. Placing elderly patients with above-knee amputations or fractured hips on wheelchairs during the day is an effective measure to prevent pneumonia but tends to result in flexion contracture of the hip joint.

Another important factor affecting the "environmental body" is the condition of the objects with which it has direct contact. Materials that are rough surfaced, rigid, and minimally ventilated also predispose the host to secondary disability.

The most intriguing part in epidemiologic observation of secondary disability is identification of the agent. The agent is sometimes mechanical force, which may be either excessive or totally absent. Excessive and concentrated force to the skin area may result in decubitus, and the absence of force may cause demineralization of bone or disuse atrophy of muscle. At times this force may simply be the natural presence of gravity. Equinus deformity in flaccid foot drop and subluxation of the shoulder joint in hemiplegics are some examples of secondary disability related to gravity. The concept of the natural history of secondary disability specifies that the three causative factors (agent, host, and environment) must interact frequently or for a prolonged period. The time element is perhaps the key to the occurrence of disability stimuli.

The characteristics of secondary disability in the period of pathogenesis are always insidious and the symptoms are non-specific, regardless of the primary disability and its causative disease or condition. The process is always progressive and if not checked can at some point become irreversible. The secondary disability is usually painless but may sometimes be fatal if allowed to develop to the ultimate. The most usual result is a severe curtailment of function. There seems to be little seasonal variation and there is no known immunity to this condition.

IMMOBILIZATION

One universally recognized condition that severely damages the disabled is immobilization. According to the United States Public Health Service, disability due to immobilization was one of ten leading preventable health problems in 1960. Merely by utilization of present knowledge such disability in the United States could be reduced by 50 to 75 per cent.[78] Correlation between the amount of damage from immobilization and the duration of the immobilization is a controversial subject.[72, 88] In general, the greater the size of the body segment and the longer the period of immobilization, the greater the intensity of the pathologic condition and the number of organ systems that become involved.

The discussion of the agent factor provides the basis for understanding the mechanism of immobilization as one of the causes of secondary disability. Undoubtedly, immobilization is associated with the absence of mechanical force, the one stimulus so essential to maintenance of proper body function. Osteoporosis, the loss of bone density, is the most commonly known pathological change due to immobilization. This change is often detected in patients after a long-term plaster cast immobilization and is also found in the lower extremities of paraplegics. If the absence of force as a stimulus is the agent factor for osteoporosis, then it should be possible to produce this pathologic condition in normal individuals in a simulated environment. This hypothesis was proved correct by the distinct decrease in bone density and increase in calcium excretion in the astronauts during the 14-day Gemini VII voyage.[61, 105]

Many experimental immobilizations have revealed similar results. Mechanical stress, such as is produced by weight-bearing and muscle tension, is necessary for maintenance of the normal skeletal mass. During prolonged bed rest or extended conditions of zero gravity, the static stress distribution and its metabolic requirements are altered. The absence of normal mechanical stress on the skeletal system removes some of the stimuli necessary to bone formation.[47] Moreover, previously discussed causative factors of secondary disablement are also applicable to immobilization. The deleterious effect of immobilization cannot be considered a primary disability.

Every pathophysiological change starts its development at the onset of immobilization, just as the aging processes begin at birth. It is interesting to review the literature that seeks to establish the exact point wherein these changes become recognizable. The cardiac rate at rest increases approximately 0.5 beat per minute per each day of immobilization, and the loss of muscle tone resulting from complete disuse is estimated to be 10 to 15 per cent of strength per week.[99] After a few days of immobilization, an increase in bone blood flow was detected by means of radioactive strontium uptake and it was suggested that this may favor bone atrophy.[87] Similarly, within six to ten days following immobilization, the nitrogen balance of healthy male subjects reverses to a negative balance.[20] Significantly, the tendon capillary bed decreases after a six-week period of immobilization, but nothing of significance was observed in the muscle capillary bed. Because of this finding it is advisable to mobilize the recently repaired or reconstructed tendon as soon as possible, consistent with the limits of healing tensile strength.[83]

Events resulting in immobilization may be classified in various ways. Inadvertent and therapeutic immobilizations[44] are probably the most inclusive classifications. Bed rest and confinement to chair or wheelchair belong to the former category. Post-traumatic or post-surgical states, acute infection or inflammation, the convalescent period from non-surgical ailments, and so forth, constitute the latter category. In either group, immobilization is artificially forced upon the patients. On the other hand, there may also occur unavoidable immobilization, such as is caused by severe pain, neuromuscular impairment, or psychiatric illness. Irrespective of the reason, the pathophysiological changes and clinical symptoms of immobilization are non-specific.

These changes and symptoms continue progressively throughout the immobilization, and reversal is not always spontaneous upon termination of the restriction. Even if the changes are reversible, the period of recovery from these effects is much longer than the period of immobilization. An experiment determined that young healthy men confined in bed for three weeks need five weeks after resumption of normal activity to regain normal cardiovascular response to the upright position.[99] It is conceivable that those who have deteriorated physically, particularly the elderly, need a longer recovery period. Besides the time element, the manpower and money required for restoration is enormous. Pathological changes of immobilization superimposed upon the primary disability often create totally dependent persons out of patients who initially would have been self-sufficient. This can be devastating to the families and the socioeconomic well-being of a community. Since total immunization against the ill effects of immobilization has not been developed, simulation of mechanical stimuli to the human body during immobilization is the most effective preventive measure.

PRIMARY DISABILITY — PAST, PRESENT, AND FUTURE

Incidence and type of primary disabilities are often a reflection of contemporary technology and the political and social cultures of the society in which the population at risk resides.

For thousands of years the simple societies of our ancestors presented few risks to life and limb. In one century we have enriched our lives through technology and we have also increased our risks a thousand-fold. The endless drive for more speed, more products, and more power has created more comfort, more leisure, and more problems.

In a primitive society, man depends solely on his two legs for his locomotion. Thus, paraplegia due to locomotive activity in such a society is most likely caused either by a falling object or by man falling. Since the development of the wheel, there has been continuous evolution in locomotive devices for comfort, convenience, and efficiency. Thus, invention of the internal combustion engine produced the automobile. As the automobile became larger, heavier, and faster, a vast network of highway systems became a part of American life. The net result was drastic increases in highway accidents, which often resulted in fatalities or left the survivors with severe disabilities. We cannot go back in time and abolish the wheel, because the quadriplegic who was a victim of wheels and technology regains his mobility by using a motorized wheelchair, which is also a product of wheels and technology.

Major political decisions are seldom made on the basis of humanity or health. However, the Federal Government reduced the speed limit on highways to 55 miles per hour to decrease fuel consumption. Inadvertently, this economic decision dramatically decreased the incidence of highway accidents. In addition, future automobiles are expected to be equipped with less powerful engines, again a measure to save fuel. Since these engines will be unable to attain high speeds, we can hope for further reduction in the number of serious accidents.

Almost daily a new machine replaces some type of skilled or unskilled labor. The skilled and educated are usually able to adapt to other occupations. The unskilled and undereducated add to the ever-increasing group of chronically unemployed. Many others learn to live by their wits, sometimes within the law and sometimes not.

An observation at a municipal hospital in New York City shows that two decades ago the major causes of traumatic paraplegia and quadriplegia were automobiles, falling, and industrial and swimming accidents. The current most common cause is the gunshot wound.[55] The circumstances that lead to this injury are often obscured, but they are usually related to some kind of illegal activity, particularly drugs.

However, the drug problem is not confined to the impoverished ghetto. Middle and upper income communities complain of drugs in their schools. Colleges report greater usage on their campuses and physicians acknowledge an increase in rhinoplasty due to a growing number of wealthy cocaine addicts. Cerebral anoxia due to overdose is commonly seen in hospital emergency rooms everywhere in this country.

Mental health has long been involved in treatment of addiction, and rehabilitation medicine has treated the victims of drug-related accidents and violence. However, if the prevalence of drug addiction persists we can expect myriad physical disabilities in these addicts if they live to reach middle age.

Technology and culture are constantly changing for better or for worse. These changes directly or indirectly influence morbidity. While some disabilities that were prevalent in the past become non-existent, disabilities due to new causes emerge. Examples of the former are disabilities caused by infections such as poliomyelitis or gonorrhea. Some examples of the latter have already been discussed. Trauma to upper and lower extremities due to skateboarding and severe injuries due to snowmobile accidents are new types of injury.

A spinal cord injury at the level of C-2, C-3 has been considered a fatal injury. However, improvement of emergency medical services and new medical and surgical techniques[3, 11] are now able to save this patient and keep him alive with the aid of a respirator. If this trend continues, an increase in the number of high quadriplegics must be expected.

The cumulative effects of low dosage but frequent and/or prolonged exposure to an agent are insidious. Noise notch, a hearing deficit at a specific frequency of sound, has been known as an occupational disability. Thus, noise control in work environments and mandatory use of ear muffs and plugs in certain occupations are a part of occupational safety measures. Ultraloud music in the discoteque and blasting hard rock music on radios and record players are part of today's youth culture. It is reasonable to assume that this will create noise notch in many of these young people.

Jogging has become very popular among all age groups in the United States in the past few years. This activity may be of benefit to cardiopulmonary function,[101] but a sedentary middle-age person may injure various organ systems[22, 65] by daily jogging on paved streets or by starting this sport without sufficient preparation. Disorders of the nipples of the breasts due to jogging have already been reported.[57, 69]

High-heel shoes are known to cause various foot disorders in women. Recent fashion promotes high-heel shoes and cowboy boots for men. The high-heel shoe simply adds one or more inches to the regular broad heel of a man's shoe. The cowboy boot, however, has a slanted narrow high heel and sharply pointed toe. Originally custom made and fitted to the wearer by a skilled bootmaker, it was designed to hook into the stirrups of a saddle and to maintain a foothold on unpaved ground. Today, thousands of young men wear a mass-produced variety on city sidewalks instead of regular shoes. It is hard to believe that men are immune to foot disorders, and we can expect to see men with the same foot problems that have heretofore been confined to women.

Contraceptive devices and pills are effective tools for population control programs that are fundamentally socioeconomic and ecological measures. Today their widespread use in industrialized countries has created the potential for an increase in disability among young women. It is well known that intrauterine devices can penetrate the uterine wall and cause catastrophic infections, whereas the pill appears relatively harmless. But now when a young woman is brought into an emergency room with symptoms of cerebral vascular accident, we suspect rupture of congenital aneurysm, embolism due to rheumatic heart disease, or prolonged intake of contraceptive pills.[19, 45]

Some say the use or misuse of population control tools and the moral implications are not within the province of medicine. Wherever the life and health of the population is involved, all the questions that arise should be our concern. We know that the health and survival of man are related to the total population that this earth can support. Medicine concerned with the future health and survival of man cannot ignore any phase of any effort to preserve earth so that it can continue to nurture the human race.

We must be concerned with earth and its population, with rehabilitation of that which has been destroyed or contaminated, and with prevention of future destruction and contamination that maims people and deforms infants, whether by nuclear war or other means. We must contribute our expertise to every dialogue and every plan to preserve the health of man and earth for future generations. We cannot limit ourselves to rehabilitation of the victims of man-made disabilities and disasters. We must also use our expertise to prevent their occurrence.

A history is taken from the patient in order to make a diagnosis and prognosis. Our future patients are living their history today. If we are alert to what is happening in their and our world we can often predict future outcomes. We need to anticipate and be prepared to cope with the disabilities of the future and prevent those that can be prevented. It is reasonable to assume that new causes of disability that cannot be imagined today will be identified in the decades to come, and we must develop our science to meet that challenge.

PREVENTIVE REHABILITATION

All clinical specialties focus their interest and effort toward restoration of man's health from the state of Overt Illness to Optimum Health. In this sense, if the definition of rehabilitation is accepted, all clinicians practice "the act of rehabilitation."[41] Care provided through rehabilitation medicine consists of restoration of function and prevention of disability. Diverse therapeutic exercises are instrumental in anatomic and physiological restoration of function. Though this type of physical rehabilitation is ideal, the outcome depends heavily upon natural recovery from the lesion responsible for the disability, and this goal is not always attainable. When anatomic and physiological restoration has failed, a compensatory body mechanism or an orthotic or prosthetic device substitutes for the lost function. Although the goals of nursing and physical and occupational therapy are primarily directed toward complete restoration or functional substitution, in actuality this may mean that they predominantly engage in prevention of secondary disability. As the greater portion of the time and energy of rehabilitation professionals is devoted, intentionally or unintentionally, to prevention of secondary disability, rehabilitation medicine should certainly become more emphatically involved in the epidemiologic approach and its application to preventive measures.

The term "Preventive Rehabilitation" has been introduced in response to this need.[41, 43, 46] Until the mid-twentieth century, the stigmatizing deformities commonly seen in patients with Hansen's disease were believed to be primary disabilities. Careful and painstaking clinical investigation and epidemiologic analysis revealed the natural history of these disabilities: they are secondary disabilities caused by trauma and infection. They result from the neglect and ignorance of both patients and medical professionals. Modifications in activities of daily living, simple self-administered daily exercise, early case finding, and regular, adequate specific chemotherapy can prevent these disabilities. Heretofore, the only alternative was reconstruction by skilled plastic surgery after these disabilities had become irreversible. "Preventive Rehabilitation" became a component of conventional rehabilitation in leprosy-control programs.[71]

In recent years epidemiologists have become progressively involved in the clinical epidemiology of diseases that result in physical disabilities, and clinicians have become increasingly aware of the epidemiologic approach to clinical problems. Feinstein[26] characterized clinical epidemiology as being not restricted by type of disease, age, locale, or any particular form of data collection. Clinical epidemiology may be viewed as ecologic medicine, social medicine, or community medicine. The concept of health and the model for the natural history of disease were derived from experience in transmissible disease, and they are essential to any analysis of non-infectious diseases or conditions such as disability. The fundamental purpose of epidemiology is the prevention and eradication of diseases and conditions through a better understanding of causation. If complete prevention or total eradication is not possible, containment is the second choice.

In pursuit of the philosophy of Preventive Rehabilitation, medical and paramedical specialists in rehabilitation must develop keen sensitivity to the relationship between social, economic, cultural, and political environment and disability. Recreational use of motorcycles and mopeds is increasing, and unchecked operation of these vehicles may cause primary disability not only to the drivers but also to pedestrians.[6] Motorcycles are becoming a popular mode of transportation among the young population. In many states, drivers are obliged to wear a crash helmet to prevent fatal head injury in an accident. The helmet may decrease fatality but does not necessarily prevent spinal cord injury.

Various investigators have estimated the cost of care for decubitus ulcers. Calculation of the cost differs from one study to another, and the more recent the study the higher the cost because the inflationary factor is taken into consideration. Weinstein[103] estimated that a minimun cost for prevention and treatment of the ulcer in the United States was 357 million dollars as of 1970 to 1973. Lee,[54] on the other hand, calculated the total cost of treatment of decubitus ulcers in the United States at an 883 million dollar minimum in 1977.

Public education is often offered as a method of preventing disability. Instituting educational programs does not necessarily mean that the intended goal is achieved. For example, high school driver education has not decreased the incidence of fatal automobile accidents.[79] What is needed now are aggressive public relations programs rather than educational programs.

The pioneers of rehabilitation utilized the public relations technique, presenting successfully rehabilitated cases and the economic value of rehabilitation programs in order to justify expenditures for this new specialty. While this campaign was obviously effective, the public began to place too much trust in the capability of the rehabilitation program. People are often careless and take unnecessary risks believing that surgery and rehabilitation can correct any injury or disability. There is a tendency to believe that rehabilitation can work miracles. Glorification of rehabilitation medicine is no longer necessary. Rather, the public must be informed of the not-so-glamorous parts of rehabilitation — the high cost, the plight of the disabled, and the grim statistics of unsuccessful cases. The emphasis of the new public relations campaign must be placed on prevention of primary disability. In doing so, we must learn to reach business, government, economists, legislators, bureaucrats, and the general public.

In this new concept of Preventive Rehabilitation, the scope of expertise and the role of the physiatrist must be enlarged. Prevention of disability does not start at birth or after a primary disability occurs. Disability due to genetic defects or genetic incompatibility can be prevented by means of genetic counseling. The potentials of genetic engineering in this regard must be seriously considered. During the early gestation period, expectant mothers must be protected from rubella and from certain pharmaceutical products. Amniotic fluid analysis may provide vital information pertinent to the discovery of potentially disabling diseases in the newborn.

These are measures to prevent primary disability. However, artificial termination of pregnancy to eliminate the fetus with suspected deformities should not be considered as prevention of primary disability. The justification for advocating artificial abortion in these cases is preponderantly psychosocial and economic and not medical. Cerebral palsy due to intracranial damage in a high forceps delivery should concern the physiatrist as much as it involves the obstetrician. Although modern health care provides many deterrents to primary disability (Fig. 10–3), prevention has mainly involved public health specialists and allied health professionals but not the physiatrist.

Current population growth, particularly a rapid increase of the aged, predicts a sharp rise in our disabled population in the near future. It is well documented that there is a great shortage of medical and paramedical professionals to care for the disabled and we cannot even meet present demands.

In recent years, specialists in neurology, orthopedic surgery, and pediatrics are increasingly involved and have a vital role in the field of rehabilitation medicine. This phenomenon should not be interpreted as an invasion of the field by other specialists but rather it signifies recognition of the importance of rehabilitation medicine. The additional expertise of specialists in public health and preventive medicine is also a welcome contribution to the further enrichment of rehabilitation medicine.

Unless more effective methods of specific prevention are developed to protect the population from primary disability in the future, the newly disabled will face a critical situation. The cumulative shortage of health manpower will cause them to be without benefit of rehabilitation services, and superimposed secondary disabilities will render them totally dependent. This will not only result in insurmountable personal tragedy, but will create infinite economic problems for families, communities, and nations.

Exploration into the epidemiology of disability, the causative factors, the natural history of secondary disability, the epidemiology of immobilization, and the importance of functional diagnosis exposes the urgency for a reassessment of rehabilitation medicine. Our professionals, medical and para-

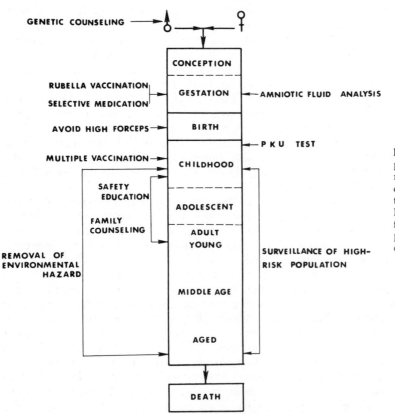

FIGURE 10–3. Prevention of primary disability in the life of man. Items on the left side of the column indicate specific protection against primary disability, Measures on the right side are for early detection and probable prevention of potential primary disability.

medical, have played rather passive roles in clinical medicine and comprehensive health care.* Although rehabilitation medicine has pioneered in vocational and legislative areas and contributed immeasurably to the welfare of the handicapped, it has not played the same spectacular role in the delivery of health care. Further, we need to focus our attention on research, health planning, and health education. Laymen, through the efforts of rehabilitation medicine, are now sensitive to and aware of the social and vocational needs of the disabled, and many laymen are now capable of furthering the principles that we initiated. It is now time for the science-oriented medical rehabilitation community to develop and promote its more scientific aspects, to explore every phase of disability and disability prevention, and to contribute epidemiologic investigation that will make it possible for those engaged in rehabilitation to prevent epidemics of disability in much the same manner that we are now able to prevent communicable disease.

---

*Comprehensive health care is defined as care that is provided to the patient according to his needs in appropriate, continuous and dynamic pattern.[24]

REFERENCES

1. Abramson, J. H., Mann, K. J., Nizan, A., and Goldberg, R.: Epidemiology of disability after work injuries. Arch. Environ. Health, 9:572–580, 1964.
2. Alba, A., Trainor, F. S., Ritter, W., and Dacso, M. M.: A clinical disability rating for Parkinson patients. J. Chron. Dis., 21:507–522, 1968.
3. Albin, M. S.: Resuscitation of spinal cord. Crit. Care Med., 6:270–276, 1978.
4. American Public Health Association: Report after Love Canal — Thousand areas are potential hazard. Nation's Health, 8:1–6, 1978.
5. Askergreen, A., and Szamosi, A.: Relation between radiological pleuropulmonary changes, clinical history and weight index of construction workers. Scan. J. Work Environ. Health, 4:179–183, 1978.
6. Balcerak, J. C., Pancione, K. L., and States, J. D.: Moped, minibike and motorcycle accidents. Associated injury problems. N.Y. State J. Med., 78:628–633, 1978.
6a. Banhuys, A., Schoenberg, J. B., Beck, G. J., and Schilling, R. S. F.: Epidemiology of chronic lung disease in a cotton mill community. Lung, 154:167–186, 1977.
7. Boyd, H. B., and George, I. L.: Fracture of the hip. Result following treatment. J.A.M.A., 137:1196–1199, 1948.
8. Brown, M. E.: Daily activity inventory and progress record for those with atypical movement. I. Am. J. Occup. Ther., 4:195–204, 1950.
9. Brown, M. H.: Love Canal, U.S.A. New York Times Magazine, pp. 23, 38, 41–44, 21 Jan., 1979.
10. Bruett, T. L., and Overs, R. P.: A critical review of 12 ADL scales. Phys. Ther., 49:857–862, 1969.
11. Burke, D. C.: Early management of spinal cord injury. Med. J. Aust., 1:145–148, 11 Feb., 1978.
12. Buchwald, E.: Physical Rehabilitation for Daily Living. New York, McGraw-Hill Book Co., 1952.
13. Burns, R. M.: Rating of industrial disabilities. Lancet, 58:17–20, 1939.
14. Carbone, A.: Agonist-antagonist theory: New pain killer. Hosp. Formulary, 13:877–881, 1978.
15. Carson, R.: Silent Spring. Boston, Houghton Co., 1962.
16. Carter, R. M.: Estimation of disability. Industr. Med., 8:52–54, 1939.
17. Carroll, D.: The disability in hemiplegia caused by cerebrovascular disease. J. Chron. Dis., 15:179–188, 1962.
18. Clark, E. G.: The epidemiological approach and contribution to preventive medicine. In Leavell, H. R., and Clark, E. G. (Eds.): Preventive Medicine for the Doctor in His Community. New York, McGraw-Hill Book Co., 1965, Chapter 3.
19. Collaborative Group for Study of Stroke in Young Women: Oral contraception and increased risk of cerebral ischemia or thrombosis. N. Engl. J. Med., 288:871–878, 1973.
20. Deitrick, J. E., Whedon, G. D., and Shorr, E.: Effects of immobilization upon various metabolic and physiologic functions of normal men. Am. J. Med., 4:3–32, 1948.
21. Dennerstein, A. S., Lowenthal, M., and Dexter, M.: Evaluation of a rating scale of ability in activities of daily living. Arch. Phys. Med., 46:579–584, 1965.
22. Deutsch, M. E.: More on jogger's ailment. N. Engl. J. Med., 298:405, 1978.
23. Dristine, M. J.: Disability evaluation. Principles of quantitative diagnosis. Northwest Med., 61:1041–1042, 1962.
24. Division of Chronic Disease, Public Health Service: The concept of comprehensive care. In Lilienfeld, A. M., and Gifford, A. J. (Eds.): Chronic Disease and Public Health. Baltimore, Johns Hopkins Press, 1966.
25. Division of Epidemiology, Columbia University, School of Public Health and Administrative Medicine: Principles, Methods and Uses of Epidemiology. New York, 1965.
26. Feinstein, A. R.: Clinical epidemiology, I. The populational experiments of nature and of man in human illness. Ann. Intern. Med., 69:807–820, 1968.
27. Fowler, C. H., and DePuy, W. H.: Home and Health and Home Economics. New York, Phillips and Hunt, 1880.
28. Fracastoro, G.: De contagione et contagiosis morbis et eorum curatine, Libri III. Translated and notes by Wilmer Cave Wright. New York, G. P. Putnam's Sons, 1930.
29. Fukuji, M.: Studies of the cause that the causative agent of Minamata disease was formed, especially on the accumulation of the mercury com-

pound in the fish and shellfish of Minamata Bay. J. Kumamoto Med. Soc., *37*:494–521, 1963.

30. Goldberger, J., Wheeler, G. A., and Sydenstricker, W.: A study of the relation of diet to pellagra incidence in seven textile-mill communities of South Carolina in 1916. Pub. Health Rep., *35*:648–713, 1920.

31. Goodwin, W. M.: Meaning of functional disabilities. Int. J. Surg., *37*:540–548, 1924.

32. Gorden, E. E., and Kohn, K. H.: Evaluation of rehabilitation methods in the hemiplegic patient. J. Chron. Dis., *19*:3–16, 1966.

33. Gordon, B. L.: Medieval and Renaissance Medicine. New York, Philosophical Library, Inc., 1959, Chapter XXII.

34. Gordon, J. E., and LeRiche, H.: The epidemiologic method applied to nutrition. Am. J. Med. Sci., *219*:312–345, 1950.

35. Greenseid, D. Z., and McCormack, R. M.: Functional hand testing. A profile evaluation. Plast. Reconstr. Surg., *42*:567–571, 1968.

36. Hammond, E. C., Selikoff, I. J., and Churg, J.: Neoplasia among insulation workers in USA with special reference to intra-abdominal neoplasia. Ann. N.Y. Acad. Sci., *132*:519–525, 1965.

37. Hoberman, M., Cicenia, E. F., and Stephenson, G. R.: Daily activity testing in physical therapy and rehabilitation. Arch. Phys. Med.,*33*:99–108, 1952.

38. Hoff, W. I., and Mead, S.: Evaluation of rehabilitation outcome. An objective assessment of the physically disabled. Am. J. Phys. Med.,*44*:113–121, 1965.

39. Huddleston, O. L., Moore, R. W., Rubin, D., Humphrey, T. L., Campbell, J. W., and Balanchetter, R.: Evaluation of physical disabilities by means of patient profile chart. Arch. Phys. Med.,*42*:250–257, 1961.

40. Ingles, T.: St. Christopher's Hospice. Nursing Outlook, *22*:759–763, 1974.

41. Itoh, M., and Lee, M. H.: The future role of rehabilitation medicine in community health. Med. Clin. North Am., *53*:719–733, 1969.

42. Itoh, M., and Dacso, M. M.: Rehabilitation of patients with hip fracture. A clinical study of 126 cases. Postgrad. Med., *28*:134–139, 1960.

43. Itoh, M.: Preventive rehabilitation for leprosy — A new approach to an old problem. Rehab. Rev., *19*:13–14, 1968.

44. Jebsen, R. H.: Therapeutic exercise in motion problems, I. Northwest Med., *65*:742–747, 1966.

45. Jick, H., Porter, J., and Rothman, J.: Oral contraceptives and non-fatal stroke in healthy young women. Ann. Intern. Med.,*89*:58–60, 1978.

46. Karat, S.: Preventive rehabilitation in leprosy. Leprosy Rev., *39*:39–44, 1968.

47. Kazasian, L. E., and Von Gierker, H. E.: Bone loss as a result of immobilization and chelation. Preliminary results in *Macaca mulatta*. Clin. Orthop.,*65*:67–75, 1969.

48. Kelman, H. R., and Muller, J. N.: Rehabilitation of nursing home residents. Geriatrics, *17*:402–411, 1962.

49. Knapp, M. E.: Disability evaluation, 1. Postgrad. Med.,*46*:184–186, 1969.

50. Knapp, M. E.: Disability evaluation, 2. Postgrad. Med.,*46*:201–203, 1969.

51. Krusen, E. M.: Rehabilitation of the elderly. Southern Med. J., *51*:225–228, 1958.

52. Lawton, E. B.: Activities of daily living: Testing training and equipment. New York, Institute of Physical Medicine and Rehabilitation, New York University Bellevue Medical Center, Monograph No. 10, 1956.

53. Leavell, H. R., and Clark, E. G.: Levels of application of preventive medicine.*In* Leavell, H. R., and Clark, E. G. (Eds.): Preventive Medicine for the Doctor in His Community. New York, McGraw-Hill Book Co., 1965, Chapter 2.

54. Lee, M.: The Decubitus Ulcer Patient — Statement of the Problem. Presented at the Conference on Current Trends in the Care and Treatment of Decubitus Ulcer. Goldwater Memorial Hospital, New York, Oct. 4, 1977.

55. Lee, M. H., Novey, J., and Rusk, H. A.: An Experiment in the Care and Rehabilitation of Severely Disabled Young Adults in a Long Term Hospital. Paper presented at Amer. Cong. Rehab. Med., Nov., 1978. Also appeared in RT-1 Report 1978, New York Univ. Med. Center.

56. Lerner, J.: Disability evaluation in psychiatric illness and the concept of hysteria. Canad. Psychiatr. Ass. J., *11*:350–355, 1966.

57. Levit, F.: Jogger's nipples. N. Engl. J. Med., *297*:1127, 1977.

58. Liegner, L. M.: St. Christopher's Hospice, 1974. Care of dying patient. J.A.M.A.,*234*:1047–1048, 1975.

59. Linn, M. W.: A rapid disability rating scale. J. Am. Geriat. Soc., *15*:211–214, 1967.

60. Lilienfeld, B. E.: Epidemiologic methods and inferences. *In* Hilleboe, H. E., and Larimore, G. W. (Eds.): Preventive Medicine. Philadelphia, W. B. Saunders Company, 1965, Chapter 43.

61. Lutwak, L.: Chemical analysis of diet. Urine, feces and sweat parameters relating to the calcium and nitrogen balance studies during Gemini VII flight (Exp. M7). NASA Contractor Report, NAS 9-5375, 1966.

62. Lysman, A. G.: Drug therapy in terminally ill patients. Am. J. Hosp. Pharmacy, *32*:270–276, 1975.

63. Mahoney, F. I., Wood, O. H., and Barthel, D. W.: Rehabilitation of chronically ill patients. Influence of complication of chronically ill patients. Southern Med. J., *51*:605–609, 1958.

64. Mann, K. J., Abramson, J. H., Nizan, A., and Goldberg, R.: Epidemiology of disabling work injuries in Israel. Arch. Environ. Health (Chicago), *9*:505–513, 1964.

65. Massey, E. W., and Pleet, A. B.: Neuropathy in joggers. Am. J. Sports Med., *6*:209–211, 1978.

66. McBride, E. D.: Disability evaluation — Principles of treatment of compensable injuries, 4th Ed. Philadelphia, J. B. Lippincott Co., 1942.

67. Milby, T. H.: Pneumoconioses. *In* Occupational Diseases, A Guide to Their Recognition. Washington, D.C., U.S. Dept. of Health, Education and Welfare, Public Health Service. Public Health Service Publication No. 1097, 1964, Section V.

68. Moskowitz, E., and McCann, C. B.: Classification of disability in chronically ill and aging. J. Chron. Dis., 5:342–346, 1957.

69. Nequin, N. D.: More on jogger's ailment. N. Engl. J. Med., 298:405–406, 1978.

70. Noordeen, S. K., and Srinivasan, H.: Epidemiology of disability in leprosy, I. A general study of disability among male patients above fifteen years of age. Int. J. Leprosy, 34:159–169, 1966.

71. Pan American Health Organization: Consolidated Report on Item III, Determination of Objectives and Preparation of Timetables, 1968.

72. Patel, A. N.: Disuse atrophy of human skeletal muscles. Arch. Neurol., 20:413–421, 1969.

73. Paul, J. R.: Clinical Epidemiology. Chicago, The University of Chicago Press, 1966.

74. Pederson, E.: A rating system for neurological impairment in multiple sclerosis. Acta Neurol. Scand., 41(Suppl. 13):557–558, 1965.

75. Plant, J.: Finding a home for hospice care in the United States. Hospitals, 51:53, 55, 57–58, 1977.

76. Pool, D. A., and Brown, R. A.: A functional rating scale for research in physical therapy. Texas Rep. Biol. Med., 26:133–136, 1968.

77. Price, L.: Medical disability standards. J. Occup. Med., 8:542–547, 1966.

78. Public Health Service: Public Health Service Hearing before the House Subcommittee on Appropriations, Eighty-sixth Congress, Second Session, 1960, pp. 1205–1212.

79. Robertson, L. S., and Zador, P. L.: Driver education and fatal crash involvement of teenaged drivers. Am. J. Pub. Health, 68:959–965, 1978.

80. Robey, L. R.: Intertrochanteric and subtrochanteric fracture of the femur in the Negro. J. Bone Joint Surg., 38A:1301–1312, 1956.

81. Rogers, E. S.: Human Ecology and Health. Introduction for Administrators. New York, Macmillan Co., 1960.

82. Rosen, G.: A History of Public Health. New York, MD Publications, 1958.

83. Rothman, R. H., and Slogoff, S.: The effect of immobilization on the vascular bed of tendon. Surg. Gynecol. Obstet., 124:1064–1066, 1967.

84. Rusk, H. A., and Hilleboe, H. E.: Rehabilitation. In Hilleboe, H. E., and Larimore, G. W. (Eds.): Preventive Medicine, Philadelphia, W. B. Saunders Company, 1965, Chapter 33.

85. Ryder, C. F., and Daitz, B.: Prevention of disability. In Selle, W. A. (Ed.): Restorative Medicine in Geriatrics. Springfield, Ill., Charles C Thomas, Publisher, 1963, Chapter 14.

86. Schoening, H. A., and Iverson, I. A.: The Kenny Selfcare Evaluation: A Numerical Measure of Independence in Activity of Daily Living. Minneapolis, Kenny Rehabilitation Institute, 1965.

87. Semb, H.: Effect of immobilization on bone blood flow estimated by initial uptake of radioactive strontium. Surg. Gynecol. Obstet., 127:275–281, 1968.

88. Sevitt, S., and Gallagher, N.: Venous thrombosis and pulmonary embolism. Br. J. Surg., 48:475–489, 1961.

89. Smillie, W. G.: Preventive Medicine and Public Health. New York, Macmillan Co., 1952, Chapter 18.

90. Snyder, H.: Opiate receptors and internal opiates. Sci. Am., 236:43–56, 1977.

91. Snyder H.: The opiate receptor and morphine like peptides in the brain. Am. J. Psychiatry, 135:645–652, 1978.

92. Sokolow, J., Silson, J., Taylor, E. J., Anderson, E. T., and Rusk, H. A.: A method for the functional evaluation of disability. Arch. Phys. Med. Rehab., 40:421–428, 1959.

93. Sokolow, J., and Taylor, E. J.: Report of a national field trial of a method for functional disability evaluation. J. Chron. Dis., 20:896–909, 1967.

94. Solomon, M., Itoh, M., Clarke, C. P., and Goldstein, J. M.: Telemetric electrocardiogram as a tool for dynamic cardiac evaluation in physical therapy. Arch. Phys. Med. Rehab., 15:730, 1970.

95. Spencer, W. A., and Vallbona, C.: A preliminary report on the use of electronic data processing technics in the description and evaluation of disability. Arch. Phys. Med., 43:22–35, 1962.

96. Srinivasan, H., and Noordeen, S. K.: Epidemiology of disability in leprosy. Int. J. Leprosy, 34:170–174, 1966.

97. Stinson, M.: Medical care and rehabilitation of the aged. Geriatrics, 8:266–299, 1953.

98. Stoddard, S.: The Hospice Movement. A Better Way of Caring for the Dying. New York, Random House, 1978.

99. Taylor, H. L., Henschel, A., Brozek, J., and Key, A.: Effects of bedrest on cardiovascular function and work performance. J. Appl. Physiol., 2:223–239, 1949.

100. Van Demark, E. G., and Van Demark, R. E.: Hip nailing in patients of eighty years or older. Am. J. Surg., 85:664–668, 1953.

101. Vaisrub, S.: Joyful jogging (editorial). J.A.M.A., 240:1385, 1978.

102. Vorwald, A. J., Robin, E. D., Gordon, B. L., Moteley, L., and Noonan, T. B.: Evaluation of disability. Arch. Environ. Health, 8:889–897, 1964.

103. Weinstein, B.: The cost of decubitus ulcer. A statistical approximation (mimeographed report). Personal Communication. Rehab. Unit, University of Rochester, N.Y.

104. Welch, W. H.: Institute of hygiene. In Rockefeller Foundation Annual Report, New York, 1916, pp. 415–427.

105. Whedon, C. D., Lutwak, L., and Neuman, W.: Calcium and Nitrogen Balance. In a review of medical results of Gemini VII and related flights. J. F. Kennedy Space Center, Florida, NASA SP-121, 1967.

106. World Health Organization: Constitution of the World Health Organization. Geneva, World Health Organization, 1964.

107. World Health Organization: Manual of the International Statistical Classification of Diseases, Injuries and Causes of Death. 1965 Revision, Vol. 1. Geneva, World Health Organization, 1967.

108. World Health Organization: Classification of disabilities resulting from leprosy, for use in control program. Bull. W.H.O., 40:609–612, 1969.

109. Wylie, C. M.: Administrative research in the rehabilitation of stroke patient. Rehab. Lit., 25:2–7, 1964.

110. Wylie, C. M., and White, B. K.: A measure of disability. Arch. Environ. Health, 8:834–839, 1964.

111. Yamshon, L. T.: Industrial injury. Practical need for evaluation of capacity. J.A.M.A., 165:934–938, 1957.

11

THE NEUROPHYSIOLOGY OF MOTOR FUNCTION

FREDERIC J. KOTTKE

There is a lack of agreement regarding the neurophysiological mechanisms resulting in the organization of motor function in man. The differences in interpretation of existing scientific data are profound. For this reason, at the outset it is worth emphasizing that essentially the same data are interpreted quite differently by different authorities depending on each individual's concept of the organization of the nervous system. The overly simplistic conventional presentation is that voluntary muscular coordination is initiated in the motor cortex and transmitted over uninterrupted axons that cross through the medullary pyramids to synapse on motor neurons in the contralateral anterior horn of the spinal cord and provide a direct connection for control of each of the muscles in the coordination pattern. Most textbooks of physiology imply, even if they do not directly state, that movements originate in a limited region of the cortex or arise there in response to stimuli from other regions of the brain and that each movement is encoded in the cortex as a pattern of nerve impulses transmitted over the corticospinal tract to the appropriate motor neurons to produce the desired motor pattern. It was even sug-

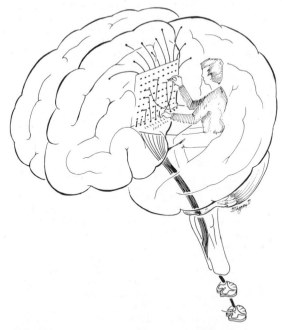

FIGURE 11–1. Coordination is far more complex than selecting and exciting neurons in the motor cortex which have genetically encoded patterns of motor activity. (From Kottke, F. J., Halpern, D., Easton, J. K. M., Ozel, A. T., and Burrill, C. A.: Training of coordination. Arch. Phys. Med. Rehabil., 59:567–572, 1978.)

gested very early that each neuron of the premotor cortex contains a pattern of coordination and that this area of the cortex serves as a keyboard from which appropriate combinations of activities are selected by some unidentified area of the brain to produce the desired coordination[15] (Fig. 11–1). Another hypothesis is that subcortical structures in the basal ganglia, thalamus, and brain stem ganglia act as the organizers or integrators to combine into coordinated patterns the sensorimotor relationships stored in the cortex.[50] Still others hypothesize that the pyramidal system and the extrapyramidal system monitor motor activities in different segments of the extremities or that the pyrami-

dal tract is responsible for fast actions and the extrapyramidal tract for initiating slow or postural responses.

Likewise there are markedly different concepts regarding the involvement of the reflexes in normal coordination. One concept is that reflexes are residuals of an ancient nervous system and are redundant because of the more direct pathways that have developed from the brain. Another hypothesis is that the reflexes exist in a parallel relationship to motor coordination so that initiation of reflexes can facilitate and amplify the magnitude of the voluntary response. Still another hypothesis, which is the thesis of this chapter, is that the reflexes form the

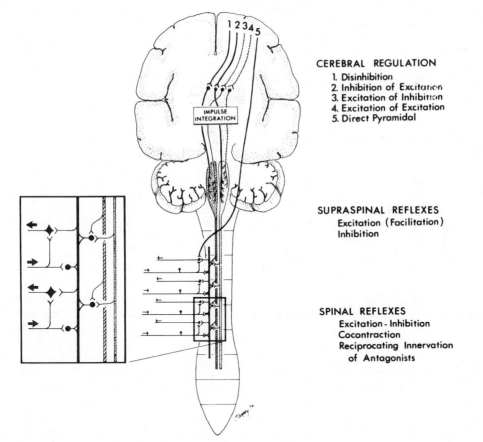

CEREBRAL REGULATION
1. Disinhibition
2. Inhibition of Excitation
3. Excitation of Inhibition
4. Excitation of Excitation
5. Direct Pyramidal

SUPRASPINAL REFLEXES
Excitation (Facilitation)
Inhibition

SPINAL REFLEXES
Excitation - Inhibition
Cocontraction
Reciprocating Innervation
of Antagonists

FIGURE 11–2. The central nervous system is organized into three hierarchic levels. The spinal reflexes, representing the lowest level, have stereotyped pathways in which only the degree of spread of activity varies according to the intensity of excitation and inhibition. The supraspinal reflexes and the reticular facilitatory and inhibitory centers at the middle level act by modifying the spinal reflexes. Cerebral regulation at the highest level also acts through modification of the activities of the lower levels. Cerebral coordination is achieved by activating engrams of facilitation and inhibition transmitted in the extrapyramidal system through the middle and lowest levels. Direct corticospinal control makes variation of the activity of a prime mover possible by localized excitation directly on the lowest level. (Modified from Kottke, F. J.: From reflex to skill: The training of coordination. Arch. Phys. Med. Rehabil., 61:551–561, 1980.)

basic organized pathways in the spinal cord, and regulation from higher centers is accomplished by excitation and inhibition imposed on these reflex pathways (Fig. 11–2). To prevent undesired activity the higher centers must maintain an inhibitory control over the spinal reflexes. To produce motor activity the higher centers must release the inhibition or stimulate excitation. Without the millions of sensory impulses entering the central nervous system each instant, the level of irritability of the internuncial neurons and anterior horn cells will not be high enough to allow any excitation from supraspinal motor centers. Over 100 years ago Hughlings Jackson hypothesized this concept as the application of the theory of evolution to the nervous system.[29] A scientific basis for this hypothesis was laid with the fundamental studies of the spinal reflexes by Sherrington.[53] Subsequent research has added further details. Today this hypothesis appears to provide the best fit for the data developed from the research of many investigators.

ORGANIZATION OF THE SPINAL CORD

The spinal reflexes are the basic units in the organization of the nervous system. These reflex pathways are activated and maintained by external stimuli, which initiate millions of sensory impulses each instant. There is a continual interaction between the sensory inflow, internuncial excitation through spinal and supraspinal pathways, and motor outflow (Fig. 11–3). These basic sensorimotor units continue throughout life as the units of neurological function. The effect of the activities of the higher centers is to modify and regulate the activities of the spinal reflexes but not to displace them.

The typical spinal reflex arc consists of a sensory neuron, one or more internuncial neurons, and the motor neuron with an axon and branches to the muscle fibers of the motor unit. The reflex pathway can become increasingly more complex at spinal and supraspinal levels to produce complex rather than simple responses. The greater the number of internuncial neurons in the pathway, the slower will be the spread of excitation through that pathway and the more complex the pathway may become. Since

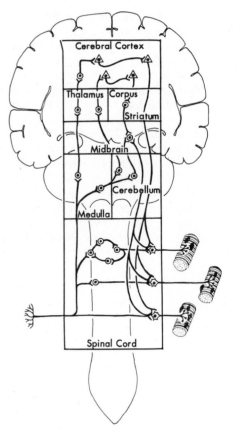

FIGURE 11–3. The entire central nervous system is a sensorimotor system at all levels with all activity driven by sensory excitation. In these schematic diagrams internuncial neurons of the spinal cord and brain are represented by circles; major cells of the cortices of the cerebrum and cerebellum are represented by pyramids; and anterior horn cells are represented as stellate.

internuncial neurons have many dendritic synapses for excitation and many axonal branches for transmission, recirculation of impulses through an internuncial pool occurs and provides a mechanism for prolonged re-excitation as well as for maintenance of a *high level of activity at all times* in the central nervous system (Fig. 11–4).

This high level of activity is important because each neuron reaches its excitatory threshold only when it is stimulated by a large number of excitatory stimuli. Each neuron has many dendritic synapses, some of which transmit excitatory impulses and others of which transmit inhibitory impulses. The sum of the excitatory impulses must exceed the number of inhibitory impulses sufficiently so that the threshold of excitabili-

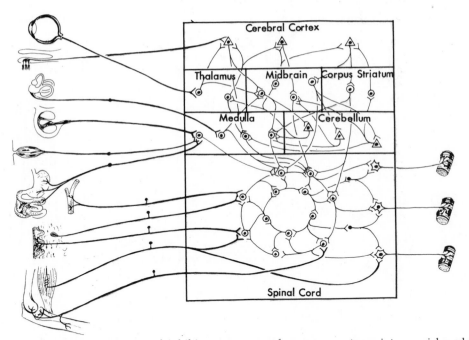

FIGURE 11-4. The many excitatory and inhibitory synapses of neurons create an internuncial pool through which nerve impulses may recirculate repeatedly. Sensory impulses from all types of receptors contribute to the high level of activity of the internuncial pool in proportion to the intensity of excitation. Sensory input is essential to maintain internuncial activity at a continually high level. The primary inhibitory center in the brain stem modulates the activity of internuncial neurons and decreases the excitability of motoneurons in the anterior horn below the discharge threshold so that a few more impulses of reflex or volitional origin are sufficient to excite a motor response.

ty of that neuron is exceeded in order for it to discharge an impulse over its axon. When motor neurons are investigated electrophysiologically, it is found that the intraneuronal potential at rest is approximately 70 millivolts of negative potential in relation to the extracellular fluid. Each excitatory impulse decreases this negative potential, whereas each inhibitory impulse increases the negative potential (Fig. 11-5). In nature there is a continual flow both of excitatory impulses and of inhibitory impulses to each neuron. When the excitatory impulses exceed the arriving inhibitory impulses so that the intraneuronal negative potential is reduced to the excitatory threshold, which is at about -50 millivolts, the neuron discharges an impulse. When the threshold is exceeded there is an abrupt rise of positive charges within the neuron, caused by inflow of sodium ions through the cell membrane. The neuron becomes positively charged to approximately +30 millivolts, and an impulse is generated which is transmitted over the axon and all of its branches to excite

the axonal synaptic endings. Electrophysiologically, therefore, the level of activity of each neuron in the neuron pool can be described in terms of positive and negative charges associated with excitation, quiescence, or inhibition of that neuron.

There are four aspects of neuron inhibition that influence spinal reflexes. Postsynaptic inhibition occurs when an axonal ending makes an inhibitory synapse with the cell membrane of another neuron. Transmission of an impulse across this inhibitory synapse increases the intracellular or postsynaptic, negative potential and decreases the excitability of that neuron (Fig. 11-6). Presynaptic inhibition, which occurs in reciprocal excitation-inhibition of spinal reflexes, apparently acts proximal to the synaptic junction on the presynaptic axon terminal, preventing it from discharging to excite the dendritic receptor.[10] This blocking action isolates the neuron from excitation without postsynaptic depression of excitability. Instead, the temporary isolation of the neuron from excitation because of presynaptic inhi-

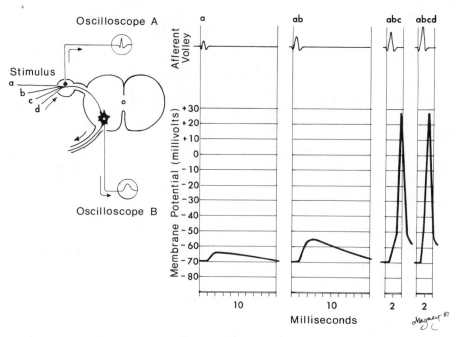

FIGURE 11–5. A neuron at rest has an intracellular potential of −70 millivolts in relation to that of the extracellular fluid. Excitatory stimuli reduce this potential and when it falls below the threshold there is reversal of the intraneuronal potential and an axonal impulse is generated.

bition results in increasing membrane instability. Therefore, postsynaptic inhibition decreases the excitability of a neuron, whereas presynaptic inhibition increases the subsequent excitability of that neuron. Recurrent inhibition occurs when an impulse transmitted over an axon spreads through a collateral branch and back through a Renshaw cell to

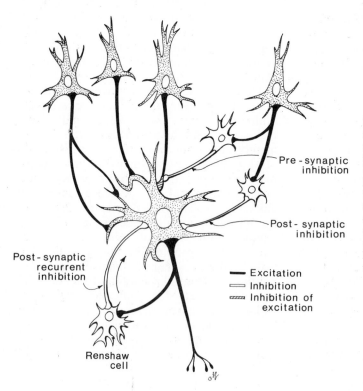

FIGURE 11–6. Inhibition is a positive neurophysiologic phenomenon. Presynaptic inhibition prevents excitatory impulses from reaching the neuron but does not decrease neuronal excitability. Postsynaptic inhibition increases the internal negative potential of the neuron and decreases neuronal excitability. Recurrent inhibition results after excitation of a motoneuron as impulses are conducted through axon collaterals to the Renshaw cell, which imposes postsynaptic inhibition on the excited motoneuron.

inhibit the excited motor neuron and adjacent motor neurons. Recurrent inhibition is a physiological mechanism that produces self-monitoring inhibition of motor neurons and by doing so limits the maximal rate of discharge. In the same way there can be recurrent inhibition of inhibition to antagonists so that excitation of an impulse in an agonist motor neuron spreads through the recurrent collaterals to block inhibitor impulses to the antagonist.

The net result of the continuous sensory inflow into the central nervous system is the establishment of a very high level of continual activity in the internuncial pool. All excitation of the central nervous system is derived from these external sensory stimuli. No cells have been identified in the central nervous system which can spontaneously generate impulses. Fundamentally, therefore, the entire nervous system is built upon and dependent upon reflex activity. The background of activity of the internuncial pool, derived from sensory stimuli, raises the level of excitability of the motor neurons, and in the normal central nervous system a mechanism is present through which inhibition is adequate to suppress the level of excitability of each motor neuron below its threshold until that activity is required. Therefore, although a person may remain motionless the activity of the nervous system is continually at an extremely high level and needs very little change in excitation in order to generate muscular activity. In conditions such as spinal shock in which the flow of impulses to the internuncial pool is suddenly reduced, excitability of motoneurons soon falls far below the threshold level and the person becomes flaccid and areflexic.

Internuncial circuits are organized unilaterally. They probably are organized in even more restricted arrangements than that, but these have not been successfully identified (Fig. 11–7). As a result of the unilateral organization, however, patients may show unilateral hypotonia or hypertonia. When the activity of the internuncial pool is reduced, a diffuse increase of sensory input is effective to increase the level of excitability.[8] Conversely, if there is excessive stimulation, e.g., nociceptive stimulation from skin irritation such as ulcers, tight shoes, rubbing braces, bladder infections, fractures, or sprains, there is an increase of uncontrolled reflex activity.

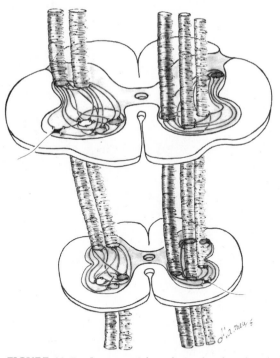

FIGURE 11–7. Internuncial pools in the dorsal and ventral horns of the spinal cord provide preferential reverberating connections between neurons at segmental and intersegmental levels.

THE MUSCLE SPINDLE

The muscle spindle is an elaborate and complex sensory mechanism[2, 43] (Fig. 11–8). It is composed of two specialized types of muscle fibers enclosed in a fibrous capsule innervated by two types of sensory fibers and two types of gamma motor neurons. Muscle spindles are usually located at or near the ends of fascicles in the muscle, attaching to tendon, aponeurosis, or perimysium at one end and running parallel to the extrafusal muscle fibers to attach to the connective tissue surrounding those muscle fibers at the other end. The nuclear bag intrafusal muscle fibers have all of their nuclei collected at the equatorial region of the fiber, and although this concentration of nuclei results in little or no enlargement of the muscle fiber it still has been labeled a "nuclear bag." Myofibrils run through the two polar ends but not through the nuclear bag. Consequently the nuclear bag is more distensible than the rest of the fiber and is stretched when the myofibrils of that cell contract. Approximately the central one sixth of the nuclear bag fiber is surrounded

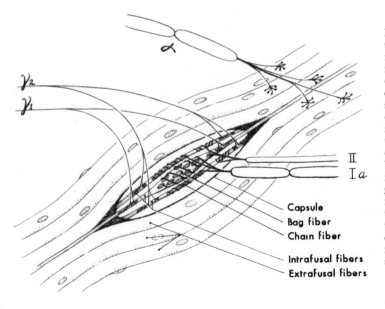

FIGURE 11–8. Schematic representation of the components of a typical muscle spindle. Group Ia sensory fibers have stretch sensitive endings on both the nuclear bag and the nuclear chain muscle fibers. Group II sensory fibers have stretch sensitive endings on the nuclear chain muscle fibers and a flower spray ending of unknown function on the region adjacent to the nuclear bag of the nuclear bag muscle fibers. Gamma$_1$ axons innervate nuclear bag fibers, while gamma$_2$ axons innervate nuclear chain muscle fibers. The motor end plates of the α motor neurons, which innervate the extrafusal muscle fibers, are located at the midregion of those fibers rather than close to the muscle spindle, as the illustration suggests.

by the connective tissue capsule of the spindle, which is filled with a lymph-like fluid. There may be from one to six nuclear bag fibers in a muscle spindle.

The nuclear chain muscle fibers are much smaller than the nuclear bag fibers, are contained entirely within the spindle capsule, and are attached to the spindle capsule at either end of the muscle fiber. The number of nuclear chain muscle fibers is more variable than is the number of nuclear bag fibers per spindle. From none to ten nuclear chain fibers may be found in a muscle spindle. The row of nuclei scattered along the central portion of the fiber gives the nuclear chain fiber its name. There are myofibrils concentrated in the polar regions of the nuclear chain fiber but also running through the central portion where the nuclei are located. The arrangement of myofibrils in the nuclear chain muscle fibers has not been demonstrated, but it appears that contraction of the nuclear chain fiber stretches and discharges the sensory endings surrounding it.[2]

The muscle spindle is innervated by two types of sensory fibers. The group I afferent or Ia fiber is a large myelinated fiber conducting impulses at 70 to 100 meters per second. It has large annulospiral endings around the bag portion of nuclear bag muscle fibers and partially if not completely circular endings around the central portion of nuclear chain muscle fibers in an arrangement that responds to distention by generation of a sensory impulse. It appears that the tension

necessary to discharge the annulospiral endings on a nuclear bag is only about 40 per cent of that necessary to discharge the endings on nuclear chain fibers. There is only one Ia sensory fiber per muscle spindle. This fiber branches so that there may be sensory endings on multiple nuclear bag and nuclear chain muscle fibers within that spindle, but all are branches from the same Ia sensory neuron. Each muscle spindle, therefore, initiates impulses in only one Ia sensory neuron. There is no evidence that Ia sensory neurons have endings on more than one muscle spindle.[43]

The other type of sensory fiber on muscle spindles is the group II or secondary sensory fiber. Two types of endings have been described for this fiber also. The more complex ending is a partially circumferential, stretch-sensitive ending on the nuclear chain muscle fibers. There is another plaque-like or flower-spray ending on the nuclear bag fiber adjacent to the region of the bag but overlying myofibrils; it is not clear what function is played by this flower-spray ending. The group II afferent fibers are smaller and less myelinated than the Ia fibers and conduct impulses at 40 to 70 meters per second. Their endings are less sensitive to stretch but appear to produce a more prolonged discharge when they are excited.

Each type of intrafusal muscle fiber appears to have innervation from a specialized gamma motor neuron.[2] Gamma$_1$ (γ_1) axons innervate the nuclear bag muscle fibers. The axons to the nuclear chain muscle fibers, labeled gamma$_2$ (γ_2) axons, appear to be slightly smaller and conduct more slowly than the γ_1 axons to the nuclear bag fibers. On these intrafusal muscle fibers it has been reported that there are some well-developed, large, space-occupying motor endplates similar to those found on extrafusal muscle fibers, which would appear to cause spreading excitation and contraction of the entire intrafusal muscle fiber. There are also small multiple endings in a line or trail, similar to endings of autonomic nerve fibers on smooth muscle, which may be small enough to cause only localized rather than spreading excitation. The possibility that trail-ending excitation might cause localized and sustained partial contraction such as occurs in smooth muscle fibers adds a further dimension of flexibility to the potential responses of the muscle spindle.

The two types of intrafusal muscle fibers, each with two types of motor innervation and two types of sensory innervation, provide the muscle spindle with the possibility for complex responses in the excitation of reflex activity of the muscle.

THE SPINAL REFLEXES

The Primary Stretch Reflex

The muscle spindle stretch reflexes can be divided into the primary sensory fiber stretch reflex, the secondary sensory fiber stretch reflex, and the fusimotor reflexes. The primary stretch reflex, the Ia sensory fiber reflex, can be subdivided again into the dynamic response, also called the phasic or clonic stretch reflex response, which appears to arise from stretch of the highly sensitive annulospiral endings on the nuclear bag, as opposed to the static, tonic, or tetanic reflex response arising from stretching the endings on the nuclear chain muscle fibers. Both of these endings will be stretched if the entire muscle is stretched. If the nuclear bag fibers are stimulated to contract by the γ_1 motor neurons, the sensitivity of the endings on the nuclear bags will be enhanced. On the other hand, if the nuclear chain muscle fibers are contracted in response to stimuli from the γ_2 motor neurons, discharge from the static endings will be increased. In order for the muscle spindle to be effective to facilitate the contraction of a muscle, it is necessary that the intrafusal muscle fibers contract as much as or to a greater extent than the contraction of the extrafusal motor units. This generally occurs in muscular contractions from resting fiber length down to about 70 per cent of resting length. As muscles shorten to less than 70 per cent of their resting length, it is observed that strength falls off rapidly, owing, in part, to loss of facilitation from the muscle spindles[43] (Fig. 11–9).

The pathway in the central nervous system for the primary stretch reflex (the Ia sensory neuron reflex) will be the same whether

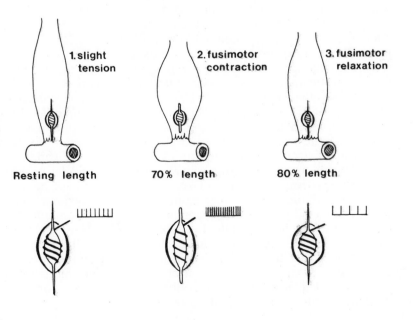

FIGURE 11–9. The major function of gamma motoneurons is to excite contraction of the intrafusal muscle fibers to maintain or increase tension on the stretch-sensitive endings of the muscle spindle so that spindle activity continues to facilitate the strength of contraction as the muscle shortens.

1. slight tension — Resting length

2. fusimotor contraction — 70% length

3. fusimotor relaxation — 80% length

impulses arise from sensory endings of that neuron on the nuclear bag or on the nuclear chain fibers (Fig. 11–10). If the stimulus is minimal, only the monosynaptic pathways will be excited. Whether or not an alpha motoneuron with a monosynaptic pathway from a Ia spindle sensory fiber reaches the threshold of excitation depends on the number of excitatory synaptic terminals converging on the motoneuron from that sensory neuron.[12, 26, 27, 46] When a stronger stimulus results in a greater discharge of impulses, multisynaptic pathways will also be excited. The extent of spread of the muscular response will depend on the intensity of excitation and relates to the number of synaptic resistances that must be overcome. There are short monosynaptic or multisynaptic connections to other motor units in the muscle stretched, to a few motor units in synergists of the muscle stretched, and a few even to the antagonists. The longer multisynaptic connections are to other motor units in the synergists and antagonists and to motor neurons on the opposite side of the cord, where there is a reversal of pattern so that the homologous muscle is inhibited and its antagonist is facilitated. In every neuron the excitatory threshold must be exceeded before an impulse is discharged over the axon. However, a lesser number of stimuli that do not reach the threshold level still increase the excitability of that neuron, or facilitate it, so that fewer excitatory stimuli from other sources become adequate to achieve threshold excitation. Conversely, inhibitory stimuli decrease neuronal excitability and increase the number of excitatory stimuli necessary to exceed the threshold level. The summation at any instant of excitatory stimuli from all sources minus the inhibitory stimuli that reduce excitability determines whether the threshold of excitation will be exceeded and an impulse generated over the axon. This reflex is concentric in that the greatest effect is centered close to the excited muscle spindle and the intensity of response diminishes progressively with the distance from the point of excitation. Stretching of the nuclear bag ending produces a burst of impulses that accommodates rapidly. On the other hand, the Ia endings on the nuclear chain muscle fibers have a higher threshold so that they do not begin to discharge until a certain degree of stretch has been exceeded and then they continue to discharge for the duration of the stretch at a

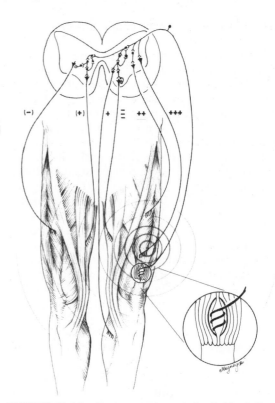

FIGURE 11–10. Representation of the field of distribution of the primary sensory stretch reflex, Ia. It is monosynaptic and strongest to motor units lying close to the muscle spindle in the muscle. It has more synapses in the pathways and, therefore, is less excitable to more distant motor units or to synergists. The intensity of inhibition of antagonists also depends on the number of synapses in the pathway. The pathway crosses to the opposite side to produce a reversal of the pattern. The intensity of excitation decreases from maximal muscle response +++ to minimal facilitation of neuron excitability (+). The intensity of inhibition decreases from complete blocking of muscular excitation ≡ to decreasing the threshold of excitation of the motoneuron (−).

rate that increases slowly with any further increase in stretch. It is evident, therefore, that because of the functional organization of the spindle the primary sensory fiber may generate either dynamic (clonic) or static (tetanic) discharges. A change of the response can be produced by varying the rate of discharge of the γ_1 motor neurons or of the γ_2 motor neurons. Often it is possible during the examination of a patient to vary spasticity from clonus to rigidity or the reverse merely by manipulation of the extremity, which changes the relative excitability of the gamma motoneurons and therefore the relative amount of contraction of the nuclear bag fibers compared to the nuclear chain fibers.[3, 11, 43]

Secondary Sensory Neuron Reflex

The reflexes initiated from the muscle spindle over the secondary sensory neuron (secondary spindle reflexes) are not nearly as well known as the primary sensory reflexes. It has proved to be much more difficult to isolate and study them. As a result there is disagreement and confusion surrounding this topic. On the basis of his research, Hunt[28] postulated that the secondary spindle reflexes caused contraction only in the flexor muscles regardless of whether that spindle was located in a flexor or an extensor. On other less direct bases, it has been hypothesized that the broadly responsive multi-extremity postural reflexes described by Sherrington,[53] Marie and Foix,[42] and others are initiated by stimulation of the sensory endings of the secondary sensory fibers in muscle spindles.[34]

The effective stimulus for initiation of the secondary spindle reflexes is the stretch of the secondary sensory nerve endings on the nuclear chain intrafusal fibers by stretch of the whole muscle, by stretch of the nuclear chain fibers when contraction of the extrafusal muscle fibers compresses the spindle capsule (Fig. 11–11), and by contraction of nuclear chain myofibrils in response to γ_2 motor neuron stimulation. The pathway of this reflex is multisynaptic, slowing recruiting, and long persisting, and spreads broadly to cause patterns of flexion synergies or patterns of extension synergies. Stimulation of secondary sensory endings in flexors initiates flexion synergies. Stimulation of secondary sensory endings in extensors causes extensor synergies. The reflex spreads by multisynaptic segmental pathways to alpha and gamma motor neurons and also has a pathway up to the spinal cord to the reticular formation of the brain stem, which results in marked augmentation due to the excitation returning through the reticulospinal pathway. This recurrent reticulospinal excitation enters the internuncial pool of the spinal cord to cause alpha and gamma motor neuron activation of the stretched muscle and its synergists and overflow of impulses to cause

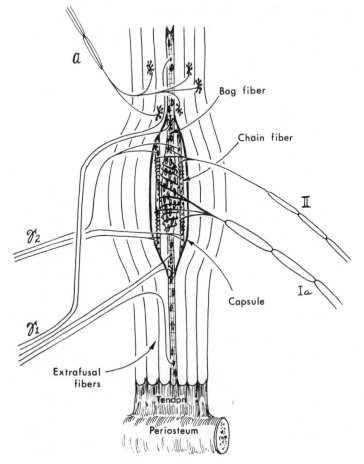

FIGURE 11–11. Compression of the spindle capsule as a muscle contracts may stretch the sensory ending on nuclear chain fibers of the muscle spindle and increase their rate of discharge.

some cocontraction of antagonists. This strong contraction of synergists with weaker cocontraction of antagonists is typical of supraspinal facilitation.[16]

The patterns produced by the secondary spindle reflexes were described during early studies of the spinal reflexes, although at that time they were not specifically identified as originating from muscle spindles. Unfortunately, because the original investigators in describing these responses used terminology relating to the position of the joints, these reflexes often are thought of as originating from the joints rather than from the muscles. The reflexes are the long spinal reflex, the crossed extension-flexion reflex and the extensor thrust reflex of Sherrington,[53] and the flexion reflex of Marie and Foix.[42] These reflexes might also be identified as the proximal muscle synergies and the distal muscle synergies. The long spinal reflex and the crossed extension-flexion reflex are two parts of the same proximal muscle synergy, while the extensor thrust reflex represents a distal muscle extensor synergy, and the Marie-Foix reflex represents a distal muscle flexor synergy. When the secondary sensory endings of muscle spindles in flexors are

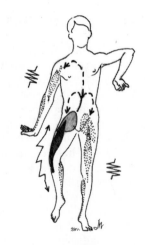

■ Extensor muscle spindles stretched
▨ Extensor reflex contraction

FIGURE 11–13. Stretch of the secondary sensory endings in any of the extensor muscles of proximal joints produces reflex contraction of extensor muscles (1) of the same extremity, local synergies; (2) of the ipsilateral extremity, long spinal component; and (3) of the opposite extremity, crossed extension component.

stretched, the spread of excitation is to flexor muscles in the synergic distribution. When the secondary sensory endings of muscle spindles in extensor muscles are stretched, there is spread of excitation to the extensor muscles in the synergic distribution.

The proximal muscle flexor synergy is excited when secondary muscle spindle endings are stretched in flexor muscles of the hip or knee and result in reflex activation of the flexors of that extremity, the flexors of the hip and knee of the opposite extremity, and the flexors of the shoulder and elbow of the same side (Fig. 11–12). The same response occurs if there is stretch of the secondary sensory endings of the proximal flexor muscles (shoulder and elbow) of the upper extremity — excitation of flexion in that extremity, in the opposite extremity, and in the ipsilateral lower extremity. Stretch of the secondary sensory endings in any of the extensor muscles of the proximal joints of the upper or lower extremity causes reflex excitation of extensors of that extremity, of the extensor muscles of the contralateral extremity, and of the extensors of the ipsilateral extremity (Fig. 11–13).

The long spinal reflex refers to the response of the secondary spindle reflex in

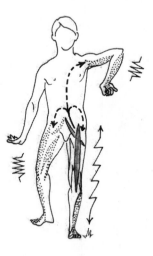

■ Flexor muscle spindles stretched
▨ Flexor reflex contraction

FIGURE 11–12. When any of the flexor muscles of the proximal joints are stretched, impulses from the secondary sensory endings produce reflex contractions of the flexor muscles (1) of the same extremity, local reflex components; (2) of the ipsilateral extremity, long spinal component; and (3) of the opposite extremity, crossed flexion component.

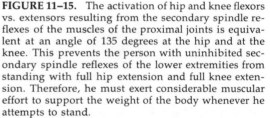

FIGURE 11–14. The secondary sensory spindle reflex posture becomes more evident both in its long spinal and in its crossed extension-flexion components as intensity of effort increases from slow walking to running to hurdling.

muscles of the ipsilateral extremity, whereas the crossed extension-flexion reflex refers to the response seen in the contralateral extremity. The long spinal reflex is the unilateral component of the secondary spindle stretch reflex, in that stretch of proximal extensor muscles in the upper extremity generates impulses that cause contraction of extensor muscles in the lower extremity and vice versa. The same rule applies to the stretching of flexor muscles of the proximal joints in one extremity to cause reflex flexion in the other extremity on the same side. This long spinal reflex component of the secondary spindle reflex augments interaction between the two extremities on the same side and is seen with increasing clarity as a person progresses from a slow walk to a fast walk, to running, to hurdling (Fig. 11–14).

The other component of the secondary sensory fiber reflex synergy of the muscle spindles of the proximal muscles was called the crossed extension-flexion reflex by Sherrington. When an extensor muscle of a proximal joint is stretched there is reflex contraction of the extensors in the same extremity and simultaneously reflex contraction of extensors in the contralateral extremity. The same rule applies to flexor muscles: stretch of secondary endings of muscle spindles of flexors causes the contraction of flexor muscles in the extremity stretched and in the contralateral extremity. This applies both to the upper and to the lower extremities. When the flexor synergy is inadequately inhibited, stretch of the hip flexors or knee flexors not only increases contraction in the flexors on the same side of the body but also increases contraction of the flexors of the hip and knee on the opposite side of the body, which interferes with full extension of both hips and both knees during standing. This reflex syn-

ergy interferes with normal relaxed standing with minimal effort because it causes partial flexion of the hips and of the knees bilaterally, and continual muscular contraction is necessary to counteract the force of gravity. This reflex produces flexion of the hips and of the knees to an angle of approximately 135 degrees, which is the angle at which joint flexors and joint extensors receive equal reflex excitation.[23] This reflex interferes seriously with prolonged standing and walking in patients with loss of secondary spindle reflex inhibition (Fig. 11–15). Any assumption that extension of the hips to the normal maximal angle of 170 degrees[48] and extension of the knees to 180 degrees is the physiologically neutral and quiescent position is not correct. Since this synergy also spreads to

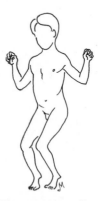

FIGURE 11–15. The activation of hip and knee flexors vs. extensors resulting from the secondary spindle reflexes of the muscles of the proximal joints is equivalent at an angle of 135 degrees at the hip and at the knee. This prevents the person with uninhibited secondary spindle reflexes of the lower extremities from standing with full hip extension and full knee extension. Therefore, he must exert considerable muscular effort to support the weight of the body whenever he attempts to stand.

the contralateral extremity, flexion of one hip or knee will decrease the flexor tone and increase the extensor tone in the muscles of the opposite extremity. This fact has been applied practically for thousands of years by societies all over the world in using a variety of stances in which the hip and knee on one side are flexed to facilitate full extension for easy standing on the opposite extremity (Fig. 11–16).

The major difference between the distal synergic reflexes arising from the secondary sensory endings of muscle spindles and the proximal synergies is that the distal synergic responses appear to be limited to the extremity to which the stimulus is applied. Secondary spindle reflexes arising from extensor (elongator or plantar-extensor) muscles of the toes or ankle produce reflex contraction of the toe plantar flexors, ankle plantar flexors, knee and hip extensors, adductors, and internal rotators of that extremity in the patient with a transected spinal cord (Fig. 11–17). If the gamma loop to the reticular formation is intact, the reflex pattern called the positive supporting reaction occurs in which there is weak cocontraction of the flexor antagonists together with the strong contraction of the extensors, changing the lower extremity into a solid pillar of support. The distal flexor synergy has been called the Marie-Foix reflex (Fig. 11–18). It is initiated

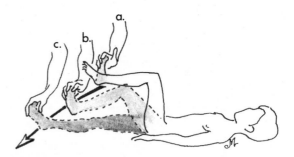

FIGURE 11–17. The extensor thrust reflex is produced by stretch of the plantar extensor muscles of the toes and ankle. This is the distal synergic reflex from the secondary sensory endings of muscle spindles in those muscles, causing toe and ankle plantar extension, knee extension, and hip extension, adduction, and internal rotation.

by stretching the muscle spindles in the dorsiflexor muscles of the toes and results in synergic contraction of the dorsiflexors of the toes, dorsiflexors of the ankle, flexors of the knee, and flexors, abductors, and external rotators of the hip. Marie and Foix also reported that pressure on the ball of the foot facilitates this reflex.[42] Pressure on the ball of the foot initiates the cutaneous-gamma reflex to cause intrafusal fiber contraction in the muscle spindles of the dorsiflexors of the toe. Bechterew also described a component of this reflex synergy: stretch of the dorsiflexors of the ankle facilitates the flexor synergy at the hip and knee.

The extensor thrust and Marie-Foix reflexes operate in the upper extremities also. Stretch of secondary sensory endings of muscle spindles of the flexors of the fingers and of the wrist (which phylogenetically are elongators of the upper extremity) produce reflex contraction of those muscles, of the extensors of the elbow, and of the protractors of the shoulder (Fig. 11–19). The Marie-Foix maneuver of the upper extremity is produced by stretching the finger and wrist dorsiflexors (which are phylogenetic shorteners or flexors) resulting in cocontraction of those muscles, the flexors of the elbow, and the flexors and retractors of the shoulder (Fig. 11–20). Terminology and adapted anatomy for prehension make these muscle synergies confusing if one forgets that the relationships developed phylogenetically when the extremities were used for support, at which time the muscles of the wrist and hand which we now call flexors were elongators of

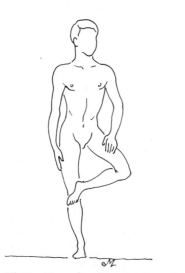

FIGURE 11–16. Nomadic plainsmen have developed the habit of standing on one leg with the opposite foot on the knee. The stretch of proximal extensors in the flexed extremity facilitates extension of the supporting extremity through the secondary spindle reflex.

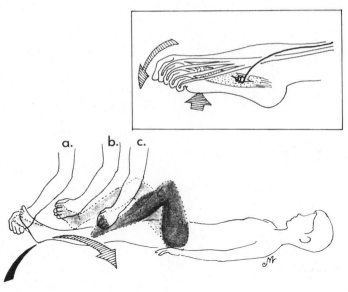

FIGURE 11–18. The Marie-Foix flexion reflex is produced by stretch of the toe dorsiflexors and initiates a flexor response of the ankle, knee, and hip.

the extremity and the muscles which we now call extensors were used to shorten or withdraw the extremity. If that relationship is kept in mind then the rule exists that excitation of secondary sensory endings in muscle spindles of flexors (shorteners) spreads to flexors and excitation of secondary spindle reflexes in extensors (elongators) spreads to extensors.

The neural pathway postulated for the secondary sensory fiber reflex from the mus-

cle spindles appears to have a spinal intersegmental component and also a supraspinal component through the reticular formation of the brain stem (Fig. 11–21). The spinal intersegmental pathway is multisynaptic, long, and slow. Stretch of flexors radiates reflex activity to flexors in the synergic distribution. Stretch of extensors radiates reflex activity to extensors in the synergic distribution. The spinal intersegmental pathway appears to extend to both alpha and gamma motor neurons in that synergic pattern. Impulses that travel upward to synapse in the

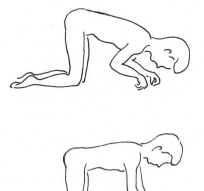

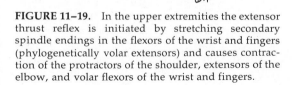

FIGURE 11–19. In the upper extremities the extensor thrust reflex is initiated by stretching secondary spindle endings in the flexors of the wrist and fingers (phylogenetically volar extensors) and causes contraction of the protractors of the shoulder, extensors of the elbow, and volar flexors of the wrist and fingers.

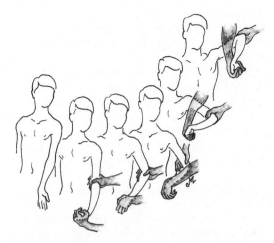

FIGURE 11–20. The Marie-Foix flexion reflex is produced in the upper extremity by flexing the fingers and wrist and causes flexion of the elbow, pronation of the forearm, and flexion, abduction, and internal rotation of the shoulder.

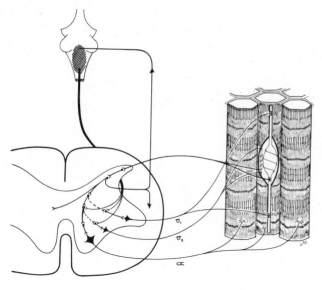

FIGURE 11–21. The components of the secondary sensory fiber reflex from the muscle spindle appear to be a spinal intersegmental multisynaptic pathway to alpha and gamma motoneurons and a stronger but slower supraspinal pathway through the reticular formation.

reticular formation result in a much stronger outflow to the internuncial pool of the spinal cord, producing a slower but much more prolonged and powerful reflex response with some overflow of excitation to antagonists as well as stronger activation of agonists in the pattern. If this postulated pathway from the secondary endings of muscle spindles back to gamma motor neurons is correct, it represents a positive feedback mechanism that should progressively and increasingly re-excite itself unless there is continuous inhibition to control and regulate the system. It is of interest that athetoid patients who show inability to inhibit these reflex patterns also frequently show a progression from areflexia or hyporeflexia to normal reflexia, to hyper-reflexia, and finally to a dystonia in this posture as inhibition becomes progressively less adequate.

The feedback of excitation to intrafusal muscle fibers through gamma motor neurons causes activation of the primary sensory neurons of the muscle spindle as well as the secondary sensory neurons, and consequently the Ia stretch reflex will be superimposed on the pattern of the group II spindle reflex.

The reflexes from the secondary sensory neurons of muscle spindles become very complex in their patterns of response because of the regional spread of excitation to the many muscles of the synergic distribution rather than being concentrically specific to one or very few muscles. Whereas the primary stretch reflex has its major impact on motor units of the muscle that is stretched (Fig. 11–10), the response to stimulation of the secondary spindle reflex is a generalized diffuse regional response. Moreover, the spindles of all muscles have secondary sensory endings that discharge impulses when stretched to produce these diffuse synergic reflex responses. Contraction of a flexor muscle results in stretch of the extensor antagonists with stimulation of the secondary spindle endings in those extensors, which initiates competing extensor reflexes. As a consequence a large number of augmenting or competing reflexes are set up in the muscles of each joint as they deviate from the physiologically neutral position, with the result that a pure flexor or pure extensor reflex pattern rarely occurs throughout the whole extremity. Rather, the posture assumed is the summation of multiple flexor and extensor synergies. In any pathological state in which normal inhibition is diminished, the result of these competing reflexes will be an agonist-antagonist hypertonia with shifting dominance depending on the relative amounts of stimulation summated from the multiple sensory endings. When inhibition is lacking, these competing secondary spindle flexion and extension synergies result in prolonged dystonic postures.

Each secondary sensory spindle reflex, when maximally stimulated and not opposed, produces a target posture of the body because it activates multiple muscles across multiple joints. For the secondary spindle reflex, in contradistinction to the primary spindle reflex, it is not sufficient to think merely of contraction of the stretched muscle, but rather one must consider the posture produced by contraction of all muscles in that flexion synergy or extension synergy. If there is maximally effective stimulation of a proximal flexion synergy without competing or interfering extensor reflex contractions, what will be the posture produced by that reflex, i.e., the "target posture" of that reflex synergy? As the reflex response diminishes in intensity or is opposed by other reflexes, one or more of the muscles will be insufficiently excited to produce a maximal response and therefore the posture will show a progressive deviation from the target position as the intensity of the reflex diminishes. It is necessary to know the target posture produced by maximal effective stimulation of a reflex in order to recognize the various components of that reflex. In a number of joints we are dealing not only with flexion and extension but also with abduction, adduction, internal rotation, and external rotation. We need to know how these other motions also are involved in the reflex patterns. Kabat[30] pointed out in 1952, as have others, that many joint motions involve rotation and abduction or adduction as well as flexion and extension, producing what he called diagonal patterns. However, previous investigators have not defined the precise target posture produced by each of the secondary spindle reflex synergies when acting in isolation.

In the secondary spindle reflex synergy of the upper extremity, flexion of the shoulder is associated with abduction and internal rotation so that the maximal target posture is flexion, abduction, and internal rotation of the shoulder. Flexion of the elbow is associated with pronation of the forearm. The reflex is completed by flexion of the wrist and flexion of the fingers producing a posture similar to that which results if one attempts to tuck his fist into his axilla (Fig. 11–22). Logic suggests that the posture of the "extension" reflex synergy should be essentially opposite the flexion posture, and investigation demonstrates that to be the case. In the extension synergy of the upper extremity the shoulder is extended, adducted, and externally rotated. If extension occurs before adduction the arm will be behind the plane of the torso, but if the adduction component is initiated before the extension component the

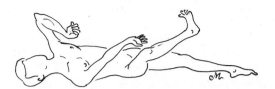

FIGURE 11–22. The target postures produced when the responses of the extremities to the secondary spindle flexor or extensor reflexes of the muscles of the proximal joints are unopposed. In this figure the flexed extremities show the unopposed flexion synergic posture and the extended extremities show the unopposed extension synergy. (From Kottke, F. J.: Neurophysiologic therapy for stroke. *In* Licht, S. (Ed.): Stroke and Its Rehabilitation. Baltimore, E. Licht, Publisher, 1975.)

torso will block and maintain the adducted, extended, and externally rotated arm crossing diagonally in front of the body. The elbow is extended with the forearm in supination. The wrist and fingers are extended. Components of these reflex synergies can be seen in any part of the range from full extension to full flexion. In athetoid and dystonic patients there is simultaneous activation of components of both extensor synergies and flexor synergies, since activation of one will stretch and excite muscle spindles in the antagonists, and the resulting posture will shift along the range depending upon the relative excitation of the opposing antagonists. Therefore, it is only rarely and fleetingly that the maximal target posture of either synergy will be seen. Kabat[31] and Brunnstrom[4] have advocated the use of these synergies in retraining of upper extremity function. When a synergy is in its maximal target posture the muscle spindles of the muscles of that synergy will be at minimal length with minimal stimulation to maintain that position. As the extremity deviates from the target posture the spindle endings will be stretched progressively, augmenting the discharge of impulses to increase the strength of the reflex contraction to return the extremity to the target posture. The position assumed, therefore, will be at the point of balance between the forces produced by reflex activation of the synergy in one direction and the opposing forces produced by gravity, opposing reflexes, or other muscular contractions tending to move the extremity away from the target posture. Similarly, the abductor, adductor, and rotator muscles also contain spindles that contribute to the reflex synergies just as the spindles of the extensors and flexors do. Consequently, stretching an adductor or an external rotator of the shoulder will facilitate extension of the shoulder and elbow. Conversely, stretching an abductor or internal rotator will facilitate the flexion synergy in the upper extremity. This reflex excitation will also be exerted in the lower extremity as the long spinal reflex and in the contralateral extremity as the crossed extension-flexion reflex. Because of the multiple muscles from which muscle spindles initiate these synergies and the multiple muscles which respond, the contraction of any muscle may be maintained strongly in spite of procedures to decrease spindle activity in that muscle. Within an extremity it may be observed that full flexion of one joint will cause stretch of spindles in the extensor muscles to produce reflex extension at the next joint, and that extension in turn stretches flexor spindles, which then produce flexion in the joint beyond. For that reason in athetoid and dystonic patients in whom the secondary sensory reflex synergies frequently are evident, it is not unusual to see alternating flexion and extension in successive joints in an extremity.

There are similar target postures in the lower extremity resulting from the secondary spindle reflexes. The maximal target posture of the flexion synergy consists of flexion, abduction, external rotation of the hip, flexion of the knee, dorsiflexion of the ankle, and dorsiflexion of the toes. The extension synergy consists of extension, adduction, internal rotation of the hip, extension of the knee, plantar flexion and inversion of the ankle, and plantar flexion of the toes. The toe dorsiflexors are part of the flexion synergy and the toe plantar flexors are part of the extension synergy. Gellhorn observed that the same synergic combinations of muscular responses were elicited by electrical stimulation of the premotor cortex as were elicited by excitation of a reflex from its sensory receptor, i.e., cortical stimulation excited the existing spinal reflex patterns.[17] The total reflex pattern in the maximal target position in man resulting from the secondary sensory fiber reflex of the proximal muscle spindles is illustrated in Fig. 11-22. Since these extreme postures of the extremities initiate counterreflexes by stretch of the muscle spindles of antagonist muscles, we rarely and only fleetingly see a near-maximal response; however, components of these responses occur regu-

larly in normal individual activities and become more evident in persons who have impairment of inhibition.

Fusimotor Reflexes

The fusimotor reflexes cause contraction of the intrafusal muscle fibers. These reflexes are mediated through the gamma motor neurons, which apparently can activate the nuclear bag fibers or the nuclear chain fibers separately, and by doing so, selectively increase the response of the sensory endings on the respective fibers. When the γ_1 neurons discharge, causing contraction of nuclear bag fibers, there is an increase in the dynamic response of the primary spindle reflex and little if any change of response of the secondary spindle reflex. On the other hand, when the γ_2 motor neurons excite contraction of the nuclear chain muscle fibers, there is a prolonged static response of the primary stretch reflex and excitation of the secondary spindle reflex synergy. Since the muscle spindle reflexes are the major facilitators of voluntary muscular contractions, the major fusimotor function is to cause cocontraction of intrafusal muscle fibers equal to or exceeding the contraction of extrafusal motor units so that reflex facilitation from the muscle spindle is maintained throughout the period of voluntary contractions of muscles.[21] Intrafusal muscle fiber contraction can maintain stretch on the sensory endings, causing reflex facilitation of motor units, until shortening of the muscle reaches approximately 70 per cent of its resting length. When a muscle contracts to less than 70 per cent of its resting length, the muscle spindle discharge falls off rapidly. When a muscle shortens maximally to 60 per cent of resting length, the sensory endings of the spindle are scarcely stimulated and reflex facilitation from the muscle spindles essentially ceases.

Although in some cases reflexes are defined by the sites or types of the sensory receptors, in the case of the fusimotor reflexes we are classifying reflex activity of a specific group of motor neurons, the gamma motor neurons, to cause contraction of intrafusal muscle fibers. All of the teleceptors — the retina, olfactory organ, taste endings, organ of Corti, labyrinths — supply sensory input to activate the fusimotor reflexes. Much of this activity is through multi-

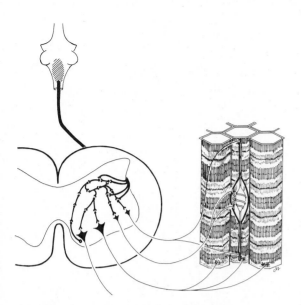

FIGURE 11–23. Reticulospinal excitation from the primary excitatory center in the brain stem causes strong facilitation of fusimotor reflexes.

synaptic pathways into the excitatory center of the reticular formation of the brain stem and is referred to generally as reticular excitation because of the difficulty in isolating specific pathways from the multiple sensory endings through the reticular formation to the gamma motor neurons (Fig. 11–23). Supraspinal excitation into the reticular formation is mingled with cutaneous and proprioceptive spinal excitation. However, excitation of gamma motor neurons occurs from the excitatory center of the reticular forma-

tion and persists even after all of the dorsal roots of the spinal cord of the cat are cut, demonstrating the great influence of the supraspinal input to raise the level of excitation of the internuncial pool of the spinal cord through which impulses flow to the alpha motor neurons. However, in addition to the diffuse reticular excitation, specific reflex stimulation of fusimotor activity can also be demonstrated. The static labyrinthine reflex has been demonstrated to activate gamma motor neurons of the antigravity flexor muscles of the upper extremities and the extensor muscles of the lower extremities and back when the head is upright or supine.[19] The cutaneous fusimotor reflex demonstrated first on human patients by Kenny[32] and verified by Hagbarth[22] in the animal laboratory is initiated by stimulating the skin overlying the belly of the muscle and the tendon of insertion (Fig. 11–24). Irritation of the skin by stroking, touching, pulling hairs, pricking, slapping, or icing results in a cutaneous-gamma activity proportional to the intensity of the stimulation.[13, 22, 51, 52] This reflex is localized, producing alpha motoneuron and fusimotor activity and reflex activation of the muscle underlying the stimulated skin. The cutaneous-gamma motor neuron reflex appears to have a weak, multisynaptic spinal segmental pathway and a much slower but stronger supraspinal pathway. This reflex may be confused with or obscured by the nociceptive flexion reflex. In the spinal or decerebrate cat or in normal man both

FIGURE 11–24. The cutaneous fusimotor reflex is initiated by stimulation of the skin overlying the belly of the muscle and the tendon of insertion and results in localized facilitation.

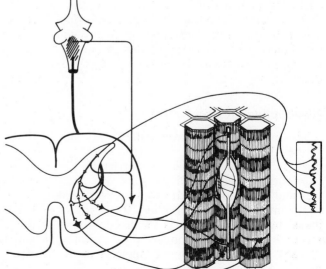

gamma and alpha motoneurons are activated by cutaneous stimulation, but the fusimotor activity has a lower threshold than does the pathway directly to the alpha motoneuron.[13] When there is loss of supraspinal inhibition, the nociceptive flexion reflex becomes more sensitive with prolonged and dominant muscular contractions that may also extend to the opposite side of the body.[9] Fusimotor activity is initiated also by the tonic neck reflexes. Finally, it appears that fusimotor activity is increased by stimulation of the secondary sensory fiber endings on the nuclear chain muscle fibers of the muscle spindle.

Tendon Organ of Golgi Reflex

Golgi described specialized sensory endings at the musculotendinous junction which enfold a number of collagen bundles in such a way that tension in the muscle causes stretch of these endings. Stretching of the Golgi tendon organ causes inhibition of the alpha and gamma motor neurons to the muscle stretched and release from inhibition of the antagonist[20] (Fig. 11–25). The response of these tendon organ endings is reported to be about one tenth to one thirtieth as sensitive to stretch as are the sensory endings in muscle spindles. Inhibition induced by stretching has been used by many therapists[1] for treatment of hypertonia and represents the initiation of this tendon organ inhibitory reflex to decrease undesired muscular contraction. Tendon organ endings are sensitive enough that they are activated by normal muscular contractions that are of greater than moderate intensity. It is probable that they provide a reflex mechanism to protect the body from mechanical disruption by preventing excessively strong muscular contractions.

Nociceptive Flexion Reflex

The nociceptive flexion reflex was described by Sherrington.[53] In response to a noxious stimulus of the distal part of the extremity there is contraction of flexor muscles and inhibition of extensors proportional to the intensity of the stimulus. If the stimulus is slight the response is localized. As the stimulus becomes stronger the response spreads progressively to the muscles of the more proximal joints, and the speed of flexion withdrawal increases. The reflex path-

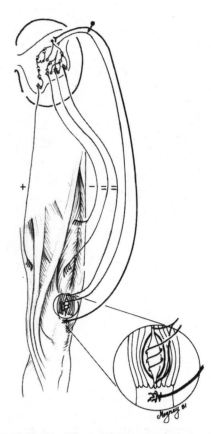

FIGURE 11–25. The inhibitory tendon organ reflex of Golgi produces inhibition of alpha and gamma motoneurons to the stretched muscle and facilitation of the antagonist. It also facilitates reversal of the pattern on the opposite side of the body.

way extends to alpha motor neurons as well as to gamma motor neurons, although the reflex time is longer than that of the monosynaptic stretch reflex. Megirian restudied the nociceptive reflex from multiple skin sites.[45] He found that when the stimulus was applied to the skin of the proximal part of the extremity rather than the distal, the contraction occurred in the muscles underlying the area of stimulated skin and served to move the part away from the source of the stimulus (Fig. 11–26). If the stimulus was on an extensor surface the underlying extensor muscles contracted, arching the body away. If the stimulus was on a flexor surface the flexor muscles contracted. This again appears to be the mixing of the more sensitive cutaneous-gamma reflex with the less sensitive nociceptive flexion reflex.[9] The Babinski reflex represents the release of the nociceptive flexion reflex from inhibition when there has been damage to the inhibitory center or pathways. When there is severe loss of inhibition and of extensor facilitation from the supraspinal centers, nociceptive stimulation may cause the mass flexion reflex of Riddoch with simultaneous flexion bilaterally of extremities, neck, and trunk, spreading to autonomic discharge with evacuation of bowel and bladder, flushing of the skin, sweating, and piloerection (Fig. 11–27).

It appears that this list of reflexes is relatively limited until one considers all of the possible combinations of responses that may be accomplished by manipulation of portions or all of these reflexes. It then becomes apparent that any muscular function may be activated by one or more of these reflexes. As will be discussed in detail later, it appears that activities of the higher centers of the nervous system are superimposed on the existing spinal reflexes so that supraspinal motor responses are achieved by the changes that are induced through the spinal reflexes. The one exception to this is the pyramidal pathway from Brodmann's area 4 gamma in the precentral cortex with each axon extend-

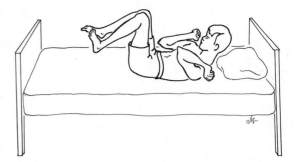

FIGURE 11–27. The mass flexion reflex of Riddoch.

ing down through the spinal cord to the region of the motor neurons of prime movers, which allows excitation of individual or very small groups of motor neurons under direct, conscious supervision.

THE SUPRASPINAL REFLEXES

The supraspinal reflexes consist of the tonic neck reflexes, both symmetrical and asymmetrical, and the static and kinetic labyrinthine reflexes. The positive supporting reaction and negative supporting reaction, which are frequently listed as supraspinal reflexes, are merely reticular facilitation of the extensor thrust and Marie-Foix spinal reflexes. The righting reflexes are not separate reflexes, but rather, combinations of the previously listed reflexes which assist the patient to assume and maintain the upright position.

Tonic Neck Reflexes

The tonic neck reflexes originate from sensory endings located beneath the ligaments around the joints between the occiput, the atlas, and the axis.[44] The sensory fibers enter the central nervous system through the first, second, and third posterior cervical roots of the spinal cord to centers in the upper two cervical segments and the lower medullary reticulum. The reflex activity appears to be initiated through the gamma neurons to increase spindle activity in the muscles stimulated.

The asymmetrical tonic neck reflex is initiated when the head is rotated or tilted to one side.[24] The side toward which the head is rotated or tilted is referred to as the chin side and the opposite is called the skull side. On rotation of the head the chin shoulder is

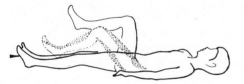

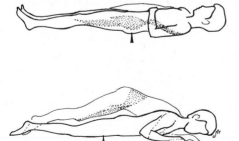

from Megerian

FIGURE 11–26. The nociceptive flexion reflex or withdrawal reflex shows a flexor response proportional to the intensity of the stimulus when the extremity is stimulated distally. When the skin of the proximal part of the extremity is stimulated, the reflex contraction occurs in the muscles underlying the area of the stimulus similar to the cutaneous-fusimotor reflex.

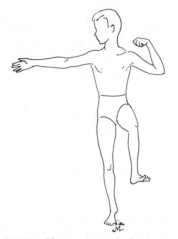

FIGURE 11–28. The asymmetrical tonic neck reflex, caused by turning or tilting the head to one side, produces extension in the chin extremities and flexion in the skull extremities.

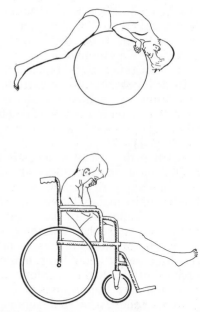

FIGURE 11–29. The symmetrical tonic neck flexion reflex produces flexion in the upper extremities with the fists under the chin, flexion of the back, and extension of the lower extremities without reference to the orientation of the head with relation to gravity.

abducted and the elbow extended; the chin leg also is extended (Fig. 11–28). The skull shoulder is abducted and the elbow flexed. The skull lower extremity also flexes. The tonic neck reflexes are not affected directly by gravity. However, when the head is erect so that the labyrinthine reflexes are active, the latter may oppose and therefore diminish or mask the tonic neck reflex response. Although some of the literature reports that the tonic neck reflexes are aberrant in cerebral palsied children, Hellebrandt[25] found that the responses were consistent during strong effort. The aberrations that have been reported apparently have been due to confusion of the effects of the tonic neck reflexes with effects produced by other reflexes.

The symmetrical tonic neck flexion reflex is produced by flexing the neck forward in the sagittal plane. This reflex is unaffected by gravity, but the static labyrinthine reflex may interfere with its response when the head is oriented in a position that stimulates the latter. Neck flexion increases flexor tone and grasp and decreases extensor tone in the upper extremities[40] (Fig. 11–29). It also decreases the activity of the erector spinae muscles. Neck flexion increases the extensor muscle activity and decreases flexor activity in the lower extremities. Conversely, neck extension increases the activity of the extensor muscles in the upper extremities and trunk and decreases flexor tone and grasp in the upper extremities, while it increases flexor tone and decreases extensor tone in the lower extremities (Fig. 11–30).

When the patient is in the quadruped position there is usually a mixed response with reflex activity from the tonic neck reflexes competing with static labyrinthine reflexes. In the quadruped position, neck flexion causes the arms to be brought to the sides with flexion of the elbows, wrists, and fingers (Fig. 11–31). In the lower extremities extensor tone is increased. The erector spinae relax and the back flexes. When the neck is extended this produces extension of the shoulder to 90 degrees, with protraction of

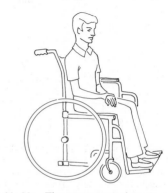

FIGURE 11–30. The symmetrical tonic neck extension reflex increases the tone of the extensor muscles of the upper extremities and back and of the flexor muscles of the hips, knees, and ankles.

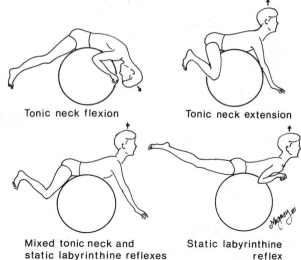

Tonic neck flexion

Tonic neck extension

Mixed tonic neck and
static labyrinthine reflexes

Static labyrinthine
reflex

FIGURE 11–31. Postures produced by the unopposed tonic neck flexion, tonic neck extension, and static labyrinthine reflexes compared to the posture resulting from the competing tonic neck extension and static labyrinthine reflexes.

the scapulae, extension of the elbows, and increased extensor tone in the wrists and fingers. There is increased erector spinae contraction with increasing lordosis. The hips, knees, and ankles are flexed. When the patient is on his hands and knees with neck extended, the symmetrical neck extension reflex plus the extensor thrust reflex from stretch of the finger flexors produces a stronger extensor response in the upper extremities than the flexor response produced by the static labyrinthine reflex. In the lower extremities the competing reflexes produce incomplete flexion of the hips and knees.

The tonic neck reflexes extend to the jaw and face in responses that are less well recognized. Extension of the neck causes opening of the lower jaw, while flexion of the neck is associated with clenching of the jaw. The asymmetrical tonic neck reflexes appear to cause asymmetrical changes in facial muscle responses which have not been precisely defined.

The tonic neck reflexes can act only on a background of spinal reflex activity. Unless the central nervous system excitation is great enough to approach the threshold for motor response, the tonic neck reflexes will not be manifest. During the practice of relaxation training or during sleep the general level of excitation in the central nervous system will be reduced enough so that the tonic neck reflexes may not be evident. However, as soon as the patient assumes antigravity activity or other activity that increases excitation in the internuncial pool the tonic neck

reflexes will reappear. Prolonged relaxation training does not develop the capacity for inhibition of the tonic neck reflexes during activity, i.e., generalized relaxation and specific inhibition of undesired reflex activity during voluntary muscular contraction are not the same phenomenon.

Static Labyrinthine Reflexes

The labyrinthine reflexes or vestibular reflexes (the terms will be used as synonyms in this chapter) may be divided into the static labyrinthine reflexes and the kinetic labyrinthine reflexes. The static labyrinthine reflexes are produced by the force of gravity acting on the receptors in the utricle of the inner ear.[38] The maximal effect occurs when the head is tilted back in the supine, semireclining position at an angle of 60 degrees to the horizontal (Fig. 11–32). Minimal stimulation occurs when the head is in the diametrically opposite position, prone with the head down 60 degrees below the horizontal. Stimulation of the static labyrinthine reflex produces increased flexor tone in the upper extremities with the shoulders abducted to 90 degrees and externally rotated, the elbows flexed, and the fingers flexed so that the hands are up beside the head. The back is extended. The lower extremities are extended in competition with the crossed extension-flexion component of the secondary spindle reflex. As a consequence of these competitive reflexes, if the person is suspended in the upright position there is incom-

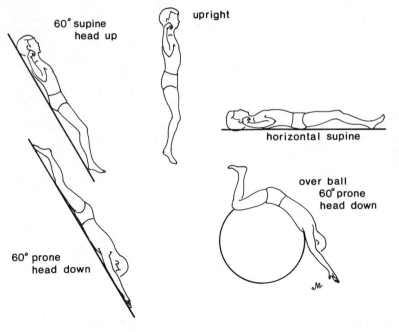

FIGURE 11–32. The static labyrinthine reflex is maximal in the upright 60-degree semireclining position and diminishes to minimal effect when the head is prone and down 60 degrees.

plete extension of hip and knee. If the feet are in firm contact with the floor the static vestibular reflex plus the extensor thrust reflex result in full extension of hip and knee. The static vestibular reflex, therefore, assists the upright standing position by facilitating lower extremity extension, back extension, and neck extension. When extensor contraction is weak, maintaining the head in the upright position rather than allowing the patient to look at his feet increases extension in the lower extremities. Conversely, if there is inadequate inhibitory control, the overactive static labyrinthine reflex causes bilateral extension of the lower extremities and interferes with the walking pattern. Since adduction and internal rotation are components of the extensor synergy of the hip, an inadequately inhibited static labyrinthine reflex will activate extension, adduction, and internal rotation at the hip.

When the patient is upright the static labyrinthine reflex facilitates abduction, flexion, and external rotation of the arm, bringing the hand up beside the head and out of the line of sight. This interferes seriously with hand activity, since the patient cannot bring his hands down in front of him into his line of vision nor to the midline for hand-to-hand activities. It appears that the static labyrinthine reflex is the major reflex interfering with bringing the hand to the midline or across the midline. The static labyrinthine reflex also interferes with moving the hand

down to the side so that the patient may push down on the arm of his chair or push down on the handle of his crutch or cane for support (Fig. 11–33). The static labyrinthine reflex is responsible for the floating hand that is held out to the side in mid-air rather than relaxing onto a supporting surface or hanging at the side.

The so-called aversive reaction is a manifestation of an inadequately inhibited static labyrinthine reflex. Reflexes are dynamic and exert their effect in proportion to the distance that the extremity is from the target position. Consequently, the farther toward

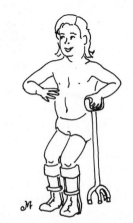

FIGURE 11–33. The effect of the static labyrinthine reflex to flex and abduct the upper extremities makes it difficult for the patient to push down on the handle of a crutch or cane for support.

the midline or the farther toward the floor the patient attempts to reach, the stronger will be the dynamic effect of the labyrinthine reflex. As a person reaches toward an object the initial ballistic motion is strong and fast, exceeding the strength of the static labyrinthine reflex. The final approach, though, is under direct volitional control and is relatively weak as well as precise. At the transition between the forceful ballistic engram and the less forceful final directed approach the static labyrinthine reflex becomes stronger than the volitional effort, and the patient's hand is reflexly withdrawn (Fig. 11–34). The farther the hand is moved from the target position of the labyrinthine reflex, the stronger the aversive response becomes. The response occurs repeatedly without any apparent compensatory learning because the person does not perceive any sensory change prior to the reflex withdrawal. Training a patient with an aversive reaction due to the static labyrinthine reflex to perform the appropriate precise motion to make the correct contact with his target object is difficult.

During sitting the increased extensor tone at the hips and knees due to the static labyrinthine reflex causes the patient to slide forward in the wheelchair or to stand on the foot plates of the chair. If the patient is startled, which overloads the capacity to inhibit the static labyrinthine reflex response, the sudden extension of his lower extremities and back may cause him to "vault" backward over the back of the chair.

When the patient is lying in the supine position there is strong stimulation of the static labyrinthine reflex, somewhat less than when the head is upright. When the patient lies prone the labyrinthine reflexes are markedly diminished in proportion to the deviation of the orientation of the head from the 60-degree semireclining supine position (Fig. 11–32). The strength of the reflex response diminishes progressively to a minimum when the patient is prone and head down at an angle of 60 degrees. There is a misconception expressed in some of the literature that there is a prone labyrinthine reflex. That is incorrect. There is merely absence of the static labyrinthine reflex which is stimulated when the head is in the upright position. If the patient is prone with the neck extended so that the head is upright, then the static labyrinthine reflex will again appear in proportion to the approach of the head to the orientation for maximal stimulation. When the patient lies on his side the labyrinthine reflex appears to be as much reduced as when the patient lies prone. It is of interest to speculate whether people normally sleep on one side or turn on the side or face down as they fall asleep to diminish the stimulation of the static labyrinthine reflex on the excitatory center in the reticular formation.

When a patient is on hands and knees with his head up, or over a beach ball with his head up, the net result of competition for dominance by the tonic neck extension reflex and the static labyrinthine reflex is to cause extension and protraction of the upper extremities supporting the quadruped position, strong extension of the back, flexion of the hips to approximately 110 degrees (which is inadequate for stable support), strong flexion of the knees to less than 90 degrees, and sharp dorsiflexion of the ankles (Fig. 11–31). If the vestibular reflex is inadequately inhibited, the legs tend to suddenly extend out

FIGURE 11–34. The aversive reaction causing withdrawal of the reaching hand occurs at the point where the pull of the static vestibular reflex becomes stronger than the precisely directed but relatively weak volitional approach to the target.

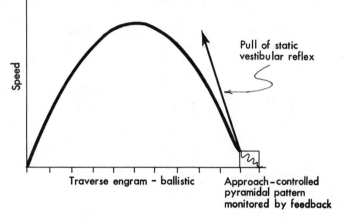

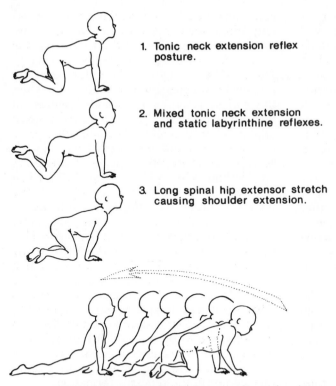

1. Tonic neck extension reflex posture.

2. Mixed tonic neck extension and static labyrinthine reflexes.

3. Long spinal hip extensor stretch causing shoulder extension.

4. Vestibular shoot from hand-knee posture due to inadequately inhibited static vestibular reflex as head is raised to erect position.

FIGURE 11–35. Variations of kneeling posture influenced by reflexes. (1) The tonic neck extension reflex causes flexion of the knees to an angle less than 90 degrees, lifting the feet and legs off the floor and reducing lateral stability of the hip. (2) The mixed tonic neck extension and static vestibular posture result in hip extension beyond 90 degrees so that the patient is likely to go into a vestibular shoot (4). (3) The long spinal reflex interferes with flexion of the shoulder when the hip extensors are stretched.

behind the patient in a "vestibular shoot" as the head comes up (Fig. 11–35).

The equilibrium reaction or response to slow tilt is a mixture of the static labyrinthine reflex effected through the gamma system on muscle spindle sensitivity and a proprioceptive response to stretch. As a person tilts in one direction the static labyrinthine receptors on the "down side" increase their discharge to antigravity muscle spindles on that side with an increased antigravity response of extension and adduction. On the "up side" the diminished labyrinthine activation of the muscle extensor spindles results in flexion and abduction (Fig. 11–36). When the sitting person tilts forward the back and neck extend and the arms and legs are retracted toward the body, which maintains the center

of gravity in the center of the base of support (Fig. 11–37). When a sitting person tilts backward, the opposite reaction occurs with flexion of the neck and back and extension forward of the extremities, which again maintains the center of gravity in the center of the base of support. When a person on hands and knees is tilted forward the neck and back extend, the upper extremities extend, and the lower extremities flex, pushing the person backward toward the center of the base of support (Fig. 11–38). When the person tilts backward, the neck, back, and upper extremities flex and the hips and knees extend, moving the center of gravity toward the center of the base of support. When there is damage to one labyrinth there is decreased antigravity tone in the upper and lower ex-

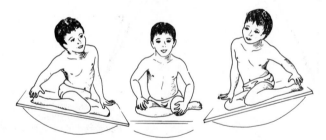

FIGURE 11–36. The reaction to slow tilt is a mixture of static labyrinthine and proprioceptive stretch reflexes. Slow tilt sidewards causes extension and adduction of the arm and leg on the downtilting side and flexion and abduction of the uptilting side with rotation of the head and trunk toward the uptilting side.

FIGURE 11–37. Forward tilt in the sitting position causes extension of the trunk and neck, with retraction of the upper and lower extremities. Backward tilt causes flexion of the neck and trunk and forward thrusting of the upper and lower extremities. (From Kottke, F. J.: Neurophysiologic therapy for stroke. *In* Licht, S. (Ed.): Stroke and Its Rehabilitation. Baltimore, E. Licht, Publisher, 1975.)

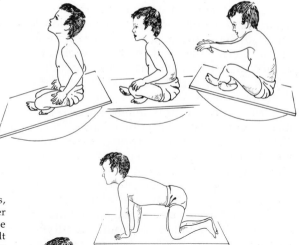

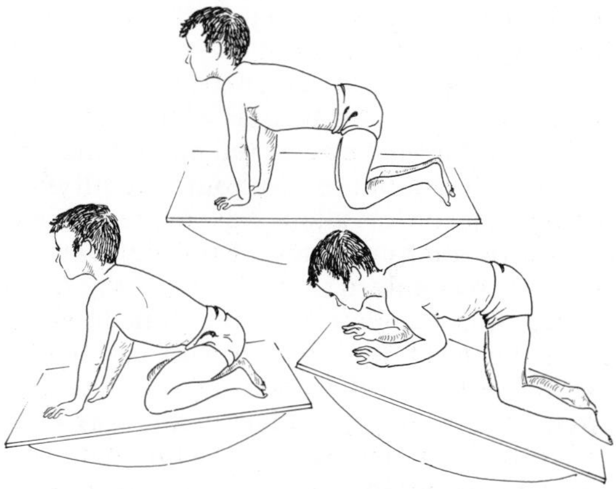

FIGURE 11–38. When patient is on hands and knees, forward tilt causes extension of neck, back, and upper extremities and flexion of the lower extremities in the tonic neck extension reflex posture. Backward tilt causes flexion of the neck, back, and upper extremities and extension of the lower extremities, the tonic neck flexion reflex posture. (From Kottke, F. J.: Neurophysiologic therapy for stroke. *In* Licht, S. (Ed.): Stroke and Its Rehabilitation. Baltimore, E. Licht, Publisher, 1975.)

tremity on the side of damage, and even tilting of the head toward that side is not performed to the extent that bilaterally equal antigravity tone is restored. The equilibrium reactions are seen only when the shift in position is slow, since if the shift occurs rapidly enough to stimulate the kinetic labyrinthine reflexes, then movements of protective extension become predominant.

Kinetic Labyrinthine Reflexes

The kinetic labyrinthine reflexes are initiated by angular acceleration of the head, stimulating the acceleration-sensitive mechanism of the semicircular canals. These kinetic labyrinthine reflexes produce upper and lower extremity responses, which are referred to clinically as protective extension. The three pairs of semicircular canals initiate reflex responses in the muscles of the extremities and trunk of the same side of the body in response to rotation occurring in the plane of each canal. The horizontal semicircular canals are oriented in the head in such a position that they are horizontal when the normal line of sight is directed 30 degrees below the horizontal plane. Rotation of the head around a vertical axis causes maximal stimulation of the horizontal semicircular canals, with flexion of the arm, trunk, and leg

on the side toward which the head is rotating, i.e., the axial side, and extension of the arm, trunk, and leg on the side away from which the head is rotating, i.e., the peripheral side (Fig. 11–39). The strong reflex response occurs rapidly and ceases as soon as the head ceases turning. The stimulus is produced by the inertia of the fluid in the

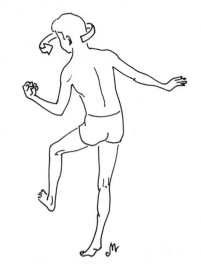

FIGURE 11–39. Rotation of the head around the axis through the vertex stimulates the horizontal semicircular canals causing flexion of the arm, trunk, and leg on the axial side and extension on the peripheral side.

semicircular canals distorting the neural cristae in the direction opposite to the rotation of the head. When the head stops after rotation, inertia causes the fluid in the semicircular canals to continue in the same direction, which distorts the cristae in the opposite direction and produces a reversal of the pattern. Therefore, it is important to recognize whether any description of the effect of stimulation of a canal is a response occurring during angular acceleration or the response after angular acceleration has ceased because opposite responses will be described in the two cases. Unfortunately, these opposing descriptions have occurred many times in the clinical literature without identifying whether the observation was made during rotation or after cessation of rotation. Temple Fay[14] recognized that flexion of the arm and leg was facilitated on the side toward which the head was turning and extension was facilitated on the opposite side and referred to this as the salamander crawling pattern or the homologous crawling pattern. It should be noted that the reflex response from the horizontal semicircular canal when the head is turned is just the reverse of the slower response initiated by the asymmetrical tonic neck reflex.

The plane of each anterior or superior semicircular canal is oriented vertically and directed forward and outward at an angle of 45 degrees to the sagittal plane. Any vector motion in the forward direction rotating around a transverse axis will stimulate the cristae of these canals bilaterally. Maximal stimulation occurs when rotation is in the plane of the canal and diminishes as the rotation deviates from that plane. However,

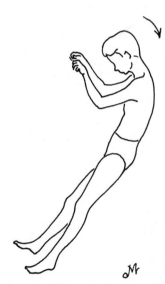

FIGURE 11–41. Falling backward stimulates the posterior semicircular canals, causing flexion of the upper extremities, neck, and trunk and extension of the lower extremities.

falling directly forward stimulates the cristae of both of the superior canals, causing reflex elevation of the arms above the head, with extension of the elbows, extension of the neck and back, and flexion of the lower extremities in the typical "belly flop" dive (Fig. 11–40). The plane of the posterior semicircular canals is oriented vertically, projecting backward and outward 45 degrees from the sagittal plane. Motion of the head rotating backward around a transverse axis stimulates the cristae of these canals. When a person falls backward the kinetic reflex of the posterior semicircular canals causes flexion of the upper extremities, flexion of the neck and back, and extension of the lower extremities (Fig. 11–41).

When a person falls sideward there is excitation of the superior and posterior semicircular canals on the side toward which he is falling and diminution of stimulation on the opposite side. The stimulation of the superior semicircular canal causes reflex extension of the arm while stimulation of the posterior semicircular canal causes reflex extension of the leg on the side toward which the person is falling, with flexion of the arm and leg occurring on the side away from which he is falling (Fig. 11–42).

All of the postures just described can be recognized as the protective extension responses of the extremities to rapid motion of the head. The effect of these responses is to

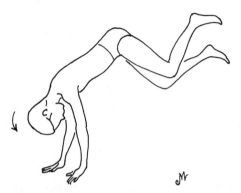

FIGURE 11–40. Forward falling stimulates the superior semicircular canals, causing extension of the upper extremities, neck, and back and flexion of the lower extremities.

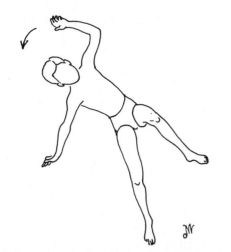

FIGURE 11–42. Falling sideways stimulates both the superior and posterior semicircular canals on the side toward which one falls, producing extension of the arm and leg on that side and flexion of the arm and leg on the opposite side.

broaden the base of support and protect against a fall. It is not known why protective extension, based on these reflexes, increases with practice.

Positive and Negative Supporting Reactions

The positive supporting reaction is provided by reticular facilitation of the spinal extensor thrust reflex. Although this has been described as a brain stem reflex, it appears that facilitation, resulting in a stronger response of the extensor thrust reflex plus some supraspinal overflow causing cocontraction of the flexors of the hips and knees to convert the lower extremity into a rigid pillar of support, is the only change that occurs (see Fig. 11–17). This reflex has also been called the magnetic reaction, since pressure properly applied to the ball of the foot initiates the positive supporting reaction and then slow withdrawal allows the reflex extension in the lower extremity to keep up with the stimulating hand as though drawn by a magnet. The negative supporting reaction represents facilitation from the reticular formation of the brain stem of the Marie-Foix flexion reflex (see Fig. 11–18). The stretch of the toe dorsiflexors is more effective to produce dorsiflexion of the toes and ankles, flexion of the knees, and flexion, abduction, and external rotation of the hip when there is also strong excitation from the

reticular formation to the gamma motor neurons to increase the sensitivity of the secondary sensory endings of the muscle spindles. The negative supporting reaction, therefore, often appears considerably stronger than the Marie-Foix spinal flexion reflex.

Righting Reflexes

The righting reflexes were studied and described by Magnus in 1924.[39] He was looking for those reflexes or combinations of reflexes that assist an animal to assume and maintain the upright position. He described these responses as reflexes prior to the time that some of the other reflexes had been fully defined. It will be seen as these reflexes are reviewed that most of them are combinations of the reflexes that have just been discussed.

The optical righting reaction is not a reflex but rather a conscious learned reaction of orienting the head upright in response to visual recognition of the surrounding environment (Fig. 11–43). It is necessary that the pathway to the visual cortex be intact and that the animal be conscious and able to recognize objects in the environment for this reaction to occur. In the environment there are numerous cues signifying vertical and horizontal orientation. Through experience the normal individual learns to recognize when the head is in the vertical position and observes the relationships that he sees in this

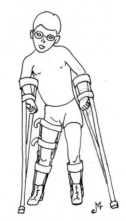

FIGURE 11–43. The optical righting reaction requires conscious recognition of cues in the environment by which to orient the head in the upright position. When visual perception is distorted, causing the head to be tilted, the entire balance is disturbed.

position. The person learns through proprioceptive and other perception that it is easier and less fatiguing to maintain the head in the upright position than to maintain it in any position that deviates from upright. From this he learns to use his visual righting reaction. On the other hand, an environment that does not provide vertical and horizontal cues makes this optical righting reaction useless. A person in complete darkness, in a dense fog, or in any other situation in which orienting cues are absent cannot use the optical righting reaction. The learned response to visual cues is used in the amusement park funhouse where a room is built so that the apparently vertical and horizontal cues do not coincide with the pull of gravity. In that case the optical righting reaction and the labyrinthine righting reflex provide contradictory information, in which case the observer becomes confused and loses his balance. In the same way, when there is damage to the visual system so that perception of the upright position is distorted, the patient tries to correct for this by tilting the head, which in turn competes with the responses of the labyrinthine reflexes.

The labyrinthine righting reflex is produced by the stimulation of the force of gravity on the receptor endings in the utricle. This reflex requires an intact pathway through centers in the midbrain. In response to stimulation the head is oriented upright in space regardless of the orientation of the body (Fig. 11–44). If there is damage to the labyrinth on one side there is less stimulation from that side and the head tilts toward that side, apparently to balance the input from the two sets of receptor organs. Damage to the labyrinthine righting reflex diminishes the sense of verticality and makes it difficult

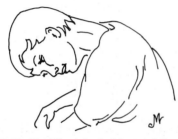

FIGURE 11–44. The labyrinthine righting reflex allows the head to be held upright automatically. When this reflex pathway is damaged, patients can maintain the head erect only by conscious effort and then cannot attend to other activities simultaneously.

Body Righting Reflex Acting on Head

Stimulus - unilateral pressure of body lying on one side.
Center - midbrain.

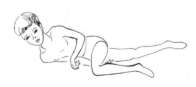

Response - head lifted and rotated to upright position.

FIGURE 11–45. Body righting reflex acting on the head. (From Kottke, F. J.: Neurophysiologic therapy for stroke. *In* Licht, S. (Ed.): Stroke and Its Rehabilitation. Baltimore, E. Licht, Publisher, 1975.)

for the patient to maintain the head easily oriented in the upright position. Patients lacking the labyrinthine righting reflex have to concentrate on holding the head upright. When they pay attention to another complex task they are unable to simultaneously hold the head erect and carry out the complex activity. A partially damaged labyrinthine righting reflex appears to be trainable to increase its responsivity. On the other hand, it may be that the training results in improved proprioception rather than a change in the response of the labyrinthine righting reflex.

The body righting reflex acting on the head arises from stimulation of cutaneous receptors and requires a pathway to a center in the midbrain. When the body is lying on one side so that there is stimulation from pressure only on one side of the body, the response is the lifting of the head away from the side of pressure and rotating it toward the upright position (Fig. 11–45).

The neck righting reflex acting on the body requires an intact pathway as high as the midbrain. When the body is recumbent and because of the labyrinthine reflex the head is raised erect so that there is rotation or tilting of the neck, a sequence of responses occurs which appears to be typical tonic neck reflex responses (Fig. 11–46). The chin shoulder retracts and extends. The skull shoulder protracts and flexes, which rotates the shoulders into the neutral position in relation to the head. The rotation of the shoulders produces stretch reflex responses in the muscles of the

Neck Righting Reflex Acting on the Body

Stimulus - neck rotated or bent (with head in normal position).
Center - midbrain

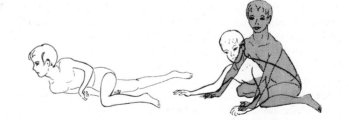

FIGURE 11–46. Neck righting reflex acting on the body. (From Kottke, F. J.: Neurophysiologic therapy for stroke. *In* Licht, S. (Ed.): Stroke and Its Rehabilitation. Baltimore, E. Licht, Publisher, 1975.)

Normal response -
Chin shoulder retracted and extended; skull shoulder protracted and flexed.

Rotates thorax into neutral position vs. head with neck straight.
Contraction of lumbar muscles to rotate lumbar spine and pelvis to neutral vs. thorax.
Chin leg extended and skull leg flexed to orient lower extremities to neutral vs. thorax and head.

thorax so that the thorax rotates to a balanced position under the shoulders. The lumbar muscles rotate to a balanced position under the thorax. The pelvis rotates to a balanced position below the lumbar spine. The chin leg is extended and the skull leg is flexed as a result of the asymmetrical tonic neck reflex, which assists to orient the pelvis and the lower extremities in a prone and straight position in relation to the head. Then as the labyrinthine righting reflex orients the head in an upright position, which extends the neck, the tonic neck extension reflex causes extension of the upper extremities, extension of the trunk, and flexion of the lower extremities, bringing the patient to the squatting position. All of these responses are consistent with a progressive display of the asymmetrical tonic neck reflex, the muscle spindle stretch reflexes, and the tonic neck extension reflex under the persistently upright head.

The body righting reflex acting on the body can occur when there is a pathway only as high as the medulla. The effective stimulus is pressure on the underside of the body as it lies on one side. The response is a cutaneous fusimotor reflex with extension of the arm and leg on the side of pressure and flexion of the trunk, arm, and leg on the upper or unstimulated side (Fig. 11–47). This results in overbalancing the body forward so that

Body Righting Reflex Acting on the Body

Stimulus - unilateral pressure of body lying on one side.
Center - medulla.

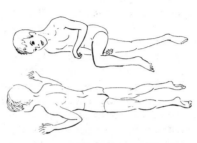

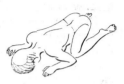

FIGURE 11–47. Body righting reflex acting on the body. (From Kottke, F. J.: Neurophysiologic therapy for stroke. *In* Licht, S. (Ed.): Stroke and Its Rehabilitation. Baltimore, E. Licht, Publisher, 1975.)

Normal response- uppermost leg and arm flexed; lowermost leg and arm extended.
Rotation of uppermost side of pelvis forward toward prone position.
Successive rotation of pelvis, lumbar trunk, thoracic trunk and forequarters to prone position.

In the absence of ability to extend the neck, patient pulls knees under hips and gets up rear end first.

the patient rolls face down. Stimulation of the skin over the thighs and lower abdomen causes flexion of the hips and knees so that the body is raised rear end first. In this case the lack of facilitation from the midbrain prevents effective use of the tonic neck reflexes to raise the shoulders. Consequently the individual rises to the hand-knee position by flexing his hips and knees to shift the weight of the torso backward below the knees and then balancing on his knees and legs while he extends his hips enough to lift his trunk and shoulders to a horizontal crawling position.

Reflexes to the Muscles of the Face and Tongue

There are a number of reflexes affecting the face which are seen particularly in the young infant or in the brain-damaged patient. Generally these are cutaneous reflexes and probably exert their function by cutaneous fusimotor facilitation. The rooting reflex is initiated by touching the skin around the mouth of the infant, causing the infant to turn toward the side of stimulation. In this case we see activation of neck muscles for head turning as well as activation of muscles of the face. The snout reflex is another cutaneous, probably fusimotor, reflex arising from stimulation of the skin of the lips which causes contraction of the orbicularis oris and protrusion of the lips. Pressure on the gums or on the teeth causes the response of closing the jaw and tongue retraction, which produces sucking. Whether this is a superficial fusimotor reflex or a stretch reflex of the muscles of mastication has not been fully investigated. Touching the tip of the tongue produces the spitting reflex with tongue protrusion. When this reflex is uninhibited, the tongue is protruded when it is touched and consequently feeding is impaired.

The jaw responses to neck or head motions may interfere with feeding or speaking functions. When the neck is extended the jaw opens. When the neck is flexed the jaw is closed and the teeth are gritted together while the lips are compressed in a grinning grimace. Jaw motion and facial motion also occur when the head is turned. It has not been identified whether these responses are secondary to motion in the neck or to stimulation of the semicircular canals. However, in patients with athetosis, motion of the head and neck is associated with involuntary motion of the muscles of the face.

CEREBRAL COORDINATION OF MOTOR FUNCTION

The organization of the forebrain for control of neuromuscular function is not understood, and every concept which has been proposed is open to challenge. The tremendous complexity of the system, which has a capacity exceeding by a number of magnitudes that of even the largest computer, has made all hypotheses of consciousness, thought processing, motor planning, and motor execution impossible to verify up to the present time. Recent research in neurophysiology seems increasingly to support the hypothesis of Jackson[29] that higher centers produce motor action by modifying the lower centers to increase or decrease performance. According to this schema in which the higher centers can function only by modification of the lower centers, the basic spinal reflexes provide the foundation for all motor function. Sensorimotor interaction occurs continually at the lowest level of function in the nervous system. Spinal reflexes are maintained at a level of activity just below threshold by supraspinal inhibition in order that excitatory impulses from supraspinal centers can act on them to produce movement.[37, 41] Cerebral regulation is accomplished by modifying the supraspinal or spinal activity. Even the pyramidal tract running directly from the motor cortex to the region of the anterior horn cells is not truly independently active but rather facilitates a highly localized response only because the anterior horn cells have been aroused to the subthreshold level of function by reflex activation. It appears, therefore, that the basis for all motion is modification of the basic reflex patterns.

The cerebrum regulates the lower centers through any combination of mechanisms, which can be placed in five categories: (1) disinhibition, or inhibition of supraspinal inhibition, releases spinal reflex activity so that motion occurs; (2) inhibition of supraspinal excitation decreases spinal reflex activity and decreases the motor response; (3) excitation of supraspinal inhibition decreases reflex activity and decreases motor response; (4) excitation of supraspinal excitation increases spinal reflex activity and increases the motor response. These four pathways all are integrated through the basal ganglia of the cerebrum and the brain stem nuclei through the extrapyramidal system. It is through this mechanism for integration of components of excitation and inhibition that engrams of activity can be formed, developed, and by repetition be made automatic so they do not require constant conscious monitoring. The highest level of motor coordination — if by highest we mean the most complex, quickest, most specific, and strongest responses developed as patterns of multimuscular activity — is, therefore, extrapyramidal. Normal coordination appears to be extrapyramidal automatic activity. Patterns of neuromuscular activity are programmed in the extrapyramidal system by repetition millions of times in the course of development.[6] Development of these programs of activity requires that a fifth pathway be used, the corticospinal pyramidal pathway running from Brodmann's area 4 gamma motor cortex to the immediate region of the motor neurons in the anterior horn of the spinal cord. This direct corticospinal tract is used to excite the desired activity repeatedly, which programs extrapyramidal pathways until those patterns become automatic engrams. In normal infants this programming begins at birth and engrams develop only as the result of repeated practice of the correct pattern. At first only simple patterns can be performed and those with frequent errors. As they are perfected by repetition into engram units those units can be combined or chained and then the more complex patterns can be practiced. Although in many ways this need to practice patterns of activity has been noted in our society, the concept of maturation of genetic potential with age[5, 18] has caused many investigators to ignore the importance of this practice as "only play." Moreover, the tacit acceptance by investigators that cognitive recognition of an activity was the major component of motor learning and that the remaining factor in the development of automatic motor engrams was maturation has caused them to overlook the fact that hundreds of thousands or millions of repetitions are necessary to develop each automatic motor engram.[6, 36] Improvement of skills is usually tested after 10 to 100 repetitions, rarely after many hundreds, and practically never after thousands. Yet that is only the beginning of the forma-

tion of an engram.[35] This beginning of training might be thought of as the facilitation of a specific reflex activity by the corticospinal pyramidal tract until the extrapyramidal engram begins to develop.

In addition, the pyramidal tract can impose single pathway modification on established extrapyramidal engrams as they are being carried out but only at a maximal rate· of shift of attention of two to three per second. However, the ability to impose pyramidal influence on extrapyramidal engrams results in an ability to produce a whole spectrum of performances of a trained coordinated activity.

Consciousness, initiation of neuromuscular function, and coordination of neuromuscular function all arise from subcortical regions in the forebrain rather than being initiated in some area of the cortex. Penfield[50] and others demonstrated that any portion of the cerebral cortex can be extirpated without abolition of these functions. The cortical switchboard, hypothesized by Ferrier[15] to contain patterns of activity localized in the neurons of the precentral cortex, with each neuron or neuron group producing a coordinated pattern of performance when it was excited, has never been demonstrated to exist even after nearly a century of exquisitely precise investigation by numerous neurophysiologists. There is no center in the premotor cortex which when stimulated will produce a highly coordinated performance of a neuromuscular pattern. Rather, what emerges is the elicitation of relatively primitive excitation of spinal and supraspinal reflexes. Although the patterns emerging appear to have a somewhat purposeful appearance, there is never the highly precise and coordinated multimuscular pattern and sequence that any normal person can very easily produce.[50] These data collectively provide the basis for the premise that coordination is not a function localized in the neurons of the cerebral cortex.

Consciousness was localized by Penfield in a subcortical area that he called the centrencephalic center but did not otherwise define anatomically.[50] It probably includes the forebrain structures of the thalamus, basal ganglia, and possibly hypothalamus. From that center emanate impulses that activate the sensorimotor associations stored in the neurons of the motor and premotor cortices to produce activity coordinated through the integrating function of the cerebral basal ganglia and the brain stem ganglia. Just how this integration of coordination occurs still must be defined. Nevertheless, the observation in athetoid cerebral palsy that damage to the cerebral basal ganglia results in inability to develop engrams of motor coordination supports the hypothesis that the integrative action occurs at that level.[7, 49] The studies of Magoun,[41] Moruzzi,[47] and others demonstrated that the primary inhibitory center is located in the brain stem reticular formation and the paleocerebellum intermingled with the cells of the primary excitatory or arousal center. Impulses integrated through the basal ganglia apparently act selectively on this excitatory-inhibitory system to evoke the patterns of coordination that are produced.

In the discussions of neuromuscular function the terms *control* and *coordination* are used with different meanings by different authors and often without meaningful distinction. Since physiologically there are two distinct mechanisms of neuromuscular excitation these terms will be applied specifically to differentiate these mechanisms. Control refers to the excitation of the corticospinal pathway from the 4 gamma motor cortex under direct attention and volition to activate a few motor units of a single muscle in the anterior horn of the spinal cord to produce an isolated contraction of that selected muscle. Since this is a purely excitatory pathway there is no inhibition of other neurons and the conscious activity can occur in isolation only if the person is otherwise relaxed and adequately supported and the excitation is maintained at a noneffortful level by carrying out the activity slowly and against minimal resistance. A person cannot monitor a control activity to cause isolated contraction of a prime mover and maintain relaxation of all other muscles unless the activity is slow. If the activity is rapid or against increased resistance the increased effort causes irradiation of impulses transcerebrally and through internuncial synapses to produce cocontraction of other muscles. Control, therefore, is the activation imposed on one muscle voluntarily through the corticospinal pyramidal pathway.

Coordination refers to a more complex neuromuscular activity in which some muscles are excited and others are inhibited in patterns and sequences to produce the functional motions of the body. Volition is re-quired to excite, maintain, and discontinue the coordinated activity, but the individual elements of that activity are not consciously monitored. Coordination requires the integrating activity of the basal cerebral ganglia and the brain stem ganglia acting on the excitatory and inhibitory centers to produce these patterns. Coordination develops only as the result of prolonged precise practice of the elementary units of each pattern of activity. The neuromuscular phenomenon involved in the development of each pattern is called an engram. Simple engrams, as they are developed by practice, can be combined by further practice to produce larger and more complex engrams. When an engram has been developed it can be executed faster than the person can perceive all of the activity that is occurring. One essential component of coordination is the capacity to inhibit those muscles that should not be activated at the same time that the desired muscles are contracting. With continued correct practice the capacity for inhibition increases and then the effort to produce a faster, stronger, more complex engram can be increased without irradiation of excitation to muscles that should not be active. Normal activity is mainly coordination on which control of one prime mover at a time can be imposed by directed attention to provide almost infinite variations of performance.

Both the learning of control and the learning of coordination require sensory feedback. It appears that the major pathway for sensory feedback is through the spinocerebellar system. The most important proprioceptive and stereognostic feedback arise from sensory endings around the joints. Small motions or change in tension on joints produces spinocerebello-cerebral feedback, which produces awareness of the relationship between activation of the corticospinal pathway and the response obtained. In the same way, as patterns of activity evolve, the spinocerebellar feedback reports how accurately the pattern is performed. Modifications of excitation make corrections for errors that have occurred. In addition there is interaction between the cerebellum and the basal ganglia to automatically adjust for errors of performance without that correction coming to consciousness.

The conscious control of motor activity is limited. We can consciously attend to only one activity, one position, one movement, or one muscle at a time and shift our attention only two to three times per second. Stimulus-response time to a naive performance is about 300 milliseconds when a person is rested and slows to about 500 milliseconds per stimulus-response as the activity is prolonged.[21]

The fastest stimulus-response time to patterns of activity integrated into engrams is only about 100 to 150 milliseconds. However, the greater value of the extrapyramidal engram mechanism is that multiple channels can be utilized simultaneously so that complex performances of trained engrams may be carried out. Conscious monitoring of engrams consists of retrospective recognition that an error has occurred. Engrams are preprogrammed in a feed-forward pattern. Automatic sensorimotor integration provides for automatic maintenance of patterns. When the performer wishes to consciously monitor the components of an activity, that activity must be slowed down to allow the attention to be shifted from one component to another at a rate no faster than three times per second. In normal skilled performers we always see this slowing in the performance when there is conscious checking of the components of the performance.

The cerebral cortex, instead of being the central ganglion for the initiation of all of the patterns of activity which occur in coordinated functions, is, rather, an association storage site for sensory and sensorimotor relationships that can be called upon by the center for initiation of activity and the center for integration of performance. The integrative center for neuromuscular performance may be likened to a computer. The mechanism for integration is complex but need not be massive in size. On the other hand, the size of a computer must enlarge as the number of "byts" of information stored there is increased. The great expansion of the cerebral cortex in the human relates to the capacity to store and recall the billions of sensorimotor associations that can be used in integrated performance. If we compare man to other animals, we find that it is not the speed of performance that is increased in man. There are many animals that can run faster or carry out muscular activity with greater speed or skill than man. However, man is unique in the vast variety of performances that he can consistently execute in a coordinated manner, especially the performance required for speech and for manual manipulation. The variability of the repertory of man is vastly superior to that of other animals, and the capacity for expanding that repertory by training is likewise very great due to the capacity for storage of sensorimotor relationships in the cerebral cortex.

REFERENCES

1. Bobath, K., and Bobath, D.: Spastic paralysis; Treatment of by use of reflex inhibition. Br. J. Phys. Med., 13:121–127, 1950.
2. Boyd, I. A.: Nuclear-bag fibre and nuclear-chain fibre systems in muscle spindles of cat. In Barker, D. (Ed.): Symposium on Muscle Receptors: Proceedings of a Meeting Held in September 1961 as Part of the Golden Jubilee Congress of the University of Hong Kong. Hong Kong, Hong Kong University Press, 1962, pp. 185–188.
3. Brown, M. C., and Matthews, P. B. C.: On the subdivision of the efferent fibres to muscle spindles into static and dynamic fusimotor fibers. In Andrew, B. L. (Ed.): Control and Innervation of Skeletal Muscle. Dundee, Thomson, 1966.
4. Brunnstrom, S.: Movement Therapy in Hemiplegia. A Neurophysiological Approach. New York, Harper and Row, 1970.
5. Coghill, G. E.: Anatomy and the Problem of Behavior. Cambridge, Cambridge University Press, 1929.
6. Crossman, E. R. F. W.: A theory of acquisition of speed-skill. Ergonomics, 2:153–166, 1959.
7. Denny-Brown, D.: Diseases of the Basal Ganglia and Subthalamic Nuclei. Oxford, Oxford University Press, 1946.
8. Denny-Brown, D.: The Cerebral Control of Movement. Springfield, Ill., Charles C Thomas, Publisher, 1966.
9. Dimitrijevic, M. R., and Nathan, P. W.: Studies of spasticity in man. 3. Analysis of reflex activity evoked by noxious cutaneous stimulation. Brain, 91:349–368, 1968.
10. Eccles, J. C.: Presynaptic inhibition in the spinal cord. Prog. Brain Res., 12:65–91, 1964.
11. Eccles, J. C.: Central connections of muscle afferent fibers. In Barker, D. (Ed.): Symposium on Muscle Receptors. Hong Kong, Hong Kong University Press, 1962.
12. Eccles, J. C., Eccles, R. M., and Lundberg, A.: The convergence of monosynaptic excitatory afferents onto many different species of alpha motorneurones. J. Physiol., 137:22–50, 1957.
13. Eldred, E., and Hagbarth, K. E.: Facilitation and inhibition of gamma efferents by stimulation of certain skin areas. J. Neurophysiol., 17:59–65, 1954.
14. Fay, T.: The neurophysical aspects of therapy in cerebral palsy. Arch. Phys. Med. Rehabil., 29:327–334, 1948.
15. Ferrier, D.: The Functions of the Brain. New York, G. P. Putnam's Sons, 1876.

16. Fulton, J. F.: Physiology of the Nervous System, 3rd ed. New York, Oxford University Press, 1949, p. 179.

17. Gellhorn, E.: The validity of the concept of multiplicity of representation in the motor cortex under conditions of threshold stimulation. Brain, 73:267–274, 1950.

18. Gesell, A.: The Embryology of Behavior. New York, Harper & Brothers, Publishers, 1945.

19. Gilman, S., and Van Der Meulen, J. P.: Muscle spindle activity in dystonic and spastic monkeys. Arch. Neurol., 14:553–563, 1966.

20. Granit, R.: Receptors and Sensory Perception. New Haven, Yale University Press, 1955.

21. Granit, R.: The Purposive Brain. Cambridge, Mass., The MIT Press, 1977.

22. Hagbarth, K. E.: Excitatory and inhibitory skin areas for flexor and extensor motoneurones. Acta Physiol. Scand., 26(Suppl. 94):1–58, 1952.

23. Halpern, D.: Unpublished data.

24. Hellebrandt, F. A., Houtz, S. J., Partridge, M. J., and Walters, C. E.: Tonic neck reflexes in exercises of stress in man. Am. J. Phys. Med., 35:144–159, 1956.

25. Hellebrandt, F. A., and Waterland, J. C.: Expansion of motor patterning under exercise stress. Am. J. Phys. Med., 41:56–66, 1962.

26. Henneman, E., Somgen, G., and Carpenter, D. O.: Functional significance of cell size in spinal motoneurons. J. Neurophysiol., 28:560–580, 1965.

27. Henneman, E., Somgen, G., and Carpenter, D. O.: Excitability and inhibitability of motoneurons of different sizes. J. Neurophysiol., 28:599–620, 1965.

28. Hunt, C. C., and Perl, E. R.: Spinal reflex mechanisms concerned with skeletal muscle. Physiol. Rev., 40:538–579, 1960.

29. Jackson, J. H.: On some implications of dissolution of nervous system. Med. Press Circular, 2:411, 433, 1882.

30. Kabat, H.: Studies on neuromuscular dysfunction. XV. The role of central facilitation in restoration of motor function in paralysis. Arch. Phys. Med. Rehabil., 33:521–533, 1952.

31. Kabat, H.: Proprioceptive facilitation in therapeutic exercise. In Licht, S.: Therapeutic Exercise, 2nd Ed. New Haven, E. Licht, Publisher, 1965.

32. Knapp, M. E.: Exercises for poliomyelitis. In Licht, S.: Therapeutic Exercise, 2nd Ed. New Haven, E. Licht, Publisher, 1965.

33. Kottke, F. J.: Neurophysiologic therapy for stroke. In Licht, S. (Ed.): Stroke and Its Rehabilitation. Baltimore, E. Licht, Publisher, 1975.

34. Kottke, F. J.: Reflex patterns initiated by secondary sensory fiber endings of muscle spindles: Proposal. Arch. Phys. Med. Rehabil., 56:1–7, 1975.

35. Kottke, F. J.: From reflex to skill: The training of coordination. Arch. Phys. Med. Rehabil., 61:551–561, 1980.

36. Kottke, F. J., Halpern, D., Easton, J. K. M., Ozel, A. T., and Burrill, C. A.: Training of coordination. Arch. Phys. Med. Rehabil., 59:567–572, 1978.

37. Llinos, R., and Terzuolo, C. A.: Mechanism of supraspinal actions upon spinal cord activities. Reticular inhibition mechanism on alpha extensor motoneurons. J. Neurophysiol., 27:579–591, 1964.

38. Lorente de No, R.: Ausgewahlte Kapitel aus der vergluchenden Physiologie des Labyrinthes. Die Augenmuskelneflexe beim Kaninchen und ihre Grundlagen. Ergebnisse der Physiologie, 32:75–237, 1931.

39. Magnus, R.: Croonian lecture — animal posture. Proc. R. Soc. Lond. (Biol.), 98:339–353, 1925.

40. Magnus, R.: Cameron prize lectures on some results of studies in physiology of posture. Lancet, 2:531–536, 1926.

41. Magoun, H. W., and Rhines, R.: Spasticity. The Stretch Reflex and Extrapyramidal Systems. Springfield, Ill., Charles C Thomas, Publisher, 1947.

42. Marie, P., and Foix, C.: Reflexes d'automatisme medullaire et reflexes dits de defense. Le phenomene des raccourcisseurs. La Semaine Medicale, 33:505–508, 1913.

43. Matthews, P. B. C.: Mammalian Muscle Receptors and Their Central Actions. Baltimore, Williams and Wilkins Co., 1972.

44. McCouch, G. P., Deering, I. D., and Ling, T. H.: Location of receptors for tonic neck reflexes. J. Neurophysiol., 14:191–195, 1951.

45. Megirian, D.: Bilateral facilitatory and inhibitory skin areas of spinal motoneurons of cat. J. Neurophysiol., 25:127–137, 1962.

46. Mendell, L. M., and Henneman, E.: Terminals of single Ia fibers: Location, density and distribution within a pool of 300 homonymous motoneurons. J. Neurophysiol., 34:171–187, 1971.

47. Moruzzi, G.: Problems in Cerebellar Physiology. Springfield, Ill., Charles C Thomas, Publisher, 1950.

48. Mundale, M. O., Hislop, H. J., Rabideau, R. J., and Kottke, F. J.: Evaluation of extension of the hip. Arch. Phys. Med. Rehabil., 37:75–80, 1956.

49. Oppenheim, H., and Vogt, C.: Nature et localization de la paralysie pseudobulbaire congenetale et infantile. Psychol. Neurol., 18:293–300, 1911.

50. Penfield, W.: Mechanisms of voluntary movement. Brain, 77:1–17, 1954.

51. Rood, M. S.: Neurophysiological reactions as a basis for physical therapy. Phys. Ther. Rev., 34:444–449, 1954.

52. Rood, M. S.: Neurophysiological mechanisms utilized in the treatment of neuromuscular dysfunction. Am. J. Occup. Ther., 10:220–225, 1956.

53. Sherrington, C. S.: The integrative action of the nervous system. New York, Charles Scribner's Sons, 1906. Second edition, New Haven, Yale University Press, 1947.

12

HEALTH ACCOUNTING — FUNCTIONAL ASSESSMENT OF THE LONG-TERM PATIENT

CARL V. GRANGER

DEFINITION OF FUNCTIONAL ASSESSMENT

Functional assessment is a method for describing abilities and limitations in order to measure an individual's use of the variety of skills included in performing tasks necessary to daily living, leisure activities, vocational pursuits, social interactions, and other required behaviors. For a comprehensive functional assessment, selected diagnostic descriptors, performance (skill/task) descriptors, and social role descriptors are used to assemble the information desired. The technique includes coding the component skills and tasks according to categories of activities required in daily living. The data are used to help formulate judgments as to how well these essential skills are used and to gauge the degree to which tasks are accomplished and social role expectations are being met. A clinician who is proficient in using functional assessment can obtain a performance-oriented data base that can be analyzed with diagnostic descriptions of pathological conditions and impairment states. This integration of medical status, status in performance of tasks and fulfillment of social roles, together with knowledge of the individual's level of social supports, allows for the construction of a set of data that profiles the whole person. Given this profile derived from functional analysis of related sources of data,

problems and areas of need can be identified more accurately and interventions and long-range coordination strategies (e.g., case management) can be developed that maximize personal independence and dignity. This type of data base provides a framework for an orderly review of needs at the organ, person, and societal level, which is important for development of skills, accomplishment of tasks, and fulfillment of social roles and for a satisfactory quality of life.

It is possible to compare changes in status over periods of time by assessing function at appropriate intervals to determine whether social roles have been influenced by the professional interventions of health care, rehabilitation, education, and/or psychological and social counseling. The measures can describe changes both for individuals and for groups of individuals.

Utilizing the example of the problem-oriented medical record described by Weed,[1, 2] functional assessment represents the extension of the defined data base beyond the traditional components of the history, the physical examination, and the laboratory data. Functional assessment provides a framework for an orderly review of those biological and psychological, as well as physical and social, environmental systems important to fulfillment of social roles and for a satisfactory quality of life. Conceptual underpinnings for functional assessment are provided through the "disability models" proposed by Nagi[3, 4] and Wood.[5, 6] Nagi proposes PATHOLOGY → IMPAIRMENT → FUNCTIONAL LIMITATIONS → DISABILITY. Pathology is the interruption of normal processes and the simultaneous efforts of the organism to restore a normal state. Impairment is the anatomical, physiological, mental, or psychological loss or abnormality. Functional limitations reflect reductions in functioning of the whole person to account for ways in which impairment contributes to disability. Disability is used to mean inability or limitation in performing social roles and activities such as in relation to work, family, or independent living.

Wood proposes IMPAIRMENT → DISABILITY → HANDICAP. Wood and Nagi agree on the use of impairment. Wood considers disability to be the representation of reductions in composite activities and behaviors that are generally considered to be essential components of everyday life. Wood thus considers functional limitations, rather, to be manifestations of impairment. Handicap is used to represent the values attached to an individual's situation when it departs from the social norm. Social norms are defined in the World Health Organization (WHO) document[7] within six key roles or dimensions of experiences in which competence is expected of the individual for survival: orientation, physical independence, mobility, occupation, social integration, and economic self-sufficiency. In order to satisfy these social roles, the individual employs a variety of functional skills that result in complex behaviors and performances of tasks.

Certain fundamental accomplishments or behaviors related to the existence and survival of man as a social being are expected of the individual in virtually every culture:

1. The individual is expected to receive signals from surroundings (such as seeing, listening, smelling, or touching), assimilate these signals, and express response to what is assimilated.

2. He/she is expected to maintain a customarily effective independent existence in regard to the more immediate physical needs of his/her body, including feeding, personal hygiene, and various other activities of daily living.

3. He/she is expected to move around effectively in his/her environment.

4. He/she is expected to occupy his time in a fashion customary to his/her sex, age, and culture, including following an occupation, such as tilling the soil, laboring for others, running a household, bringing up children, and carrying out activities such as play or recreation.

5. He/she is expected to participate in and maintain social relationships with others.

6. He/she is expected to sustain socioeconomic activity and independence by virtue of his/her labor or exploitation of material possessions like natural resources, livestock, or crops. This economic self-sufficiency customarily includes obligations to sustain others, such as members of the family.

Chronic diseases have increased in prevalence and now have displaced infectious diseases as prime public health problems. Estimation of health status relies on symptoms, signs, and other indicators more directly related to those biologic responses that are associated with morbidity or proneness to morbid conditions. Measurement of health and well-being of a population must include mental health, social health, and functional limitations as related to disability.[8-10] Measures used by the National Center for Health Statistics to account for disability are life years, institutional days, activity limitation days, presence of acute or chronic illness, bed disability days, and days lost from work due to illness.[11] Yet these measures rely upon symptomatology and rates of utilization of health and medical services by the population and are, therefore, still measuring health status or morbidity rather than disability. Measures of disability for a population[12] are extremely difficult to construct, since they require descriptions of task performances and behaviors in the context of "normally" expected social roles, which themselves are difficult to define precisely.

Stewart et al.[8, 9] studied functional limitations in a household sample using domains of mobility or traveling, physical activity including working and bending, and social activity including work, play, self care, and leisure time activities. They found strong associations between all three scales; in particular, social dysfunction nearly always occurred along with mobility limitations, whereas the opposite was not true. A major weakness of population studies was noted in this study in that 90 per cent or more of individuals did not have functional limitations on most of the items and scales. Thus, it would require very large samples to detect any differences in health according to functional limitation assessments. The authors also noted in their study that considerable overlap was present in the measures that they used.

DESIRABLE FEATURES OF A FUNCTIONAL ASSESSMENT INSTRUMENT

A functional assessment instrument should meet certain objectives such as those summarized by Donaldson et al.[13]: (1) objective description of functional status at a given point in time, (2) serial repetition allowing detection of changed functional status, (3) data collected through observation relevant to and useful in monitoring the treatment program, (4) enhancement of communication among treatment team members and between referral agencies, and (5) comparable clinical observations compatible with research questions. Other researchers (1) emphasize using a classification that is "composed of a set of descriptive terms that are patient-oriented, multidimensional in content, objectively stated, precisely defined, and relative to the goals of long-term care"[14]; (2) stress compacting a wide range of data "that is unobtrusive to the service provider, is adaptable to the particular clinical setting, that reinforces the goals of the service program by identifying problems and needs and by aiding comprehensive planning, and that utilizes standard expressions"[15]; and (3) advocate methods for quality assurance by using the data to perform program evaluation, program audit, and analyses of outcomes and benefits as well as cost-effectiveness.[11, 16]

DEVELOPMENT OF FUNCTIONAL ASSESSMENT INSTRUMENTS

Deaver and Brown[17] summarize the basic goals of medical rehabilitation as (1) max-imum use of the hands, (2) ambulation, (3) independence in self care, (4) communication, and (5) the appearance of being normal. Lists of tasks have been compiled by many rehabilitation workers and are called the activities of daily living (ADL). They are usually used for teaching patients how to take care of themselves.[18] Over the past 30 years many different scales have emerged to tabulate those activities performed independently versus those performed through assistance of another person or with a mechanical aid. These are used as measures of functional independence. Donaldson et al.[13] performed a survey of the English language literature from 1950 to 1970 and determined that 25 scales met two of three criteria: (1) had a mechanism for scoring, (2) had been used in a survey or other type of research, and (3) were applicable to a general rehabilitation population. They devised and tested a new, expanded instrument that permitted concurrent scoring of the Katz, Barthel, and Kenny scales.[19-21] Their conclusions were that (1) the new scale was more useful than prior scales because of clear criteria for mutually exclusive categories, and (2) 92 of 100 pairs of pre-test and post-test scores showed comparability of Kenny, Barthel, and Katz scores, with the Kenny being the most sensitive to change and the Katz the least sensitive.

The Functional Life Scale (FLS), developed by Sarno et al.,[22] recognizes that knowing the actual performance of skills is a better measure of degree of disability than knowing the elements that constitute performance. For example, a scale should indicate the adequacy of locomotion rather than whether range of motion and muscle power of the legs are normal or not. The Functional Life Scale as reported in 1973 is composed of 44 items designed for application outside of the hospital setting based upon an interview technique. Normal behavior is used as the standard for comparison. Items assessed were judged for self-initiation, frequency, speed, and overall efficiency and were numerically rated along a continuum from 0 to 4, yielding a series of subscores. Test-retest reliability, inter-rater reliability, internal consistency, and validity testing were generally satisfactory and in some cases yielded high correlation values.

The Long-Range Evaluation System (LRES) developed by Granger and others[15] has some features in common with other ADL scales. In the first place it incorporates the scoring methodology of the Barthel index and the PULSES profile,[23] and as such, the domain of personal care depends heavily upon independent functioning in self care, mobility, and bladder and bowel sphincter control. Abilities in active use of the limbs, in communication and vision, the need for physician and/or nursing services, and the level of social supports are described through the ESCROW profile.[24] The three scales together form the backbone of the Long Range Evaluation System. This system has several features that are unique: (1) there is a series of descriptive modules that are inserted or left out as appropriate to the informational needs relevant to the particular population being evaluated; (2) the method has been computerized to provide feedback summaries for incorporation into the patient's medical record; (3) the data stored in the computer are used to compile a variety of management reports that reflect the characteristics of the population on whom the data have been collected; (4) each record entered into the system has been designed for the particular encounter for which it is used and is time-oriented with respect to date of entry and whether it represents an admission, an interval, a discharge, or a follow-up report; (5) the system is designed to track individuals over time through a series of service facilities, whether inpatient or outpatient; and (6) a method of program evaluation is accommodated whereby results or outcomes of care can be compared with predetermined standards in measurable terms.

Other functional assessment scales are under constant development.[25–27] For further background, the reader is referred to an updated summary of functional assessment scales and bibliography which appeared in a recent publication entitled "Functional Limitations: A State of the Art Review."[28]

PURPOSES AND USES OF FUNCTIONAL ASSESSMENT

Functional assessment is primarily a method for integrating data on diagnostic descriptions of pathologic conditions and impairment states with data related to limitations or residual abilities in the performance of social roles. By constructing a set of data that profiles the whole person, it becomes possible to better understand how a handicapped person functions. Given this understanding, problems and areas of need can be identified more accurately and interventions can be developed that are more appropriate for enhancing personal independence and autonomy in fulfilling social roles.

In particular, functional assessment and analysis are useful in the following ways:

1. Systematically developing a patient problem list that includes limitations in functioning.

2. Determining clinical care changes in patients or clients by comparing measures of function before and after treatment interventions.

3. Relating needs of a defined population through assessment and analysis of function measured from samples of individuals representative of that population.

4. Determining the benefits of clinical care in analyzing cost-benefits and cost-effectiveness.

5. Manpower studies that can relate needs for various numbers and kinds of health care personnel to levels of severity of disability in the patients being served.

6. Utilization review for necessity of given levels of care and alternative levels of care and to justify costs.

7. Prioritization of needs should it become necessary to ration scarce resources.

8. Program evaluation, quality assurance, and medical care audit studies in order to detect deficiencies in care and then to improve care.

9. Tracking patients through a system of care in order to determine the strengths and weaknesses of the system.

10. Establishing comparability of groups of patients for research studies and for policy planning.

11. Facilitating case management in order to assure that a program of care is addressing issues that are most likely to maximize the quality of life for the disabled person.

Kottke[29] presents a spectrum of the stages of recovery (Figs. 12–1 and 12–2) based on a scheme of growth and development. This scheme can guide the responses of the rehabilitation team professionals toward helping the patient achieve and maintain an optimal quality of life. The survival of organs is the

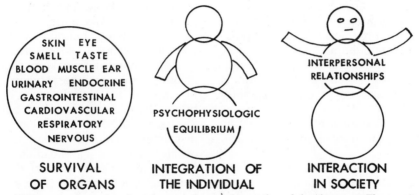

FIGURE 12–1. The stages of recovery based on a scheme of growth and development. The survival of organs is the first concern of acute medical care. The activities of the rehabilitation professionals are most intense during establishment of psychophysiologic equilibrium and reintegration. They continue support through interpersonal relationships in order to enhance interactions with society. (From Kottke, F. J.: Philosophical Considerations of Quality of Life for the Disabled. Presented at the 56th Annual Session of the American Congress of Rehabilitation Medicine, November 11, 1979, Honolulu, Hawaii.)

first concern of acute medical care. The hazard is that in preserving an organ the physician may lose sight of the whole patient and thus unwittingly continue to reinforce the patient's passive ("sick") role in the recovery process. The activities of the rehabilitation professionals are most intense during establishment of psychophysiologic equilibrium and reintegration. Their strategy includes bringing the patient out as a total being. The rehabiliation professionals continue to support and encourage the patient through the next stage. At the same time the personality of the patient takes on a more important role if he or she is to be more effective in interpersonal relationships and interactions with society. The following stage (Fig. 12–2) requires that the patient "dare to succeed," meaning that he moves away from comfortable supports and overdependence upon professional help. By now

the patient should have learned how to utilize most self-help resources and begun to organize his or her life toward productive and constructive efforts. The final growth stage is represented by less dependence on routine although productive endeavors and more participation in creative performances. In actuality the final stage is also the first stage because all along the way, medical and rehabilitation professionals should be encouraging the patient to assume personal responsibility for his or her activities and to move forward constructively toward personal goals. Application of functional assessment through the stages of recovery can document the recognized accomplishments of the rehabilitation process. Through feedback to the patient, motivation and personal progress can be enhanced.

The uses of functional assessment are applicable to medical rehabilitation inpatient

FIGURE 12–2. Further stages of recovery. The patient moves away from overdependence upon professional help and organizes his or her life toward productive and constructive efforts. Finally, the patient participates in creative performances, being less dependent upon routine endeavors. (From Kottke, F. J.: Philosophical Considerations of Quality of Life for the Disabled. Presented at the 56th Annual Session of the American Congress of Rehabilitation Medicine, November 11, 1979, Honolulu, Hawaii.)

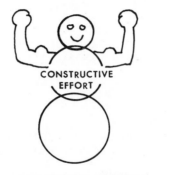

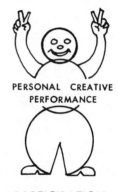

and outpatient programs, nursing home care, and other long-term care facilities, day hospital and day care programs, vocational rehabilitation programs, home care programs, and other service programs for the handicapped. In addition, functional assessment is the means for estimating levels of disability within a community population for purposes of epidemiological studies related to judging needs and for allocation of manpower and other resources.

In hospital rehabilitation programs, the majority of patients are discharged to home settings in the community, while the minority are discharged to nursing home long-term care facilities. One of the major aims of the hospital rehabilitation programs[30] is to maximize the percentage of patients discharged home. A number of studies have assessed the usefulness of functional assessment and other patient data for predicting the course of rehabilitation treatment. High assessment scores in physical functioning at discharge for populations with multiple diagnoses and with stroke were found to be important correlates[15,31-33] with the private home for discharge placement and continued living site. Such areas as self-care, mobility, and sphincter control were components of the overall functional assessments. Age appeared in several studies as a predictor of placement, younger patients tending to be sent home rather than to institutions,[15, 31, 33-35] with the qualification that family support may be an intervening variable.[33, 34] Other predictors of home rather than institutional placement in stroke patients were absence of associated heart, pulmonary, and vascular disease; absence of intellectual, emotional, and perceptual deficits; presence of spouse or other family member; and competent family support and involvement.[31, 33, 34] Functional status as measured by admission and discharge scores on functional assessment instruments (Barthel index and PULSES profile), together with hospital length of stay for stroke patients, predicted whether patients returned home or were placed in long-term care facilities.[36]

LONG-RANGE EVALUATION SYSTEM (LRES)

The Long-Range Evaluation System (LRES) is a functional assessment system designed, tested, and used in clinical settings, including medical rehabilitation for inpatients and outpatients, patients in day care and home care programs, and residents of long-term care facilities. It is a measurement tool for describing areas of service need, severity of handicap, and change in individuals over a period of time, and for comparing the status of groups of individuals treated at different times and in different locations. An example of one type of form used to collect functional assessment data on outpatients is shown in Table 12–1.

The modified Barthel index was studied in

Text continued on page 263

TABLE 12–1. INSTITUTE FOR REHABILITATION AND RESTORATIVE CARE — LONG-RANGE EVALUATION SYSTEM

Name:_____ Date:_____ Number:_____

To the Patient:

Fill in your name and date above. Mark "X" in the appropriate bracket column ( ).

For each item listed, please check the one best choice:

BECAUSE OF HEALTH-RELATED PROBLEMS, HOW OFTEN ARE YOU VISITING OR BEING VISITED BY A PHYSICIAN *OR* NURSE (DO NOT INCLUDE VISITS FOR PHYSICAL OR OCCUPATIONAL THERAPY):
1 ( ) Infrequently, no more than every 3 months.
2 ( ) Moderately frequently, at least every 3 months.
3 ( ) Very frequently, at least once a week.
4 ( ) At least daily.

WHEN YOU SPEAK TO ANOTHER PERSON, DO YOU SPEAK:
1 ( ) Without any help from anyone and no difficulty in saying words.
2 ( ) With some difficulty with saying words but without help from anyone else.
3 ( ) With some help from another person (such as a coach or translator) or can communicate by using sign language, or another symbolic equivalent (writing, communication board, etc.).
4 ( ) Unable to communicate verbally, needing complete assistance from another person.

Table continued on opposite page

**TABLE 12–1. INSTITUTE FOR REHABILITATION AND RESTORATIVE CARE–
LONG-RANGE EVALUATION SYSTEM (Continued)**

WHEN A PERSON SPEAKS TO YOU, DO YOU HEAR:
1 ( ) Normally with both ears.
2 ( ) With partial impairment or use of an assistive device (such as a hearing aid).
3 ( ) With some help from another person to speak extra loudly; or you can understand sign language,
        lip reading, or written communication.
4 ( ) Unable to hear and needing complete assistance from another person (meaning profoundly deaf and
        not able to understand sign language or lip reading).

CAN YOU:
1 ( ) See normally with both eyes.
2 ( ) See with partial impairment such as use of eyeglasses or eye medication.
3 ( ) Not see well due to either partial blindness or legal blindness and you use a cane, guide dog, or
        some help from another person.
4 ( ) Not see at all due to blindness, with complete dependence upon another person for assistance.

LIMB FUNCTIONING: Which of the following choices best describes use of your four limbs:

If you have an amputation of the upper limb above the wrist or of the lower limb above the ankle, then check accordingly below (*):	UPPER LIMBS Shoulder, Elbow, Wrist, Fingers		LOWER LIMBS Hip, Knee, Ankle		
	Right	Left	Right	Left	
Have normal strength including full coordinated and painless movement of all joints.	( )	( )	( )	( )	GOOD
Have ordinary use in spite of some reduced strength or incoordination or else some pain or restriction of motion.	( )	( )	( )	( )	FAIR
Have very limited use because of poor strength or incoordination or else too much pain or stiffness to permit any more use than as a helping limb, or (*) if amputated, you wear and use a prosthesis daily.	( )	( )	( )	( )	POOR
Have no use because of too much pain, stiffness, or paralysis, or (*) if amputated, you do not wear a prosthesis daily.	( )	( )	( )	( )	NULL

Personal Activities of Daily Living

For each task listed, please check the one choice
that best describes how you perform the task.

EATING   When you eat and drink, do you usually feed yourself:

1 ( ) Without use of assistive devices.
2 ( ) With use of assistive devices such as spork, rocker knife, or extended straw.

        With help from another person (if so, which below):
2 ( ) Helped by cutting meats, buttering bread, or pouring liquids.
3 ( ) Helped with more than cutting meats, buttering bread, or pouring liquids, meaning that someone else
        helps to bring food to your mouth.

4 ( ) Or you are fed by a tube into the stomach.

DRESSING   Which choice best describes how you usually get dressed, including bra, slip,
                    pull-overs, front-opening shirts and blouses, as well as undergarments, slacks,
                    socks, nylons, and shoes, plus managing zippers, buttons, snaps, and laces?

1 ( ) By yourself without the use of assistive devices.
2 ( ) By yourself with the use of assistive devices such as long-handled reachers, elastic laces,
        or Velcro closures.
3 ( ) With some help from another person.
4 ( ) With complete assistance from another person.

4 ( ) Or you do not get dressed.

DON BRACE OR   Which choice best describes how you usually put on and take off, if applicable,
PROSTHESIS   a prescribed sling, splint, brace (orthosis), corset, or artificial limb (prosthesis)?

1 ( ) By yourself with reasonable ease.
2 ( ) By yourself but taking a while to do it.
3 ( ) With some help from another person.
4 ( ) Not applicable because you do not wear a brace or prosthesis.

Table continued on following page

**TABLE 12–1. INSTITUTE FOR REHABILITATION AND RESTORATIVE CARE–
LONG-RANGE EVALUATION SYSTEM** *(Continued)*

GROOMING   How do you generally take care of things such as brushing hair, shaving, cleaning teeth or dentures, and applying makeup?

1 ( ) By yourself.
2 ( ) By yourself with the use of assistive devices.
3 ( ) With some help from another person.
4 ( ) With complete assistance from another person.

BATHING   How do you bathe or take sponge baths?

1 ( ) Able to wash and dry your entire body including back and feet by yourself without use of assistive devices.
2 ( ) By yourself with the use of assistive devices such as long-handled brush or sponge.
3 ( ) With some help from another person.
4 ( ) With complete assistance from another person.

BLADDER CONTROL   With respect to bladder control, do you usually:

1 ( ) Have no accidents and have complete control.
2 ( ) Have no accidents but use special devices such as a catheter or urinary collecting device which you are able to clean and maintain yourself.
3 ( ) Have occasional accidents *or* need help from another person for any reason.
4 ( ) Have frequent accidents.

BOWEL CONTROL   With respect to bowel control, do you usually:

1 ( ) Have no accidents and have complete control.
2 ( ) Have no accidents but use special techniques such as stool softeners, suppository, enemas, or laxatives by yourself.
3 ( ) Have occasional accidents *or* need some help from another person for any reason.
4 ( ) Have frequent accidents.

TOILETING   How well are you able to clean yourself and adjust your clothing after using the toilet:

1 ( ) By yourself without the use of assistive devices.
2 ( ) By yourself with the use of assistive devices.
3 ( ) With some help from another person.
4 ( ) With complete assistance from another person.

4 ( ) Or you do not always have help available.

HAND SKILLS   How well are you able to write your name, turn a doorknob, turn a key in a lock, handle money, manipulate lamp and wall light switches, dial a telephone, turn a radio or TV on and off, turn a faucet handle, and open a jar?

1 ( ) By yourself without difficulty with any of these.
2 ( ) By yourself with difficulty with some of these.
3 ( ) With some help from another person.
4 ( ) With complete assistance from another person.

TRANSFERRING   Which best describes how you usually get to and from a chair (including a wheelchair if applicable) to a bed and return or to stand and walk?

1 ( ) By yourself without the use of assistive devices.
2 ( ) By yourself with the use of assistive devices.
3 ( ) With some help from another person.
4 ( ) With complete assistance from another person.

   Which best describes how you usually get on and off a toilet?

1 ( ) You use a toilet with fixed plumbing by yourself without the use of assistive devices.
2 ( ) You use a toilet by yourself with the use of assistive devices (such as grab bars or elevated seat) or else you use a commode which you empty by yourself.
3 ( ) You use either a toilet or commode with some help from another person.
4 ( ) You are unable to use a toilet or commode.

   Which best describes how you get in and out of a tub or shower?

1 ( ) By yourself without the use of assistive devices.
2 ( ) By yourself with the use of assistive devices (such as grab bars).
3 ( ) With some help from another person (includes supervision).
4 ( ) With complete assistance from another person.

4 ( ) Or you are given sponge baths only.

Table continued on opposite page

TABLE 12–1. INSTITUTE FOR REHABILITATION AND RESTORATIVE CARE– LONG-RANGE EVALUATION SYSTEM *(Continued)*

Which best describes how you enter and leave an automobile safely?

1 ( ) By yourself without the use of assistive devices.
2 ( ) By yourself with the use of assistive devices such as a sliding board or lift.
3 ( ) With some help from another person.
4 ( ) Heavy lifting required or with complete assistance from another person.

AMBULATION   How do you walk on a level surface of 50 yards or more?

1 ( ) By yourself without the use of assistive devices such as cane or leg brace.
2 ( ) By yourself with the use of assistive devices such as a cane, walker, or brace.
3 ( ) With some help from another person.
4 ( ) Not able to walk as far as 50 yards with or without help.

How do you climb up and go down stairs (at least one full flight)?

1 ( ) By yourself without the use of assistive devices or a handrail.
2 ( ) By yourself with the use of assistive devices (such as a handrail or cane).
3 ( ) With some help from another person.
4 ( ) Not able to climb a full flight of stairs.

How do you walk outdoors for a distance of 50 yards (about one block)?

1 ( ) By yourself without the use of assistive devices such as a cane or leg brace.
2 ( ) By yourself with the use of assistive devices such as a cane, walker, or brace.
3 ( ) With some help from another person.
4 ( ) Not able to walk as far as 50 yards with or without help.

WHEELCHAIR   Answer this question only if you use a wheelchair. How do you usually propel and maneuver a wheelchair to turn corners or get close to the bed?

1 ( ) By yourself.
2 ( ) By yourself with the use of a power source such as a battery.
3 ( ) With help from another person.

Null
( ) Or you do not use a wheelchair every day.

ENVIRONMENT (*E* OF ESCROW) — ARCHITECTURAL BARRIERS Check according to one of the following descriptions:

1 ( ) Irrelevant — you have access into and out of home, to all levels if multi-story, and to all rooms without safety hazard or requiring assistance, or else not relevant to problem.
2 ( ) Minor — you have access into and out of home, to all essential levels if multi-story, and to all rooms essential to well-being and participation in family activities. Some nonessential rooms may not be accessible or else inconvenience may be imposed by thresholds, narrow passages, or awkward arrangement of furniture. However, you are able to manage without assistance.
3 ( ) Major — you are not able to manage without assistance in getting into or out of home or in gaining access to rooms essential to well-being and/or participation in family activities. Family does not wish to move because of these problems.
4 ( ) You live in housing with major problems and desire to move because of them.

SOCIAL INTERACTION (*S* OF ESCROW) Check according to one of the following descriptions:

1 ( ) You maintain a balance of social contacts by way of visiting, telephone calls, hobbies and interests, etc.
2 ( ) Your social contacts are restrictive.
3 ( ) You or someone else in the family unit occasionally requires assistance at home from a person or agency from the outside such as the visiting nurse association, home care, counseling services, etc.
4 ( ) You or someone else in the family unit is consistently dependent upon assistance at home from a community agency at least weekly.

CLUSTER OF FAMILY MEMBERS (*C* OF ESCROW) Check according to one of the following descriptions: *Do not answer if you live alone.*

1 ( ) Your family consists of at least one member besides yourself related by marriage, kinship, or else a close personal companion; as a unit the family is sufficiently competent physically and mentally to provide adequate support to you at home at this time and under foreseeable circumstances.
2 ( ) Your family is as above but under particular conditions of stress they may not be able to support you either physically or mentally, or else particular circumstances such as a job require a crucial family member to be away from the home part of the day.
3 ( ) The impact of the disability has been such as to change either the work effort, pattern of socialization, interests and hobbies, or other important activities of some family member.
4 ( ) The impact of the disability has been such as to produce severe strain or disruptions of relationships between family members.

Table continued on following page

**TABLE 12–1. INSTITUTE FOR REHABILITATION AND RESTORATIVE CARE–
LONG-RANGE EVALUATION SYSTEM (Continued)**

HOUSEHOLD CONSTELLATION:
- ( ) Alone
- ( ) Spouse
- ( ) Children
- ( ) Parent(s)
- ( ) Other relatives
- ( ) Friend(s)
- ( ) Other:_____

RESOURCES (R OF ESCROW) Check according to one of the following descriptions:

1 ( ) Your family is able to absorb the costs of the disability without increased indebtedness.
2 ( ) Your family is required to incur debts to handle costs of the disability.
3 ( ) Your family requires some form of public assistance to cover medically related costs
      (Medicaid or Medical Assistance).
4 ( ) Your family requires public assistance to cover medical and subsistence costs (Welfare or
      SSI – Supplemental Security Income).

OUTLOOK (O OF ESCROW): Describe how you feel about making decisions that affect your own well-being:
1 ( ) You are able to make decisions easily.
2 ( ) You are able to make decisions but with moderate difficulty.
3 ( ) You are not able to make decisions except with great difficulty.
4 ( ) You only make very few decisions or none at all.

VOCATIONAL STATUS:
- ( ) Homemaker
- ( ) Student
- ( ) Competitive employment
- 3 ( ) Sheltered workshop
- 4 ( ) Unemployed or Retired for disability or Disabled (not yet age 60)
- ( ) Retired for age (age 60 or more)

FOR COMPETITIVE EMPLOYMENT, HOMEMAKER, OR STUDENT (W OF ESCROW):

1 ( ) You have no work or educational or homemaking restrictions. You essentially devote full time
      to major activity(ies). Time lost does not exceed one day per month on the average.
2 ( ) You may have a work or educational or homemaking restriction or require some modification such as
      part-time, light work, etc. Time lost does not exceed more than 2 to 5 days per month on the average.
3 ( ) Work or education is attended in a special facility adapted for the handicapped or else time lost may
      exceed one week per month on the average. If a homemaker, assistance is needed from outside the
      home to perform household tasks.

FOR RETIRED DUE TO AGE (NOT DUE TO DISABILITY) (W OF ESCROW):

1 ( ) You fulfill usual and customary tasks and roles, other than earning an income, in the household
      and/or community.
2 ( ) You fulfill usual and customary tasks and roles, other than earning an income, in the household
      and/or community in a limited way.
4 ( ) You do not fulfill usual and customary tasks and roles, other than earning an income, in the
      household or community.

REMARKS:

ANSWERED BY: _____

two sets of patient populations. When administered at the time of discharge of 10 stroke patients, it had high interjudge reliability of 0.97 (two different nurses made judgments on the same patient). When administered at admission to 100 rehabilitation patients, there was a high internal consistency reliability (an alpha coefficient of 0.92), indicating good scalability of the items in the index. The total score was found to be discriminating and valid, and changes over time deemed to be a reliable measure of observed functional change.[37] In another study using modified versions of the PULSES profile and the Barthel index, the scales highly correlated with each other from rehabiliation hospital admission to discharge to follow-up. Test-retest reliability was high at 0.87 and 0.89, respectively, and intercoder reliability was above 0.95 on both scales.[38]

Other workers[39, 40] with extensive experience in collecting clinical data regard an interjudge reliability coefficient of 0.85 or better as acceptable. Further, they find it rather easy to train and attain the criterion of 0.85 reliability for measures of physical functioning, including the Barthel index, compared with greater difficulty in attaining this criterion level using measures of psychosocial functioning.

Basic profile dimensions are based upon the following domains: active motion of limbs, verbal communication, hearing ability, visual ability, self-care ability, mobility, need for physician or nursing services, intellectual and emotional adaptability, adequacy of the home setting, the level of social interactions or dependence upon home service agencies, the level of support from the family unit, the financial resources, and educational or vocational status. The data collection forms are descriptive checklists prepared for computer entry with allowance for free text descriptions as well. The forms are intended for use by clinicians serving the patient. Mutually exclusive definitions have been developed for the descriptive criteria, thus reducing ambiguity in rating. Educational material has been developed, and workshops* are conducted regularly to teach the uniform criteria to potential users of the system. Following entry of the data into the computer, scores are generated according to the modified versions of the Barthel index (Table 12–2) and the PULSES profile (Table 12–3) and are used to represent physical dependence with regard to personal care. A recent study has shown a strong correlation between the Barthel index score and independent performance of personal care tasks such as those typically performed by home health aides within a home care–visiting nurse program.[24] The level of social support is measured by the ESCROW profile (Table 12–4). It is a newer scale, and its reliability and validity are still being tested. It is postulated that the physically disabled person

---

*Evaluation of Functional Abilities: A Workshop for Health Professionals. Sponsored by the Institute for Rehabilitation and Restorative Care, Program in Medicine, Brown University, Providence, Rhode Island.

TABLE 12–2. MODIFIED BARTHEL INDEX SCORING

Independent		Dependent		
I Intact	II Limited	III Helper	IV Null	
10	5	1	1	Drink from cup/Feed from dish
5	5	3	0	Dress upper body
5	5	2	0	Dress lower body
0	0	−2	0	Don brace or prosthesis
5	5	0	0	Grooming
4	4	0	0	Wash or bathe
10	10	5	0	Bladder continence
10	10	5	0	Bowel continence
4	4	2	0	Care of perineum/clothing at toilet
15	15	7	0	Transfer, chair
6	5	3	0	Transfer, toilet
1	1	0	0	Transfer, tub or shower
15	15	10	0	Walk on level 50 yards or more
10	10	5	0	Up and down stairs for 1 flight or more
15	5	0	0	Wheelchair/50 yds—Only if *not walking*

TABLE 12–3. "PULSES" PROFILE (ADAPTED)

P — Physical condition including diseases of the viscera (cardiovascular, gastrointestinal, urologic, and endocrine) and neurologic disorders:
1. Medical problems sufficiently stable that medical or nursing monitoring is not required more often than 3-month intervals.
2. Medical or nurse monitoring is needed more often than 3-month intervals but not each week.
3. Medical problems are sufficiently unstable as to require regular medical and/or nursing attention at least weekly.
4. Medical problems require intensive medical and/or nursing attention at least daily (excluding personal care assistance only).

U — Self-care activities (drink/feed, dress upper/lower, brace/prosthesis, groom, wash/bathe, perineal care) dependent mainly upon upper limb function:
1. Independent in self care without impairment of upper limbs.
2. Independent in self care with some impairment of upper limbs.
3. Dependent upon assistance or supervision in self care with or without impairment of upper limbs.
4. Dependent totally in self care with marked impairment of upper limbs.

L — Mobility activities (transfer chair/toilet/tub or shower, walk, stairs, wheelchair) dependent mainly upon lower limb function:
1. Independent in mobility without impairment of lower limbs.
2. Independent in mobility with some impairment in lower limbs; such as needing ambulatory aids, a brace or prosthesis, or else fully independent in a wheelchair without significant architectural or environmental barriers.
3. Dependent upon assistance or supervision in mobility with or without impairment of lower limbs, or else partly independent in a wheelchair, or else there are significant architectural or environmental barriers.
4. Dependent totally in mobility with marked impairment of lower limbs.

S — Sensory components relating to communication (speech and hearing) and vision:
1. Independent in communication and vision without impairment.
2. Independent in communication and vision with some impairment such as mild dysarthria, mild aphasia, or need for eyeglasses or hearing aid, or needing regular medication.
3. Dependent upon assistance, an interpreter, or supervision in communication or vision.
4. Dependent totally in communication or vision.

E — Excretory functions (bladder and bowel):
1. Complete voluntary control of bladder and bowel sphincters.
2. Control of sphincters allows normal social activities despite urgency or need for catheter, appliance, suppositories, etc. Able to care for needs without assistance.
3. Dependent upon assistance in sphincter management or else has accidents occasionally.
4. Frequent wetting or soiling from incontinence of bladder or bowel sphincters.

S — Intellectual and emotional adaptability (*O* of ESCROW), support from family unit (*C* of ESCROW), financial ability (*R* of ESCROW), and social interaction (*S* of ESCROW):
1. Fulfills usual role(s) and performs customary tasks.
2. Must make some modification in usual role(s) or performance of customary tasks.
3. Dependent upon assistance, supervision, encouragement, or assistance from a public or private agency due to any of the above considerations.
4. Dependent upon long-term institutional care (chronic hospital, nursing home, etc.) excluding time-limited hospitalization for specific evaluation, treatment, or active rehabilitation.

TABLE 12–4. CRITERIA FOR ESCROW FUNCTIONAL SCALE
(Not for Persons Living in Institutions)

E — ENVIRONMENT

1 ( ) Irrelevant — has access into and out of home, to all levels if multi-story, and to all rooms without safety hazard or requiring assistance, or else not relevant to problem.
2 ( ) Minor — has access into and out of home, to all essential levels if multi-story, and to all rooms essential to well-being and participation in family activities. Some nonessential rooms may not be accessible, or else inconvenience may be imposed by thresholds, narrow passages, or awkward arrangement of furniture. However, able to manage without assistance.
3 ( ) Major — not able to manage without assistance in getting into or out of home or in gaining access to rooms essential to well-being and/or participation in family activities. Family does not wish to move because of these problems.
4 ( ) Lives in housing with major problems and desires to move because of them.

Table continued on opposite page

TABLE 12-4. CRITERIA FOR ESCROW FUNCTIONAL SCALE *(Continued)*
(Not for Persons Living in Institutions)

S—SOCIAL INTERACTION

1. Maintains a balance of social contacts by way of visiting, telephone calls, hobbies and interests, etc.
2. Social contacts are restrictive.
3. The patient or someone in the family unit occasionally requires assistance at home from a person or agency from the outside such as the visiting nurse association, home care, counseling services, etc.
4. The patient or someone in the family unit is consistently dependent upon assistance at home from a community agency at least weekly.

C—CLUSTER OF FAMILY MEMBERS
(Do Not Answer if Patient Lives Alone—if so, a rating of 4 is given)

1. The family unit consists of at least one member besides the patient related by marriage, kinship, or else a close personal companion; as a unit the family is sufficiently competent physically and mentally to provide adequate support to the patient at home at this time and under foreseeable circumstances.
2. The family unit is as above but under particular conditions of stress they may not be able to support the patient either physically or mentally, or else particular circumstances such as a job require a crucial family member to be away from the home part of the day.
3. The impact of the disability has been such as to change either the work effort, pattern of socialization, interests and hobbies, or other important activities of some family member.
4. The impact of the disability has been such as to produce severe strain or disruptions of relationships between family members.

R—RESOURCES

1. The family is able to absorb the costs of the disability without increased indebtedness.
2. The family is required to incur debts to handle costs of the disability.
3. The family requires some form of public assistance to cover medically related costs (Medicaid).
4. The family requires public assistance to cover medical and subsistence costs (Welfare or SSI).

O—OUTLOOK

1. The individual functions independently without impairment in the following areas: problem-solving, regard for others, perceptual motor ability, judgment, reliability, and self-esteem. The individual feels *able to make decisions easily.*
2. The individual functions independently with mild impairment in some area(s) mentioned above or else has *moderate difficulty making decisions.*
3. The individual is observed to function appreciably better with assistance, supervision, cuing, coaxing, or structured environment due to one or more of the problems mentioned above or else *has great difficulty making decisions.*
4. The individual is not particularly benefited by assistance with problems mentioned above or else actually *makes very few, if any, decisions.*

W—WORK/SCHOOL/RETIREMENT STATUS

FOR COMPETITIVE EMPLOYMENT, HOMEMAKER, STUDENT:
1. There are no work or educational or homemaking restrictions. Essentially devotes full time to major activity(ies). Time lost does not exceed one day per month on the average.
2. The individual may have a work or educational or homemaking restriction or require some modification such as part-time, light work, etc. Time lost does not exceed more than 2 to 5 days per month on the average.
3. Work or education is attended in a special facility adapted for the handicapped *or else* time lost may exceed one week per month on the average. If a homemaker, assistance is needed from outside the home to perform household tasks.

FOR RETIRED DUE TO AGE (NOT DUE TO DISABILITY):
1. Fulfills usual and customary tasks and roles, other than earning an income, in the household or community.
2. Fulfills usual and customary tasks and roles, other than earning an income, in the household or community in a limited way.
4. Not able to fulfill usual and customary tasks and roles, other than earning an income, in the household or community.

with a marginal level of independence in personal care is more likely to have potential for independent living if social supports are high as represented by the ESCROW scale.

RATIONALE FOR QUALITY ASSURANCE AND PROGRAM EVALUATION

Codman[41] first described auditing to improve quality of medical care in what he described as "end result analysis." Donabedian[42-44] expressed the differences between measures of quality of medical care based upon judging (1) input or structural characteristics, (2) process characteristics, and (3) outcome characteristics or results. For example, input characteristics include certification of professional health care providers, and process characteristics include adherence to accredited treatment procedures. It has been assumed that quality of treatment results could be approximated by assuring conformity to standards according to input and/or process features. With rising costs of medical care and other human service programs, it has become necessary to measure, or at least estimate, efficacy, effectiveness, and efficiency. Of course none of these are measurable without agreement on the benefits of care that has been rendered. Determination of outcomes is not only more difficult than documenting input or process characteristics, but it is essential to do in order to measure benefits.

In the report of a study by the Institute of Medicine, in reference to long-term care it is stated that "methods for assessing the quality of care should include all sources of care and should consider the impact of care on the patient's expected and actual ability to function in daily life." It also stated that "an assessment of quality based on diagnostic-specific criteria is often inappropriate, and functional status is a more relevant measure."[45]

Two recent volumes are recommended to the reader on this topic — *Assessing and Improving Health Care Outcomes* by J. W. Williamson and *Health Program Evaluation* by S. M. Shortell and W. C. Richardson. Williamson[11] suggests the following operational definitions:

1. **Efficacy** — the extent to which health care intervention can be shown to be beneficial under optimal conditions of care.
2. **Effectiveness** — the extent to which benefits achievable under optimal conditions of care are actually achieved in clinical practice. (Lack of effectiveness would be identified when achievable benefits were not obtained.)
3. **Efficiency** — the proportion of total cost (e.g., money, scarce resources, and time) that can be related to actual benefits achieved.

He further suggests prerequisites for measuring outcomes:

1. Outcomes should be defined clearly and objectively, including the process used and the time duration of the process. (Broadly speaking, outcomes are not solely confined to patient function or health status but can encompass any aspect of the patient and his/her health problems or of providers and their interactions. Choosing the most relevant outcome for measurement is a basic requirement.
2. A causal relationship between outcome and process should be made explicit and be analyzed for validity. (There should be reasonable attribution of outcome to the care provided even though in most situations medical care is based upon implicit assumptions of causality. Validity of these assumptions must be supported by reasonable evidence, including consideration of the several factors involved, such as compliance of the patient.)
3. The value of the outcome should be analyzed for helpful and harmful effects — for the individual and for the social group — within a given time and under given circumstances. (Since life is a continuum and its several phases are subject to intrinsic influences as well as any medical care interventions, the number of different outcomes is almost infinite. Therefore, the time range over which change is expected to occur must be specified.)

Williamson summarizes by stating "the first can be established by consensual definition; the second requires valid scientific evidence; and the third requires value clarification."

Shortell and Richardson[16] state that

... attempting to evaluate a social program is at best risky and at worst treacherous. In few other activities are the ambivalent tendencies of society so clearly revealed. On the one hand is society's desire to learn more so that the quality of life may be improved, while on the other hand is the ubiquitous fear of what might be found.

They identify the following deficits that characterized early efforts to evaluate the process of service delivery:

1. Neglect of outcome measures of program effectiveness.
2. Use of objectives based on untested, unstated, and frequently erroneous assumptions.
3. Reliance on biased data and samples of unknown representation.
4. Failure to follow principles of sound experimental design.
5. Inadequate attention given to the accuracy, reliability, and validity of measurement.
6. Inability to draw causal inferences regarding program effects.

They summarize that

. . . program evaluation helps to answer basic questions concerning whether the program is any good; helps to ensure accountability to oneself, one's staff and one's clients; helps to keep the emphasis on end-results; contributes to the development of analytical processes; promotes the training of staff, and fosters the development of professional attitudes and behavior.

The medical rehabilitation facility or any facility providing care for the long-term patient or client that uses a reliable and valid functional assessment method has a tool that will greatly assist in accomplishing quality assurance and program evaluation.

TECHNIQUES FOR FUNCTIONAL ASSESSMENT AND PROGRAM EVALUATION

The functional assessment must cull out appropriate descriptors (often by proxy) that address relevancies within the concepts of pathology, impairment, functional limitations, disability and handicap as defined by Nagi[3, 4] and Wood.[5-7] Diagnosis of pathology is usually considered to be the linchpin of medical characterization and classification; however, it may not necessarily be the most important variable to describe various states of disability. As noted by Sherwood et al.,[46] diagnostic classification for those with chronic illness is not simple. Diagnostic data come from several sources — the physician,

a hospital record, the patient. The physician-specialist may emphasize certain terms and omit others more distant to his/her sphere of interest. Hospital data may be distorted by the need to satisfy third-party requirements for reimbursement. The patient may not be fully informed of important diagnoses, may have been supplied with euphemistic terms, or may have suppressed discomforting information. Diagnoses tend to wax and wane in importance with the passage of time; a stroke of 20 years ago has different implications than one which occurred one month previously. As one condition appears, others may become less important or may be resolved. Diagnostic designations, therefore, often are not permanent, nor does the same diagnosis necessarily have the same implication in different circumstances. Identical diagnoses may have variable impact on the patient; in the absence of assessment of functional status, that impact cannot be quantified. A diagnosis of rheumatoid arthritis may reflect mild stiffness in a few joints or total incapacitation requiring a bed-to-chair existence. With regard to diagnostic terminology one must realize the following points:

1. Diagnosis may be serving a labeling function rather than transmitting real information.
2. Severity and prognosis cannot be presumed from most diagnoses alone but may require accurate descriptions of functional status.
3. Psychosocial implications and needs consequent to diagnostic conditions may be entirely missed without supplying specific supplemental information.
4. Diagnostic terminology may not be relevant to the cluster of problems to be resolved from the perspective of functions of daily living.

The standard International Classification of Diseases, 9th Revision — Clinical Modification (ICD9-CM)[47] coding is widely used by hospital medical record departments to describe the pathology and etiologies of various conditions and is sometimes useful to identify impairments. Wood[7] has proposed an exhaustive classification scheme which details each of the three concepts of impairment, disability, and handicap that he has outlined. These proposals to supplement the International Classification of Diseases are intended as a way to code data in order to reduce the amount of detail of a case into a standardized numerical form. This would facilitate retrieval of records and analysis of statistical data. The Long-Range Evaluation System employs auxiliary coding systems to identify the "major handicapping condition" and organ system that is mainly responsible for bringing the patient for rehabilitation or long-term care considerations. A version of the classification system for the major handicapping condition is shown in Table 12–5.

Another coding system is employed to identify complications that have arisen during the course of rehabilitation that significantly interferred with care or progress. At any rate there exist well-developed methods for identifying pathologies, etiologies, morbid and co-morbid conditions, complications, and impairments.

Methods for describing functional limitations and disability are much less well devel-

TABLE 12–5. GROUPING OF MAJOR HANDICAPPED CONDITIONS

Musculoskeletal Disorders
> Consists of musculoskeletal disorders which, if they result in functional limitation, do so by misalignment of bones, restriction of joints, or poor control of muscles, either mechanically or because of inflammation and/or pain.

Cardiorespiratory and Vascular Disorders
> Consist of cardiorespiratory and vascular disorders which, if they result in functional impairment, do so by impairing stamina, exercise tolerance, general vigor, or peripheral vascular supply.

Central and Peripheral Neuromuscular Disorders
> Consist of neurological disorders which, if they result in functional limitation, do so by impairing motor, sensory, or some other modality of limbs or trunk; also language skills.

Special Sensory Disorders
> Consist of disorders characterized by deficiencies of sight or hearing.

Diffuse Brain Disorders
> Consist of central nervous system disorders which are characterized by integrative deficiencies, e.g., senility, mental retardation, etc.

Gastrointestinal Disorders
> Consist of gastrointestinal problems, such as cirrhosis, which may impair function in variable and often nonspecific fashion.

Hematological and Metabolic Disorders
> Consist of hematological, metabolic, and other disorders which, if they result in functional limitation, do so by virtue of their general toxicity and/or disturbance of biochemical equilibrium; this type of impairment is generally not localized, focal, or specific.

Psychiatric and Psychological Problems
> Consist of psychiatric and psychological problems in which the individual may be distressed in his/her personal or social role(s) or possibly a danger to society or oneself (in the legal as well as the clinical sense of that phrase).

Genitourinary Disorders
> Consist of renal and genitourinary tract problems which may be, but not necessarily are, associated with sphincter incontinence, but more usually, if they impair function, do so in variable and often nonspecific fashion.

Tumors (including Cancer)
> Consist of malignant or benign growths.

Growth and Development Disorders
> Consist of the various developmental disorders of birth or early childhood that impair the normal sequence of physical, psychological, and emotional maturation and limit the options for necessary experiences of growth and development.

Amputations
> Consist of congenital or acquired amputations of limbs.

Skin Disorders
> Consist of chronic dermatoses or scarring (as from body burns) that restrict mobility by constraining joint movement, or cause cosmetic disfigurement, or else threaten health because of the presence of or tendency for infection.

Oral-Dental-Facial Disorders
> Consist of disorders resulting in facial disfigurement, or impairment of the masticatory apparatus or articulatory apparatus for speech.

oped, understood, or accepted and are infrequently practiced. Functional limitations and residual abilities of an individual are identified by systematically taking an inventory of the repertoire of skills and task performances that are considered necessary to fulfill expected social roles. Such lists can be literally endless and hopelessly detailed, on the one hand, or else too skimpy and insufficiently comprehensive, on the other hand. Instead of "laundry lists" it is more useful to employ a conversion to a numerical scoring method for representing defined domains in the continuum between intactness and deficiency. This means that the items that make up the score are scalable. Disability is represented by the sum of interactions between the person and his/her environment that fail to meet expected social roles. Thus, functional assessment concentrates on displaying the presence or absence of key performances and behaviors, within those domains, that define expected social roles. These are usually translated to mean an individual's basic strengths and weaknesses, which are then presented in a concise and synoptic format. Some social roles can be readily identified as separate although interdependent domains, such as work or educational pursuits; maintenance of independent living circumstances; roles with family and a close circle of friends; roles with the larger community (social, professional, business, and political); management of one's personal affairs; leisure time activities; or else roles as defined by Wood in the World Health Organization publication,[7] noted earlier in this chapter.

The Long-Range Evaluation System collects functional assessment data on a worksheet coded for computer entry, appropriate for the point in time, whether admission, discharge, or follow-up, for example. Mutually exclusive categories for descriptive choices are guided by explicit criteria. The computer generates feedback reports that contain the scores calculated for the Barthel, PULSES, and ESCROW scales for incorporation into the patient's medical record. Another score is generated called the BPI (Barthel-PULSES Index — calculated as Barthel score $\times$ 10 $\times$ 6/PULSES score), which is a combination measure of level of physical dependence and is used in the calculations for program evaluation. All data are stored in the computer for management reporting, including program evaluation, and for tracking individual patients. One method for display of data, only for illustrative purposes, according to the Barthel, PULSES, and ESCROW scales, is shown in a hypothetical case in Figure 12–3.

John W. is a 23-year-old married graduate student, with an infant daughter, who was injured in an automobile accident six weeks prior to ad-

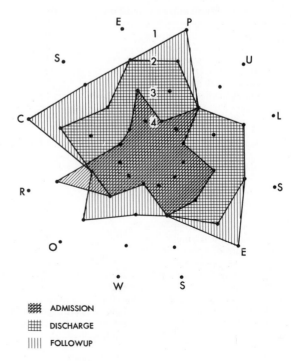

FIGURE 12–3. Progressive expansion of "life space" of disabled patient from admission to discharge to follow-up as quantified by each of the components of PULSES and ESCROW.

▨ ADMISSION

▦ DISCHARGE

|||| FOLLOWUP

mission for hospital rehabilitation. He suffered a closed head injury and was in a coma for three weeks. He entered rehabilitation with a left-sided hemiplegia, severe dysarthria, confusion and perceptual-motor deficits, depression, and bladder and bowel incontinence.

At the time of admission John W. and his family were living in a rented trailer and had inadequate insurance for a catastrophic event. At discharge from rehabilitation six weeks after admission, arrangements had been made for living accommodations with other relatives. In the home of his relatives stairs imposed a minor barrier. By this time he had secured eligibility of the medical assistance program (Medicaid). At the time of follow-up reporting, 10 months after hospital discharge, John's wife was more confident in meeting his needs and she had secured a driving license. John was independent in personal care except for need for minimal assistance in dressing. His depressive mood and problem-solving abilities had improved and he had begun an evaluation and counseling program with the state vocational rehabilitation agency. The circular display of PULSES and ESCROW scores is intended to reflect widening of "life-space" as functional improvement toward independence occurs from admission to follow-up. The more independent score (1) is represented by the outer orbit and the most dependent score (4) is represented by the inner orbit.

Aggregated data representing all patients served by a rehabilitation facility may be displayed in many different ways. One example is shown below using data from the Comprehensive Service Needs Study (CSNS).[38] The format of Table 12–6 allows easy comparison of key characteristics of patients served from one year to the next for a given facility or to compare one facility with others.

While the display in Table 12–6 is useful for understanding the performance of a rehabilitation program, such a display does not meet the requirements for program evaluation. The key elements of program evaluation are a written purpose statement for the facility, and specific goals and objectives. The objectives must be measurable, and are related to intake, process, and results. The Commission of Accreditation of Rehabilitation Facilities (CARF) requires that accredited facilities have an ongoing system for program evaluation.[48] Program evaluation measures the results achieved by patients after they have received the services of the rehabilitation program. The example that is presented reflects results at discharge; a more advanced modification will incorporate

TABLE 12–6. COMPARATIVE REHABILITATION PROGRAM REPORT*

| Major Handicapped Condition | Type of Discharge* | | | | |
	Home	Acute Hospital	LTCF	Other	Total
Focal cerebral disorders	105	2	22	5	134
Spinal cord disorders	84	4	6	1	95
Other neuromuscular disorders	16	—	2	—	18
Musculoskeletal/skin disorders	22	1	1	—	24
Lower limb amputation	27	—	5	—	32
Other medical/psychiatric disorders	3	—	—	1	4
Totals	257	7	36	7	307
Percentage	84%	2%	12%	2%	100%
Males/Females	147/110	4/3	21/15	5/2	177/130
Averages					
Age	49	50	59	45	50
Admission Barthel score	41	32	31	26	39
Discharge Barthel score	76	65	53	49	72
Change in Barthel score	+35	+33	+22	+23	+33
Length of stay in weeks	9.3	11.2	6.8	7.7	9.0

*An example taken from the Comprehensive Service Needs Study data (N = 307).

†The type of discharge is explained by *home* (those who returned to community settings either alone or more commonly with relatives and/or friends); *acute hospital* (those who were discharged to the acute hospital because of a medical/surgical complication and did not return to the inpatient hospital program); *long-term care facility*—LTCF (those who were discharged to a nursing home or chronic hospital setting); and *other* (those who transferred to complete the rehabilitation program at another facility).

follow-up data to reflect results some time after receipt of services.

The illustration that follows is a first-generation effort and therefore measures objectives achieved between admission and discharge and does not extend to follow-up data. In order to implement program evaluation, each facility must establish its own goals and objectives and then go about obtaining data that demonstrate the degree to which the organization is achieving its goals. By a process of consensus among members of the facility staff, measurable objectives must be determined and a standard value set for each objective. An example of five objectives (I through V) and standard values is shown in Table 12–7.

The first objective, I, to maximize the percentage of patients discharged home from the inpatient program, is consistent with the rehabilitation goals of returning people to the community at the highest levels of independence possible. The effectiveness ratio, II, is derived by dividing the average discharge Barthel-PULSES Index (BPI) score by the average admission BPI score as a measure of general improvement in functional independence. The ratio of dependence, III, is an equation using BPI to identify the "severely and profoundly" handicapped on admission and on discharge. This measure credits the facility for the percentage of patients admitted and raised from severe and profound dependence to a level of less dependence. Minimizing length of stay, IV, is consistent with the goal of maximizing independence in the shortest time possible. Maximizing the change in Barthel score, V, is a measure of program effectiveness. Thus, a facility that discharges 75 per cent of its patients to home has an average effectiveness ratio of 1.5, a

dependence ratio of 2.0, an average length of stay of six weeks, and a positive change in Barthel score of 20 points would meet all of the standard values and, hence, would have met its goals.

In order to develop this methodology for program evaluation, the objective must be identified in *measurable* (i.e., numerical) terms as *standard values*. The actual results from the rehabilitation facility program must be compared with the standard value for each objective, and then an overall score is developed that represents whether or not the facility has met its goal, again in numerical terms. One method for doing this, described by Kay,[49] is to set up a matrix that assigns each *standard value* to an *index value of 100*. Thus, when the *actual value* equals the *standard value*, the *index value* is 100. This relationship is shown in Table 12–8, where the actual value of 75 per cent (which equals the standard value for objective I in Table 12–7) matches the index value of 100. Next, a range of values must be anticipated for the results within each objective that would contain the majority (perhaps about two-thirds) of expected results. The lower and upper limits of this range must be "equidistant" from the *standard value* and are assigned *index values* of 50 and 150, respectively. This is shown in Table 12–8, where actual values of 65 per cent and 85 per cent for objective I are assigned to index values of 50 and 150, respectively.

The next step is to assign a *weight value* to each *100 index value* apportioned in such a way that the *sum of each weight value* for all of the objectives *equals 100*. The weight value of 40 that is assigned to objective I is shown in Table 12–8 to match with the actual value of 75 per cent and the index value of 100. The apportionment of weight to each of the objectives in order to form a total value of 100 is shown in Table 12–9 under the "Expected Weight" column. Then, in similar fashion, the lower and upper limits of the *index values,* 50 and 150, respectively, are assigned weight values that also represent an "equidistant" spread down and up from the *weight value* assigned to the *100 index value.* This is shown in Table 12–8 by the weights of 20 and 60 that are assigned to the index values of 50 and 150, respectively, for objective I. Thus, the sum of weight values for all the objective index values of 50 equals a *score of 50* and the sum of index values of

TABLE 12–7. PROGRAM EVALUATION OBJECTIVES

	Objectives	Standard Values
I	Patients discharged home	75%
II	Effectiveness ratio: $\dfrac{\text{Discharge B-P index}}{\text{Admission B-P index}}$	1.5
III	Ratio of dependence	2.0
IV	Length of stay in weeks	6.0
V	Change in Barthel score	20

TABLE 12-8. AN EXAMPLE OF MATCHING RESULT, INDEX, AND WEIGHT VALUES FOR OBJECTIVE I

ACTUAL VALUE	65%	67%	69%	71%	73%	75%	77%	79%	81%	83%	85%
INDEX VALUE	50	60	70	80	90	100	110	120	130	140	150
WEIGHT VALUE	20	24	28	32	36	40	44	48	52	56	60

The standard value was set at an index value of 100 (in this case 75%), which also corresponds to the weight value (in this case 40). If an actual value less than the standard had been attained, the index value would have been less than 100 and the corresponding weight value would have been less. The opposite applies when the standard value has been exceeded. The ranges of the indices are controlled in order that they not exceed 150 or go below 50.

150 equals a *score of 150*. Finally, the calculations are adjusted in order that regardless of an actual value, the index value never goes below 50 nor does it exceed 150.

It is important to realize that assignment of standard values to the objective is arbitrary and is not arrived at scientifically (at least not at this stage of development), and neither are the assignments of the weighted scores. Nevertheless, as an illustration of the methodology, data derived from the Comprehensive Service Needs Study,[38] are used in Table 12–8 to show the matching of actual, index, and weight values for objective I. Table 12–9 displays the summary report of expected standards and weights and the actual results, indexes, and weights using data from the Comprehensive Service Needs Study.

In the program evaluation report shown in Table 12–9, objective I exceeded the standard and carried a weight of 56. Objective II exceeded the standard and carried a weight of 15. Objective III exceeded the standard and carried a weight of 30. Objective IV did not meet the standard and carried a weight of 12. Objective V exceeded the standard and carried a weight of 15. The evaluation shows that only objective IV failed to meet the standard, reaching an index value of only 60.

However, the cumulative score weight of 128 places the total score of the Comprehensive Service Needs Study sample above the standards established for this illustration. This illustration should not be taken as a general standard to be applied to any specific facility or population because of the biases operating in the selection of the Comprehensive Service Needs Study sample for that particular study.

When a program evaluation system is first begun, initial results may be disappointing. However, with continued use and increased staff experience, the facility should soon approach maximum results. A program that is both effective and efficient in achieving its goals will be beneficial to the patients served by that rehabilitation facility. The patients will have achieved significant improvements following discharge. Also, with program evaluation it is possible to have a meaningful presentation of a report that reflects the total program effort. The report measures actual results against expected objectives. In this way, it becomes an invaluable tool for the manager of the facility. The person making the decisions needs information, and this method provides the raw material for decisions and actions. The manager will know

TABLE 12-9. PROGRAM EVALUATION USING THE COMPREHENSIVE SERVICE NEEDS STUDY SAMPLE TO COMPARE EXPECTED WITH ACTUAL RESULTS

| | Objectives | Expected | | Actual | | |
		Standard	Weight	Result	Index	Weight
I	Patients discharged home	75%	40	83%	140	56
II	Effectiveness ratio	1.5	10	4.5	150	15
III	Dependence ratio	2.0	20	4.2	150	30
IV	Length of stay in weeks	6.0	20	9.0	60	12
V	Change in Barthel score	20	10	33	112	15
	Total		100			128

whether or not a program is achieving its objectives, and any possible problem areas will be highlighted. The facility that can show better information on results achieved can successfully compete for the limited monies that are available to conduct rehabilitation service programs. That facility will be in a better position to justify, maintain, or expand funding and to gain community support.

This type of evaluation method is based upon outcomes of care and provides a measure of benefits derived from medical rehabilitation. Given data of this type about a facility, the managers and staff of a facility have the means to objectively study effectiveness and efficiency, monitor quality of care in an ongoing and complete fashion, and obtain objective data to support decisions for improving care or for containing costs.

Acknowledgment

I am indebted to Julianna Barrett, Donna Dryer, Marilyn Kaplan, and Sylvia Pendleton for their kind assistance in preparing this chapter.

REFERENCES

1. Weed, L.: Medical Records, Medical Education and Patient Care. Cleveland, Case Western Reserve University, 1970.
2. Weed, L.: Medical records that guide and teach. N. Engl. J. Med., 278:593–600, 652–657, 1968.
3. Nagi, S. Z.: Disability concepts and prevalence. Mershon Center, Ohio State University. Presented at the First Mary Switzer Memorial Seminar, Cleveland, Ohio, May, 1975.
4. Nagi, S. Z.: An epidemiology of disability among adults in the United States. Milbank Memorial Fund Quarterly; Health & Society, 54(4):439–467, 1976.
5. Wood, P. H. N., and Badley, E. M.: An epidemiological appraisal of disablement. *In* Bennett, A. E. (Ed.): Recent Advances in Community Medicine. Edinburgh, Churchill Livingstone, 1978.
6. Wood, P. H. N., and Badley, E. M.: Setting disablement in perspective. Int. Rehabil. Med., 1:32–37, 1978.
7. World Health Organization (WHO): International Classification of Impairments, Disabilities, and Handicaps. Geneva, World Health Organization, 1980, p. 184.
8. Stewart, A., Ware, J. E., and Brook, R. H.: The meaning of health: Understanding functional limitations. Medical Care, 15:939–952, 1977.
9. Stewart, A., Ware, J. E., and Brook, R. H.: The meaning of health: Understanding functional limitations. Unpublished manuscript.
10. Health Services Research, Volume 11, Number 4, Winter, 1976. (A range of health status scales is presented and discussed; see Ware, J. E. 11(4):396–415, 1976.)
11. Williamson, J. W.: Assessing and Improving Health Care Outcomes: The Health Accounting Approach to Quality Assurance. Cambridge, Mass., Ballinger Publishing Company, 1978.
12. Knight, R., and Warren, M. D.: Physically Disabled People Living at Home: A Study of Numbers and Needs. Department of Health and Social Security, Her Majesty's Stationery Office, London, 1978.
13. Donaldson, S. W., Wagner, C. C., and Gresham, G. E.: Unified ADL evaluation form. Arch. Phys. Med. Rehabil., 54:175–179, 185, 1973.
14. Jones, E. W.: Patient Classification for Long-term Care: User's Manual. DHEW Publication No. HRA 74-3107, Washington, D.C., U.S. Government Printing Office, 1973.
15. Granger, C. V., and Greer, D. S.: Functional status measurement and medical rehabilitation outcomes. Arch. Phys. Med. Rehabil., 57:103–109, 1976.
16. Shortell, S. M., and Richardson, W. C.: Health Program Evaluation. St. Louis, C. V. Mosby Company, 1978.
17. Deaver, G. G., and Brown, M. E.: Physical Demands of Daily Life. New York, Institute for the Crippled and Disabled, 1945.
18. Lawton, E. B.: Activities of Daily Living for Physical Rehabilitation. New York, McGraw-Hill Book Company, 1963.
19. Katz, S., Downs, T. D., Cash, H. R., et al.: Progress in development of index of ADL. Gerontologist, 10:20–30, 1970.
20. Mahoney, F. I., and Barthel, D. W.: Functional evaluation: Barthel index. Md. State Med. J., 14:61–65, 1965.
21. Schoening, H. A., and Iversen, I. A.: Numerical scoring of self-care status: A study of Kenny self-care evaluation. Arch. Phys. Med. Rehabil., 49:221–229, 1968.
22. Sarno, J. E., Sarno, M. T., and Levitz, E.: The functional life scale. Arch. Phys. Med. Rehabil., 54:214–220, 1973.
23. Moskowitz, E., and McCann, C. B.: Classification of disability in the chronically ill and aging. J. Chronic Dis., 5:324–346, 1957.
24. Fortinsky, R. H., Granger, C. V., and Seltzer, G. B.: The use of functional assessment in understanding home care needs. Medical Care, 19:489–497, 1981.
25. Breckenridge, K.: Medical rehabilitation program evaluation. Arch. Phys. Med. Rehabil., 59:419–423, 1978.
26. Grauer, H., and Birnbom, F.: A geriatric functional rating scale to determine the need for institutional care. J. Am. Geriatrics Soc., 23:472–476, 1975.
27. Duke University Center for the Study of Aging and Human Development: Multidimensional functional assessment. The OARS methodology, 2nd Ed. Durham, N. C., Duke University, 1978.
28. Muzzio, T. C., and Burris, C. T.: Functional Limitations: A State of the Art Review. 1979 Indices Inc., 5827 Columbia Pike, Falls Church, VA 22041.
29. Kottke, F. J.: Philosophical Considerations of Quality of Life for the Disabled. Arch. Phys. Med. Rehabil., 63:60–62, 1982.

30. Granger, C. V., Kaplan, M., Barrett, J., and Lunger, D.: Trends in outcome analysis: A program evaluation model. *In* Proceedings of the Seminar on Medical Rehabilitation Model Delivery Systems. February 23–24, 1978, Association of Rehabilitation Facilities, 5530 Wisconsin Ave., Suite 955, Wash., D.C. 20015.

31. Granger, C. V., Greer, D. S., Liset, E., Coulombe, J., and O'Brien, E.: Measurement of outcomes of care for stroke patients. Stroke, 6:34–41, 1975.

32. Scranton, J. A., Fogel, M. L., and Erdman, W. J., II: Evaluation of functional levels of patients during and following rehabilitation. Arch. Phys. Med. Rehabil., 51:1–21, 1970.

33. Eggert, G. M., Granger, C. V., Morris, R., and Pendleton, S. F.: Caring for the patient with long-term disability. Geriatrics, 32:102–114, 1977.

34. Lehmann, J. F., Delateur, B. J., Fowler, R. S., et al.: Stroke rehabilitation: Outcome and prediction. Arch. Phys. Med. Rehabil., 56:383–389, 1975.

35. Kerstein, M. D., Zimmer, H., Dugdale, F. E., and Lerner, E.: What influence does age have on rehabilitation of amputees? Geriatrics, 30:67–71, 1975.

36. Granger, C. V., Sherwood, C. C., and Greer, D.S.: Functional status measures in a comprehensive stroke care program. Arch. Phys. Med. Rehabil., 58:555–561, 1977.

37. Annual Progress Report, Tufts Medical Rehabilitation Research and Training Center (RT–7), 1975–1976. 185 Harrison Avenue, Boston, MA 02111.

38. Granger, C. V., Albrecht, G. L., and Hamilton, B. B.: Outcome of comprehensive medical rehabilitation: Measurement by PULSES profile and the Barthel index. Arch. Phys. Med. Rehabil., 60:145–154, 1979.

39. Mor, V., Sherwood, C. C., and Wieners, C. N.: Developing inter-rater reliability among social workers and public health nurses in the assessment of long term care needs (manuscript). Department of Social Gerontological Research. Hebrew Rehabilitation Center for the Aged, Boston, MA 02131.

40. Sherwood, S.: Personal communication. Department of Social Gerontological Research, Hebrew Rehabilitation Center for the Aged. Boston, MA 02131.

41. Codman, E. A.: A Study in Hospital Efficiency: As Demonstrated by the Case Report of the First Five Years of a Private Hospital. Boston, Thomas Todd Company, 1916. (This work was reproduced in 1972 by University Microfilms, Ann Arbor, MI.) See also Christoffel, J. D.: Medical care evaluation: An old new idea. Hosp. Med. Staff, 5(10):11–16, 1976.

42. Donabedian, A.: A Guide to Medical Administration, Volume II: Medical Care Appraisal — Quality and Utilization. New York (now Washington): American Public Health Association, 1969. (176 pages plus Annotated Selected Bibliography by A. J. Anderson.)

43. Donabedian, A.: Needed Research in the Assessment and Monitoring of Quality of Medical Care. DHEW publication No. (PHS) 78-3219. Research Report Series, 1978.

44. Donabedian, A.: Evaluating the quality of medical care. Milbank Memorial Fund Quarterly, 44 (Suppl.):166–206, 1966.

45. Institute of Medicine: Assessing Quality in Health Care: An Evaluation. National Academy of Science, Washington, D.C., 1976.

46. Sherwood, S., Greer, D. S., Morris, J. N., Mor, V., et al.: An Alternative to Institutionalization: The Highland Heights Experiment. Cambridge, MA, Ballinger Publishing Company, 1981, p. 86.

47. International Classification of Diseases, 9th Edition — Clinical Modification (ICD9-CM). Commission on Professional and Hospital Activities, Ann Arbor, MI, 48105, July, 1978.

48. Commission on Accreditation of Rehabilitation Facilities: Program Evaluation in Inpatient Medical Rehabilitation Facilities. Tucson, Arizona, 1979.

49. Kay, H. B.: Goodwill Industries of North Florida, Inc. (Unpublished material.)

13

DIATHERMY AND SUPERFICIAL HEAT AND COLD THERAPY

JUSTUS F. LEHMANN
BARBARA J. DE LATEUR

THERAPEUTIC HEAT

The following discussion will be limited to local applications of heat. The various types of heating modalities used in therapy can be subdivided into those that heat the superficial tissues and those that heat the deeper structures (Table 13–1). They can also be subdivided according to the primary modes of heat transfer into the tissues, which are conduction, convection, and the conversion of other forms of energy into heat by absorption. Heat therapy by conversion of other forms of energy includes radiant heat and the three deep-heating modalities: shortwaves, microwaves, and ultrasound. Not every modality that heats by conversion is a deep-heating modality. It should be noted that radiant heat is a superficial heating agent in spite of the fact that it heats by converting photons into heat by absorption. However, the photons penetrate only into the more superficial layers of the tissues. While all heating modalities produce the desirable therapeutic responses primarily by tempera-ture elevation, the rationale for their use derives from the fact that they selectively heat different areas in the body, with the peak temperatures in different locations. Therapeutic heat application is not a cure for any one of the indications for which it is used but is, rather, a valuable adjunct to other therapies if properly used with adequate equipment.

FACTORS DETERMINING THE EXTENT OF BIOLOGIC REACTIONS

The temperature of the tissues is a most important factor in the physiologic response to heat. Figure 13–1 shows the percentage of hyperemia plotted against the tissue temper-ature measured in a series of 560 experimen-tal animals.[134] The duration of the tissue temperature elevation was kept constant. Below a certain temperature threshold no reactions were observed. The curve of reac-

This chapter is in part based on research supported by Research Grant #G008003029 from the National Institute of Handicapped Research, Department of Education, Washington, D.C. 20202.

TABLE 13–1. THERAPEUTIC HEATING MODALITIES

Primary Mode of Heat Transfer	Modality	Depth
Conduction	Hot packs Paraffin bath	
Convection	Fluidotherapy Hydrotherapy Moist air	Superficial Heat
Conversion	Radiant heat Microwaves Shortwaves Ultrasound	Deep heat

From Lehmann, J. F., and de Lateur, B. J.: Therapeutic heat. *In* Lehmann, J. F. (Ed.): Therapeutic Heat and Cold, 3rd Ed. Baltimore, Williams and Wilkins, 1982.

tions is S-shaped, with the most rapid increase in reactions in the mid-range. In the upper portion of the curve, destructive changes are inevitably associated with the therapeutically desirable hyperemia. Thus, the therapeutic temperature range is a rather narrow one and extends in this particular reaction from approximately 43° C (109.4° F) to 45° C (113° F). It is apparent that within the therapeutic range a minor change in tissue temperature produces a major change in the degree of the physiologic response and that the margin of effectiveness and safety is narrow. In order to produce a limited response, it is necessary to obtain tissue temperatures in the lower portion of the curve; if vigorous effects are desired, the temperatures have to be within the upper half of the effective range. Thus, the control of the technique of application and the use of available dosimetry are essential for success in the therapeutic situation.

In a similar type of experiment, it was found that the duration of the tissue temperature elevation was important in determining the extent of the biologic reaction (Fig. 13–2).[134] For this reaction a minimal effective duration of exposure was five minutes, whereas maximal reactions were obtained after exposure of approximately 30 minutes. The tissue temperature was kept constant throughout the experiment.

The rate of temperature increase also played a role in determining the extent of biologic responses. Depending on the rate of increase, effective temperature levels will be reached sooner or later. Thus, a modality that rapidly raises the temperature to biologically effective levels will produce a more pronounced effect than a modality that raises the tissue temperature more slowly, provided that both modalities are applied over the same period of time.

In addition, it has been noted that some

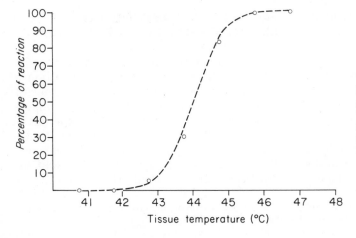

FIGURE 13–1. Dependence of hyperemia on tissue temperature (Lehmann, J. F.: The biophysical basis of biologic ultrasonic reactions with special reference to ultrasonic therapy. Arch. Phys. Med. Rehabil., 34:139–152, 1953).

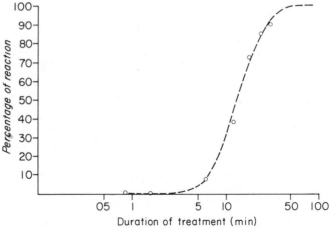

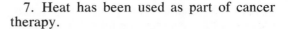

Duration of treatment (min)

FIGURE 13–2. Dependence of hyperemia on duration of treatment (Lehmann, J. F.: The biophysical basis of biologic ultrasonic reactions with special reference to ultrasonic therapy. Arch. Phys. Med. Rehabil., 34:139–152, 1953).

responses of temperature receptors seem to be more pronounced when the rate of the tissue temperature change is rapid.[46, 47, 98, 99, 141] The extent of reflex phenomena may also depend on the size of the area treated.[72]

In summary, the major factors determining the number and intensity of the physiologic reactions to heat are:

1. The level of tissue temperature. The approximate therapeutic range extends from 40 to 45.5° C (104 to 113.9° F).
2. The duration of the tissue temperature elevation. The approximate therapeutic range is 3 to 30 minutes.
3. The rate of temperature rise in the tissues.
4. The size of the area treated.

PHYSIOLOGIC EFFECTS OF THERAPEUTIC SIGNIFICANCE

General Indications and Contraindications

In general, the physiologic responses that are accepted as a basis for the most common therapeutic application of heat are as follows:

1. Heat increases the extensibility of collagen tissue.
2. Heat decreases joint stiffness.
3. Heat produces pain relief.
4. Heat relieves muscle spasm.
5. Heat increases blood flow.
6. Heat assists in the resolution of inflammatory infiltrates, edema, and exudates.

7. Heat has been used as part of cancer therapy.

There are also special safeguards to be observed when heat is applied. Heat application is either contraindicated or should be used with special precautions over anesthetic areas or in an obtunded patient. For most heat therapy, the sensation of pain is a warning signal that safe limits are exceeded. In the absence of pain sensation, dosimetry is not accurate enough in most of the modalities to reliably avoid excessive temperatures. Heating of tissues with inadequate vascular supply is contraindicated, since the elevation of the temperature increases metabolic demand without adequate vascular response. The result may be an ischemic necrosis. Any bleeding tendency is markedly increased by heating because of the increase of blood flow and vascularity. If one suspects the presence of malignancy in the area to be heated, one should generally not apply heat, since temperatures below those therapeutic for cancer may accelerate tumor growth[95] or increase the likelihood of formation of metastases resulting from the increase of blood flow and vascularity. At temperatures of 44 to 45° C, Child et al.[33] did not find an increase in the formation of metastases; these temperatures were produced by ultrasound application for 5 to 10 minutes. Also, heating of the gonads or the developing fetus should be avoided.[44, 45, 60–62, 81, 94, 187, 192, 197, 243]

Local Effects

Local effects are produced partly through a direct effect of the elevated temperature on the tissues. These physiologic responses

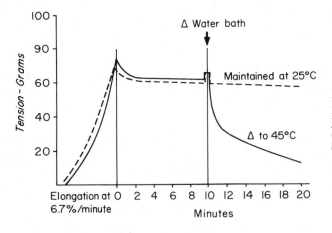

FIGURE 13–3. The effect of temperature elevation on tendon extensibility (Lehmann, J. F., Masock, A. J., Warren, C. G., and Koblanski, J. N.: Effect of therapeutic temperatures on tendon extensibility. Arch. Phys. Med. Rehabil., 51:481–487, 1970).

may occur to varying degrees depending on the conditions of heating. In part, they are produced by direct action of the temperature elevation on tissue and cellular function, by the production and accumulation of metabolites and carbon dioxide, by the reduction of oxygen tension, and by the production of histamine-like substances and bradykinin. Temperature receptors may play an important role.[72]

With the heat, there is a marked alteration of the physical properties of fibrous tissues as found in tendons, joint capsules, and scars;[79] these tissues yield much more readily to stretch when heated.[163] This effect is illustrated in Figure 13–3. In this experiment, the tendon was loaded with 73 grams in a 25° C (77° F) bath. The length of the tendon was maintained, and the tension decreased slightly. When the temperature of the bath changed from 25° C to 45° C (113° F), the tension deteriorated rapidly. Figure 13–4 shows the residual increase in length when various loads were applied at 45° C. It shows clearly that at 45° C a marked increase in length could be obtained, which increased in

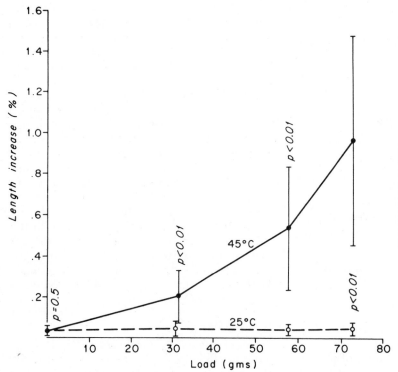

FIGURE 13–4. Residual tendon length as measured after loading at the indicated levels of 45°C and 25°C baths (Lehmann, J. F., Masock, A. J., Warren, C. G., and Koblanski, J. N.: Effect of therapeutic temperatures on tendon extensibility. Arch. Phys. Med. Rehabil., 51:481–487, 1970).

proportion to the load. Heat alone, without stretch, did not produce any length increase. In contrast to this, the controls at 25° C did not show such an elongation. It can be concluded, therefore, that heating produces a greater extensibility of fibrous collagen tissues. The optimal condition for obtaining this effect is the combination of heat and stretch application. Prolonged, steady stretch is more effective than intermittent or short-term stretch. This is of great significance in the management of joint contractures, as they occur as a result of tightness of the joint capsule and ligaments or fibrosis of muscle and scarring.

Investigations by Bäcklund and Tiselius[11] and by Wright and Johns[118, 283, 284] have shown that the subjective complaints of stiffness on the part of the rheumatoid patient coincide with changes in the measurements of the visco-elastic properties of joints.[11] The joint stiffness, assessed both subjectively and by objective measurement, could be influenced by treatment with drugs such as cortisone and by physical therapy such as the application of heat and cold. Heat application markedly decreases stiffness and the patient's discomfort. Cold application increases stiffness and the patient's complaints.

Application of heat to a peripheral nerve causes an increase in the pain threshold in the area supplied by the nerve. Also, one may elevate the pain threshold, as measured by the Hardy-Wolff-Goodell method,[91] by heating other tissues such as skin.[141]

Heating of tissues has been shown to affect the gamma fiber activity in muscle.[72] The resulting decrease in the sensitivity of the muscle spindle to stretch, as well as reflexes triggered through temperature receptors, may be the physiologic basis for the clinically observed relaxation of muscle spasm following the use of heat. Mense[186] found that, in a prestretched muscle, warming increased the firing rate of the group 1A afferents. He distinguished between two types of secondary afferents; those with a high background discharge responded as the 1A afferents, whereas those with low initial discharge rate showed a depression or cessation of firing by warming. The majority of the secondary endings showed the latter behavior when heated. Also, the Golgi tendon organs increased their firing rate when the temperature was increased. Therefore, one

may speculate that, if the secondary muscle spasm is to a degree a tonic phenomenon, the selective cessation of the firing from the secondary endings may reduce muscle tone, an effect which would be augmented by the greater inhibitory impulses from the Golgi tendon organs.

The blood flow is increased owing to arteriolar and capillary dilatation. These physiologic changes are produced by a direct effect of the temperature elevation and by reflex mechanisms.[1, 2, 38, 89, 114, 211, 235] The reflex mechanisms range from simple axon reflexes to complex phenomena occurring as part of the core temperature control. The rate of filtration and of diffusion across biologic membranes is increased. Thus, there may be a greater capillary membrane permeability with a resulting escape of plasma proteins. Vigorous heating may result in cellular responses associated with an inflammatory reaction, ranging from mild to severe.[134, 135] As a result of the temperature elevation, tissue metabolism is initially increased. However, if temperatures are elevated extensively for a prolonged period of time, tissue metabolism may be decreased.[158, 206, 286] Associated with the changes in metabolic rate are changes in enzyme reactions.[72] These may be speeded up by moderate tissue temperature elevation and may be gradually abolished at higher temperatures. This may be explained by the fact that the rate of chemical reaction is increased by temperature elevation, while the protein component of the enzyme system is destroyed at higher temperatures. Proteins may be denatured and the resulting products, such as polypeptides and histamine-like substances, may in turn become biologically active.

A detailed review of hyperthermia as part of cancer therapy is presented elsewhere.[200] Hyperthermia in malignancies is primarily used in combination with other forms of therapy, for instance, where it increases the effectiveness of ionizing radiation or reduces the radiation dose required to obtain the same results. Figure 13–5 may serve as an example of this.

This brief review of the most significant local reactions to heat application indicates not only that a large number of physiologic responses can be elicited, but also that many of them can be produced to any desired degree, that is, vigorous responses can be readily produced.

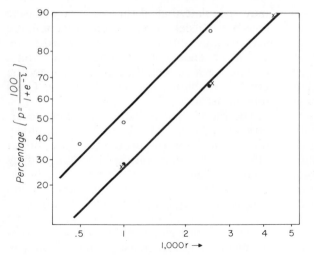

FIGURE 13–5. The percentage of mice in which a regression of tumor growth occurred is plotted against the dose of x-rays (scale according to Berkson[16]). Each point represents the percentage in 30 to 50 animals. Key: x's, treated with x-rays only; circles, treated with ultrasonic energy at 30° C and x-rays; and dots, treated with ultrasonic energy at 5 to 10° C and x-rays (Lehmann, J. F., and Krusen, F. H.: Biophysical effects of ultrasonic energy on carcinoma and their possible significance. Arch. Phys. Med. Rehabil., 36:452–459, 1955).

Reactions Occurring Distant from the Site of Tissue Temperature Elevation

Reactions distant from the site of tissue temperature elevation are usually produced by elevating the surface temperature of the body.

If the skin of one part of the body (e.g., over one extremity) is heated, a consensual response in terms of blood flow increase is observed in other parts of the body (e.g., the opposite extremity). The consensual reaction is always less pronounced than the local response to heat application, and its intensity is dependent on the size of the area treated,[72] that is, on the extent of neural input.

If the skin is heated without heating the muscle, the vessels of the musculature beneath show no increase in diameter or may even show a vasoconstriction,[72] which is consistent with the body temperature regulatory mechanism that diverts the flow to the skin for heat exchange and reduces flow to inactive organs.

If the skin of the abdominal wall is heated, it has been observed that a blanching of the gastric mucosa occurs and gastric acidity is reduced.

Relaxation of the smooth musculature of the gastrointestinal tract during superficial heat application has also been observed. This is evidenced by a decrease in peristalsis,[19, 72] which is the basis for relief of gastrointestinal cramps. Also, smooth musculature of the uterus relaxes, which in turn reduces menstrual cramps.

Heating of the superficial tissues produces marked relaxation of the skeletal muscles, and even protective muscle spasms may be resolved. The reaction may be reflex in nature and triggered by the effect on the temperature receptors in the skin. In addition, it has been shown[72] that stimulation of the skin in the neck region decreases gamma fiber activity resulting in a decreased spindle excitability. This could explain why superficial heating agents decrease muscle spasm. Heating of the skin may have a psychologic component as well.[72]

Some reactions may be produced by an elevation of the core temperature of the body, which in turn produces all those reactions commonly found as part of the mechanism regulating body temperature. Heat also has been applied as a counterirritant stimulus to the skin to provide pain relief. The explanation for the pain relief may be based on the gate theory of Melzack and Wall[185] or on the action of endorphins.[76]

In summary, thermal reactions occurring distant from the site of temperature elevation are limited in number, site, and extent. They are always less pronounced than the corresponding reactions occurring locally at the site of temperature elevation.

VIGOROUS VERSUS MILD HEATING

If vigorous heating effects are therapeutically desirable, the highest temperature must be produced at the site of the pathologic lesion. Thus, the vigorous local responses can be utilized. The tissue temperature is elevated close to tolerance level; the effective elevation of the tissue temperature is maintained for a relatively long period of time, and the rate of rise of the tissue temperature is rapid.

With mild heating, a relatively small temperature elevation is obtained in the tissues at the site of the pathologic lesion, or the highest temperature is produced in a tissue that is superficial to, and therefore distant from, the site of the lesion. Effective local tissue temperature is usually maintained for a relatively short period of time, and the rate of increase of temperature in the tissues is often slow.

Vigorous heating is appropriately used for chronic disease processes. Mild heating may be used in subacute disease processes. The following examples may illustrate the use of vigorous heating versus mild heating. Vigorous heating is used for treatment of joint contractures when scarring and tightening of the joint capsule and the periarticular structures have occurred. It will increase the temperature in the scar tissues to a level at which they become more extensible and thus more amenable to therapy designed to increase the range of motion. However, with an acute synovial inflammatory response as it occurs in rheumatoid arthritis, an aggravation can be produced by vigorous and selective heating of the area. Chronic pelvic inflammatory disease represents another indication for vigorous heating.[126, 127, 217] A marked increase in vascularity is produced which may assist in the resolution of the pathologic process or may render antibiotic therapy more effective. On the other hand, vigorous heating is contraindicated in an acute inflammatory process, since it will superimpose another inflammatory reaction that ultimately may lead to undesirable effects, such as tissue necrosis or perforation of an abscess into the abdominal cavity.[237]

An example of a mechanical problem is an acutely protruded intervertebral disk impinging upon a nerve root in the intervertebral foramen. This condition represents a contraindication to vigorous heating, since any marked temperature elevation at the site of the encroachment will produce an increase in vascularity and edema, which are space-occupying processes and may aggravate the symptoms. On the other hand, superficial heating with resulting relief of secondary muscle spasm may subjectively benefit the patient without changing the pathology at the level of the nerve root.

Selection of Modality

In order to produce vigorous heating, the tissue temperature must be elevated close to tolerance levels at the site of the pathologic lesion. This means that one must select the modality that will produce the highest temperature at the site of the lesion without exceeding tolerance levels in either the overlying or the underlying tissues. In order to select the proper modality for this purpose, it is important to know the temperature distribution produced by the available heating devices. In order to use the proper techniques of application with the selected modality, the factors that may modify this tissue temperature distribution and the actual temperature levels obtained must be understood.

If mild heating is desired in the depth of the tissues, there is a choice among superficial heating agents, such as infrared, hot packs, paraffin baths, and others that produce only mild reflex responses in the deeper tissues, and a deep-heating modality that is applied in such a way as to limit the rise of the tissue temperature to moderate levels at the site of the lesion. However, if small parts of the body such as the fingers are treated, even a superficial heating agent may produce a marked elevation of the temperatures in the deeper tissues, resulting in vigorous heating effects that may or may not be desirable, depending upon whether the lesion is chronic or acute.

DEEP HEATING OR DIATHERMY MODALITIES

For therapeutic purposes, diathermy is defined as deep heating.

Factors Determining Temperature Distribution

The relative amount of energy converted into heat at any given point throughout the tissues is important and is called the pattern of "relative heating." The amount of energy converted into heat at the level of the interface between the subcutaneous fat and the musculature or at the interface between the musculature and the bone is customarily set as one. The pattern of relative heating depends on factors that will be discussed for the individual diathermy modalities, since these factors vary from one deep-heating agent to another.

The tissue temperature distribution depends not only upon the pattern of "relative heating," but upon such tissue properties as specific heat as well. The temperature distribution is also modified by the thermal conductivity of the tissues if heating extends over a period of time long enough to allow for heat exchange to occur.

A temperature distribution thus produced in tissues of a live organism will finally be modified by physiologic factors such as preexisting temperature distribution and blood flow changes. Usually, the skin surface is relatively cool and the core temperature relatively high. Any temperature elevation produced by diathermy application is superimposed upon this pre-existing physiologic temperature distribution. As the diathermy is applied, an increase in the blood flow may occur locally as a result of the tissue temperature elevation; since the blood temperature is usually cooler than that of the heated tissue, the inflowing blood may act as a cooling agent. A modification of the temperature distribution can be produced in this fashion.

Shortwave Diathermy

EQUIPMENT

Shortwave diathermy is the therapeutic application of high-frequency currents. In spite of many variations, shortwave diathermy machines have three basic components of the circuitry that are common to all. They are power supply, oscillating circuit, and the patient's circuit. The frequency of the oscillating circuit, and thus that of the patient's circuit, is rigorously controlled to comply with the tolerance specified by the Federal Communications Commission (FCC). The frequencies that are allowed for shortwave diathermy operations are 13.66, 27.33, and 40.98 megahertz.[69] Wavelength is determined by the formula

$$\lambda = V/N$$

where λ is the wavelength, N is the frequence of oscillation, and V is the velocity of light. The wavelengths corresponding to the allowed frequencies are 22, 11, and 7.5 meters, respectively. Most of the commercially available diathermy machines operate at a frequency of 27.33 MHz and hence at a wavelength of 11 meters.

It is worth noting that in all machines, regardless of the technique of application, the patient's electrical impedance becomes part of the impedance of the patient's circuit. It is necessary for any given therapeutic application to retune the patient's circuit to resonance after the patient has been inserted into the circuit. Thus the frequency of the patient's circuit is made equal to the frequency of the oscillating circuit of the machine. Tuning is often accomplished by adjusting a variable capacitor (Figs. 13–6 and 13–7). The power meter on the panel of the machine will indicate maximal flow of current when the resonance frequency is obtained in the patient's circuit. Some machines have eliminated the need for tuning by an automatic device or by designing the machine so that

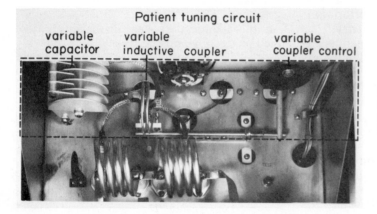

FIGURE 13–6. Patient tuning circuit of a typical shortwave diathermy machine. (Courtesy of the Birtcher Corporation.)

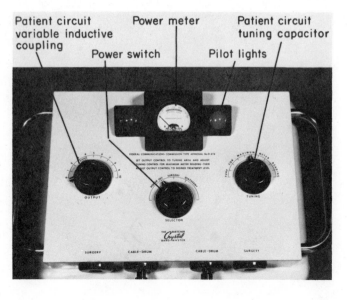

FIGURE 13–7. Typical control panel of a shortwave diathermy machine. (Courtesy of the Birtcher Corporation.)

the patient's electrical impedance has a negligible effect on the overall impedance of the patient's circuit. After the machine has been tuned, the current flow through the patient's circuit can be regulated. One way of doing this is to change the inductive coupling of the patient's and high-frequency oscillating circuits.

DOSIMETRY

At present it is not possible to measure the high-frequency current flow through the body of the patient. The meter on the panel does not give this information. The dosimetry still depends largely on biologic factors — the therapist is guided by the feeling of warmth on the part of the patient. When the dose applied is high, the patient's feeling of warmth goes up to tolerance; when the dose is medium, the patient feels comfortably warm; and when minimal the patient just barely feels warmth. Although these are guidelines, it is obvious that they are unreliable for accurate dosimetry and depend on intact sensation and alertness on the part of the patient. However, in the application of pelvic diathermy with an internal electrode it is possible to obtain measurements of the biologically effective dose. Since the electrode is placed in the area of highest temperature elevation in the body, it rapidly assumes the tissue temperature owing to the high conductivity of the metal. Therefore, if a thermometer is inserted into the electrode, a reading of the tissue temperature elevation

can be obtained. The duration of the tissue temperature elevation can be readily controlled by a timing device.

TECHNIQUE OF APPLICATION[233]

Condenser Technique

The part of the patient to be treated is placed between two capacitor plates. Four modifications of this technique are used: (1) Space plates are capacitor plates enclosed in rigid plastic material. A plastic ring surrounding the condenser plate is adjustable and provides proper spacing between body surface and condenser plates. (2) The capacitor plates are covered by a glass envelope. In order to avoid sweat accumulation and selective heating of the area, the glass cover should not be in direct contact with the skin. The position of the condenser plate within the glass envelope, and thus the distance between the body surface and the condenser plates, is adjustable. (3) The capacitor plates are flexible and are enclosed in rubber or plastic materials called condenser pads. Proper spacing between the skin and the electrode is provided by a 1- to 2-inch layer of terry cloth between the skin and the pads (Fig. 13–8). (4) Internal metal electrodes (Fig. 13–9) are inserted into the vagina or rectum after applying a water-soluble lubricant. The vaginal electrode is inserted so that the concave part comes to rest under the cervix and in the upper portion of the posterior fornix of the vagina. The rectal electrode

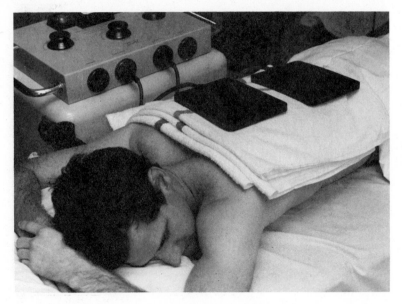

FIGURE 13–8. Shortwave diathermy application with condenser pads to back, with spacing between skin and electrodes provided by layers of terry cloth.

is inserted to fit the slightly concave part over the prostate. A large belt-like electrode is applied over the abdomen, thus producing a high current density around the internal electrode. The largest internal electrodes that fit should be used, to provide complete contact with the surrounding tissues. If the contact is partial, current concentrations may occur and lead to burns.

Techniques of Application to Specific Parts of the Body

— To the shoulder: Condenser plates may be used (Fig. 13–10).

— To the hip: The usual method is application with pads.

— To the elbows, knees, ankles, arms, feet, and hands: Condenser plates and pads are commonly used (Figs. 13–11 and 13–12).

— To the hands: The method of choice is usually the application of condenser plates in the form of pads or space plates.

— To the back: Condenser plates or pads are used (see Fig. 13–8).

— To the neck: Condenser plates or pads are used.

— To the pelvic organs: The method of choice is application with internal electrodes.

The temperature elevation is measured with a thermometer inside the electrodes. Temperatures up to 45°C (113°F) have been recommended, and duration of application

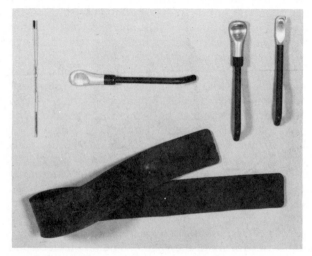

FIGURE 13–9. Internal vaginal and rectal electrodes with external belt and alcoholic thermometer. (Courtesy of the Burdick Corporation.)

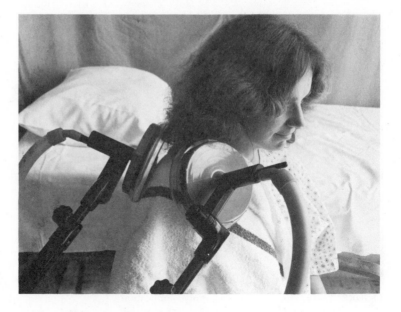

FIGURE 13–10. Condenser plates applied to the shoulder.

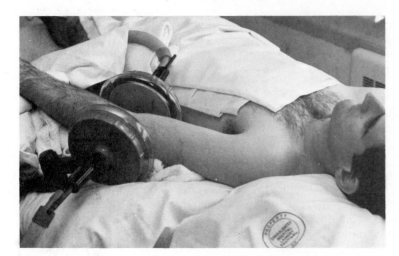

FIGURE 13–11. Condenser plates applied to the elbow.

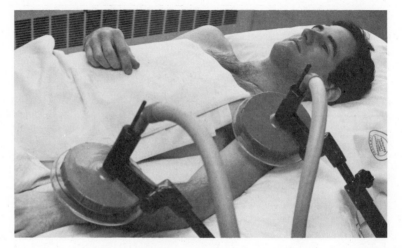

FIGURE 13–12. Shortwave diathermy application to the arm with condenser plates. Spacing is provided by space plates.

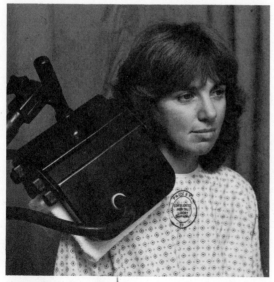

FIGURE 13–13. Shortwave diathermy application with induction coil (drum applicator).

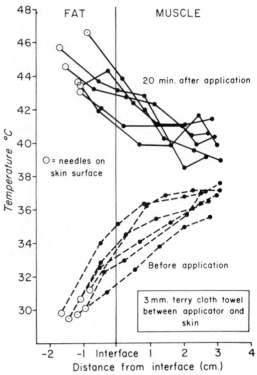

FIGURE 13–15. Temperature distribution in the human thigh at the completion of 20 minutes of exposure to shortwave (27.12 MHz) applied with the monode with 3 mm of terry cloth inserted between applicator and skin (Lehmann, J. F., de Lateur, B. J., and Stonebridge, J. B.: Selective heating by shortwave diathermy with a helical coil. Arch. Phys. Med. Rehabil., 50:117–123, 1969).

varies from 5 to 30 minutes. Often it is advisable to start with a lower temperature and shorter duration and observe the tolerance of the patient. It is most important to realize that the more acute the process to be treated, the less the tissue temperature elevation should be and the shorter the duration of the treatment.

Induction Coil Application

Another mode of application is with the induction coil. The induction coil may be applied with the so-called "drum" (Fig. 13–13). The coil is enclosed in a plastic container that is flexible at hinges and can be molded to

fit the body. This plastic housing provides proper spacing between the skin and loops of the cable. Another applicator of this type is the "monode," which operates on the same

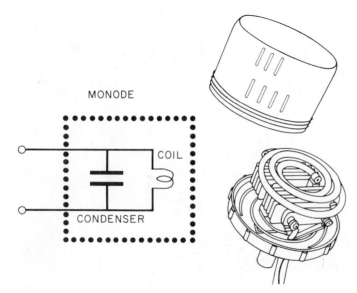

FIGURE 13–14. Monode applicator with wiring diagram. (Courtesy of Siemens-Reiniger Werke Ag.)

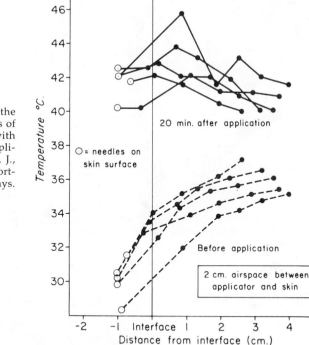

FAT | MUSCLE

20 min. after application

○ = needles on skin surface

Before application

2 cm. airspace between applicator and skin

Temperature °C.

Distance from interface (cm.)

FIGURE 13–16. Temperature distribution in the human thigh at the completion of 20 minutes of exposure to shortwave (27.12 MHz) applied with the monode with 2 cm of air space between applicator and skin (Lehmann, J. F., de Lateur, B. J., and Stonebridge, J. B.: Selective heating by short-wave diathermy with a helical coil. Arch. Phys. Med. Rehabil., 50:117–123, 1969).

basic principle but is not flexible (Fig. 13–14). Precautions should be taken to avoid direct contact between the plastic housing and the skin, since it interferes with the heat exchange. The result of direct contact application in human volunteers is shown in Figure 13–15, where the deep-heating agent is converted into an agent producing the highest temperature on the skin, whereas the same applicator with appropriate air space of 2 cm between skin and plastic housing produces the highest temperatures in the superficial musculature (Fig. 13–16). A heavily insulated cable can be shaped to any desired form of applicator, such as the "pancake" coil (Fig. 13–17), or it may be wrapped around a joint (Fig. 13–18). Spacers are used to keep the loops apart. Special precautions

FIGURE 13–17. Shortwave diathermy application to back with induction coil (pancake coil). Spacing between coil and skin is provided by layers of terry cloth. (Courtesy of the Burdick Corporation.)

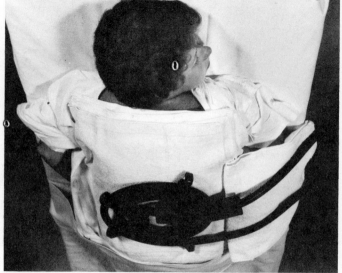

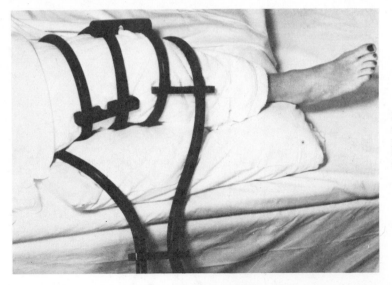

FIGURE 13–18. Induction coil application to knee, with spacing provided by layers of terry cloth. (Courtesy of the Burdick Corporation.)

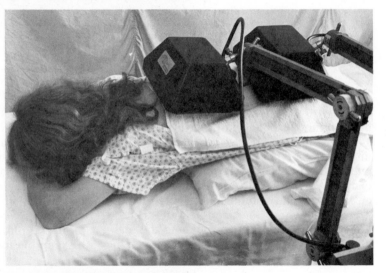

FIGURE 13–19. Induction coil applicators (IME) applied to the back.

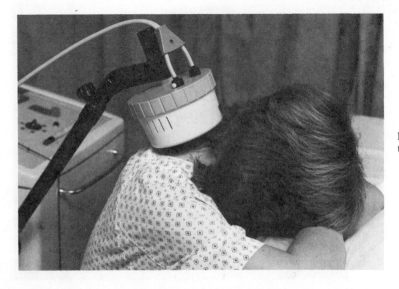

FIGURE 13–20. Monode applied to the neck.

must be taken to insure that the cable turns do not cross each other; if this is inevitable, a special separator must be inserted between the turns of the cable. In all these cases of cable application, the proper spacing between the skin and the loops of the cable is provided by an insertion of an approximately 2-inch thickness of terry cloth between the skin and the cable.

Techniques of Application to Specific Parts of the Body

— To the shoulder: The drum or monode may be used (see Fig. 13–13).

— To the elbows and knees: Wraparound coils or the monode is used (see Fig. 13–18).

— To the hands and feet: The method of choice is usually the application of the monode or drum.

— To the back: The pancake coil or the drum is used (see Figs. 13–17 and 13–19).

— To the neck: The drum or monode (Fig. 13–20).

— To the hip: The drum or pancake coil.

— To the knees and ankles: Wrap-around coil.

TEMPERATURE DISTRIBUTION AS MODIFIED BY TECHNIQUE OF APPLICATION

For both the condenser type and induction coil applications, the specific absorption rate (H) is proportional to the square of the induced electrical current (I) and inversely proportional to the electrical conductivity of the tissues (G).[228]

$$H = I^2/G$$

The current distribution in a given part of the anatomy will depend on the mode of application and on the properties of the tissues such as geometry (anatomy) and conductivity (reciprocal of resistance). Tissues can be considered to be in series or in parallel as they are traversed by the high-frequency current. If they are in parallel, it can be assumed that the greatest current flow will occur in the tissue with the greatest conductivity, that is, the tissues with the least resistance, and therefore this tissue will be heated most, since heating occurs with the square of the current. If the tissues are in series, the tissue with the greatest resistance will be heated most, since the current through all of them is the same and especially since the ratio of capacitance to resistance in each of the tissue layers is essentially constant. The conductivity of the tissues is closely related to the water content.

Capacitive Coupling

The higher the water content, the better the conductivity.[232] Guy et al.[89] reviewed the characteristics of shortwave diathermy applicators. Capacitor (condenser) applicators have the fundamental characteristic of inducing greater power absorption in subcutaneous fat than in deep muscle tissue, except in situations in which capacitive fields need only pass through thin layers of fat. In some situations, however, capacitive electrodes can be effective in heating deeper tissues, that is, pelvic diathermy with internal electrodes. Figure 13–21 shows schematically the current density in the tissues as the capacitor plates are applied over the skin of the back. The greatest current density is found in the subcutaneous fat under the electrodes and in the superficial musculature between the electrodes. In the first location the tissues are in series. In the second they are resistors in parallel. Therefore under the electrodes the subcutaneous fat is heated most, and between the electrodes the superficial musculature is heated most. Another example of how fields in the subcutaneous fat can be made significantly smaller in amplitude than in the deeper tissues to be treated is the use of capacitive applicators for heating the pelvic organs, using an internal electrode of small diameter and an external electrode of large surface area over the abdomen (Fig. 13–22). The resulting temperatures in the pelvic organs can be readily controlled and brought into the therapeutic range, whereas this is not possible by using microwave or ultrasound applicators (Fig. 13–23). Internal fields, which are much greater than those in the subcutaneous fat, can be produced because of the concentration of fields at the small electrode. Also, when small cylindrical, spherical, or ellipsoidal tissue shapes with thin fat layers, such as hands, wrists, ankles, and feet, are treated, relatively uniform heating due to the induced internal fields can be expected. It is a prerequisite that the parts of the body be

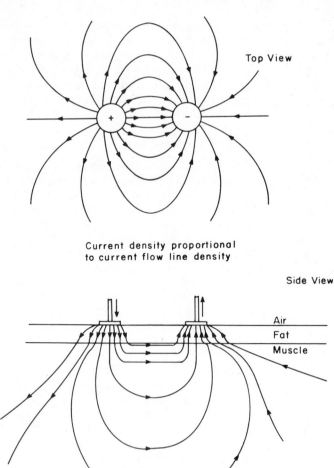

Top View

Current density proportional
to current flow line density

Side View

Air
Fat
Muscle

Current density proportional
to current flow line density

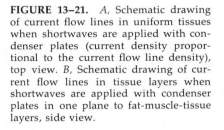

FIGURE 13–21. *A,* Schematic drawing of current flow lines in uniform tissues when shortwaves are applied with condenser plates (current density proportional to the current flow line density), top view. *B,* Schematic drawing of current flow lines in tissue layers when shortwaves are applied with condenser plates in one plane to fat-muscle-tissue layers, side view.

small as compared to the wavelength. Finally, in areas where the subcutaneous fat thickness is minimal, a condenser applicator may be used for heating the deeper structures.

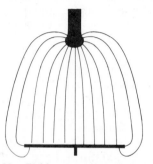

FIGURE 13–22. Field pattern that might be expected with the use of an internal electrode (Lehmann, J. F., and de Lateur, B. J.: Therapeutic heat. *In* Lehmann, J. F. (Ed.): Therapeutic Heat and Cold, 3rd Ed. Baltimore, Williams and Wilkins, 1982).

Inductive Coupling

Inductive coil applicators have been shown both theoretically and experimentally to produce higher power absorption in the deeper high-water-content tissues than in the subcutaneous fat.[89] Circular electrical fields or eddy currents are induced in the tissues by the applied magnetic fields. If the magnetic field is directed normal (perpendicular) to the tissue interfaces, the electrical field is tangential to tissue interfaces and not as much modified by tissue boundaries as in the case of capacitive electrode applicators. Since the electrical conductivity of muscle is an order of magnitude greater than that of fat, the power absorption density will be an order of magnitude greater than in the fat.[230, 231] Thus, inductive applicators are preferred over condenser applicators if muscle heating is desired. Schematically, the anticipated current distribution in the tissues is shown in Figure

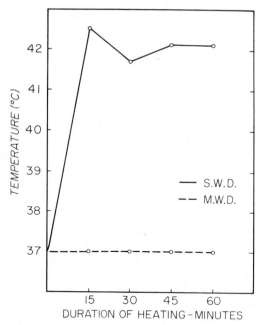

FIGURE 13–23. Mean rectal temperature during intrapelvic heating with shortwave diathermy or low abdominal heating with microwave diathermy (Kottke, F. J.: Heat in pelvic diseases. *In* Licht, S. (Ed.): Therapeutic Heat and Cold, 2nd Ed. Baltimore, Waverly Press, 1965, pp. 474–490).

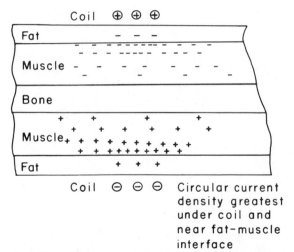

FIGURE 13–25. Longitudinal cross section of thigh with wrap-around coil showing current flow at coil and near fat-muscle interface. Direction of instantaneous flow and current density indicated by pluses and minuses (Lehmann, J. F., and de Lateur, B. J.: Therapeutic heat. *In* Lehmann, J. F. (Ed.): Therapeutic Heat and Cold, 3rd Ed. Baltimore, Williams and Wilkins, 1982).

13–24, when the "pancake" coil is applied to the back. Pluses and minuses indicate the direction of current flow. Their density indicates the relative amount of current in a given area. Figure 13–25 shows the relative current distribution in the tissue layers when a wrap-around coil is used in the area of the thigh. The temperature distribution produced by the monode is shown in Figure 13–16.[146] Hollander and Horvath[107] observed temperature rises up to 101° F (38° C) when the knee joint was heated with a wrap-around coil. On the other hand, joints with a considerable amount of soft tissue cover, such as the hip joint, cannot be effectively heated by shortwave diathermy application using the induction coil, even when the output of the equipment produces a first-degree burn and discomfort in the superficial tissue (see Fig. 13–47).[164]

NONTHERMAL EFFECTS AND PULSED SHORTWAVE DIATHERMY

The potential use of pulsed shortwave diathermy has been extensively reviewed.[155] Initially, pulsed shortwave diathermy was used to minimize the heating effect, which is in proportion to the average output, in the hope that the peak intensities during the pulses may produce therapeutic nonthermal effects. Later, some other investigators[9, 10, 97, 101, 102, 228, 248, 252] tried to show the

FIGURE 13–24. Schematic drawing of current flow in tissue with superficial induction (pancake) coil applicator. Direction of instantaneous flow and current density indicated by pluses and minuses (Lehmann, J. F., and de Lateur, B. J.: Therapeutic heat. *In* Lehmann, J. F. (Ed.): Therapeutic Heat and Cold, 3rd Ed. Baltimore, Williams and Wilkins, 1982).

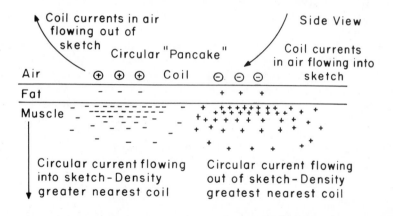

existence of nonthermal effects to document their presence as a potentially hazardous side effect of shortwave diathermy application. The significance of the findings resulting from this type of investigative approach can be summarized as follows: while the existence of nonthermal effects can be documented, none of them has been proven to be clearly of therapeutic advantage over continuous wave application and none of them has been shown to produce any significant side effects during therapeutic application. The hope of distinguishing between thermal and nonthermal effects by comparing the responses obtained from pulsed wave application with those from continuous wave application has not been completely realized because, as in the pearl-chain formation of particles, many of the nonthermal effects respond to the average of the pulsed output, as do the heating effects, and not to the peak values during the pulses. Thus, at present, there is no specific therapeutic indication for the use of pulsed output.[24, 36, 67, 70, 82, 96, 120, 143, 155, 172, 189, 195, 198, 221, 240, 241, 249, 250, 253, 273-275, 280]

STANDARDS FOR EQUIPMENT

Standards need to be developed to assure effectiveness and safety of shortwave diathermy equipment. The standard should, first, assure the user that the equipment is powerful enough to produce vigorous heating effects; second, that the user has adequate information as to where the highest temperature will be produced in the tissues when the various available applicators are used; and, third, that the equipment be built to assure safety both to the patient treated and to the personnel administering the treatment.

Tissue substitute substances with electrical properties equal to those found in the human have been developed by Guy and associates[85, 89] and can be modeled to conform to comparable anatomic structures. The tissue substitute models allow identification of the location of the peak tissue temperature with different applicators without great difficulty. In pre-split models, the two halves can be readily separated for thermographic screening after short exposure. From the linear portion of the initial temperature rise in any part of the model, the specific absorption rate can be calculated and, on this basis,

temperature distribution can be predicted in human application. Research is being developed to overcome the electromagnetic discontinuity at the site of the split of the model. On this basis, it has been predicted that in order to get a temperature increase adequate to produce vigorous therapeutic responses, an approximate absorbed power of the order of 170 watts/kg is required. Since at this point blood flow increase with resulting cooling is triggered, an additional absorbed power of more than 100 watts/kg will be necessary to overcome the cooling effect of the blood flow. Therefore, the equipment should be powerful enough under those circumstances to produce, probably, an absorbed power in the tissues of more than 200 watts/kg. Much of the available equipment does not fulfill these requirements. Safety features of the equipment should include an adequate timer. Concern has also been voiced about stray radiation to which the therapist and parts of the patient's body not treated are exposed.[143, 189]

PRECAUTIONS

Special precautions must be taken with all techniques of application. All metallic objects, such as watches or jewelry, should be removed. The patient should be positioned on a wooden plinth or chair. These precautions are necessary, since selective heating of metal parts could occur because of current concentration. For the same reason the accumulation of sweat beads should be prevented by using terry cloth. Tuning of the patient circuit should always be done at the low output level to prevent excessive heating from an uncontrolled surge of current through the patient. The tuning of the patient circuit should be optimal. Then the output of the machine should be adjusted to the desired level. If this procedure is not followed, small movements of the patient may change the impedance of the circuit in such a fashion that resonance occurs and the current flow may be greatly increased without the therapist's being aware of it. An increase in dose, and possibly burns, may result.

Metallic implants, including surgical implants, cardiac pacemakers, and electrophysiologic braces, should not be exposed to shortwave diathermy because the device may be destroyed or made to malfunction or selectively heated with a resulting burn. Surgical implants, however, represent a contraindication only if it is anticipated that any significant current would reach the site of implant. Intrauterine devices (IUD) containing copper or other metals should represent a contraindication to the use of shortwave diathermy until proven otherwise.[224] Finally, contact lenses should be removed, since they may cause hot spots.

It should be noted that shortwave diathermy applied to the low back has been observed to increase menstrual flow, and patients should be advised of that possibility or therapy should be discontinued during the menstrual period. Pregnant women should not be treated with pelvic diathermy using internal electrodes because of possible damage to the fetus.[243] There is also some controversy about treatment of children around the bone growth zones and of the possibility of other side effects, which are summarized by Michaelson[189] and Lehmann.[143] By and large, for the short-term exposure as in therapy, the main concern should be to avoid temperatures that produce burns. The existence of stray radiation as an occupational hazard to the therapist is also controversial. Based on microwave studies, it has been suggested that in the absence of more accurate measures, intensity of long-term exposure should be held below 5 to 10 mW/cm^2.[143, 155]

Microwaves

Microwaves are a form of electromagnetic radiation[73] with frequencies of 2456 and 915 MHz approved for medical use. As with other electromagnetic waves, microwaves travel at the speed of light and can be propagated through a vacuum. They can be reflected, scattered, refracted, or absorbed. The medical use of microwaves is primarily based on the fact that they are selectively absorbed in tissues with high water content and thus allow selective heating of certain tissues such as the musculature.

EQUIPMENT

Therapeutic equipment ideally should be able to heat musculature selectively and evenly. The equipment should be able to raise the tissue temperature to tolerance levels and potentially to overcome the cooling resulting from increased blood flow. The equipment should be capable of demonstrating a vigorous physiologic response with a minimum of stray radiation exposing sensitive organs of the patient and of the therapist. The meter should show, quantitatively, the flow of power into the tissues; that is, it should measure the total forward output minus reflected power. An accurate timer should be available. It has been shown that the use of the lower frequency of 915 MHz would be advantageous over 2456 MHz.[86, 88, 156] Direct-contact applicators provide better coupling and less stray radiation than the standard noncontact applicators. Such direct-contact applicators also can be equipped with air cooling with the air blown through porous dielectric with which the cavity is loaded. A thin plastic radome with the proper distribution of air channels assures even cooling of the skin and eliminates selective heating of the surface and at the applicator edges. Applicators may have a fixed direction of the E field vector; that is, they are linearly polarized (Fig. 13–26). Others are circularly polarized with the rotating E field vector (Fig. 13–27).

The noncontact applicators operating at 2456 MHz that are still in clinical use include the A, B, C, and E directors. The A director consists of an antenna with a hemispherical

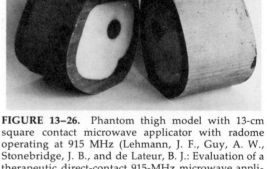

FIGURE 13–26. Phantom thigh model with 13-cm square contact microwave applicator with radome operating at 915 MHz (Lehmann, J. F., Guy, A. W., Stonebridge, J. B., and de Lateur, B. J.: Evaluation of a therapeutic direct-contact 915-MHz microwave applicator for effective deep-tissue heating in humans. IEEE Trans. Microwave Theory & Tech. MTT, 26:556–563, 1978).

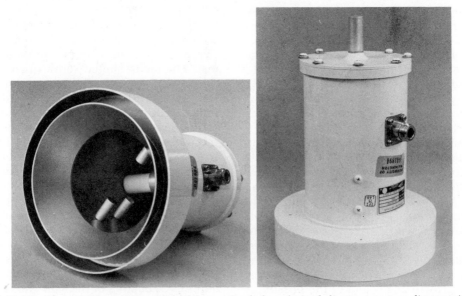

FIGURE 13–27. Nine-hundred-fifteen MHz Transco circularly polarized direct contact applicator with circular quarter wavelength choke around applicator edge (Lehmann, J. F., and de Lateur, B. J.: Therapeutic heat. *In* Lehmann, J. F. (Ed.): Therapeutic Heat and Cold, 3rd Ed. Baltimore, Williams and Wilkins, 1982).

reflector (diameter 9.3 cm). The B director consists of an antenna rod with a hemispherical reflector with a diameter of 15.3 cm. Both produce a beam having a cross section pattern with the highest intensity in the shape of a ring, with the intensity in the center being approximately half of the value of the intensity in the ring. The size of the total therapeutic field is approximately equal to the diameter of the reflector. The C and E directors have an antenna rod with a corner reflector. The dipole antenna of the C director has a length of half the wavelength. The E director has a full-wave, 12.2 cm dipole antenna. Both produce an oval high-intensity zone in the center of the cross section of the beam with a useful therapeutic field of a size approximately similar to that of the opening of the corner reflector. All of these applicators have poor beaming properties because the wavelength is comparable to the antenna size. They therefore should be applied at a distance of approximately 1 to 2 inches from the skin.

To assess the therapeutic effectiveness of the equipment, tissue substitute models, as

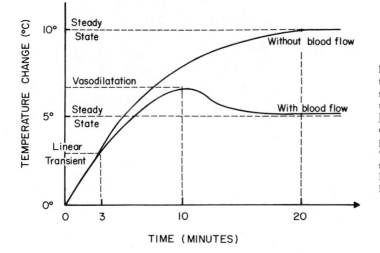

FIGURE 13–28. Schematic representation of linear transient and steady-state temperatures for a typical tissue under diathermy exposure (Lehmann, J. F., Guy, A. W., Stonebridge, J. B., and de Lateur, B. J.: Evaluation of a therapeutic direct-contact 915-MHz microwave applicator for effective deep-tissue heating in humans. IEEE Trans. Microwave Theory & Tech. MTT, 26: 556–563, 1978).

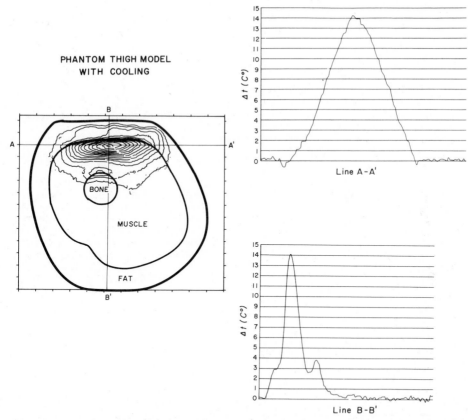

FIGURE 13–29. Isotherms produced in phantom thigh model after exposure to a 13-cm square direct-contact microwave applicator operating at 915 MHz with radome and cooling (Lehmann, J. F., Guy, A. W., Stonebridge, J. B., and de Lateur, B. J.: Evaluation of a therapeutic direct-contact 915-MHz microwave applicator for effective deep-tissue heating in humans. IEEE Trans. Microwave Theory & Tech. MTT, 26:556–563, 1978).

described under Shortwave Diathermy[65] (Figs. 13–27 to 13–29), can be used to measure the linear transient of the temperature rise with short exposure from which absorbed power can be calculated at any given point in the model. Similar temperature measurements have been made in the human volunteer with temperature probes in place. Good agreement has been found between values of the specific absorption rate obtained in the model and those in the human volunteer (Fig. 13–30). In the human volunteer, also, the physiologic responses in terms of blood flow can be estimated so that certain levels of specific absorption rates can be related to effectiveness, that is, to production of vigorous responses in terms of human blood flow change.[236] The values of specific absorption rates in the human thigh are shown and compared with the calculated change in blood flow rate they produce in Table 13–2. From these measurements it can

be concluded that, at a specific absorption rate of up to 170 watts/kg, blood flow increases of up to 30 ml/100 g tissue/minute were obtained. This increase in blood flow represents a vigorous physiologic response, since blood flow increases under extensive exercise conditions are of the order of 30 to 35 ml/100 g tissue/min. With this information, tissue substitute models can be used for quick determination of maximum specific absorption rate in the muscle, and one can predict whether the absorption rate is adequate to produce a vigorous physiologic response. It has been shown that direct-contact applicators can produce these vigorous responses with relatively little stray radiation (Fig. 13–31). Stray radiation was tested both in the model and in the human shoulder. It was found that stray radiation was considerably less with the direct-contact applicators.[169, 170] In addition, stray radiation was greatest in the area where the contact

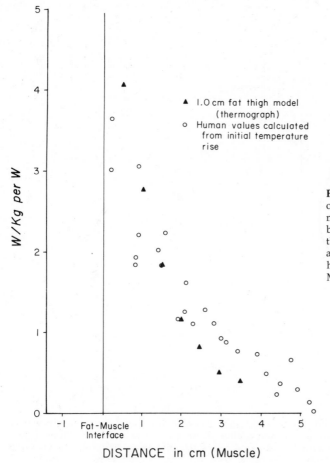

FIGURE 13–30. Comparison of the calculates of the SAR in thighs of human beings and models (Lehmann, J. F., Guy, A. W., Stonebridge, J. B., de Lateur, B. J.: Evaluation of a therapeutic direct-contact 915-MHz microwave applicator for effective deep-tissue heating in humans. IEEE Trans. Microwave Theory & Tech. MTT, 26:556–563, 1978).

could not be maintained. If a linearly polarized applicator was used, the stray radiation was greatest in the direction of the E vector. That implies that one should avoid having the E field vector pointing at the sensitive organ and one should avoid losing contact in the direction of the sensitive organ.

PROPAGATION AND ABSORPTION OF MICROWAVES IN TISSUES

As with other modalities, most therapeutic effects of microwaves are due to heating; however, the temperature distribution in the tissues treated is specific for this modality and is influenced by the frequency used. It is

TABLE 13–2. HEAT THERAPY TO HUMAN MUSCLE

Calculated Values of Absorbed Power in Human Muscle		Calculated Values for Blood Flow in Human Muscle†	
Run	SAR*	Run	ml/100 g/min
1	121.60	1	28.90
2	78.17	2	28.91
3	118.70	3	25.00
4	75.27	4	23.64
5	167.93	5	29.69

*Specific Absorption Rate (SAR) in W/kg in Musculature (1-2 cm)—at 555.55 mW/cm² maximum power density of incident radiation. (From Lehmann, J. F., Guy, A. W., Stonebridge, J. B., and de Lateur, B. J.: Evaluation of a therapeutic direct-contact 915 MHz microwave applicator for effective deep-tissue heating in humans. IEEE Trans. Microwave Theory & Tech. MTT, 26:556–563, 1978).

†Calculated Blood-Flow Rate in Muscle. (From Lehmann. J. F., Guy, A. W., Stonebridge, J. B.: and de Lateur, B. J.: Evaluation of a therapeutic direct-contact 915 MHz microwave applicator for effective deep-tissue heating in humans. IEEE Trans. Microwave Theory & Tech. MTT, 26:556–563; 1978).

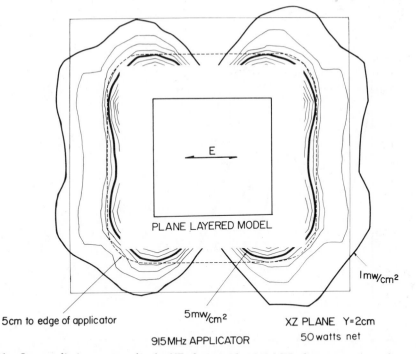

FIGURE 13–31. Stray radiation pattern for the XZ plane, with a 915-MHz direct-contact applicator on the plane-layered model. Graduated in 1 mW/cm² increments at 50 watts net input power (Lehmann, J. F., Stonebridge, J. B., and Guy, A. W.: A comparison of patterns of stray radiation from therapeutic microwave applicators measured near tissue-substitute models and human subjects. Radio Science, 14:271–283, 1979).

on this basis that this modality is selected. The temperature distribution, in turn, depends on the propagation and absorption characteristics of the tissues traversed by the beam.[85-87, 106] Several workers have studied the absorption of microwave energy in biologic media.[35, 37, 229, 231] It is apparent that the dielectric properties of the medium and the specific resistance or conductivity are responsible for the energy absorption. Tissues with high water content, such as musculature, and fluid media, such as found in the eye or in sweat beads, are likely to absorb more microwave energy than bone.

The reflection of microwaves at the body surface and at the tissue interfaces can be calculated if the dielectric properties and the conductivities of the tissues are known. Schwan[228] has pointed out that a large and variable amount of energy may be reflected at the skin surface under therapeutic conditions. It is possible to have variable losses of more than 50 per cent of the energy irradiated from the director, and thus it is difficult to reproduce the biologic effects in a reliable fashion. This reflection is minimized by using the lower available frequency of 915 MHz

and by using a direct-contact applicator, filling the cavity of the applicator with substances of matched dielectric properties.

Schwan[228] calculated a pattern of relative heating for homogeneous tissues with plane and parallel interfaces. Lehmann and associates[153] obtained the pattern of relative heating by actual measurements of the distribution throughout a specimen consisting of skin, subcutaneous fat, and musculature with typical anatomic and biologic interfaces. They confirmed Schwan's calculations that an appreciable reflection of microwave energy occurred at the interface between subcutaneous fat and musculature, with the result that a large amount of energy was converted into heat in the subcutaneous tissues (Fig. 13–32A). Also, in agreement with Schwan, they found that the depth of penetration was poor in muscle tissues if the frequency of 2450 MHz was used. The intensity available at the surface of the muscle dropped to a 50 per cent level at a depth of approximately 1 cm. By contrast, the amount of energy converted into heat in the subcutaneous tissues was much less and the depth of penetration (approximately 3 cm) in

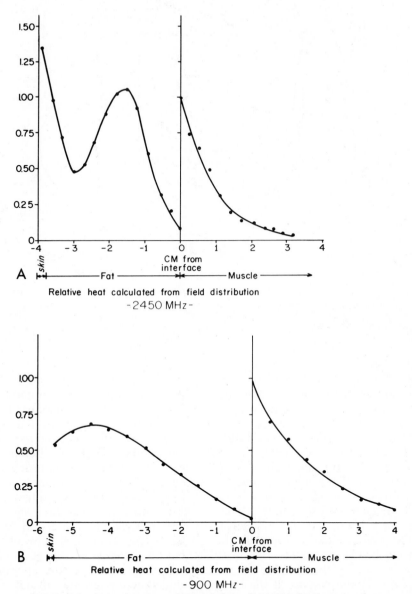

FIGURE 13–32. *A,* Pattern of relative heating calculated from field distribution at a frequency of 2450 MHz. *B,* Pattern of relative heating calculated from field distribution at a frequency of 900 MHz (Lehmann, J. F., Guy, A. W., Johnston, V. C., Brunner, G. D., and Bell, J. W.: Comparison of relative heating patterns produced in tissues by exposure to microwave energy at frequencies of 2,450 and 900 megacycles. Arch. Phys. Med. Rehabil., 43:69–76, 1962).

the musculature was much better if microwave frequency of 900 MHz was used (Fig. 13–32B). The resulting temperature distribution in the live human was modified not only by such constants as specific heat, specific weight, and thermal conductivity, but also by physiologic responses such as change in the blood flow, as illustrated in Figure 13–33.[140] After a peak temperature is reached, blood flow cooling reduces tissue temperature in spite of continuous microwave application. As shown in Figure 13–33, the new experimental 915-MHz direct-contact applicator provides simultaneous cooling of the surface temperatures.[141] Even heating of the muscle can be obtained from the most superficial musculature to a depth of approximately 4 cm, that is, to the tissues adjacent to the bone (Fig. 13–34). Whereas the temperature distribution of microwaves operating at a frequency of 2456 MHz in most instances can be duplicated by shortwave application, the 915-MHz direct-contact applicator is a unique tool for selective heating of the musculature.[156]

The conclusion for therapy is that the application of microwaves at the commercially available frequency of 2456 MHz would result in a relatively high, if not the highest, temperature in the subcutaneous tissues unless application is made to an area where skin and subcutaneous fat are of minimal thickness, as was demonstrated by Rae and coworkers[215] with dogs. Also, Hollander and Horvath[107] were able to elevate the joint temperature above the skin temperature in elbows and knees, both joints having a minimal soft-tissue cover. Their temperature differential was less pronounced in patients with rheumatoid arthritis. The application of microwaves at or below the frequency of 900 MHz to a person with a moderate amount of subcutaneous fat would result in a temperature distribution in which the highest temperature would occur in the muscle; also, the muscle could be evenly heated down to the bone.

Lehmann and associates[165] later studied a pattern of relative heating and the actual temperature distribution produced in specimens with more complex geometry, similar to that encountered in the treatment of joints, for the frequencies of 2456 and 900 MHz (Fig. 13–35). It was found that, during exposure to a frequency of 2456 MHz, a heating pattern indicative of energy reflec-

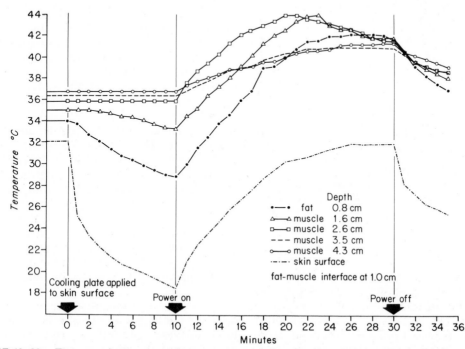

FIGURE 13–33. Temperature in a typical experiment at various depths of tissue resulting from application of microwave with a 915 MHz contact applicator (From de Lateur, B. J., Lehmann, J. F., Stonebridge, J. B., Warren, C. G., and Guy, A. W.: Muscle heating in human subjects with 915 MHz microwave contact applicator. Arch. Phys. Med. Rehabil., 51:147–151, 1970).

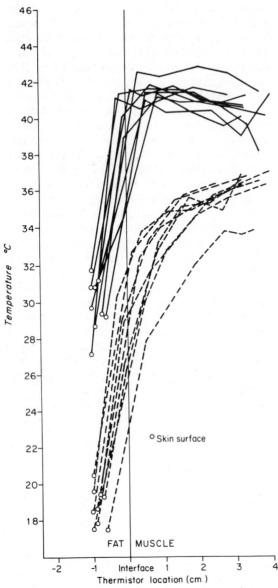

FIGURE 13–34. Temperature distribution in all volunteers with less than or equal to 1 cm of subcutaneous fat before(_ _ _ _)and 20 minutes after (_____) microwave application (From de Lateur, B. J., Lehmann, J. F., Stonebridge, J. B., Warren, C. G., and Guy, A. W.: Muscle heating in human subjects with 915 MHz microwave contact applicator. Arch. Phys. Med. Rehabil., 51:147–151, 1970.)

tion and production of a pattern of standing waves at the muscle-bone interface was observed. The development of undesirable "hot spots" can be the result. This possibility seems to be less at or below frequencies of 900 MHz. The difference between the frequencies with regard to the development of "hot spots" in front of the bone may be explained by the fact that the bone repre-

sents a reflecting obstacle for wave propagation at the higher frequency, since its diameter is relatively large as compared with the wavelength in muscle tissue. Thus, in Figure 13–35 the relation between bone diameter and wavelength is reversed at the low frequency, and the waves of high frequency are reflected to a greater extent than those of the low frequency. Consistent with these conclusions, Worden and coworkers[282] observed burns over the femurs of dogs (Fig. 13–36), which appeared to be the result of energy reflected at the bone surface. Engel and associates[66] reported that horse flesh was heated to a higher degree if bone was present under the flesh at a depth of 1 cm. Most recently, Addington and others[4] found that the hollow viscera heat differentially and that the stomach and liver may be considered "hot spots." Selective burns in these areas were observed in dogs. Also, the tissues overlying the thoracic cage were selectively burned[110] and the anterior cardiac surface was selectively heated.[174, 181] Selective absorption can also occur if metallic implants are present in tissues that can be reached by an appreciable amount of microwave energy.[71] A dramatic illustration of this can be given by igniting steel wool in the microwave field in air.

This review of the investigations using different frequencies strongly suggests that the microwave machines used at present do not operate at the most effective frequency. They were introduced into therapy because generators operating at these frequencies were available for medical application after World War II, and not because 2456 MHz was considered to be the best frequency for medical use. The data now suggest that the optimal frequency would be at 900 MHz or below, minimizing the heating effect in the subcutaneous tissues and heating the underlying tissues more adequately. The development of "hot spots" as a result of reflection from bone is prevented to a large degree. These frequencies also have a better depth of penetration. FCC regulations have allocated the frequency of 915 MHz for medical purposes.

These investigations also suggest that, because of the large amount of reflection at the bone surface, very little energy reaches the area beyond the bone at either frequency, 2456 or 900 MHz. This is indicated by the difference in temperature between the area in front of and behind the bone when ex-

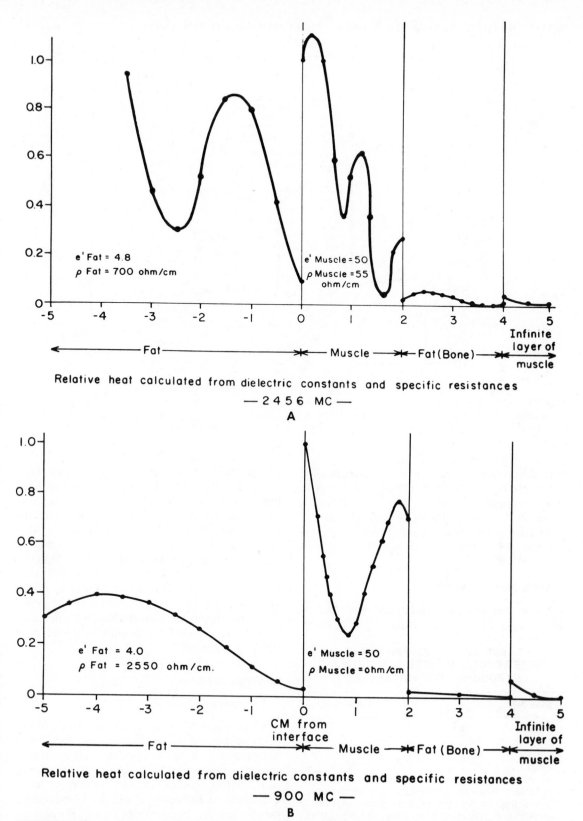

FIGURE 13–35. *A,* Pattern of relative heating calculated from dielectric constants and specific resistances in a complex specimen at a frequency of 2456 MHz. *B,* Pattern of relative heating calculated from dielectric constants and specific resistances in a complex specimen at a frequency of 900 MHz (Lehmann, J. F., McMillan, J. A., Brunner, G. D., and Guy, A. W.: A comparative evaluation of temperature distributions produced by microwaves at 2,456 and 900 megacycles in geometrically complex specimens. Arch. Phys. Med. Rehabil., 43:502–507, 1962).

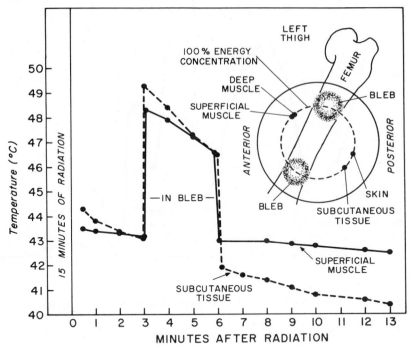

FIGURE 13–36. Development of burns from reflection, where high-intensity field crosses bone, and temperature measurement across the bleb (Worden, R. E., Herrick, J. F., Wakim, K. G., and Krusen, F. H.: The heating effects of microwaves with and without ischemia. Arch. Phys. Med., 29:751–758, 1948).

posed to microwaves (Table 13–3). Though this difference is less when a frequency of 900 MHz is used, it is still too great to allow full therapeutic exposure of a joint through bone. If it is the purpose to heat the entire joint, the joint should be exposed from all aspects, as is the case in ultrasonic therapy.[140, 219]

PHYSIOLOGIC RESPONSES

Since microwave diathermy was introduced into physical medicine,[128, 216] exten-

TABLE 13–3. TEMPERATURE DIFFERENCES IN TISSUE FOLLOWING EXPOSURE TO MICROWAVES

2456 MHz	900 MHz
6.4°C	5.1°C
4.6°C	1.7°C
9.2°C	3.6°C
6.0°C	2.4°C

Difference in temperatures indicated by measurements in front of and behind bone after exposure to microwaves at frequencies of 2456 and 900 MHz. (From Lehmann, J. F., McMillan, J. A., Brunner, G. D., and Guy, A. W.: A comparative evaluation of temperature distributions produced by microwaves at 2,456 and 900 megacycles in geometrically complex specimens. Arch. Phys. Med. Rehabil., 43:502–507, 1962.

sive studies have been conducted on the physiologic effects produced by this new type of radiation. A large number of physiologic, pathologic, and biochemical reactions were studied. In some instances the mechanism by which they were produced was also investigated. A recent complete review of the literature has been done by Michaelson.[189] The result of these studies indicated that the microwave heating effects were responsible for the vast majority of the reactions of potential therapeutic significance. However, nonthermal reactions could also be demonstrated.

HEATING EFFECTS

Therapeutic Effects

Since microwave energy is absorbed in the body and is effective in elevating the tissue temperature, it is obvious that all reactions that can be produced by temperature elevation in the tissues can be observed after exposure to microwave energy of adequate power levels. From a therapeutic point of view it is important to recognize that microwaves may selectively (see Fig. 13–34) and evenly heat the musculature. It also can selectively heat joints covered with little soft tissue.

Side Effects

The heating effects are also important, since they can create hazards if the temperature is raised selectively in sensitive organs. The effects of microwaves on the eye, among other organs, have been studied extensively.[25, 27, 39, 40, 188, 220, 271, 287] It has been found that it may be possible to heat selectively the fluid media of the eye, including the lens. It is most likely that lenticular cataracts are produced by the heating effect of microwaves. Below a power density of 0.112 watt/cm^2, opacities have not been observed even after prolonged exposure.[26, 90] Other heat-sensitive organs include the testicles,[64, 83, 115, 189] which are easily exposed to stray radiation during therapeutic application. In contrast to the testicles, the ovaries are covered with such a thick layer of soft tissue that it is difficult to expose them to any significant amount of radiation.[125, 256] Other investigations have included the study of the effects of microwaves on bone growth. Wise et al.[276] found, after the application of high dosage of microwaves, a decrease in bone growth, probably related to the heating effect. On the other hand, lower dosage of shortwave diathermy applied by Doyle and Smart[49] produced a stimulation of bone growth. Granberry et al.,[84] however, found no effect on bone growth without associated sensation of pain. Finally, it has been established that temperature increases above 38.9° C[94, 243] in the pregnant uterus may produce congenital anomalies in the fetus. Specifically, Rubin and Erdman[223] reported on four women treated with microwave diathermy for pelvic inflammatory diseases. These women were or became pregnant during the course of therapy. They were treated with frequencies of 2450 MHz and 100 W total output, using a nondirect-contact applicator. Three women delivered normal infants and one aborted on day 67 but delivered a normal baby following a subsequent pregnancy, even though she again received microwave therapy. In these cases, however, it is doubtful that there was a significant temperature rise in the uterus. Microwaves were also used to ease parturition without injury to the newborns, who were followed for one year after delivery. As discussed also, reflection over bone may enhance energy levels to the point that burns occur, a point that should be considered in therapeutic application. Finally, sweat beads may be selectively heated and produce superficial skin burns, a problem totally avoided by air-cooled direct-current applicators.

Nonthermal Effects

Most of the biologic reactions of therapeutic significance are due to the heating effect resulting from microwave absorption in the tissues. There are, however, some effects that are nonthermal in nature. The significance of these effects for therapeutic purposes is still inadequately understood. These effects have been reviewed by Michaelson[189] and Lehmann.[143] It is not known how many of these would actually occur in the live organism under therapeutic conditions. Therefore, for therapeutic purposes, this discussion is limited to the heating effect of microwave energy. However, it is possible that in the future there may be unveiled some specific reactions that are nonthermal in nature and that may add to the specificity of the therapeutic results.

DOSIMETRY

The dose can be defined as the product of applied energy times duration of action. As in the other diathermies, the actual tissue temperature is more important than the applied energy for determining the biologic results, since most of the reactions to microwaves are thermal in nature. Even though we have information on the relative distribution of temperature in the organism exposed to microwaves, we do not at present have a way to assess the absolute level of the temperatures obtained in the tissue. However, major improvement in new equipment is possible. With direct contact applicators, the proposed federal Food and Drug Administration (FDA) standard for this equipment requires a meter indicating the forward power to the patient, that is, the total output minus the reflected power. From a previous study it can be anticipated that vigorous effects can be produced with forward power of the order of 50 watts,[161] with an average intensity of 500 mW/cm^2. The air-cooled applicators are preferable because they avoid undesirable temperature increases in the skin and subcutaneous fat. However, to safeguard against exceeding tolerance levels, pain should still be used as a warning signal and vigorous exposure avoided in the absence of such pain sensation.

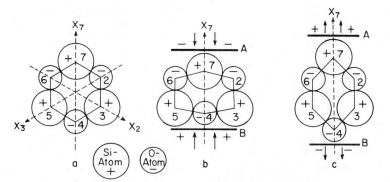

FIGURE 13–37. Quartz crystal lattice demonstrating the piezoelectric effect. *a*, Natural state of the crystal with electrical neutrality of the surfaces. *b*, Compressed crystal with greater proximity of the two negative charges to surface A and the two positive charges to surface B, producing corresponding changes of the surface charges. *c*, With crystal extended, proximity of the positive charge to the surface producing a positive charge at A and closer proximity of the negative charge producing negative surface charge at B (Bergmann, L.: Der ultraschall und seine Anwendung in Wissenschaft und Technik. Stuttgart, S. Hirzel, Verlag, 1949).

Ultrasound

EQUIPMENT

The therapeutic ultrasound machine consists of a generator that produces a high-frequency alternating current of about 0.8 to 1 MHz. The high-frequency electric current is then converted by a transducer into mechanical, i.e., acoustic, vibrations. The transducer consists basically of a crystal inserted between two electrodes. The conversion of the high-frequency alternating voltage into mechanical vibrations is accomplished by reversal of the piezoelectric effect, which is shown in Figure 13–37.[15] If an alternating electrical charge is applied to the surfaces of the crystal, the crystal will be deformed, depending on the sign of the charges. The three basic components of the electrical generator usually found in the therapeutic machines are the power supply, the oscillating circuit (radio frequency generator) producing the high-frequency current, and the transducer circuit. The power supply of therapeutically acceptable machines has full-wave rectification and filtering to provide for a steady output not appeciably (within 1 per cent) modified by the 60 Hz alternating line current. Federal standard proposes that variations exceeding ±20 per cent for all emanations greater than 10 per cent of the maximum emission are not acceptable. The capacitance and inductance of the oscillating circuit are selected to produce an alternating current of the same frequency as the mechanical resonance frequency of the quartz crystal in the transducer. Adjustment of the

frequency is made possible by tuning, usually by adjusting a variable capacitor. Some manufacturers have eliminated tuning by controlling the oscillating frequency.

The sound beams produced by therapeutic applicators are almost cylindrical in shape. The beaming properties of any sound applicator depend on its diameter and the wavelength. The sine of the angle of divergence, γ, is in proportion to the ratio of the wavelength to the diameter of the applicator. Thus, a transducer operating at therapeutic frequencies will produce a beam with a greater angle of divergence if the diameter of the transducer is small than if it is large (Fig. 13–38).[213]

The sound intensity across the beam produced by a therapeutic transducer is not uniform. If measurements are made of the sound intensity along the central axis of the beam produced by a therapeutic applicator, the intensity distribution shows maxima and minima near the applicator and then a gradual decline beyond the last maximum of intensity (Figs. 13–39 and 13–40).[159] The "interference" or "near field" is the area in the ultrasound beam extending from the applicator surface to the location of the most distant intensity maximum. In this area, maxima and minima of intensity are located close to each other. Beyond this point, the beam has a more uniform intensity, and this area is called the "far" or "distant field."[213] Figure 13–41 shows the distance between transducer surface and the last intensity maximum, dependent on the diameter of the radiating surface of the applicator.

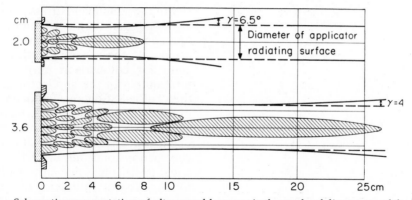

FIGURE 13–38. Schematic representation of ultrasound beam; γ is the angle of divergence of the beam; shaded areas are zones of high ultrasound intensity (Pohlman, R.: Die ultraschalltherapie. Stuttgart, Georg Thieme Verlag, 1951).

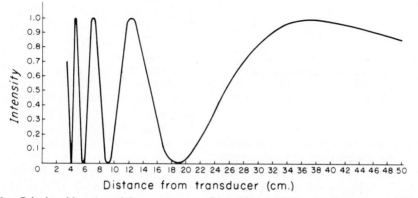

FIGURE 13–39. Calculated location of the maximum and minimum of intensity along the axis of the sound beam produced by a transducer with a diameter of 8 cm operating at a frequency of 0.35 MHz in water (Born, H.: Zur Frage der Absorptionsmessungen im Ultraschallgebiet. Zeitschrift Phys., 120:383, 1943).

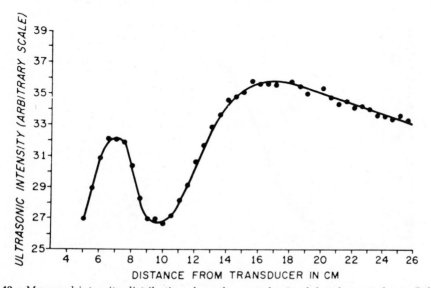

FIGURE 13–40. Measured intensity distribution along the central axis of the ultrasonic beam (Lehmann, J. F., and Johnson, E. W.: Some factors influencing the temperature distribution in thighs exposed to ultrasound. Arch. Phys. Med. Rehabil., 39:347–356, 1958).

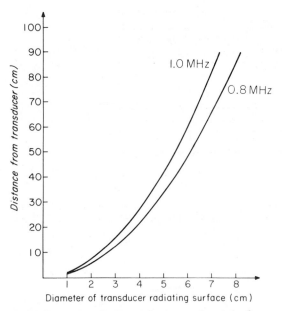

FIGURE 13–41. Distance between the transducer surface and the last interference maximum dependent on the diameter of the radiating surface of the applicator for the therapeutic frequency of 0.8 and 1 MHz (Pohlman, R.: Die Ultraschalltherapie. Stuttgart, Georg Thieme Verlag, 1951).

The sound applicators produce an ultrasonic field in the vicinity of the applicator which shows a characteristic interference pattern. In the far field, the intensity distribution across the beam shows a bell-shaped distribution curve (Fig. 13–42).[159] The inten-

sity of the sound field drops gradually to zero at the edge of the distribution. Therefore, a procedure has been developed to determine accurately the radiating surface of an applicator for comparison purposes. First, the total output of the applicator is determined, then baffles of decreasing diameter are used in front of the applicator which cut out the edge of the ultrasonic beam. The size of the opening of that baffle which cuts out 10 per cent of the total output of the applicator is equal to the radiating surface of the applicator. An arbitrary reduction of the total output to 10 per cent is commonly used to determine the radiating surface of the applicator for comparison purposes. A preferable applicator for therapeutic purposes should have a radiating surface area that is only slightly smaller than the total applicator surface. This minimizes the problem of maintaining full contact between the skin and the applicator surface, at the same time utilizing the total surface of the applicator for therapeutic irradiation. The ultrasonic intensity is expressed in watts/cm², referring to the average intensity of the field. This average intensity is obtained by measuring the total output of the applicator (watts) and then dividing it by the size of the radiating surface of the applicator (cm²). In order to be able to produce vigorous therapeutic effects in the depth of the tissues, the therapeutic applicator should be able to produce ultrasonic average inten-

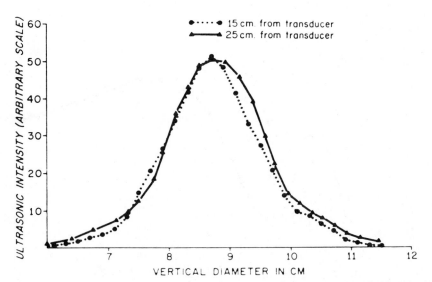

FIGURE 13–42. Intensity distribution in the vertical cross section of the ultrasonic far field (Lehmann, J. F., and Johnson, E. W.: Some factors influencing the temperature distribution in thighs exposed to ultrasound. Arch. Phys. Med. Rehabil., 39:347–356, 1958).

sities of 3 to 4 watts/cm². For an applicator with a radiating surface area of 10 cm², the maximal total output would be between 30 and 40 watts. The peak intensity, in the bell-shaped distribution curve, should be not more than approximately four times the average intensity. The peak intensity in the far field over average intensity is also a reasonable measure of the uniformity of the beam. This means that a therapeutically acceptable transducer has a broad-based, bell-shaped intensity distribution curve, in contrast to an undesirable applicator, which produces a pencil-shaped type of beam with either one or several high-intensity peaks in the field distribution. Multiple high peaks with a nonuniform distribution are commonly encountered in so-called mosaic crystals. Therefore a single quartz or synthetic crystal is to be preferred. Machines with a nonuniform beam may be dangerous because undesirable side effects may be produced by the high intensities in the peaks of the distribution curve.

The losses in the therapeutic applicator should be kept to a minimum in order to avoid excessive heating during application, which may modify those therapeutic results dependent on temperature. Since the total output of an applicator is a product of average intensity (watts/cm²) and the total radiating surface area (cm²), it is desirable to have larger applicators. The angle of divergence of the beam is less if an applicator with a large diameter is used. It is for this reason that applicators smaller than 5 cm² are not acceptable for therapeutic purposes. It is also difficult to treat the deep tissues in an area of limited size with a beam of small diameter. On the other hand, if the radiating surface of the applicator is too large, it may be difficult to maintain contact with the surface of the body at all times. Therefore, an applicator with a radiating surface of 7 to 13 cm² is most convenient and effective for therapeutic application. If the equipment produces pulsed output, the shape of the pulses should preferably be rectangular with an accurate statement as to intensity during the pulses, the rate of the pulses, and the duration of the pulses — that is, the duty cycle. The shape of the pulses should be known to avoid excessive temporal intensity peaks that may produce undesirable side effects.

MEASUREMENT OF ULTRASOUND[75]

If ultrasound is incident on a totally reflecting surface, a pressure is exerted on the surface.[213] Figure 13–43 shows a schematic arrangement of the so-called sound-pressure balance. The balance is usually calibrated in watts. Similarly, if a floating reflector with its stem immersed in a heavier fluid, such as carbon tetrachloride, could be used, the stem would be calibrated and as a result of the sound pressure would be driven deeper into the heavy fluid. Also, small probes have been developed to determine sound intensities in small areas of the field.[15, 134, 213]

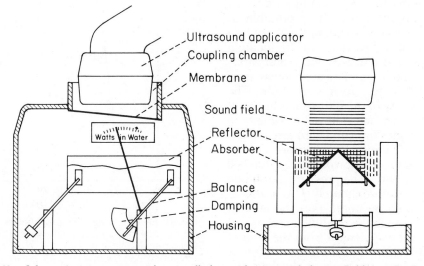

FIGURE 13–43. Schematic arrangement of a so-called sound-pressure balance (Pohlman, R.: Die Ultraschalltherapie. Stuttgart, Georg Thieme Verlag, 1951).

PHYSICS[15, 51, 75, 136, 143]

Ultrasound is defined as a form of acoustic vibration occurring at frequencies too high to be perceived by the human ear. Thus, frequencies under 17,000 Hz are usually called *sound*, whereas those above this level are designated *ultrasound*. With the exception of the differences in frequencies, the physics of ultrasound is in no way different from that of audible sound. Sound and ultrasound are propagated in the form of longitudinal compression waves. The movement of the particles in the medium occurs parallel to the direction of the wave propagation. In the case of a cylindrical ultrasound beam, the propagation also occurs parallel to the axis of the beam. Hence, the propagation of sound depends on the presence of a medium capable of being compressed. It follows that sound cannot be transmitted through a vacuum.

Ultrasonic frequencies used for therapeutic purposes range between 0.8 and 1 MHz. The sound velocity in water and in tissues is approximately 1.5×10^5 cm/sec. The wavelength is approximately 0.15 cm. Thus, many tissue structures are large as compared with the wavelength, although they are small as compared with the wavelength of audible sound. The result is that biologic interfaces and structures that are transparent to audible sound waves may reflect or scatter ultrasound.

The primary reactions occurring within an ultrasonic beam at therapeutic intensities of the order of 1 to 4 watts/cm² are directly related to the particle movement as a result of the wave propagation. It is possible to assess quantitatively the amplitude of the displacement of the particles in the medium as rarefaction and compression occur alternately. The amplitude of displacement is of the order of 1×10^{-6} to 6×10^{-6} cm. The maximum velocity of the particles is approximately 10 to 26 cm/sec. The accelerations to which the particles are subjected are about 5×10^7 to 16×10^7 cm/sec². This represents an acceleration that is approximately 100,000 times that of gravity. The pressure amplitude in the waves is approximately 1 to 4 atmospheres. It should be noted that the area of maximal pressure in the medium is separated by just one-half wavelength from the area of maximal rarefaction. Thus, a great difference in pressure occurs over a relatively short distance.

These powerful mechanical forces can create secondary reactions in the tissues. Since dissolved gases are always present in biologic media, the phenomenon called gaseous cavitation may occur. Gas-filled cavities may be produced in the fluid medium during the phase of rarefaction in the sound waves. During the following phase of compression, these cavities may collapse, creating a high-energy concentration in the form of shock waves. Or the gas bubbles may become larger. The growth of the bubbles can be explained by the following mechanism. During the phase of compression, when the surface of the gas bubble is relatively small, the gas moves out of the bubble into the surrounding fluid. During the following phase of rarefaction, when the bubble is expanded and its surface is relatively large, the gas moves out of the fluid into the cavity. The amount of gas passing into or out of the bubble is in proportion to the bubble surface; thus, there is a net gain of gas moving into the bubbles. Electrical and chemical phenomena have been described as results of cavitation. Mechanical destruction also may be produced when the cavities collapse or

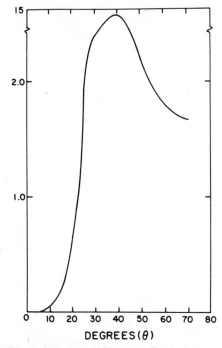

FIGURE 13–44. Ratio of heating due to shear wave to heating due to longitudinal wave (Chan, A. K., Sigelmann, R. A., and Guy, A. W.: Calculations of therapeutic heat generated by ultrasound in fat-muscle-bone layers. IEEE Trans. Biomed. Eng. BME, 21:280–284, 1973).

TABLE 13–4.   ULTRASONIC ATTENUATION IN PIG TISSUES

Tissue	Number of Samples	Attenuation in db/cm	Standard Deviation
Whole bone	13	8.4	± 1.2
Skeletal muscle	30	0.8	± 0.1
Subcutaneous fat	28	1.8	± 0.1

From Lehmann, J. F., and Johnson, E. W.: Some factors influencing the temperature distribution in thighs exposed to ultrasound. Arch. Phys. Med. Rehabil., 39:347–356, 1958.

when gas bubbles grow large enough to vibrate in resonance with the sound waves.[132, 263, 268] The occurrence of gaseous cavitation can be prevented by application of external pressure of sufficient magnitude.

As sound is propagated through the tissues, it is gradually absorbed and converted into heat. The surface intensity is attenuated exponentially. The depth of penetration is commonly defined as that depth of the tissues at which the intensity drops to one half of its value at the surface.

The absorption of ultrasound in uniform tissues has been investigated by Hüter,[111, 112] Dussick et al.,[52] and Lehmann and Johnson.[159] Tissue with a very high coefficient of absorption will also show selective rise of temperature in its more superficial portion. Bone may serve as an example.

Carstensen et al.,[28] Piersol et al.,[212] and Smith[242] have demonstrated that ultrasonic absorption occurs primarily in the tissue proteins, although such structural elements as cellular membranes are responsible for a minor degree of absorption. Hüter[111, 112] has shown that attenuation of ultrasound in muscle tissue depends on whether or not the ultrasonic beam is parallel to myofascial interfaces, thus demonstrating a selective absorption at interfaces that can be explained on the basis of scattering, which, in turn,

results in an increased absorption at irregular surfaces. It is also possible that the longitudinal ultrasound waves may be converted into transverse, that is, shear waves, which are quickly attenuated. Chan et al.[29, 30] showed that the portion of ultrasonic heating resulting from shear waves is significant and depends on the angle of incidence (Fig. 13–44). In addition, as a result of absorbing ultrasound, a special gradient of acoustic energy is created, producing a streaming in a viscous medium.

BIOPHYSICS[51, 189]

The propagation of ultrasonic energy in tissues depends mainly on two factors: absorption (Table 13–4) characteristics of the biologic media and reflection of ultrasonic energy at tissue interfaces (Table 13–5). Whole bone absorbs approximately 10 times more energy than skeletal muscle.

Reflection can occur at interfaces between tissues of different acoustic impedance. The impedance was measured and reflection at tissue interfaces determined by Lehmann and Johnson.[159] The results shown in Table 13–5 indicate that very little reflection occurs between soft tissues, but a great deal occurs at the surface of the bone where up to 30 per cent of energy may be reflected. Surgical

TABLE 13–5.   EXPERIMENTAL AND CALCULATED REFLECTION OF ULTRASONIC ENERGY AT TISSUE INTERFACES

Interface	Observed Reflection (% of Incident Energy)	Calculated Reflection (% of Incident Energy)
Water-fat (pig)	0	0.2
Water-muscle (pig)	0	0.3
Fat-muscle (pig)	—	1.1
Water-bone (pig)	30	30
Muscle-bone (pig)	—	26.8

From Lehmann, J. F., and Johnson, E. W.: Some factors influencing the temperature distribution in thighs exposed to ultrasound. Arch. Phys. Med. Rehabil., 39:347–356, 1958.

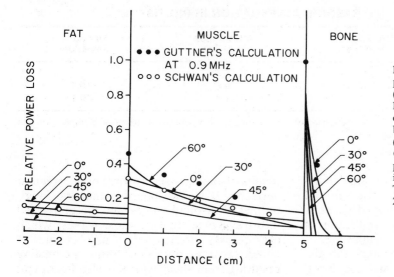

FIGURE 13–45. Relative heating pattern in a three-layered system (fat-muscle-bone). Frequency: 1 MHz. Schwan's and Guttner's calculated values are superimposed, but these values are renormalized (Chan, A. K., Sigelmann, R. A., and Guy, A. W.: Calculations of therapeutic heat generated by ultrasound in fat-muscle-bone layers. IEEE Trans. Biomed. Eng. BME, 21:280–284, 1973).

metallic implants constitute artificial interfaces. Acoustic impedance of stainless steel, vitallium, and titanium was found to be greatly different from that of bone or soft tissues. Thus, it could be anticipated that the major problem encountered with surgical metallic implants in the ultrasonic field might be that of reflection leading to an intense increase in ultrasonic energy due to the production of a pattern of standing waves and focusing.

THERAPEUTIC TEMPERATURE DISTRIBUTION

Once the absorption coefficient of the tissues and reflection at tissue interfaces are known, it is possible to calculate the so-called pattern of relative heating. This was done for therapeutic ultrasonic frequencies by Schwan[228] and Chan[29] (Fig. 13–45). The data indicate that relatively little energy is converted into heat in the subcutaneous fat and not much more energy is converted into

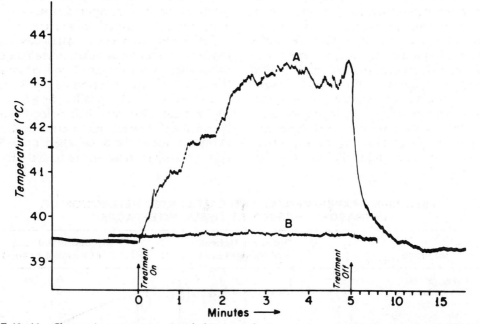

FIGURE 13–46. Change in temperature inside hip joint during exposure to (A) ultrasound and (B) microwave (Lehmann, J. F., McMillan, J. A., Brunner, G. D., and Blumberg, J. B.: Comparative study of the efficiency of shortwave, microwave and ultrasonic diathermy in heating the hip joint. Arch. Phys. Med. Rehabil., 40:510–512. 1959).

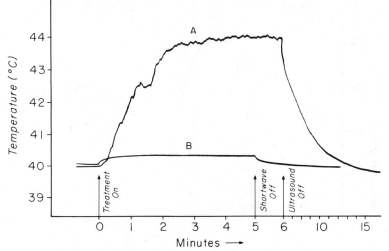

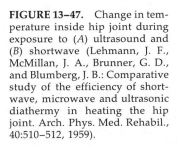

FIGURE 13–47. Change in temperature inside hip joint during exposure to (*A*) ultrasound and (*B*) shortwave (Lehmann, J. F., McMillan, J. A., Brunner, G. D., and Blumberg, J. B.: Comparative study of the efficiency of shortwave, microwave and ultrasonic diathermy in heating the hip joint. Arch. Phys. Med. Rehabil., 40:510–512, 1959).

heat in the musculature. The depth of penetration of the ultrasonic energy in the musculature is therefore very satisfactory. One half of the intensity at the muscle surface is still available at a depth of approximately 3 cm. Most of the energy is converted into heat at the bone interface.

The temperature distribution produced by ultrasound is unique among deep-heating modalities. Ultrasound causes comparatively little temperature elevation in the superficial tissues and has a greater depth of penetration in the musculature and other soft tissues than do shortwave and microwave diathermy. Ultrasound selectively heats interfaces between tissues of different acoustic impedance because of reflection, formation of shear waves, and the high selective absorption in the superficial layers of tissue with high coefficient of absorption. Thus, biophysical research suggests that ultrasound is the most effective deep-heating agent. The temperature in joints covered by heavy masses of soft tissues can be raised to therapeutic and even tolerance levels without any deleterious effects elsewhere in the tissues.[164] It was found by comparison that neither shortwave nor microwave diathermy produced any therapeutic rise of temperature in the hip joint, even though a first-degree burn was obtained in the superficial tissues with either modality (Figs. 13–46 and 13–47). The high degree of reflection of ultrasound on the surface of the bone, as well as the high coefficient of absorption in bone tissue, eliminates the possibility of heating the distant side of the bone or joint.[164] A practical conclusion evolving from this research is that

when treating an entire joint, one should utilize a multiple field technique, exposing all joint surfaces directly to the ultrasonic beam if the joint is to be heated uniformly throughout.

Experiments in pigs have shown that the structures of the knee joint can be selectively heated. As shown in Figure 13–48, the temperature was measured in the capsular tissues and bone just above the knee joint and at the level of the joint space through the capsular tissues and meniscus. The resulting temperature distributions are shown in Figure 13–49.[148]

It is characteristic of ultrasound that a selective increase in temperature may occur at the interface between tissues of different

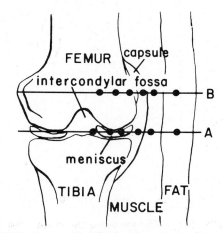

FIGURE 13–48. Needle location in the knee joint (*A*) and 2 cm proximal (*B*) (Lehmann, J. F., de Lateur, B. J., Warren, C. G., and Stonebridge, J. B.: Heating of joint structures by ultrasound. Arch. Phys. Med. Rehabil., 49:28–30, 1968).

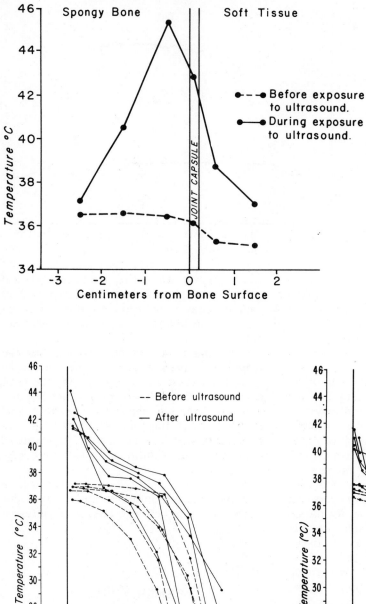

FIGURE 13–49. Temperature distribution 2 cm proximal to the joint space (Lehmann, J. F., de Lateur, B. J., Warren, C. G., and Stonebridge, J. B.: Heating of joint structures by ultrasound. Arch. Phys. Med. Rehabil., 49:28–30, 1968).

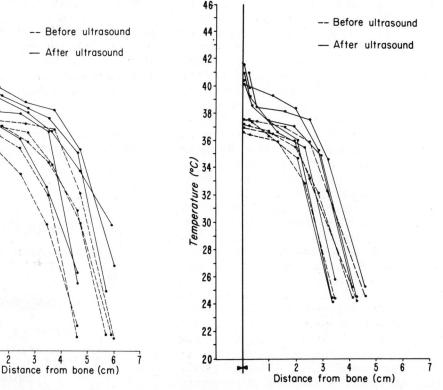

FIGURE 13–50. Comparison of temperature distributions in five human thighs before and after exposure to ultrasound, using a mineral oil coupling medium at 18°C (Lehmann, J. F., de Lateur, B. J., and Silverman, D. R.: Selective heating effects of ultrasound in human beings. Arch. Phys. Med. Rehabil., 47:331–339, 1966).

FIGURE 13–51. Comparison of temperature distribution in five human thighs before and after exposure to ultrasound, using degassed water coupling medium at 24°C (Lehmann, J. F., de Lateur, B. J., and Silverman, D. R.: Selective heating effects of ultrasound in human beings. Arch. Phys. Med. Rehabil., 47:331–339, 1966).

acoustic impedance. Such a selective temperature increase occurs in the human being as shown in Figure 13–50.[144] In addition, it has been documented that the temperature distribution in the human largely depends on the type and temperature of the coupling medium used.[144] For instance, if water, which has a high thermal conductivity and high heat-carrying capacity, is used as a coupling medium, an adequate selective temperature increase in front of the bone still can be obtained at a temperature of 24° C (Fig. 13–51). This is not so with the use of mineral oil (Fig. 13–52). Also, for practical purposes, the temperature of the applicator itself should be kept low. These studies, both in animals and in humans, indicate clearly that it is possible to selectively heat joint structures, such as capsules, synovia, and others, with ultrasound. However, it must also be recognized that the temperature obtained in

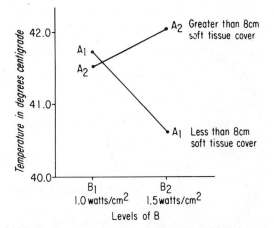

FIGURE 13–53. Temperature recorded at the periosteum of the femur at the moment of pain (Lehmann, J. F., de Lateur, B. J., Stonebridge, J. B., and Warren, C. G.: Therapeutic temperature distribution produced by ultrasound as modified by dosage and volume of tissue exposed. Arch. Phys. Med. Rehabil., 48:662–666, 1967).

the superficial bone will be slightly higher than those in the capsular tissues in front of the bone.[148]

If the therapeutic objective is to heat the capsular synovial tissues of the joint, the technique of application should be modified so as to minimize the difference between the peak temperature in the superficial bone and the temperature in the adjacent soft tissue structures.[147] This is illustrated in Figure 13–53, where the temperature was measured in front of the bone when the first pain was perceived. It should be noted that in individuals with less than 8 cm soft tissue cover of the bone, higher temperatures were obtained at lower wattage. Also, at higher wattage the temperature in front of the bone, at pain, was markedly higher in the individual with thick absorbing tissue cover of the bone than in the thin individual. This discrepancy was explained on the basis that if higher wattage was used in the thin individual the temperature of the superficial bone rose very rapidly and selectively, and thus insufficient time was available for thermal conduction to take place which would minimize the temperature difference between superficial bone and the site of measurement. Pain occurred earlier in these cases, whereas in the slim individual with lower dosage the treatment was tolerated longer without pain; therefore, heat conduction from the superficial bone into the soft tissues in front of the bone substantially elevated the tissue temperature in front of

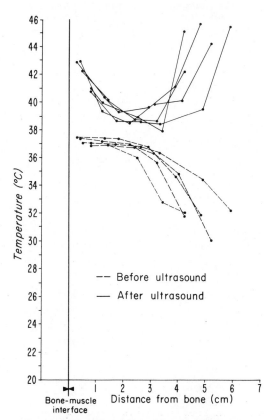

FIGURE 13–52. Comparison of temperature distribution in human thighs before and after exposure to ultrasound, using a mineral oil coupling medium at 24°C (Lehmann, J. F., de Lateur, B. J., and Silverman, D. R.: Selective heating effects of ultrasound in human beings. Arch. Phys. Med. Rehabil., 47:331–339, 1966).

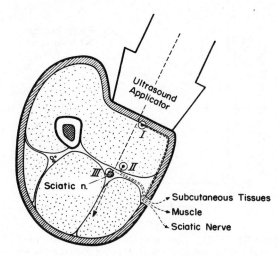

FIGURE 13–54. A cross section through the thigh exposed to ultrasound with thermocouples in, I, subcutaneous tissues; II, muscle tissue; III, sciatic nerve (Rosenberger, H.: Ubert den Wirkungmechanismus der Ultraschallbehandlung, insbesondere bei Ischias und Neuralgien. Chirurg, 21:404, 1950).

TABLE 13–6. CHANGE OF ULTRASONIC INTENSITY RESULTING FROM THE PRESENCE OF METALLIC IMPLANTS

Type of Metal Implant	Mode of Application of Ultrasound and Location of Probe	Factor by Which Ultrasonic Intensity Is Changed (Mean Value)	Standard Deviation of the Mean
Stainless steel disc	Probe in front of disc, ultrasound beam incident at angle of 90°	1.9	± 0.06
Stainless steel disc	Probe behind disc, ultrasound beam incident at angle of 90°	0.03	± 0.22
Vitallium hip cup (diameter 5 cm)	Ultrasound beam incident perpendicularly at opening of cup, probe in focal area	6.2	± 0.10
Vitallium hip cup (diameter 5 cm)	Ultrasound beam incident at convex side of cup, measurements within cup	0.086	± 0.007
Vitallium hip cup (diameter 5 cm)	Ultrasound beam incident at side of cup, measurements within cup	0.1	± 0.00
Vitallium hip cup (diameter 3.1 cm)	Ultrasound beam incident perpendicularly at opening of cup, probe in focal area	6.4	± 0.06
Smith-Petersen nail	Ultrasound beam incident between 2 flanges of the nail, probe in focal area	2.7	±0.07
Smith-Petersen nail	One flange pointing toward ultrasound applicator, probe in focal area	2.7	± 0.001
Kuntscher nail	Ultrasound beam incident at groove of nail, probe in focal area	3.7	± 0.18

From Lehmann, J. F., Lane, C. E., Bell, J. W., and Brunner, G. D. Influence of surgical metal implants on distribution of the intensity in the ultrasonic field. Arch. Phys. Med. Rehabil., 39:756–760, 1958.

the bone at the site of measurement. Similarly, at high wattages temperature rose rapidly to the pain threshold in the superficial bone in the thin individual, and it took a longer period of time in the more obese individual.

The therapeutic application of these findings is that one should treat over a longer period of time, at least over 5 to 10 minutes per field, to obtain optimal heating of joint tissues located right in front of the bone.

There is also evidence that other biologic interfaces are selectively heated by ultrasound.[100, 109, 166, 203, 222] Pätzold and Born[203] demonstrated that myofascial interfaces, as they occur in the musculature, are selectively heated. Rosenberger[222] found a selective rise of temperature in the sciatic nerve of experimental animals (Fig. 13–54). Herrick[100] and associates were able experimentally to destroy the sciatic nerve in dogs without affecting the histologic structure of surrounding musculature or the tissues.

On the other hand, ultrasound can be utilized safely in the presence of surgical metallic implants. Marked reflection occurs resulting in the development of patterns of standing waves. Focal concentrations of energy may occur in the vicinity of the implant. This causes a large increase in ultrasonic intensity close to the metal (Table 13–6). Lehmann et al.[139] studied the distribution of temperature throughout specimens with metal implants and found that, when exposed to ultrasound, no selective rise of temperature occurred in these areas (Fig. 13–55). Often the temperature in the specimen close to metal was lower than the temperature measured in the same place without

metal present. This was explained by the fact that the metal implants have a very high thermal conductivity. Thus, the heat energy is removed from the areas of increased intensity more rapidly than it is absorbed. The experimental findings obtained in specimens were later confirmed in live pigs.[138] Temperatures in the focal areas and in the standing waves close to the implants were within the therapeutic range and could be well controlled (Fig. 13–56). In another series, identical implants were inserted bilaterally into live pigs. One side served as a control and the other was exposed to ultrasound. After the pigs were killed, histologic examinations showed no evidence of any retardation of the healing process or callus formation or any other untoward effects on the side treated with ultrasound. In conclusion, ultrasonic energy seems to be the only type of diathermy that can be used with metallic implants in the treatment field, a finding consistent with previous observations by Gersten.[78]

TECHNIQUE OF APPLICATION

Before ultrasound can be applied, the machine must be tuned and the output must be set. Proper coupling between the applicator and the skin surface must be provided. Coupling media that produce adequate transmission are shown in Figure 13–57.[260] It is important, however, that the coupling media do not contain any gas bubbles that would significantly reflect and scatter ultrasound, with resulting drop in transmission (Fig. 13–58). Also, gas bubbles may stick to the skin and may produce a significant amount of loss in

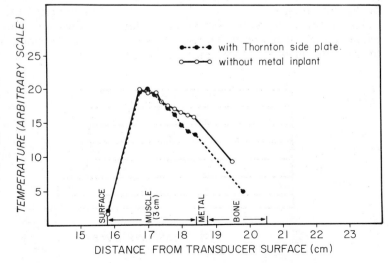

FIGURE 13–55. Temperature distribution in a specimen consisting of muscle and bones with and without a Thornton side plate inserted in front of the bones (Lehmann, J. F., Brunner, G. D., and McMillan, J. A.: The influence of surgical implants on the temperature distribution in thigh specimens exposed to ultrasound. Arch. Phys. Med. Rehabil., 39:692, 1958).

CHANGE IN TEMPERATURE BETWEEN FLANGES OF STAINLESS STEEL SMITH-PETERSEN NAIL DURING EXPOSURE TO ULTRASOUND

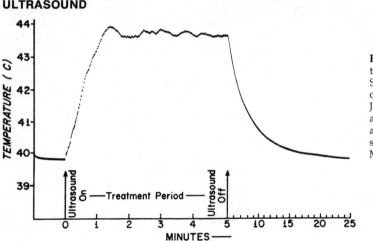

FIGURE 13–56. Change in temperature between flanges of stainless steel Smith-Petersen nail during exposure of a live pig to ultrasound (Lehmann, J. F., Brunner, G. D., Martinis, A. J., and McMillan, J. A.: Ultrasonic effects as demonstrated in live pigs with surgical metallic implants. Arch. Phys. Med. Rehabil., 40:483–488, 1959).

transmission, according to Pätzold and associates.[204] These bubbles could be removed by using a wetting agent, such as a detergent, prior to treatment; this must be carefully rinsed off to prevent skin irritation. The skin irritation is likely due to the fact that with ultrasound some of these agents may penetrate the skin.

Two types of application have been developed. The sound head may be held stationary or it may be moved slowly in a back-and-forth stroking motion. The stationary technique is rarely used because it produces a rapid rise of temperature in a very small area, which is rather difficult to control. "Hot spots" are produced in the interference field and in the far field where the highest intensity is found in the center of the beam. These "hot spots" are likely to heat small areas excessively while the rest of the tissues are not heated adequately for therapeutic purposes.

The stroking technique is most commonly employed. Strokes are comparatively short, of the order of one inch in length, and each stroke partially overlaps the area of another, with the applicator gradually moving in a direction perpendicular to the strokes. Circular strokes may be used, but they are somewhat more difficult to control. The temperature increase produced by this technique is rather smooth with little ripples and can be well controlled, as seen in Figure 13–47 and 13–56. The temperatures obtained in the tissues will depend on the total output of the applicator, the time of application, and the size of the field treated. For most therapeutic applicators it will be necessary to treat a field of approximately 3 to 4 sq in. If vigorous results are to be obtained it is necessary to produce temperatures that are just below the maximally tolerated level. In order to find this level it is suggested to go briefly to pain and then either to reduce the output of the applicator slightly or to increase the field size, that is, the volume of tissue treated, maintaining the same output. With this procedure one uses the warning signal of pain to test tolerance limits. However, the patient should be instructed to indicate pain immedi-

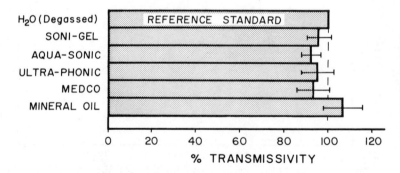

FIGURE 13–57. Per cent transmissivities of several coupling agents using ultrasound generator without transducer voltage control circuit (Warren, C. G., Koblanski, J. N., and Sigelmann, R. A.: Ultrasound coupling media: their relative transmissivity. Arch. Phys. Med. Rehabil., 57:218–222, 1976).

FIGURE 13–58. Per cent transmissivities for several common coupling media in aerated and non-aerated forms using ultrasound generator without voltage control circuit (Warren, C. G., Koblanski, J. N., and Sigelmann, R. A.: Ultrasound coupling media: their relative transmissivity. Arch. Phys. Med. Rehabil., 57:218–222, 1976).

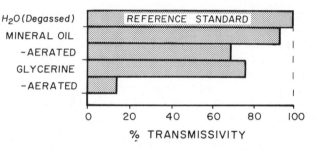

ately so that damage is avoided. Mild to moderate effects can be obtained by lowering the ultrasonic output substantially below the pain threshold.

The temperature distribution in the tissues will also be modified by the temperature of the coupling medium or the temperature of the surface of the metal applicator.[144] The cooler the temperature of the coupling medium or the applicator, the greater the heat loss at the skin and the deeper the peak temperatures found in the tissues. These investigations suggest that if ultrasound is prescribed for deep-heating purposes, it is important to state the temperature of the coupling medium if water is used. Also, it is important to use an applicator with minimal electrical and mechanical losses which maintains a fairly constant temperature during treatment.[168] If the applicator warms up noticeably after one field is treated, it should be quickly placed in tap water to cool it before the next field is treated.

When a major joint covered with a large amount of soft tissue is treated with ultrasound, it has been shown in animal experimentation that the most superficial bone is heated most.[144] In human volunteers it was found that the temperature reached in the tissue in front of the bone — for example, joint structures — depended not only on the thickness of the soft tissue and the intensity of ultrasound, but also on the interaction between these two factors. Thus if the intensity was too high in a thin individual, tolerance levels in the superficial bone will be exceeded before conduction of heat to the tissues in front of the bone can occur. The experimental evidence indicates that 5 to 10 minutes of ultrasound application per field is necessary to produce adequate heating of the joint structures in front of the bone.[147]

Joints such as the shoulder or the hip are typically treated with three fields of application: an anterior, a lateral, and a posterior field, since effective treatment through the interposed bone is not possible. In case of the hip joint, special care should be taken that the lateral field of application is located so that one avoids aiming the sound beam at the greater trochanter.[164] It is also essential that any exercise or stretching procedure immediately follow the ultrasound treatment or be applied simultaneously with ultrasound; e.g., the anterior aspect of the hip joint could be treated with ultrasound and stretched in the Thomas position. A special technique has been developed so that one part of the shoulder joint is treated and subsequently stretched.[184] After this another field is exposed and again the treated structures are stretched immediately, until the entire shoulder joint has been treated and stretched.

To avoid the occurrence of gaseous cavitation and its destructive effects,[143] stroking technique can be used with intensities up to 4 watts/cm^2 and a total output of 40 watts at a frequency of 1 MHz. Cavitation is under those circumstances inhibited by the high viscosity of tissue fluids such as blood serum and the high volume concentration of cells in blood and tissues. However, cavitation can occur much more readily in the fluid media of the eye, the amniotic fluid, and the synovial fluid in joint effusions. Therefore the eye, the pregnant uterus, and joints with effusions should not be treated with therapeutic intensities and frequencies.[135] For the stationary technique, the cavitation threshold is approximately between 1 and 2 watts/cm^2. These intensities applied in this fashion also produce burns. Because of the threshold for cavitation, ultrasonic equipment should not produce high temporal or spatial peak intensities that may exceed cavitation thresholds.

PULSED APPLICATION

The pulsing frequencies in most applications of pulsed ultrasound are so high that the temperature rise will be equal to that produced by continuous-wave application of the same average output. Therefore, all thermal reactions can be equally and less expensively produced by continuous-wave application. Also, many nonthermal reactions such as streaming are equal to the average output just as the thermal reactions are. There is no evidence that nonthermal reactions selectively produced by the high intensity during the pulses have any therapeutic significance.[143]

Equipment is also available which combines an electrical stimulator with an ultrasound generator. There is no evidence that this equipment does anything therapeutically that could not be produced equally by these two modalities contained in separate pieces of equipment.

DOSIMETRY

The factors that determine the biologic response to ultrasound are mainly the temperature obtained in the tissues and the duration of the temperature elevation. It would be ideal if it were possible to measure and control these factors accurately, permitting a quantitative control of the biologic response. However, only the ultrasonic energy entering the tissues and the duration of the treatment can be measured, and thus the resulting tissue effect can only be estimated, provided that information is available on the temperature distribution in the organism as well as an understanding of how it can be modified by the technique of application. For therapeutic purposes it is necessary to determine the total ultrasonic output (watts) and the average intensity (watts/cm^2). Therapeutic machines can be tuned adequately in water and then applied to the patient without retuning. The output of the machine can be preset in a water bath utilizing a meter on the front panel of the machine which indicates total output (watts) and average intensity (watts/cm^2). Some machines do not require tuning. The output can be preset by pressing a contact button, activating a simulated load. The output indicated on the meter will be transmitted to the tissues, provided that reflection at the skin surface is prevented by proper use of a coupling medium.

Some machines are equipped with a protective system. The moment that contact with the body is partially lost and the load of the applicator is therefore changed, a feedback to a control system reduces the output. This is indicated by the meter on the panel and a buzzing device. Its disadvantage is that no ultrasonic energy is applied to the body when poor coupling is inevitable because of uneven body surfaces where full contact cannot be maintained. Intensities found useful in therapy range from 0.5 to 4 watts/cm^2, usually applied with a moving applicator. If the applicator is kept stationary, intensities less than 1 watt/cm^2 are tolerated. The increase in temperature of the tissues is determined by the technique of application. The duration of the treatment is usually 5 to 10 minutes per field. Applications usually are repeated on a daily basis. Sometimes treatment is given twice a day or three times a week.

In order to obtain vigorous results in deep-heated structures such as the hip joint, intensities up to 4 watts/cm^2 with a total output of 40 watts may be needed. For mild heating, intensities of 2 watts/cm^2 with a total output of 10 to 20 watts may be used. For applicators with smaller radiating surface area, allowances will have to be made. For very mild treatment or very superficial structures, average outputs of 0.1 to 1 watt/cm^2 are used, with a total output of 1 to 10 watts. Adjustment has to be made from these suggested outputs for more superficially located structures. The output should be reduced. It should be emphasized that the maximally tolerated output, which can be assessed by a brief occurrence of pain, can be used as a guide, especially for vigorous heating.

PHYSIOLOGIC EFFECTS OF ULTRASOUND[143]

A large number of biologic and therapeutic responses have been investigated.[136] In this chapter the results of an extensive research effort in this area will be summarized briefly. Reactions due to heating of the tissues and nonthermal reactions will be discussed.

Reactions Due to Heating

Since physiologically effective temperature elevations can be produced in the tissues, it is logical to assume that all those reactions which are known to occur as a result of temperature elevation in the tissues will also be produced by ultrasound. Three groups of researchers[3, 17, 205] found that the peripheral arterial blood flow is increased as a result of ultrasound application. The tissue metabolism can be changed, according to Lehmann and coworkers[158] and Pauly and Hug.[206] Experimental evidence has been furnished that these reactions are quantitatively due to the heating effect of ultrasonic energy.[134, 135] It has been observed that reactions such as hyperemia and inflammatory responses characterized by an increase in vascularity, edema, and tissue necrosis all can be quantitatively explained on the basis of the heating effect of ultrasonic energy. It was also found experimentally that a marked increase in permeability of biologic membranes and change of membrane potentials can be produced and is to a large degree the result of the temperature elevation in the tissues during exposure to ultrasound.[134, 135, 137] However, part of the effect is also due to nonthermal mechanisms. The effects of ultrasonic energy on nerve tissues have been studied extensively, and most of them have been found to be due entirely to the heating effect.[113, 130, 132, 178]

It is of interest for therapeutic purposes to note that conduction velocity in peripheral nerves can be altered and temporary blocks can be produced. Different types of fibers show differences in sensitivity to ultrasound; the smallest, C fibers, are most sensitive. An increase or decrease of spinal reflexes can also be produced, depending on dosage.[6, 76, 238] Some of these effects on the spinal cord function are nonthermal in nature.[79, 143] The pain threshold can be elevated by application of ultrasonic energy to the peripheral nerve or to the area of the free nerve endings.[141] "Muscle spasm" as found in poliomyelitis can be relieved by ultrasonic application.[74, 244] An increase in vascularity and skin temperature can be produced by ultrasonic radiation applied to the sympathetic nerves.[227, 246] Careful investigations of the action of ultrasonic energy on bone showed that if therapeutic dosage is applied, no detrimental effects are observed in either the growing or the adult bone.[12, 116] On the other hand, no beneficial influence on the healing of fractures or callus formation could be demonstrated.[8, 179] Excessive dosage led to pathologic fractures.[7]

Nonthermal Reactions

A review of the biologic reactions indicates that most of these reactions clearly are due to the temperature elevation resulting from exposure to ultrasound.[259] In some instances, however, the entire reaction could not be explained on the basis of the heating effects of ultrasonic energy. The reaction was due in part to nonthermal effects. In only a few instances have nonthermal effects been studied in detail. It has been found that the permeability of biologic membranes is altered not only by the heating effect of ultrasonic energy, but also by nonthermal effects occurring during exposure to ultrasound which speed up the rate of diffusion of ions across the membrane.[173] Lehmann[134, 135] and Lehmann and Biegler[137] showed that this nonthermal reaction can be explained on the basis of streaming of fluids in the ultrasonic field and the resultant stirring effect, that is, an increase in the gradient of concentration of ions across the biologic membrane which accelerates the rate of diffusion. Quantitatively, the thermal effect was definitely the dominant one. The stirring effect could also be demonstrated in living cells. Membrane potentials were similarly affected by the mechanical effect of ultrasonic energy. Gersten[77, 79, 80] pointed out that neither the effect on tendon extensibility produced by ultrasound nor the effects on musculature or the spinal cord could be explained entirely on the basis of thermal reactions alone.

There are numerous reactions to gaseous cavitation; most of them, however, occur in the test tube only.[133] Typically destructive reactions such as hemolysis occur only if there is a low concentration of cells and the viscosity of the medium is low as compared with therapeutic conditions.[134, 135] Cavitation also was studied in the live organism.[157] The histologic appearance of the cavitation reaction was characteristic: the destruction of cells was spotty and led to petechial hemorrhages. This appearance could be explained by the spotty occurrence of gas bubbles in the tissues (Fig. 13–59). Intensity thresholds of 1 to 2 watts/cm^2 were required to produce these lesions. The reactions could be prevented by the application of external pressure, proving that they were due to cavitation. It was noted that under conditions similar to those in therapy (i.e., at intensities of 1 watt/cm^2 or below applied with the stationary technique), the destructive effects of cavitation did not occur. It was observed that when stroking technique commonly used in therapy was simulated, intensities up to 4 watts/cm^2 were tolerated without the appearance of destructive effects of cavita-

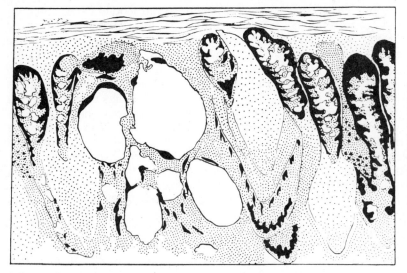

FIGURE 13–59. Destruction of mucous membrane in the intestine with hemorrhage and formation of gas bubbles (Lehmann, J. F., and Herrick, J. F.: Biologic reactions to cavitation, a consideration for ultrasonic therapy. Arch. Phys. Med. Rehabil., 34:86–98, 1953).

tion. It also could be demonstrated that the danger of producing cavitation under therapeutic conditions is increased if unsuitable equipment is used. Animals were irradiated with the stationary applicator with an ultrasonic intensity of 1.5 watts/cm^2 and a total output of the applicator of 15 watts. The machine had a power supply with full-wave rectification. In one series of irradiations, filters were used to produce a steady ultrasonic output; in another series, the filters were removed, producing a greatly modulated ultrasonic output. In the animals treated with the steady output, a few reactions to cavitation were observed, whereas when ultrasound was applied with the same machine with the same average output but with the filtering removed, cavitation effects were observed in 55 per cent of the animals. These experiments demonstrate that peak ultrasonic intensities resulting from the lack of filtering of the rectified line voltage may be potentially dangerous.

Dyson et al.[53, 59] showed that if ultrasound was applied with the stationary technique, blood cell aggregates formed in the vessels in the wave nodes which occurred when a pattern of standing waves was set up; this led to a temporary stasis of blood flow. However, this effect could be avoided when stroking technique was used.

Zarod and Williams,[288] Chater and Williams,[31] and Williams et al.[262, 265-267, 269, 270] observed *in vitro* platelet aggregation and increase in recalcification time of platelet-rich plasma; *in vivo* Zarod et al. found platelet aggregation following ultrasound expo-

sure. The authors felt that hydrodynamic shear stresses, which can be produced by ultrasound, could be responsible. However, there is no evidence that the same phenomena occur under therapeutic conditions *in vivo*. These phenomena are less likely to be observed when the ultrasound is applied by stroking technique. The mechanism is not clearly understood but is likely related to the occurrence of cavitation.

Dyson and associates[55] found clear evidence that varicose ulcers treated with ultrasound healed faster than those treated with mock insonation (Fig. 13–60). An ultrasonic frequency of 3 MHz with an average intensity of 1 watt/cm^2 and a duty cycle of 20 per cent was used. The mechanism by which ultrasound stimulates the healing is uncertain. According to Dyson, the mechanism may be thermal or nonthermal. According to Dyson and Pond,[54, 56, 57] the therapeutic effect may be related to the stimulation of tissue regeneration and accelerated collagen deposition and also to remodeling of the scar collagen.

A large number of other effects have been investigated and are reviewed elsewhere.[51, 143] In most of the cases the exact mechanism is unknown, and the conditions under which these physiologic or destructive effects are observed are significantly different from those of therapeutic application.

In conclusion, this brief review of the physiologic reactions to ultrasound indicates that those reactions of potential therapeutic significance are due primarily to the temperature elevation resulting from absorption of ultrasonic energy. In addition, a few non-thermal effects have been demonstrated, such as the acceleration of diffusion processes across biologic membranes, which may be therapeutically useful and are nonthermal in nature. These effects are also dependent on temperature and occur at a faster rate if they are associated with temperature elevation. Fortunately the destructive effects due to cavitation have not been observed under therapeutic conditions if the proper equipment is used and a therapeutic dosage is applied with proper technique. A more detailed investigation of the nonthermal effects would be most desirable, since they could potentially lead to new specific indications for ultrasonic therapy. Investigation has also shown that there are marked differences between thermal reactions produced by ultrasound and those produced by other heating modalities. These discrepancies have been attributed mainly to the differences in temperature distribution produced by ultrasound and other heating modalities. Therefore, it is important to obtain information on those reactions which ultimately produce the temperature distribution characteristic of ultrasound application.

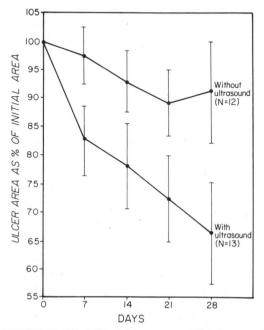

FIGURE 13–60. Effect of treatment with ultrasound on varicose ulcer area (Dyson, M., Franks, C., and Suckling, J.: Stimulation of healing of varicose ulcers by ultrasound. Ultrasonics, 14:232–236, 1976).

CONTRAINDICATIONS TO ULTRASOUND THERAPY

Ultrasound is a very powerful and effective heating agent. Therefore, it must be applied with the proper precautions, in the proper dosage, and with the correct technique of application. There are, however, only a very few specific contraindications. Ultrasound should not be applied to the eye in therapeutic dosage range, since cavitation will most likely occur in the fluid media and may lead to irreversible damage. The pregnant uterus should not be treated because of the possibility of cavitation in the amniotic fluid which may occur at therapeutic intensities and because of danger of producing malformation of the fetus as a result of thermal damage.[51, 94, 243] Usually this is not a problem, since the uterus is not reached by any appreciable amount of energy in any of the common therapeutic applications. Because of the good beaming properties of ultrasound applicators, it is also easy to avoid aiming the beam at the uterus. Special precautions in adjusting the dosage should be taken when the area of the spinal cord is treated after laminectomy. After the covering tissues have been removed, it is likely that higher energy levels may be obtained in the spinal cord.[52] Again, because of the good beaming properties of most applicators, the facet joints, for instance, could be treated without exposing the spinal cord. Ultrasound should be applied with caution over anesthetic areas. Since dosimetry is better developed in ultrasound than in shortwave or microwave diathermy, it is possible to use ultrasound in such cases, if special precautions are taken to insure that the dose is below the damaging level. Recent investigations determined that methyl methacrylate and high density polyethylene, materials commonly used in total joint replacements, will absorb significantly more ultrasound than will soft tissue. In addition, the absorption in methyl methacrylate depends largely on the conditions of mixing of the plastic and the ultimate air bubble content.[170] Whether or not this selective absorption by these materials would lead to overheating or even melting of the plastics has at the present time not been determined. Therefore at the present materials of this type in the sound field should be considered a contraindication to therapy.

The heart should not be directly exposed

to ultrasound because Mortimer[196] showed it would change the action potential and contractile properties. Other investigators have shown change in conduction properties. In addition, Williams[264, 266, 269] showed, in animal experiments, that hemolysis, probably through development of gas bubbles, may occur in the heart as a result of the turbulence of blood flow in that area.

Ultrasound should not be applied to areas where a malignant tumor could be reached by an unknown quantity of ultrasonic energy, since Hayashi[95] has shown that both by such ultrasound and by shortwave exposure tumor growth may be accelerated. The increase or retardation of growth or the destruction of tumors by this type of heat therapy, according to Hayashi, depends on the dosage. Thus, if the dose is uncontrolled, hyperthermia may not necessarily have a beneficial effect.

Sound should not be applied over areas of vascular insufficiency because the blood supply would be unable to follow the increase in metabolic demand, and necrosis might result. During the International Congress in Erlangen in 1949,[108, 218] it was agreed that ultrasonic energy could not be used for treatment of tumors, since a regression of growth could be obtained in a few cases only and the well-established x-ray therapy produced results far superior to those obtained with ultrasonic energy. In some cases exposure to ultrasonic energy caused an even more rapid growth and such exposure was, therefore, considered to be potentially dangerous.[108, 210] Finally, all general contraindications to heat therapy should be observed carefully.

SUPERFICIAL HEATING AGENTS

The hallmark of all these modalities is that they produce temperature distributions, with the highest temperature usually at the surface of the body. Consequently these superficial heating agents may produce mild or vigorous therapeutic responses if the pathology is located in the most superficial tissues. The extent of the reaction will depend on the temperature at the site. For any pathology located deep in the tissue, these modalities can produce only a mild or moderate response. In the superficial tissue they may produce physiologic changes either by local changes of the tissue or cellular function or by triggering reflex mechanisms. Virtually all responses deep in the organism are produced indirectly through reflexes. The mode of heat transfer of these modalities, however, varies. They may heat by conversion, conduction, and/or convection.

Superficial Heat by Conversion: Radiant Heat

Mode of Heat Transfer. For heating purposes the portion of the visible light from yellow to red and the near and far infrared are used. The portion of the visible light used for radiant heating purposes extends over the wavelength from 5,500 to 7,000 Å units and for the infrared from 7,000 to 120,000 Å. The infrared is subdivided into the near infrared with wavelengths from 7,000 to 14,000 Å and the far infrared with wavelengths from 14,000 to 120,000 Å.

The energy content of the photon is expressed by the formula

$$E = hF$$

where h represents Planck's constant and F is the frequency of radiation. Basically, the higher the energy content of the photon, the shorter the photon wavelength and, in turn, the greater the depth of penetration in the tissues.[145] However, practically, these differences have no significant influence on the temperature distribution. Once the photons have penetrated into the tissues they are absorbed and converted into heat. However, all of them penetrate only into the most superficial tissues.

Technique of Application. One of the advantages of these modalities is that the heat can be applied without touching the body and the skin stays dry. Heat lamps are used for application. Heating elements are made out of carbon-metal alloys or special quartz tubes. Also, simple light bulbs with either carbon or tungsten filaments are used, such as a 250 watt Mazda lamp. A number of light bulbs are also used in the heat cradle. The quality of the lamp should be judged primarily by how large the skin area is which is evenly heated. This, in turn, will largely depend on the quality of the design of heating element and reflector. A simple test will allow a check of the evenness of the heating effect. Carbon-blackened paraffin is poured into a pan and allowed to solidify. Once the lamp is turned on, the area where the paraffin begins to melt evenly is an indication of the area with similar intensity of the incident light (Fig. 13–61). Second, the capability of such lamps to produce a vigorous effect over the area heated will depend on the total light output which, in turn, is most readily assessed by the electrical wattage rating of the heating elements. Finally, the quality of the stand, its versatility with regard to adjustment, and its stability are all features to be considered.

The large high-output commercial lamps usually produce more infrared than do light bulbs. As mentioned, the differences in depth of penetration of various types of lamps with the difference in output in the visible light and the infrared spectrum is of no significance with regard to the temperature distributions they produce. Figure 13–62 shows clearly that the temperature distributions in the human are identical with three different lamps.

The advantage of the 250-watt bulb with built-in reflector is that it is inexpensive, that it can be clamped onto chairs or other furniture, and that it can be used as a home

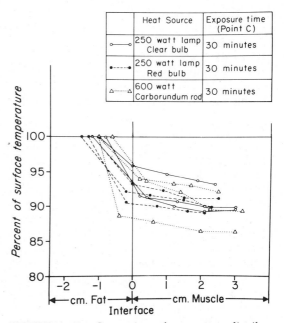

	Heat Source	Exposure time (Point C)
o——o	250 watt lamp Clear bulb	30 minutes
•----•	250 watt lamp Red bulb	30 minutes
△······△	600 watt Carborundum rod	30 minutes

FIGURE 13–62. Comparison of temperature distribution in the human thigh during exposure to infrared radiation in nine individuals using three modalities (Lehmann, J. F., Silverman, D. R., Baum, B. A., Kirk, N. L., and Johnston, V. C.: Temperature distributions in the human thigh, produced by infrared, hot pack and microwave applications. Arch. Phys. Med. Rehabil., 47:291–299, 1966).

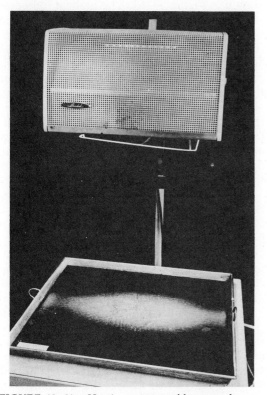

FIGURE 13–61. Heating pattern of lamp as demonstrated by melting of blackened paraffin (Lehmann, J. F., and de Lateur, B. J.: Therapeutic Heat. *In* Lehmann, J. F. (Ed.): Therapeutic Heat and Cold, 3rd Ed. Baltimore, Williams and Wilkins, 1982).

heating device. However, its limitations are due to the fact that it heats only a very small area evenly and that it has a limited total wattage. The commercial lamps have a higher wattage of the order of 500 watts and heat a larger area evenly. Also their stand is much more versatile. This is important, since it is preferred that the light be incident perpendicular on the skin. For heating a larger part of the body, the preferred apparatus is the heat cradle, which contains numerous light bulbs with either tungsten or carbon filaments, a switch to dial the number of bulbs to be lit, and a reflector. When two cradles are used, the trunk, arms, and legs can be covered. A blanket usually covers the cradle in order to retain the heat.

Dosimetry. Heat lamps may have switches to change the wattage output and thus the heat output. The light intensity can also be varied by varying the distance from the lamp to the skin. The lamps with their reflectors produce a divergent beam. Increasing the distance reduces the light intensity to which the skin is exposed. Guidance is given by the subjective feeling of warmth. This physiologic guide is adequate, since the skin, with its temperature receptors, is the area of highest temperature elevation. In the heat cradle the number of bulbs lit may alter the heating effect. If two heat cradles are used, it should be remembered that under normal circumstances, the amount of heat the human body can transfer to the outside is 0.01 watt/cm^2 body surface. This may be raised about tenfold under favorable circumstances, including evaporative cooling by sweating. The amount of radiant heat absorbed without causing a core temperature increase is possible only to the degree the body in turn can get rid of heat absorbed. This limit is reached if the heat input exceeds a value between 100 and 1000 watts. A normal heat cradle with an output of 300 watts is therefore not likely to raise body temperature. A double heat cradle, however, may do so. Studies by Evans and Mendelssohn[68] have shown that heat cradles and lamps do not reach maximum power output for one hour. The patient under the cradle, for instance, will receive three times as much radiation after one hour as at the beginning of the treatment. This is due to secondary radiation from bulb, envelope, and reflector.

Temperature Distribution. Temperature distribution is mentioned and is shown in Figure 13–62. The highest temperature values are found at the skin surface, with a rapid drop and no significant temperature elevation in the musculature.

Superficial Heating by Conduction

Hydrocollator and Related Packs

Mode of Heat Transfer. The main mode of heat transfer is by conduction. There may be some additional heat transfer by infrared radiation and convection. The amount of heat (H) which flows through the body by conduction is directly proportional to the time of flow (t), the area through which it flows (A), the temperature gradient (ΔT), and the thermal conductivity (k). It is inversely proportional to the thickness of the layer ΔL.

$$H = k \, At \, (\Delta T/\Delta L)$$

The practical application of this formula is that in order to reduce the heat flow from the pack to the skin, the heat transfer can be slowed by inserting material with poor thermal conductivity, such as terry cloth toweling, between the pack and the skin. Slowdown of the heat flow in turn could be markedly reduced if the patient were lying on the pack and the water were coming out of the pack and thoroughly wetting the toweling, increasing the thermal conductivity. Even without the water seeping through the toweling, the thickness of the toweling would be compacted, reducing its insulating value.

Technique of Application. The most common commercially available packs are the Hydrocollator packs, which contain silicate gel in a cotton bag. They are heated in a thermostatically controlled water bath where the gel absorbs and holds a large amount of water with its high heat content. The temperature of the pack when applied is about 160 to 175°F or 71 to 79°C. Application is done drip-dry over layers of terry cloth for 20 to 30 minutes.

Dosimetry. Dosimetry with the pack at a constant temperature is done primarily by varying the thickness of the terry cloth, which in turn slows down the heat transfer. Temperatures produced by the pack are as shown in Figure 13–63. The highest temperatures were found in the skin of the human volunteer, with a rapid drop of the temperature to the subcutaneous fat. Deeper tissues such as musculature are not heated significantly.[143, 167] Repeated packing does not alter the temperature distribution significantly, since first the skin blood flow increase is triggered, which not only reduces the temperature in the skin but also creates an additional barrier for heat transfer into the deeper tissues.[167]

Hot Water Bottle

Frequently a rubber hot water bottle can be used in the same fashion as the Hydrocollator pack. This heat application is preferred for home use. However, it must be realized that in this case the heat transfer into the tissues will also depend on the temperature of the water in the bottle, which is not necessarily thermostatically controlled as in the Hydrocollator pack. For hospital use hot packs of this type contain a thermostatically controlled fluid that is pumped through the pad to assure the avoidance of burns. In this case again the transfer is somewhat different, since the pack temperature remains constant, in contrast to both the

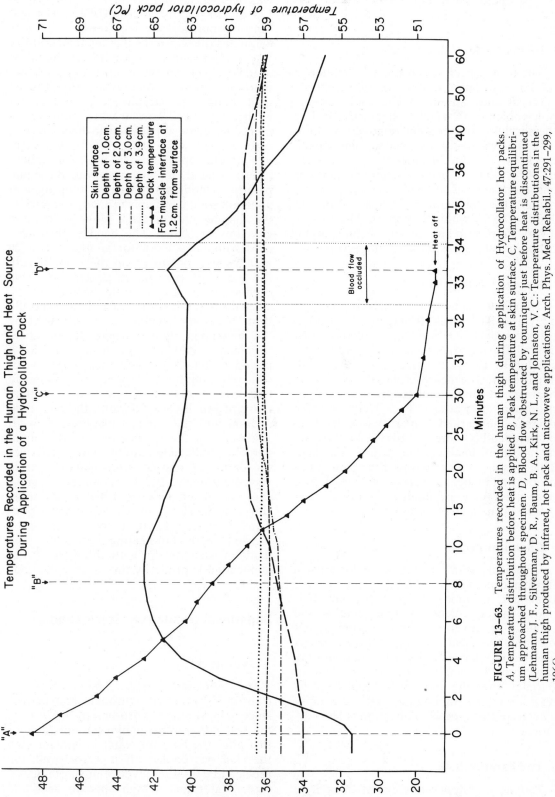

FIGURE 13–63. Temperatures recorded in the human thigh during application of Hydrocollator hot packs. *A,* Temperature distribution before heat is applied. *B,* Peak temperature at skin surface. *C,* Temperature equilibrium approached throughout specimen. *D,* Blood flow obstructed by tourniquet just before heat is discontinued (Lehmann, J. F., Silverman, D. R., Baum, B. A., Kirk, N. L., and Johnston, V. C.: Temperature distributions in the human thigh produced by infrared, hot pack and microwave applications. Arch. Phys. Med. Rehabil., 47:291–299, 1966).

Hydrocollator pack and the hot water bottle.

Kenny Packs[415]

The Kenny pack was originally developed primarily for polio patients to relieve muscle soreness and "spasms." The pack consists of a woolen cloth which is steamed and then the surplus water content removed by spinning. The relatively dry pack is then applied quickly to the skin, usually at a temperature of 140°F (60°C). Since it contains little water and therefore has a small heat-carrying capacity, the temperature drops rapidly to 100°F (37.8°C) within 5 minutes. Thus this is a very short-term but vigorous heating application, producing a marked reflex response.

Electric Heating Pads

The electric heating pad can be used dry as a Hydrocollator pack. It may also be used, if properly insulated by plastic, over a moist cloth. The heat transfer is significantly greater to the skin using the moist pack application. The heat output of the electric heating pad can be adjusted by increasing or decreasing its wattage. The electric heating pad has one marked danger; that is, the heat output steadily increases over a long period of time until finally equilibrium is reached. This is especially dangerous if the patient lies on the pad or falls asleep with the pad. The heat itself may be analgesic enough that severe burns may be produced.

Chemical Packs

Chemical packs currently available are in a flexible container in which, by moving the container, a compartment is broken. This allows the ingredients to come together and produce an elevation of temperature by exothermic chemical reaction. All these packs are poorly controlled as to the temperature produced. The ingredients are irritating or harmful when the outer pack breaks and its content comes in contact with the skin. Therefore this type of application is least desirable.

The Paraffin Bath

Technique of Application and Mode of Heat Transfer. For therapeutic purposes paraffin wax with a melting point of approximately 125 to 130°F (51.7 to 54.5°C)[126, 245] is used. The thermostatically controlled container maintains the wax at its melting temperature. For safety reasons a thermometer should be used to check on the temperature; another indication of the correct temperature is when melted and solid paraffin are found together in the container. Paraffin wax is most commonly used for application to hands, arms, and feet. The wax is applied with two methods. If the dip method is used the patient inserts a hand, for instance, into the liquid paraffin, withdraws it when a thin layer of adherent solid paraffin is formed, and repeats the dipping until a thick glove of paraffin envelops the hand. The hand is then covered with terry cloth for another 10 to 20 minutes in order to retain the heat. Finally the glove of paraffin is peeled off. This produces a relatively mild heating effect, since the paraffin has a relatively low specific heat. Vigorous heating can be obtained by the immersion method where, for instance, the hand is immersed in the paraffin for a period of up to 20 to 30 minutes. The glove of solid paraffin forms around the immersed hand and because of the low thermal conductivity of this layer of paraffin the heat conduction into the hand is markedly slowed. Without this the temperature of the liquid paraffin would be too hot to be tolerated over this period of time. This technique produces vigorous effects. It also produces a significant rise of temperature in the small joints, since the layer of soft tissue cover is thin. Thus this method can be considered also a vigorous method of heating these joints. The mode of heat transfer with either method of application is primarily through conduction.

Superficial Heating by Convection

Hydrotherapy

Mode of Heat Transfer. The mode of heat transfer is primarily through convection, since in most of the hydrotherapy application the water is moved, achieving agitation, so that after the layer of water in contact with the skin has cooled off it is removed and replaced by another layer of higher temperature. Water has a high specific heat and therefore great heat-carrying capacity.

Technique of Application. For total immersion, hydrotherapy is usually done in a whirlpool bath. The water is usually agitated. The Hubbard tank, in its special configuration, allows exercising of arms and legs, with the buoyancy of the water eliminating the effects of gravity. The agitators in turn allow cleansing of wounds such as decubiti. However, the entire equipment has to be sterilized after such a procedure. This includes the agitator, which may be difficult to sterilize.[143] Special wading tanks and therapeutic pools are available where ambulation is possible with elimination of the force of gravity.

Temperature Distribution. The temperature distribution produces the highest temperature at the skin, with a rapid drop-off unless the core temperature is elevated and an artificial fever produced.

Dosimetry. With total body immersion most of the temperature regulatory mechanisms of the body are disabled. An exchange from the skin to the surrounding environment by infrared radiation and sweating and convective cooling can occur only around the part that is not immersed. Panting, unlike its action in the dog, is not very effective in man. In contrast to normal circumstances, the skin vasodilatation response to heating does not serve to transfer heat from the core to the outside, but rather picks up more heat from the surrounding water bath. Therefore it is advisable under these circumstances to monitor the oral temperature. Such monitoring should occur with total body immersion at water temperatures above 100°F (37.8°C). Usually water temperatures above 105°F (40.6°C) are not used. For partial immersion, for instance of a limb, temperatures up to 115°F (46.1°C) are applied.

Moist Air Cabinet

The moist air cabinet may apply heat to a part or to the entire body using water vapor–saturated air that is thermostatically controlled and blown over the patient. The recommended temperatures are the same as for Hubbard tank therapy. The possibilities of raising body core temperature also exist in this application.

Contrast Bath

A contrast bath produces hyperemia by alternating submersion in hot water and in cold water. The hot water is kept at a temperature between 105° and 110°F (40.6° and 43.3°C) and the cold water is between 59° and 68°F (15° and 20°C). This method has been used to treat rheumatoid arthritis of the fingers, feet, and ankles,[182, 214, 281] resulting in subjective relief of pain and stiffness. Hyperemia may be produced by submersing the affected part in hot water for ten minutes, then in cold water for one minute, followed by cycles of four minutes in hot water and one minute in cold water, until a total of 30 minutes has elapsed.

Fluidotherapy

Mode of Heat Transfer and Technique of Application. The heat transfer occurs by convection. Thermostatically controlled hot air is blown through a pad of finely divided solids, e.g., glass beads.[21, 143] This produces a dry, warm semifluid mixture into which hand, foot, or part of the extremity can be immersed. The sterilization of the particles can be obtained by an auxiliary 300 watt heater that is used in addition to the 200 watt heater in the air line. In this application the skin stays dry; heat exchange through sweating can occur.

Temperature Distribution. It must be assumed that the highest temperatures are found in the most superficial tissues, as in any type of convective heat therapy applied to part of the body.[22] Borrell, when he applied fluidotherapy at 118°F (47.8°C), observed temperature increases of 16.2°F (9°C) in the capsules of the small joints of the hands and feet. He compared these temperature increases with those obtained by mild application of heat with a dip method of paraffin wax and with the water bath treatment at 102°F (32.9°C). He found with these two methods smaller temperature increases in the joints. However, the conclusion that therefore fluidotherapy is a more effective heating agent seems not to be warranted by the experimentation, since the application of heat at higher water bath temperatures or with immersion paraffin technique is also likely to produce higher temperatures in the joint. It is more likely that the joint temperatures will depend in this case not so much on the modality as on the temperature at which the modality is applied.

The following will not deal with total body hypothermia; only local cold application for therapeutic purposes will be discussed. This type of cold application is also frequently called cryotherapy. The rationale for the use of cryotherapy is primarily based on physiologic changes that have been documented and supported by a few clinical studies. The details of these studies are reviewed elsewhere.[142]

PHYSIOLOGIC AND THERAPEUTIC EFFECTS, INCLUDING CLINICAL STUDIES

The physiologic and therapeutic effects in conjunction with some clinical studies form the rationale for the use of cold in (1) muscle spasm and spasticity, (2) mechanical trauma, (3) burns, (4) pain relief, and (5) arthritides.

The Use of Cold in Muscle Spasm and Spasticity

Physiologically, muscle tone and spasticity and muscle spasm seem to be reduced by an effect on the muscle spindle itself, provided that the muscle temperature is lowered.[63, 175, 190, 201]

These physiologic observations are consistent with a documented reduction of spasticity and muscle clonus in patients (Fig. 13–64).[122, 208, 209]

Knutsson[123] found that not only was the clonus abolished, but that the strength of the protagonist, freed from the influence of the hyperreflexic antagonist, was enhanced by more than 50 per cent in 11 of 29 cases. It is important to note that Miglietta[191] documented that the clonus disappeared only if the

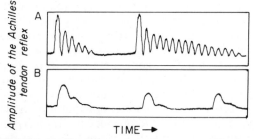

FIGURE 13–64. Effect of cooling on amplitude of ankle clonus recorded by photomotograph, (A) before and·(B) after 20 minutes of cold application with water at 13°C in a spinal-cord-injured patient (Petajan, R. H., and Watts, N.: Effect of cooling on the triceps surae reflex. Am. J. Phys. Med., 41:240–251, 1962).

muscle temperature was lowered. Miglietta, as well as Hartviksen,[93] also demonstrated that the effect on the muscle temperature as well as on the spasticity lasted for a long period of time. The reason is that the insulating fat layer with the vasocontraction slowed down the rewarming of the muscle from the outside, and because of the vasoconstriction the rewarming from the inside was also delayed. This is in contrast to the quick reversal of the temperature elevation with heating, where the increased blood flow rapidly cools the muscle. Thus the effect of the reduction on the muscle spasticity can be used for therapeutic purposes for range-of-motion exercises and for skill-training such as ambulation without interference of the spasticity. Temperatures that reduce spasticity do not affect sensory feedback to such a degree[142] that skill-training would be grossly interfered with. In addition, cooling may also affect the gamma fibers, the nerve conduction through the peripheral nerve, both sensory and motor, and the transmission of the nerve impulses through the myoneural junction, but the sensitivity of these structures to the lower temperature is significantly less than that of the spindles; therefore, it is questionable how much the effect on these structures and their function contributes to the relief of spasticity.

Muscle spasms secondary to underlying joint or skeletal pathology or nerve root irritation are relieved by the same mechanism.

Use of Cold in Muscle Re-education

Studies by Knutsson and Mattsson[124] and Urbscheit and Bishop[255] assessed the effect of cooling on both the H response and the tendon jerk. These authors showed that initially there was an increase of the H response as a result of increase of facilitation of the alpha motor neuron when cold was applied to the skin. Both Hartviksen[93] and Miglietta[191] showed also that when the H response was facilitated the clonus was increased. On continuous cooling the tendon jerk decreased as the muscle temperature dropped.[191] These findings are summarized elsewhere,[142] and they suggest that cooling of the skin alone may increase spasticity, clonus, and tendon jerk. This probably is produced reflexly through excitation through the exteroceptors of the skin. On the other hand, cooling of the muscle reduces the spasticity and muscle tone. These findings can be considered a basis for facilitation technique.[34] These techniques use ice massage of the skin over the muscle whose function should be enhanced as part of a muscle re-education effort.

Use of Cold in Mechanical Trauma

Cold applied in acute but not severe trauma such as sprains produces desirable effects by vasoconstriction, which in turn reduces swelling and bleeding. Pain may be reduced directly through an effect on the sensory endings and pain fibers or by relieving muscle spasm. Indirectly it may be reduced by prevention of the swelling and bleeding. Pain also may be reduced indirectly by relieving muscle spasm. The vasoconstriction is produced reflexly via the sympathetic fibers and also by direct effect on the blood vessels by lowering the temperature.[208] Only Matsen[183] and Marek[180] found, contrary to the above, that in experimental fractures swelling was increased by cold application. However, Matsen's measured differences in swelling were not statistically significant. Schmidt's work[226] supported the traditional view; he reduced edema by application of ice and gel packs.

The physiologic effect of cold application on mechanical trauma has been confirmed in a clinical study by Basur et al.,[13] who treated ankle sprains. Both in the control group and in the patients treated with ice compression, bandages were used. Exact outcome measures were not used. In more serious injuries, Moore and Cardea[194] found a reduction of compartment pressures in the anterior, lateral, and posterior compartments of the leg. However, this study was not well-controlled, since the treated group received not only ice application but also an intermittent compression program. Schaubel[225] found in post-surgical cases a reduction of swelling as indicated by the reduction of need for cast splitting and also by reduction of pain as indicated by lesser usage of prn narcotics and sedatives.

Use of Cold in Burns

Zitowitz and Hardy[289] in animal experiments and Shulman[239] in patients with burns

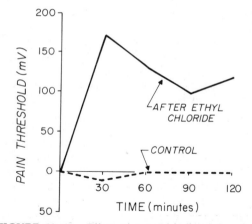

FIGURE 13–65. Effect of a pain induced by ethyl chloride spray on the pain threshold of normal human subjects (Parsons, C. M., and Goetzl, F. R.: Effect of induced pain on pain threshold. Proc. Soc. Exp. Biol. Med., 60:327–329, 1945).

showed that immediate ice application reduced the effect of the burns only if required therapy was applied shortly after the thermal trauma. If it was applied late, it retarded healing or aggravated the tissue damage.

Use of Cold as an Analgesic

Cryotherapy can not only relieve pain indirectly by reducing painful spasms, spasticity, or swelling from trauma or inflammatory reaction, but cold can also be used as a counterirritant to relieve pain.[201] The experimental findings in which cold application to any part of the body increased the pain threshold when stimulating the tooth pulp can be explained either on the basis of the gate theory of Melzack and Wall[185] or by the production of endorphins (Fig. 13–65).

Use of Cold in Arthritis

The benefit from cold application to a joint with inflammatory reaction or to the inflamed bursa is due in part to the vasoconstriction with reduction of edema. Pain is indirectly relieved in this way, and also by direct effect on the nerve fibers. The application of ice to joints has been popularized by findings of Harris and McCroskery.[92] They showed that destructive enzyme activity such as that of collagenase was significantly lowered at 30° to 35°C, yet Wright and Johns[283, 284] and Bäcklund and Tiselius[11] clearly demonstrated by objective measurement that joint stiffness in patients with rheumatoid arthritis was increased by cold application and decreased by heat application. The subjective complaints of joint stiffness correlated highly with the objective measurements. Experimental studies in arthritis as performed by Schmidt et al.[226] showed variable results of heat and cold application depending on the experimental methodology and especially depending on the mode of producing the joint inflammatory reaction. Clinical studies in man unfortunately are all poorly controlled, with questionable outcome measurements. However, there seems to be a consensus that if painful joints are cooled enough, pain will be reduced because the pain threshold is elevated.[202] Kirk and Kersley[122] found that when heat and cold were compared in a small number of cases of rheumatoid arthritis, both modalities improved pain and stiffness.

Similarly, Landon[131] found in 117 patients with low back pain an improvement by both modalities. However, as measured by the length of hospital stay, the acute cases stayed for a shorter period in the hospital when treated with heat as compared with cold, whereas in the chronic pain patients the hospital stay was shorter when they were treated with cold. No differences between the hospital stay in patients treated with heat or cold were observed if he did not differentiate between acute and chronic cases.

TECHNIQUES OF COLD APPLICATION

The most commonly used technique of application is by melting ice together with water. The temperature of this mix is 32°F (0°C). The part may be treated by immersion in this ice water, or compresses may be used as applied to other parts of the body that cannot be easily submersed. Also, terry cloth dipped in water with ice shavings, then rung out and applied rapidly, is used for cooling larger portions of the body. Finally, ice massage has been used, moving a block of ice over the surface to be cooled. The result of any one of these applications is a rapid drop of skin temperature and a much slower reduction of muscle temperature. The slowness of the drop of the muscle temperature depends largely on the thickness of fat. From the experiments shown in Figures 13–66 to 13–69, it becomes apparent that if

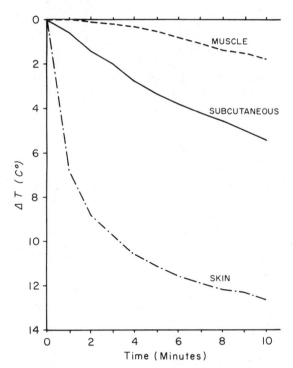

FIGURE 13–66. Change of skin. subcutaneous, and muscle temperatures during topical (thigh) ice application in a person with less than 1 cm of subcutaneous fat (Lehmann, J. F., and de Lateur, B. J.: Therapeutic heat. *In* Lehmann, J. F. (Ed.): Therapeutic Heat and Cold, 3rd Ed. Baltimore, Williams and Wilkins, 1982).

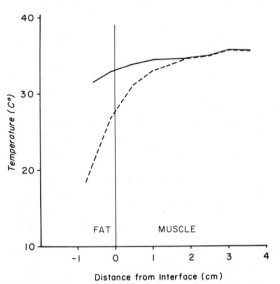

FIGURE 13–67. Temperature distribution before (solid line) and after (dashed line) topical (thigh) application for 10 minutes in a person with less than 1 cm of subcutaneous fat (Lehmann, J. F., and de Lateur, B. J.: Therapeutic heat. *In* Lehmann, J. F. (ed.): Therapeutic Heat and Cold, 3rd Ed. Baltimore, Williams and Wilkins, 1982).

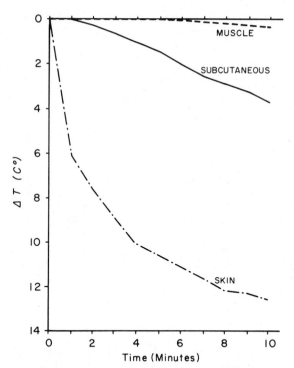

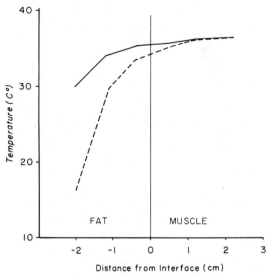

FIGURE 13–68. Change of skin, subcutaneous, and muscle temperatures during topical (thigh) ice application in a person with greater than 2 cm of subcutaneous fat (Lehmann, J. F., and de Lateur, B. J.: Therapeutic heat. *In* Lehmann, J. F. (Ed.): Therapeutic Heat and Cold, 3rd Ed. Baltimore, Williams and Wilkins, 1982).

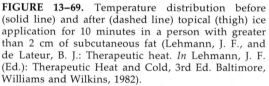

FIGURE 13–69. Temperature distribution before (solid line) and after (dashed line) topical (thigh) ice application for 10 minutes in a person with greater than 2 cm of subcutaneous fat (Lehmann, J. F., and de Lateur, B. J.: Therapeutic heat. *In* Lehmann, J. F. (Ed.): Therapeutic Heat and Cold, 3rd Ed. Baltimore, Williams and Wilkins, 1982).

the muscle is to be cooled — to reduce spasticity, for instance — it will take at least 10 minutes to begin to cool the muscle in a thin individual and probably half an hour to do the same in a more obese person. Clinically one can best judge whether a desirable effect is obtained by checking, for instance, in case of spastic calf muscles, the ankle jerk. The therapeutic effect is achieved when the clonus or the tendon jerk is abolished. In other joints of the body, the decreased resistance to rapid motion will indicate that relief of spasticity is obtained. Short cooling with such a technique as ice massage affects only the skin and is frequently used for muscle re-education as described. In this case facilitation of the alpha–motor neuron occurs only when the skin is cooled without significantly cooling the musculature.

Once the muscle is cooled enough to relieve spasticity, this effect usually lasts long enough to be of therapeutic value. When cooling is applied in trauma it should be applied early before substantial swelling and hemorrhage have developed. This can be done with simultaneous compression of the injured part. This type of cooling is usually extended for 4 to 6 hours by renewing ice packing or adding ice to the water bath. Once swelling and bleeding are prevented and are not likely to recur, further cooling serves no purpose. Lundgren et al.[177] have shown that cooling over an excessive period of time may retard healing. They showed that the retardation of wound healing seems to be secondary to the vasoconstriction. Sympathectomy in experimental animals prevented this retardation of wound healing.

Evaporative cooling spray is done by spraying the skin with ethyl chloride from a distance of 1 m with a stroking motion.[18] Chlorofluoromethanes have been used[251] to replace the more flammable ethyl chloride. This type of cooling produces pain relief as a counterirritant via the mechanism described above.

Newer modalities of cold application use chemicals in an envelope that can be broken within the package to react with another agent to produce an endothermal reaction. These packs are not as effective and not as safe as the conventional methods of cooling, since the temperature they develop is poorly controlled and if the outer envelope is broken the chemicals in contact with the skin may be irritating.

Refrigeration units used as cold applicators must be very well thermostatically controlled to prevent frostbite.[278, 279]

COMPARISON BETWEEN THERAPEUTIC EFFECTS OF HEAT AND COLD[142]

From the review of the literature on effects of heat and cold it becomes apparent that in many cases similar effects are obtained between the two ends of the temperature spectrum. In other cases, cold does the opposite of that which heat application will produce. There are a number of reactions in which heat and cold produce similar effects. Muscle spasm secondary to underlying joint or skeletal pathology can be effectively reduced by either modality. In this case it is often necessary to break the vicious circle continuing the painful muscle spasm. In upper motor neuron lesions with spasticity, cold is very effective in reducing the spasticity, an effect that lasts long enough to be of therapeutic value. While heat may also reduce spasticity, this effect is of very short duration, since the muscle tone is rapidly restored by the fact that the blood flow to the musculature is increased, cooling the heated tissue.

Pain may be reduced by both modalities if it is secondary to muscle spasms. The pain threshold also seems to be elevated by direct effect of both heat and cold on the free nerve endings and of the pain-killing fibers.

Other reactions show a different behavior when the tissues are exposed to heat or cold. The blood flow is increased with heat application and decreased after cold application. Therefore the tendency to bleed is increased with heat application and decreased with cold application. Edema resulting from trauma is increased with heat application and most literature references claim it is decreased in its development by cold application. Swelling associated with inflammatory reactions shows the same behavior. Burns are aggravated by heat application, but the tissue damage is reduced with cold application immediately following the thermal trauma. Joint stiffness, as objectively measured, is decreased with heat application and increased with cold application.

THE CLINICAL USE OF HEAT AND COLD IN VARIOUS CONDITIONS

In the following section examples of some of the usage of heat and cold therapy in common clinical conditions will be discussed. It should be remembered that therapeutic heat and cold are not curative in these disease entities, but are a valuable adjunct when properly used in conjunction with other treatment. The other treatment procedures may include not only other physical therapy such as immobilization, stretch, and exercise, but also medications and surgical procedures.

It is essential for successful therapeutic application of these modalities that the correct diagnosis first be made. The local condition to be treated is assessed and a judgment is made as to whether or not it is treatable with heat or cold. The localization of the pathological process is clearly identified and correspondingly the modality is selected. It is essential that there is clear understanding of what physiologic effect can be achieved, and finally it is equally important that the application be done with appropriate techniques.

THE TREATMENT OF MUSCLE SPASMS AND/OR MUSCLE PAIN

Skeletal Muscle[186]

Skeletal muscle spasms, often associated with a significant amount of pain, are often observed secondary to other pathology. Muscle spasm and guarding may occur as a result of intervertebral disc protrusion with or without nerve root irritation. In this type of condition, relaxation of the painful muscle spasm can be achieved by the use of various heat modalities. Specifically, shortwave diathermy can be applied either with induction coil applicators or with condenser pads. Treatment should occur on a once- or twice-daily basis for 20 to 30 minutes. The advantage of shortwave diathermy is that it is capable of heating musculature itself as well as skin and subcutaneous tissues, and thus this application may have an effect directly on the spindle mechanism in addition to a muscle relaxation triggered reflexly through excitation of exterocepters of the skin. For a more limited area of muscle spasm, specially designed induction coils like the International Medical Electronics (IME) applicator, the monode, as well as microwave applicators, can be used.

The relaxation of such muscle spasm can also be achieved by superficial heating agents including hot packs, such as Hydrocollator packs, or radiant heat application with the heat lamp or the heat cradle. Applications should be for a period of 20 to 30 minutes. With these modalities the muscle relaxation is achieved primarily through reflexes by heating the skin. Muscle spasm can also be relieved by cold application in the form of ice packs or ice massage. The objective is to cool the musculature and decrease the muscle spasm via reducing the spindle sensitivity. That implies that ice application probably should be continued for more than 10 minutes. The clinical study of Landon[131] on 117 patients with low-back pain showed that heat and cold application were equally effective. However, there seemed to be a difference between acute and chronic conditions. In the acute conditions heat application reduced the hospital stay as compared with ice application. In chronic conditions, ice was more effective in reducing the hospital stay than was heat application. It should be noted that neither in the application of shortwaves nor in superficial heating agents is the underlying pathology such as disc protrusion affected at all. The treatment is symptomatic in order to reduce the painful muscle spasm. In contrast to the use of superficial heat, one should not use just brief superficial ice application without cooling the muscle, since this would lead to facilitation of the alpha–motor neuron discharges.[255] Secondary muscle spasm due to underlying joint pathology can be treated in the same fashion as described above.

In the acute or subacute phases of such joint diseases as rheumatoid arthritis, if heat is applied, the intent is not to heat the joint but just to relieve the secondary symptomatology. Therefore in joints covered with relatively little soft tissue such as knee, ankle, small joints of hands and feet, and the elbow, shortwave or microwave diathermy applications are frequently undesirable. Vigorous ultrasound treatment is contraindicated in such joints.

In myofibrosis or so-called trigger points, local application of both heat and cold as described can be used. In addition, the use of ultrasound in low to medium dose applied to the painful area has been found to be clinically effective. In all the above-mentioned conditions as follow-up to heat therapy, a deep sedative massage often enhances the subjective well-being of the patient. In the case of myofibrositis more vigorous massage, sometimes in the form of friction massage, seems to be more effective.

In tension states with electromyographically documented increase of muscle activity, the discomfort and pain can be relieved by heat application either by shortwave diathermy or by superficial heat application with radiant heat or hot packs. In these cases the heat application should be followed with deep sedative massage. This treatment is also used in conjunction with biofeedback to relieve the muscle tension.

The muscle soreness often called "spasm" in poliomyelitis responds very well to Kenny hot packs. Repeated packing of this type not only reduces the pain and soreness but also may eliminate to a large degree any need for analgesic drugs.

In all these cases where heat or cold may be applied it is likely that these applications produce pain relief not only by reducing the muscle tension, but also through direct effect on the nerve fibers that transmit pain and on free nerve endings in the tissues.[48] There also is good evidence that these modalities may represent a counterirritant and would reduce pain as explained on the basis of the gate theory.[185, 202]

Smooth Muscle

Exaggerated peristalsis leads to cramping of the smooth musculature of the gastrointestinal tract and pain. These painful cramps are frequently observed in gastrointestinal upsets. The discomfort and the peristalsis can be reduced by superficial heat application in the form of hot packs or a hot water bottle to the abdominal wall. Also, the electric heating pad can be used with proper precautions. This leads to a measurable reduction of the peristalsis.[19, 72, 193] The reduction of the cramps is associated with reduction of blood flow to the mucous membranes of the gastrointestinal tract and reduction of hydrochloric acid secretion in the stomach. The mechanism is reflex responses triggered by the heat receptors of the skin. Cold application to the abdominal wall does just the opposite of the heat application and aggravates the patient's condition.

Similarly, menstrual cramps respond well to superficial heat application.

CONTRACTURES

In the treatment of contractures in general it is essential to selectively heat the fibrous tissues that limit motion. It is essential that the temperatures be brought close to tolerance levels. It is also important for success that mobilization of the joint or other structures be done by stretch or range of motion exercise immediately after heat application or, if possible, during heat application.

Fibrous Muscular Contractures

In fibrous contracture of the musculature it is desirable to heat the musculature evenly throughout and to elevate the temperature to tolerance levels while stretching the muscles.[42] The ideal heating modalities for this purpose are microwaves applied with direct contact applicators, preferably operating at a frequency of 915 MHz for 30 minutes. This modality is most effective if there is a diffuse fibrosis of the muscle. If the skin can be cooled at the same time, subcutaneous fat heating is essentially prevented. The temperature distribution that is achieved is shown in Figure 13–34. Skin cooling becomes even more important if the subcutaneous fat layer is greater than 1 cm. There is some limited evidence that this type of therapy is effective (Fig. 13–70). If microwaves are not available for this purpose the best alternative is to use shortwave induction coil applicators. However, uniform muscle heating cannot be achieved in this fashion; only the more superficial musculature will be heated selectively. If, for instance, due to electrical burns, a fibrous strand within the musculature produces the contracture, ultrasound would be the better heating modality, since it selectively heats such tissues. Application for at least 10 minutes would be necessary per field, best combined with simultaneous static stretching.

Joint Contractures

The treatment of joint contractures — whether the result of shortening of the capsular or periarticular tissues or of thickening and scarring of the synovium by a rheumatic

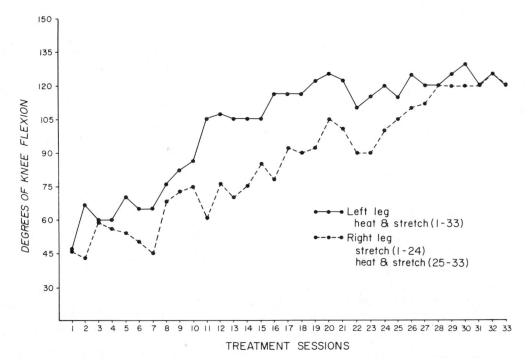

FIGURE 13–70. The degrees of knee flexion due to residual elongation of the right and left rectus femoris muscles before each treatment session (de Lateur, B. J., Stonebridge, J. B., and Lehmann, J. F.: Fibrous muscular contractures: treatment with a new direct contact microwave applicator operating at 915 MHz. Arch. Phys. Med. Rehabil., 59:488–490, 1978).

TABLE 13–7. GAIN IN RANGE OF MOTION AFTER ULTRASONIC AND MICROWAVE TREATMENT

Gain	Treatment	
	Ultrasound	Microwaves
Forward flexion	27.4° ± 2.3°*	16.1°
Abduction	32.6° ± 2.5°	21.2° ± 2.1°
Rotation	45.4° ± 2.8°	17.3° ± 4.0°

*Standard error of the mean.

From Lehmann, J. F., Erickson, D. J., Martin, G. M., and Krusen, F. H.: Comparison of ultrasonic and microwave diathermy in the physical treatment of periarthritis of the shoulder. Arch. Phys. Med. Rehabil., 35:627–634, 1954.

process, the result of limitation of the joint range due to ligamentous and capsular tightness associated with degenerative joint disease, or the result of trauma or prolonged immobilization of the joint — is always the same. However, it is important that a careful clinical evaluation of the patient be done to rule out any persisting acute or subacute process or, in degenerative joint disease of the hip, for instance, a limitation of the range of motion resulting from bony spurs. In any one of these cases the treatment involves selective heating of the contracted tissues, capsules, ligaments, and scarred synovium, raising the temperatures to maximally tolerated levels in conjunction with the use of either simultaneous or immediately applied stretch, range-of-motion exercises, or other joint mobilization techniques. This type of approach would aggravate any persistent inflammatory reaction and would be totally ineffective in the presence of bony spurs limiting the motion.

In all joints covered with a significant amount of soft tissue, the modality of choice is ultrasound, usually applied with a multiple field technique at relatively high dosage using stroking technique. Ultrasound can also be used for small joints such as the interphalangeal joints of the fingers, toes, and the metacarpophalangeal or metatarsophalangeal joints. However, these joints also can be effectively heated by application of shortwave, microwave, or paraffin wax using the immersion method. In larger joints with little soft tissue cover such as the elbow or the knee, the alternative to heating with ultrasound would be using induction coil applicators, including wrap-around coils for shortwave diathermy, as second choice.

A controlled clinical study of periarthritis of the shoulder[150] has shown that ultrasound is more effective than microwaves in gaining range of motion, since microwaves alleviate only the secondary muscle spasms (Table 13–7). Similarly, in a controlled clinical study it was shown that in patients with hip fractures treated with insertion of Richard's screws, the gain in range of motion with ultrasound was greater than with infrared application, and the ambulatory potential of the patients improved (Table 13–8). Other studies had similar results. Hintzelmann[104, 105] found (Fig. 13–71) that in chronic ankylosing spondylitis ultrasound treatment to the costovertebral joints combined with deep breathing exercises increased chest expansion and vital capacity. No control subjects were presented in this study. Pain relief was an associated benefit. There is no reason why this type of treatment could not be repeated frequently. Other clinical studies are reviewed elsewhere.[143]

Skin

In scleroderma contractures may primarily be produced by the tightness of the skin rather than by the periarticular structures. The contracture most frequently involves the hands early, limiting the range of motion at interphalangeal and metacarpophalangeal joints. Also, ischemic necrosis of the finger tips is observed. Ultrasound[254] has been used for this condition in conjunction with stretch and range-of-motion exercises. Also, temporary healing of the sores of the finger tips has been observed. However, since there was no controls and since the ultimate course of the disease was not changed, this is a condition in which ultrasound is of suggested value only. An alternative to the treatment of this condition is the use of the paraffin bath with either the dip or immersion method. Also

TABLE 13–8. COMPARISON OF AMOUNT OF CHANGE IN RANGE OF MOTION AFTER ONE WEEK OF TREATMENT*

	Ultrasound			Infrared				
	N	Mean	S.D.	N	Mean	S.D.	t	p
Hip								
Flexion	15	21.67	9.7	15	5.40	11.4	4.057	0.01
Extension	15	10.40	8.2	15	−3.20†	7.7	4.503	0.01
Abduction	15	6.33'	7.4	15	−1.67†	5.6	3.225	0.01
Adduction	15	9.67	6.6	15	−1.20†	6.0	4.567	0.01
External Rotation	14	12.86	7.9	15	0.20	7.9	4.178	0.01
Internal Rotation	14	10.93	7.6	15	−1.60†	8.8	3.965	0.01
Knee								
Flexion	15	18.33	14.9	15	10.33	13.3	1.498	0.20
Extension	15	3.60	3.9	15	−3.47†	4.8	4.259	0.01

*Ultrasound and infrared groups compared using independent samples method.
†When the mean is expressed as a negative value, range of motion has been lost during treatment.
From Lehmann, J. F., Fordyce, W. E., Rathbun, L. A., Larson, R. E., and Wood, D. H.: Clinical evaluation of a new approach in the treatment of contracture associated with hip fracture after internal fixation. Arch. Phys. Med. Rehabil., 42:95, 1961.

treatment with shortwave diathermy and microwave could be tried.

Joint contractures as a result of superficial scars, for instance due to electrical burns,[18] are usually treated with ultrasound in conjunction with exercise and stretch.

Dupuytren's Disease

Dupuytren's disease is a contracture of the palmar fascia of unknown, probably in part genetic, origin. The nonsurgical treatment of the fibrous contracture of the palmar fascia is mostly done with ultrasound (Fig. 13–72).

Peyronie's Disease

Peyronie's disease is a condition associated with sclerosing lesions in the tunics of the corpora cavernosa of the penis, the septum, and Buck's fascia. Induration interferes with complete erection and often produces a lateral curvature of the penis. Patients complain of pain ·and interference with intercourse. The condition is self-limited, with resolution in approximately four years.[272] It is also associated with Dupuytren's contractures in 10 per cent of the cases. The condition has been treated with ultrasound at an intensity

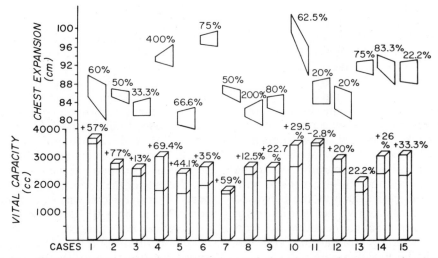

FIGURE 13–71. Chest expansion and vital capacity before and after ultrasound treatment of patient with ankylosing spondylitis (Hintzelmann, U.: Ultraschalltherapie rheumatischer Erkrankungen. Dtsch. Med. Wochenschr., 72:350, 1947; 74:869, 1949).

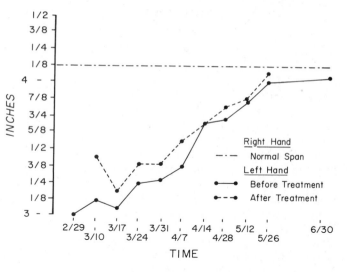

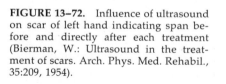
FIGURE 13–72. Influence of ultrasound on scar of left hand indicating span before and directly after each treatment (Bierman, W.: Ultrasound in the treatment of scars. Arch. Phys. Med. Rehabil., 35:209, 1954).

of approximately 1.5 w/cm² with stroking technique over a period of 5 minutes. Several authors[50, 103, 119, 173, 234] suggest that daily treatments may reduce the time to resolution. Subjectively patients noted better filling during erection and more satisfactory intercourse, with relief of erectile pain. No control studies are available, however.

JOINT STIFFNESS AND PAIN

Joint Stiffness in Collagen Diseases

Stiffness and discomfort, especially in the morning, are common bothersome symptoms of patients with rheumatoid arthritis and other collagen diseases. Wright and Johns[118, 283, 284] and Bäcklund and Tiselius[11] were able to produce an objective measurement of joint stiffness and found a high correlation between measured stiffness and complaints on the part of the patient. They also found that heat as well as corticosteroids measureably reduced the joint stiffness. Cold application aggravated it. Heat was applied with superficial heating modalities. Clinically both radiant heat and a hot tub bath are commonly used for this purpose. Modalities that selectively heat joints are usually not used in this condition, since it is frequently associated with activity of the rheumatoid process in the joint. For small joints in hands and feet, whirlpool bath or the mild heat application with the dip method of paraffin application is used. The use of im-

mersion of small joints, i.e., hands and feet, in a water bath may be useful, but temperatures should not exceed 105° F (40.6° C) to produce a mild effect. If total immersion in a Hubbard tank or in a tub is used, it is equally important to limit the temperature to less than 102° F (38.9° C) and assure avoidance of artificial fever by taking oral temperatures. Immersion of the limbs in the water eliminates most of the forces of gravity by buoyancy, and therefore range of motion exercises can be performed simultaneously with less pain and greater ease. Finally, for relief of stiffness in hands and feet the contrast bath is used. The measured benefit of this application is a very marked increase in blood flow to the part.[182]

If superficial heat application is used in the form of radiant heat, the heat lamp is used but can cover only a limited number of joints. In more generalized stiffness the heat cradle or double baker is recommended.

In spite of the fact that Johns and Wright[118] and Bäcklund and Tiselius[11] showed that joint stiffness is measurably increased by cold application, ice application to joints to relieve stiffness has been advocated. The suggestion to use ice has been based both on the fact that it numbs pain and on the findings of Harris and McCroskery[92] that the activity of destructive enzymes such as collagenase is reduced. Controlled clinical studies of enzyme activity or joint stiffness are not available, not even of medication schedules, which makes questionable any conclusion on therapeutic effectiveness in a disease such as rheumatoid arthritis.[207]

Reflex Sympathetic Dystrophy Including Shoulder-Hand Syndrome and Sudeck's Atrophy

In the shoulder-hand syndrome, pain and joint stiffness can be treated in the same fashion as joint contractures in other conditions.[18, 129, 199, 258, 277] However, this type of therapy, which includes the selective heating of periarticular structures in combination with stretch and exercise to increase range of motion, has to be appropriately integrated with other therapeutic regimens. If sympathetic (that is, stellate) ganglion blocks are used, it is essential that the physical therapy with heat, stretch, and mobilization exercise follow the block immediately. Woeber[277] has also advocated treatment of the sympathetic outflow with ultrasound. Woeber claimed that ultrasound exposure of the sympathetics gave results similar to those obtained by stellate ganglion block. However, the study was not controlled. It is also important that this type of therapy be given in conjunction with therapeutic measures to reduce swelling; this would include elevation of the limb for postural drainage, manual or mechanical massage, and elastic wrapping, especially of fingers, from distal to proximal, and active exercise of the wrapped hand above heart level.

EPICONDYLITIS, BURSITIS, AND TENOSYNOVITIS

In acute calcific bursitis, such as is commonly found in the subdeltoid or subacromial bursa, there is acute pain due to swelling pressure within the content of the bursa and an inflammatory reaction. Selective heating of the bursa is therefore contraindicated. Ice application may greatly alleviate the acute pain, especially if used in conjunction with removal of the bursal content and injection of hydrocortisone preparations combined with a local anesthetic. Since this condition occurs frequently in combination with calcific tendinitis of the supraspinatus or biceps tendons and also is associated with tight capsules that limit the range of motion of the shoulder joint, treatment in the chronic stage is with ultrasound in conjunction with the corresponding stretch and range of motion exercises. There is no evidence, however, that large calcium deposits in the bursa, which may mechanically interfere with motion by impinging upon the greater tuberosity of the humerus or coracoacromial ligament, are more readily resolved with ultrasound treatment. As a matter of fact, it has been demonstrated that spontaneous resolution of the calcium deposit occurs as frequently with as without ultrasound.[5, 14, 285] In the rare instance of calcium deposits large enough to mechanically interfere with motion, surgical removal may be the only effective therapy.

As in the subacromial or subdeltoid bursa, closed sacks lined with cellular membranes resembling synovium are found in other localities to facilitate motion of tendons and muscles over bony prominences. Local pain and nonspecific inflammation are found as a result of friction or repeated trauma. Common sites of this type of bursitis include, in addition to the subdeltoid bursa, the olecranon, the trochanteric, the anserine, and several bursae in the patellar area. Treatment is as described under subdeltoid bursa. However, in these locales ice may be used. Often injection of local anesthetics in combination with hydrocortisone preparations and with superficial heating and immobilization are preferred. Important are rest and removal of the irritating factors. In all bursitis the local therapy is used combined with systemic application of anti-inflammatory agents such as butazolidine and indomethacin.[257]

In lateral epicondylitis, or tennis elbow, there is an inflammatory reaction in the area of the common origin of the extensor tendon upon the lateral epicondyle of the humerus. In the acute stage, treatment should be primarily that of rest and splinting combined with ice application. If pain persists, superficial heat application may be useful. Mild shortwave diathermy administration could also be used. This treatment is often combined with injection of hydrocortisone preparations and of a local anesthetic. Ultrasound selectively raises the temperature of the common tendon of origin and the extensor aponeurosis. However, ultrasound is contraindicated in the acute stage but may be helpful in the presence of prolonged pain, especially when the patient is unable or unwilling to follow the prescribed regimen of immobilization. If in such cases ultrasound is used in the chronic stage it should be given in low dosage, approximately 0.5 w/cm².

Tenosynovitis is treated in similar fashion if it occurs as an overuse injury.[257]

FIGURE 13–73. Compartment pressure changes in mm Hg (plotted as mean and range) after distal tibial fracture in 10 patients treated conventionally. Horizontal axis represents days after fracture. Shaded area represents range of normal values obtained from uninjured legs (Moore, C. D., and Cardea, J. A.: Vascular changes in leg trauma. South. Med. J., 70: 1285–1286, 1977).

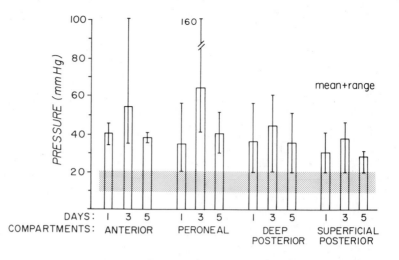

TRAUMA

Surgical Trauma and Fractures

In major trauma such as in surgical procedures leading to subsequent casting, Schaubel[225] found that cold application materially reduced the necessity for recasting due to swelling. He treated 207 cases with cooling and compared the results obtained in 312 cases without ice application. With ice application the necessity of splitting the cast was reduced from 42.3 per cent to 5.3 per cent. Unfortunately, because of the nonuniformity of the surgical procedures and the presenting pathology, further clinical studies will be needed to confirm the results. The procedures included knee surgery, surgery of the foot, and the hip, fractures, tendon repair, bone grafts, osteotomy, fusions, and others.

Schaubel also found that the requirement for narcotics to produce pain relief was markedly decreased when ice was applied. Moore and Cardea[194] found in fractures of the distal tibia and fibula measured increases in the anterior, lateral, superficial posterior, and deep posterior compartments. Five patients were treated conventionally and five patients were treated with the application of a water-cooled jacket that also produced intermittent compression. These authors observed a rapid return of the compartment pressures to normal as compared with the conventional treatment (Figs. 13–73 and 13–74). There is only one contradictory study, which is by Matsen et al.[183] They found that local cooling in femoral fractures of rabbits increased edema. However, the differences of the results were not statistically significant.

FIGURE 13–74. Compartment pressure changes in mm Hg (plotted as range and mean) during prototype boot application in five patients. Horizontal axis represents days after fracture. Shaded area represents range of normal values obtained from uninjured legs (Moore, C. D., and Cardea, J. A.: Vascular changes in leg trauma. South. Med. J., 70:1285–1286, 1977).

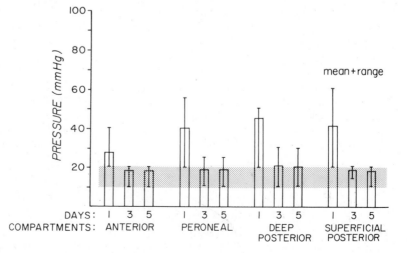

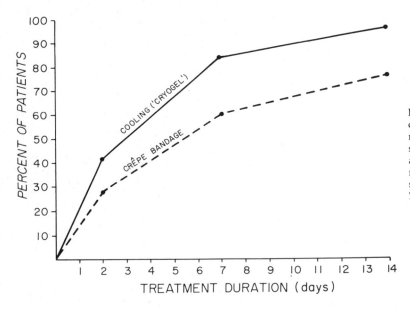

FIGURE 13–75. Percentage recovery at various stages of treatment with cooling and compression (Basur, R. L., Shepherd, E., and Monzas, G. L.: A cooling method in the treatment of ankle sprains. Practitioner, 216:708–711, 1976).

Mechanical

Minor trauma such as sprains have also been treated with cold application in order to produce vasoconstriction with reduction of swelling and bleeding. Basur et al.[13] treated 60 patients with ankle sprains without evidence of bone trauma. Two groups were compared. One group of patients was treated with compression bandages only. The other received additional ice therapy. They found that recovery of function occurred earlier in the group treated with ice (Fig. 13–75).

Marek et al.[180] treated post-traumatic edema by mild cooling, and Jezdinský[117] observed no inhibitory effect on the development of edema. In fact, he found a tendency toward increase in edema after cold application. However, the standard procedure for such minor injuries usually combines cold application, compression, elevation, and immobilization. It must be remembered, however, that this application of ice should be extended only over a period long enough to prevent the swelling and the bleeding. Usually this can be accomplished with repeated ice packing for several hours, whereas prolonged ice application over more than one day may retard healing.[257]

Thermal

Shulman[239] confirmed the results of animal experimentation by Zitowitz and Hardy[289] that in superficial burns the ice pack application relieved pain and reduced the extent of redness and blistering if ice application oc-

curred early after the thermal injury. These authors recommended that cooling be continued for several hours, and packs were reapplied if pain recurred after discontinuation of cold application. His findings were confirmed by Demling et al.[43] In addition, Demling pointed out that timing of the ice application after thermal injury is critical. In his experiments he found that cold treatment beginning two minutes after the burn did not decrease edema formation and did impair resorption.

INFLAMMATION ASSOCIATED WITH INFECTIONS

Furuncles and Other Skin Infections

The time-honored way to treat such superficial skin infections as isolated folliculitis, furuncles, carbuncles, and paronychia is with hot soaks or hot pack application with the intent to increase hyperemia and speed up abscess formation (''pointing''), pus evacuation, and healing. Obviously this method of treatment, while commonly used, is just an adjunct to other therapy.

Chronic Pelvic Inflammatory Disease

In chronic pelvic inflammatory disease the pelvic diathermy applied with vaginal or rectal electrodes is capable of selectively heating this area, with full control of the temperature in the tissue surrounding the internal electrode. Treatment of this type will increase blood flow and vascularity and thus assist the resolution of the process. Prior to the availability of antibiotics, Krusen et al.[126, 127, 217] found that in 86.5 per cent of a series of 37 patients with chronic pelvic inflammatory disease the cultures became negative and remained so. An additional benefit may be derived from the therapy in that the poor vascularity in the inflamed tissues may prevent adequate antibiotic levels from reaching this area, a situation that potentially could be improved by the increase in vascularity and blood flow. In the acute stage of the disease, vigorous therapy with internal electrodes is contraindicated. Abscess formation and perforation of the tubal abscess, for instance, could be precipitated. Therefore only chronic pelvic inflammatory disease should be treated, and it is imperative to start with short exposure at relatively low temperatures. The temperature and time of exposure may then be gradually increased as tolerated.

VASCULAR DISEASE

Peripheral Arterial Insufficiency

Peripheral arterial insufficiency is commonly the cause of arteriosclerosis and commonly found in the lower extremities. Heat application above the level of the lesion has resulted in increased blood flow below the level of the lesion. However, the measurements used to document the increase in flow may have been responsive primarily to skin blood flow change. There is no documentation that the muscle blood flow is also increased.[2] Erdman[67] used shortwave diathermy to the pelvic area to achieve the increase in vascularity in the lower extremity in normal subjects. Significantly increasing the temperature in the deep tissues below the level of the lesion is contraindicated. The increase in metabolic demand without the ability to increase the blood flow to fulfill this demand may lead to tissue necrosis.

Peripheral Venous Insufficiency and Varicose Ulcers

Dyson et al.[55, 58] showed in a controlled study that ultrasound improves the rate of healing of varicose ulcers (see Fig. 13–60). Dyson used an ultrasonic frequency of 3 MHz with average intensities of 1 w/cm². Some of the applications were pulsed, with a 20 per cent duty cycle. The duration of the pulses was 2 msec. The treatment was applied primarily to the edge of the healing ulcer with a commercial gel coupling medium. Treatments were repeated three times a week for a minimum of four weeks.

Pressure Sores

Decubiti resulting from vascular occlusion due to pressure in patients with loss of sensation or obtunded consciousness have been conventionally treated in the Hubbard tank. This therapy is especially helpful, since cleansing of the undermined edges can be readily obtained by the use of agitators. Water additives such as detergents and antibacterial agents, e.g., Betadine, have been advocated. It is most important to recognize that this treatment can be considered only as an adjunct to pressure relief and surgical debridement and repair through plastic surgery.

Ultrasound has also been tried as described in varicose ulcer therapy; however, there is no clinical study available demonstrating any evidence that the therapy is of value.

Thrombophlebitis

In superficial thrombophlebitis one adjunct to therapy may be the application of hot packs and/or hot moist packs or the heat cradle with resulting relief of inflammation and discomfort.

Raynaud's Disease

In Raynaud's disease, the digital arteries respond excessively to vasospastic stimuli producing the characteristic bilateral symmetrical pallor and cyanosis of the skin of the digits followed by redness. The attack is precipitated usually by cold and relieved by warmth. Abnormalities of the sympathetic nervous system seem to play a role. A number of authors[23, 247, 277] have advocated ultrasound application locally and to the sympathetics in an attempt to reduce the manifestations of the disease. Their empirical clinical findings seem to confirm this. However, more controlled clinical investigations will be necessary. The treatment for Raynaud's phenomenon was similar.

PAIN SYNDROMES

In the preceding discussion, it has been shown that heat or cold application may relieve pain in many conditions either by a direct influence on pain fibers or free nerve endings or secondarily by relieving the painful conditions, such as inflammation, muscle spasm, and others. Ultrasound has been used specifically with two painful conditions: the painful amputation neuroma and postherpetic pain. In both cases it has been documented that the peripheral nerve embedded in myofascial interfaces is selectively heated, and thus pain sensation could be altered.

Specifically in amputation neuromas it is most important first to assess whether the pain actually originates in the amputation neuroma and to assure that one does not deal with a painful phantom limb resulting from other causes. If it is a local amputation neuroma that is irritated due to scarring, treatment should be with ultrasound applied over a very small field with relatively high intensities, with the intent to decrease the nerve function. While there is no clear statistical evidence that this treatment is effective, clinical observations suggest its usefulness and in the absence of any side effects it may be tried before surgical revision is considered.

The treatment of postherpetic pain is based on the same assumption and, since this is a condition difficult to deal with, a trial is worthwhile even though it is based purely on a clinical, empirical basis. In this case the involved peripheral nerve should be treated.

MISCELLANEOUS

There are a number of conditions in which ultrasound has been of suggested value empirically, and in the absence of side effects ultrasound could be given a trial.

In plantar warts[32, 121] a relatively high dosage of ultrasound is applied to the limited area of the wart on a daily basis. Since the plantar warts represent a difficult problem and ultrasound has no significant side effects in this application, a trial with this therapy may be worthwhile. Unlike ionizing radiation this type of radiation can be repeated, and unlike surgery it does not produce scars.

Superficial radiant heat is also sometimes used as part of good nursing care, especially in paralyzed individuals, to dry out superficial lesions that occur with moisture accumulation in the perineal area. In this case it is most important that the heat application be very mild to prevent superficial burns.

In summary, while the various modes of heat and cold application can be used in many conditions, they are considered only an adjunct to proper therapy, but an adjunct that can significantly improve the therapeutic results and accelerate restoration to normal.

REFERENCES

1. Abramson, D. I.: Physiologic basis for the use of physical agents in peripheral vascular disorders. Arch. Phys. Med. Rehabil., 46:216–244, 1965.
2. Abramson, D. I., Bell, Y., Tuck, S., Jr., Mitchell, R., and Chandrasekharappa, G.: Changes in blood flow, oxygen uptake and tissue temperatures produced by therapeutic physical agents: III. Effect of indirect or reflex vasodilatation. Am. J. Phys. Med., 40:5–13, 1961.
3. Abramson, D. I., Burnett, C., Bell, Y., Tuck, S., Jr., Rejal, H., and Fleischer, C. J.: Changes in blood flow, oxygen uptake and tissue temperature produced by therapeutic physical agents: I. Effect of ultrasound. Am. J. Phys. Med., 39:51–62, 1960.
4. Addington, C. H., Osborn, C., Swartz, G., Fischer, F. P., Neubauer, R. A., and Sarkees, Y. T.: Biological effects of microwave energy at 200 mc. Biological Effects of Microwave Radiation. Proc. 4th Ann. Tri-Service Conf. on the Biological Effects of Microwave Radiation. New York, Plenum Press, 1961, vol. 1, pp. 177–186.
5. Aldes, J. H., and Klaras, T.: Use of ultrasonic radiation in the treatment of subdeltoid bursitis with and without calcareous deposits. West. J. Surg., 62:869, 1954.
6. Anderson, T. P., Wakim, K. G., Herrick, J. F., Bennett, W. A., and Krusen, F. H.: An experimental study of the effects of ultrasonic energy on the lower part of the spinal cord and peripheral nerves. Arch. Phys. Med., 32:71–83, 1951.
7. Ardan, N. I., Janes, J. M., and Herrick, J. F.: Changes in bone after exposure to ultrasonic energy. Minn. Med., 37:415–420, 1954.
8. Ardan, N. I., Janes, J. M., and Herrick, J. F.: Ultrasonic energy and surgically produced defects in bone. J. Bone Joint Surg., 39A:394–502, 1957.
9. Bach, S. A.: Biological sensitivity to radiofrequency and microwave energy. Fed. Proc., 24(Suppl. 14):S-22–S-26, 1965.
10. Bach, S. A., Luzzio, A. J., and Brownell, A. S.: Effects of radio-frequency energy on human gamma globulin. Proc. 4th Ann. Tri-Serv. Conf. on the Biological Effects of Microwave Radiation, 1:117–133, 1960.
11. Bäcklund, L., and Tiselius, P.: Objective measurement of joint stiffness in rheumatoid arthritis. Acta Rheum. Scand., 13:275–288, 1967.
12. Barth, G., and Bülow, H. A.: Zur Frage der

Ultraschallshadigung jugendlicher Knochen. Strahlentherapie, 79:271–280, 1949.

13. Basur, R. L., Shephard, E., and Mouzas, G. L.: A cooling method in the treatment of ankle sprains. Practitioner, 216:708–711, 1976.

14. Bearzy, H. J.: Clinical applications of ultrasonic energy in treatment of acute and chronic subacromial bursitis. Arch. Phys. Med. Rehabil., 34:228, 1953.

15. Bergmann, L.: Der Ultraschall und seine Anwendung in Wissenschaft und Technik. Stuttgart, S. Hirzel Verlag, 1949.

16. Berkson, J.: A statistically precise and relatively simple method of estimating the bio-assay with quantal response, based on the logistic function. J. Am. Stat. Assoc., 48:565, 1953.

17. Bickford, R. H., and Duff, R. S.: Influences of ultrasonic radiation of temperature and blood flow in the human skeletal muscle. Circ. Res., 1:134, 1953.

18. Bierman, W.: Ultrasound in the treatment of scars. Arch. Phys. Med. Rehabil., 35:209, 1954.

19. Bisgard, J. D., and Nye, D.: The influence of hot and cold application upon gastric and intestinal motor activity. Surg. Gynecol. Obstet., 71:172–180, 1940.

20. Born, H.: Zur Frage der Absorptionsmessungen im Ultraschallgebiet. Zeitschrift Phys., 120:383, 1943.

21. Borrell, R. M., Henley, E. J., Ho, P., and Hubbell, M. K.: Fluidotherapy: evaluation of a new heat modality. Arch. Phys. Med. Rehabil., 58:69–71, 1977.

22. Borrell, R. M., Parker, R., Henley, E. J., Masley, D., and Repinecz, M.: Comparison of in vivo temperatures produced by hydrotherapy, paraffin wax treatment, and fluidotherapy. Phys. Ther., 60:1273–1976, 1980.

23. Buchtala, V.: The present state of ultrasonic therapy. Br. J. Phys. Med., 15:3, 1952.

24. Cameron, B. M.: Experimental acceleration of wound healing. Am. J. Orthod., 3:336–343, 1961.

25. Carpenter, R. L.: Experimental radiation cataracts induced by microwave radiation. Proc. 2nd Tri-Serv. Conf. Biologic Effects Microwave Energy. Rome Air Dev. Center, Air Res. and Dev. Command, Rome, N.Y., ASTIA Doc. AD-131–477, July, 1958, p. 146.

26. Carpenter, R. L., Biddle, D. K., and van Ummerson, C. A.: Annual report of work in progress at Tufts University. January, 1958.

27. Carpenter, R. L., Biddle, D. K., and van Ummerson, C. A.: Progress report. Investigator's Conf. Biol. Effects of Electronic Radiating Equipment. Rome Air Dev. Center, Air Res. and Dev. Command, Rome, N.Y., ASTIA Doc. AD-214693, January, 1959, p. 12.

28. Carstensen, E. L., Li, K., and Schwan, H. P.: Determination of the acoustic properties of blood and its components. J. Acoust. Soc. Am., 25:286–289, 1953.

29. Chan, A. K., Sigelmann, R. A., and Guy, A. W.: Calculations of therapeutic heat generated by ultrasound in fat-muscle-bone layers. IEEE Trans. Biomed. Eng. BME, 21:280–284, 1973.

30. Chan, A. K., Sigelmann, R. A., Guy, A. W., and Lehmann, J. F.: Calculation by the method of finite differences of the temperature distribution in layered tissues. IEEE Trans. Biomed. Eng. BME, 20:86–90, 1973.

31. Chater, B. V., and Williams, A. R.: Platelet aggregation induced in vitro by therapeutic ultrasound. Thromb. Haemost., 38:640–651, 1977.

32. Cherup, N., and Bender, L. E.: Treatment of plantar warts with ultrasound. Arch. Phys. Med. Rehabil., 43:371, 1962.

33. Child, S. Z., Vives, B., Fridd, C. W., Hare, J. D., Linke, C. A., Davis, H. T., and Carstensen, E. L.: Ultrasonic treatment of tumors — II. Moderate hyperthermia. Ultrasound Med. Biol., 6:341–344, 1980.

34. Clendenin, M. A., and Szumski, A. J.: Influence of cutaneous ice application on single motor units in humans. Phys. Ther., 57:166–175, 1971.

35. Cole, K. S., and Cole, R. H.: Dispersion and absorption in dielectrics. I. Alternating current characteristics. J. Chem. Phys., 9:341, 1941.

36. Constable, J. D., Scapicchio, A. P., and Opitz, B.: Studies of the effects of diapulse treatment of various aspects of wound healing in experimental animals. J. Surg. Res., 11:254–257, 1971.

37. Cook, H. F.: A comparison of the dielectric behavior of pure water and human blood at microwave frequencies. Br. J. Appl. Phys., 3:249, 1952.

38. Crockford, G. W., and Hellon, R. F.: Vascular responses of human skin to infrared radiation. J. Physiol., 149:424–432, 1959.

39. Daily, L., Jr., Wakim, K. G., Herrick, J. F., and Parkhill, E. M.: The effects of microwave diathermy on the eye. Am. J. Physiol., 155:432, 1948.

40. Daily, L., Jr., Wakim, K. G., Herrick, J. F., Parkhill, E. M., and Benedict, W. L.: The effects of microwave diathermy on the eye of the rabbit. Am. J. Ophthalmol., 35:1001–1017, 1952.

41. de Lateur, B. J., Lehmann, J. F., Stonebridge, J. B., Warren, C. G., and Guy, A. W.: Muscle heating in human subjects with 915 MHz microwave contact applicator. Arch. Phys. Med. Rehabil., 51:147–151, 1970.

42. de Lateur, B. J., Stonebridge, J. B., and Lehmann, J. F.: Fibrous muscular contractures: treatment with a new direct contact microwave applicator operating at 915 MHz. Arch. Phys. Med. Rehabil., 59:488–490, 1978.

43. Demling, R. H., Mazess, R. B., and Wolberg, W.: The effect of immediate and delayed cold immersion on burn edema formation and resorption. J. Trauma, 17:56–60, 1979.

44. Dietzel, F., and Kern, W.: Kann hohes mütterliches Fieber beim Kind auslösen. Originalmitteilungen ist ausschliesslich der Verfasser verantwortlich. Naturwissenschaften, 2:24–26, 1971.

45. Dietzel, F., and Kern, W.: Kann hohes mütterliches Fieber Missbildungen beim Kind auslösen? Geburtshilfe Frauenheilkd., 31:1074–1079, 1971.

46. Dodt, E., and Zotterman, Y.: Mode of action of warm receptors. Acta Physiol. Scand., 26:345–357, 1952.

47. Dodt, E., and Zotterman, Y.: The discharge of specific cold fibres at high temperatures (the paradoxical cold). Acta Physiol. Scand., 26:358–365, 1952.

48. Douglas, W. W., and Malcolm, J. L.: The effect of

localized cooling on conduction in cat nerves. J. Physiol., 130:53–71, 1955.

49. Doyle, J. R., and Smart, B. W.: Stimulation of bone growth by shortwave diathermy. J. Bone Joint Surg., 45-A:15–24, 1963.

50. Dugois, P.: The action of ultrasonics in Peyronie's diseases, accelerated by alpha-chymotrypsin. Lyon Med., 93:238, 1961.

51. Dunn, F., and Frizzell, L. A.: Bioeffects of ultrasound. In Lehmann, J. F. (Ed.): Therapeutic Heat and Cold, 3rd Ed. Baltimore, Williams and Wilkins, 1982.

52. Dussick, C. T., Fritch, D. J., Kyraizidan, M., and Sear, R. S.: Measurement of articular tissues with ultrasound. Am. J. Phys. Med., 37:160–165, 1958.

53. Dyson, M.: Alterations in fibroblast activity in response to ultrasound. Presented 9/11/81 at "An International Symposium on Therapeutic Ultrasound," Winnipeg, Manitoba, Canada.

54. Dyson, M.: The effect of ultrasound on the rate of wound healing and the quality of scar tissue. Presented 9/11/81 at "An International Symposium on Therapeutic Ultrasound," Winnipeg, Manitoba, Canada.

55. Dyson, M., Franks, C., and Suckling, J.: Stimulation of healing of varicose ulcers by ultrasound. Ultrasonics, 14:232–236, 1976.

56. Dyson, M., and Pond, J. B.: The effect of pulsed ultrasound on tissue regeneration. Physiotherapy, 56:136–142, 1970.

57. Dyson, M., Pond, J. B., Joseph J., and Warwick, R.: The stimulation of tissue regeneration by means of ultrasound. Clin. Sci., 35:273–285, 1968.

58. Dyson, M., and Suckling, J.: Stimulation of tissue repair by ultrasound: a survey of the mechanisms involved. Physiotherapy, 64:105–108, 1978.

59. Dyson, M., Woodward, B., and Pond, J. B.: Flow of red blood cells stopped by ultrasound. Nature, 232:572–573, 1971.

60. Edwards, M. J.: Congenital defects in guinea pigs. Arch. Pathol., 84:42–48, 1967.

61. Edwards, M. J.: Influenza, hyperthermia, and congenital malformation. Lancet, 1:320–321, 1972.

62. Edwards, M. J., Mulley, R., Ring, S., and Wanner, R. A.: Mitotic cell death and delay of mitotic activity in guinea-pig embryos following brief maternal hyperthermia. J. Embryol. Exp. Morphol., 32:593–602, 1974.

63. Eldred, E., Lindsley, D. E., and Buchwald, J. S.: The effect of cooling on mammalian muscle spindles. Exp. Neurol., 2:144–157, 1960.

64. Ely, T. S., Goldman, D., Hearon, J. Z., Williams, R. B., and Carpenter, H. M.: Heating Characteristics of Laboratory Animals Exposed to Ten Centimeter Microwaves. Bethesda, Md., U.S. Nav. Med. Res. Inst.(res. Rep. Proj. NM 001–050. 13.02), IEEE Trans. Biomed. Eng., 11:123–137, 1964.

65. Emery, A. F., Stonebridge, J. B., Sekins, K. M., and Lehmann, J. F.: Experimental and numerical studies of the elevated temperatures induced in a human leg by microwave diathermy with surface cooling. Radio Science, 14(6S):297–314, 1979.

66. Engel, J. P., Herrick, J. F., Wakim, K. G., Grindlay, J. H., and Krusen, F. H.: The effect of microwaves on bone and bone marrow on adjacent tissues. Arch. Phys. Med., 31:453–461, 1950.

67. Erdman, W. J., II: Peripheral blood flow measurements during application of pulsed high-frequency currents. Am. J. Orthod., 2:196–197, 1960.

68. Evans, D. S., and Mendelssohn, K.: The physical basis of radiant heat therapy. Proc. R. Soc. Med., 38:578–586, 1945.

69. Federal Communications Commission: Rules and Regulations, vol. 2, subpart A, section 18.13, 1964.

70. Fenn, J. E.: Effect of pulsed electromagnetic energy (Diapulse) on experimental hematomas. Can. Med. Assoc. J., 100:251–254, 1969.

71. Feucht, B. L., Richardson, A. W., and Hines, H. M.: Effect of implanted metal on tissue hyperthermia produced by microwaves. Arch. Phys. Med., 30:164–169, 1949.

72. Fischer, E., and Solomon, S.: Physiological responses to heat and cold. Chapter 4, pp. 126–169. In Licht, S. (Ed.): Therapeutic Heat and Cold, 2nd Ed. Baltimore, Waverly Press, 1965.

73. Food and Drug Administration, US DHEW: Performance standard for microwave diathermy products. Fed. Reg., 40:23877–23878, 1975.

74. Fountain, F. P., Gersten, J. W., and Sengir, O.: Decrease in muscle spasm produced by ultrasound, hot packs, and infrared radiation. Arch. Phys. Med. Rehabil., 41:293–298, 1960.

75. Frizzell, L. A., and Dunn, F.: Biophysics of ultrasound. In Lehmann, J. F. (Ed.): Therapeutic Heat and Cold, 3rd Ed. Baltimore, Williams and Wilkins, 1982.

76. Gammon, G. D., and Starr, I.: Studies on the relief of pain by counterirritation. J. Clin. Invest., 20:13–20, 1941.

77. Gersten, J. W.: Changes in spinal cord thresholds following the application of ultrasound. Paper given at Fourth Annual Conference, Amer. Inst. Ultrasonics in Med., Detroit, 1955.

78. Gersten, J. W.: Effect of metallic objects on temperature rises produced in tissues by ultrasound. Am. J. Phys. Med., 37:75, 1958.

79. Gersten, J. W.: Effect of ultrasound on tendon extensibility. Am. J. Phys. Med., 34:362–369, 1955.

80. Gersten, J. W.: Ultrasonics and muscle disease. Am. J. Phys. Med., 33:68, 1954.

81. Ghietti, A.: Embriopatia da onde corte. Minerva Nipiologica, 5:7–12, 1955.

82. Ginsberg, A. J.: Pulsed shortwave in the treatment of bursitis with calcification. Int. Record Med., 174:71–75, 1961.

83. Gorodetskaya, S. F.: The effect of centimeter radiowaves on mouse fertility. Fiziol. Zh., 9:394, 1963.

84. Granberry, W. M., and Janes, J. M.: The lack of effect of microwave diathermy on rate of growth of bone of the growing dog. J. Bone Joint Surg., 45A:4:773–777, 1963.

85. Guy, A. W.: Analyses of electromagnetic fields induced in biological tissues by thermographic studies on equivalent phantom models. IEEE MTT, 19:205–214, 1971.

86. Guy, A. W.: Electromagnetic fields and relative

heating patterns due to a rectangular aperture source in direct contact with bilayered biological tissue. IEEE MTT, 19:214–223, 1971.

87. Guy, A. W., and Lehmann, J. F.: Comparative evaluation of electromagnetic diathermy modalities in 433 MHz to 2450 MHz. 21st ACEMB — Shamrock Hilton Hotel, Houston, Texas, Nov. 18-21, 1968.

88. Guy, A. W., and Lehmann, J. F.: On the determination of an optimum microwave diathermy frequency for a direct contact applicator. IEEE BME, 13:76–87, 1966.

89. Guy, A. W., Lehmann, J. F., and Stonebridge, J. B.: Therapeutic applications of electromagnetic power. Proc IEEE, 62:55–75, 1974.

90. Guy, A. W., Lin, J. C., Kramar, P. O., and Emery, A. F.: Effect of 2450-MHz radiation on the rabbit eye. IEEE Trans. Microwave Theory Tech. MTT, 23:492–498, 1975.

91. Hardy, J. D., Wolff, H. G., and Goodell, H.: Studies on pain. A new method for measuring pain threshold: observations on spatial summation of pain. J. Clin. Invest., 19:649–657, 1940.

92. Harris, E., Jr., and McCroskery, P. A.: The influence of temperature and fibril stability on degradation of cartilage collagen by rheumatoid synovial collagenase. N. Engl. J. Med., 290:1–6, 1974.

93. Hartviksen, K.: Ice therapy in spasticity. Acta Neurol. Scand., 38 (Suppl. 3):79–84, 1962.

94. Harvey, M. A. S., McRorie, M. M., and Smith, D. W.: Suggested limits of exposure in the hot tub and sauna for the pregnant woman. J. Can. Med. Assoc., 125:50–53, 1981.

95. Hayashi, S.: Der Einfluss der Ultraschallwellen und Ultrakurtzwellen auf den malignen Tumor. J. Med. Sci. Biophysics Japan, 6:138, 1940.

96. Hedenius, P., Odeblad, E., and Wahlstroem, L.: Some preliminary investigations on the therapeutic effect of pulsed shortwaves in intermittent claudication. Curr. Ther. Res., 8:317–321, 1966.

97. Heller, J. H.: Reticuloendothelial Structure and Function. New York, The Roland Press Co., 1960, Chap. 12.

98. Hensel, H.: Temperaturempfindung und intracutane Wärmebewegung. Pflügers Arch., 252:165–215, 1950.

99. Hensel, H., and Zotterman, Y.: Quantitative Beziehungen zwischen der Entladung einzelner Kaltefasern und der Temperatur. Acta Physiol. Scand., 23:291–319, 1951.

100. Herrick, J. F.: Temperatures produced in tissues by ultrasound: experimental study using various technics. J. Acoust. Soc. Am., 25:12–16, 1953.

101. Herrick J. F., Jelatis, D. G., and Lee, G. M.: Dielectric properties of tissues important in microwave diathermy. Fed. Proc., 9:60, 1950.

102. Herrick, J. F., and Krusen, F. H.: Certain physiologic and pathologic effects of microwaves. Elec. Eng., 72:239–244, 1953.

103. Heslop, R. W., Oakland, D. J., and Maddox, B. T.: Ultrasonic therapy in Peyronie's disease. Br. J. Urol., 39:415, 1967.

104. Hintzelmann, U.: Ultraschalltherapie rheumatischer Erkrankungen. Dtsch. Med. Wochenschr., 72:350, 1947.

105. Hintzelmann, U.: Ultraschalltherapie rheumatischer Erkrankungen. Dtsch. Med. Wochenschr., 74:869, 1949.

106. Ho, H. S., Guy, A. W., Sigelmann, R. A., and Lehmann, J. F.: Microwave heating of simulated human limbs by aperture sources. IEEE MTT, 19:224–231, 1971.

107. Hollander, J. L., and Horvath, S. M.: The influence of physical therapy procedures on the intra-articular temperature of normal and arthritic subjects. Am. J. Med. Sci., 218:543–548, 1949.

108. Horatz, K.: Erfahrungen bei der Tumorbeschallung. Ultraschall Med., 1:149–154, 1949.

109. Horvath, J.: Experimentelle Untersuchungen über die Verteilung der Ultraschallenergie in menschlichen Gewebe. Ärztliche Forsch., 1:357, 1947.

110. Howland, J. W., Thomson, R. A. E., and Michaelson, S. M.: Biomedical aspects of microwave irradiation of mammals. Biological Effects of Microwave Radiation. Proc. 4th Ann. Tri-Service Conf. on the Biological Effects of Microwave Radiation, 1:261–285, 1961.

111. Hüter, T.: Messung der Ultraschallabsorption in tierischen Geweben und ihre Abhängigkeit von der Frequenz. Naturwissenschaften, 35:285, 1948.

112. Hüter, T., and Bolt, F. H.: An ultrasonic method for outlining the cerebral ventricles. J. Acoust. Soc. Am., 23:160, 1951.

113. Hüter, T., Dyer, J., Ludwig, G. D., and Kyrazia, D.: Thresholds of damage in nervous tissues. MIT Q. Prog. Rep., October, 1950.

114. Imig, C. J., Randall, B. F., and Hines, H. M.: Effect of ultrasonic energy on blood flow. Am. J. Phys. Med., 53:100–102, 1954.

115. Imig, C. J., Thomson, J. D., and Hines, H. M.: Testicular degeneration as a result of microwave irradiation. Proc. Soc. Exp. Biol., 69:382–386, 1948.

116. Janes, J. M., Herrick, J. F., Kelly, P. J., and Peterson, L. F. A.: Long-term effect of ultrasonic energy on femora of the dog. Proc. Staff Meet. Mayo Clin., 35:663–671, 1960.

117. Jezdinský, J., Marek, J., and Ochonský, P.: Effects of local cold and heat therapy on traumatic oedema of the rat hind paw. I. Effects of cooling on the course of traumatic oedema. Acta Univ. Olomuc Fac. Med., 66:185–201, 1973.

118. Johns, R. J., and Wright, V.: Relative importance of various tissues in joint stiffness. J. Appl. Physiol., 17:824–828, 1962.

119. Kaczynski, A., Litwak, A., and Mika, T.: Remarques sur l'action de Pultrason et de la microonde dans le traitement de l'induration plastique due penis. Urol. Int., 20:236, 1965.

120. Kaplan, E. G., and Weinstock, R. E.: Clinical evaluation of diapulse as adjunctive therapy following foot surgery. J. Am. Pod. Assoc., 58:218–221, 1968.

121. Kent, H.: Plantar wart treatment with ultrasound. Arch. Phys. Med. Rehabil., 40:15–18, 1959.

122. Kirk, J. A., and Kersley, G. D.: Heat and cold in the physical treatment of rheumatoid arthritis of the knee. Ann. Phys. Med., 9:270–274, 1968.

123. Knutsson, E.: Topical cryotherapy in spasticity. Scand. J. Rehabil. Med., 2:159–163, 1970.

124. Knutsson, E., and Mattsson, E.: Effects of local cooling on monosynaptic reflexes in man. Scand. J. Rehabil. Med., 1:126–132, 1969.

125. Kottke, F. J.: Heat in pelvic diseases. *In* Licht, S. (Ed.): Therapeutic Heat and Cold, 2nd Ed. Baltimore, Waverly Press, 1965, pp. 474–490.

126. Krusen, F. H.: Physical Medicine. Philadelphia, W. B. Saunders Company, 1942.

127. Krusen, F. H., and Elkins, E. C.: Investigations in fever therapy. Arch. Phys. Ther., 20:77–84, 1939.

128. Krusen, F. H., Herrick, J. F., Leden, U., and Wakim, G.: Microkymatotherapy: preliminary report of experimental studies of the heating effect of microwaves ("radar") in living tissues. Proc. Staff Meet. Mayo Clin., 22:209–224, 1947.

129. Kuhler, E.: Der Einfluss des Ultraschalls auf das Sudeck'sche Syndrome. Strahlentherapie, 87: 575, 1952.

130. Lambert, E. H., Treanor, W. J., Herrick, J. F., and Krusen, F. H.: Comparative study of the effects of heat and ultrasound on nerve conduction. Fed. Proc., 10:78, 1951.

131. Landon, B. R.: Heat or cold for the relief of low back pain? Phys. Ther., 47:1126–1128, 1967.

132. Lehmann, J. F.: Beitrag zur Ultraschallhämolyse. Strahlentherapie, 70:533–542, 1950.

133. Lehmann, J. F.: Die Therapie mit Ultraschall und ihre Grundlagen. *In* Ergebnisse physikalischdiatetischen Therapie. Dresden, Verlag Steinkopff, 1951.

134. Lehmann, J. F.: The biophysical basis of biologic ultrasonic reactions with special reference to ultrasonic therapy. Arch. Phys. Med. Rehabil., 34:139–152, 1953.

135. Lehmann, J. F.: The biophysical mode of action of biologic and therapeutic ultrasonic reactions. J. Acoust. Soc. Am., 25:17–25, 1953.

136. Lehmann, J. F.: Ultrasound therapy. *In* Licht, S. (Ed.): Therapeutic Heat and Cold, 2nd Ed. Baltimore, Waverly Press, 1965, pp. 321–386.

137. Lehmann, J. F., and Biegler, R.: Changes of potentials and temperature gradients in membranes caused by ultrasound. Arch. Phys. Med. Rehabil., 35:287–295, 1954.

138. Lehmann, J. F., Brunner, G. D., Martinis, A. J., and McMillan, J. A.: Ultrasonic effects as demonstrated in live pigs with surgical metallic implants. Arch. Phys. Med. Rehabil., 40:483–488, 1959.

139. Lehmann, J. F., Brunner, G. D., and McMillan, J. A.: The influence of surgical implants on the temperature distribution in thigh specimens exposed to ultrasound. Arch. Phys. Med. Rehabil., 39:692, 1958.

140. Lehmann, J. F., Brunner, G. D., McMillan, J. A., Silverman, D. R., and Johnson, V. C.: Modification of heating patterns produced by microwaves at the frequencies of 2456 and 900 mc by physiologic factors in the human. Arch. Phys. Med. Rehabil., 45:555–563, 1964.

141. Lehmann, J. F., Brunner, G. D., and Stow, R. W.: Pain threshold measurements after therapeutic application of ultrasound, microwaves, and infrared. Arch. Phys. Med. Rehabil., 39:560–565, 1958.

142. Lehmann, J. F., and de Lateur, B. J.: Cryotherapy. *In* Lehmann, J. F. (Ed.): Therapeutic Heat and Cold, 3rd Ed. Baltimore, Williams and Wilkins, 1982.

143. Lehmann, J. F., and de Lateur, B. J.: Therapeutic heat. *In* Lehmann, J. F. (Ed.): Therapeutic Heat and Cold, 3rd Ed. Baltimore, Williams and Wilkins, 1982.

144. Lehmann, J. F., de Lateur, B. J., and Silverman, D. R.: Selective heating effects of ultrasound in human beings. Arch. Phys. Med. Rehabil., 47:331–339, 1966.

145. Lehmann, J. F., de Lateur, B. J., and Stonebridge, J. B.: Heating patterns produced in humans by 433.92 MHz round field applicator and 915 MHz contact applicator. Arch. Phys. Med. Rehabil., 56:442–448, 1975.

146. Lehmann, J. F., de Lateur, B. J., and Stonebridge, J. B.: Selective heating by shortwave diathermy with a helical coil. Arch. Phys. Med. Rehabil., 50:117–123, 1969.

147. Lehmann, J. F., de Lateur, B. J., Stonebridge, J. B., and Warren, C. G.: Therapeutic temperature distribution produced by ultrasound as modified by dosage and volume of tissue exposed. Arch. Phys. Med. Rehabil., 48:662–666, 1967.

148. Lehmann, J. F., de Lateur, B. J., Warren, C. G., and Stonebridge, J. B.: Heating of joint structures by ultrasound. Arch. Phys. Med. Rehabil., 49:28–30, 1968.

149. Lehmann, J. F., de Lateur, B. J., Warren, C. G., and Stonebridge, J. B.: Heating produced by ultrasound in bone and soft tissue. Arch. Phys. Med. Rehabil., 48:397–401, 1967.

150. Lehmann, J. F., Erickson, D. J., Martin, G. M., and Krusen, F. H.: Comparison of ultrasonic and microwave diathermy in the physical treatment of periarthritis of the shoulder. Arch. Phys. Med. Rehabil., 35:627–634, 1954.

151. Lehmann, J. F., Fordyce, W. E., Rathbun, L. A., Larson, R. E., and Wood, D. H.: Clinical evaluation of a new approach in the treatment of contracture associated with hip fracture after internal fixation. Arch. Phys. Med. Rehabil., 42:95, 1961.

152. Lehmann, J. F., Guy, A. W., de Lateur, B. J., Stonebridge, J. B., and Warren, C. G.: Heating patterns produced by shortwave diathermy using helical induction coil applicators. Arch. Phys. Med. Rehabil., 49:193–198, 1968.

153. Lehmann, J. F., Guy, A. W., Johnston, V. C., Brunner, G. D., and Bell, J. W.: Comparison of relative heating patterns produced in tissues by exposure to microwave energy at frequencies of 2,450 and 900 megacycles. Arch. Phys. Med. Rehabil., 43:69–76, 1962.

154. Lehmann, J. F., Guy, A. W., Stonebridge, J. B., and de Lateur, B. J.: Evaluation of a therapeutic direct-contact 915-MHz microwave applicator for effective deep-tissue heating in humans. IEEE Trans. Microwave Theory Tech. MTT, 26:556–563, 1978.

155. Lehmann, J. F., Guy, A. W., Stonebridge, J. B., and Warren, C. G.: Review of evidence for indications, techniques of application, contraindications, hazards, and clinical effectiveness of shortwave diathermy. Report No. FDA/HFK-75-1, to Office of DHEW/Public Health Service, Food and Drug Administration, 1/1/74 to 12/31/74, Contract Number FDA 74-32.

156. Lehmann, J. F., Guy, A. W., Warren, C. G., de

Lateur, B. J., and Stonebridge, J. B.: Evaluation of microwave contact applicator. Arch. Phys. Med. Rehabil., 51:143–147, 1970.

157. Lehmann, J. F., and Herrick, J. F.: Biologic reactions to cavitation, a consideration for ultrasonic therapy. Arch. Phys. Med. Rehabil., 34:86–98, 1953.

158. Lehmann, J., and Hohlfeld, R.: Der Gewebestoffwechsel nach Ultraschall und Wärmeeinwirkung. Strahlentherapie, 87:544–549, 1952.

159. Lehmann, J. F., and Johnson, E. W.: Some factors influencing the temperature distribution in thighs exposed to ultrasound. Arch. Phys. Med. Rehabil., 39:347–356, 1958.

160. Lehmann, J. F., Johnston, V. C., McMillan, J. A., Silverman, D. R., Brunner, G. D., and Rathbun, L. A.: Comparison of deep heating by microwaves at frequencies 2456 and 900 megacycles. Arch. Phys. Med. Rehabil., 46:307–314, 1965.

161. Lehmann, J. F., and Krusen, F. H.: Biophysical effects of ultrasonic energy on carcinoma and their possible significance. Arch. Phys. Med. Rehabil., 36:452–459, 1955.

162. Lehmann, J. F., Lane, C. E., Bell, J. W., and Brunner, G. D.: Influence of surgical metal implants on the distribution of the intensity in the ultrasonic field. Arch. Phys. Med. Rehabil., 39:756–760, 1958.

163. Lehmann, J. F., Masock, A. J., Warren, C. G., and Koblanski, J. N.: Effect of therapeutic temperatures on tendon extensibility. Arch. Phys. Med. Rehabil., 51:481–487, 1970.

164. Lehmann, J. F., McMillan, J. A., Brunner, G. D., and Blumberg, J. B.: Comparative study of the efficiency of shortwave, microwave and ultrasonic diathermy in heating the hip joint. Arch. Phys. Med. Rehabil., 40:510–512, 1959.

165. Lehmann, J. F., McMillan, J. A., Brunner, G. D., and Guy, A. W.: A comparative evaluation of temperature distributions produced by microwaves at 2,456 and 900 megacycles in geometrically complex specimens. Arch. Phys. Med. Rehabil., 43:502–507, 1962.

166. Lehmann, J. F., and Nitsch, W.: Uber die Frequenzabhangigkeit biologischer Ultraschallreaktionen mit besonderer Berucksichtigung der spezifischen Temperaturverteilung im Organismus. Strahlentherapie, 85:606, 1951.

167. Lehmann, J. F., Silverman, D. R., Baum, B. A., Kirk, N. L., and Johnston, V. C.: Temperature distributions in the human thigh, produced by infrared, hot pack and microwave applications. Arch. Phys. Med. Rehabil., 47:291–299, 1966.

168. Lehmann, J. F., Stonebridge, J. B., de Lateur, B. J., Warren, C. G., and Halar, E.: Temperatures in human thighs after hot pack treatment followed by ultrasound. Arch. Phys. Med. Rehabil., 59:472–476, 1978.

169. Lehmann, J. F., Stonebridge, J. B., and Guy, A. W.: A comparison of patterns of stray radiation from therapeutic microwave applicators measured near tissue-substitute models and human subjects. Radio Science, 14:271–283, 1979.

170. Lehmann, J. F., Stonebridge, J. B., Wallace, J. E., Warren, C. G., and Guy, A. W.: Microwave therapy: stray radiation, safety and effectiveness. Arch. Phys. Med. Rehabil., 60:578–584, 1979.

171. Lehmann, J. F., Warren, C. G., Wallace, J. E., and Chan, A.: Ultrasound: Considerations for use in the presence of prosthetic joints. Arch. Phys. Med. Rehabil., 61:502, 1980.

172. Levy, H.: Pulsed shortwaves in sinus and allied conditions in childhood. Western Med., 2:246, 1961.

173. Liakhovitskii, N. S.: Experience in the use of ultrasonics in the therapy of plastic induration of the penis. Urology, 25:61, 1960.

174. Linke, C. A., Lounsberry, W., and Goldschmidt, V.: Effects of microwaves on normal tissues. J. Urol., 88:303–311, 1962.

175. Lippold, O. C. J., Nicholls, J. G., and Redfearn, J. W. T.: A study of the afferent discharge produced by cooling a mammalian muscle spindle. J. Physiol., 153:218–231, 1960.

176. Lota, M. J., and Darling, R. C.: Change in permeability of the red blood cell membrane in a homogeneous ultrasonic field. Arch. Phys. Med. Rehabil., 36:282–287, 1955.

177. Lundgren, C., Muren, A., and Zederfeldt, B.: Effect of cold vasoconstriction on wound healing in the rabbit. Acta Chir. Scand., 118:1–4, 1959.

178. Madsen, P. W., and Gersten, J. W.: The effect of ultrasound on conduction velocity of peripheral nerve. Arch. Phys. Med. Rehabil., 42:645–649, 1961.

179. Maintz, G.: Tierexperimentelle Üntersuchungen uber die Wirkung der Ultraschallwellen auf die Knochenregeneration. Strahlentherapie, 82:631–638, 1950.

180. Marek, J., Jezdinský, J., and Ochonský, P.: Effects of local cold and heat therapy on traumatic oedema of the rat hind paw. III. Effects of various kinds of compresses on the course of traumatic oedema. Acta Univ. Olomuc Fac., 66:203–228, 1973.

181. Marks, J., Carter, E. T., Scarpelli, D. G., and Eisen, J.: Microwave radiation to the anterior mediastinum of the dog (II). Ohio Med. J., 57:1132–1135, 1961.

182. Martin, G. M., Roth, G. M., Elkins, E. C., and Krusen, F. H.: Cutaneous temperature of the extremities of normal subjects and of patients with rheumatoid arthritis. Arch. Phys. Med., 27:665, 1946.

183. Matsen, F. A., III, Questad, K., and Matsen, A. L.: The effect of local cooling on post fracture swelling. Clin. Orthop., 109:201–206, 1975.

184. McGee, M., and Freshman, S.: Ultrasound and stretch: a decreased range of motion. A slide-tape presentation. Health Sciences Learning Resources Center, University of Washington, 1978.

185. Melzack, R., and Wall, P. D.: Pain mechanisms: a new theory. Science, 150:971–979, 1965.

186. Mense, S.: Effects of temperature on the discharges of muscle spindles and tendon organs. Pflügers Arch., 374:159–166, 1978.

187. Menser, M.: Does hyperthermia affect the human fetus? Med. J. Australia, 2:550, 1978.

188. Merola, L. O., and Kinoshita, J. H.: Changes in the ascorbic acid content in lenses of rabbit eyes exposed to microwave radiation. Proc. 4th Ann. Tri-Service Conf. on the Biological Effects of Microwave Radiation, 1:285–291, 1961.

189. Michaelson, S. M.: Bioeffects of high frequency currents and electromagnetic radiation. *In* Leh-

mann, J. F. (Ed.): Therapeutic Heat and Cold, 3rd Ed. Baltimore, Williams and Wilkins, 1982.

190. Michalski, W. J., and Seguin, J. J.: The effect of muscle cooling and stretch on muscle spindle secondary endings in the cat. J. Physiol., 253:341–356, 1975.

191. Miglietta, O.: Action of cold on spasticity. Am. J. Phys. Med., 52:198–205, 1973.

192. Moayer, M.: Die morphologischen Veränderungen der Plazenta unter dem Einfluss der Kurzwellen-durchflutung. Tierexperimentelle Untersuchungen. Strahlentherapie, 142:609–614, 1971.

193. Molander, C. O.: Physiologic basis of heat. Arch. Phys. Ther., 22:335–340, 1941.

194. Moore, C. D., and Cardea, J. A.: Vascular changes in leg trauma. South Med. J., 70:1285–1286, 1977.

195. Morrissey, L. J.: Effect of pulsed short-wave diathermy upon volume blood flow through the calf of the leg: plethysmographic studies. J. Am. Phys. Ther. Assoc., 46:946–952, 1966.

196. Mortimer, A. J., Roy, O. Z., Taichman, G. C., Keon, W. J., and Trollope, B. J.: The effects of ultrasound on the mechanical properties of rat cardiac muscle. Ultrasonics, 16:179–182, 1978.

197. Mussa, B.: Embriopatie da cause fisiche. Minerva Nipiologica, 5:69–72, 1955.

198. Nadasdi, M.: Inhibition of experimental arthritis by athermic pulsing shortwave in rats. Am. J. Orthop., 2:105–107, 1960.

199. Newman, M. K., Kill, M., and Frampton, G.: Effects of ultrasound alone and combined with hydrocortisone injections by needle or hypospray. Am. J. Phys. Med., 37:206, 1958.

200. Oleson, J. R., and Gerner, E. W.: Hyperthermia in the treatment of malignancies. In Lehmann, J. F. (Ed.): Therapeutic Heat and Cold, 3rd Ed. Baltimore, Williams and Wilkins, 1982.

201. Ottoson, D.: The effects of temperature on the isolated muscle spindle. J. Physiol., 180:636–648, 1965.

202. Parsons, C. M., and Goetzl, F. R.: Effect of induced pain on pain threshold. Proc. Soc. Exp. Biol. Med., 60:327–329, 1945.

203. Pätzold, J., and Born, H.: Behandlung biologischer Gewebe mit gebundeltem Ultraschall. Strahlentherapie, 76:486, 1947.

204. Pätzold, J., Guttner W., and Bastir, R.: Beitrag zum Dosisproblem in der Ultraschalltherapie. Strahlentherapie, 86:298–305, 1954.

205. Paul, W. D., and Imig, C. J.: Temperature and blood flow studies after ultrasonic irradiation. Am. J. Phys. Med., 34:370–375, 1955.

206. Pauly, H., and Hug, O.: Untersuchungen über den Einfluss von Ultraschallwellen und von Wärme auf den Stoffwechsel überlebender Gewebe. Strahlentherapie, 95:116, 1954.

207. Pegg, S. M. H., Littler, T. R., and Littler, E. N.: A trial of ice therapy and exercise in chronic arthritis. Physiotherapy, 55:51–56, 1969.

208. Perkins, J. F., Li, M.-C., Hoffman, F., et al.: Sudden vasoconstriction in denervated or sympathectomized paws exposed to cold. Am. J. Physiol., 155:165–178, 1948.

209. Petajan, R. H., and Watts, N.: Effect of cooling on the triceps surae reflex. Am. J. Phys. Med., 41:240–251, 1962.

210. Pezold, F. A.: Zur Frage des Ultraschallschadens. Ultraschall Med., 4:1–28, 1952.

211. Pickering, G. W.: The vasomotor regulation of heat loss from the human skin in relation to external temperature. Heart, 16:115–135, 1932.

212. Piersol, G. M., Schwan, H. P., Pennell, R. B., and Carstensen, E. L.: Mechanism of absorption of ultrasonic energy in blood. Arch. Phys. Med., 33:327–332, 1952.

213. Pohlman, R.: Die Ultraschalltherapie. Stuttgart, Georg Thieme Verlag, 1951.

214. Polley, H. F.: Physical treatment of arthritis. In Krusen, F. H. (Ed.): Physical Medicine and Rehabilitation for the Clinician. Philadelphia, W. B. Saunders Company, 1951.

215. Rae, J. W., Jr., Herrick, J. F., Wakim, K. G., and Krusen, F. H.: A comparative study of the temperatures produced by microwave and shortwave diathermy. Arch. Phys. Med., 30:199–211, 1949.

216. Rae, J. W., Martin, G. M., Treaner, W. J., and Krusen, F. H.: Clinical experience with microwave diathermy. Proc. Staff Meet. Mayo Clin., 24:441, 1950.

217. Randall, L. M., and Krusen, F. H.: A consideration of the Elliott treatment of pelvic inflammatory disease of women. Arch. Phys. Ther., 18:283–287, 1937.

218. Rech, W., and Matthes, K.: Bericht über die medizinische Ultraschall-Arbeitstagung in Erlangen. Ultraschall Med., 1:366, 1949.

219. Reinike, A., and Alm, H.: Untersuchungen über die Tiefenwirkung der Mikrowellenbestrahlung im Bereich der Nasennebenhohlen und des Ohres. Z. Laryn. Rhinol. Otol., 35:556–566, 1956.

220. Richardson, A. W., Duane, T. D., and Hines, H. M.: Experimental lenticular opacities produced by microwave irradiation. Arch. Phys. Med., 29:765–769, 1948.

221. Romero-Sierra, C., and Tanner, J. A.: Biological effects of nonionizing radiation: an outline of fundamental laws. Ann. N.Y. Acad. Sci., 238:263–272, 1974.

222. Rosenberger, H.: Über den Wirkungsmechanismus der Ultraschallbehandlung, insbesondere bei Ischias und Neuralgien. Chirurg, 21:404, 1950.

223. Rubin, A., and Erdman, W. J.: Microwave exposure of the human female pelvis during early pregnancy and prior to conception. Am. J. Phys. Med., 38:219–220, 1959.

224. Sandler, B.: Heat and the I.U.C.D. Br. Med. J., 25:458, 1973.

225. Schaubel, H. J.: The local use of ice after orthopedic procedures. Am. J. Surg., 72:711–714, 1946.

226. Schmidt, K. L., Ott, V. R., Rocher, G., et al.: Heat, cold and inflammation. Rheumatology, 38:391–404, 1979.

227. Schroeder, K. P.: Effect of ultrasound on the lumbar sympathetic nerves. Arch. Phys. Med. Rehabil., 43:182–185, 1962.

228. Schwan, H. P.: Biophysics of diathermy. In Licht, S. (Ed.): Therapeutic Heat and Cold, 2nd Ed. Baltimore, Waverly Press, 1965, pp. 63–125.

229. Schwan, H. P., and Li, K.: Hazards due to total body irradiation by radar. Proc. I. R. E., 44:1572, 1956.

230. Schwan, H. P., and Piersol, G. M.: The absorption of electromagnetic energy in body tissues. Part

1, Biophysical aspects. Am. J. Phys. Med., 33:371–404, 1954.

231. Schwan, H. P., and Piersol, G. M.: The absorption of electromagnetic energy in body tissues. Part 2, Physiological and clinical aspects. Am. J. Phys. Med., 34:425–448, 1955.

232. Scott, B. O.: Heating of fatty tissues in a short-wave field. Ann. Phys. Med., 2:48–52, 1952.

233. Scott, B. O.: Shortwave diathermy. In Licht, S. (Ed.): Therapeutic Heat and Cold, 2nd Ed. Baltimore, Waverly Press, 1965, pp. 279–309.

234. Scott, W. W., and Scardino, P. L.: A new concept in the treatment of Peyronie's disease. South. Med. J., 41:173, 1948.

235. Sekins, K. M., de Lateur, B. J., Dundore, D., Emery, A. F., Esselman, P., Lehmann, J. F., and Nelp, W. B.: Local muscle blood flow and temperature responses to 915 MHz diathermy as simultaneously measured and numerically predicted. Submitted to Arch. Phys. Med. Rehabil., 1982.

236. Sekins, K. M., Dundore, D., Emery, A. F., Lehmann, J. F., McGrath, P. W., and Nelp, W. B.: Muscle blood flow changes in response to 915 MHz diathermy with surface cooling as measured by Xe[133] clearance. Arch. Phys. Med. Rehabil., 61:105–113, 1980.

237. Selke, O. O.: Complications of heat therapy. Am. J. Orth., 4:168–169, 1962.

238. Shealy, C. N., and Henneman, E.: Reversible effects of ultrasound on spinal reflexes. Arch. Neurol., 6:374–386, 1962.

239. Shulman, A. G.: Ice water as primary treatment of burns. J.A.M.A., 173:1916–1919, 1960.

240. Silverman, D. R.: A comparison of the continuous and pulsed shortwave diathermy resistance to bacterial infection of mice. Arch. Phys. Med. Rehabil., 45:491–499, 1964.

241. Silverman, D. R., and Pendleton, L.: A comparison on the effects of continuous and pulsed short-wave diathermy on peripheral circulation. Arch. Phys. Med. Rehabil., 49:429–436, 1968.

242. Smith, A., and Schwan, H. P.: Ultrasonic absorption and velocity of sound of cell nuclei. National Biophysics Conf., Columbus, 1957. Abstract, p. 66.

243. Smith, D. W., Clarren, S. K., and Harvey, M. A. S.: Hyperthermia as a possible teratogenic agent. J. Pediatr., 92:878–883, 1978.

244. Stillwell, D. M., and Gersten, J. W.: Effect of ultrasound on spasticity. Am. Inst. Ultrasonics in Med. Proc. 4th Ann. Conf. on Ultrasonic Therapy, 124–131, 1955.

245. Stillwell, G. K.: General principles of thermotherapy. In Licht, S. (Ed.): Therapeutic Heat and Cold, 2nd Ed. Baltimore, Waverly Press, 1965, pp. 232–239.

246. Stuhlfauth, K.: Neurological effects of ultrasonic waves. Br. J. Phys. Med., 15:10, 1952.

247. Sulzberger, M. B., Wolf, J., Witten, V. H., and Kopf, A. W.: Dermatology, Diagnosis and Treatment. Chicago, Year Book Publishers, 1961.

248. Takashima, S.: Studies on the effect of radio-frequency waves on biological macromolecules. IEEE Trans. Biomed. Eng. BME, 13:28–31, 1966.

249. Taylor, K. J. W.: Ultrasonic damage to spinal cord and the synergistic effect of hypoxia. J. Pathol., 102:41–47, 1970.

250. Taylor, R. G.: The effect of diapulse (pulsed high frequency energy) on wound healing in humans. Cited by Lehmann.[155]

251. Tennenbaum, J. I., and Lowney, E.: Localized heat and cold urticaria. J. Allergy Clin. Immunol., 51:57–59, 1973.

252. Texeira-Pinto, A. A., Nejelski, L. L., Cutler, J. L., and Heller, J. H.: The behavior of unicellular organisms in an electromagnetic field. Exp. Cell Res., 20:548–564, 1960.

253. Trojel, H., and Lebech, P. E.: Intermitterende kortbolge (Diapulse) i behandlingen af inflammatoriske underlivslidelser. Nordisk Med., 81:307–310, 1969.

254. Uchman, L. S.: Role of ultrasound in scleroderma. A preliminary report of two cases. Am. J. Phys. Med., 35:118, 1956.

255. Urbscheit, N., and Bishop, B.: Effects of cooling on the ankle jerk and H-response in hemiplegic patients. Phys. Ther., 51:983–988, 1971.

256. VanDemark, W. R., and Free, J. R.: Temperature effects. In Johnson, A. D., et al. (Eds.): The Testis, Vol. III. New York, Academic Press, Inc., 1973, pp. 233–312.

257. Vinger, P. F., and Hoerner, E. F. (Eds.): Sports Injuries, The Unthwarted Epidemic. Littleton, Mass., John Wright·PSG·Inc., 1982.

258. Wachsmuth, W.: Ultraschall bei Sudeckscher Krankheit. Ultraschall Med., Zurich, 1949.

259. Wakim, K. G.: Special review: ultrasonic energy as applied to medicine. Am. J. Phys. Med., 32:32–46, 1953.

260. Warren, C. G., Koblanski, J. N., and Sigelmann, R. A.: Ultrasound coupling media: their relative transmissivity. Arch. Phys. Med. Rehabil., 57:218–222, 1976.

261. Whyte, H. M., and Reader, S. P.: Effectiveness of different forms of heating. Ann. Rheum. Dis., 10:449–452, 1951.

262. Williams, A. R.: Intravascular mural thrombi produced by acoustic microstreaming. Ultrasound Med. Biol., 3:191–203, 1977.

263. Williams, A. R.: Release of serotonin from human platelets by acoustic microstreaming. J. Acoust. Soc. Am., 56:1640–1643, 1974.

264. Williams, A. R.: The effects of therapeutic ultrasound on platelets and the blood coagulation system. Presented 9/11/81 at "An International Symposium on Therapeutic Ultrasound." Winnipeg, Manitoba, Canada.

265. Williams, A. R., Chater, B. V., Allen, K. A., and Sanderson, J. H.: The use of β-thromboglobulin to detect platelet damage by therapeutic ultrasound in vivo. J. Clin. Ultrasound, 9:145–151, 1981.

266. Williams, A. R., Chater, B. V., Allen, K. A., Sherwood, M. R., and Sanderson, J. H.: Release of beta-thromboglobulin from human platelets by therapeutic intensities of ultrasound. Br. J. Haematol., 40:133–142, 1978.

267. Williams, A. R., Hughes, D. E., and Nyborg, W. L.: Hemolysis near a transversely oscillating wire. Science, 169:871–873, 1970.

268. Williams, A. R., and Miller, D. L.: Photometric detection of ATP release from human erythrocytes exposed to ultrasonically activated gas-

filled pores. Ultrasound Med. Biol., 6:251–256, 1980.

269. Williams, A. R., O'Brien, W. D., and Coller, B. S.: Exposure to ultrasound decreases the recalcification time of platelet rich plasma. Ultrasound Med. Biol., 2:113–118, 1976.

270. Williams, A. R., Sykes, S. M., and O'Brien, W. D., Jr.: Ultrasonic exposure modifies platelet morphology and function *in vitro*. Ultrasound Med. Biol., 2:311–317, 1976.

271. Williams, D. B., Monahan, J. P., Nicholson, W. J., and Aldrich, J. J.: Biologic effects of microwave radiation. USAF School of Aviation Medicine Report No. 55-94, Washington, 1955.

272. Williams, J. L., and Thomas, G. G.: The natural history of Peyronie's disease. J. Urol., 103:75, 1970.

273. Wilson, D. H.: Treatment of soft-tissue injuries by pulsed electrical energy. Br. Med. J., 2:269–270, 1972.

274. Wilson, D. H.: Comparison of shortwave diathermy and pulsed electromagnetic energy in treatment of soft tissue injuries. Physiotherapy, 60:309–310, 1974.

275. Wilson, D. H., Jagadeesh, P., Newman, P. P., and Harriman, D. G. F.: The effects of pulsed electromagnetic energy on peripheral nerve regeneration. Ann. N.Y. Acad. Sci., 238:575–585, 1974.

276. Wise, C. S., Castleman, B., and Watkins, A. L.: Effect of diathermy (shortwave and microwave) on bone growth on the albino rat. J. Bone Joint Surg., 31A:487–500, 1949.

277. Woeber, K.: Biological basis and application of ultrasound in medicine. Ultrasonics Biol. Med., 1:9, 1956.

278. Wolf, S. L., and Basmajian, J. V.: A rapid cooling device for controlled cutaneous stimulation. Phys. Ther., 53:25–27, 1973.

279. Wolf, S. L., and Basmajian, J. V.: Intramuscular temperature changes deep to localized cutane-ous cold stimulation. Phys. Ther., 53:1284–1288, 1973.

280. Wong, C., and Ehrlich, H. P.: A preliminary report on pulsed high frequency energy (diapulse therapy) in wound healing. Cited by Lehmann et al.[151]

281. Woodmansey, A., Collins, D. H., and Ernst, M. M.: Vascular reactions to the contrast bath in health and in rheumatoid arthritis. Lancet, 2:1350–1353, 1938.

282. Worden, R. E., Herrick, J. F., Wakim, K. G., and Krusen, F. H.: The heating effects of microwaves with and without ischemia. Arch. Phys. Med., 29:751–758, 1948.

283. Wright, V., and Johns, R. J.: Physical factors concerned with the stiffness of normal and diseased joints. Bull. Johns Hopkins Hosp., 106:215–231, 1960.

284. Wright, V., and Johns, R. J.: Quantitative and qualitative analysis of joint stiffness in normal subjects and in patients with connective tissue diseases. Ann. Rheum. Dis., 20:36–46, 1961.

285. Wulff, D.: Behandlungsergebnisse mit Ultraschall. Ultraschall Med., 7:111, 1954.

286. Zankel, H. T.: Effect of ultrasound on leg blood flow. Scientific Proc. Seventh Ann. Conf. Am. Inst. Ultrasonics in Med., August, 25, 1962, pp. 7–17.

287. Zaret, M. M., and Eisenbud, M.: Preliminary results of studies of the lenticular effects of microwaves among exposed personnel. Biological Effects of Microwave Radiation. Proc. 4th Ann. Tri-Service Conf. on the Biological Effects of Microwave Radiation, 1:293–308, 1961.

288. Zarod, A. P., and Williams, A. R.: Platelet aggregation *in vivo* by therapeutic ultrasound. Lancet, 1:1266, 1977.

289. Zitowitz, I., and Hardy, J. D.: Influence of cold exposure on thermal burns in the rat. J. Appl. Physiol., 12:147–154, 1958.

14

ULTRAVIOLET THERAPY

G. KEITH STILLWELL

PHYSICAL PRINCIPLES

Quantum theory states that the energy contained in the individual quanta is greater at higher frequencies of electromagnetic radiation (Fig. 14–1). The amount of this energy, q, is expressed (in ergs) by the equation

$$q = hv \qquad (1)$$

in which h = Planck's constant, which is 6.6236×10^{-27} erg seconds, and v = frequency of the wave emanation in waves per second. While lower quantum energies (infrared) are able only to increase the molecular and atomic motion, which is heat, the higher quantum energies can produce changes in the electronic structure of the atoms or molecules. Some ultraviolet energies may be able to separate an electron from the atom, producing an ion. The very high quantum energies of radiation at wavelengths shorter than the ultraviolet (for example, x-rays and gamma rays) may produce more drastic and irreversible effects upon the atoms and molecules. Ultraviolet may be subdivided into "far" and "near" with respect to its relationship to the visible spectrum, with the division occurring at 2900 Angstroms. More commonly it is subdivided into UV-A 3150–4000 Angstroms, UV-B 2800–3150 Angstroms, and UV-C 2000–2800 Angstroms.

When an atom absorbs a quantum of energy in the ultraviolet range, it becomes temporarily excited or activated. It then changes to a state of lesser excitation in one

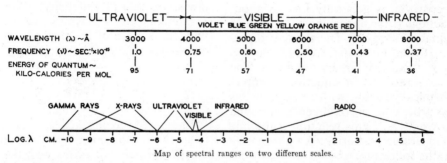

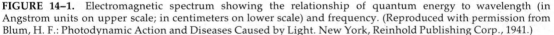

Map of spectral ranges on two different scales.

FIGURE 14–1. Electromagnetic spectrum showing the relationship of quantum energy to wavelength (in Angstrom units on upper scale; in centimeters on lower scale) and frequency. (Reproduced with permission from Blum, H. F.: Photodynamic Action and Diseases Caused by Light. New York, Reinhold Publishing Corp., 1941.)

351

or more stages, releasing (emitting) quanta of energy in the process.

The atoms of any particular element can absorb or emit only certain specific quanta of energy (that is, certain specific wavelengths of electromagnetic energy). The energy released in the process of degradation from an excited state may be transferred to another molecule, consumed in a chemical reaction or liberated as ultraviolet energy, visible light (fluorescence), or heat. Ordinarily the emitted quanta are smaller than the absorbed quanta, and some of the energy appears as heat.

Mercury vapor excited by the passage of an electric current will emit energy of several specific wavelengths, which correspond to the wavelengths that mercury vapor can absorb. These have been correlated with the several different levels of excitation that the mercury atom may possess.

The photochemical process of the absorption of a quantum is independent of oxygen and is not influenced much by temperature. Subsequent reactions may require oxygen and have a Q_{10} between 2 and 3. The reactions may be indicated by the following equations,

$$M + h\nu \longrightarrow M_r \qquad (2)$$
$$M_r + X \longrightarrow X^1 + M \qquad (3)$$
$$X^1 + O_2 \longrightarrow X_{ox} \qquad (4)$$

in which M is the substance that absorbs the quantum, $h\nu$, and becomes an activated or excited substance, M_r. M may be some substance normally present in the system or a photosensitizing drug or dye. In equation 3, M_r delivers some or all of this energy of the absorbed quantum to substance X, which becomes excited or activated as X^1. This process may actually be repeated several times through a series of molecules. However, the most that is generally known about these reactions is the absorbing substance M and the final product X_{ox}. The changes represented in equation 3 last for only a few microseconds and are largely unknown. The excited substance X^1 in equation 4 enters into a chemical reaction with oxygen in this example, producing an oxidized compound of X^1 shown as X_{ox}. This reaction is the one that is temperature sensitive. An alternative might be the following,

$$X^1 + Y \longrightarrow XY \qquad (5)$$

which does not involve oxygen but may be affected by temperature.[1, 2]

Absorption Spectra and Action Spectra

An action spectrum for a particular photochemical reaction is determined by measuring which parts of the spectrum are most effective in energizing the reaction. The action spectrum should correspond with the absorption spectrum of the substance M of equation 2. However, the absorption spectra of many of the proteins present in biologic systems are similar. The precise determination of the substance M by the relationship between action and absorption spectra may not be possible.

It is apparent that the spectrum is not sharply delimited in its photobiologic effects. As one moves from the infrared through the visible spectrum and into the ultraviolet, the quantum energy increases and the potential for photochemical reactions increases. The wavelengths that are effective in the ordinary course of events will be secondarily influenced by the following factors: (1) the wavelengths available (for example, the spectrum of sunlight as modified by passage through the earth's atmosphere); (2) the absorption or reflection of certain wavelengths at the surface of the skin, which in turn may be modified by moisture, ointments, or other substances on the skin; and (3) the thickness of the stratum corneum of the skin.

Dosage Factors

Several factors which influence the transfer of energy by radiation are of importance in ultraviolet radiation. The inverse square law states that the intensity of the radiation, I, falling on the surface, S_2, varies inversely with the square of the distance, d, between the source, S_1, and the surface:

$$I \propto \frac{1}{d^2} \qquad (6)$$

Lambert's cosine law is also applicable (Fig. 14–2). The intensity of radiation falling on the surface, S_2, varies with the cosine of the angle, a, between the incident beam and the perpendicular to the surface. In addition,

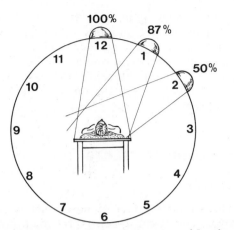

FIGURE 14–2. Graphic representation of Lambert's cosine law of energy exchange by radiation. (From Krusen, F. H.: Physical Medicine. Philadelphia, W. B. Saunders Company, 1941, p. 236.)

the reflection and scatter of radiation are more pronounced with increasingly oblique rays, and this will further decrease their effectiveness.

With the powerful sources of ultraviolet radiation used in some clinical situations, in which erythema may be produced in the skin by exposure at a distance of 30 inches for 15 seconds, *the factors of distance and time are critical and must be governed very closely*. All other factors being equal, the duration of exposure will be determined by the distance from the lamp to the part of the patient that is closest to it.

Minimal Erythema Dose (M.E.D.)

The sensitivity of the human skin to ultraviolet radiation varies considerably because of variation in the thickness of the stratum corneum and in the amount of superficial pigmentation. The dose of ultraviolet radiation that will produce, within a few hours, a minimal erythema in the average Caucasian skin is called the minimal erythema dose. For the high-pressure mercury arc in a quartz burner, this dose is usually in the order of 15 seconds of exposure at a distance of 30 inches. It is determined by observation on several subjects, usually on the volar aspect of the forearm. It is necessary to determine this dose two or three times yearly, since the ability of the quartz envelope to transmit ultraviolet emanation deteriorates with age. A very old lamp may be emitting principally heat and visible light.

The minimal erythema dose may be used as a dosage unit in the prescription of ultraviolet irradiation. It is usually possible to increase progressively the number of M.E.D.s used in each treatment of a given patient as the stratum corneum thickens and the sensitivity to ultraviolet radiation decreases. Pigmentation of the skin also influences the sensitivity to ultraviolet radiation. Brunettes are less sensitive than blondes, and reddish-blondes are more sensitive. The M.E.D. is an *average* quantity, and the dosage for an individual patient in fractions or multiples of the M.E.D. should be prescribed with respect to the probable sensitivity of this individual in relationship to average sensitivity.

Further Degrees of Erythema. The M.E.D. has also been called a first degree erythema. A second degree erythema is caused by a dose of about 2½ M.E.D. It has a latency of four to six hours, may be a little painful and subsides in two to four days. It is followed by desquamation. Third degree erythema is caused by about 5 M.E.D. and has associated edema. The latency may be as brief as two hours. It is followed by marked desquamation. Such a dose cannot, of course, be safely applied to a large part of the body surface. Fourth degree erythema, which is produced by about 10 M.E.D., is characterized in addition by the development of a superficial blister.

Precautions

Photo-ophthalmia. The eye is highly sensitive to ultraviolet radiation, and therefore the eyes of both the patient and the operator of the lamp *must be shielded* at all times. Shielding can be accomplished by the use of spectacles of ordinary glass or, in the case of the patient, of pledgets of cotton or gauze soaked in water and placed over the eyes.

In addition to conjunctivitis, keratotic changes in the cornea may occur (usually, but not always, reparable). With massive doses of ultraviolet radiation, lenticular opacities may be produced.

Other Susceptible Regions. If there is a significant difference in the distance between the source of the radiation and the various parts of the patient, excessive irradiation of the closer parts may occur. This is most likely to affect the buttocks of the prone patient or the breasts of the supine female patient. In the latter instance, it is often necessary to drape the breasts in order to be able to employ adequate doses of ultraviolet radiation to the face and upper anterior part of the chest, as in the treatment of acne.

Photosensitizing Drugs. Abnormal sensitivity to ultraviolet radiation may occur in some persons when they are taking certain chemicals. As the number and variety of drugs used in medicine increase, the incidence and variety of these cases may be expected to increase also.[3] Photosensitization to wavelengths longer than 3200 Angstroms has been reported with the use of various dyes (eosin, rose bengal, fluorescein), coal tar derivatives, and some plant materials. Lipstick cheilitis is probably related to absorption of the fluorescein dye from the lipstick into the skin of the lips.

Protective Factors. The principal protection against erythema (see the next section) is the thickness of the stratum corneum. Pigmentation is located too deeply to provide much protection, except in the Negro skin. Areas of "thin skin," for example, healed indolent ulcers, scars, and some skin grafts, are therefore more readily burned than is the rest of the surface. Such areas may be screened from the ultraviolet radiation by wet towels or dressings.

Modification of the transmission of all ultraviolet by the stratum corneum has been reported.[4] Chemical sunscreens containing light-absorbing agents may be highly effective. The most commonly used are para-aminobenzoic acid or its esters, cinnamates, salicylates, and anthranilates. They are mainly effective in blocking UV-B radiation. Opaque physical screens are also used for small areas.[5]

PHYSIOLOGIC EFFECTS

Erythema

The sunburn effect of ultraviolet is well known. The action spectrum for the production of erythema has two maxima, at 2500 Angstroms and at 2970 Angstroms. No erythema is produced by wavelengths longer than 3300 Angstroms. The spectrum of sunlight at the surface of the earth is cut off at 2900 Angstroms, and only a very small fraction of sunlight is erythemogenic. Window glass cuts off all wavelengths shorter than 3200 Angstroms and provides complete protection against sunburn (Fig. 14–3).

The primary phenomenon in the production of erythema is believed to be absorption of the specific quanta by protein(s) in the prickle cell layer of the skin. This denatures the protein and thereby damages the cells. This photochemical reaction is not affected by temperature, and the threshold time of

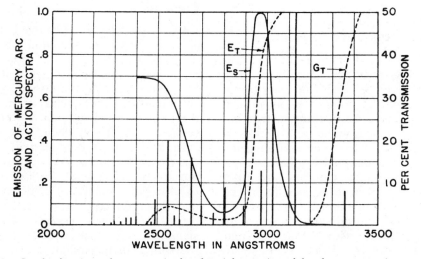

FIGURE 14–3. Graph of various phenomena in the ultraviolet portion of the electromagnetic spectrum. E_S is the action spectrum of the erythema of sunburn (after Coblentz and Stair, corrected for relative number of quanta). E_T is the curve for transmission of human epidermis 0.08 mm thick, cleared to diminish scattering (after Lucas). G_T is the transmission through window glass. Vertical lines at the bottom show the position and relative intensity of lines of "hot quartz" mercury-vapor lamp. Ordinate units for action spectrum and energies of mercury lines arbitrarily chosen. (Reproduced with permission from Blum, H. F.: Radiation: Photophysiologic and photopathologic processes. *In* Glasser, O.: Medical Physics. Chicago, Year Book Publishers, Inc., 1944, vol. 1, pp. 1145–1157.)

exposure is not affected by temperature. The damaged cells release a vasodilator substance at a rate that *is* sensitive to temperature, and this substance diffuses to the subdermal level, where it causes vasodilatation. The latent period for this process may be several hours. The chemical mediators of the erythema from UV-A, UV-B, and UV-C may not be the same.[6, 7] There may be a variety of entities within the UV-A spectrum. Combining the erythema action spectrum and the solar spectrum suggests that the peak wave length for solar erythema is 3060 Angstroms. However, because of the relatively large amount of UV-A in sunlight, about 15 per cent or more of solar erythemogenesis is due to UV-A. As a sequel to the erythema the stratum corneum thickens, and this change provides some protection from the erythemogenic effects of subsequent exposure.

Pigmentation

Melanogenesis. While this phenomenon, also known as "delayed tanning," is not usually apparent until about 72 hours after the exposure to ultraviolet radiation, the process begins earlier. It involves an increase in the number of *functioning* melanocytes and in their size and melanogenesis and an increased transfer of melanosomes from the melanocytes to the keratinocytes. The major action spectrum is the same as for sunburn, although it can be induced by shorter or longer wavelengths.

Immediate tanning begins within a few minutes, reaching a maximum within an hour if exposure continues. It is believed to involve photo-oxidation of preformed melanin along with changes in the melanocytes and an increase in the transfer of melanosomes to the keratinocytes and a change in their distribution there. The action spectrum extends from 3000 Angstroms to 4400 Angstroms, with a maximum at 3400 Angstroms. Little of the emission of a mercury vapor arc is in this spectral region.

Antirachitic Effect

The irradiation of ergosterol and some closely related sterols will lead to the formation of antirachitic substances. In human skin, this reaction occurs as the conversion of 7-dehydrocholesterol to vitamin D_3.[8] The action spectrum for the antirachitic effect is compatible with the absorption spectrum for 7-dehydrocholesterol, which extends from about 2400 to 3000 Angstroms with a maximum at 2830 Angstroms. This maximum corresponds to a minimum in the action spectrum for erythema. It has been proposed that most of the energy at this wavelength is absorbed in superficial layers of the skin where the vitamin D is produced and that it does not penetrate deeply enough to participate in the production of erythema.

Diseases Caused by Light

Chemical Photosensitivity. There are many photosensitizing chemicals in the modern environment, particularly medications and cosmetics.[3, 6] The abnormal responses are classified as phototoxic or photoallergic.

In phototoxicity the radiation may be absorbed by the sensitizing chemical or a compound derived from it, leading to subsequent oxidative reactions with cellular damage as a result. The sensitizing chemical may at the end of the process be bound so that it is no longer sensitizing, or it may return to its original ground state. The reaction resembles sunburn, and theoretically anyone can react.[6] Psoralens and chlorpromazine have been studied most.

Photoallergy is mediated by immunologic processes and is uncommon.[9, 10] The product of the irradiated photosensitizing chemical may combine with a protein carrier to form an antigen; or an irradiated protein molecule may be rendered able to combine with the photosensitizer. There is an incubation period subsequent to the exposure to the chemical, and repeated exposures to the radiation are required. The reaction may extend beyond the irradiated area. Generally the active spectrum is in the UV-A range.[10]

Other Diseases. Blum[1] divided these into diseases caused by irradiation of wavelengths shorter or longer than 3200 Angstroms. Parrish et al.[6] list the following conditions (pp. 149–151):

(a) Persistent light reactivity
(b) Actinic reticuloid
(c) Polymorphous light eruption
(d) Solar urticaria
(e) Porphyrias and other endogenous photosensitization syndromes
(f) Melasma (chloasma) and ephelides (freckles)

There is, in addition, an established role in the etiology of basal cell and squamous cell carcinoma and malignant melanoma.[1, 2, 6] This is mainly an effect of UV-B and may be enhanced by phototoxic substances. Ultraviolet probably also enhances or accelerates the process of aging in human skin.[6]

METHODS OF ULTRAVIOLET IRRADIATION

Therapeutic Devices

Mercury-Vapor Arcs. Mercury vapor enclosed in a quartz envelope is activated by an electric current. The arc emits a continuous spectrum through the visible range into the infrared. In addition, relatively more intense emanations occur at various points in the ultraviolet and the blue end of the visible spectrum, and these are specific for mercury. Most of this portion of the spectrum is not present in sunlight, which has no wavelengths shorter than 2900 Angstroms at the earth's surface. The spectrum emitted is affected by the pressure of the mercury.

"HOT QUARTZ" LAMPS (Fig. 14–4). These lamps operate with a relatively high pressure of mercury and produce a modified mercury emission spectrum with high intensity lines at 2652, 2967, 3025, 3130, and 3660 Angstroms, plus some energy on each side of the 2537 Angstrom line. The M.E.D. of a lamp in good condition may be of the order of 15 seconds of exposure at a

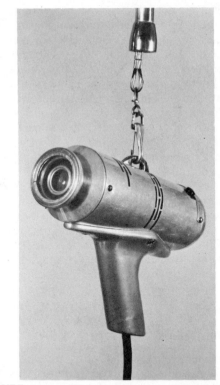

FIGURE 14–5. "Hot quartz" air-cooled ultraviolet source which may be used with orificial applicators or for small areas.

distance of 30 inches. Smaller lamps of this type may be cooled by a water jacket or an air blower (Kromayer type) so that they can be used close to the surface of the patient without causing thermal burns (Fig. 14–5). They can also be adapted for orificial appli-

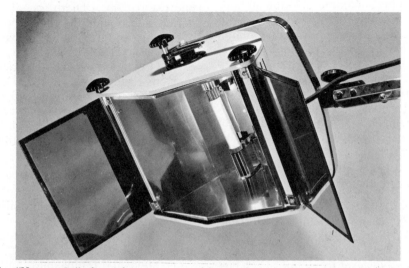

FIGURE 14–4. "Hot quartz" ultraviolet source, stand lamp, showing the burner and reflector. The wings of the reflector can be folded to close it, but amounts of ultraviolet sufficient to harm the eyes can still escape through the cracks.

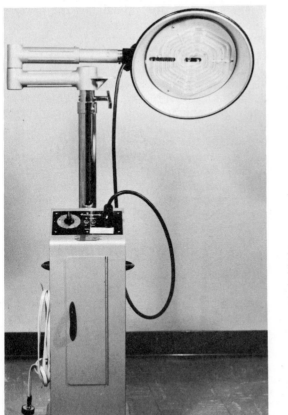

FIGURE 14–6. "Cold quartz" ultraviolet source, stand lamp. (Courtesy of Dr. F. J. Kottke.)

cation. The M.E.D. of such lamps may be of the order of 5 seconds of exposure at a distance of 2 inches.

A new high-pressure mercury vapor water-cooled lamp has been reported by Alsins et al.[11] In addition, a super-pressure mercury vapor lamp with a flexible light guide to replace the Kromayer lamp is described by Plewig et al.[12]

"COLD QUARTZ" LAMPS (Figs. 14–6 and 14–7). These lamps have a relatively low mercury pressure and contain, in addition, a rare gas such as argon or neon to initiate the arc. Almost all the transmitted ultraviolet emission is at 2537 Angstroms, which is in the lower maximum of the erythema action spectrum. The surface of the envelope is warmed only to about 60° C. The emission at 1849 Angstroms, which generates ozone in air, is not transmitted by the fused quartz burners used in these lamps.

"SUN LAMPS." "Sun lamps" contain a tungsten filament with which to heat the lamp and vaporize the mercury so that a mercury arc can be established between tungsten electrodes. The envelope is a glass that will transmit ultraviolet radiation. The M.E.D. is usually measured in minutes.

Xenon Arcs. High-pressure xenon arc lamps are sometimes alluded to as "solar simulators." They emit a spectrum ranging from 1700 Angstroms to the infrared. Lower pressure confined-arc xenon flash tubes operate at lower temperatures with less danger of explosion.[6]

Carbon Arcs. The carbon arc produces a continuous spectrum ranging from the far ultraviolet to the infrared. The relative intensity in the near or far ultraviolet portion of the spectrum can be modified by the use of carbon rod electrodes having different metallic salt cores. Carbon arcs consume the

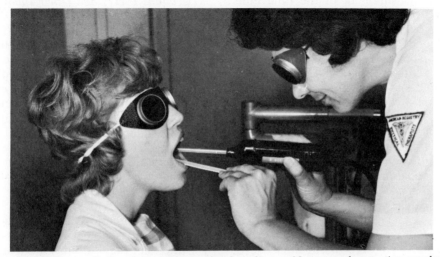

FIGURE 14–7. "Cold quartz" ultraviolet source, orificial applicator. Note use of protective goggles by patient and therapist. (Courtesy of Dr. F. J. Kottke.)

carbon and must have a reliable automatic feed mechanism to maintain the size of the gap between the electrodes so that sparks and sputtering will be minimized and the spectrum emitted will be reasonably constant.

The production of ozone is slightly annoying, but the concentrations produced are not hazardous in a well-ventilated room.

"Black-Light" Lamps. For diagnostic procedures involving the observation of fluorescence, a glass filter may be employed to eliminate the visible emanation from the lamp. With a low-pressure mercury-arc lamp, a black phosphate glass may be used. With a high-pressure mercury-arc lamp, Wood's nickel oxide glass is used.

Technique of Application

The technique of igniting the arc of the burner should be found in the instruction manual for the particular device being employed. The dosage of ultraviolet radiation must be regulated within very narrow limits. In general, the procedure is as follows:

1. Patient and operator must be screened from the ultraviolet source except during the actual time of the therapeutic exposure.

2. The eyes should be shielded at all times by glass or wet gauze. This applies also to scattered reflected radiation from the walls and other structures.

3. The M.E.D. of the source must be known. If it is not known, it should be determined before the lamp is used on a patient.

4. The timing device used must be capable of accurate measurement of the time units being employed (a good second hand on a watch may be used if the M.E.D. is measured in seconds).

5. The distance from the source to the nearest part of the patient must be measured, not estimated.

6. Draping of the patient to screen some portions of the body from the radiation must be essentially identical in subsequent treatments if the dosage is being increased. It is customary, though perhaps not essential, to drape the genital area.

INDICATIONS FOR ULTRAVIOLET THERAPY

For the most part the therapeutic use of ultraviolet irradiation, in the U.S.A., at least, is now in the domain of the dermatologist rather than the physiatrist. The literature published on the subject for the last several years has been almost exclusively in dermatology publications. A physician who intends to use ultraviolet in the treatment of dermatologic disorders should take steps to maintain familiarity with this component of the dermatology literature. The physiatrist has often used ultraviolet therapy for acne vulgaris, but doubt has been cast on its value for this.[13]

Psoriasis. The Goeckerman technique for psoriasis, involving the use of a crude coal tar ointment in addition to ultraviolet radiation, may act through a photochemical or photosensitizing mechanism. It is often more effective than the use of either coal tar or ultraviolet radiation alone. Since little or none of the ultraviolet radiation penetrates through the medicament to the skin, relatively large doses of ultraviolet radiation are used. The steps in the technique are as follows:

1. The crude coal tar ointment is applied to the skin in the evening in a thick layer over the psoriatic patches.

2. Before ultraviolet irradiation, the next day, the bulk of the coal tar ointment is wiped off with olive oil.

3. Immediately after this, the stained patches are exposed to ultraviolet radiation. The usual initial dosage is 4 M.E.D. with the mercury-vapor lamp, with daily increases by 2 M.E.D. as long as the reaction of the skin is favorable.

4. Following the ultraviolet irradiation, the patient bathes.

Decubitus Ulcers and Other Indolent Ulcers (Fig. 14–8). It is, of course, most difficult to evaluate the relative merits of various steps one may take to attempt to heal such ulcers. Ultraviolet therapy may be expected to be beneficial because of its bactericidal effects (particularly of the far ultraviolet emanation at 2537 Angstroms from the mercury-vapor arc) and its erythemogenic effect at the margins of the ulcer. Because the usual erythema of ultraviolet radiation is dependent on an initial reaction occurring in skin (see the section on Erythema in this chapter under Physiologic Effects), it cannot be expected to occur in the floor of the ulcer itself. No vasodilating effect of ultraviolet radiation in granulation tissue has been documented.

Ultraviolet radiation has a bactericidal effect on superficial ulcers. Two M.E.D. of

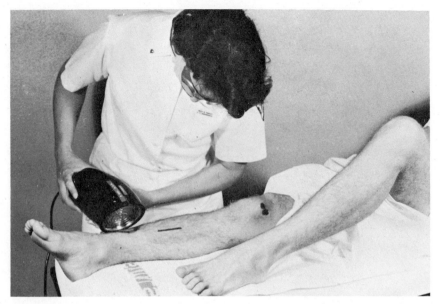

FIGURE 14–8. "Cold quartz" ultraviolet source being used in treatment of chronic ulcer. (Courtesy of Dr. F. J. Kottke.)

cold quartz ultraviolet is effective to destroy any motile forms of bacteria on the surface of the ulcer.[14] Since the bacteria in a wound are superficial rather than within the tissues, ultraviolet radiation is effective to kill the motile pathogens in the wound. Although the spores of spore-forming bacteria are resistant to ultraviolet, they have no effect until they develop into the motile form. Therefore, daily ultraviolet radiation is effective as a bactericidal agent for superficial wounds. Cold quartz ultraviolet, up to 5 M.E.D. daily by a grid source, or by orificial applicator for fistulas or undermined ulcers, is effective in causing bacteriostasis without tissue destruction. Cold quartz irradiation of more than 5 M.E.D. will delay epithelial formation. Ultraviolet irradiation greater than 10 M.E.D. may cause tissue destruction.

Disinfection of Air. The use of ultraviolet radiation for this purpose in operating rooms, nurseries, schools, and other areas is variable in its efficacy. There is no doubt of the bactericidal effect, particularly of the 2537 Angstrom band from the "cold quartz" mercury burner, but the application of this phenomenon is difficult.

REFERENCES

1. Blum, H. F.: Photodynamic Action and Diseases Caused by Light. New York, Hafner Publishing Co., 1964.
2. Urbach, F.: The Biologic Effects of Ultraviolet Radiation (With Emphasis on the Skin). New York, Pergamon Press, 1969.
3. New sunlamp standards and photosensitivity. F.D.A. Drug Bull., 10:14–15, 1980.
4. Fusaro, R. M., and Johnson, J. A.: Photoprotection of patients sensitive to short and/or long ultraviolet light with dehydroxyacetone/naphthoquinone. Dermatologica, 148:224–227, 1974.
5. Sunscreens. Med. Lett. Drugs Ther., 21:46–48, 1979.
6. Parrish J. A., Anderson, R. R., Urbach, F., and Pitts, D.: UV-A: Biological Effects of Ultraviolet Radiation with Emphasis on Human Responses to Longwave Ultraviolet. New York, Plenum Press, 1978.
7. Warin, A. P.: The ultraviolet erythemas in man. Br. J. Dermatol., 98:473–477, 1978.
8. Beadle, P. C.: Sunlight, ozone and vitamin D. Br. J. Dermatol., 97:585–591, 1977.
9. Epstein, J. H.: Photoallergy. Australas. J. Dermatol., 18:51–56, 1977.
10. Emmett, E. A.: Drug photoallergy. Int. J. Dermatol., 17:370–379, 1978.
11. Alsins, J., Claesson, S., Fischer, T., and Juhlin, L.: Development of high intensity narrow-band lamps and studies of the irradiation effect on human skin: Irradiation with high intensity lamps. Acta Derm. Venereol. (Stockh.), 55:261–271, 1975.
12. Plewig, G., Hofmann, C., Braun-Falco, O., Nath, G., and Kreitmair, A.: A new apparatus for the delivery of high intensity UVA and UVA+UVB irradiation, and some dermatological applications. Br. J. Dermatol., 98:15–24, 1978.
13. Mills, O. H., and Kligman, A. M.: Ultraviolet phototherapy and photochemotherapy of acne vulgaris. Arch. Dermatol., 114:221–223, 1978.
14. Koller, L. R.: Ultraviolet Radiation. New York, John Wiley and Sons, 1952.

15

ELECTROTHERAPY

G. KEITH STILLWELL

ELECTRICAL STIMULATION

Physics

An electric current may be considered to be a flow of electrons. This may be a flow of free electrons, as in a solid conductor, or of electrons carried by ions and delivered at some point, as with the solution of an electrolyte in water. The force which causes the electrons to be moved is the difference in electrical potential between the point at which electrons are being injected into the system and the point at which they are being removed; this is measured in volts. The rate of delivery of the electrons is called the current flow and is measured in amperes. The opposition to the movement of electrons through a conductor is called the resistance of the conductor and is measured in ohms.

The relationship among these three factors is expressed in Ohm's law,

$$E = I R$$

in which E is the electrical potential, I is the amperage, and R is the resistance.

An electric current flowing through a solid conductor causes a magnetic field to be developed around the conductor. The strength of this field varies with the strength of the current. Conversely, changes in a magnetic field around a conductor will induce a flow of electrons in the conductor.

Currents in which the direction of flow of the electrons alternates between two poles are called alternating currents. Many complex concepts are involved in the transfer of energy by alternating currents, but these cannot be adequately considered here.

Physiologic Effects

Nature of Stimulus. Any change in the environment of an irritable tissue may be regarded as a stimulus. If the stimulus fails to elicit a response from the tissue, it is subliminal. If it elicits the maximal response from the tissue, it is said to be a maximal stimulus. Any greater stimulus is supramaximal. Because electric currents are highly effective in stimulating nerve and muscle, and can be accurately measured and finely gradated, they are more suitable than other types of stimulation in producing contraction of muscles directly or by way of nerves for diagnostic or therapeutic purposes.

The factors influencing the effectiveness of a stimulus are the magnitude of the change, the rate of the change, and the duration of the altered condition. The relationship between the magnitude of the change and the duration of the change resulting from electrical stimulation is shown in Figure 15–1. Similar curves are obtained whether the strength of the stimulus is measured in volts or in milliamperes. The curve characteristic of muscle is labeled "denervation," while the curve characteristic of nerve is labeled "normal." It will be noted that, in each instance, as the duration of the stimulus decreases, the strength increases. The minimal effective duration for muscle is much longer than that for nerve.

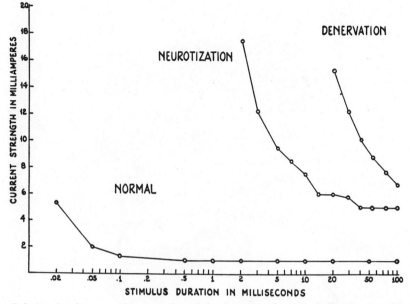

FIGURE 15–1. Relationship between the strength and the duration of minimal effective stimulus for denervated, neurotized, and normally innervated muscle. (From Rose, D. L.: Electrodiagnostic methods: Evaluation and interpretation. *In* Krusen, F. H.: Physical Medicine and Rehabilitation for the Clinician. Philadelphia, W. B. Saunders Company, 1951, pp. 95–108.)

The rate of change of the stimulus is important because of the phenomenon of accommodation. Nerve accommodates relatively well and may not be stimulated by a change of several volts if the change occurs gradually over a period of 0.2 second or so. Muscle does not accommodate nearly as well and probably loses much of what little accommodation it possesses in the atrophy of denervation.

Types of Electrical Stimulus. Various electrical changes may be produced by available stimulators. The prototypes are shown in Figure 15–2. From the remarks made earlier about the nature of a stimulus, it follows that the effectiveness of a stimulus, although influenced by the "wave form," is not dependent entirely upon it.

Technique of Electrical Stimulation

The technique of the use of any stimulating device, if unfamiliar to the operator, should be reviewed in the operating manual for the device. Certain points are generally applicable.

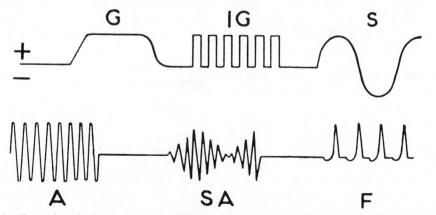

FIGURE 15–2. Examples of voltage changes in different forms of stimuli. G, Galvanic or direct current; I G, interrupted galvanic; S, sinusoidal or alternating current; A, a more rapidly alternating form; S A, surging alternating current; F, faradic or induced current. (From Kovacs, R.: Physical therapy: Low-frequency currents. *In* Glasser, O.: Medical Physics. Chicago, Year Book Publishers, Inc., 1944, vol. 1, pp. 1068–1073.)

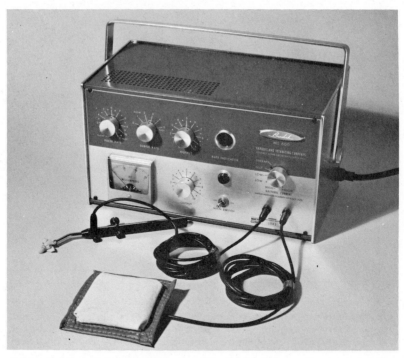

FIGURE 15–3. Table-model electrical stimulator capable of generating galvanic or faradic types of current. The galvanic current can also be used for ion transfer. Note the milliammeter for measurement of the flow of direct current, the small "active" electrode (with a contact switch on its handle), and the larger "indifferent" electrode pad.

1. Good contact should be maintained between the skin and the electrodes. The use of a conductive solution or jelly diminishes the resistance at this point. Sodium chloride solution, soap suds, electrode jelly, and other conductive substances may be used. Whatever is employed should not in itself be irritating to the skin.

2. Usually (but not always) "active" and "indifferent" electrodes are employed (monopolar technique), the latter being larger. The density of current flow at the indifferent (larger) electrode is less, and stimulation can be selectively produced at the "active" electrode (Fig. 15–3).

3. In the stimulation of innervated muscle, the active electrode is placed over the motor point of the muscle.

4. Denervated muscle does not have a motor point. The active electrode may be placed at the point giving the best response, or two electrodes of about the same size may be placed one at each end of the muscle so that the current will pass through the muscle and stimulate all of it (bipolar or longitudinal technique).

5. The two electrodes should generally be placed on the same side of the body, particularly to avoid passage of the current through the thorax or the genital area.

6. With unidirectional current (direct current, galvanic current), the active electrode may be the cathode or the anode, the choice depending upon which is more effective. Following prolonged stimulation with one pole, adverse cutaneous effects may be noted from the passage of the current. Some believe it is advisable to counteract this by the subsequent passage of a current of reversed polarity for a while, or to reverse the polarity periodically during the treatment.

Clinical Uses of Electrical Stimulation

Stimulation of Denervated Muscle

PURPOSE. One purpose of stimulating denervated muscle is to retard the progression of atrophy.[1] Since the rate of development of denervation atrophy declines exponentially with time, most of the atrophy takes place early. Therefore, steps to prevent it must be taken early if they are to be effective. Atrophy of denervation has been demonstrated to be retarded by appropriate electrical stimulation in rabbits, rats, and dogs, but not in cats. There is no solid evidence that it retards atrophy in humans. Supramaximal stimulation in rats seems to impair regeneration of muscle fibers.[2] Another purpose of stimulation is to diminish intrafascicular and interfascicular agglutination and sclerosis of areolar tissue. Stimulation may be of help in this respect even if begun late in the period of denervation. Stimulation is also used to improve the circulation and nutrition of the muscle. Muscular contraction is helpful in moving venous blood and lymph out of the muscle.

TYPE OF CURRENT. Direct current, either square wave or nearly so, is effective. Sinusoidal alternating current is effective if it is not too high in frequency. The effective frequencies range as high as 7000 cycles per second, but the optimal frequency is in the neighborhood of 25 c.p.s. or less. The slowly increasing stimulus may be able to stimulate denervated muscle without simultaneous stimulation of nerve (or even innervated muscle) in the field.

Impulses briefer than 10 or 20 milliseconds may not be able to cause a contraction of denervated skeletal muscle except at very high intensities. Impulses of a duration of about 100 milliseconds are more satisfactory. The principal spike of a faradic current stimulus has a duration of only about 1 millisecond.

STRENGTH OF CONTRACTION. Strong contractions should be produced. Denervated muscle may become fatigued rapidly so that only 25 to 50 strong contractions can be obtained at one session. A strong contraction against resistance may be of more benefit, since the development of tension in the muscle seems well correlated with the retardation of atrophy.

SCHEDULE OF TREATMENT. Work on experimental animals suggests that three or four treatment sessions each day may be required to retard the progress of atrophy. This regimen is generally feasible if the patient has his own stimulator and is taught to use it by himself. A battery stimulator for home use is shown in Figure 15–4.

SUPPLEMENTAL HEAT. It is helpful but not essential to apply heat before the stimulation. Care must be taken, of course, not to burn insensitive areas.

DURATION OF TREATMENT. After the patient is able to produce reasonably good active contractions of the muscle, there is no value in continued stimulation.

Stimulation of Innervated Muscle. Innervated muscle is stimulated by way of its nerve supply. The minimal effective duration of stimulus is about 0.02 millisecond if the voltage is high enough. Innervated muscle is easily stimulated by impulses as brief as 1 millisecond. This method of treatment may be helpful in producing relaxation of muscle in "spasm," for example subsequent to trauma; in preventing atrophy of disuse in a muscle which the patient cannot contract well voluntarily, for example the quadriceps, after injury to the knee; in reeducation of muscles when other methods of reeducation

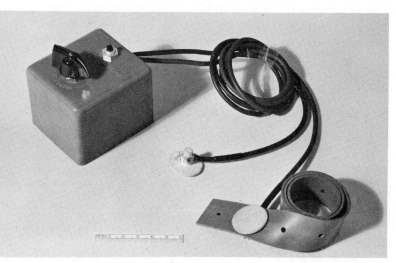

FIGURE 15–4. Battery stimulator suitable for use in the home. It produces galvanic current only, with no measurement of current flow.

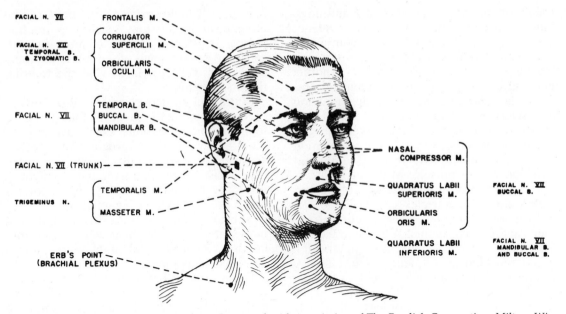

FIGURE 15–5. Motor points of the face. (Reprinted with permission of The Burdick Corporation, Milton, Wisconsin.)

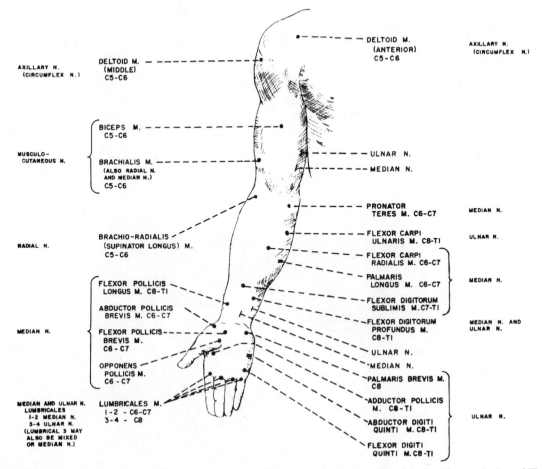

FIGURE 15–6. Motor points of the anterior aspect of the upper extremity. (Reprinted with permission of The Burdick Corporation, Milton, Wisconsin.)

fail; in reducing spasticity in spastic paralysis, particularly that due to injury of the spinal cord; and in stimulation of the calf muscles in the immediate postoperative period to prevent phlebothrombosis.

Electrical stimulation of the abdominal wall and diaphragm as an aid to ventilation has been used ("electrolung"). More frequent currently is the use of electrical stimulation of the phrenic nerves for artificial respiration in patients with lesions of the spinal cord above C4. This "diaphragmatic pacing" or "electrophrenic respiration" is accomplished with implanted stimulators. Stimulation of a single phrenic nerve causes

descent of the ipsilateral hemidiaphragm with some shift of the mediastinum to that side. There is ventilation of both lungs despite a slight ascent of the contralateral hemidiaphragm.[3] "Motor points" are the areas for optimal stimulation of skeletal muscles. They are usually located at the area where the motor nerve penetrates the epimysium. The threshold stimulus for the muscle will be lowest at that point. Motor point charts (Figs. 15–5 to 15–11) show their approximate locations, but some local exploration needs to be done for precise location in the individual.

Functional electrical stimulation for con-

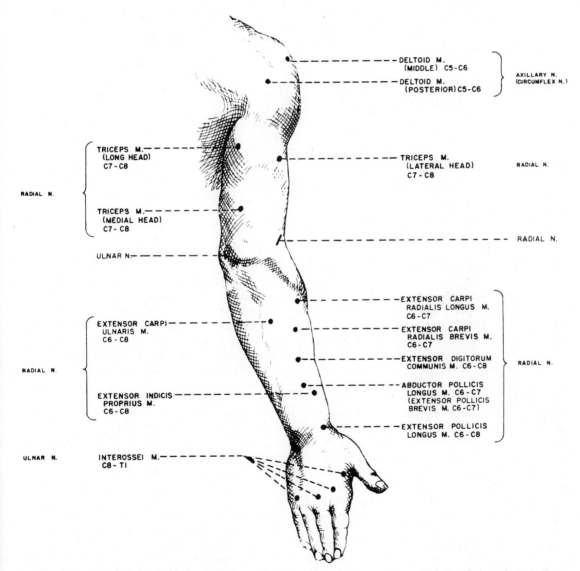

FIGURE 15–7. Motor points of the posterior aspect of the upper extremity. (Reprinted with permission of The Burdick Corporation, Milton, Wisconsin.)

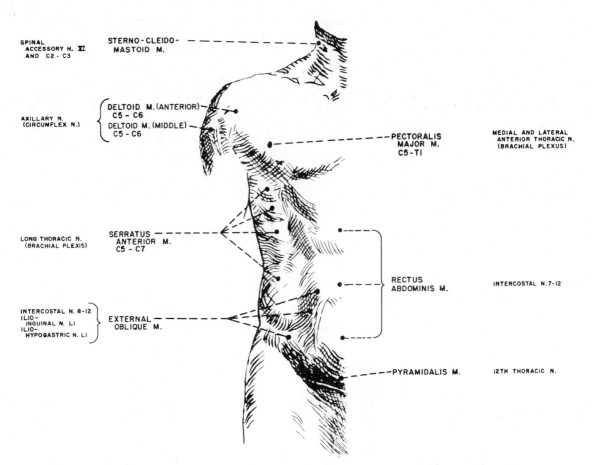

SPINAL ACCESSORY N. XI AND C2 - C3

STERNO - CLEIDO - MASTOID M.

AXILLARY N. (CIRCUMFLEX N.)

DELTOID M. (ANTERIOR) C5 - C6

DELTOID M. (MIDDLE) C5 - C6

PECTORALIS MAJOR M. C5 - TI

MEDIAL AND LATERAL ANTERIOR THORACIC N. (BRACHIAL PLEXUS)

LONG THORACIC N. (BRACHIAL PLEXIS)

SERRATUS ANTERIOR M. C5 - C7

RECTUS ABDOMINIS M.

INTERCOSTAL N. 7-12

INTERCOSTAL N. 8-12
ILIO - INGUINAL N. LI
ILIO - HYPOGASTRIC N. LI

EXTERNAL OBLIQUE M.

PYRAMIDALIS M.

12TH THORACIC N.

FIGURE 15–8. Motor points of the anterior aspect of the trunk. (Reprinted with permission of The Burdick Corporation, Milton, Wisconsin.)

trol of the locomotor system is covered in Chapter 16 of this volume.

Electrical Stimulation for Analgesia. The gate control theory of pain presented by Melzack and Wall[4] proposed that input into the spinal cord via the larger "A" fibers could close a gate in the substantia gelatinosa of the dorsal horn of the gray matter. This would block transmission beyond that point of painful input arriving via the small "C" fibers. A wide variety of forms of stimulation of the skin might close the gate, and the theory provided an explanation for the analgesic effects of many physical methods of treatment. Wall and Sweet[5] reported on the use of electrical stimulation through the skin or with needle electrodes for the relief of pain and noted that there may be a relatively long-lasting effect.

Shealy[6] theorized that electrical stimulation of the dorsal columns of the spinal cord would be more effective for patients with disabling chronic pain. However, there were

77 complications occurring in 48 of the 80 patients with implanted stimulators. He now feels that "implantation should only be undertaken as an extreme last resort," since transcutaneous electrical stimulation has been effective in 50 per cent of his patients. Transcutaneous electrical nerve stimulation is a valuable component in the selection of patients for implantation.[7]

In the last decade there has developed a widespread clinical use of transcutaneous electrical nerve stimulation for chronic or acute pain. It is not clear whether the mechanism is a gating one in the spinal cord[8] or an endogenous analgesic neurohumeral one in the brain or cord.[9-11] Brief periods of intense stimulation[12, 13] or longer periods of lower-intensity stimulation[14, 15] have both been shown to be more effective than placebo treatment. Stimulation with short trains of impulses at a frequency of 3 to 5 per second and an intensity three to five times perception threshold has been called

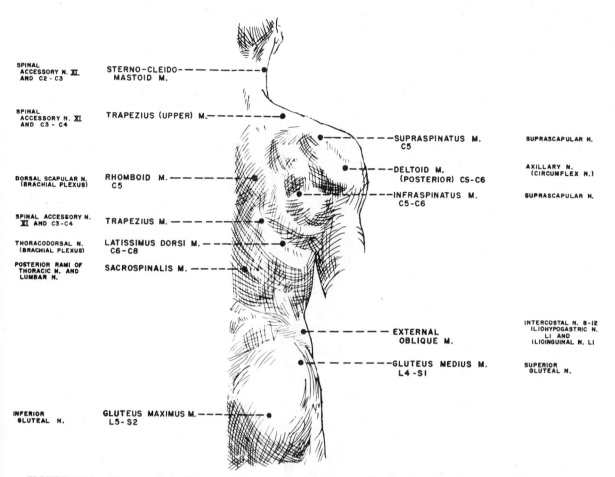

SPINAL ACCESSORY N. XI AND C2-C3 — STERNO-CLEIDO-MASTOID M.

SPINAL ACCESSORY N. XI AND C3-C4 — TRAPEZIUS (UPPER) M.

DORSAL SCAPULAR N. (BRACHIAL PLEXUS) — RHOMBOID M. C5

SPINAL ACCESSORY N. XI AND C3-C4 — TRAPEZIUS M.

THORACODORSAL N. (BRACHIAL PLEXUS) — LATISSIMUS DORSI M. C6-C8

POSTERIOR RAMI OF THORACIC N. AND LUMBAR N. — SACROSPINALIS M.

INFERIOR GLUTEAL N. — GLUTEUS MAXIMUS M. L5-S2

SUPRASPINATUS M. C5 — SUPRASCAPULAR N.

DELTOID M. (POSTERIOR) C5-C6 — AXILLARY N. (CIRCUMFLEX N.)

INFRASPINATUS M. C5-C6 — SUPRASCAPULAR N.

EXTERNAL OBLIQUE M. — INTERCOSTAL N. 8-12 ILIOHYPOGASTRIC N. LI AND ILIOINGUINAL N. LI

GLUTEUS MEDIUS M. L4-SI — SUPERIOR GLUTEAL N.

FIGURE 15–9. Motor points of the posterior aspect of the trunk. (Reprinted with permission of The Burdick Corporation, Milton, Wisconsin.)

''acupuncture-like.'' Its analgesic effect may be blocked by naloxone, suggesting that it works through an endorphin mechanism. It is effective in some cases of chronic pain in which the high-frequency (100 stimuli per second) stimulation at two to three times perception threshold is not. The analgesic effect of the high-frequency stimulation, which often occurs more promptly than that from low frequency, is not blocked by naloxone.[16]

Transcutaneous electrical nerve stimulation has been used with varying degrees of success for pain associated with various neuropathies,[12, 17] rheumatoid arthritis,[18] the first stage of obstetric labor,[19, 20] dental work,[21] postoperative incisional pain,[22–25] spinal cord injury,[26] and a variety ot other neuromusculoskeletal conditions. In some patients its efficacy may persist for months or years, while in others it diminishes in a few weeks.

Experimentation may be required to find the optimum placement of the electrodes. Usually this is at or near the site of the pain, but spots with lower resistance to the flow of electrical current or acupunctural analgesia points may prove better. In the applications for postoperative pain and pain after spinal cord injury, relatively large electrodes have been used. It may be that too much effort is expended trying to find small discrete spots for the electrical input. Resistance to current flow may be reduced by various solutions, pastes, and adhesives. Localized skin reactions to these substances may occur, rather than to the current iself. This would seem to be the only adverse physical effect of transcutaneous electrical nerve stimulation. Burton has suggested the following, however:

Reasonable cautions include avoidance of (1) use in patients with demand cardiac pacemakers, (2) placement of the electrodes over the carotid

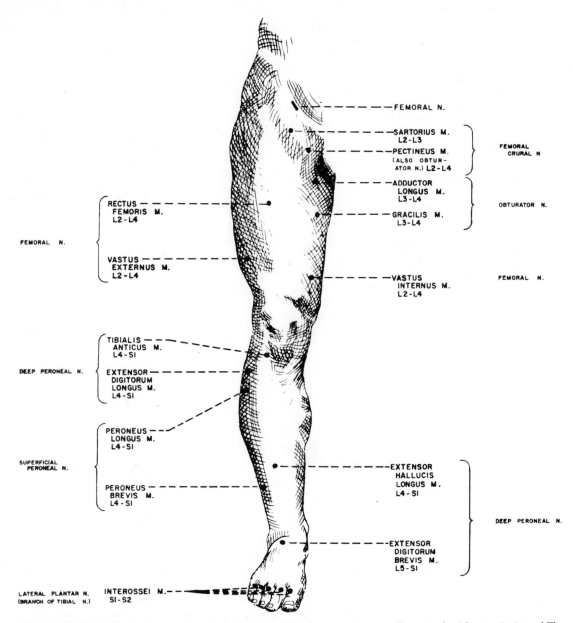

FIGURE 15–10. Motor points of the anterior aspect of the lower extremity. (Reprinted with permission of The Burdick Corporation, Milton, Wisconsin.)

sinuses (to avoid vagovagal reflexes), and (3) use in patients during the first trimester of pregnancy. All patients should be warned to avoid sudden movement of the pulse generator controls, to avoid a ''startle'' response that could have adverse consequences during operation of a motor vehicle or a potentially dangerous piece of machinery.[27]

Miscellaneous Applications. Electrical stimulation has been used to enhance urinary continence.[28, 29] It has generally been less

than successful in causing detrusor action when stimulation was applied to the bladder wall.[30] Activation of the detrusor through stimulation of the conus medullaries with an implanted device has worked well in selected patients.[31] Electric currents have shown promise for treatment of fractures with delayed healing. This may be accomplished by electromagnetically induced currents[32, 33] or by the percutaneous insertion of four cathodic electrodes near the nonunion site.[34]

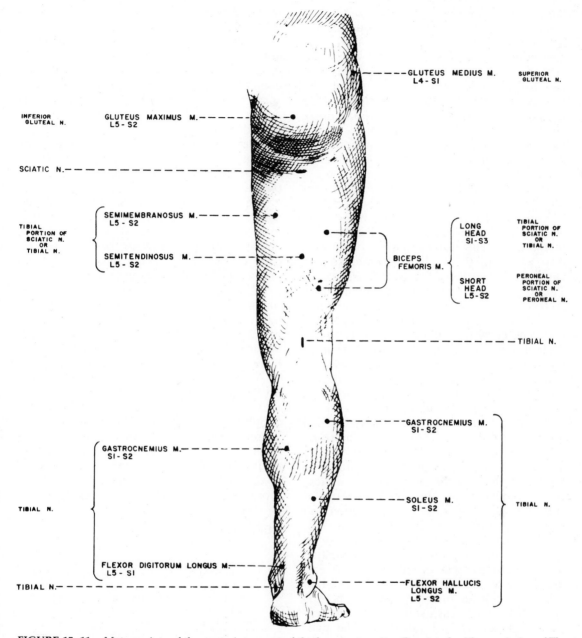

FIGURE 15–11. Motor points of the posterior aspect of the lower extremity. (Reprinted with permission of The Burdick Corporation, Milton, Wisconsin.)

IONTOPHORESIS

Iontophoresis is the process of transferring ions into the body by an electromotive force. Ions bearing a positive charge may be driven into the skin at the anode and those with a negative charge at the cathode.[35] Positively charged ions, zinc, copper, and alkaloids such as the vasodilating drugs, histamine and mecholyl, are introduced into the skin and mucous membranes from the positive pole. Skin anesthesia can be produced by iontophoresis of local anesthetic drugs using the positive pole. Negative ions such as iodine, chlorine, and salicylic acid are introduced into the tissues from the negative pole. Other drugs for general metabolic or specific hormonal effects can be driven into the circulating blood by iontophoresis, but most physicians employ simpler methods for administering these drugs. The greatest concentration is moved into the skin where the skin is broken, or along sweat glands and hair follicles. Ions transferred through the skin are taken up by the circulation and do not proceed through the tissues to the other electrode. As a rule ions used for medicinal purposes cannot be made to migrate far below the surface of the skin or mucous membranes.

The velocity of movement of the transferred ions is directly proportional to the voltage applied. The quantity transferred is affected by the current flow and the duration of the flow. The usual intensity of current flow is 0.1 to 0.5 milliampere per square centimeter of surface of the active electrode. The apparatus should include a milliammeter so that the flow can be measured. The duration of treatment is usually 15 minutes or less. The current is turned up slowly to the desired level, maintained as long as desired, *provided that the patient is comfortable and that there are no adverse systemic effects,* and then slowly turned off again (or occasionally reversed for one minute or so).

Any direct current generator may be used for iontophoresis. The electrodes must be connected to the correctly identified positive and negative terminals of the generator. For treatment through the skin the active electrodes should be an absorptive material of sufficient thickness to hold the solution and keep moist during treatment. Gauze 6 millimeters thick, cotton, or filter paper may be used. For the introduction of vasodilating drugs, blotting paper or filter paper is employed, covered by a felt pad soaked in saline beneath the metal electrode. There is no advantage in using a solution at a concentration greater than 1 per cent. The pad, saturated in solution at a comfortable temperature, is firmly applied to the area to be treated. A metal plate somewhat smaller than the pad is placed on the pad; no metal edges should touch the skin, since even a minute direct contact between the metal and the skin may lead to a chemical burn. Breaks in the skin may also concentrate ion flow and cause electrical burns.

For treatment of mucous surfaces, a metal electrode, solution, or packing containing the ions is placed in direct contact with the walls of the cavity and serves as the active electrode.

The dispersive electrode is a pad considerably larger than the active electrode, soaked in warm saline solution and placed in firm contact with a convenient part of the body surface. Alternatively the foot, hand, or arm may be placed in a saline bath to provide a dispersive electrode of large area.

After treatment the pads should be thoroughly cleaned and rinsed in order to remove secondary chemical products near the metal plate.

The technique has the advantage of concentrating a relatively large amount of a drug in a local area of the skin when this is desired. The drug will not be delivered locally to structures deeper than the skin but may be taken up by the circulation.

Disadvantages include the difficulty of estimating the dosage of the drug and, particularly, of estimating how much of the drug may act systemically. Severe reactions may occur in allergic persons, for example when histamine is administered by iontophoresis.

The method has been of interest to many investigators as a research tool. Its therapeutic value is limited. It has been employed for a multitude of conditions in the past but with a great paucity of evidence to establish its value. Anyone interested in using the method is referred to an excellent critical review of the matter by Harris which also provides more detailed information on technique.[36]

REFERENCES

1. Stillwell, G. K.: Clinical electric stimulation. *In* Licht, S. (Ed.): Therapeutic Electricity and Ultraviolet Radiation, 2nd Ed. New Haven, Connecticut, Elizabeth Licht, Publisher, 1967, pp. 105–Licht, Publisher, 1967, pp. 105–155.
2. Schimrigk, K., McLaughlin, J., and Grüninger, W.: The effect of electrical stimulation on the experimentally denervated rat muscle. Scand. J. Rehabil. Med., 9:55–60, 1977.
3. Sarnoff, S. J., Gaensler, E. A., and Maloney, J. V., Jr.: Electrophrenic respiration. IV. The effectiveness of contralateral ventilation during activity of one phrenic nerve. J. Thorac. Surg., 19:929–937, 1950.
4. Melzack, R., and Wall, P. D.: Pain mechanisms: A new theory. Science, 150:971–979, 1965.
5. Wall, P. D., and Sweet, W. H.: Temporary abolition of pain in man. Science, 155:108–109, 1967.
6. Shealy, C. N.: From dorsal column implants to external transcutaneous neurostimulator devices: Comparison and appraisal of the development of

the technique. *In* Ersek, R. A. (Ed.): Pain Control with Transcutaneous Electrical Neuro Stimulation (T.E.N.S.). St. Louis, Warren H. Green, Inc., 1981, pp. 54–61.

7. Miles, J.: Transcutaneous electrical neuro stimulation in the assessment of patients for electrical stimulator implant. *In* Ersek, R. A. (Ed.): Pain Control with Transcutaneous Electrical Neuro Stimulation (T.E.N.S.). St. Louis, Warren H. Green, Inc., 1981, pp. 118–128.

8. Kerr, F. W.: Pain: A central inhibitory balance theory. Mayo Clin. Proc., 50:685–690, 1975.

9. Almay, B. G. L., Johansson, F., Von Knorring, L., Terenius, L., and Wahlström, A.: Endorphins in chronic pain. I. Differences in CSF endorphin levels between organic and psychogenic pain syndromes. Pain, 5:153–162, 1978.

10. Fields, H. L., and Basbaum, A. I.: Brainstem control of spinal pain-transmission neurons. Annu. Rev. Physiol., 40:217–248, 1978.

11. Editorial: Endorphins through the eye of a needle? Lancet, 1:480–482, 1981.

12. Melzack, R.: Prolonged relief of pain by brief, intense transcutaneous somatic stimulation. Pain, 1:357–373, 1975.

13. Jeans, M. E.: Relief of chronic pain by brief, intense transcutaneous electrical stimulation: A double-blind study. Adv. Pain Res. Ther., 3:601–606, 1979.

14. Thorsteinsson, G., Stonnington, H. H., Stillwell, G. K., and Elveback, L. R.: The placebo effect of transcutaneous electrical stimulation. Pain, 5:31–41, 1978.

15. Long, D. M., Campbell, J. N., and Gucer, G.: Transcutaneous electrical stimulation for relief of chronic pain. Adv. Pain Res. Ther., 3:593–599, 1979.

16. Sjölund, B. H., and Eriksson, M. B. E.: The influence of naloxone on analgesia produced by peripheral conditioning stimulation. Brain Res., 173:295–301, 1979.

17. Thorsteinsson, G., Stonnington, H. H., Stillwell, G. K., and Elveback, L. R.: Transcutaneous electrical stimulation: A double-blind trial of its efficacy for pain. Arch. Phys. Med. Rehabil., 58:8–13, 1977.

18. Mannheimer, C., and Carlsson, C.-A.: The analgesic effect of transcutaneous electrical nerve stimulation (TNS) in patients with rheumatoid arthritis: A comparative study of different pulse patterns. Pain, 6:329–334, 1979.

19. Robson, J. E.: Transcutaneous nerve stimulation for pain relief in labour. Anaesthesia 34:357–361, 1979.

20. Stewart, P.: Transcutaneous nerve stimulation as a method of analgesia in labour. Anaesthesia 34:361–364, 1979.

21. Chapman, C. R., Wilson, M. E., and Gehrig, J. D.: Comparative effects of acupuncture and transcutaneous stimulation on the perception of painful dental stimuli. Pain, 2:265–283, 1976.

22. VanderArk, G. D., and McGrath, K. A.: Transcutaneous electrical stimulation in treatment of postoperative pain. Am. J. Surg., 130:338–340, 1975.

23. Hymes, A. C., Yonehiro, E. G., Raab, D. E., Nelson, G. D., and Printy, A. L.: Electrical surface stimulation for treatment and prevention of ileus and atelectasis. Surg. Forum, 25:222–224, 1974.

24. Cooperman, A. M., Hall, B., Mikalacki, K., Hardy, R., and Sadar, E.: Use of transcutaneous electrical stimulation in the control of postoperative pain: Results of a prospective, randomized, controlled study. Am. J. Surg., 133:185–187, 1977.

25. Bussey, J. G., and Jackson, A.: Post surgical analgesia with T.E.N.S. *In* Ersek, R. A. (Ed.): Pain Control with Transcutaneous Electrical Neuro Stimulation (T.E.N.S.). St. Louis, Warren H. Green, Inc., 1981, pp. 151–159.

26. Davis, R., and Lentini, R.: Transcutaneous nerve stimulation for treatment of pain in patients with spinal cord injury. Surg. Neurol., 4:100–101, 1975.

27. Burton, C.: Transcutaneous electrical nerve stimulation to relieve pain. Postgrad. Med., 59:105–108, 1976.

28. Erlandson, B.-E., Fall, M., and Sundin, T.: Intravaginal electrical stimulation. Part III. Clinical experiments on urethral closure. Scand. J. Urol. Nephrol. (Suppl.) 44:31–39, 1977.

29. Godec, C., and Cass, A. S.: Electrical stimulation for voiding dysfunction after spinal cord injury. J. Urol., 121:73–75, 1979.

30. Jonas, U., and Hohenfellner, R.: Late results of bladder stimulation in 11 patients: Followup to 4 years. J. Urol., 120:565–568, 1978.

31. Nashold, B. S., Jr., Grimes, J., Friedman, H., Semans, J., and Avery, R.: Operative stimulation of the neurogenic bladder. Neurosurgery, 1:218–220, 1977.

32. Watson, J., and Downes, E. M.: Clinical aspects of the stimulation of bone healing using electrical phenomena. Med. Biol. Eng. Comput., 17:161–169, 1979.

33. De Haas, W. G., Watson, J., and Morrison, D. M.: Non-invasive treatment of ununited fractures of the tibia using electrical stimulation. J. Bone Joint Surg. (Br.), 62:465–470, 1980.

34. Brighton, C. T., Black, J., Friedenberg, Z. B., Esterhai, J. L., Day, L. J., and Connolly, J. F.: A multicenter study of the treatment of non-union with constant direct current. J. Bone Joint Surg. (Am.), 63:2–13, 1981.

35. Gangarosa, L. P., Park, N. H., Fong, B. C., Scott, D. F., and Hill, J. M.: Conductivity of drugs used for iontophoresis. J. Pharm. Sci., 67:1439–1443, 1978.

36. Harris, R.: Iontophoresis. *In* Licht, S. (Ed.): Therapeutic Electricity and Ultraviolet Radiation, 2nd Ed. New Haven, Connecticut, Elizabeth Licht, Publisher, 1967, pp. 156–178.

16

FUNCTIONAL ELECTRICAL STIMULATION

FRANJO GRACANIN

Functional electrical stimulation (FES) has been described as a stimulation of muscles, both smooth and striated, which have been deprived of nervous control, with a view to providing muscular contraction producing a functionally useful movement.[16] The method was first described as functional electrotherapy in 1961[28] and was termed *functional electrical stimulation* in 1962.[33] In both cases it signified the stimulation of individual muscles or nerves in a hemiplegic person during gait. Application of FES in the control of muscle contraction has broader significance in medicine. It is used in the control of rhythmic functions like heart beat, of respiration through stimulation of the phrenic nerve, of urinary bladder function using implant systems, of gastrointestinal motility, and of other functions. Control of motor output and movements in paralyzed extremities represents a special area within FES. In the beginning, FES was used to alleviate spasticity and other symptoms of release phenomena.[26, 27] Later, it was applied in the direct control of movements[28] like dorsiflexion and eversion in a hemiplegic person with footdrop. Today, FES represents a clinically effective method in the rehabilitation of patients with a lesion of the upper motor neuron — whether FES be part of a therapeutic program or be intended for independent use at home as an orthotic aid with a therapeutic effect.[13]

From the therapeutic point of view there are some advantages of FES over other known neurotherapeutic methods. Functional electrical stimulation makes possible a selective, repetitive, and reproducible input of programmed information for activation of reflex mechanisms that are indispensable in organizing motor activity and movements that are impaired to various degrees or practically absent in patients with damaged upper motor neurons.[10]

NEUROPHYSIOLOGIC AND ORTHOTIC ASPECTS OF FES

The neurophysiologic mechanisms involved include contractions and tension of muscle as the result of motor neuron activity in response to reflex stimulation, to volition, or to FES through activation of proprioceptive and musculocutaneous reflex mechanisms.[16] Gait and other reciprocal movements of the extremities are integrated chiefly in the spinal cord, and most of the response is determined by the afferent inflow from the limbs at segmental and intersegmental levels.[34]

Application of efferent FES for direct control of muscle contraction is due to electrical excitation of the motor nerve fibers, neuromuscular transmission, and the ability of the muscles to contract. Stimulation of afferent nerve fibers to exert an indirect influence on the muscle contraction via spinal reflex mechanisms is termed afferent FES.[12] The results of afferent FES are overshadowed by direct muscle contraction as a result of depolarization of motor nerve fibers and by an additional inflow from muscle receptors and Golgi's tendon organs, which contribute to the processes of excitation, facilitation, and inhibition of motor pools of the same extremity. This results in establishing spinal reflex mechanisms whose basic characteristics are excitation of the agonist with inhibition of antagonist, co-contraction of synergists, and sequential reciprocating innervation of agonist and antagonist.[22] Effects of facilitation and inhibition produced by afferent FES may be explained by the investigations of Lloyd,[29] who stated that the afferent inflow via group Ia fibers facilitates motor activity in synergistic muscles and inhibits it in the antagonists (especially with stimulation of afferent fibers to flexors). Additional explanation of the effects produced by FES (bilateral alternating FES in particular) may be found in Sherrington's studies of double reciprocal innervation and of rhythmically alternating stepping movements as the result of electrical stimulation of the peroneal nerves.[5] By application of these procedures we can control mechanisms like flexor and extensor synergies, which are parts of the gait mechanisms. The influence of FES is apparent in the immediate control of movement and affects reflex motor activity such as clonus, but the effects lasting hours or even permanently after discontinuing FES cannot be explained solely by mono- and oligosynaptic reflex mechanisms or by the specific properties of peripheral nerves or muscles themselves.

The degree of improvement of impaired motor functions achieved through the application of FES undoubtedly depends on the location of the lesion in relation to the level of the sensory-motor integration, on the extent of the lesion, on the potentialities for developing cerebral motor functions, and on the eventual use of equipotential empty areas of the minor hemisphere. Doubtless, a programmed, artificial afferent inflow of information into the central nervous system and an adequate triggering of proprioceptive mechanisms with the motor pattern repeated thousands of times contribute to establishing engrams that become manifest in a perma-

nent effect of the FES on gait and posture and an improvement of voluntary control of movements. We can presume that the long-term effects of FES are the result of a process of learning through functional reorganization of interneuron networks at the segmental and suprasegmental levels and of the afferent inflow impinging on the reticular formation. There is considerable influence on subcortical excitatory and inhibitory mechanisms and on cerebral and cerebellar mechanisms for control of motor function when the pathways are preserved.

From the orthotic aspect, systems for FES have an advantage over the usual passive orthotic aids. FES systems represent an active orthotic aid. In a large number of patients they have a therapeutic effect whose functioning during walking integrates with the mechanisms of sensory-motor organization. But FES systems require more maintenance and their daily application is more demanding. Application itself requires the cooperation of a trained staff and prolonged training of patients for continued use at home. Patient use requires adequate maintenance service and the possibility of consultation when necessary. These requirements limit applications to patients who have the necessary medical and technical services readily available.

INDICATIONS

FES may be indicated for upper motor neuron paralysis. This includes cases with a clinical picture of hemiplegia, paraparesis, and cerebral palsy and some cases of multiple sclerosis. The goals of functional electrical stimulation are to alleviate spasticity, to assist the reorganization of motor activity in the early phase after such lesions, to accelerate spontaneous neurologic recovery of voluntary control of movement, to influence reestablishment of the basic motor mechanisms integrated at the level of the spinal cord, and to substitute electrical control for simple movements such as dorsiflexion of the foot or extension of the fingers.

FES can be applied as an isolated therapy, in conjunction with other therapeutic methods, or as a functional orthotic aid for direct substitution of absent motor functions.

1. Hemiplegia. For persons who have suffered a cerebrovascular insult, cerebral

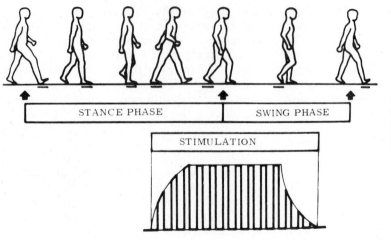

FIGURE 16–1. In the usual sequence of FES the peroneal nerve is stimulated by the closing of a switch as the ipsilateral heel breaks contact with the floor.

trauma, extirpation of a brain tumor, or other cerebral disease with a clinical picture of hemiplegia, FES may be used to retrain and assist gait. In general FES is indicated as a therapeutic treatment in all persons with a clinically present paralysis or paresis. While the patient is still immobile, electrical stimulation of the peroneal nerve or of corresponding muscles is performed with controls that cycle automatically. Once the patient starts walking, electrical stimulation is triggered at some phase of the gait, as shown on Figure 16–1. Under these conditions FES not only activates the ankle dorsiflexors but also inhibits spasticity in the plantar-flexors.

In properly selected cases FES may be used as the orthosis of choice. It is efficient as an orthotic aid in 25 to 30 per cent of hemiplegics who meet certain criteria. There should be no changes in osteoarticular structures such as contractures and deformities, nor strongly spastic equinovalgus. Inequality of extremity length or extreme weakness of the hip, knee, or ankle joint decreases the likelihood of effective use. The lower motor neuron pathway must be intact and the muscles should exhibit good contractile properties. The peroneal nerve should demonstrate normal excitability. There should be no difficulties in locating the exact points of transcutaneous stimulation. There should be normal response to normal intensity of stimulation. The patient should be able to understand and use the system for FES independently. Brain lesions causing severe physical or psychological changes may make this impossible[11] (Fig. 16–2). When the motor deficit is displayed predominantly as footdrop and spasticity is of slight or moderate degree, FES

provides a functional pattern of walking. However, the patient must have the understanding and tolerance to accept the greater degree of attention required by the more complicated electronic system.

FES for control of finger and wrist exten-

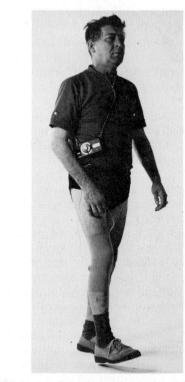

FIGURE 16–2. Gait of a patient with a right hemiplegia, during FES. Adequate control of dorsal flexion of the foot is achieved. (From Vodovnik, L., Gračanin, F., and Strojnik, P.: Functional electrical stimulation for control of locomotor systems. CRC: Critical Review of Bioengineering, Sept., 1981, pp. 63–131.)

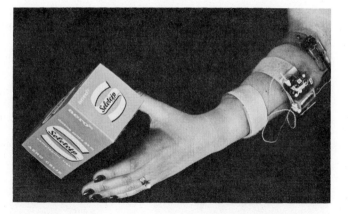

FIGURE 16–3. Stimulation of the finger and wrist extensors in a patient who has preserved ability for grasp enables her to use the hand for ADLs. The bracelet containing the control switch is seen near the elbow. The stimulator, batteries, and electrodes are attached to the arm by Velcro tape.

sion may be indicated for patients in whom the possibility for grasping is preserved but who are unable to do so because of extensor paralysis. Application of electrical stimulation to the radial nerve or corresponding muscles may result in functional use of the fingers. Such electrical stimulation for retraining is applied during the rehabilitation program or in the course of occupational therapy. Indications for continuing use of FES as an orthotic aid beyond the therapeutic period exist for only a small number of patients[12] (Fig. 16–3).

2. Multiple Sclerosis. In multiple sclerosis FES is applicable in cases in which the clinical manifestations of the motor deficit are similar to those in hemiplegic patients with footdrop or paralysis of finger and wrist extensors. For patients with paralysis of other muscles FES has rarely been useful. Normal electrical excitability of the spinal motor neurons must be retained. Practically, this means that systems for FES can be applied using standard parameters of electrical stimuli. From the functional point of view, application brings benefits only if the progress of the disease is relatively slow.

3. Cerebral Palsy. FES is indicated in children who display an impaired walking pattern. The child's cooperation and acceptance of FES are indispensable if FES is to be applied therapeutically or as an orthotic aid.

The location of the electrodes for optimal stimulation may be slightly different for a child. Likewise the timing of the stimulus must be adjusted to the faster gait. In cases of hemiplegia application of bilateral FES is efficacious. A combination of afferent stimulation to the unaffected side and efferent stimulation to the affected side is possible. In some children FES creates patterns of flexion synergy in both the swinging leg and the supporting leg (the secondary spindle reflex flexion synergy), which reduce the ability to sustain the erect posture on the supporting leg. In such cases the peroneal nerve is stimulated during the swing phase and the tibial nerve during the stance phase. FES is applicable in clinical cases of monoplegia, hemiplegia, bilateral hemiplegia, diplegia, and quadriplegia, provided the child is capable of standing erect either alone or supported so that stepping can be induced. The major obstacles are contractures that do not allow foot dorsiflexion or a strong valgus deformation.

Children show skin hypersensitivity, usually of an eczematous nature, to daily electrical stimulation more often than adults. In our studies 2.6 per cent of children developed dermatitis, and in 1.7 per cent of all children treated by surface FES the treatment had to be discontinued in spite of its benefit because of persistent dermatitis.

Because of the specific benefits in gait in children we have introduced additional modes of sequence control of stimulation: contralateral control and a more successful contralaterally controlled alternating FES (CCA FES) (Fig. 16–4). Here, both peroneal nerves and their branches are stimulated. If this stimulation fails to achieve an optimal dorsiflexion in a developed valgus deformity or when there is severe spasticity of the triceps surae muscle, peroneal nerve and tibial muscle are stimulated. These variations may achieve functional control of the mechanisms of gait.

Because application of FES systems for hand control demands a higher level of cooperation, it is rarely performed in small chil-

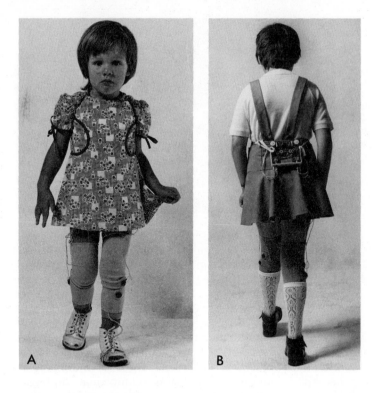

FIGURE 16–4. Gait of children with cerebral palsy using bilateral FES of the peroneal nerves. In both cases successful prevention of equinus position of the foot and reduction of internal rotation and adduction at the hip were achieved. (From Vodovnik, L., Gračanin, F., and Strojnik, P.: Functional electrical stimulation for control of locomotor systems. CRC: Critical Review of Bioengineering, Sept., 1981, pp. 63–131.)

dren. For children of preschool age and school age who will tolerate the stimulation, FES is applied during the program of physical or occupational therapy.

4. Miscellaneous. FES is indicated for patients with paraparesis that has resulted from lesions or diseases of the spinal cord but in whom the electrical excitability of spinal motor neurons is preserved to such a degree that standard parameters of electrical stimuli enable an adequate control of dorsiflexion and eversion of the foot during gait. Beside improving the gait during stimulation, FES may also show permanent improvement of the impaired motor pattern to a greater extent than in cases of hemiplegia.

Conditions Preventing a Wider Application of FES

Although FES may cause motor responses in many cases of upper motor neuron dysfunction, it is practical for application only to a small proportion of these cases. Application is limited by certain contraindications.[10, 39, 44] Dyskinesia with or without dystonia or hyperkinetic hypertonic syndromes impairs control of movement. When there is flaccid paralysis of central origin, movement is limited to that produced by the FES, and

no permanent therapeutic effect can be expected. In such cases there is no indication for FES either as an orthotic aid or a therapy.

FES units are relatively complicated and expensive. They require frequent adjustments and repairs. The patient and family must be willing to take extra time and effort to apply and maintain them. In addition unsolved interface problems, breakdown of equipment, and delay in repairs and servicing prevent broader usage. Despite these disadvantages, FES often makes it possible to restore or substitute for impaired motor function. Therefore, FES should be regarded as a new and applicable rehabilitation method for appropriately selected patients.

SYSTEMS OF FUNCTIONAL ELECTRICAL STIMULATION

Control of Movements of Lower Extremities. In the last 30 years many systems for FES have been developed, the majority in the form of electronic walking aids, intended for improvement of gait.[4, 7, 9, 14, 17, 18, 20, 25, 30, 31, 37, 40, 41, 43, 44] Only a few of these studies have been applied to large groups of patients. Among these are the Ljubljana Functional Electronic Peroneal Brace type FEPA-10

TABLE 16–1. MODES OF CONTROLLING THE STIMULATION OF NERVES AND LEG MUSCLES, RESPECTIVELY

Modes of Control	Characteristics
1. Unilateral one-channel stimulation	
a. Ipsilateral control	Electrical stimulation starts with heel-off in the phase of support and lasts during the whole swing phase until heel-strike. The variants are the so-called preset, when the stimulation interval is defined in advance, and "walking rate," when the stimulation time is regulated by the walking speed. These time intervals are usually shorter than the heel-off to heel-strike interval.
b. Contralateral control	Electrical stimulation begins with the stance phase and lasts until the beginning of swing phase of the non-stimulated leg. Variants preset and walking rate are possible.
2. Bilateral one-channel stimulation	Stimulation sequence are partly overlapping themselves.
a. Ipsilateral control	Characteristics are the same as in 1.a and 1.b.
b. Contralateral control	
c. CCA FES (contralaterally controlled alternating functional electrical stimulation)	Stimulation of left and right legs is reciprocally related and the stimulation sequences do not overlap themselves.
3. Two-channel stimulation	
a. Unilateral	Represents stimulation of two nerves or stimulation of the corresponding antagonistic muscles of one joint, or the stimulation of synergistic muscles of two or more joints.
b. Bilateral	Stimulation of two nerves of the corresponding antagonistic muscles of both legs produces reciprocally dependent synergy in flexion (swing phase) and extension (support phase of gait).
4. Multichannel stimulation	Stimulation of many muscles or muscle groups and nerves with application of stimulation sequences desired to produce the motor pattern.

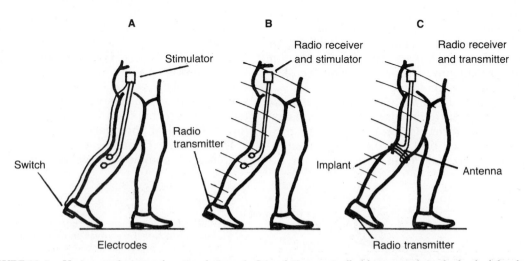

FIGURE 16–5. Various techniques for stimulation. *A,* Stimulation controlled by a switch in the heel of the shoe with wire connections to stimulator at hip and to surface electrodes. *B,* A radio link from a switch in the insole to stimulator with wire connections to surface electrodes. The insole contains both the switch and the transmitter. *C,* A radio link from a switch in the insole to implanted receiver, stimulator, and electrodes.

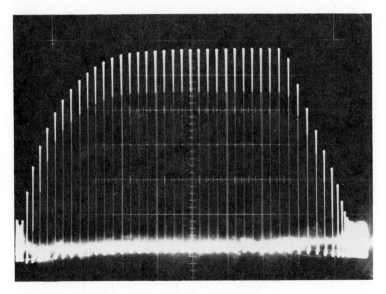

FIGURE 16–6. Amplitude modulation of the train of electrical pulses recruits a smoother movement.

with numerous modifications such as FEPA-11 (with a radio link), FEPA-12 (radio link and implant), FEPA-14 (CCA FES). Medtronic's Neuromod and ENA-2 of the Mensor Corporation, both from U.S.A.; LIC from Sweden; and STIPEL and BISTIPEL from France all work on the same or similar principles. Some systems are constructed so that electrical stimulation is performed with surface electrodes. Some have a radio link from the switch either to an external stimulator or to an implanted stimulator[21, 45] (Fig. 16–5).

Identical features in all systems are an impulse generator (stimulator); stimulation electrodes (surface or implant); a switch built into the insole or the shoe itself; and wires for connection between the impulse generator, the electrodes, and the switch, or, in case of a radio link, a wire for connection with the antenna that is placed on the skin above the implanted receiver.

Electrical Impulse Generator (Stimulator). It generates impulses of exponential or rectangular form. Current parameters provide a duration of 0.3 to 0.6 ms; frequency, 20 to 100 Hz; and train duration up to 1.8

secs. The train of impulses usually has amplitude modulation that provides a slow increase in amplitude at the beginning and a slow decrease of amplitude at the end of the train. In case of frequency modulation, frequency increases at the beginning and decreases at the end of the stimulation (Fig. 16–6). The output may be based on either constant voltage or constant current.

The Electrode. Electrodes differ from those for electrocardiography and range from silver tape to artificial foam. To enable constant conductivity, the electrode in the Ljubljana FEPB has a small water container that allows the liquid to ooze out slowly through the gauze. The side opposite the skin is protected with a plastic cover. The contact surface is slightly curved so as to allow firm contact regardless of minor anatomical unevenness (Fig. 16–7). For permanent stimulation, in order to minimize the irritation of the skin, plain water is used rather than saline solution or the various conducting jellies and creams used in detection of biological electrical potentials.

The Switch. There are several varieties of switches. A commonly used type is a tape

GAUZE

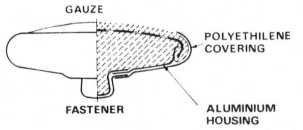

POLYETHILENE
COVERING

FASTENER

ALUMINIUM
HOUSING

FIGURE 16–7. Surface electrode used for the Ljubljana functional electrical peroneal brace. The design affords prolonged moistening of the electrode.

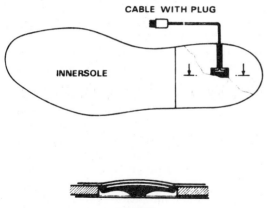

FIGURE 16–8. A switch designed for insertion into the insole.

switch (gilded and encased in a plastic foil) that can be built into the heel, midfoot, or toe area of a common insole in the shoe (Figs. 16–8 to 16–10).

Control of Motor Function and Movements of the Upper Extremity. The systems applied today in external control of hand, wrist, and finger movements are still experimental. The Ljubljana Functional Electronic Radial Brace (FERB) operates either as an "on-off" response to a pressure switch or on adjustable stimulation time. The wrist and finger extensor brace (FESE H3) system can be set with proportional electrical stimulation that is under the volitional control of the user[36]

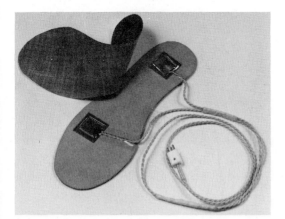

FIGURE 16–9. A switch built into the insole. At the beginning of training, because of spasticity of the triceps surae muscle, the child walks with a toe-strike or hits the ground with the lateral edge of the foot. After walking with FES, he soon strikes the heel first. Two switches, placed under the forefoot and under the heel, assure timely triggering of the electrical stimulus.

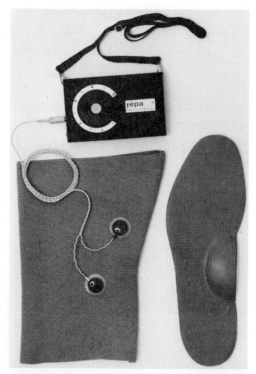

FIGURE 16–10. The equipment for radio-linked functional electrical stimulation, FEPA-11. The switch and radio transmitter built into the medial part of the insole activate the stimulator without need for a direct wire connection between the switch and the stimulator.

(Fig. 16–11). For a therapeutic program, universal portable stimulators with variable parameters (AM5 ZR1, Fig. 16–13) can be used.

Application of the Systems for FES and Training of the Patient in Independent Use of the System

Selection of the Parameters of the Electrical Stimulus for Functional Electrical Stimulation. Functional electrical stimulation is not a natural stimulation and can cause pain and irritation of the skin. For these reasons, it is necessary to use the minimal energy expenditure (amplitude, frequency) that achieves an adequate movement. The stimulator may use constant voltage or constant current output. The pulse duration is adjusted to be as short as possible to minimize sensory stimulation and yet obtain an effective motor response.

To produce a smooth movement in patients with upper motor neuron lesions the pulse repetition rate should be slower than

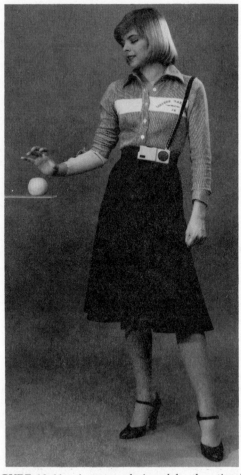

FIGURE 16–11. A system designed for the stimulation of finger and wrist extensors, FESE-H3. Continuous control of the stimulus intensity is maintained through a slide potentiometer that is controlled by shoulder movements of the unaffected side. (From Vodovnik, L., Gračanin, F., and Strojnik, P.: Functional electrical stimulation for control of locomotor systems. CRC: Critical Review of Bioengineering, Sept., 1981, pp. 63–131.)

that for healthy individuals. As motor function improves, the pulse repetition rate may be increased gradually. The amplitude of the pulse is modulated by a gradual increase of the amplitude at the beginning of the train to provide progressive recruitment of the contraction. The duration of each train, regardless of the method of stimulation, usually depends upon the patient's walking rate.

Determination of the Skin Motor Points for Stimulation. When applying an FES system the exact sites for placing the electrodes should be located. The best sites for placing the electrodes are those at which a stimulus of minimal intensity produces optimal movement. For lower extremity flexion the typical

points of stimulation in almost all patients are in the popliteal fossa close to the medial edge of the biceps femoris muscle, which is over the common peroneal nerve, and distally behind the head of the fibula (Fig. 16–12).

The diameter of the distal area is somewhat larger, since the point of stimulation is determined by stimulation of one of the branches of the peroneal nerve, depending upon the kind of movement to be evoked. Attention should be given to the polarity of the electrodes. *When the cathode is proximal a secondary spindle flexor synergy pattern is elicited,* whereas when the cathode is distal an efferent motor response predominates. Determination of electrode placement is made with the patient in a sitting position with the knee semiflexed. The lower part of the patient's leg must be supported so that the foot is free to move as shown in Figure 16–13.

Fixing of the Electrodes During the Patient's Gait Training with FES. At the time that training is initiated it is best to fix the electrodes with Velcro or similar tape (Fig. 16–13). The patient walks while the physical

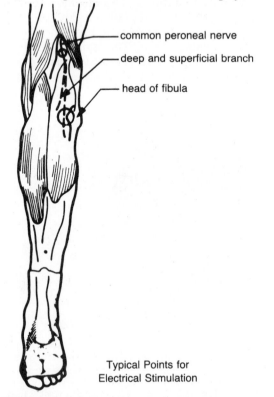

— common peroneal nerve

— deep and superficial branch

— head of fibula

Typical Points for
Electrical Stimulation

FIGURE 16–12. Typical points for electrical stimulation to obtain a flexor response of the lower extremity.

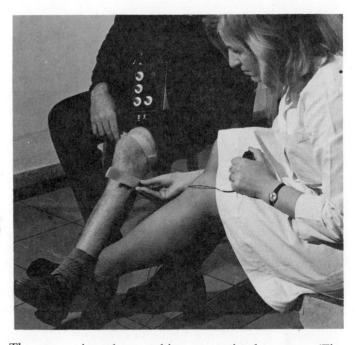

FIGURE 16–13. Determining the proper sites for electrical stimulation.

therapist controls the stimulation. The optimal duration of the train of stimuli is usually 0.8 to 1.0 sec. During this practice time the physical therapist can make small changes in the position of either electrode as necessary

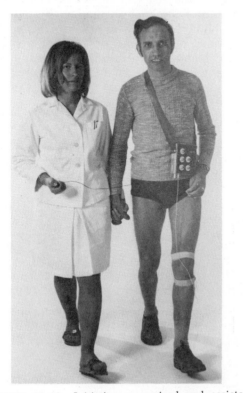

FIGURE 16–14. Initiating supervised and assisted gait training.

in order to achieve an optimal response (Fig. 16–14).

Gait Training of the Patient with an FES System and Adjustment of Stimulus Parameters. It must be remembered that the patient has not used his paretic muscles actively for a long time. The muscles have lost strength and endurance. For this reason it is necessary at the start to exercise several times daily for about 10 minutes and to increase the time as endurance improves. When the optimal points for location of the electrodes have been determined they may be applied attached to an elastic knee support. It was found that the elastic knee support should be of a size that will be comfortable for the patient after hours of use while concomitantly holding the electrodes close to the skin. The choice of the appropriate size is of great importance. Figure 16–15 provides European measurements as an indication of the size of suitable knee support. When marking points for fastening the electrodes on the knee support, it is best to pull the knee support over the electrodes while they are held in place by Velcro, and then mark the corresponding points on the knee support. At the beginning of the training with FES, stimulation can be strong enough to achieve slight over-correction of dorsiflexion and eversion of the foot. The physical therapist holds the patient's unaffected hand to assist balance and support. No other devices (canes, crutches, etc.) are

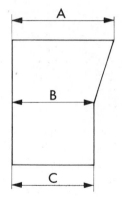

size	6	8	10	12
A cm	17	18	19	21
B cm	13	14,5	15,5	17
C cm	13	14,5	15,5	17

FIGURE 16–15. Dimensions of elastic knee supports for European standard sizes.

recommended. The physical therapist walks along with the patient and triggers the stimulator in the middle of the stance phase (Fig. 16–14). It is recommended that a metronome be used to control the time and regular rhythm of the gait. If extensor spasticity is severe, stimulation could be triggered at the beginning of the stance phase in order to achieve optimal movement during the swing phase. By adjustment of the duration of the train of stimuli, the desired motor response is obtained. The duration of the train of stimuli is adjusted to the walking rate of each patient by the physical therapist. In the Ljubljana FEPA-10 this is done by removing the cover of the stimulator, placing the switch for stimulation mode on preset (PS), and rotating the duration control "ts" to the desired duration of the stimulation train. If necessary, the frequency can be adjusted similarly, i.e., by rotating the knob f (Hz) (Fig. 16–16). PS means preset duration, in which mode the duration of the train of stimuli is constant. WR means walking rate, in which mode the duration of the stimulation time depends on the speed of gait and shortens as the speed of

walking increases. Control of the stimulation by a heel switch may be commenced when the patient becomes familiar with the technique, regardless of whether he still needs the physical therapist's assistance for balance or not.

Training of the Patient for Independent Use of the Device. The patient should learn to use the FES system during his rest periods as well as during walking. He should learn how to put on the elastic knee support with the electrodes on the inside and positioned correctly. One indication of correct orientation is when the seam of the stocking is in the midline of the back of the leg (Fig. 16–17). He should learn how to place the insole into the shoe, put the shoe on the foot, and plug the cables of the electrodes and insole into the stimulator. He should learn to regulate the stimulator. The equipment is always put on with the stimulator turned off, The patient should learn to turn on the stimulator and increase the intensity of stimulus to achieve the appropriate dorsiflexion and eversion of the foot. He also should be taught how to recognize equipment malfunctions.

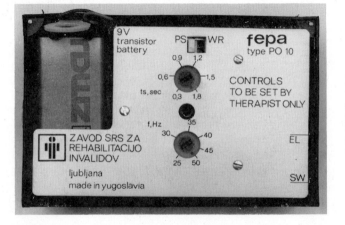

FIGURE 16–16. Control surface on the reverse side of the stimulator, with the cover removed. The physical therapist can determine the train duration (ts), the frequency of electrical impulses in the train (f,Hz), and the preset (PS) or walking rate (WR) stimulation modes.

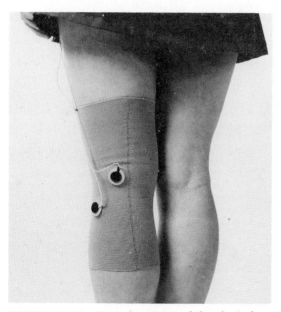

FIGURE 16–17. Typical position of the elastic knee support and electrodes.

Functional Electrical Stimulation in Research, Feasibility Studies, and Sporadic Applications Using Similar Techniques

Striving for control of more complex movements of the lower extremities by means of simultaneous or sequential stimulation of a number of muscles has led to the development of multichanneled electronic FES systems. Today we have a two-channel FES system for activation of antagonist muscles of the ankle joint[31] or for the stimulation of the femoral and inferior gluteal nerve during gait.[28] Three-channel and multichannel stimulators for gait control during the execution of a therapeutic program have also been developed.[1, 27, 29, 30, 31] However, use of this equipment is limited because of the difficulties experienced in the application and because of the unsolved interface problems. Several publications on the subject testify to the interest in the development of these systems. We now have at our disposal a 6-channel stimulator with programmed optimal stimulation sequences.[38, 42] It is evident from these publications that the goal is a functional orthosis rather than a therapeutic method. Among the problems interfering with practical application of these systems is the fact that the optimal anatomical structures for stimulation may not be accessible. There are unresolved difficulties of interface

linkage between the patient and the FES system. The systems now available to be applied and used independently are too complex for the patient. There is inadequate knowledge about the influence of prolonged simultaneous and sequential generation of nerve impulses on the organization of motor activity, on postural mechanisms, and on the responses of the vegetative nervous system. Feasibility studies have shown that a paraplegic patient can be maintained in an upright posture between parallel bars by stimulation of certain muscle groups. It has also been shown that stepping similar to the swing phase of gait can be stimulated.[23] The research, tests, and feasibility studies mentioned here represent work from groups around the world over a number of years. A group from Cleveland has combined stimulation of individual muscles with the use of classic mechanical aids in an attempt to improve hand function of a quadriplegic patient who has lower motor neuron damage as well as upper motor neuron damage.[35]

The application of FES for reducing the deformity in idiopathic scoliosis has shown remarkable results. Not only has there been a reduction of the curvature but also a complete change of the motor activity pattern of paravertebral muscles during functional loading of the spine.[2, 3, 6, 15, 16]

Some authors seem to confuse functional electrical stimulation with the classic form of electrotherapy of innervated and denervated muscles as described elsewhere in this text, or give FES the role of a mere orthotic aid. From our experience in applying FES programs with or without use at home for more than 2000 hemiplegics, more than 50 patients with multiple sclerosis and paraparesis of various origins, and more than 400 children with cerebral palsy, and after having distributed approximately 3000 FES systems to various rehabilitation centers around the world, we can critically compare indications, advantages, and disadvantages for this method with other neurotherapeutic methods and classic orthotic aids. FES is more than a muscle stimulator. From advances in knowledge of neurophysiology today, we know that systematically repeated sensory input to the central nervous system through afferent pathways with the resulting proprioceptive and reflex responses influences the organization of motor activity in man. Appropriately applied stimuli result in improved multimuscular performance. Although there are limitations due to current technology and serious deficiencies in the development of the interfacing between the patient and equipment, still FES has become a successful method in reestablishing motor functions to control motor output and movements. By applying an FES system to a patient we give him a functional orthotic aid that is an immediate substitute for the impaired functions, and at the same time this enables him to repeat the motor pattern thousands of times, which is of great importance for the therapeutic effect.

A special approach to the control of motor functions with the objective of reducing the neurologic deficit is the so-called dorsal column stimulation (DCS, spinal cord stimulation, epidural stimulation), introduced by Cook et al. in 1973 for multiple sclerosis patients with moderate to severe motor deficits, insufficiency of bladder control, and other signs of impaired nervous functions. Clinical research indicates that the method is still in the development phase, and further research is needed to explain the effect of dorsal column stimulation on the organization of motor activity.[8] This will enable a more selective choice of patients and help to establish criteria for assessing the degree of improvement of motor functions by this method.

REFERENCES

1. Ačimović, R., Stanič, U., Gros, N., and Bajd, T.: Correction of hemiplegic gait pattern by multichannel surface stimulation during swing and stance phase. *In* Komi, P. V. (Ed.): Biomechanics V-A. Baltimore, University Park Press, 1976.
2. Axelgaard, J., McNeal, D. R., and Brown, J. C.: Lateral electrical surface stimulation for the treatment of progressive scoliosis. *In* Proc. Int. Symp. External Control of Human Extremities, Dubrovnik, Yugoslavia, 1978, p. 63.
3. Bobechko, B. P.: Electrostimulation in Scoliosis, Report of Workshop on Functional Neuromuscular Stimulation. Bethesda, Md., National Academy of Sciences, 1972, p. 145.
4. Canzoneri, J., and Koenig, D. E.: A biomedical engineering report on functional electric peroneal activators based on two years of clinical experience. *In* Proc. Int. Symp. External Control of Human Extremities, Dubrovnik, Yugoslavia, 1972, pp. 1–32 (appendix).
5. Creed, R. S., Denny-Brown, D., Eccles, J. C., Liddell, E. G. T., and Sherrington, C. S.: Reflex Activity of the Spinal Cord. Oxford, Oxford University Press, 1932.
6. Crivelini, M., Divieti, C., Fillipi, V., and Sibilla, P.: Electrical stimulation for scoliotic patients. *In* Supplement of Proc. Int. Symp. External Control of Human Extremities, Dubrovnik, Yugoslavia, 1978, p. 125.
7. Dillner, S., Georgiev, G., and Korsznia, A.: Proposed Requirement Specification for Peroneal Muscle Stimulators, EFTO Report 9/77, Jönköping, Sweden, 1977.
8. Gračanin, F.: Use of Functional Stimulation in Rehabilitation of Hemiplegic Patients, Report 19-P-58395-F-012–66. Washington, D.C., Department of HEW, 1972.
9. Gračanin, F.: Functional electrical stimulation in cerebral palsy children as an orthotic walking aid with a neurotherapeutic effect. *In* Abstracts of the Congress Intl. Soc. Prosthetists Orthotists, Montreux, Switzerland, 1974, p. 77.
10. Gračanin, F.: Use of electrical stimulation in external control of motor activity and movements of human extremities. Med. Progr. Technol., 4:149, 1977.
11. Gračanin, F.: Functional electrical stimulation in control of motor output and movements. Electroencephalogr. Clin. Neurophysiol. (Suppl.), 34:355, 1978.
12. Gračanin, F., and Dimitrijević, M. R.: An electronic brace for externally controlled movement in wrist and fingers of the hemiparetic patients. *In* Proc. Symp. Electronics in Medicine, Ljubljana, Yugoslavia, 1968, p. 9.
13. Gračanin, F., and Dimitrijević, M. R.: Application of Functional Electrical Stimulation in Rehabilitation of Neurological Patients. *In* The Use of Reflex Mechanisms in Reeducation of Mobility. Ed. Baluca, Praha, 1968, p. 91.
14. Gračanin, F., Benedik, M., Jeglič, A., Vavken, E., and Vrabič, M.: Instruction Manual for Usage of Ljubljana FEPA 12. Ljubljana, Zavod Rehabil. Invalidov, Publ., 1966.
15. Gračanin, F., and Bizjak, F.: Omogucaj ulozi posturalnih refleksnih mehanizama u nastojanju deformacije kraljesnice. *In* Kovacic, S. (Ed.): Proc. Symp. Scoliosis and Kyphosis, Zagreb, Yugoslavia, 1977, p. 261.
16. Gračanin, F., Bizjak, F., and Preseren-Štrukelj, M.: Po men elektrofizioloskih analiz za dolocanje optimalnega terapevtskega programa pri bolnikih z idiopatsko skoliozo. *In* Proc. Symp. Scoliosis and Kyphosis, Skopje, Yugoslavia, 1979 (in press).
17. Gračanin, F., Kralj, A., and Reberšek, S.: Advanced version of "the Ljubljana functional electronic peroneal brace" with walking rate controlled tetanization. *In* Proc. Int. External Control of Human Extremities, Dubrovnik, Yugoslavia, 1969, p. 487.
18. Gračanin, F., and Marinček, I.: Development of new systems for functional electrical stimulation. *In* Proc. Int. Symp. External Control of Human Extremities, Belgrade, Yugoslavia, 1970, p. 495.
19. Gračanin, F., and Vrabič, M.: Instruction Manual for Usage of Ljubljana FEPA 10. Ljubljana, Zavod Rehabil. Invalidov, Publ., 1974, p. 19.
20. Gračanin, F., and Dimitrijević, M. R.: Application of functional electrical stimulation in rehabilitation of the neurological patient. *In* The Use of Reflex Mechanisms in Reeducation of Mobility. Praha, Balnea, 1968, p. 91.

21. Jeglič, A.: Two-channel implant approach to an orthotic device. *In* Proc. Int. External Control of Human Extremities. Dubrovnik, Yugoslavia, 1972, p. 647.

22. Kottke, F. J.: Facilitation and inhibition as fundamental characteristics of neuromuscular organization. *In* Buerger, A. A., and Tobis, J. S. (Eds.): Neurophysiologic Aspects of Rehabilitation Medicine. Springfield, Ill., Charles C Thomas, Publisher, 1976, pp. 251–279.

23. Kralj, A., and Grobelnik, S.: Functional electrical stimulation — a new home for paraplegic patients. Bull. Prosthet. Res., 10–20:75–102 (Fall), 1973.

24. Gračanin, F., Bizjak, F., and Prešeren-Štrukelj, M.: Electrophysiological Analyses in Determining Optimal Therapeutic Program of Idiopathic Scoliosis Patients. *In* Proceedings of the VIIth Symposium on Scoliosis and Kyphosis. Skopje, 1979.

25. Prospectus for Stimulateur Peronier Electronique "STIPEL" Grenoble, France, Lectronique.

26. Levine, M. G., Knott, M., and Kabat, H.: Relaxation of spasticity by electrical stimulation of antagonist muscles. Arch. Phys. Med. Rehabil., 33:668–673, 1952.

27. Lee, W. J., McGovern, J. P., and Duvall, E. N.: Continuous tetanizing (low voltage) currents for relief of spasm: A clinical study of twenty-seven spinal cord injury patients. Arch. Phys. Med. Rehabil., 31:766–771, 1950.

28. Liberson, W. T., Holmquest, H. J., Scot, D., and Dow, M.: Functional electrotherapy: Stimulation of the peroneal nerve synchronized with the swing phase of the gait of hemiplegic patients. Arch. Phys. Med. Rehabil., 42:101–105, 1961.

29. Lloyd, D. P. C.: Integrative pattern of excitation and inhibition in two-neuron reflex arcs. J. Neurophysiol., 9:439–444, 1946.

30. Matejčič, E.: Development of a miniature electronic peroneal brace. *In* Functional Electrical Stimulation of Peroneal Muscles, Report to the Boris Kidric Fund, Ljubljana, Yugoslavia, 1966, p. 22.

31. Maležič, M., Trnkoczy, A., Reberšek, S., Ačimovič, R., Gros, N., Strojnik, P., and Stanic, U.: Advanced cutaneous electrical stimulators for paretic patient's personal use. *In* Proc. Int. Symp. External Control of Human Extremities, Dubrovnik, Yugoslavia, 1978, p. 233.

32. Milner, M., Basmajian, J. V., and Quanbury, A. O.: Locomotion of the paralyzed by ordered electrostimulation of the available musculature — the concept and various problem areas. Proc. Conf. on Medical and Biological Engineering, 1969.

33. Moe, J. H., and Post, H.: Functional electrical stimulation for ambulation in hemiplegia. Lancet, 82:285–288, 1962.

34. Monnier, M.: Functions of the nervous system, Vol. 2. Amsterdam, Elsevier Publishing Company, 1970, p. 352.

35. Mortimer, J. T., and Peckham, P. H.: Intramuscular electrical stimulation. *In* Fields, W. S., and Leavitt, L. (Eds.): Neural Organization and Its Relevance to Prosthetics. New York, Intercontinental Medical Book Corp., 1973, p. 131.

36. Reberšek, S., and Vodovnik, L.: Proportionally controlled functional electrical stimulation of hand. Arch. Phys. Med. Rehabil., 54:378–382, 1973.

37. Thomas, D.: La stimulation électrique fonctionelle appareillage et technique de facilitation. Ann. Kinésith., 5:437, 1978.

38. Stanič, U., Ačimovič, R., Gros, N., Trnkoczy, A., Bajd, T., and Kljajic, M.: Multichannel electrical stimulation for correction of hemiplegic gait. Scand. J. Rehabil. Med., 10(2):75–92, 1978.

39. Takebe, K., Kukulka, C., Narayan, M. G., Milner, M., and Basmajian, J. V.: Peroneal nerve stimulator in rehabilitation of hemiplegic patients. Arch. Phys. Med. Rehabil., 56:237–243, 1975.

40. Trnkoczy, A., Stanič, U., and Jeglič, A.: Electronic peroneal brace with a new sequence of stimulation. Med. Biol. Eng., 13:570–576, 1975.

41. Vodovnik, L., Dimitrijević, M. R., Prevec, T., and Logar, M.: Electronic walking aids for patients with peroneal palsy. World Med. Electron., 4(2):58, 1966.

42. Vodovnik, L., Bajd, T., Kralj, A., Gračanin, F., and Strojnik, P.: Functional electrical stimulation for control of locomotor systems. CRC: Critical Review of Bioengineering, Sept., 1981, pp. 63–131.

43. Vredenbregt, J., and Vanleeuwen, J.: A muscle stimulator for hemiplegic patients. *In* Medicine and Sport, Vol. 6: Biomechanics II, Basel, Switzerland, Karger, Publisher, 1971, pp. 285–287.

44. Milner, M., Quanbury, A. O., and Edwards, E. P.: Human locomotion by ordered electrostimulation of the available musculature. Report LTR-CS-11, National Research Council, Ottawa, Canada, 1969.

45. Wilemon, W. K., Mooney, V., McNeal, D., and Reswick, J.: Surgically implanted neuroelectric stimulation: Two years experience at Rancho Los Amigos Hospital. Presented to Committee on Prosthetics Research and Development, Houston, Texas, 1970.

17

MASSAGE

MILAND E. KNAPP

Definition. *Massage* is a term used to signify a group of systematic and scientific manipulations of body tissues which are best performed with the hands "for the purpose of affecting the nervous and muscular system and the general circulation."

HISTORY

Massage is probably the oldest of all remedies, since it is instinctive, not only in man but in the lower animals as well. The oldest written record of massage was made 3000 years ago by the Chinese. The ancient Hindus, Persians, and Egyptians used manipulation in some form and some of the movements of massage for rheumatic ailments. The Greeks recognized gymnastics as an institution which was an auxiliary to the development of the people both socially and politically. Hippocrates wrote important papers on massage, for instance, about the use of friction after sprains and dislocations and about kneading in case of constipation. About two centuries ago the Chinese books on massage were translated into French, which accounts for the French terminology so common in massage texts. At the beginning of the nineteenth century Peter Henry Ling, a fencing master of Stockholm, Sweden, introduced a system of movement which he had not originated but had systematized. It consists of, first, massage (manipulation of the soft tissues) and, sec-ond, medical gymnastics (exercise of the joints). During the last century, Lucas-Championnière championed treatment of fractures by mobilization including massage and exercise. And more recently, during the years 1917 to 1940, James B. Mennell of England systematized massage movements and applied them to the treatment of a great many conditions.

PHYSIOLOGIC EFFECTS OF MASSAGE

Unfortunately, most of the teaching of massage in the past has been done by lay persons who did not understand physiology in the modern sense so that many statements made in massage texts are obviously untrue insofar as physiologic effects of massage are concerned. The effects may be classified as reflex and mechanical.

Reflex Effects. Reflex effects are produced in the skin by stimulation of the peripheral receptors, which then transmit impulses through the spinal cord to the brain and produce sensations of pleasure or relaxation. Peripherally these impulses cause relaxation of muscles and dilatation or constriction of arterioles. Sedation is one of the very important physiologic effects of massage. It is obtained when the massage is given in a monotonously repetitive manner without sharp variations in pressure or irritating changes in the method of application.

These pleasant effects result in relaxation of muscle as well as reduction of mental tension.

Mechanical Effects. The mechanical effects consist of (1) measures that assist return flow circulation of blood and lymph because the massage is given with the greatest force in the centripetal direction, and (2) measures that produce intramuscular motion. They may be effective in stretching adhesions between muscle fibers and mobilizing accumulations of fluid.

Massage does *not* develop muscle strength and should *not* be used as a substitute for active exercise.

TECHNIQUE

Proficiency in the performance of massage movements is not easily acquired. It requires long and diligent practice. Massage is an art rather than a science. One individual may learn to administer acceptable massage quickly and after only a minimum of practice while another may never give acceptable massage even after many months of assiduous effort. Natural ability is an important factor. However, as with other arts, improvement will be gained by practice.

I am not in favor of trying to teach the patient or his family to give massage at home except under unusual circumstances, because this kind of training is usually inadequate and the resulting treatment may produce harmful effects as easily as helpful results.

Description of technique is difficult, but certain principles may be stated:

1. The patient must be relaxed and comfortable. Clothing should not be tight, especially proximal to the area to be treated. Clothing should be removed from the area to be treated but the patient should not be uncovered unnecessarily to avoid embarrassment and needless cooling.

2. The therapist should also be relaxed and comfortable and should stand in a position such that the entire stroke can be performed without change of stance or undue movement.

3. Skill is required rather than strength. Pain and apprehension must not be produced if deep effects are desired. A relaxed muscle has the physical properties of a liquid enclosed in a membrane, and pressure exerted on any portion of it will be transmitted equally in all directions. Pressure is thus transmitted to the deeper muscles. On the other hand, a tense, contracted muscle has the properties of a solid and does not transmit the force evenly.

4. A lubricating oil, powder, or cream facilitates good technique. Heavy mineral oil is suitable.

Stroking (Effleurage). Stroking massage is performed by running the hand lightly over the surface of the skin. The force of the stroke starts distally and progresses proximally to assist return flow circulation. The hands may be lifted off the part at the end of the stroke and returned to the point of beginning if the motion is rhythmic and the contact and release are performed gently, without abruptness. It is probably better, however, to return to the point of beginning with the hands in contact with the skin but producing little or no actual pressure.

Stroking may be superficial or deep. In superficial stroking the direction of the force is not important, since the pressure is so light that mechanical effects are not produced. In deep stroking the direction of force is important because the usual major objective is to assist return flow circulation. Therefore, the force of the stroke definitely should be centripetal.

Compression (Pétrissage). Compression includes kneading, squeezing, and friction. Kneading may be described as a motion in which the soft tissues are picked up between the fingers and manipulated in an alternating fashion so that there is motion within the muscle itself. It does not proceed in any particular direction but is used to mobilize the tissue fluids and create intramuscular motion to stretch adhesions. Squeezing is performed with larger portions of the muscle, squeezing the part either between the two hands or between the hand and a solid object such as the table or bone. Friction is a circular motion performed by placing a small part of the hand on the area. This portion of the hand is usually the thumb, the heel of the hand, or the finger tips. The movement is in circular loops and is done fairly rapidly with increasing pressure.

Percussion (Tapôtement). Percussion movements are alternating movements performed to produce stimulation. Hacking is usually done with the outer border of the hand or the relaxed fingers, bouncing the hands alternately off the part to be treated. It may also be used in a kind of whipping motion using the fingers as the flexible portion of the whip. Clapping is done with the palms of the hand in a similar manner. If the hands are cupped the deeper sound produced may be of some psychologic benefit. Beating is performed with the clenched fist by a similar technique. The therapist produces vibration by placing his finger tips in contact with the skin and shaking his entire arm. This transmits a trembling movement to the patient. The therapeutic value of this type of movement is questionable, although it is pleasant when performed expertly.

The movements of massage are not done in sequence but are intermingled, using varying techniques for different purposes. The compression techniques are used to mobilize tissue deposits and to stretch adhesions. They may be followed by stroking massage to remove the deposits or edema fluid. Friction is used to treat very limited areas, particularly nodules such as fibrositic nodules, and this again is followed by stroking massage. The percussion movements are ordinarily used at the end of the treatment. It is my opinion that they are used primarily for psychologic effects rather than for any real physical benefit.

Numerous mechanical devices have been invented and manufactured for the application of massage movements. Rollers of various types operated manually or by electric motors have tried to simulate kneading and stroking types of massage. Perhaps the most common machines are those that produce vibration. They are attached to the hand or incorporated in pads of various kinds and on tables. While they may produce pleasurable effects, it is generally conceded that they are not therapeutically effective.

INDICATIONS

Massage is useful in any condition in which relief of pain, reduction of swelling, or mobilization of contracted tissues is desired. Probably its greatest single indication is to overcome the swelling and induration that frequently follow trauma (see Chapter 33). Fractures, dislocations, joint injuries, sprains, strains, bruises, and tendon and nerve injuries may be benefited by massage at certain stages of recovery. Arthritis, periarthritis, bursitis, neuritis, fibrositis, low back pain, and paralytic conditions such as hemiplegia, paraplegia, quadriplegia, cerebral palsy, and multiple sclerosis may present problems that can be relieved by massage.

Psychoneurotic patients and occasionally even patients with psychoses may be helped by massage. However, such treatment should be prescribed only after careful consideration of its psychologic effects because harmful psychologic trends may be intensified by physical treatment.

Abdominal massage has been advocated and described in the past but is not used to any great extent at the present time. It is also ineffective for weight reduction.

Massage is not a substitute for exercise. It does not increase muscle strength. Strength develops in muscles contracting actively, preferably against resistance.

A masseur once told me he was giving an alcoholic patient massage equivalent to a three-mile hike. Perhaps he was, but the hike was being performed by the masseur, on his hands. The patient was getting rest in bed.

CONTRAINDICATIONS

The greatest contraindications to massage are infections, because of the likelihood of spreading the infection through the tissues and breaking down barriers to the spread of infection; malignancies, because tumor tissues similarly may be spread beyond confined limits and promote metastases or extension of the malignancy; and skin diseases (which might be communicated to the masseur), when irritation is contraindicated or when lesions might be spread by contact. Massage should be given with caution in debilitated individuals and in areas where the skin has been damaged by burns or where it is thin for other reasons. In thrombophlebitis massage may be dangerous because thrombi may be broken into emboli.

REFERENCES

1. Krusen, F. H.: Physical Medicine. Philadelphia, W. B. Saunders Co., 1941.
2. Mennell, J. B.: Physical Treatment by Movement, Manipulation and Massage, 4th Ed. Philadelphia, The Blakiston Co., 1940.
3. Tidy, N. M.: Massage and Remedial Exercises in Medical and Surgical Conditions, 3rd Ed. Baltimore, William Wood and Co., 1937.
4. Wood, E. C., and Becker, P. D.: Beard's Massage, 3rd Ed. Philadelphia, W. B. Saunders Company, 1981.

18

THERAPEUTIC EXERCISE TO MAINTAIN MOBILITY

FREDERIC J. KOTTKE

Therapeutic exercise may be defined as the prescription of bodily movement to correct an impairment, improve musculoskeletal function, or maintain a state of well-being. Therapeutic exercise may vary from highly selected activities restricted to specific muscles or parts of the body, to general and vigorous activities used to restore a convalescing patient to the peak of physical condition. The prescription for therapeutic exercise will vary with the purpose for which it is used. This, in turn, is directly dependent upon the condition of the patient. An adequate medical evaluation is essential before therapeutic exercise is prescribed. Therapeutic exercise prescribed without competent medical evaluation and supervision may be not only inadequate but actually detrimental to the patient.

Knowledge of the biophysical and physiologic aspects of kinesiology and the basic principles of therapeutic exercise is needed by the physician who plans to prescribe and supervise a program of therapeutic exercise for his patient. Therapeutic exercises have local and general effects on the physiology of the body. These responses occur in the muscular, skeletal, nervous, circulatory, and endocrine systems in particular. Metabolism may be altered significantly. The prescription of an exercise to produce a desired response is just as specific as, and often more

involved than, the prescription of a pharmaceutical compound. An adequate program of therapeutic exercise requires that the prescription be modified as the condition of the patient changes.

This chapter contains the principles of therapeutic exercise to maintain mobility and information concerning the general types of exercises used in medical practice. Because the exercise program for each patient is developed according to his needs on the basis of the medical evaluation of his disability, no attempt is being made here to provide a "cookbook" of exercises, since for any part of the body, exercises may be designed in a number of ways depending upon the desired goal and the equipment at hand.

EXERCISES TO INCREASE OR MAINTAIN MOBILITY OF JOINTS AND SOFT TISSUES

Physiology of Fibrous Connective Tissue

There is a continual turnover of the components of connective tissue by breakdown and replacement and by reorganization of the attachments of the various components. The connective tissue of the body provides the connection between all cells and around and

389

between all organs. The fibers are made up of reticulin and collagen, which do not appear to be essentially different in their ultramicroscopic structure; elastic fibers, which differ from collagen in their physical and chemical characteristics as well as their metabolic response; and fibrin, which is a temporary connective tissue element extremely important in the process of repair. In addition, there is the amorphous ground substance, which is structureless but which plays an important role in binding the structural elements together. It appears that the attachments between fibers produced by the ground substance can shift as the result of prolonged tension or can develop as the result of prolonged contact.

Although metabolic studies have not clearly defined the rate at which collagen is removed, altered, or replaced under ordinary circumstances, there is considerable information regarding the rapid response of fibrous connective tissue in areas where trauma has occurred. Newly formed collagen fibrils are abundant around proliferating fibroblasts within five days.[1, 2] Recent studies indicate that in normal connective tissue, a small percentage of collagen is turned over rapidly, while the remainder of the collagen fibers show a very slow rate of metabolic change.[3]

The collagen fibril is an aggregation of tropocollagen rods in staggered array, forming the characteristic 640 Å bands. The most soluble collagen is that most recently formed. Chemical bonding between parallel tropocollagen molecules leads to increasing insolubility and increased tensile strength. However, the process may be reversible and soluble collagen may result from the breakdown of insoluble collagen as well as from the synthesis of collagen.

Connective tissue is usually described in relation to the arrangement of the fibrous elements.

Organized Connective Tissue. Tendons and ligaments are made up of organized connective tissue composed of dense bundles of coarse collagen between which columns of fibrocytes are interspersed. Collagen fibers are arranged linearly in the long axis of the tendon or ligament and present a uniform appearance (Fig. 18–1). More fibrocytes are present in columnar arrangement in tendons than in ligaments. These fibrocytes are stellate with processes extending between the bundles of collagen fibers. It appears that this organization is a response to the tension produced by muscular contraction.

TENDON HEALING. Buck[1] sectioned the Achilles tendon of the rat and allowed it to retract without suturing (Fig. 18–2). A fibrin coagulum was laid down in the defect between the cut ends of the tendon, oriented longitudinally with the tendon. Fibroblasts began to grow into the coagulum from the periphery within three days, and reticulin fibers and collagen fibers were laid down within four days. The collagen fibers were oriented parallel to the fibrin threads in the long axis of the tendon. Within two weeks, the entire length of the tendon up to the muscular insertion was invaded by fibroblasts. The reaction as indicated by proliferation of collagen, and the persistence of fibroblasts throughout the tendon lasted for four months.

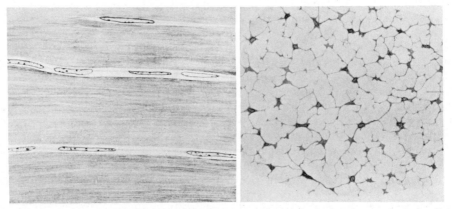

FIGURE 18–1. Drawing of the histology of a tendon in longitudinal and cross section to show the distribution of fibrocytes between the bundles of collagen fibers. (From Maximow and Bloom.)

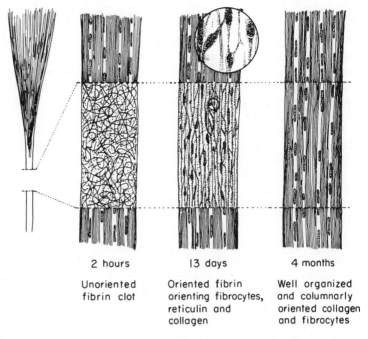

FIGURE 18–2. Diagram of healing of Achilles tendon of rat when cut and not sutured. (From data of Buck.[1])

2 hours

Unoriented
fibrin clot

13 days

Oriented fibrin
orienting fibrocytes,
reticulin and
collagen

4 months

Well organized
and columnarly
oriented collagen
and fibrocytes

When the muscle was denervated at the time the tendon was cut, the fibrin did not organize in a uniform longitudinal pattern and the collagen fibers, likewise, developed in a random orientation rather than in parallel bundles.

It appears that the regular pattern of fibers produced in the healing tendon is due to the exertion of tension on the fibrin coagulum to produce a linear pattern and that collagen is organized on this matrix.[2]

ADHESION FORMATION. The increasing strength of new connective tissue is correlated with the formation and maturation of collagen fibers.[4] After injury collagen fibrils can be detected by using the electron microscope as early as the second day, by biochemical means on the third day, and by use of the light microscope only a day or two later, when molecular accretion has occurred. Within four to five days, collagenous adhesions begin to form between a sutured tendon and the surrounding structures. Watson-Jones[5] observed collagen fibers at fracture sites within five days. Gentle passive or active motion of the sutured tendon begun the day after surgery will prevent adhesions to surrounding structures without producing significant tension on the suture. Motion may be re-established in this manner before inflammation has weakened the tendon. By two weeks after suture, the inflammatory reaction within a tendon has greatly reduced its tensile strength. This inflammatory reaction lasts for at least four months. Early gentle motion preserves the gliding motion of the tendon without force and shortens the functional recovery time, i.e., the time required for the tendon to be healed and free to move.

Loose Connective Tissue. Loose or areolar connective tissue forms between organs and other structures, such as joint capsules, fascia, intermuscular layers, and subcutaneous tissue, where movement occurs repeatedly. It will allow movement through limited distances, adapt by shortening and fixation if there is no motion, or elongate slowly under prolonged tension.

Histologically, networks of collagen and reticular fibers run in all directions without a regular pattern. These fibers form a loose mesh which allows flexibility for movement. When these fibers are laid down or replaced, their length and mobility between attachments depend upon the motion of the part during the period of formation.

Thousands of reticulin fibers are attached over the entire external surface of the sarcolemma of each muscle fiber so that resistance to motion is provided not only through the heavy fibrous attachments at the ends of each muscle fiber but also through the reticular fibers to the surrounding connective tissue. The proportionate force of the muscular contraction transmitted through these reticular fibers is not known, but in conditions of fibrosis it is increased significantly.

When a part is immobilized, the collagenous and reticular networks become contracted and the distance between attachments in the network is shortened so that the tissue becomes dense and hard and loses the suppleness of normal areolar tissue.

Dense Connective Tissue. In areas where motion does not occur, such as in fascial planes and the capsules of muscles or organs, collagen is laid down as dense meshworks, sheets, or bands. This type of connective tissue is also laid down in scars. If motion is maintained during healing of a wound, connective tissue of the areolar type develops. If the wound is immobilized, dense contracted scar forms. In areas immobilized by edema dense connective tissue will also develop. It is imperative if motion is to be maintained in a part that the motion be initiated early and carried on during the period of healing so that areolar rather than dense collagen networks form. Except in the case of necessary immobilization of a fracture or of an open draining wound, gentle passive or active assistive motion under proper supervision should be begun immediately after surgery or trauma to insure that supple areolar connective tissue rather than dense scar develops in sites in which motion should occur.

Histologic evidence of fibrosis may occur in as short time as four days.[1, 6] Gross evidence of restriction of motion begins to occur in approximately four days and develops progressively from that time. Immobilization of a normal joint for four weeks results in diminution or loss of motion because of formation of dense connective tissue. Immobilization of an injured joint for two weeks results in connective fiber fusion and loss of motion at that joint.

The following indicates the effect of limitation of motion on development of restrictive connective tissue after injury to the shoulder.[7] If the shoulder is not immobilized, recovery occurs in 18 days. If the shoulder is immobilized 7 days, recovery occurs in 52 days. If the shoulder is immobilized 14 days, recovery occurs in 121 days. If the shoulder is immobilized 21 days, recovery occurs in 300 days.

Factors promoting the formation of dense fibrosis are immobilization, edema, trauma, and impaired circulation. *Immobilization* allows deposition of collagen and reticulin as a dense network instead of a loose areolar network. *Edema* increases the tendency to fibrosis. Whether this is due to increased tissue fluid protein, impaired metabolism, increased metabolites, or other causes is not known. Probably all of these factors are important in the formation of both the edema and the fibrosis. *Trauma* causes capillary damage and increases the loss of protein into the tissue. Fibrinogen precipitates as a fibrin meshwork in the tissue spaces, forming a matrix on which collagen fibers are laid down. *Impaired circulation* appears to augment the rate of development of fibrosis.

The Normal Maintenance of Mobility

Motion in joints and soft tissues is maintained by the normal movement of the parts of the body, including joint capsules, muscles, subcutaneous tissue, and ligaments, through full range of motion many times each day. In the course of the day, these movements traverse the full range of motion. If for any reason the range is restricted, tightness develops and restricts the arc of motion.

It is easier to prevent tightness by frequently repeated activity than to correct it after it has developed.

Limitation of the range of motion is of the greatest importance when it interferes with habitual postures or activities. (For the normal range of motion of various joints see pages 24 to 33 in Chapter 2.)

Tightness that prevents normal standing without muscular support is disabling. In the normal relaxed standing posture, extension of the back, the hip, and the knee is maintained by positioning the center of gravity of the body above these joints so that the weight of the body holds the joints extended against restricting ligaments and the extensor muscles are relaxed. Muscular activity is used for balance or motion rather than to support the weight of the body. Electromyographic studies of patients during normal quiet standing reveal no continuously active contraction of the muscles in the back, the extensors of the hip, or the extensors of the knee.[8] Maintenance of balance is provided mainly by activity of the soleus muscles and intermittent counterbalancing activity of the anterior tibial muscles. During relaxed standing, the center of gravity of the head, arms, and trunk falls slightly posterior (0.5 to 1.0 cm.) to the center of motion of the acetabulum, far anterior (3 to 5 cm.) to the of the weight of the body during quiet standing. Therefore, the patient fatigues more rapidly and has less endurance for standing or ambulatory activity than does a person with normal mobility. The contraction of muscles to hold the body erect places more compressive stress on the joint surfaces, resulting in more rapid wear and more likelihood of joint pain.

Mechanics of Ambulation

HIP. During relaxed standing the hip is fully extended, forming an angle of 160 to 175 degrees between the long axis of the pelvis and the femur[10] (Fig. 18–4). Maximal forced

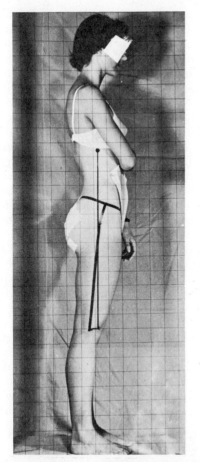

FIGURE 18–3. During normal relaxed standing the hip is fully extended. The center of gravity falls just posterior to the center of the acetabulum, well in front of the knee and through the tarsal arch. The longitudinal and transverse axes of the pelvis and the longitudinal axis of the femur are marked. The subject is standing behind a two-inch grid. (From Kottke and Kubicek.[9])

center of motion of the knee, and through the center of the tarsal arch approximately midway between the points of contact of the heel and heads of the metatarsals[9] (Fig. 18–3).

During relaxed standing, the hip and the knee are fully extended. There is no free extension of the hip or knee beyond this standing position. Further extension is possible only to the extent that connective tissues can be stretched.[10]

Methods purporting to measure hyperextension of the hip beyond the standing position are erroneous because of inaccurate evaluation of the orientation of the innominate bone.

If tightness prevents complete extension of these weight-bearing joints, relaxed standing cannot occur. When the joints are not fully extended, muscles must support a part

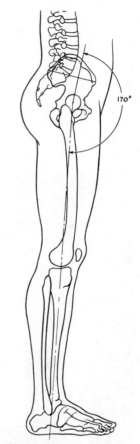

FIGURE 18–4. Diagram of the relationships of the lumbar spine, pelvis, and lower extremity in normal relaxed stance. The transverse axis of the pelvis is defined by a line drawn between the anterior and the posterior superior iliac spines. The longitudinal axis of the pelvis is a perpendicular to this line dropped through the center of the acetabulum. The longitudinal axis of the femur is defined by a line from the center of the head of the femur to the center of weight-bearing at the knee. The pelvifemoral angle is formed by the longitudinal axes of the pelvis and the femur. (From Kottke and Kubicek.[9])

extension may add approximately 5 degrees to this angle. Therefore, it should be remembered that no free range of extension of the hip can occur beyond the position assumed during normal standing. The hyperextension that appears to occur is due to forward rotation of the pelvis with simultaneous extension of the lumbar spine and flexion of the opposite hip.

The act of walking exerts repeated stretch on the ligaments, fascia, muscles, and connective tissue across the flexor aspect of the hip. Unless a person is standing and walking frequently each day, the normal reaction of fibrous connective tissue to shorten and fuse together results in a progressive limitation of extension. As extension of the hip becomes more limited, the extension of the lumbar trunk usually increases in a compensatory manner. Because of this compensatory extension in the trunk, the limitation of motion of the hip may develop insidiously until suddenly the patient is observed to stand and walk with an excessive lumbar lordosis or he loses the ability to stand (Fig. 18–5). Compensatory lordosis does not exceed the range of extension of the lumbar spine (Fig. 18–6). In children, who normally have lumbar ex-

tension of 80 to 90 degrees, compensatory lordosis may be that great. The range of lumbar extension is decreased in adulthood, and adults who develop flexion contractures of the hips do not develop as marked compensatory lumbar lordosis as is seen in children.

Habitual sitting makes flexion contractures of the hips likely unless they are prevented by appropriate stretching exercises. The difficulty in visualizing the change in position of the short innominate bone buried beneath thick soft tissues makes it possible for contractures of the flexors of the hips to develop to a severe degree before they are recognized.

During walking, in addition to full extension of the ipsilateral hip, the pelvis is tilted anteriorly and the lumbar spine is extended in order to bring the leg into the trailing position (Fig. 18–7). If the lumbar spine cannot extend enough to compensate for the anterior tilting of the pelvis, the center of gravity of the torso is shifted forward with the tilt of the pelvis and greater muscular work is required to support the weight of the body. The farther the center of gravity of the head, arms, and trunk is ahead of the ace-

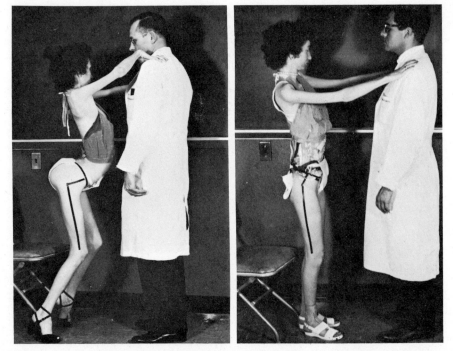

FIGURE 18–5. A patient with severe contractures of the hip flexors secondary to muscular dystrophy. Pelvifemoral angles have been marked as defined in Figure 18–4. Lumbar extension partially compensates for fixed hip flexion. Release of the contracted connective tissues and prolonged stretching increased the extension of the hips from 95 degrees to 150 degrees and made it possible for the patient to balance on her lower extremities again.

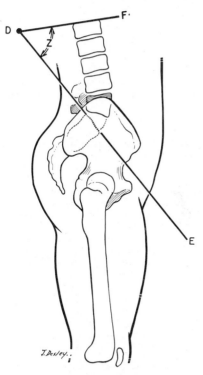

DE = PLANE OF SUPERIOR SURFACE OF S_1.
DF = PLANE OF SUPERIOR SURFACE OF L_1.
Z = ANGLE OF LUMBAR LORDOSIS.

FIGURE 18–6. Lumbar lordosis is measured as the angle between the plane of the superior surface of the first sacral segment and the plane of the superior surface of the first lumbar vertebra.

tabulum, the greater the muscular work required to support the torso.

Since the center of gravity falls ahead of the acetabulum during walking, weight can be borne on the trailing leg only if the extensor muscles of the hip are contracted. If the hip extensors are weak, the trailing leg may not be able to support the weight of the body. The amount of muscular strength needed to support the body on the trailing leg may be lessened by several compensatory mechanisms. The stride may be shortened. The lumbar spine may be extended further to keep the center of gravity over the acetabulum. The knee may be flexed to allow the foot to trail farther behind the pelvis at the expense of a stronger contraction of the quadriceps femoris.

When there is a flexion contracture of the hip, one or more of the compensatory mechanisms must be utilized to allow stable walking. If lumbar extension is limited and the quadriceps femoris or hip extensors or both are weak, the hip becomes unstable in the

trailing position. As the weight of the body moves ahead of the acetabulum, the knee flexes and collapses because the femur cannot extend further at the hip. Patients with a flexion contracture of the hip often can stand successfully when the leg on the side of the contracture is forward or in a mid-position but are unable to maintain the knee extended when the leg is trailing during walking (Fig. 18–8). Consequently, the attention is directed to the knee and the conclusion may be drawn that the major problem is weakness of the quadriceps femoris or abnormality of the knee when, in fact, the primary problem is the flexion contracture of the hip.

When a flexion contracture develops at the hip, the iliotibial band becomes progressively tighter, producing a flexion, abduction, external rotation deformity (Fig. 18–9). This progressive contracture may produce a pelvic obliquity and a secondary scoliosis.

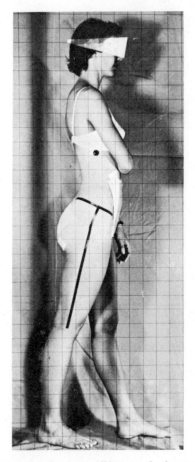

FIGURE 18–7. During walking, as the leg trails, the pelvis is tilted forward and the center of gravity of the head, arms, and trunk falls in front of the acetabulum. (From Kottke and Kubicek.[9])

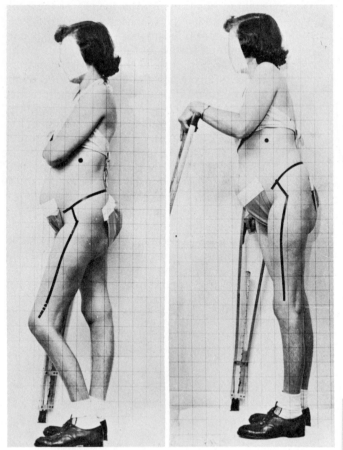

FIGURE 18–8. The combination of tightness of the flexor structures of the hip and weakness of the extensor muscles of the hip produces instability of both the hip and knee. During relaxed standing the left thigh is flexed forward because tightness of the flexor ligaments and fascia prevents further extension of the left hip. The center of gravity is over the pelvis but all weight is borne on the right lower extremity. If the left knee is forced into extension, the fixed flexion contracture of the left hip causes the pelvis to tilt forward and the center of gravity of the body is shifted ahead of the acetabulum. Since the extensor muscles of the hip are weak, the hip will collapse if anterior support is not provided. Attempts to center the weight of the body behind the acetabulum so that the hip becomes stable result in flexion of the knee because of the limitation of extension of the hip. Consequently either the hip or the knee is always in a position of instability. (From Kottke and Kubicek.[9])

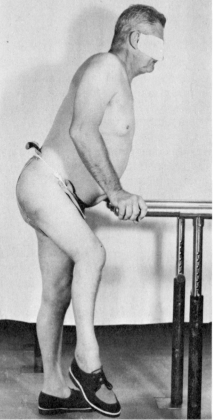

FIGURE 18–9. Typical postural deformity of flexion, abduction, and external rotation of the hip due to paresis and flexion contractures of the hip.

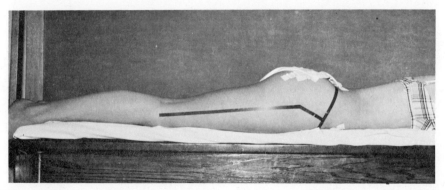

FIGURE 18–10. Normal hip extension when lying prone or supine on a flat surface is 10 to 20 degrees less than when standing.

When a patient lies on a flat, hard surface, extension of the hip is not as great as when he stands erect. The average extension when a patient is lying prone or supine on a hard surface is 155 degrees (Fig. 18–10), while the average extension during relaxed standing is 170 degrees. The extension of the hip when the patient is lying in bed varies from 135 to 150 degrees. The greater extension when standing is due to the greater extensor torque created by the weight of the torso centered slightly posterior to the hip joint. Patients who must remain in bed, even though they are positioned properly, will develop progressive hip flexion contractures unless they receive daily stretching of the hip flexors (Fig. 18–11).

KNEE. Tightness causing flexion of the knees develops in the hamstring and gastrocnemius muscles and the posterior capsule of the joint if the knees are not stretched to full extension by standing and walking each day. When a patient has a paretic or painful disability and habitually sits or lies with the knees flexed, contractures develop rapidly with progressive limitation of extension of

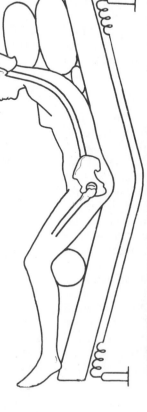

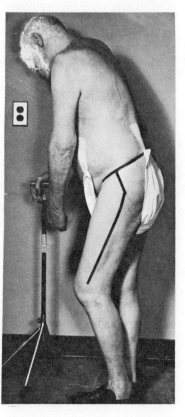

FIGURE 18–11. The prolonged bedfast position without maintenance of the normal range of motion results in a kyphosis of the spine and flexion contractures of the hips, knees, and ankles.

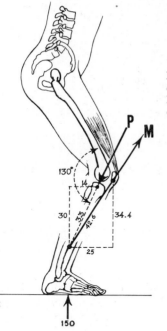

FIGURE 18–12. The compressive force, P, exerted on the flexed knee is a combination of the weight of the body and tension exerted by the quadriceps, M. If a patient weighing 150 pounds walks with the knee extended to 130 degrees, the calculated compressive force on the knee is:

$$\Sigma\ F_x = 0$$
$$P \cdot \frac{14}{33}\ M \cdot \frac{25}{42.6} = 0$$
$$P = 1.38M$$
$$\Sigma\ F_y = 0$$
$$150 + P \cdot \frac{30}{33} - M \cdot \frac{34.4}{42.6} = 0$$
$$150 + \frac{30}{33} \cdot 1.38M - \frac{34.4}{42.6}\ M = 0$$
$$M = 342\ \text{lb.}$$
$$P\ = 472\ \text{lb.}$$

the knees. For arthritis patients or patients with neurologic diseases, the placing of pillows under the knees results in the rapid development of contractures of the knees. The compressive force that must be exerted on the flexed knee during walking is considerably greater than the force exerted when the knee is extended and, consequently, patients with arthritis in the knees have far less tolerance for standing and walking when there are flexion contractures than when the knees can extend fully (Fig. 18–12).

ANKLE. When a patient lies in bed without the support of a footboard or sits with the feet plantar-flexed much of the time, progressive tightness develops in the muscles of the calf and may become great enough so that the sole of the foot cannot assume a position perpendicular to the long axis of the tibia. Thus the patient cannot bear weight on the heel when standing. Even before this degree of tightness has been reached, tightness in the gastrocnemius increases stress on the longitudinal arch of the foot and the heads of the metatarsal bones when the patient walks. For patients who are chronically ill with painful or paretic disease, tightness in the triceps surae is accentuated by lack of a footboard on the bed, lack of foot support when sitting, and lying prone with the feet plantar-flexed.

Mobility Exercises to Maintain the Range of Motion

Twice daily all joints should be carried through the full range of motion three times. (See the normal ranges of motion on pages 24 to 33 in Chapter 2.) The patient should perform mobility exercises actively after he has been taught the proper procedures. Exercises must be carried on with assistance to the patient if he is weak or has pain.

The greater the inflammation and pain, the more gentle the exercise must be. For cases of acute rheumatoid arthritis, passive motion should be carried out with the patient completely relaxed. Joint inflammation requires more gentle motion than does muscular tightness. The therapist, nurse, or member of the family should gently move the part through the full range of free motion but not force motion or cause pain. The joint must be moved very slowly and gently. For patients with acute joint involvement it is highly desirable to have a skilled therapist carry out the passive motions. As the patient improves the range can be increased slowly with gradual progression to active assistive exercise and then to active exercise. Improper exercise or over-exercise may impede rather than help recovery in the acute stage. If motion is not maintained in the presence of inflammation, contractures occur rapidly and may become irreversible.

The therapists, nurses, or family should be taught any stretching procedures that are desired. Repeated examinations and supervision of the procedures are essential to assure that the proper motions are obtained. The difference between properly supervised and unsupervised exercise is usually the difference between adequate and inadequate care.

Stretching to Increase Range of Motion

A tight muscle can be stretched vigorously unless there is inflammation, when the stretching must be much more mild. For conditions such as poliomyelitis or Guillain-Barré syndrome, stretching should be past the point of pain, but there should be no residual pain when the stretching is discontinued. When performing manual stretching, hold momentarily at the point of maximal stretch. This type of stretching should be done by a trained therapist. The therapist must use caution in cases of prolonged disuse, paralysis, or anesthesia, because osteoporosis may have occurred and vigorous stretching may cause fractures. In the presence of paralysis or hypesthesia, overstretching commonly occurs, causing bleeding into the disrupted connective tissue and subsequent ectopic calcification and ossification. In quadriplegic patients this is seen most frequently in the flexor muscles of the hips and the elbows.

Stretching of tight joints must be less vigorous than stretching of muscles. The motion should be slow and gentle with the patient completely relaxed, and it should stop short of the point that produces pain in the joint, although the patient may experience discomfort from stretch of the soft tissues. Inflamed joints tolerate vigorous stretching less well than joints that are not acutely inflamed. Edematous tissue is more likely to be torn than normal tissue, resulting in residual pain, swelling, and soreness. Inflammation in any joint may reduce the tensile strength of the capsule and collateral ligaments to as little as 50 per cent of the normal tensile strength.[11]

Certain principles apply to all techniques of stretching. The body segments on each side of the joint to be stretched must be properly stabilized so that the maneuver is under complete control. The force must be applied in the precise direction that produces tension in the appropriate connective tissues. Prolonged moderate stretching is more effective than momentary vigorous stretching; connective tissue shows the plastic property of "creeping" in response to prolonged tension, although it will resist a much greater momentary force. The plastic "creeping" of connective tissue under moderate stretch increases as the tissue temperature increases up to the maximal tolerated temperature, which is approximately 43°C for tissues with normal circulation.[12] Therefore, thermotherapy to raise the temperature close to 43°C during the period of stretching will increase the effectiveness of the treatment. Connective tissue at a temperature of 20 to 30°C requires about three times as much tensile force to effect a specified elongation as is necessary at 43°C.[13]

Stretching must be held within the pain tolerance of the patient; during brief manual stretching there may be pain when the stretch is applied, with relief of pain as soon as stretch ceases; prolonged stretching should remain within the patient's pain threshold to avoid tearing of blood vessels. Stretching should be repeated in less time than is required for connective tissue to "set" in a shortened position, daily or more often. Inflammation indicates decreased tensile strength of connective tissue, which must be stretched cautiously. Special procedures are used for prolonged stretching of joints that do not respond well to a manual stretch (Fig. 18–13).

Hip Flexors. The patient, lying prone, is strapped snugly to a padded plinth by a strap run through C-clamps on either side of the hips and across the ischial tuberosities. A sling under the distal end of the thigh is attached by a rope through overhead pulleys to a weight that provides a constant tension. A stretching weight of 30 to 50 pounds is added to the weight necessary to counterbalance the lower extremity. Only one hip is stretched at a time because it is not possible to immobilize the pelvis adequately to stretch both hip flexors simultaneously. The contralateral hip and knee are flexed and the leg is supported on the seat of a chair or cushion of appropriate height. This stretch is maintained for 20 minutes each day.

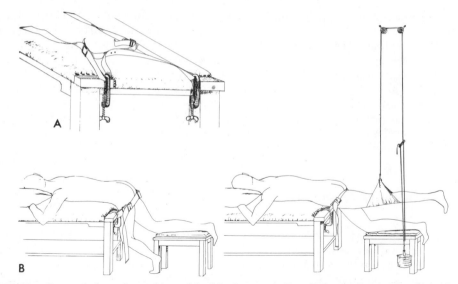

FIGURE 18–13. Counterbalanced stretching of the hip flexors. *A*, Two C-clamps fastened to the end of a padded table at hip width provide attachment for a double-ended stretching strap. *B*, The pelvis is immobilized by a strap fastened over the ischial tuberosities while the hips are flexed. A sling under the distal end of the thigh is attached by rope and overhead pulley to counterbalanced weights, which exert a continuous force on the hip flexors. Thirty to 50 pounds plus the weight counterbalancing the lower extremity are applied for 20 minutes.

Knee Flexors. Contractures of the knees can be stretched by placing the patient prone on a firm surface with a pad under the knee and the leg extending unsupported. A 5- to 15-pound sandbag or weight is placed across the heel for 20 minutes (Fig. 18–14).

Alternatively, the patient sits with the knee extended, the heel supported at seat level, and the thigh and leg unsupported, and a sandbag weighing 10 to 15 pounds is placed across the knee for 20 minutes.

Triceps Surae. The patient sits on an Elgin table or other apparatus to which an exercise boot with a toe extension may be attached. The foot is strapped to the exercise boot and 10 to 30 pounds of tension is exerted at the end of the toe extension bar for 20 minutes (Fig. 18–15).

Alternatively, to dorsiflex the ankle, the patient stands at arm's length from a wall with the feet on a wedgeboard that elevates the front of the foot 20 degrees above the

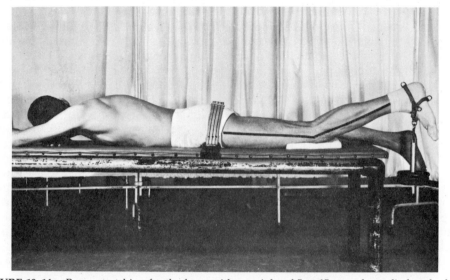

FIGURE 18–14. Prone stretching for the knee with a weight of 5 to 15 pounds applied at the heel.

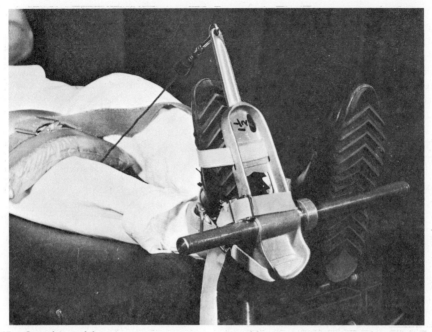

FIGURE 18–15. Stretching of the triceps surae on an exercise table using a toe extension boot. A weight of 10 to 30 pounds is applied for 20 minutes.

horizontal. He leans forward against the wall for one to five minutes three to five times each day. This exercise is the most convenient to do at home. To be effective, the knees must be kept extended and the heels kept in contact with the floor. The same stretch may be obtained by placing the patient on a tilt table (Fig. 18–16).

Elbows. Only active motion is used for mobilizing the elbow because stretch applied through the long lever of the forearm to the relatively weak ginglymus joint results in overstretching and tearing of connective tissue, which increases the contracture rather than relieving it. It has been reported that mild, prolonged spring tension, which allows frequent motion but maintains tension during the intervals of relaxation, is effective to stretch flexion contractures of the elbows.

Fingers. Stretching of fingers in flexion and extension without first mobilizing the soft tissues around the joint is inadequate. These joints have limited motion in other directions, including rotation, anteroposterior sliding, lateral sliding, and lateral bending, as well as flexion and extension.[14] General mobility of these joints must be re-established by gentle manipulatory

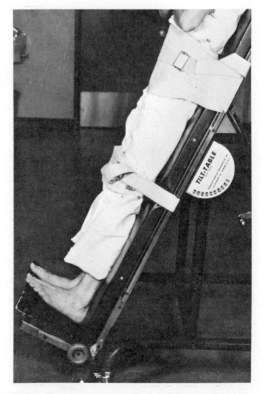

FIGURE 18–16. Prolonged stretching of the triceps surae using a tilt table and wedge board.

stretching before full flexion and full extension are possible. All motions are carried out gently a number of times daily. The connective tissue around the joints of the fingers tends to gel rapidly if there is no motion. Splinting devices which hold the hand in one position are not entirely effective because they do not provide the repeated motion necessary to restore suppleness to the connective tissues around the joints. Joint capsules of immobilized hands quickly become edematous and sclerotic. Effective manipulation of fingers is difficult and is best carried out by a skilled therapist.

REFERENCES

1. Buck, R. C.: Regeneration of tendon. J. Pathol. Bacteriol., 66:1–18, 1953.
2. Fernando, N. V. P., and Movat, H. Z.: Fibrillogenesis in regenerating tendon. Lab. Invest., 12:214–229, 1963.
3. Lindstedt, S., and Prockop, D. J.: Isotopic studies on urinary hydroxyproline as evidence for rapidly catabolized forms of collagen in the young rat. J. Biol. Chem., 236:1399–1403, 1961.
4. Viljanto, J.: Biochemical basis of tensile strength in wound healing. An experimental study with viscose cellulose sponges in rats. Acta Chir. Scand. (Suppl.), 333:1–101, 1964.
5. Watson-Jones, R.: Fractures and Joint Injuries, Vol. I, 4th Ed. Baltimore, Williams and Wilkins Co., 1952, p. 5.
6. Jackson, D. S., Flickinger, D. B., and Dunphy, J. E.: Biochemical studies of connective tissue repair. Ann. N.Y. Acad. Sci., 86:943–947, 1960.
7. Perkins, G.: Rest and movement. J. Bone Joint Surg., 25B:521–539, 1953.
8. Kelton, I. W., and Wright, R. D.: The mechanism of easy standing by man. Aust. J. Exp. Biol. Med. Sci., 27:505–515, 1949.
9. Kottke, F. J., and Kubicek, W. G.: Relationship of the tilt of the pelvis to stable posture. Arch. Phys. Med., 37:81–90, 1956.
10. Mundale, M. O., Hislop, H. J., Rabideau, R. J., and Kottke, F. J.: Evaluation of extension of the hip. Arch. Phys. Med., 37:75–80, 1956.
11. Lippmann, R. K.: Arthropathy due to adjacent inflammation. J. Bone Joint Surg., 35A:967–979, 1953.
12. Warren, C. J., Lehmann, J. F., and Koblanski, J. N.: Elongation of rat tail tendon: Effect of load and temperature. Arch. Phys. Med. Rehabil., 52:465–474, 1971.
13. Gersten, J. W.: Effect of ultrasound on tendon extensibility. Am. J. Phys. Med., 34:362–369, 1955.
14. Mennell, J.: The Science and Art of Joint Manipulation, Vol. I: The Extremities, 2nd Ed. Philadelphia, The Blakiston Co., 1949, pp. 51–69.

19

THERAPEUTIC EXERCISE TO DEVELOP NEUROMUSCULAR COORDINATION

FREDERIC J. KOTTKE

The development of the ability to regulate multiple muscles simultaneously or in sequence to perform apparently simple or complex activities is the aspect of therapeutic exercise that is most difficult to understand. There has been continuing controversy regarding both the neurophysiologic mechanisms involved and the functional process that is used to activate single or multiple muscles to perform a task. There is lack of agreement regarding what part of neuromuscular activity is voluntary, what part is based on automatic patterns, what part is purely the result of heredity, what part has to be learned, and when learning is necessary what the fundamentals of that process may be. This chapter will attempt to deal with these issues.

As used in this chapter, *control* is defined as the conscious activation of an individual muscle or the conscious initiation of a preprogrammed engram. Control involves conscious awareness and intentional guidance of an activity. Control of the individual muscle involves the volitional activation and conscious regulation of the intensity and duration of that contraction. For an engram, control means the selection and initiation of a specific engram of activity, maintenance for the period desired, and termination when wished. *Coordination* is the process that results in the combination of activities of a number of muscles into the smooth patterns of cocontraction and the sequences of contraction and relaxation seen under normal conditions. Coordination of multimuscular activity occurs as the result of the organization of functional networks of internuncial neurons, or engrams, in the extrapyramidal system rather than by seriatim excitation of muscles by consciously directed volitional control transmitted over the corticospinal pathway. An engram represents the neurological organization of a preprogrammed pattern of muscular activity. Once an engram has been developed, each time it is excited it automatically produces the same pattern. In this automatic activity produced by an enram, not only must all of the involved muscle be excited in the correct sequence and at the right intensity, but also, all muscles not required for the activity must be inhibited if the pattern is to be produced smoothly with minimal expenditure of energy. The activities of the component mus-

403

cles of a well-coordinated motion are automatic in that they are not consciously perceived or selected. Only the accomplishment of the activity is perceived.[1] Except for very light and unusual activity, most muscular activity occurs as the synchronized activation and inhibition of a number of muscle groups rather than the isolated contraction of a single prime mover. When exercise occurs against resistance there is always cocontraction of synergists and stabilizers. The greater the resistance, the greater the spread of activity to produce cocontraction in more distant muscles, both ipsilateral and contralateral.[2]

Because it is possible after engrams have been developed to select and activate sequences of preprogrammed patterns and at any time to superimpose on the preprogrammed pattern an additional controlled muscular activity to modify the response, it has been difficult to understand the difference between coordination and control. Most of our common activities are initiated by willing an automatic preprogrammed motor pattern (a coordination pattern) to occur. The pattern may be limited or extensive but occurs as it was preprogrammed by previous practice. In addition, an individual muscle can be activated, i.e. controlled, by directing attention to that specific muscular action. When a muscular action is being voluntarily controlled, the neuromuscular process occurs more slowly than when the action is preprogrammed. Only one muscular action can be observed at a time. Attention may be switched from the control of one activity to the control of another only at the rate of two to three times per second. In rapid, strong multimuscular activities, all components must be integrated into a timed sequence of interrelated responses, most of which are performed automatically. The goal of coordination training is to develop the ability to reproduce at will automatic multimuscular motor patterns that are faster, more precise, and stronger than those that can be produced when only voluntary control of each individual muscle is used.

If a muscle is of major importance in performing a motion of a joint, it is called a prime mover or agonist. Other muscles that assist that motion are called synergists. Muscles that oppose the motion are called antagonists. Muscles of the same or adjacent joints that maintain position to allow the

motion and are used synchronously with the prime mover are called stabilizers. Neuromuscular education or control training refers to the teaching of the discrete control of a prime mover of a motion under the direct consciousness of the patient. Coordination training refers to the training that develops preprogrammed automatic multimuscular patterns or engrams.

When a muscle is contracting against a load that is very light relative to the total voluntary strength of that muscle, it is possible to limit activity to that muscle voluntarily. As the load becomes heavier, synergists as well as the prime mover begin to contract. When the load becomes still heavier, the stabilizer muscles in the extremities and also in the trunk establish stability and balance in relation to gravity. With even heavier loading, antagonists and distant muscles that serve no useful purpose become active during the motion because the amount of activity excited in the internuncial pool exceeds the capacity for selective inhibition. Prolonged activity causes fatigue of any muscle and increases the proportionate resistance that a constant load imposes on the available strength of the prime mover.

Coordination Results from Engrams of Automated Movement

The development of coordination depends upon repetition. When training for coordination is first carried out, the movement must be simple and the rate slow enough that the person can consciously monitor all components of the activity. As the activity is repeated precisely many times, an engram is formed. The activity then can be performed with greater effort without the occurrence of errors in performance. The speed of performance can be increased. The conscious attention required for precise performance becomes less and there is less spread of excitation to other neurons outside of the activity pattern. Eventually the pattern can be carried on with little conscious perception of its individual components and is said to be automatic, or a preprogrammed engram.[3]

A high degree of coordination and speed does not develop until the activity pattern becomes so well developed through repeated practice that it does not require awareness of all phases of the activity. For example, a pianist when playing a piano does not need to think of the contraction of the individual muscles involved nor even the individual placement of each finger, because the symbols on a page signify a whole pattern of responses, and cerebral awareness provides the initiation of an *automatized preprogrammed pattern* without need for conscious attention to the components of that activity. During motor activity proprioceptive feedback provides both subconscious and conscious monitoring of whether or not the performance was successful rather than awareness of the precise activity of each muscle.

How the flow of nerve impulses becomes limited to specific neural pathways by repetition and how sensory feedback from precisely performed activity becomes integrated by repetition into automatic patterns of activity has not been fully defined. Nevertheless, all skilled muscular activities are developed only in this way. Repetition of activity with perceived sensory feedback to regulate performance is the basis for the development of motor skills in the infant and child. It is the mechanism by which highly skilled performance is perfected in the adult. Likewise, it is the basis for relearning coordination for the patient who has suffered injury to the neuromuscular system.

The components of skilled automatic performance are the following:

1. **Volition** — the ability to initiate the activity when it is wanted, to maintain it as long as desired, and to discontinue it at will. When an engram has been formed volition can excite, maintain, and discontinue that engram, but the engram runs as it was preprogrammed. Volition is used to select or modify the sequence of engrams and, therefore, to determine the order of the performance.

2. **Perception** — to tell whether or not the performance is occurring as desired. Coordinated activity is monitored primarily by sensory stimuli transmitted through proprioceptive pathways and reinforced by visual and tactile perception. A patient must have intact proprioception and intact subcortical centers for integrating proprioceptive impulses with motor impulses in order to achieve a high degree of coordination.[4] When there is damage to the proprioceptive pathways, visual monitoring must be substituted for proprioceptive monitoring, but the degree of coordination achieved is never as

great as when the proprioceptive pathways are intact. Conscious awareness of the components of the activities being performed is only superficial. The monitoring of position and motion for skilled motor patterns is largely automatic through interaction between the cerebellum and the cerebral basal ganglia in conjunction with the precentral cortex. Perception is processed in the central nervous system more slowly than is performance and, therefore, is a retrospective recognition of error and a correction of subsequent performance.

3. **Engram Formation** — the development of preprogrammed patterns of activity as the basis for coordination. Development of a motor engram is dependent upon the establishment of an internuncial network that programs each motor pattern. Repetition of each pattern many times at the maximal speed and force consistent with precision results in the development of a fast and forceful motor engram. Repetition involves the activation of nervous pathways to motor units which should be contracting at the same time that all other motor units are inhibited. *The only way by which automatic engrams can be developed is by voluntary repetition of the precise performance until the engram is formed.* The component units of a coordinated activity must be performed with precision several million times before peak performance is reached.[5]

Inhibition is the heart of coordination. The development of coordination results in greater preciseness of motion and greater economy of muscular effort because there is less extraneous muscular activity. This precision of motion depends upon active inhibition of motor neurons other than those involved in the desired motion. *Inhibition of undesired activity is an essential part of the automatic regulation of coordination.* In one of his lectures Karel Bobath used the metaphor, "Each motor engram is a pathway of excitation surrounded by a wall of inhibition." Precise coordination can be developed only to the extent that a person can train the inhibition of all undesired activity. Although inhibition is the heart of coordination, it cannot be trained directly, but, rather, only by the execution of precise activity and increasing the intensity of effort as precision can be maintained. There is no voluntarily controllable system by which inhibition can be imposed selectively on any anterior horn cell. As engrams develop, the capacity for inhibition also develops. Inhibition of undesired activity is more difficult to train than is the initiation of desired activity. The training of coordination results in the progressive development of selective inhibition during increasing effort. When the capacity for inhibition increases, voluntary effort can be increased to produce a stronger and faster specific motor activity, while neuronal excitation remains restricted to the desired neuromuscular pathways. Coordination of the most complex, most rapid and skillful, and most powerful contractions is an extrapyramidal automatized activity rather than a voluntary activity controlled through the corticospinal pathway.

TRAINING OF CONTROL OF INDIVIDUAL MUSCLES

Conscious Control of a Muscle

The corticospinal pathway from the 4 gamma cortex has the ability to activate small groups of motoneurons of individual muscles under the direct attention of the individual. This is the only pathway for motor control in the nervous system that does not need training other than awareness of sensory-motor relationships. However, this pathway is limited to attending to one muscle or one motion at a time, and attention cannot be shifted more rapidly than two to three times per second. In addition, this is solely an excitatory pathway with no capacity for inhibition. It appears that this controllable pathway is used by the normal infant to augment or oppose reflex responses by imposing additional neural impulses to facilitate a muscular activity and through this laborious mechanism gradually to develop multimuscular coordination. It appears that the normally coordinated adult is able to modify multimuscular activity by imposing additional muscular activities, one by one, over the corticospinal pathway.

When a patient is unable to activate even the simple combinations of muscles to produce a coordination contraction consistently without error, therapeutic exercise to teach coordination must be begun by teaching isolated control of the individual muscles under direct attention.

The patient must learn to control each muscle individually before its actions can be integrated into a coordination engram. Kenny[6] and Knapp[7] developed and described the clinical techniques for training control of individual prime movers. Simard and Basmajian[8] reported that a similar technique could be used to teach control of individual motor units using electromyographic feedback.

Requirements for Training Control

The training of control of the individual prime mover muscles is an educational process requiring intense concentration and participation. The patient must be rational, old enough to comprehend and follow instructions, and able to learn, cooperate, and concentrate on the muscular training during the exercise period. He should be alert and emotionally calm. The patient should be allowed to have frequent short rest periods. As soon as he begins to tire or become inattentive, the training session should be discontinued.

The training exercise should be carried on in a quiet room so that the patient will not be distracted. He must be positioned to be relaxed, comfortable, and securely supported. A patient who is unsteady or insecure cannot concentrate on controlling the activity of an isolated muscle. If he has generalized weakness or a problem of balance, he should be fully supported in the recumbent position. Patients with cerebral palsy may not relax fully when lying on a high or narrow table or when sitting in an erect position.

The patient must have intact proprioceptors or teleceptors to monitor muscular activity. If proprioception is normal, the patient is taught while recumbent and relaxed and the emphasis is on proprioception, because proprioceptive sensation is more rapid and precise than other sensations. If proprioception is impaired, the patient must be positioned in such a way that he can watch the activity in order to monitor it. Electromyography can be used to augment impaired sensation, either to reinforce the activity of the prime mover or to suppress undesired activity of other muscles during the training of control; however, central neurophysiological processing of the conscious monitoring by electromyography is too slow to be utilized during the performance of a coordination engram. Patients who have no mechanism available for perception of position or muscular activity cannot be taught precise control.

The patient must have a pain-free arc of motion of the joint across which the muscle is working. The sense of position and movement is derived primarily from joint receptors which are stimulated by motion of that joint.[9] A motion of approximately 10 degrees in a joint is adequate to initiate proprioceptive monitoring if that sensation is normal. In the presence of pain, inhibition of activity occurs and incoordination results. In addition, when pain is present the patient learns to anticipate the pain and restrict his activity before motion produces pain. Usually when pain may occur at both ends of the range of motion, neuromuscular education can be carried out if there is a pain-free arc of motion of about 30 degrees. This larger range affords the therapist adequate motion within the totally pain-free range in which to stimulate proprioceptive feedback.

During training there must be competent direction from a trained therapist who provides clear-cut commands for precise performance and is alert to monitor and confirm that the correct performance is occurring. If there is any substitution or incoordination, the therapist must teach the patient how to limit the activity to the desired prime mover by decreasing the effort appropriately. This may require that the activity be an assisted motion with minimal voluntary effort. In addition, the therapist encourages the patient to be working continually at the maximal level of his ability.

Technique for Training Control of Individual Muscles

Verify that there is a lower motor neuron pathway. For the hyporesponsive muscle that is not contracted by volition, the stretch reflex may be stimulated by a tendon tap or rapidly repeated lengthening and relaxation to demonstrate that the lower motor neuron pathway is intact. A minimal reaction can often be observed best by palpation of the tendon of insertion. Multiple quick short stretches or vibration using an electric vibrator may be more effective to initiate the response than a single stretch. Vibrations at 200 Hz will saturate the discharge rate from Ia sensory endings of muscle spindles. Function of the lower motor neuron may also be verified by electromyography.

Verify the upper motor neuron pathway by facilitation. For upper motor neuron diseases in which the stretch reflexes are readily elicited, the problem is to determine whether or not there is a trainable upper motor neuron pathway. It may be necessary to use one or more of the facilitation techniques to demonstrate that there is an upper motor neuron pathway over which volitional control of motor function may be transmitted.[10-12] When motor neurons cannot be activated by volition alone, facilitation is used to initiate and increase activity before control training is begun. Facilitation techniques utilize overflow of nerve impulses from one interneuronal pathway to another to reduce synaptic resistances and activate motoneurons not otherwise receiving threshold stimulation. Either reflex stimulation or mass cerebral discharge over multiple motor pathways may be used to activate inactive motoneurons. This type of facilitation can be used to demonstrate a potential pathway to a muscle. It is postulated that repeated activation of a motoneuron or motor pathway which has a high threshold in some way lowers that threshold.[13] Many of the specialized therapeutic exercises have focused on techniques for facilitation of voluntary function.[10-17] If volition is insufficient to excite contraction of a prime mover, then facilitation is necessary to attempt to achieve that goal. The less effective the volitional excitation is, the greater must be the facilitation. As volitional excitation becomes more effective, the reflex facilitation can be decreased. After it is possible to produce a voluntary contraction of the prime mover, then reflex or mass proprioceptive neuromuscular facilitation must be withdrawn before control can be used as the basis for training coordination. The ability to produce activity in a muscle by facilitation techniques does not necessarily assure that the neural pathway can be retrained to the level of useful performance. But since facilitation to activate voluntary muscular contraction followed by prolonged training to develop control and then coordination engrams is the only course available to regain useful function, a therapeutic trial is necessary.

Cutaneous reinforcement of excitation. Stimulation of the skin over the tendon of insertion and the belly of the muscle reflexly increases the sensitivity of the stretch reflex (gamma motor neuron reflex) and facilitates the contraction of the muscle.[18] This stimulus is applied immediately before each command to contract the muscle. Stroking, tapping, cold, chemical irritants, or electrical stimulation of the skin over the muscle belly may be effective to increase the motor response.[14]

Teach mental awareness of correct function. Instruct the patient in the function of each muscle, indicating the origin and insertion of the muscle, the line of pull, and the action produced by the muscle. Demonstrate the action while the patient remains passive. Instruct the patient to think of the pull as coming from the insertion and moving in the direction of the shortening muscle. Stroke the skin over the insertion in the direction of pull and tell the patient to concentrate on the sensation of motion occurring during this sensorially reinforced passive motion.

Train perception of contraction. The training of precise control of individual muscles is basically the training of awareness of the sensation produced by the isolated contraction of the prime mover so that it may be contracted independently from any other muscle. Control training or neuromuscular education begins with minimal effort against minimal resistance and is increased by small increments of intensity as the patient develops control.[6, 7] The specific sensations produced by the contraction of the prime mover are perceived only during very light effort because an isolated contraction of an individual muscle can be performed only when the muscle is contracting against a resistance that is small in relation to the total strength of that muscle. Greater effort, which would cause the spread of excitation to other motoneurons and result in the cocontraction of other muscles, should not be allowed. If such spread of excitation is allowed to occur, any stronger sensations produced by the contractions of stronger synergists and antagonists will be perceived more readily than will sensations arising from the weakly contracting prime mover. The patient then will learn to monitor the strong but incorrect motor activity and will ignore the sensations arising from the lesser activity of the prime mover. Therefore, he will not learn to control the prime mover and it will not develop its potential strength and usefulness. If this type of incoordination is allowed during therapeutic exercise, a motor pattern is developed that does not include the paretic prime mover. The final result is an uncoordinated contraction of less than the potential strength.

When the muscle is weak in relation to the weight of the part, that weight constitutes a heavy resistance for the muscle and the effort to lift the part causes irradiation of impulses and incoordination. Therefore, control exercises are begun with maximal assistance so that the muscle contracts against minimal resistance, and the resistance is increased only as ability is developed to contract the prime mover without activating other muscles.

Sequence for training neuromuscular control. For the training of control when there is an upper motor neuron lesion it is necessary first to obtain relaxation of all muscles that show a reflex hypertonia. Then the patient must limit the intensity of effort to avoid exciting irradiation of impulses beyond the prime mover. Specific control of the prime mover or unit of contraction which is controllable is trained by performance of that motion with minimal effort and as much assistance as is necessary to produce the motion. (1) The patient is instructed to think about the motion while that motion is carried out passively by the therapist in order that the patient may feel the sensations produced. The skin over the tendon of insertion is stroked in the direction of the motion to reinforce the sensation of the motion. Even this level of participation during which the patient is told only to think about the motion may result in cocontraction of other muscles as the patient tries hard to participate. If that is the case he must be taught to diminish his effort so that overflow does not occur. (2) As the second step, after stimulating the skin over the tendon of insertion the therapist carries out the motion while the patient assists only slightly by a minimal contraction of the prime mover. When the patient can limit his performance to the muscle or unit of motion being trained, he is allowed to increase participation gradually, and the assistance is decreased as the precision is maintained. (3) The patient produces increasingly stronger contractions as the therapist continues the technique of cutaneous stimulation followed by the desired movement. As the precise activity is carried on repeatedly, the patient learns how to control that prime mover without initiating other activity. Repetition begins to form the correct engram of that single activity. (4) As the patient develops the ability to produce a stronger controlled contraction of the desired motion, the therapist gradually decreases assistance until the patient is producing the correct antigravity contraction.

Progression from one step to the next should be permitted only when the first step can be performed accurately without substitution or incoordination. At the beginning of training the step being trained is carried out three to five times for each muscle or motion at each training session, depending upon the fatigability of the muscle. As the muscle gets stronger and endurance increases, the number of repetitions can be increased. Throughout control training, avoidance of substitution must be emphasized. Control of the individual muscles of a pattern should be achieved before more complex coordination training is attempted. Control of simple motions with inhibition of other activity represents the beginning of coordination.

Training of Multimuscular Coordination

Therapeutic exercise to train coordination has as its objective the development of a high level of coordination in the shortest possible time. The purpose of this training is to strengthen the selection and utilization of the best method of performance of each activity to be carried out. In order to accomplish this, the trainer must know each method to be used. This knowledge includes both the perceptual and the motor components of the coordinated performance. Then that method needs to be put into the patient's repertory by the repetition of the correct pattern of performance.[5]

For optimal learning of coordination, conditions should be set up in which the method is consistently and successfully performed. A learning environment must be established in which the patient can concentrate on the task and can carry out the necessary activity correctly under direct perception (see Training of Control of Individual Muscles, p. 406). To do this, the activity is broken down, or *desynthesized, to components that are simple enough to be performed correctly.* Desynthesis increases the consistency and frequency of correct performance and elimininates errors. The more complex the task to be learned, the more extensively it must be desynthesized to insure that each subtask can be correctly practiced. If a patient has such poor control that he has not developed any simple subunits of coordination, it is necessary to completely desynthesize the multimuscular movement and practice the contraction of the individual prime mover muscles. During training it is necessary to keep the effort low by decreasing both the speed and the resistance against which the patient must perform because as effort increases there is an increased spread of excitation to activate motor neurons that are not a part of the desired coordination pattern.

When the motor pattern is desynthesized to unit motor tasks that can be performed successfully, each task is trained by practicing it under voluntary control. The patient is instructed in the desired performance accompanied by sensory stimulation and passive movement. In the early stages of training each step of the task must be observed and modified voluntarily by the patient. It is imperative to practice slowly because it is not possible for the patient to attend to more than one unit of function at any instant. It takes time for an individual to think through the sensations and muscular response of each untrained motion. An untrained activity requires a *minimum* of 500 milliseconds per observation and response. When the activity is strange or new it may require several seconds for the patient to process the sensations generated by muscular contractions and relate them to the motion desired. At the same time the patient must sort out conflicting sensory stimuli produced by contractions of other muscles and suppress that activity. Awareness of the sensations produced by this movement is reinforced. Whatever assistance is necessary to reduce the effort to the level at which precision is maintained is provided while the patient concentrates on the sensations produced by the activity. Fatigue occurs quickly during attempts to maintain precise or isolated contractions by voluntary control. As fatigue occurs the ability of the patient to concentrate on the activity to be trained diminishes and as a consequence mistakes begin to occur. Therefore, the patient should have a short rest after each two or three repetitions to prevent cumulative fatigue. If the patient shows continuing fatigue or diminished control, that activity should be discontinued for that treat-

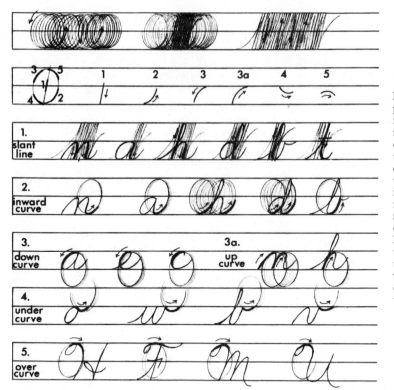

FIGURE 19–1. Repeated correct performance of simple components of a complex coordinated movement is the quickest way to develop the basic engrams, which then can be linked to practice more complex activities. Any guides that increase the awareness of correct performance or provide immediate comparison of correct performance hasten the development of coordination. As an example, in Palmer Method writing the practicing of the compact oval and vertical push-pull movements provides the pattern for the components of motions used when writing.

ment session in order that an erroneous pattern not be practiced. As the patient develops the ability to produce a precise contraction with no evidence of cocontractions, he may be allowed to exert more effort, always staying within the ability to maintain the pattern. At each step of the training, the therapist must be sure that the patient can perform independently and correctly before proceeding to more advanced activity.

Repetition of the correct performance many times causes the formation of a coordination engram in the central nervous system (Fig. 19–1). The engram that is developed is determined by the pattern that is practiced. If the practice is imprecise the engram will be imprecise. If errors are made during practice the resulting engram will show frequent errors. Therefore, one should maintain precision at all times by keeping the task within the capacity of the patient to perform it correctly. Performance of an incorrect or variable pattern not only delays the development of the correct engram but also begins to introduce an incorrect engram, which then will have to be "unlearned." It requires a longer time to "unlearn" an incorrect pattern and establish a correct pattern than it does merely to establish a correct pattern when there is no interfering engram.

Repetition of precise activity is the only way by which engrams of coordination are developed. The research that demonstrated the relationship between the number of repetitions performed and the level of skill in performance of an engram was reported by Crossman in 1959.[5] He showed that in the development of manual coordination required for an industrial task, a young adult with normal dexterity required three million repetitions of that act in order to develop maximal speed and skill (Fig. 19–2). In an investigation of other types of repetitive activities, it was found that a high level of coordination was not achieved until repetitions occurred a million or more times.[19]

Patients need to repeat the precise contraction of each movement unit many hundreds or even thousands of times each day if they are to develop precise engrams of that activity in as short a time as three years. It requires 1000 repetitions of an engram daily for three years to approximate one million repetitions. If only 100 repetitions are performed per day it requires 30 years to accumulate one million repetitions. Inadequate repetitions result in imperfect performances. Many of our daily activities have common component movements of the arms, legs, and trunk, and the practice of those components in one activity appears to have a carry-over to other activities. However, any units of activity that are specific to only one task must be practiced specifically to develop a coordination engram for that task.

As the patient develops the ability to produce the individual units of the engram easily and accurately, these are then linked into subtasks, each of which, in turn, is practiced as a unit until it too is automated as a larger engram of performance. The engrams of the subtasks as they are perfected by practice are chained progressively until the full pattern can be performed precisely with speed and force. As these engrams of subtasks and, later, full engrams are developed, the conscious regulation becomes one of selecting the sequences in which these engrams will appear. If the patterned activity is such that the same sequence of engrams will appear many times, then through practice the entire sequence can be made into a continuous engram and run automatically.

The intensity of effort is increased during practice only to the degree that precise performance can be maintained. Increasing the speed, the force, or the complexity of an activity increases the intensity of effort that is required. Attention must be paid to each of these characteristics of performance, since excessive effort always leads to incoordination. Improvement in performance is achieved by gradually increasing the force, speed, and complexity of performance within the capacity to maintain precision. Performance improves only when practicing near the peak of ability. Performance should be encouraged at the highest level at which the patient can succeed. Repeated near-maximal practice is necessary to perfect and maintain coordination.

Although each test of maximal ability exceeds the peak of performance, practice should be carried on within the range in which every repetition, insofar as possible, is correct, since engrams develop only as the result of successful performance and nothing beneficial is accomplished by performing erroneously. Therapists, therefore, should avoid setting up practice situations in which there are errors in performance. Successful performance has a dual effect. Physiologically it reinforces the strength of the engram and psychologically it rewards the patient so that he or she is more willing to continue to perform that activity.

The Role of Repetition in the Formation of Engrams

There is an interesting dichotomy of opinion that the usual activities of a normal child emerge as the result of genetic inheritance but that maximal performers of any neuromuscular act must train by practicing for years before they reach their peak skill. We usually overlook the fact that young children practice simple engrams many times each day for many months before they acquire the level of coordination necessary to begin to perform more complex activities. It requires many years of practice during play before the coordination of the child develops to the lowest level of the range of coordination found in normal adults (Fig. 19–3). Many activities are highly repetitious. Walking, a variety of forms of hand grasp, reaching, balancing — all are activities repeated thousands of times each day by all normal persons. Athletes, musicians, acrobats, and persons using finger dexterity in their occupations practice for years to perfect their skills. In recent years it has become

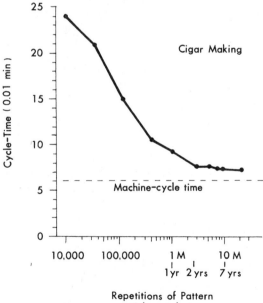

FIGURE 19–2. The development of skillful and automatic performance of a new task requires millions of repetitions to reach its peak, as demonstrated by the decrease of the unit performance time for this manual motor activity by newly employed normal young women. (From Kottke, F. J.: From reflex to skill: The training of coordination. Arch. Phys. Med. Rehabil., 61:551–561, 1980. Adapted from Crossman, E. R. F. W.: Theory of acquisition of speed-skill. Ergonomics, 2:153–166, 1959.)

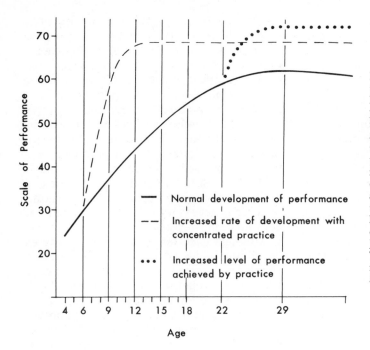

FIGURE 19–3. Under normal conditions coordination develops progressively through childhood and reaches its peak in the third decade. Concentrated training of a specific activity results in achievement of peak coordination for that activity at a much earlier age. Likewise concentrated training of an activity in adulthood results in a significant increase in the peak performance of that activity. The number of correct repetitions in each situation rather than the length of time determines the level of coordination achieved. (From Kottke, F. J., Halpern, D., Easton, J. K. M., Ozel, A. T., and Burrill, C. A.: Training of coordination. Arch. Phys. Med. Rehabil., 59:567–572, 1978.)

apparent that intense training of children in athletics or musical skills can shorten the time to reach the maximal level of performance; it is not solely a matter of maturation with age, but rather the achievement of millions of correct repetitions to perfect the necessary engrams.

Programs of therapeutic exercise should provide for as many repetitions as possible of each activity each day, since engrams do not become well developed until hundreds of thousands of repetitions have been performed. Lack of sufficient repetitions has been a major flaw in much of the programming of therapeutic exercise for the training of coordination. In a single short period scheduled for coordination training each day a child with hyperreflexia may perform only a very few repetitions of each movement. Between therapies many hours elapse during which correctly coordinated activity is not performed. Moreover, incoordinated activity may be allowed during the interval between therapies, while the therapists focus on correct performance only during the few moments of the therapy. The lack of understanding of the mechanism of formation of engrams of coordination results in failure to provide enough practice to obtain adequately developed engrams and in the tolerance of incorrect performance, which develops incoordination. Such faulty scheduling of training guarantees that the result will be poor.

For the training of the handicapped person to be successful, it needs to be organized similarly to the training of any skillful performer. Training schedules for those individuals provide each day for thousands of repetitions of specific activities. The level of practice is set and monitored so that throughout the entire schedule the performance is precise and exact. Before any performer can carry out the final complex pattern of coordination he must develop the ability to carry out each of the simple component parts. We are only now beginning to recognize that maximal skill is not attained until an engram has been practiced millions of times. The task, then, in therapeutic exercise should be to establish conditions in which patients can repeat the desired activities correctly many times each day so that as quickly as possible they have performed the hundreds of thousands or millions of repetitions that result in the development of a satisfactory coordination engram.

Factors Increasing Incoordination

There are a number of conditions that increase incoordination. Strong effort to produce a contraction causes irradiation of impulses in the central nervous system from the pathway of a coordinated activity to other motoneurons. Constant repetition of an activity in combination with the same extraneous motion will incorporate that extraneous motion into the activity pattern and produce a persistent incoordination. When a patient is insecure or fearful, there is a greater spread of excitation within the central system with activation of more motor neurons than those essential for an activity pattern. This results in a greater expenditure of effort, less precision of motion, and interference with the desired pattern of activity. If a patient has to support himself against gravity, if he is weak, or if he must overcome resistance that is great in relation to the strength of a muscle, incoordination will be increased. Excitement and strong emotions increase incoordination. Pain or increased sensory stimuli reaching the central nervous system increase irradiation from an activated pathway to other motor neurons. Fatigue increases incoordination, probably because of the inability of the inhibitory centers to restrict impulses from irradiating beyond the desired activity pathway.

Just as coordination is produced by repetition, it is lost through periods of inactivity. It is necessary to reteach coordination to muscles that have been inactive or paretic. The alienation of paretic muscles from an activity pattern occurs frequently. Only through specific training of control and coordination do these muscles again become incorporated as a part of the normal activity pattern.

Systems of Therapy

A comparison of the requirements for the training of coordination discussed above with the various "systems of therapy" that are being used throughout the United States at this time reveals that each of those systems concentrates on a limited range of the entire spectrum of need for training coordination. Each advocate of selected specified procedures of therapeutic exercise has concentrated on selected problems that must be resolved in the therapeutic program. Some methods such as those of Kabat,[10] Knott and Voss,[11] Rood,[14, 15] and Brunnstrom[12] have concentrated on reflex or mass proprioceptive neuromuscular facilitation to activate or strengthen voluntary control. For these methods the assumption appears to be that as the voluntary activity becomes stronger there will be a fading of incoordination. The major limitation of each of these methods is that after facilitation has developed activation of prime mover muscles as a part of mass activity, there are no procedures in those methods focusing on the development of inhibition of undesired activity. Continued practice of reflex facilitation or mass proprioceptive neuromuscular facilitation strengthens and perpetuates incoordination. The only way by which inhibition of undesired activity can be developed is by prolonged practice of the desired patterns in order to develop coordination engrams. Therefore, systems of reflex facilitation must be followed by coordination training if mass patterns of activity are to be converted to useful coordination.

Phelps,[20] who developed one of the early programs for cerebral palsy in the United States, was eclectic in his approach to treatment. Many components of his treatment continue to be used. Among other contributions, he recognized that a patient who learned to relax completely showed less involuntary activity during relaxation than during activity. Therefore, patients were taught prolonged relaxation. However, Phelps did not distinguish between general relaxation and inhibition of undesired muscular contraction during activity. General relaxation alone does not train inhibition during activity. Phelps recognized that repetition of a desired pattern of motion improved the performance of that pattern. He taught his patients to practice repetition of desired activities with or without assistance and accompanied by songs or jingles each day. In effect, he was using repetition to develop engrams. His insistence on the continued practice of the same basic activities indicates his awareness of the need for many repetitions before coordination begins to develop.

Temple Fay[16] recognized that motor performance was controlled by the hierarchic organization of the central nervous system and that motor coordination developed as the brain developed the capacity to inhibit and modify reflexes. He recognized that control of the basic reflexes was essential before more advanced coordination could be trained. He utilized reflex patterning and repetition as the means to begin to modify basic reflexes and referred to this as neurophysiological organization of the nervous system. Although Fay recognized that undesired reflex activity must be inhibited in any motor pattern, it is not clear to what extent he recognized the importance of training

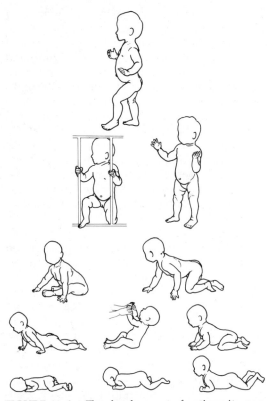

FIGURE 19–4. The development of antigravity posture shows a pyramidal contour from a broad base and low profile at birth to a progressively higher profile on a narrower base as coordination for balance and the ability to utilize and inhibit reflexes develops.

inhibition as the basis for the formation of correct engrams. It is evident that he did recognize that prolonged repetition through patterning was essential for the development of coordination engrams.[17]

Karel and Berta Bobath[21, 22] emphasized both the need for inhibition of hypertonia in patients with cerebral palsy prior to the beginning of training and the necessity for carrying out proper training in order to develop correct patterns of performance without overflow of activity to other muscles. They, like Fay, emphasize that training of posture progresses from simple activities to the more complex in a regular sequence and called this the neurodevelopmental sequence of therapy (Fig. 19–4). They utilize reflex facilitation to reinforce the motor patterns with which they are concerned, particularly in the postural activities.

Margaret Rood[14] and her students[15] have used a variety of reflex facilitatory methods to excite or inhibit motor activity. Rood, too, has focused her attention more on excitation

of prime mover function than on the inhibition of the muscles producing incoordination.

The persons who have focused our attention on incoordination resulting from effort which causes the spread of muscular activity from prime movers to other muscles to an excessive degree were Kenny[6] and Knapp.[7] Their concepts grew out of their experience in the treatment of acute anterior poliomyelitis, quite a different disease from cerebral palsy. In poliomyelitis, when a prime mover was paralyzed, the uncoordinated overuse of other muscles because of the effort exerted to activate the paralyzed muscle was a predominant finding. In the early 1940s it was presumed that the incoordination of poliomyelitis was specific to that disease. Gellhorn[23] was the first investigator to demonstrate that the incoordination of poliomyelitis was the overuse of synergists, stabilizers, and antagonists in the same typical pattern that occurred in normal individuals with increasing effort. This was the beginning of our understanding that the incoordination of motor activity is based on the normal reflex organization of the nervous system rather than being due to abnormal discharges from damaged neurons. The failure to recognize that incoordination was not a specific phenomenon peculiar to each disease but, rather, has a characteristic pattern in all diseases has delayed the development of our understanding regarding the mechanism of incoordination. Kenny and Knapp demonstrated that only when effort was decreased so that there was no irradiation of nerve impulses to other pathways could a person produce an isolated contraction of a prime mover. This is the basis for the training of control of the individual muscles.

Hypothesis of Inheritance of Motor Coordination

The hypothesis that postulates the inheritance of the basic patterns of coordination, as opposed to the learning of coordination engrams, merits presentation here because it is the widely accepted doctrine.[24-26] Many of the early students of development observed that the basic patterns of posture and movement — sitting, standing, balancing, walking, running, reaching, grasping — all appeared in a uniform sequence and time during maturation, and they assumed this to be the result of genetic endowment. A logical extension of this concept, then, was that any reflex activity that interfered with the emergence of these automatic coordination patterns was an "abnormal" reflex rather than inadequate inhibition of a normal reflex. Coordination or automatic neuromuscular activity was assumed to develop in the normal child with age as the result of maturation of neurons and myelination of nerve pathways. Elapse of time rather than prolonged practice of each activity was considered to be the essential requirement for the development of coordination for those activities common to most people. In the young, lack of muscular strength and immaturity were assumed to be the factors limiting automatic coordination. Mass movement of multiple muscles was reported to precede the development of activity of individual muscles,[27] and from this, automatic coordination of multiple muscles was assumed to precede the development of control of individual muscles. It was deduced that multimuscular automatic coordination is inherent and only later does a person learn to control individual muscles by conscious practice. This concept is the converse to that of the progressive development from reflexes to control of the individual muscle to coordination of multiple muscles as the result of repetitive practice.[3] Part of the confusion may have resulted from equating coordinated multimuscular contractions with mass reflex activity. Even mass reflex movements were shown by Windle[28] to develop in the fetus after the prior development of local reflexes. This reflex activity, either local or general, is far more rudimentary than the coordinated muscular activity with which we are concerned. However, normal infants and children in a normal environment develop motor patterns so easily and on such a regular schedule that genetic inheritance appeared adequate to explain development without invoking environment or experience.[24, 27, 29, 30] If these assumptions were accepted, it seemed quite logical also to assume that when brain damage arrested muscular performance at a low level, the impairment of function was imposed by loss of motor patterns genetically coded in the damaged neurons rather than resulting from lack of practice to develop coordination engrams.

It was only as the design of experiments changed to follow each patient and chronicle his experiences and activities, rather than evaluate performances of groups of infants at fixed ages of development, that genetic determinism appeared to be inadequate as a total explanation. Piaget[31] first, followed by others,[32-34] observed serial development of performance from the simple to the more complex as the result of many repetitions of each act. Environmental stimuli that encouraged the repetition of an activity speeded its development.[32] Prevention of activity severely delayed development.[34, 35]

Coordination Activities for the Hand and Upper Extremity

Prehension. The complex activities of pinch and grasp require multimuscular coordination for each digit. There is usually simultaneous movement of wrist, elbow, and shoulder to carry the hand to the desired place of activity. Prehension occurs most frequently as pinch between the thumb, index, and middle fingers like a three-jawed chuck (Fig. 19-5). Seventy per cent of prehensile activity is carried out by variants of this position. Power grasp, performed by approximating the four fingers toward the thenar eminence, is used in its various modifications for about 20 per cent of activities. Apposition of the thumb to the radial side of the index finger or to one fingertip occurs less frequently. Modifications of these basic patterns occur by varying the number of fingers in finger-tip grasp; abducting, adducting, or rotating at the metacarpophalangeal joints; varying the position of terminal pad contact by the amount of interphalangeal flexion; or varying the degree of closure or the number of fingers involved in the power grip (Fig. 19-6). Each of these variants of position requires the development of a multimuscular coordination engram through prolonged practice in infancy and childhood.

The activities of the multiple muscles involved in the positioning or movement of even one finger exceed the supervisory capacity of totally voluntary observation and regulation. The development of preprogrammed engrams is essential for all finger activities and in the absence of these engrams incoordination occurs even though each of the prime movers can be contracted voluntarily. This may be seen in the repeated reversal of consecutive joints of the fingers of the athetoid patient as grasp is attempted but muscles, other than the prime mover which is under immediate attention, deviate from the desired pattern. As the patient

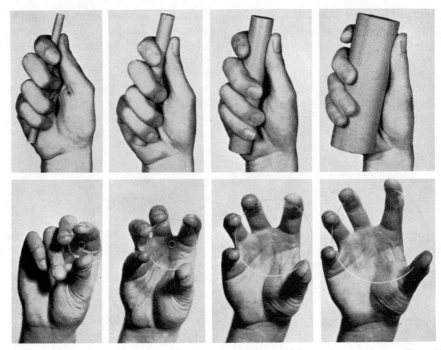

FIGURE 19–5. Prehension using the power grip or precision grip on objects of various sizes. (From Napier, J. R.: The prehensile movements of the human hand. J. Bone Joint Surg., 38B:902–913, 1956.)

shifts his attention consecutively from joint to joint, the joint receiving direct observation is brought under control, but other joints not being observed move out of position because automatic activation and inhibition are not imposed on the muscles that control them. These same patterns that are seen in the athetoid who is unable to develop engrams may be seen in the infant before engrams develop. In children or adults in whom the demands of performance exceed the engrams that have been developed, errors are more likely to result in the selection of the incorrect engram or incomplete inhibition of reflex activity.

As might be expected, the most complex patterns are the most difficult to program and require the longest period of training. Finger-thumb prehension has far too many components and too many variations to be successfully controlled by volition through the single-channelled corticospinal tract in the absence of coordination engrams. The thumb, because of its mobility at the car-

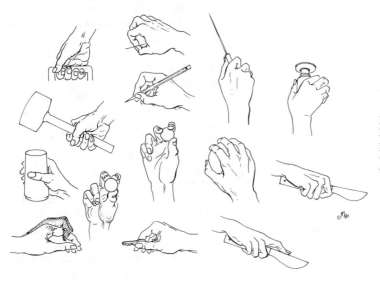

FIGURE 19–6. Although most prehensile motions are variants of the precision grip or the power grip, each position constitutes a separate engram.

pometacarpal joints, is the most mobile digit and by far the most difficult to learn to coordinate. It requires the coordinated contractions of multiple muscles to maintain one position or to move to another position. As a consequence, until the engrams of thumb coordination have developed, the thumb is a continual impediment to the use of the other fingers. Also each of the other fingers has metacarpophalangeal mobility in multiple planes: rotation, abduction-adduction, and flexion-extension. Each of these motions at each of these joints must be regulated by the appropriate contractions of the controlling muscles and inhibition of all other muscles for each of the possible variations of prehension. Coordination of all of these potential patterns requires the formation of engrams developed only by prolonged practice. In particular, the untrained thumb persistently interferes with the use of the index and middle fingers. Athetoid children learn to avoid the interfering thumb by concentrating on the use of the fourth and fifth fingers for grasp — the so-called ulnar grasp. Ulnar grasp is not a more fundamental or primitive grasp, but, rather, is the grasp that can be more successfully practiced to develop an engram because the patterns are not continually disrupted by uncontrolled motions of the thumb.

It is only after basic engrams form that useful function begins to emerge in the hand. When the activities of the normal individual without preprogrammed engrams are observed, i.e., the normal infant, as was done by White,[36] it is seen that the hand may be moved reflexly but not in a coordinated manner for the first three to four months. During that time the infant may spend minutes at a time gazing at the motionless fisted hand (probably because he has no conception of how to initiate motion in the arm). At four months there still is little prehension, and upper extremity activity is mainly swiping at an object in the visual field during which the hand may be fisted or open. It is only long after that and following practice each day throughout the waking period that the child develops crude one-handed, and later, bimanual grasp. Controlled thumb-to-index pinch does not begin to develop for about eight months, and three-finger pinch requires several more months of practice before rudimentary coordination is seen. Even then these activities are poorly programmed for integration into prehensile patterns. Two more years of daily practice are necessary before the child can integrate thumb position with arm motion and position in space to grasp a pencil and draw a simple vertical line (Fig. 19–7), and an additional 30 months of training are necessary before he can copy a triangle. The purpose in focusing attention on this long period required for the training of a normal child in the use of the hand is to demonstrate that in every normal person the development of multimuscular engrams requires millions of repetitions before they become well coordinated.

The voluntary component of normal prehension consists of the selection of the engrams to be used and of modifying activity by shifting from one engram to another in relation to the shape and position of the object being manipulated. Skillful prehension develops slowly. The slow development of the drawing and writing skills of children is a good indication of the prolonged period of practice necessary before the fundamental multimuscular patterns of manual performance begin to develop. Tests of manual manipulation show that these skills increase in a linear fashion through youth and adolescence and do not peak until the third decade of life[38] (see Fig. 19–3).

For the patient with impaired coordination, if such a complex activity as precision grip is not desynthesized to the level that each controllable subunit can be practiced accurately under direct volition, then good coordination will never be developed. When there is damage to the extrapyramidal system so that cocontraction is difficult to coordinate and automatic inhibition is slow to develop, it is essential to provide the environment and the practice routines that make the execution of performable motions possible in the correct patterns for thousands of times each day. How is this to be done?

The first criterion for repeated performance is that the patient is willing to, or better, wants to perform. The reinforcing effect of a participating and observing therapist, parent, or friend is one way to meet this criterion. However, time each day for such participation is frequently limited. An activity that provides its own rewarding feedback so that the patient wishes to perform repeatedly is a second mechanism. Such rewarding activities should be readily available so that at any time the patient wishes to practice he can do so. Musical instruments, toys, typewriters, games, and construction crafts all

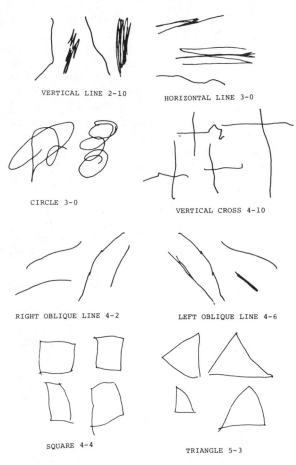

VERTICAL LINE 2-10

HORIZONTAL LINE 3-0

CIRCLE 3-0

VERTICAL CROSS 4-10

RIGHT OBLIQUE LINE 4-2

LEFT OBLIQUE LINE 4-6

SQUARE 4-4

TRIANGLE 5-3

FIGURE 19–7. It requires many months of manual activities before a child develops the ability to hold a pencil and successfully copy a figure on paper. The numerals indicate the age in years and months at which a child would be expected to perform increasingly difficult pencil-on-paper tasks on request. (From Beery, K. E.: Developmental test of visual-motor integration: Administration and scoring manual. Chicago, Follette Publishing Co., 1967.)

come to mind as conventional self-rewarding activities. For most of these currently available modes of rewarding activity, participation can occur only when prehension is well advanced. The greatest unmet need at the present time is to develop the mechanical devices that link individual prime mover contractions or the contractions of simple subunits of coordinated muscular function to self-rewarding activities. A variety of linking transducers needs to be developed to make it possible to initiate or carry out these self-rewarding activities by use of the subunit or unit engram that is to be trained. For example, it may be possible by a hinged hand splint, similar to the flexor-hinge splint for the metacarpophalangeal joints, to restrict activity to one simple agonist-antagonist pair and use this motion to control a video game, an electronic organ, or another type of self-rewarder, so that for many minutes each day the patient gains pleasure from practicing that unit of prehension. Similarly adapted splints may allow the precise practice of subunits of function of the muscles of the thumb. As these subunits are mastered by

the formation of engrams, the activities must be combined to activate other types of transducers, which requires linking of the subunits to perform a larger or more complex function. Variations of activities are necessary to prevent monotony and frustration, especially if the coordination of the patient is poor. Participation in multiple activities increases general coordination and aids in maintaining attention.

At each step when chaining small engrams into larger ones the activity must be performed more slowly than was necessary for the individual small engram in order to allow time for voluntary supervision of the linkage. As practice develops a linked engram, the speed of performance can be increased again. When the coordination of the prehensile pattern has been developed to the level of useful skill it can be combined with arm motion in a wide variety of activities for both precision grasp and palmar grasp.[39] In all of these activities at each stage the patient should have the opportunity to practice the pattern with consistent accuracy. Each stage will need to be practiced tens of thousands of

UPPER EXTREMITY MOTION

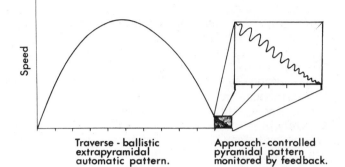

FIGURE 19–8. A reaching motion to a precise position consists of an automatic engram phase and an approach phase which is guided by voluntary control to the target.

times before significant improvement is seen. Therefore, planned rewards and reinforcers of performance are essential to maintain interest in the activity.

In contrast to the emphasis on the need for prolonged, progressive training of prehension which has just been described, it should be pointed out that very many of the so-called adaptations for hand function are substitutes or holders that make prehension unnecessary. If the patient uses one of these substitutes it dissuades him from attempting to use or improve prehension even though it may encourage the use of other arm motions.

Transfer Motions of the Arm

The arm and forearm function like a retractable derrick carrying the hand as a prehensile organ. Motions of the shoulder, elbow, and wrist to carry the hand to the site of activity normally are automatic and not under specific attention. These automated motions of reaching, moving, and positioning the upper extremity develop through practice.[40] During coordinated motion, the traversing motion of the arm is fast, strong, and automatically guided by a preprogrammed engram (Fig. 19–8). Little attention needs to be paid to that automatic pattern. In the final approach the positioning of the hand is under conscious visual and proprioceptive perception to assure accuracy of positioning and is carried out more slowly and with less force. Athetoid patients who never have been able to practice precise patterns or children who have not yet developed automatic engrams show erratically unpredictable movements of both the traverse and the approach, since automated precise engrams have not been developed and the multimuscular demands of the traverse as well as the approach exceed the ability of the single-channelled corticospinal control system to monitor them (Fig. 19–9).

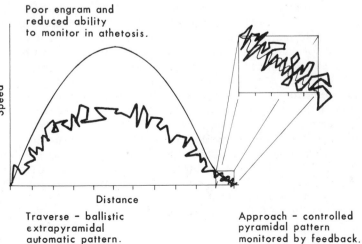

FIGURE 19–9. Children who have not yet developed coordination engrams or athetoid patients who are unable to do so show an erratic pattern of motion both in the traverse phase and in the approach phase of upper extremity motion.

Maintenance of Balance

Coordination provides automatic postural balance and antigravity support as well as the integrated activities in the extremity. To grasp with the hand, for example, prime mover responses provide motion and position for the fingers and thumb. Synergistic muscles contract with the prime movers to assist or modify those activities. Stabilizer cocontractions occur in the muscles of the wrist, elbow, and shoulder. Before this apparently primary activity can begin, a stable base must be established in relation to gravity by the properly coordinated contractions of the muscles that establish a stable posture for the body and head. To change the location of the hand requires motion produced by contraction of the muscle of the shoulder and elbow. As the arm moves there must be postural adjustments to maintain balance. The effects of these muscular contractions must be monitored by sensory feedback from the joints, musculotendinous junctions, fascia, and skin to the central nervous system. The person remains unaware of most aspects of this complex performance unless gross errors occur that require modification of the pattern. Even then the perception is of the achievement of the task rather than perception of the changes of contractions of individual muscles.

At each level of practice in the development of an engram the ability to perform against a template or target positions for comparison increases the accuracy of performance and hastens learning. As the basic subunits are trained by matching performance against that template, the correct motor pattern emerges and by practice becomes an engram. Engrams developed more rapidly in this way can be combined progressively into more and more complex patterns of performance. A template allows more frequent and more precise comparisons than would occur otherwise so that the performance becomes more precise and the repetition of the correct pattern develops the engram more quickly. As an example of the use of a guide to performance, the making of compact ovals or push-pull vertical lines in the Palmer method of penmanship provides a visual-spatial monitor of the motor activity as it occurs (see Fig. 19–1). The precision of or errors of performance can be recognized immediately. Comparison is available after each repetition. The spatial and temporal proximity of the template to the performance provides an excellent opportunity for comparison. As these basic components of the coordination engrams for writing develop, they can be selected and chained to form all of the components of the letters used in cursive writing. The development of similar types of templates for other manual activities is necessary if precise coordination is to be developed rapidly. Electromyographic feedback from the prime mover and synergists to be activated in contrast to the antagonists and other interfering muscles to be inhibited provides a close-linked means of monitoring a small number of muscles in simple patterns. Retrospective review of complex performances by video recording is of especial value in recognizing undesired reflexes or other cocontractions that must be inhibited in order to obtain the coordination pattern desired. However, the greater the delay between performance and feedback, the less effective the monitor becomes. In a similar way, repetitively retracing figures helps to develop visual-spatial-manual orientation as well as manual coordination. Spatial memory and orientation depend, at least in part, on the establishment of motor engrams in the extrapyramidal system.[41]

Occupational therapy can be used to develop varying degrees of strength and endurance at the same time that coordination is stressed. Occupational therapy is especially suited to the development of dexterity of the fingers and hand. The constructive aspects of occupational therapy aid in maintaining attention (Fig. 19–10). Similar training may also be carried on in a prevocational shop. Such activities should be designed to encourage the patient to work at the maximal rate of speed consistent with maximal precision. Modification of craft activities by incorporating artificial maneuvers or excessive resistance not only discourages the patient from participation but also interferes with the improvement of coordination.

Coordination Activities for the Lower Extremities. Ambulation training begins as training of the basic engrams of balance and recovery of balance. Early training needs to be carried out by practicing units of these patterns which are simple enough that the patient can perform each pattern correctly. Selective external stabilization may need to be provided at each stage of the training so

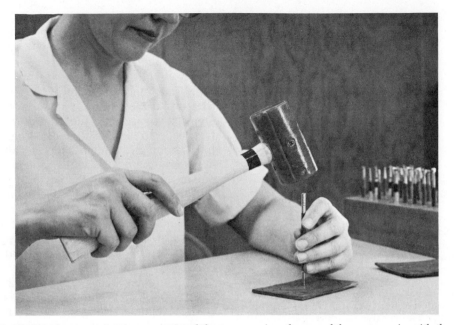

FIGURE 19–10. Leather stamping in occupational therapy requires the use of the power grip with the dominant hand and the precision grip with the nondominant hand.

that antigravity support is secure and the patient can concentrate on voluntary activation of his assigned motor patterns without the distraction of other muscular activities required to maintain balance. This training should be initiated in infants who have not gained enough coordination to make balancing of the head possible by six months of age. With adequate support provided to secure trunk and lower extremity posture, neck control and balance are practiced until automatic.[42] Training of neck control is followed in order by training of independent trunk balance and motion, training of the upper extremities for protective extension and support to balance the trunk, hip balance and motion, knee balance and motion, and free standing.

For severely involved patients, the initial upright posture may be attained on a tilt table, where control of orthostatic blood pressure may be trained at the same time that progressive training of the engrams to assure antigravity balance is begun (Fig. 19–11). As stable posture develops from the neck down, the patient can be transferred to an upright stander (Fig. 19–12) and later to the parallel bars.

The development of coordination adequate to provide stable balance, and weight-shifting and recovery, are the necessary preludes to walking. Automatic engrams for con-

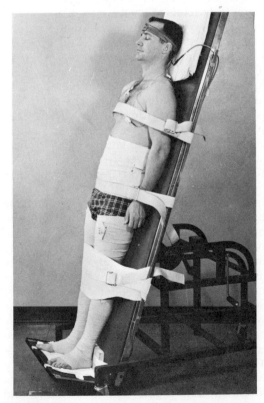

FIGURE 19–11. A tilt table may be used for stabilization of unstable joints of the lower extremities and trunk so that the patient can begin to practice controlled motion of the neck and upper trunk. At the same time he can develop cardiovascular tolerance to the upright position.

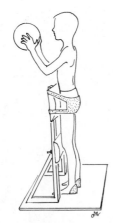

FIGURE 19–12. A standing frame provides postural stability from the floor up to the trunk so that neck, trunk, and upper extremity balance and coordination may be trained by practice. As coordination engrams develop in the upper segments the support provided by the stander may be lowered progressively to require practice of coordination of the lower trunk, hips, and knees to prepare for free standing.

trol of motion of the joints at each level or suitable bracing to make muscular activity unnecessary is essential before the patient can learn standing balance and practice weight-shifting preparatory to walking. These patterns should be practiced as lead-up drills before walking is attempted. The ability to walk with crutches does not develop if the patient attempts to walk in the parallel bars or walker before he has gained the basic skills for maintaining balance while standing. Basic balance training is initiated while standing on both feet with balance provided by both hands, then shifting weight from one foot to the other and establishing balance with the weight supported fully on one lower extremity while the hands are used only to maintain balance. Training of balance in parallel bars provides excellent stability and security but also the opportunity for misuse by pulling or pushing forward or sideways on the bars, which cannot be done when using crutches or canes. Broad-base canes provide good stability but can be used only to push in the downward direction (Fig. 19–13). If balance is not attained before walking is initiated the patient develops a lurching, falling gait that is unstable and fatiguing. Therefore, the ability to maintain balance throughout all phases of ambulation should be a fundamental component of the initial ambulation training. From full, broad, four-extremity support the patient should

practice balancing on a progressively smaller base until he can maintain weight-bearing on one foot with balance provided by only one hand. Weight-shifting from one foot to the other should become easy, reliable, and rapid as practice develops motor engrams. Shifting of weight and balance forward one step, backward one step, and during turning from side to side also needs to be practiced until automatic. Practicing lead-up drills to appropriate music provides a pleasant mechanism for monitoring the rhythm and rate of performance of the drills. Daily calisthenics of foot shifting, hand shifting, simultaneous hand and foot shifting, stepping forward or backward, knee bending and straightening, all constitute basic engrams that are coordinated in the walking pattern.

Walking requires that balance be shifted and reestablished with each step. Preservation of balance requires the automatic integration of the activities of the many muscles coordinating the motion, not only of the joints of the extremities, but also of the trunk and neck at each step. As the base of support is widened by two crutches or two broad-base canes there is decreased need for precision of balance, but engrams must be present that coordinate all four extremities and trunk (Fig. 19–13). Children under four years of age have not yet developed engrams adequate to coordinate reciprocal motion in all four extremities, which is necessary when walking in the parallel bars or when using crutches or canes. They learn to balance and walk much more readily using a stable transverse bar on

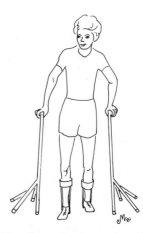

FIGURE 19–13. Canes that have a broad base enlarge the base of support during ambulation and decrease the precision of coordination which is necessary to balance and to walk.

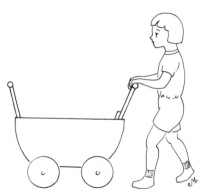

FIGURE 19–14. Until a child has developed engrams of coordination for all four extremities, he has great difficulty in consciously monitoring two legs and two crutches while learning to walk. When holding a transverse bar attached to a weighted wagon he needs to monitor only the reciprocal motion of the two lower extremities during walking. After he has developed the engrams for reciprocal motion in the lower extremities he can consciously monitor the position of the two crutches as he practices walking.

a push cart (Fig. 19–14), so that they need think only about the reciprocating motion of the two lower extremities. After they have developed their lower extremity engrams while pushing the cart, then they can begin training reciprocal motion of the upper extremities while using crutches.

Coordination Retraining for Proprioceptive or Cerebellar Dysfunction (Frenkel's Exercises). Frenkel's exercises are a series of exercises of increasing difficulty to improve proprioceptive control in the lower extremities. These exercises begin with simple movements with gravity eliminated and gradually progress to more complicated movement patterns utilizing simultaneous hip and knee motions carried on against gravity. They are especially useful when there is impairment of proprioception due to disorders in the central nervous system. Repeated practice helps to develop the usefulness of any proprioception that the patient has available to aid him. If the patient does not have adequate proprioception, he must be positioned so that he can monitor his activity by vision.

The initial exercise training is conducted under the supervision of a therapist, and the emphasis is on slow, precise motion and positioning. To avoid fatigue each exercise is performed not more than four times at each session. The first simple exercises should be accomplished adequately before progressing

to the more difficult patterns. As the patient gains the ability to perform each exercise, he is instructed to perform it every three or four hours.

Exercises While Supine. The patient lies on a bed or plinth with a smooth surface along which the heels may slide easily. The head should be supported so that the patient can see his legs and feet.

1. Flex the hip and knee of one extremity, sliding the heel along in contact with the bed. Return to the original position. Repeat with the opposite extremity.

2. Flex as in exercise 1. Then abduct the flexed hip. Return to the flexed position and then to the original position.

3. Flex the hip and knee only halfway and then return to the extended position. Add abduction and adduction.

4. Flex one limb at the hip and knee, stopping at any point in flexion or extension on command.

5. Flex both lower extremities simultaneously and equally; add abduction, adduction, and extension.

6. Flex both lower extremities simultaneously to the halfway position; add abduction and adduction to half-flexed position. Extend. Stop in the pattern on command.

7. Flex one extremity at the hip and knee with the heel held 2 inches above the bed. Return to the original position.

8. Flex as in exercise 7. Bring the heel to rest on the opposite patella. Successively add patterns so that the heel is touched to the middle of the shin, to the ankle, to the toes of the opposite foot, to the bed on either side of the knee, and to the bed on either side of the leg.

9. Flex as in exercise 7 and then touch the heel successively to the patella, shin, ankle, and toes. Reverse the pattern.

10. Flex as in exercise 7 and then on command touch the heel to the point indicated by the therapist.

11. Flex the hip and knee with the heel 2 inches above the bed. Place the heel on the opposite patella and slowly slide it down the crest of the tibia to the ankle. Reverse.

12. Use the pattern in exercise 11, but slide the heel down the crest of the opposite tibia, over the ankle and foot to the toes. If the heel is to reach the toes, the opposite knee must be flexed slightly during this exercise. Stop in the pattern on command.

13. With malleoli and knees in apposition,

flex both lower extremities simultaneously with the heels 2 inches above the bed. Return to the original position. Stop in the pattern on command.

14. Perform reciprocal flexion and extension of the lower extremities with the heels touching the bed.

15. Perform reciprocal flexion and extension of the lower extremities with the heels 2 inches above the bed.

16. Perform bilateral simultaneous flexion, abduction, adduction, and extension with the heels 2 inches above the bed.

17. Place the heel precisely where the therapist indicates with the finger on the bed or the opposite extremity.

18. Follow with the toe the movement of the therapist's finger in any combination of lower extremity motion.

Exercises While Sitting

1. Practice maintaining correct sitting posture for two minutes in an armchair with back support and the feet flat on the floor. Repeat in a chair without arms. Repeat without back support.

2. Mark time to the counting of the therapist by raising only the heel from the floor. Progress to alternatively lifting the entire foot and replacing it precisely in a marked position on the floor.

3. Make two cross marks on the floor with chalk. Alternately glide the foot over the marked cross; forward, backward, left and right.

4. Practice rising from and sitting on a chair to the therapist's counted cadence: (1) Flex the knees and draw the feet under the front edge of the seat. (2) Bend the trunk forward over the thighs. (3) Rise by extending the knees and hips and then straightening the trunk. (4) Bend the trunk forward slightly. (5) Flex the hips and knees to sit. (6) Straighten the trunk and sit back in the chair.

Exercises While Standing

1. Walking sideways. Balance is easier during sideward walking because the patient does not have to pivot over his toes or heels, which decreases his base of support. The exercise is performed to a counted cadence: (1) Shift the weight to the left foot. (2) Place the right foot 12 inches to the right. (3) Shift the weight to the right foot. (4) Bring the left foot over to the right foot. The size of the step taken to the right or left may be varied.

2. Walk forward between two parallel lines 14 inches apart, placing the right foot just inside the right line and the left foot just inside the left line. Emphasize correct placement. Rest after 10 steps.

3. Walk forward placing each foot on a footprint traced on the floor. Footprints should be parallel and 2 inches lateral to the midline. Practice with quarter steps, half steps, three-quarter steps, and full steps.

4. Turning. (1) Raise the right toe and rotate the right foot outward, pivoting on the heel. (2) Raise the left heel and pivot the left leg inward on the toes. (3) Bring the left foot up beside the right.

Exercises to Teach Relaxation

Anxiety produces a state of tension that causes increased activity in the central nervous system and affects many systems. The neuromuscular system responds by prolonged muscular contraction, causing discomfort in muscles and joints, neckache, and headache. As a result of the pain produced by prolonged muscular contraction, secondary reflex contractions also develop. The anxiety and tension of the patient are increased. Effective reversal of these secondary effects may be achieved by teaching the patient awareness of muscular tensions and how to control and inhibit them.[43]

Relaxation is taught in a quiet semidarkened room with the patient comfortably positioned on a treatment table or bed. A small pillow should be placed under the head and another pillow should be placed under the knees to relax the hip and knee musculature. The feet should be supported so that the muscles in the legs can relax. Constricting garments should be loosened.

Breath control is taught using prolonged slow breathing with proper diaphragmatic and abdominal coordination together with intercostal breathing. The patient is taught to exhale slowly through the mouth to emphasize awareness of breathing rate and breath control. As the patient gains control of breathing in the fully relaxed position, he then begins to practice breathing properly while sitting or standing.

Proprioceptive awareness of muscular contraction in the extremities is taught by having the patient flex and extend each joint in the extremity, feeling the difference between tightness and relaxation of the contracting muscles. Following a strong voluntary contraction, the patient is asked to relax and feel the difference between contraction and relaxation. Then progressively weaker contractions are alternated with complete inhibition of muscular activity so that the extremity becomes fully relaxed. Functional muscle groups at each joint are considered individually in the alternate tensing and relaxation so that the patient becomes fully aware of muscular activity in each region of the extremity. The patient should perceive the tenseness of the muscle, rather than any tension, position, or motion of a joint. Jacobson[43] emphasized that persons could learn proprioceptive awareness of tension and then use it in almost any situation to relax from a state of tension.

Electromyographic monitoring by cutaneous or intramuscular electrodes may be used to indicate whether complete relaxation has occurred. This monitoring provides auditory reinforcement of perception of tension or relaxation and hastens learning. Dropping of the completely limp arm or leg is another method used to demonstrate the difference between partial contraction and relaxation. As the patient becomes aware of the sensations associated with a muscular contraction, he becomes able to initiate or inhibit that contraction.[43]

The sequence of training is applied to all four extremities, to the shoulders by shrugging and relaxing, to the chest by tightening and relaxing the pectoral muscles, to the back by arching and relaxing, and to the facial muscles by contracting and relaxing the muscles about the mouth and eyes and on the forehead. For the tense patient, the training sessions may have to be repeated many times before the patient develops the proprioceptive awareness to know when he has relaxed completely. Patients are instructed to practice this relaxation at home or at work when they become tense during the day or in the evening at bedtime if they have difficulty in relaxing before they go to sleep. When the patient is able to inhibit muscular contraction adequately in the various segments of the body while recumbent, he is taught to reproduce the same relaxation when sitting in a fully supporting arm chair, and later when sitting in a straight chair. Training in relaxation is useful not only to relax and rest but also to enhance performance during skilled activities.

The patient should be instructed that selective muscular relaxation is possible at the same time that a person is thinking or carrying on an activity. It is not necessary for the mind "to become a perfect blank" nor for the person to forego all activity in order to inhibit muscular tension. Even in the initial training the patient will soon observe that the muscles may be relaxed, even though the mind remains active. However, disturbing stimuli or ideas make relaxation more difficult. In spite of this, the patient can learn to relax his muscles to avoid prolonged muscular tension even during periods of active cerebration.

Through controlled relaxation the individual learns to relax the muscles that do not need to be used for a specific activity and thereby decreases the energy used during ordinary activity. As a result he is less fatigued by his work. Selective relaxation of the unneeded muscles during activity avoids the pain arising secondary to prolonged muscular tension.

REFERENCES

1. Granit, R.: The Purposive Brain. Cambridge, MIT Press, 1977.
2. Ramos, M. U., Mundale, M. O., Awad, E. A., Witsoe, D. A., Cole, T. M., Olson, M., and Kottke, F. J.: Cardiovascular effects of spread of excitation during prolonged isometric exercise. Arch. Phys. Med. Rehabil., 54:496–504, 1973.
3. Kottke, F. J.: From reflex to skill: The training of coordination. Arch. Phys. Med. Rehabil., 61:551–561, 1980.
4. Skoglund, S.: Anatomical and physiological studies of knee joint innervation in the cat. Acta. Physiol. Scand., 36(Suppl. 124):58, 1956.
5. Crossman, E. R. F. W.: Theory of acquisition of speed-skill. Ergonomics, 2:153–166, 1959.
6. Knapp, M. E.: The contribution of Sister Elizabeth Kenny to the treatment of poliomyelitis. Arch. Phys. Med. Rehabil., 36:510–517, 1955.
7. Knapp, M. E.: Exercises for lower motor neuron lesions. In Basmajian, J. V. (Ed.): Therapeutic Exercise, 3rd Ed. Baltimore, Williams and Wilkins Co., 1978.
8. Simard, T. G., and Basmajian, J. V.: Methods in training conscious control of motor units. Arch. Phys. Med. Rehabil., 48:12–19, 1967.
9. Herman, R.: Electromyographic evidence of some control factors involved in the acquisition of skilled performance. Am. J. Phys. Med., 49:177–191, 1970.
10. Kabat, H.: Studies on neuromuscular dysfunction. XV. The role of central facilitation in restoration of motor function in paralysis. Arch. Phys. Med. Rehabil., 33:521–533, 1952.
11. Knott, M., and Voss, D. E.: Proprioceptive Neuromuscular Facilitation: Patterns and Techniques. New York, Paul B. Hoeber, Inc., 1956.

12. Brunnstrom, S.: Movement Therapy in Hemiplegia. New York, Harper and Row, Publishers, 1970.
13. Kabat, H.: Proprioceptive facilitation in therapeutic exercise. In Licht, S. (Ed.): Therapeutic Exercise, 2nd Ed. New Haven, Connecticut, Elizabeth Licht, Publisher, 1961.
14. Rood, M. S.: Neuromuscular mechanisms utilized in the treatment of neuromuscular dysfunction. Am. J. Occup. Therap., 10:220–225, 1956.
15. Stockmeyer, S. A.: Sensorimotor approach to treatment. In Pearson, P. H., and Williams, C. E. (Eds.): Physical Therapy Services in the Developmental Disabilities. Springfield, Ill., Charles C Thomas, Publisher, 1972, pp. 186–222.
16. Fay, T.: The neurophysiologic aspects of therapy in cerebral palsy. Arch. Phys. Med. Rehabil., 29:327–334, 1948.
17. Page, D.: Neuromuscular reflex therapy as an approach to patient care. Am. J. Phys. Med., 46:816–835, 1967.
18. Hagbarth, K. E.: Excitatory and inhibitory skin areas for flexor and extensor motoneurones. Acta. Physiol. Scand., 26(Suppl. 94):1–8, 1952.
19. Kottke, F. J., Halpern, D., Easton, J. K. M., Ozel, A. T., and Burrill, C. A.: Training of coordination. Arch. Phys. Med. Rehabil., 59:567–572, 1978.
20. Phelps, W. M.: The role of physical therapy in cerebral palsy. In Illingworth, R. S. (Ed.): Recent Advances in Cerebral Palsy. Boston, Little, Brown and Co., 1958.
21. Bobath, K., and Bobath, B.: Treatment of cerebral palsy based on analysis of patient's motor behavior. Br. J. Phys. Med., 15:107–117, 1952.
22. Bobath, K., and Bobath, B.: Cerebral palsy. In Pearson, P. H., and Williams, C. E. (Eds.): Physical Therapy Services in the Developmental Disabilities. Springfield, Ill.; Charles C Thomas, Publisher, 1972, pp. 31–175.
23. Gellhorn, E.: Patterns of muscular activity in man. Arch. Phys. Med. Rehabil., 28:568–574, 1947.
24. Gesell, A.: Maturation and infant behavior pattern. Psychol. Rev., 36:307–319, 1929.
25. McGraw, M. B.: The Neuro-Muscular Maturation of the Human Infant. New York, Columbia University Press, 1945.
26. Coghill, G. E.: Anatomy and the Problem of Behavior. London, Cambridge University Press, 1929.
27. Coghill, G. E.: Flexor spasms and mass reflexes in relation to the autogenetic development of behavior. J. Comp. Neurol., 76:463–486, 1943.

28. Windle, W. F.: Physiology of the Fetus: Origin and Extent of Function in Prenatal Life. Philadelphia, W. B. Saunders Company, 1940.
29. Gesell, A., and Halvorson, H. M.: The development of thumb opposition in the human infant. J. Genet. Psychol., 48:339–361, 1936.
30. Bullock, T. H.: The origin of patterned nervous discharge. Behavior, 17:48–59, 1961.
31. Piaget, J.: The origins of intelligence in children, 2nd Ed. Trans. by M. Cook. New York, International Universities Press, 1953.
32. White, B. L., and Held, R.: Plasticity of sensorimotor development in the human infant. In Hellmuth, J. (Ed.): Exceptional Infant, Vol. 1. Seattle, Special Child Publications, 1967.
33. Hein, A., and Held, R.: Dissociation of visual placing response into elicited and guided components. Science, 158:390–391, 1967.
34. Schneirla, T. C.: Behavioral development and comparative psychology. Q. Rev. Biol., 41:283–302, 1966.
35. Nissen, H. W., Chow, K. L., and Semmes, J.: Effects of restricted opportunity and manipulative experience on the behavior of the chimpanzee. Am. J. Psychol., 64:485–507, 1951.
36. White, B.: Experience and development of motor mechanisms. In Connelly, K. (Ed.): Mechanisms of Motor Skill Development. New York, Academic Press, 1970.
37. Beery, K. E.: Developmental test of visual-motor integration: Administration and scoring manual. Chicago, Follette Publishing Co., 1967.
38. Briggs, P. R., and Tellegen, A.: Development of the manual accuracy and speed test. Percept. Motor Skills, 32:923–943 (Monograph Suppl. 3), 1971.
39. Jebsen, R. H., Taylor, N., Trieschmann, R. B., Trotter, M. J., and Howard, L. A.: An objective and standardized test of hand function. Arch. Phys. Med. Rehabil., 50:311–319, 1969.
40. Chyatte, S. B., and Birdsong, J. H.: Methods-time measurements in assessment of motor performance. Arch. Phys. Med. Rehabil., 53:38–44, 1972.
41. Flowers, K.: Lack of prediction in the motor behavior in parkinsonism. Brain, 101:35–52, 1978.
42. Halpern, D., Kottke, F. J., Burrill, C. A., Fiterman, C., Popp, J., and Palmer, S.: Training of control of head posture in children with cerebral palsy. Develop. Med. Child. Neurol., 12:290–305, 1970.
43. Jacobson, E.: Progressive relaxation. Chicago, University of Chicago Press, 1938.

20

THERAPEUTIC EXERCISE TO DEVELOP STRENGTH AND ENDURANCE

BARBARA J. DE LATEUR

Exercise vies with heat as the most commonly applied therapeutic modality. As with heat, virtually everyone applies this modality to himself or herself regardless of whether it is prescribed by a physician or carried out under the supervision of a therapist. Some degree of muscular effort is expended to move from one spot to another. Because of this universal employment of exercise, virtually everyone considers himself to be to some degree knowledgeable if not actually expert on this topic. This familiarity has both advantages and disadvantages for one who would attempt to write scientifically about the topic. The advantage is the comfort and interest with which readers will approach the topic. The disadvantage is the misuse, in common parlance, of technical terms. An example of the latter would be the common usage of the term *tone*. Advertisements for commercial exercise establishments often speak of ''toning up your muscles,'' as though increase of tone were something that (a) resulted from an exercise program; (b) increased the firmness of muscle to palpation

or increased the definition of muscle contours; and (c) somehow reflected the strength and/or endurance of the muscles. In point of fact, muscle tone is the resistance (tension) developed in a muscle as a result of passive stretch of a muscle. This is the technical definition of tone. It cannot be determined by palpation or inspection of the muscle. It has little or nothing to do with the voluntary strength of the muscle. Thus, in order to use familiar terms in a precise way, some definitions would be useful.

DEFINITIONS

Force. A push or a pull. A force is equal to the mass of an object times the acceleration imparted to that object. $F = m \times a$. Force is a vector quantity; that is to say, it has direction as well as magnitude. In the English system a force may be expressed in pounds. In the MKS (meter-kilogram-second) system, force is expressed in newtons. A newton is that force which will give a

This chapter is in part based on research supported by Research Grant #G008200020 from the National Institute of Handicapped Research, Department of Education, Washington, D.C. 20202.

mass of one kilogram an acceleration of one meter per second per second. The term *kilopond* is also used. This is the force exerted by the mass of one kilogram on earth, i.e., the mass of one kilogram subjected to the acceleration of earth's gravity, or 9.81 m/sec². A kilopond thus equals 9.81 newtons or about 10 N.

Mass. The amount of matter contained in an object. In the MKS system this is expressed as kilograms. In the English system it is expressed as slugs. A slug is the amount of matter contained in an object that exerts the force (weight) of one pound on earth. Mass is a scalar quantity; that is, it has magnitude only, not direction.

Vector. A quantity that has both magnitude and direction, such as force; an arrow whose length represents the magnitude and whose direction represents the direction of such a quantity.

Strength. The maximum force (actually torque) that can be exerted by a muscle. This is subdivided into static and dynamic strength.

Static or Isometric Strength. The maximal force that can be exerted against an immovable or relatively immovable object. It is expressed as the MVC or maximal voluntary contraction. The term "isometric" refers to the fact that the overall length of the muscle stays essentially the same (although there is internal length change within the muscle to, for example, take up the slack in the series elastic elements). The kinesiologic function of an isometric contraction is stabilization.

Dynamic Strength. Dynamic strength has many theoretically possible subdivisions, since a muscle may vary in its rate of lengthening or of shortening as well as in the amount of force (tension) developed at any given point from beginning to end of the arc described by the moving segment of the limb. For practical purposes the most commonly used terms are *isotonic* and *isokinetic strength*.

Isotonic. The term *isotonic* is, in most circumstances, a misnomer, since it implies that either the torque exerted by the muscle or even the internal tension of the muscle remains the same throughout the arc of movement of the limb. The achievement of either of these conditions is rare. For practical purposes, in the clinical literature isotonic has been equated with kinetic or dynamic and is often expressed in such definitions as the one repetition maximum or ten repetition maximum.

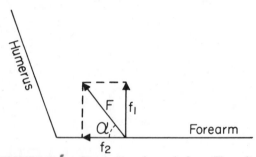

FIGURE 20–1. Resolution of muscle force (F) applied to the tendon into rotatory (f_1) and stabilizing (f_2) forces. The rotatory force acts at right angles to the lever: f_1 = F sin alpha; f_2 = F cos alpha. (From Brunnstrom, S.: Clinical Kinesiology, 2nd Ed. Philadelphia, F. A. Davis, 1966.)

One Repetition Maximum (1 RM). The highest weight that the subject can lift through the full range of motion one time only.

Ten Repetition Maximum (10 RM). The highest weight that the subject can lift through the full range of motion ten times only.

Shortening or Concentric Contraction. A muscle contraction in which the two ends of the muscle move toward each other. The kinesiologic function of such a contraction is acceleration.

Lengthening or Eccentric Contraction. A muscle contraction in which the two ends of the muscle diverge; i.e., the muscle "plays out" its length. The kinesiologic function of such a contraction is deceleration (shock absorption).

Rotatory Force. That component of the muscle tension which produces angular motion about the joint. It is equal to the product of the total muscle tension applied to the tendon times the sine of the angle of application of the tendon (Fig. 20–1).

Stabilizing Force. That component of the total muscle force which approximates the two limb segments at the joint. It is equal to the muscle tension applied to the tendon times the cosine of the angle of application of the tendon (Fig. 20–1).

Torque (moment of a force). The effectiveness of a force in producing rotation about an axis. Torque is equal to the product of a force times the perpendicular distance from the site of application to the axis (Fig. 20–2).

Isokinetic Strength. The maximum torque that can be exerted against a preset rate-limiting device. This may be defined as the peak torque that occurs at any given velocity

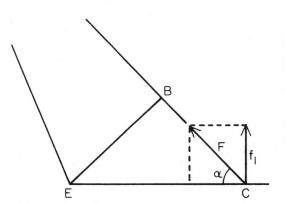

FIGURE 20–2. Two methods of computing torque. Torque equals $f_1 \times EC$ or $F \times EB$. (From Brunnstrom, S.: Clinical Kinesiology, 2nd Ed. Philadelphia, F. A. Davis, 1966.)

of contraction, regardless of the angle at which it occurs, or it may be defined as angle-specific.

Endurance. The ability to continue a specified task.

Endurance Exercise. An exercise involving the reciprocal and dynamic use of several large groups of muscles. An exercise calling upon the ability of the cardiovascular-pulmonary system to deliver oxygen to such groups of muscles.

Fatigue. The inability to continue a specified task. Fatigue has both behavioral and measurable physiologic components.

Maximal Aerobic Capacity. The maximal rate at which oxygen may be utilized (taken up) by the organism. The symbol for this is $\dot{V}O_2$ max. (The dot over a symbol always indicates a rate.) This is determined as that rate of oxygen consumption which shows no

further increase in spite of increasing mechanical work or rate of exercise performed by the subject (Fig. 20–3).

Work. Work is equal to the product of force times the distance through which the force is exerted. $W = F \times D$. Work may be expressed as newton-meters or kilopond-meters. In the older literature the latter was expressed as kilogram-meters. Energy is expended in doing work; thus, units for work are often used as units for energy. One newton-meter = one joule (see *Energy*, below).

Power. Power is the rate of performing work. It is equal to work divided by time. It is often expressed as watts or as kilopond-meters per minute (kpm/min). One watt = 1 joule/sec = 6.12 kpm/min.

Energy. Energy is equal to the product of power times the time that the power is expended. The homeowner is accustomed to the energy unit of kilowatt-hours. Energy can also be expressed as kilopond-meters or as joules. One kpm = about 10 joules. The biologic energy unit is the calorie (cal). One calorie = 4.2 joules, and therefore one K Cal (ordinarily used to express the energy content of foodstuffs) = 4.2 K joule.

THEORETICAL CONSIDERATIONS

Force-Velocity Relationships

The force-velocity relationship for mammalian muscle is described by this equation:

$$(P + a)V = b (P_o - P)$$

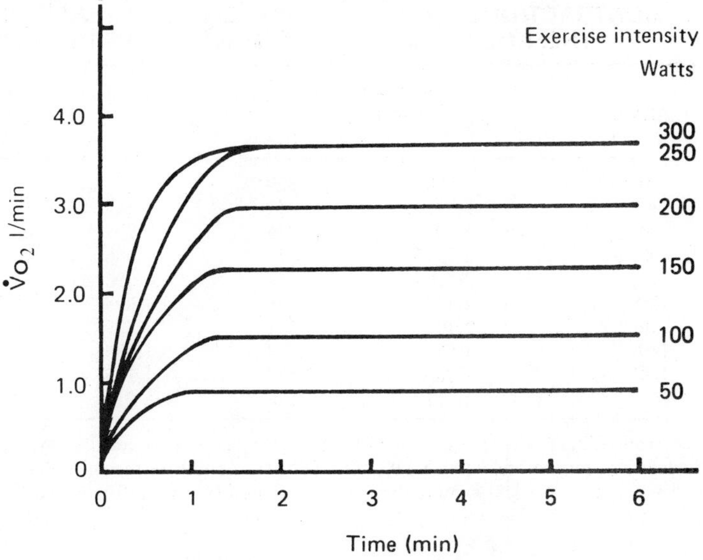

FIGURE 20–3. Relationship of oxygen uptake to various exercise intensities utilizing several muscle groups in reciprocal concentric contractions. There is no additional increase in oxygen uptake with further increase in exercise intensity (external work) once maximal oxygen uptake is reached. (From Soule, R. G.: Physiological response to physical exercise. *In* Knuttgen, H. G. (Ed.): Neuromuscular Mechanisms for Therapeutic and Conditioning Exercise. Baltimore, University Park Press, 1976, pp. 79–96. Data from Saltin, B., and Åstrand, P.O.: Maximal oxygen uptake in athletes. J. Appl. Physiol., 23:353–358, 1967.)

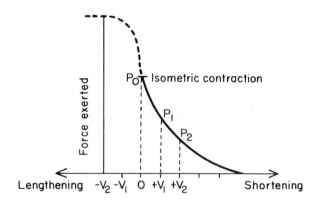

FIGURE 20–4. Force velocity curve of human muscle. Solid line: data obtained from elbow flexors of human subjects. At the time this curve was drawn, the dotted line was made by extrapolation. This portion of the curve has subsequently been confirmed experimentally (see Fig. 20–5). (From Brunnstrom, S.: Clinical Kinesiology, 2nd Ed. Philadelphia, F. A. Davis, 1966. Redrawn from Wilkie, D. V.: The relation between force and velocity in human muscle. J. Physiol., 110:249–280, 1950, and Abbott, B. C., Bigland, B., and Ritchie, J. M.: The physiological cost of negative work. J. Physiol., 117:380–390, 1952.)

FIGURE 20–5. Relationship of maximal force of human elbow flexor muscles to velocity of contraction. Velocity on abscissa is designated as per cent of arm length per second. (From Knuttgen, H. G.: Development of muscular strength and endurance. In Knuttgen, H. G. (Ed.): Neuromuscular Mechanisms for Therapeutic and Conditioning Exercises. Baltimore, University Park Press, 1976, pp. 97–118. Redrawn from Asmussen, E., Hansen, O., and Lammert, O.: The relation between isometric and dynamic muscle strength in man. Comm. Dan. Natl. Assoc. Inf. Paral., 20:11, 1965.)

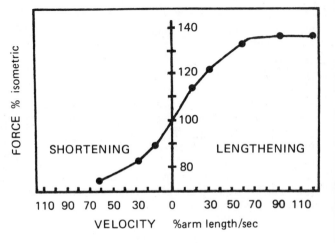

TABLE 20–1. STRENGTH (NEWTONS) OF ECCENTRIC AND CONCENTRIC CONTRACTIONS OF LOWER EXTREMITY EXTENSORS AT DIFFERENT ANGLES OF THE KNEE JOINT OF NORMAL SUBJECTS PERFORMING KNEEBENDS*

Angle	C. eccentric strength		C. concentric strength		Statistical significance[a]
	$\bar{X}$	SD	$\bar{X}$	SD	
70°	1,800	820	459	106	0.01
80°	1,899	857	543	189	0.01
90°	2,101	735	737	252	0.01
100°	2,221	576	866	347	0.01
110°	2,229	551	996	370	0.01
120°	2,157	530	1,098	442	0.01
130°	2,103	541	1,229	521	0.01
140°	1,971	524	1,236	412	0.01
150°	1,800	583	1,125	339	0.01
160°	1,321	578	918	365	0.05

*From Seliger, V., Dolejs, L., and Karas, V.: A dynamometric comparison of maximum eccentric, concentric and isometric contractions using EMG and energy expenditure measurements. Eur. J. Appl. Physiol., 45:235–244, 1980.
[a]Values of statistical significance were obtained by t test (for paired data).

where V is the speed of shortening, P_o is the maximum isometric tension, P is the load, and a and b are constants.[35] There is an inverse relationship between the rate of shortening of a muscle and the tension that it can develop (Fig. 20–4).

Figure 20–4 shows an idealized force-velocity curve. The highest tensions are developed by fast lengthening contractions. The lowest tensions are developed with fast shortening contractions. The tension developed with an isometric contraction is shown at the inflection point of the curve. One may verify this personally in a qualitative or roughly quantitative fashion by reflecting upon the fact that one can hold a weight which one cannot lift and that one can rapidly lower a weight which one cannot hold, much less lift. Such a relationship for maximal force of human elbow flexor muscles to velocity of contraction is expressed in Figure 20–5. This curve represents the performance of several human subjects at any given point in time. From Figures 20–4 and 20–5 one may infer the relationship between dynamic and static or isometric strength, but one may not necessarily conclude that a dynamic training program will improve static stength performance, or vice versa. One may anticipate that the general shape of these curves will stay the same regardless of a training program, and thus one may anticipate some degree of positive transference from one type of exercise program to the opposite type of performance, but one may not accurately predict, quantitatively, the degree of transfer. The work of Seliger et al. has comfirmed these relationships (Tables 20–1 and 20–2).[65]

They determined the maximum voluntary forces produced upon a weight-lifting rod by subjects changing from standing to squatting and from squatting to standing and during a halfway knee-bend. The rod was placed on a special stand and moved up and down at a constant speed of 8.5 m/sec by a motor. They found that at an angle of 90 degrees, with a constant angle speed of flexion (17 degrees/sec) and with a maximum voluntary effort, the muscles exerted approximately three times greater force on a load during eccentric contractions than during concentric contractions. Muscle force exerted on a load during maximum isometric contraction at an angle of 90 degrees in the knee joint was greater than during maximum concentric

TABLE 20–2. STRENGTH (IN NEWTONS) OF LOWER EXTREMITY EXTENSORS OF NORMAL SUBJECTS THROUGHOUT A 7-SECOND ISOMETRIC CONTRACTION WITH THE KNEE JOINT AT A 90° ANGLE*

Contraction Time (seconds)	Strength $\overline{X}$	SD
1	636	245
2	884	289
3	1,027	329
4	1,130	409
5	1,146	415
6	1,161	429
7	1,143	438
1–7: average	1,017	327

*From Seliger, V., Dolejs, L., and Karas, V.: A dynamometric comparison of maximum eccentric, concentric and isometric contractions using EMG and energy expenditure measurements. Eur. J. Appl. Physiol., 45:235–244, 1980.

contraction and lower than during eccentric contraction with the same angle.

The force-velocity relationships for concentric contractions have been confirmed by a number of authors with isokinetic tests.[9, 27, 41, 49, 55, 64, 68, 71] A negative exponential model characterized the decline of strength as a function of increased isokinetic velocity of angular motion.[20] Fugl-Meyer et al. found close correlations between isokinetic and static peak torques (Table 20–3). However, as would be anticipated from the force-velocity curves, the static maxima were much greater than the torques at the various speeds of contraction and could be described by a negative exponential model between the maximal plantar flexion torque and isokinetic velocity of angular motion (Fig. 20–6).

The extent to which one may alter the form of such force-velocity or torque-velocity curves underlies the question of specificity of training; the latter will be subsequently discussed in greater detail.

Absolute Muscle Strength

It has long been known that the maximal force that a muscle may develop is related to the size of the muscle, i.e., to the "physiologic" cross sectional area of the muscle. The physiologic cross sectional area of a muscle is the combined cross section of all of

TABLE 20–3. MEAN MAXIMUM ISOKINETIC PLANTAR FLEXION TORQUES FOR 135 SEDENTARY NORTHERN SWEDISH FEMALES AND MALES. MAXIMUM TORQUES MEASURED FOR THREE DIFFERENT VELOCITIES OF ANGULAR MOTION WITH THE KNEE FULLY EXTENDED (0 DEGREES)*

Age	Sex	n	Stat. max.		90°s		180°s	
			Nm	±SD	Nm	±SD	Nm	±SD
			R/L	R/L	R/L	R/L	R/L	R/L
20–29	F	15	80/87	17/16	46/55	12/11	24/29	6/8
	M	15	121/131	21/20	70/80	14/21	37/44	10/14
30–39	F	15	87/95	20/21	50/58	13/14	26/32	7/7
	M	15	126/133	19/18	74/80	12/16	37/41	9/11
40–49	F	15	74/82	15/14	41/47	11/13	18/22	7/9
	M	15	128/136	21/23	74/79	19/15	35/40	12/10
50–59	F	15	63/72	12/14	36/38	6/6	17/19	4/5
	M	15	114/118	18/14	66/74	10/13	30/36	7/11
60–65	F	9	54/60	10/13	29/33	8/7	13/14	4/7
	M	6	66/88	26/26	37/48	13/19	17/18	8/5

n: Number of subjects; NM: Newtonmeters; R: Right; L: Left
*From Fugl-Meyer, A. R., Gustafsson, L., and Burstedt, Y.: Isokinetic and static plantar flexion characteristics. Eur. J. Appl. Physiol., 45:221–234, 1980.

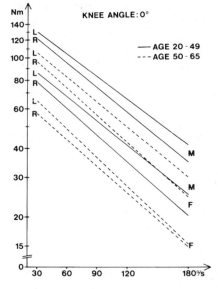

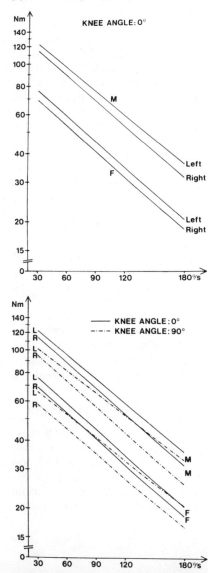

FIGURE 20–6. A negative exponential model of the relationship between maximum plantar flexion torques and isokinetic velocity of angular motion. Maximum torques given in logarithmic scale. Velocity of angular motion given on X axis. *Top left,* values for right and left maximum torques are given for 135 subjects: 69 females (F) and 66 males (M). Maneuvers performed with knees fully extended (0 degrees). *Top right,* values for subjects between ages 20 and 49 (solid lines) and for subjects between ages 50 and 65 (dotted lines) are given. R: Right; L: Left. *Bottom left,* values at fully extended (0 degrees) and flexed (90 degrees) knee positions are given. (From Fugl-Meyer, A. R., Gustafsson, L., and Burstedt, Y.: Isokinetic and static plantar flexion characteristics. Eur. J. Appl. Physiol., 45:221–234, 1980.)

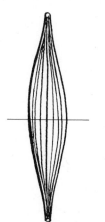

FIGURE 20–7. Parallel arrangement of muscle fibers. "Physiologic" cross section is equal to cross section of muscle belly. (From Brunnstrom, S.: Clinical Kinesiology, 2nd Ed. Philadelphia, F. A. Davis, 1966.)

its muscle fibers. Some muscles have long parallel fibers running through the belly of the muscle and the physiological cross section is the cross section of the muscle belly (Fig. 20–7). To calculate the physiological cross section of a pennate muscle, multiple sections perpendicular to the long axis of the muscle fibers must be made until all are included (Fig. 20–8). Some muscles in the

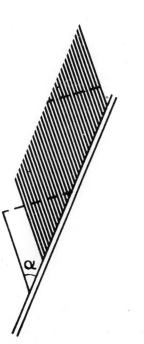

FIGURE 20–8. In pennate muscle the physiologic cross section is determined by multiple sections at right angles to the fibers until all are included (From Brunnstrom, S.: Clinical Kinesiology, 2nd Ed. Philadelphia, F. A. Davis, 1966.)

body are particularly suited to speed of contraction by their anatomic configuration. Such muscles have long parallel fibers and are placed close to the axis of rotation of the joint. Other muscles are particularly well suited to the development of large forces but with relatively small distances covered by the distal portion of the limb. Such muscles insert relatively far from the axis of motion of the joint (Fig. 20–9). The absolute muscle strength, then, is in proportion to the physiologic cross sectional area and is generally considered to be about 3.6 kilograms/cm^2 of physiologic cross sectional area.[2, 73] This is a useful and probably essentially accurate concept, although some other factors may be involved. The work of Gordon suggested that performance of high-force tasks may be improved without gross hypertrophy.[26] Progressively increasing weights were attached to the backs of the experimental animals (rats), which were then made to climb poles. Their muscles showed no overall increase in weight, but the type II (fast switch) muscles did show an increase in cross sectional area. Certainly the ability to exert large brief forces relates both to muscle cross sectional area and to motor unit recruitment patterns. In 1951 DeLorme and Watkins suggested that "the initial increase in strength on progressive resistance exercise occurs at a rate far greater than can be accounted for by morphological changes within the muscle. These initial rapid increments in strength

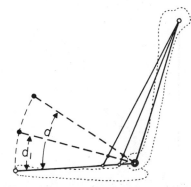

FIGURE 20–9. Relation of tendon lever arm to speed and force. If the lever arm is a short distance from the center of motion, there is greater excursion per unit of contraction but low force at the distal end of the lever. If the tendon is inserted at a greater distance from the center of motion, there is less excursion per unit of contraction but greater force at the distal end of the lever. (Redrawn from Steindler, A.: Kinesiology of the Human Body. Springfield, Ill., Charles C Thomas, Publisher, 1955.)

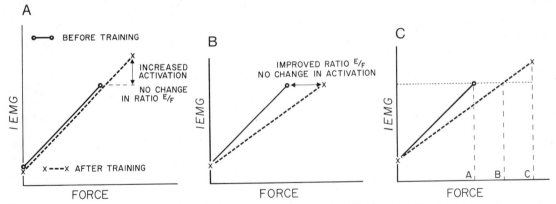

FIGURE 20–10. *A,* Increase of integrated electromyographic activity (IEMG) plotted against force of contraction as an index of strength due to neural factors gained during training. *B,* Strength gained due to hypertrophy when neural activity is maintained constant. *C,* Schema for evaluation of per cent contributions of neural factors (N.F.) versus muscular hypertrophy (M.H.) to the gain of strength through progressive resistance exercise based upon efficiency of electrical activity (EEA). Strength increase per cent (M.H.) = $(B - A)/(C - A) \times 100$. Strength increase per cent (N.F.) = $(C - B)/(C - A) \times 100$. (Redrawn from Moritani, T., and de Vries, H. K.: Neural factors versus hypertrophy in the time course of muscle strength gain. Am. J. Phys. Med., 58:115–130, 1979.)

noted in normal and disuse-atrophied muscles are, no doubt, due to motor learning. . . . It is impossible to say how much of the increase is due to morphological changes within the muscle or to motor learning."[15] Since that time, it has, indeed, become possible to tease apart the relative contribution of these two major determinants of increasing strength. Moritani and deVries, make use of

the fact that under carefully controlled conditions, the ratio of integrated electrical activity of muscle (IEMG) to the isometric force exerted by the elbow-flexors is linear throughout the entire range of forces up to and including maximal voluntary contraction.[51] Figure 20–10A shows a theoretical possibility in which all strength (force) gain is due to neural factors, i.e., "increased activation."

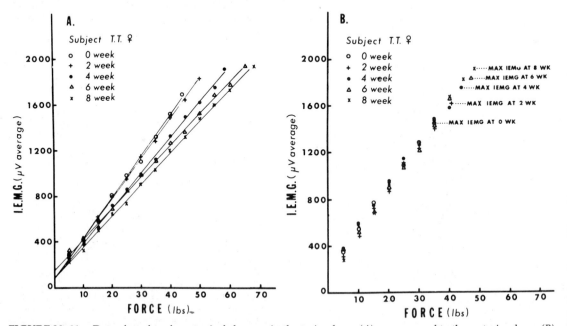

FIGURE 20–11. Data plotted to show typical changes in the trained arm *(A)* as compared to the untrained arm *(B).* Both arms gained in strength but only the trained arm showed significant changes in the E/F ratio (hypertrophy). (From Moritani, T., and de Vries, H. K.: Neural factors versus hypertrophy in the time course of muscle strength gain. Am. J. Phys. Med., 58:115–130, 1979.)

Figure 20–10B shows a scheme in which all strength gained is due to hypertrophy. In this scheme, any given force requires less EMG activity. They describe this as an improved electrical/force (E/F) ratio or efficiency of electrical activity (EEA).* Figure 20–10C shows a scheme that allows evaluation of the percentage contributions of neural factors (N.F.) and muscular hypertrophy (M.H.) to the strength gain with training. The authors actually carried out such a study on the elbow flexors of seven young healthy males and eight such females, who were subjected to an eight-week weight-training program. Figure 20–11 displays the E/F ratios obtained. This indicates that the strength increases of the first two weeks were almost entirely due to neural factors, and the strength gains of subsequent weeks were mostly due to muscular hypertrophy. Comparison of Figures 20–11A and B may explain conflicting data in the literature regarding cross-training. Unless the "untrained limb" is heavily involved in stabilization, the improvement in strength sometimes found in the unexercised limb may be due to neural factors.

Milner-Brown found elevated synchronization ratios in weight lifters[48] (Fig. 20–12). The author found that a high force training program altered synchronization ratios in previously untrained subjects. A 20 per cent increase in maximal isometric force (MVC) was associated with a doubling of the synchronization ratio (Fig. 20–13). After a further period of six weeks of no exercise, the synchronization ratio declined, but not to control levels. The synchronization ratio reflects the extent to which motor units fire simultaneously. Such synchronization occurs randomly at high levels of recruitment. However, the rate of occurrence of simultaneous firing, i.e., elevated synchronization ratios, occurs in weight lifters or in subjects whose occupation requires frequent exertion of large brief forces, as by bus drivers (Fig. 20–14). The extent to which this occurs with prolonged, low-force, static, or dynamic training is not known at present.

*Ordinarily efficiency is expressed as the ratio of mechanical output to input. In that case it would be expressed as force over electrical activity. The authors have expressed this as electrical activity over force, the opposite of the custom, but it is clear that the meaning is the same.

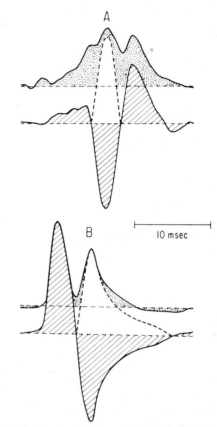

FIGURE 20–12. Average responses of 500 sweeps obtained before and after rectification of the surface EMG were used to determine the degree of synchronization. Each sweep was triggered by an impulse from a single motor unit recorded by a needle in the first dorsal interosseous muscle of (A) a weightlifter and (B) a control subject. The lower horizontal lines in each part indicate the zero voltage level and the upper horizontal lines the mean rectified surface EMG, which gives a measure of the total electrical activity in the muscle. Note that there is a substantial rise in the activity near the time of the impulses from the single motor unit in the weightlifter (dotted area), but not in the control subject. This indicates that the impulses of this unit were grouped or synchronized with those of other motor units in the muscle. The surface EMG was delayed electronically 5 or 10 msec to show the full time course of this synchronization. The only peaks observed for the control subject were those expected from the unrectified average, which represents the contribution of the single unit to the surface EMG (diagonal lines). As a measure of synchronization, Milner-Brown et al computed the ratio of the dotted area to the diagonally hatched area for a number of motor units. Any dotted area that fell below the mean rectified level was subtracted from that which exceeded this level. (From Milner-Brown, H. S., Stein, R. B., and Lee, R. G.: Synchronization of human motor units: Possible role of exercise and supraspinal reflexes. E. E. G. Clin. Neurophysiol., 38:245–254, 1975.)

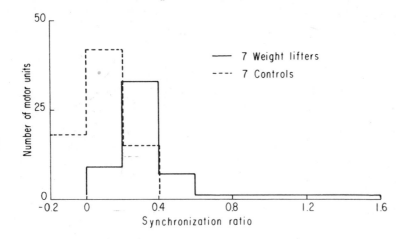

FIGURE 20–13. Synchronization ratios computed as shown in Figure 20–13 for a number of motor units from weightlifters and controls. A value greater than 0.2 was assumed to represent a significant degree of synchronization. These values were rarely observed in control subjects, but were generally found in weightlifters. (From Milner-Brown, H. S., Stein, R. B., and Lee, R. G.: Synchronization of human motor units: Possible roles of exercise and supraspinal reflexes. E. E. G. Clin. Neurophysiol., 38:245–254, 1975.)

Intensity and Endurance Relationships

The extent to which muscle endurance is related to muscle strength and the specificity of exercise programs designed to improve one or the other are subjects of controversy. Within limits strength and endurance or the intensity of activity and endurance at that activity are mathematically related. Figure 20–15, *left,* shows the relationship of endurance as total contractions of repeated flexion of the third digit to the effective force of contraction. Figure 20–15, *right,* shows the relationship of endurance (as minutes to fatigue) of cycle exercise to external power production. In both figures the intercept with the abscissa represents the exercise intensity for which the maneuver could be performed only once; this would therefore define the strength of concentric contraction. Also in both figures endurance could be specified as either the total number of contractions or minutes to fatigue. The shape of the curve, then, represents the endurance at any given intensity level. It should be noted that the curves have a very similar shape in spite of the fact that the ergograph requires the use of one muscle group and the cycle ergometer requires the reciprocal use of several large muscle groups. Figure 20–16 shows the relationships of intensity of work, in kilogram-meters, to the duration of work and the amount of work performed.[50] Figure 20–17 shows the maximal holding time as a function of force. It can be seen that there is a tight mathematical relationship over a large number of observations with various muscle groups in subjects of both sexes.[57] This may

be described as a hyperbolic curve with ends asymptotically approaching the ordinate and abscissa. It should also be noted that this experiment has not been carried out below 20 per cent of the MVC. Hill calculated that below 15 per cent of MVC an isometric contraction may be sustained indefinitely, since the rate at which the circulatory system can carry away the heat equals or exceeds the rate at which heat is generated.[34] This calculation does not take into consideration the rate of consumption and regeneration of metabolic substrate, however.

The average speed in miles per hour has been plotted against the time, in seconds, of world record runners[45] (Fig. 20–18). It is of some interest to note that even for a very different type of exercise, the acute intensity-endurance relationships remain the same, i.e., a similar hyperbolic curve.

Knuttgen suggests the physiologic significance of the curves in Figure 20–15.[12] (His comments would also apply to Figures 20–16 and 20–17.) The intercept with the abscissa, i.e., the one repetition maximum or strength is determined by the physiologic cross sectional area of the muscles involved. To the author's comment one may add that the ability to synchronize may also have an influence upon the intercept with the abscissa or one repetition maximum. Knuttgen states that the horizontal portion of the curve is determined predominantly by the capacity of the anaerobic energy release process. The vertical portion of the curve is determined by the aerobic energy release capacity as dominated by the delivery of oxygen to the muscles by the circulatory system. The portion of greatest

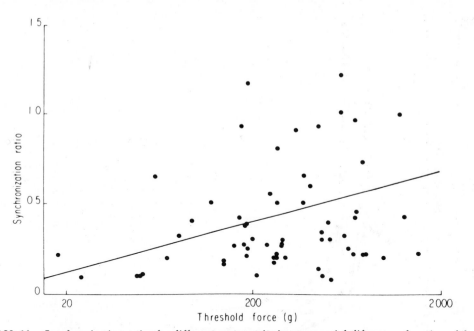

FIGURE 20–14. Synchronization ratios for different motor units in seven weightlifters as a function of the overall force in the muscle required to recruit a given unit to fire continuously (threshold force). There is a weak trend, indicated by the computed best-fitting straight line, for the higher threshold units to have larger synchronization ratios (linear correlation coefficient = 0.34). (From Milner-Brown, H. S., Stein, R. B., and Lee, R. G.: Synchronization of human motor units: Possible roles of exercise and supraspinal reflexes. E. E. G. Clin. Neurophysiol., 38:245–254, 1975.)

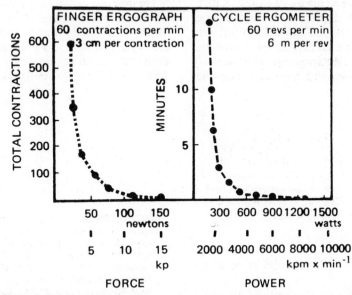

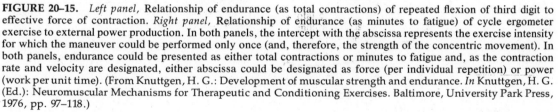

FIGURE 20–15. *Left panel,* Relationship of endurance (as total contractions) of repeated flexion of third digit to effective force of contraction. *Right panel,* Relationship of endurance (as minutes to fatigue) of cycle ergometer exercise to external power production. In both panels, the intercept with the abscissa represents the exercise intensity for which the maneuver could be performed only once (and, therefore, the strength of the concentric movement). In both panels, endurance could be presented as either total contractions or minutes to fatigue and, as the contraction rate and velocity are designated, either abscissa could be designated as force (per individual repetition) or power (work per unit time). (From Knuttgen, H. G.: Development of muscular strength and endurance. *In* Knuttgen, H. G. (Ed.): Neuromuscular Mechanisms for Therapeutic and Conditioning Exercises. Baltimore, University Park Press, 1976, pp. 97–118.)

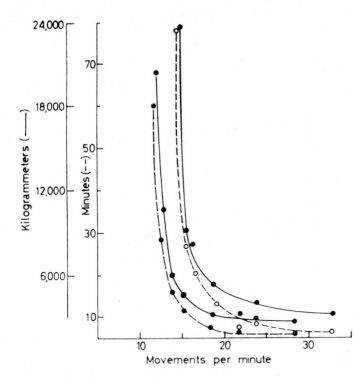

FIGURE 20–16. Endurance and intensity of work. Arm ergograph. Movements per minute plotted against duration of work and total amount of work performed. (From Monod, H., and Scherrer, J.: Capacité de travail statique d'un group musculaire synergique chez l'homme. C. R. Soc. Biol., 151:1358–1362, 1957.)

curvilinearity is related to a combination of aerobic and anaerobic power capacities. At the very high force levels at which contractions can be repeated up to 10 times, Knuttgen suggests that depletion of high-energy phosphate at the sites of contractile activity may be the limiting factor. Dissociation between integrated electromyographic activity and force in a sustained isometric contraction indicates that it is not failure of nerve impulses nor failure of the spread of excitation of the muscle membrane (Fig. 20–19).

Infante et al. demonstrated *in vitro* that when ATP resynthesis is blocked by 1-fluoro-2, 4 dinitrobenzol, frog sartorius muscle can produce only three near-maximal contractions in response to electrical stimulation before the ability of the muscle to

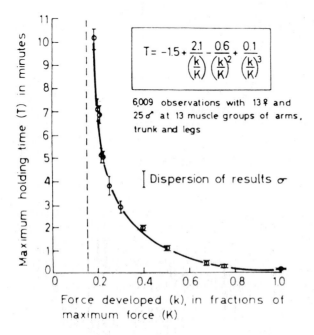

$$T = -1.5 + \frac{2.1}{\left(\frac{k}{K}\right)} - \frac{0.6}{\left(\frac{k}{K}\right)^2} + \frac{0.1}{\left(\frac{k}{K}\right)^3}$$

6,009 observations with 13 ♀ and 25 ♂ at 13 muscle groups of arms, trunk and legs

| Dispersion of results σ

FIGURE 20–17. Endurance and intensity of work. Static work: tension at fractions of maximum strength. (From Simonson, E.: Recovery and fatigue. *In* Simonson, E. (Ed.): Physiology of Work Capacity and Fatigue. Springfield, Ill., Charles C Thomas, Publisher, 1971, pp. 440–458. Redrawn from Rohmert, W.: Ermittlung von Erholungspausen für statische Arbeit des Menschen. Int. Z Angew. Physiol., 18:123–164, 1960.)

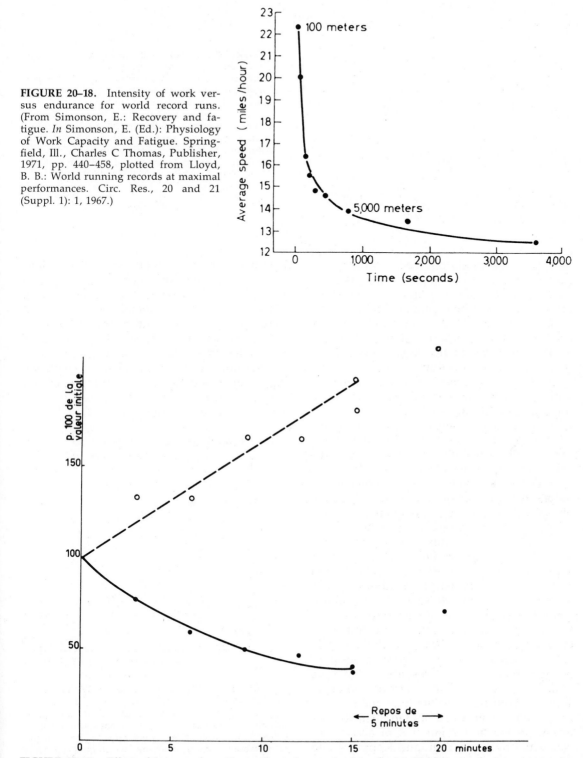

FIGURE 20–18. Intensity of work versus endurance for world record runs. (From Simonson, E.: Recovery and fatigue. *In* Simonson, E. (Ed.): Physiology of Work Capacity and Fatigue. Springfield, Ill., Charles C Thomas, Publisher, 1971, pp. 440–458, plotted from Lloyd, B. B.: World running records at maximal performances. Circ. Res., 20 and 21 (Suppl. 1): 1, 1967.)

FIGURE 20–19. Effect of intense dynamic work on the maximal isometric force of the muscle and on the integrated global EMG. Triceps, recording by surface electrodes during work to exhaustion lasting 15.1 minutes. Every three minutes the subject performed a maximal isometric contraction, whose force (in a continuous line) and integrated electrical activity (in an interrupted line) are measured. Note how the electrical activity increases again during the phase of relaxation. (From Scherrer, J., and Bourguignon, A.: Changes in the electromyogram produced by fatigue in man. Am. J. Phys. Med., 38:148–158, 1959.)

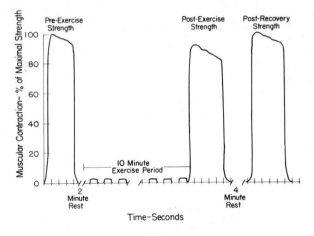

FIGURE 20–20. Maximal tension can be maintained during a voluntary maximal contraction of hand grip for less than 1 second before evidence of fatigue appears as the available supply of ATP is exhausted. Fatigue (unavailability of ATP) increases in proportion to the intensity of activity but can be demonstrated following 10 minutes of intermittent contractions at 5 per cent of maximal. (From Mundale, M. O.: The relationship of intermittent isometric exercise to fatigue of hand grip. Arch. Phys. Med. Rehabil., 51:532–539, 1970.)

contract is definitely reduced.[37] Mundale reported that during maximal voluntary isometric contractions of handgrip in man, maximal tension could not be maintained more than 1 second[53, 54] (Fig. 20–20). Anaerobic restoration of ATP occurs more slowly than it is broken down during maximal metabolic activity of muscle, resulting in a progressive decrease in muscular contractile capacity with increasing duration of activity due to the progressively diminishing supply of ATP to fuel the actin-myosin interaction in the sarcomeres. Keul, Doll, and Keppler report the relative availability of energy-supplying substrates to restore ATP during early activity.[39] The stored ATP at rest is sufficient for only 3 to 4 seconds of contraction. Creatine phosphate splitting can maintain ATP at a somewhat reduced rate of activity for approximately 20 seconds. During this time glycolytic metabolism increases to peak at approximately 40 to 50 seconds and then begins to fall. Oxidative metabolism rises slowly so that by 90 seconds the major contribution to the metabolic rate is oxidation. After 3 to 4 minutes a person on a constant exercise reaches a metabolic steady state or constant rate of consumption of oxygen. Figure 20–21 presents the relative contributions of the various energy-supplying substrates to the total energy utilization during maximal metabolism at any instant in the first 2 minutes of activity as calculated by Keul, Doll, and Keppler[39] and adapted by Kottke and Mundale according to the decreasing intensity of maximal voluntary isometric activity that occurs during that time. Glycolytic metabolism can restore ATP at only approximately 30–50 per cent of the

maximal rate of muscular metabolism, while oxidative metabolism can produce ATP at a rate of approximately 10 to 20 per cent of maximal muscular metabolism. To what extent the various kinds of training exercises cause shifts in these relative rates of metabolic activity have yet to be established.

The limit of the mechanism of oxidative phosphorylation (Krebs' cycle and electron transport system) to resynthesize ATP determines the exercise rate for the first 5 min-

Energy Sources in Relation to Duration of Contraction

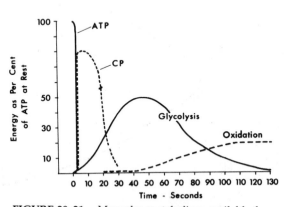

FIGURE 20–21. Muscular metabolism available from the various substrates participating in supplying energy during the first two minutes of an attempted maximal contraction. The relative contribution of each substrate at any moment is indicated.[39] The intensity of metabolic activity over the two-minute period is adjusted to the change of the isometric tension produced during a sustained voluntary maximal contraction.[52, 54] (Redrawn from Keul, J., Doll, E., and Keppler, D.: Energy Metabolism of Human Muscle. Medicine and Sport, Vol. 7. Baltimore, University Park Press, 1972.)

TABLE 20–4. COMPARISON DURING ISOKINETIC EXERCISE OF MAXIMAL ISOMETRIC STRENGTH, RELATIVE ISOKINETIC ENDURANCE, AND ABSOLUTE ENDURANCE OR ABILITY TO PERFORM WORK.

Variable	X̄	SD
Peak Torque, ft-lbs	113.65	29.19
Repetitions > 90% Peak Torque	5.88	3.46
Repetitions > 75% Peak Torque	15.29	4.88
Work > 90% Peak Torque, ft-lbs	638.82	440.95
Work > 75% Peak Torque, ft-lbs	1536.55	670.83

Repetitions at 90% or 75% of peak torque represent relative endurance. Work performed at 90% or 75% of peak torque represents absolute endurance. (From Barnes, W. S.: The relationship between maximal isokinetic strength and isokinetic endurance. Res. Q., 51:714–717, 1980.)

utes, after which oxygen delivery becomes the decisive factor. Knuttgen[42] suggests that for exercise intensities that can be maintained for extended periods (1 to 2 hours), depletion of glycogen stored in the muscle cells becomes the most likely limiting factor. Since the uptake rate of glucose from the blood is limited, depletion of the glycogen curtails both glycolytic phosphorylation and the availability of carbohydrate-provided substrate (pyruvate) for the Krebs' cycle. It should be noted that the aerobic capacity of the total individual is of great importance in the ergometer exercise but of little or no importance in the finger ergograph exercise.

The following studies shed further light on the relationship of strength and endurance. It is generally conceded that there is a significant positive correlation between maximum dynamic strength and absolute dynamic endurance.[66] Evidence is also available that this holds true of the relationship between maximum static strength and absolute static endurance.[72] These relationships are demonstrated in Figures 20–15 to 20–17. An example may serve to illustrate this relationship: if one's maximal isotonic strength of the biceps is 20 lbs, he/she will be able to lift this weight (by definition) for only one repetition. In contrast, if one's maximal isotonic strength is 40 lbs, he/she will be able to carry out the contraction at the 20-lb load for many more repetitions. By the same token, the tight mathematical relationship (with little scatter) suggests that greater strength does not improve one's *relative* endurance. Thus no matter how strong one is, 100 per cent of MVC is 100 per cent, and this will fall on the intercept with the abscissa. Barnes has studied the relationship between maximum iso-

kinetic strength and isokinetic endurance[4] (Table 20–4). When isokinetic endurance is defined as the number of repetitions performed at any given percentage of maximum isokinetic strength (i.e., relative isokinetic endurance), there is a nonsignificant correlation between strength and endurance (Table 20–5). However, when maximum isokinetic strength was correlated with isokinetic endurance, defined as the total foot-pounds of work done at any given percentage of maximum strength, the correlation coefficients were both positive and significant. This is a measure of absolute endurance. Barnes' findings support the concept that the work output of high-strength individuals is greater than that of low-strength individuals. In summary, there is no evidence that relative endurance increases as strength increases. However, there is a strong positive correlation between strength and "absolute" endurance or ability to perform work. As Barnes[4] cautions, this positive correlation between maximal

TABLE 20–5. COMPARISON OF CORRELATIONS OF ISOKINETIC STRENGTH WITH RELATIVE ISOKINETIC ENDURANCE AND WITH ABSOLUTE ENDURANCE TO DO WORK

Endurance Parameter versus	Strength "r"
Repetitions > 90% peak torque	−0.03
Repetitions > 75% peak torque	0.04
Work > 90% peak torque	0.36*
Work > 75% peak torque	0.27†

*$p < 0.01$
†$p < 0.05$
From Barnes, W. S.: The relationship between maximal isokinetic strength and isokinetic endurance. Res. Q., 51:714–717, 1980.

Length-Tension Diagrams of Total and Passive Tension

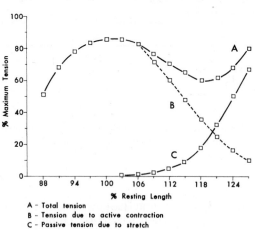

A - Total tension
B - Tension due to active contraction
C - Passive tension due to stretch

FIGURE 20–22. Length-tension diagram for passive stretch of an unstimulated muscle is shown in lower Curve C. Curve A, showing total isometric tension when the muscle was stimulated at various lengths from maximal stretch through moderate shortening, represents the summation of active contraction plus passive tension due to the stretch. Active tension due solely to muscular contraction is obtained by subtracting passive tension, C, from total tension, A, and is represented by Curve B. Normal resting length is 100 per cent. (Redrawn from Schottelius, B. A., and Senay, L. C.: Effect of stimulation-length sequence on shape of length-tension diagram. Am. J. Physiol., 186:127–130, 1956.)

strength and absolute endurance accounts for only approximately 10 to 20 per cent of the observed variance, and a major portion of endurance cannot be accounted for by strength alone. Other factors such as inherent differences in muscle fiber type, myoglobin stores, and enzymatic profiles, as well as the elusive factor of "motivation," may contribute to any given individual's endurance capacity.

Length-Tension Relationships

If a relaxed (nonstimulated) muscle is detached from its insertion and gradually stretched, a passive-length tension relationship can be determined (Fig. 20–22). The length, a tetanizing volley of electrical stimuli is delivered to the motor nerve, a new

If the length-tension relationships are again measured, but this time, at each new length, a tetanizing volley of electrical stimuli is delivered to the motor nerve, a new curve will be determined (Fig. 20–22; this figure is also referred to as the Blix diagram). The total tension at any point will be the sum of the active tension and passive tension. At all lengths below the resting length, the passive tension is, by definition, zero and there-

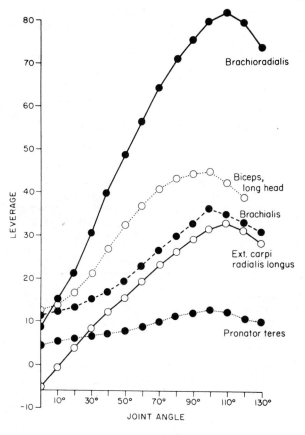

FIGURE 20–23. Leverage curves of elbow flexors. Zero degrees — elbow extended. (From Brunnstrom, S.: Clinical Kinesiology, 2nd Ed. Philadelphia, F. A. Davis, 1966; plotted from data of Braune, W., and Fischer, O.: Die Rotationsmomente der Beugemuskeln am Ellbogengelenk des Menschen. Abh. Konigl. Sachs. Wissensch. Math. Phys. Klasse, Vol. 15, 1890.)

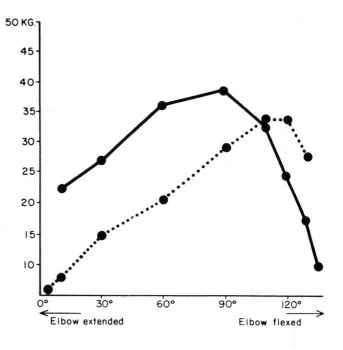

FIGURE 20–24. Torque curves for flexion and extension of right elbow, from determinations on four male subjects. Solid curve: elbow flexion curve; dotted curve: elbow extension. (From Brunnstrom, S.: Clinical Kinesiology, 2nd Ed. Philadelphia, F. A. Davis, 1966; redrawn from Bethe, A., and Franke, F.: Beitrage zum Problem der willkurlich beweglichen Armprothesen. IV. Die Kraftkurven der indirekten naturlichen Energiequellen. Munch. Med. Wochenschr., 66:201–205, 1919.)

fore at those lengths the total tension will be equal to the active tension. At all lengths beyond the resting length the active tension is determined by subtracting the passive tension from the total tension. Thus it can be seen that the greatest active tension is developed at the resting length, and the greatest total tension is developed at or slightly longer than the resting length. Kidd and Brodie have suggested superimposition of the force-velocity and active length-tension diagram to illustrate the concept that at any given velocity of lengthening or shortening there is a length-tension relationship as the muscle passes through various lengths.[40] The

classic length-tension relationship, as shown in the previous figures, is an isometric one. Thus, theoretically there would be a whole family of length-tension curves, one for each contraction velocity.

Leverage Effect

The influence of the mechanical factor of leverage, deriving from tendon location and angle of insertion, upon torque when the force of the muscle is maintained constant, varies with the sine of the angle of insertion. Figure 20–23 shows leverage curves for the elbow flexors. These are not torque curves,

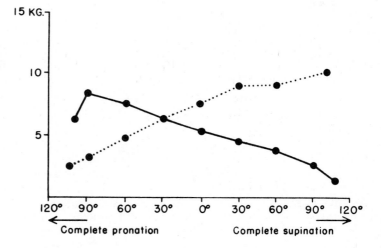

FIGURE 20–25. Torque curves for pronation and supination of right elbow, derived from determinations on four male subjects. Elbow at 90 degrees of flexion. Solid curve: supination. Dotted curve: pronation. Zero: thumb upward. (From Brunnstrom, S.: Clinical Kinesiology, 2nd Ed. Philadelphia, F. A. Davis, 1966; redrawn from Bethe, A., and Franke, F.: Beitrage zum Problem der willkurlich beweglichen Armprothesen. IV. Die Kraftkurven der indirekten naturlichen Energiequellen. Munch. Med. Wochenschr., 66:201–205, 1919.)

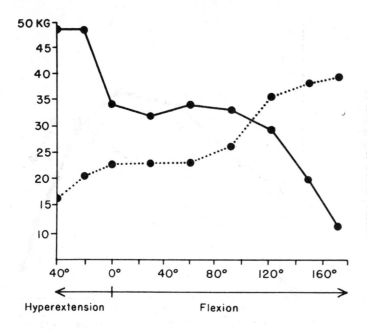

FIGURE 20–26. Torque curves for flexion and extension of right shoulder, derived from determinations on four male subjects. Solid curve: flexion. Dotted curve: extension. (From Brunnstrom, S.: Clinical Kinesiology, 2nd Ed. Philadelphia, F. A. Davis, 1966; redrawn from Bethe, A., and Franke, F.: Beitrage zum Problem der willkurlich beweglichen Armprothesen. IV. Die Kraftkurven der indirekten naturlichen Energiequellen. Munch. Med. Wochenschr., 66:201–205, 1919.)

but represent the mechanical factors contributing to torque.

Torque

As defined earlier muscle torque represents the effectiveness of a muscle's force in producing rotation about a joint. It is the net effect of the physiologic and mechanical factors. These factors do not have equal effect at all joints. In one, the mechanical effect may be more important while in another the physiologic effect of length-tension relation-

ships has greater impact upon the net torque. Figures 20–24 to 20–26 show several examples of isometric torque curves. For pronation and supination of the forearm and for flexion and extension of the shoulder, the physiologic factor of the length-tension relationship predominates, with greater tension developed at longer lengths. For elbow flexion, there is an interaction between the two factors — physiologic and mechanical. The angle of insertion of the biceps and brachialis (mechanical factor) is very favorable at 90 degrees. It remains favorable at 100 to 120

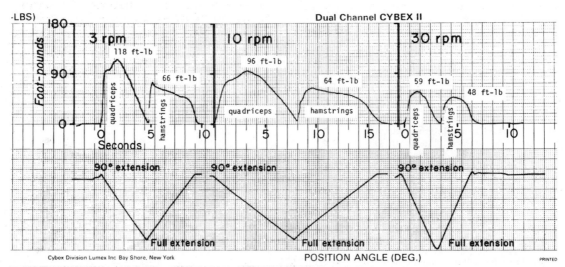

FIGURE 20–27. Torque curves of quadriceps and hamstrings throughout 90 degree range of motion and at various speeds. Note the greater strength of the quadriceps vs. the hamstrings. With the subject seated, gravity hinders the quadriceps and helps the hamstrings progressively more at higher speeds.

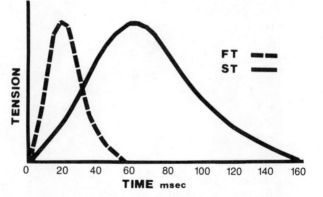

Figure 20–28. Twitch characteristics (contraction relaxation curves) of slow twitch (type I) and fast twitch (type II) muscles. (From Ianuzzo, C. D.: The cellular composition of human skeletal muscle. *In* Knuttgen, H. G. (Ed.): Neuromuscular Mechanisms for Therapeutic and Conditioning Exercise. Baltimore, University Park Press, 1976, pp. 31–53.)

degrees, but this factor is overshadowed by the physiologic factor of very short muscle length.

The Cybex II dynamometer (for description, see exercise programs and equipment) permits the measurement of torque curves throughout the range of motion and at various contraction speeds. Figure 20–27 shows examples of such measurements on the author's right quadriceps and hamstrings at the maximal torque possible at each angle from 90 degrees to 0 degrees of flexion at three contraction velocities. The angle of peak torque shifts with the increasing velocity of contraction.

Muscle Fiber Types[36]

That there might be some specialization of muscle fibers has been known at least since the "red meat" and "white meat" of fowl

were observed. Attempts have been made on the basis of various muscle characteristics to classify muscles, but in man muscle is a mosaic and not easily distinguishable on the basis of color. Attempts have been made to classify muscle types on the basis of oxidative or glycolytic capability, but the metabolic capacity of muscle is highly influenced by the state of activity and training and therefore is not a stable characteristic. Figure 20–28 shows the contraction-relaxation curves for fast twitch and slow twitch mammalian skeletal muscles. The slow twitch is also known as type I and the fast twitch is known as type II. Under ordinary circumstances, these fiber types are extremely stable. They are under control of the nerve supply. Figure 20–29 gives a diagrammatic illustration of the influence of innervation pattern.[28, 29, 60, 61] Cross-innervated muscles originally having fast twitch properties and

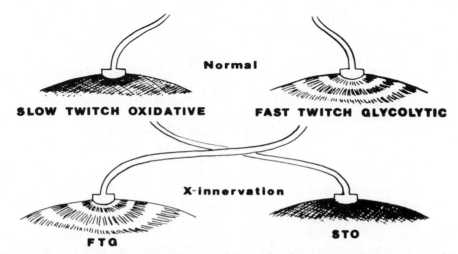

FIGURE 20–29. Cross-innervated muscles take on twitch characteristics and metabolic properties dependent on their innervation and become like the muscles of the opposite type. (From Ianuzzo, C. D.: The cellular composition of human skeletal muscle. *In* Knuttgen, H. G. (Ed.): Neuromuscular Mechanisms for Therapeutic and Conditioning Exercise. Baltimore, University Park Press, 1976, pp. 31–53.)

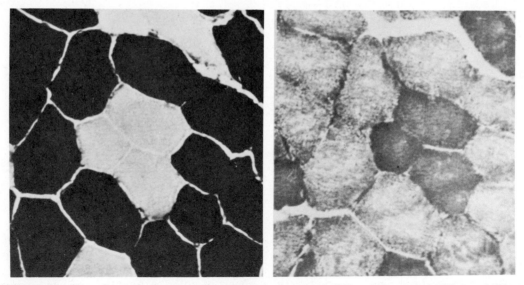

FIGURE 20–30. Histochemical micrograph illustrating the fast twitch (FT) and slow twitch (ST) muscle fibers in human skeletal muscle. The micrograph on the left has been stained for myofibrillar ATPase. The light and dark stained cells are ST and FT fibers, respectively. The micrograph at the right is from a serial section of the muscle and has been stained for DPNH-diaphorase, which indicates the aerobic potential of the fibers. These micrographs illustrate that in human skeletal muscle ST fibers have a relatively high aerobic capacity, while FT fibers have a low capacity. (From Ianuzzo, C. D.: The cellular composition of human skeletal muscle. *In* Knuttgen, H. G. (Ed.): Neuromuscular Mechanisms for Therapeutic Conditioning Exercise. Baltimore, University Park Press, 1976, pp. 31–53.)

low oxidative capacity take on slow twitch characteristics and an increased oxidative capacity, while the inverse occurs for slow twitch muscles experimentally innervated with nerves from fast muscles. In addition, the changes in the metabolic apparatus are accompanied by corresponding changes in the density of the capillaries surrounding the fibers. It has been shown that the fast twitch and slow twitch muscles have their own force-velocity relationships. The general shape of the curve is the same, but there are quantitative differences, with the rate of shortening being greater for fast twitch muscles than for slow twitch muscles with the same relative load. It should be noted, however, that the length-tension relationships of slow and fast muscles are similar when the amount of force developed is expressed per unit of cross sectional area.[10, 74] One metabolic characteristic that is relatively stable is the reaction, with supravital stain, for myofibrillar ATPase.[17] When the section of muscle is pre-incubated at pH of 9.4 (or, more recently, at pH 10.2), the type II fibers (fast twitch) will stain darkly for myofibrillar ATPase. After this technique has been used for identifying the fiber types, these muscle fibers may then be stained, on adjacent serial sections, for other enzymes reflecting other

metabolic capabilities. For example, Figure 20–30 shows adjacent serial sections from human muscle. On the left the section had been stained for myofibrillar ATPase. The darkly staining fibers are the type II or fast twitch fibers. The light fibers are the slow twitch or type I fibers. The adjacent section, shown on the right, has been stained for DPNH diaphorase, which reflects aerobic capability of the fibers. (DPNH is reduced diphosphopyridine nucleotide, or in current terminology, NADH or reduced nicotinamide adenine dinucleotide. A diaphorase is an enzyme that catalyzes the oxidation of certain nucleotides.) The slow twitch fibers are thus shown to be high in aerobic capacity. Qualitative or roughly quantitative changes resulting from training programs could be demonstrated by such stains as DPNH diaphorase, upon repeated biopsy. Such techniques have been used in recent years to study fiber typing and responses to training in athletes in various sports. It should be emphasized that the aerobic and glycolytic capabilities as well as glycogen content of muscle change, but the twitch characteristics and the myofibrillar ATPase staining remain stable. Such histochemical techniques may be supplemented by purely chemical techniques that are more quantitative but do not distinguish between fiber types. The change in enzyme activity reflects an average of both fiber types taken in the biopsy and does not distinguish the changes that may occur predominantly in slow twitch or fast twitch muscle fibers. One may also count percentages of fibers and look at the areas of individual slow twitch and fast twitch fibers (i.e., the absolute area of each), as well as the ratio of slow twitch to fast twitch fiber areas before and after training. Finally, the recruitment patterns of muscle fibers may be studied in acute experiments by repetitive biopsies during the course of various types of strenuous activity. The pattern of glycogen depletion in the fiber types may thus be followed at intervals throughout the activity.

In addition to the two basic types of muscle fibers, i.e., type I slow oxidative (SO) and type II fast glycolytic (FG), evidence is accumulating that in man there is at least one additional type, i.e., fast oxidative glycolytic (FOG), a subtype of the type II fiber. Table 20–6 summarizes the properties of these three muscle types. To this table one may add the recruitment level. The slow oxidative fibers are in motor units that have a low threshold, are recruited earlier and, therefore, contract more frequently.

Motor Unit Recruitment Patterns and the Size Principle

Evidence supports the "size principle" enunciated by Henneman.[31] There are variations in size of the motor unit and its component parts, including the soma of the neuron as well as the number and cross sectional area of the muscle fibers innervated. The smaller units are type I (slow oxidative), which have a low threshold of recruitment and generate low forces. The size principle is followed electromyographically. The electromyographer will observe that the earliest recruited motor units have smaller electrical potentials (amplitude) than units that recruit later. Although with biofeedback one can vary the order of recruitment of units of approximately the same amplitude, one cannot recruit a larger unit without first recruiting the relatively smaller one. The size principle is followed in the generation of mechanical force as well. The force generated by each motor unit varies linearly with recruitment order, so that the motor unit recruited earliest generates the least force.[48] These low-force units, recruited early, fire regularly and are relatively fatigue-resistant. The term "tonic" is often used to refer to these units (see the next paragraph). The

TABLE 20–6. A CHARACTERIZATION OF SKELETAL MUSCLE FIBERS BASED UPON THEIR METABOLIC AND MECHANICAL PROPERTIES

	Muscle Fiber Characteristics		
	Slow oxidative (SO)	Fast glycolytic (FG)	Fast oxidative glycolytic (FOG)
Major source of ATP	Oxidative phosphorylation	Glycolysis	Oxidative phosphorylation
Mitochondria	Numerous	Few	Numerous
Myoglobin content	High	Low	High
Capillarity	Dense	Sparse	Dense
Muscle color	Red	White	Red
Glycogen content	Low	High	Intermediate
Glycolytic enzyme activity	Low	High	Intermediate
Myosin ATPase activity	Low	High	High
Speed of contraction	Slow	Fast	Fast
Rate of fatigue	Slow	Fast	Intermediate
Muscle fiber diameter	Small	Large	Intermediate

*From, Kidd, G., and Brodie, P.: The motor unit: A review. Physiotherapy, 66:146–152, 1980.

type II units, recruited later and exerting higher force, fire irregularly in bursts and fatigue relatively rapidly, although the sub-type of fast oxidative glycolytic (FOG) has an intermediate aerobic capacity and fatigues less rapidly while still retaining a rapid rate of contraction.

Maton, studying single motor units in the biceps of 15 normal subjects, found that a motor unit that does not discharge for a given level of static force will discharge during the following dynamic work and can also be recruited for a higher level of static force.[47] Thus, any given motor unit activity is dependent upon the level of external force in keeping with the previous force-velocity relationships. Since higher levels of force are developed with isometric contractions, a higher level of static force is required to recruit a motor unit that would be recruited with dynamic work at the same force. Thus, the author points out that the qualifications "tonic" and "phasic" characterize the motor unit twitches and do not imply any static-dynamic differentiation. In further support of this concept, Desmedt and Godaux found that during ballistic (very rapid or steep ramp) contractions, higher order units, including type II, are recruited at lower force levels than during slow contractions.[16]

Fatigue

True fatigue may not always be easy to determine. Fatigue may be operationally defined as the inability or unwillingness to carry out the assigned task in the assigned manner under the specific conditions of reinforcement in effect and known to the subject as the result of prior activity. This is in essence a behavioral definition. However, it would be desirable to have a definite physiologic endpoint of fatigue. In at least two circumstances such a definite biologic endpoint is available. One is the maximum aerobic capacity. As defined, this is the rate of oxygen consumption ($\dot{V}O_2$), which does not increase in spite of increased performance of external work. Thus defined, this is the $\dot{V}O_2$ max, which is illustrated in Figure 20–3. This idealized figure shows that at all exercise intensities below 250 watts the subject goes to a new rate of oxygen consumption. However, when he jumps from 250 watts to 300 watts, no increase in the rate of oxygen consumption occurs in spite of an increase in exercise intensity and external work performed. This additional 50 watts of external work is being carried out anaerobically, and fatigue will quickly result in failure to continue working at that intensity. Another situation in which a good physiologic endpoint for fatigue may be determined is one in which the subject exerts a maximal isometric contraction (MVC) and the integrated electrical activity of the muscle is measured. Figure 20–19 shows the effect of intense dynamic work on maximal isometric force and on the integrated surface EMG. The fact that the integrated electrical activity *is increasing* at the time that the mechanical force is decreasing ensures that the subject is putting out a full effort but that fatigue is occurring in spite of the effort. There are concomitants of fatigue in other situations, but the endpoint is not so clear cut.

RESPONSE TO TRAINING

Are Athletes Born or Made?

Marked differences between athletes participating in different types of sports can be detected by the casual observer or the devotee of sport and in greater detail by the scientist in the human performance laboratory. The weight lifter is heavy and extremely strong. The distance runner is slight of build with very little body fat and relatively low strength but has the ability to continue running literally for hours. Definite but more subtle changes are observed between the sprinter and the distance runner. Differences in local metabolic capacity of the muscle as well as fiber type differences have been determined by large-needle biopsy.[5] Gollnick sampled the upper and lower extremity muscles of athletes participating in various sports.[22] A total of 74 trained and untrained men were studied. The quantitative chemical studies that were carried out include succinate dehydrogenase (SDH) and phosphofructokinase (PFK), representing, respectively, the oxidative and glycolytic capabilities of the muscle sample as a whole, without distinction between the fiber types. Histochemical studies included myosin adenosine tri-

TABLE 20–7. RELATIONSHIP OF EXERCISE TRAINING OF UPPER AND LOWER EXTREMITY MUSCLES TO FIBER DIAMETERS, TOTAL CROSS SECTIONAL AREAS, AND PERCENTAGES OF SLOW TWITCH AND FAST TWITCH MUSCLE FIBERS

Subject	Sample Site (Arm or Leg)		Fiber Diameter, μ		Area, μ^3		ST Fibers	% Area ST Fibers
			ST	FT	ST	FT		
PG	L	Untrained	75.2±2.9	85.8±2.0	4567.5±343.2	5843.0±273.9	34.0	28.7
CS	L	Untrained	80.3±3.3	93.2±2.2	5234.5±440.3	6902.0±329.9	30.0	24.5
MKS	L	Untrained	63.4±2.4	67.7±2.4	3057.5±273.6	3683.0±250.0	34.0	30.0
GK	A	Untrained	63.6±2.0	67.3±1.7	3234.0±181.2	3594.0±177.8	48.3	45.7
	L		72.2±3.5	75.0±1.4	4275.0±382.1	4445.0±169.1	48.6	47.6
NP	L	Sprinter	79.5±2.6	89.4±2.1	5060.5±314.0	6336.5±284.2	26.0	21.9
DM	L	Distance runner	67.1±1.7	58.0±1.3	3581.1±186.2	2668.0±1220	75.0	80.1
DS	L	Distance runner	85.1±3.5	105.2±2.5	5858.0±445.8	8776.1±408.2	70.0	50.9
DF	L	Middle-distance runner	95.5±3.2	87.9±3.4	7307.8±499.6	6235.0±448.2	55.0	58.9
RP	L	Middle-distance runner	59.2±2.7	71.6±2.5	2856.5±231.8	4118.0±295.9	47.0	38.1
BA	L	Former weight-lifter	107.1±3.8	108.9±3.4	9199.1±656.7	9482.9±666.9	24.0	23.5
MH	L	Weightlifter	85.6±4.9	110.8±3.0	6035.6±629.4	9758.1±516.6	25.3	23.5
	A		83.5±2.4	105.0±3.3	5553.5±303.8	8917.2±543.1	48.4	36.9
JR	A	Bicyclist	83.1±1.4	96.2±1.9	5467.0±187.9	7337.0±273.7	52.1	48.6
	L		104.6±2.3	112.2±2.2	8651.5±763.9	9946.6±401.5	51.3	44.0
BL	A	Canoeist	101.9±2.6	102.9±2.3	8244.0±570.3	8391.0±361.9	57.9	74.6
	L		90.5±2.7	80.3±1.5	6544.0±387.5	5100.0±190.1	69.9	57.5
SH	A	Swimmer	88.0±1.7	91.0±2.4	6124.0±233.9	6552.0±263.2	85.3	84.4
	L		79.0±2.0	93.6±1.9	4954.0±237.6	6928.0±266.9	79.7	73.7

From Gollnick, P. D., Armstrong, R. B., Saubert, C. W., IV, Piehl, K., and Saltin, B.: Enzymatic activity and fiber composition in skeletal muscle of untrained and trained men. J. Appl. Physiol., 33:312–319, 1972.

phosphatase (ATPase) for fiber-tying, as well as DPNH-diaphorase and alpha-glycerophosphate dehydrogenase for estimating (semiquantitatively only) relative (type I versus type II) oxidative and glycolytic capabilities. The distribution of glycogen was estimated (in serial sections) from the periodic acid–Schiff (PAS) reaction. Standard photographs were made so that planimetry could be used for fiber areas. In addition, each subject's maximal aerobic capacity ($\dot{V}O_2$ max) was determined while he was either running on a treadmill or pedaling a bicycle. Whereas only minor differences existed for PFK (glycolytic capacity), remarkable differences were found in local muscle oxidative capacity (SDH) and in $\dot{V}O_2$ max. The SDH and $\dot{V}O_2$ max of the weight lifters were no greater than those of the untrained men; in fact, they were slightly less. The endurance-trained athletes had much higher $\dot{V}O_2$ max and local muscle SDH activity than the untrained or the weightlifters. Of particular interest is the selective effect upon the muscles used predominantly in the sport. For instance, in the group of

bicyclists the SDH activity of the vastus lateralis (11.0 ± 1.0 micromoles/g min.) was much greater than that of the deltoid (6.1 ± 0.2), whereas in canoeists, the SDH activity of the deltoid (7.9 ± 0.6) was much higher than that of the vastus lateralis (5.8 ± 0.9). Table 20–7 shows the fiber sizes, populations, and contribution to muscle area of several individual subjects. It can be seen that in the untrained, the weight lifters, and the sprinter, the slow twitch fibers (type I) occupied a relatively small percentage of the muscle fiber area (21.9 – 30.0 per cent), whereas in the endurance-trained athletes, the slow twitch fibers occupied as much as 84 per cent of the area. This study examined the athletes as they were and did not constitute a before-and-after experiment. It might be argued that very early in their athletic careers these athletes found that they were able to compete much more effectively in one type of sport than in another and thus, because of positive reinforcement, selected the sport at which they were successful. However, there is some suggestion that the changes seen in their muscles were at least to some extent the result of training, because one would anticipate genetically a more or less constant ratio of slow twitch (ST) to fast twitch (FT) fibers in the upper and lower extremities. (This is not to say that one expects the *same* ratio of ST to FT in the deltoid and in the vastus lateralis; however, if the ratio of ST/FT is X in the deltoid and Y in the vastus lateralis in one subject, and if ST/FT in the deltoid is A and ST/FT in the vastus is B in another subject, then, if differential usage (training) has no effect, one might expect X/Y to equal A/B.) However, those athletes who used the upper or the lower extremity more in a specific sport had enhancement of the metabolic capability and a larger per cent area of the slow twitch fibers in the muscles used.

Gollnick also carried out a five-month training program with biopsy studies before and after training.[21] The training program consisted of pedaling a bicycle ergometer one hour per day for four days a week at a load requiring 75 to 90 per cent of maximal aerobic power. The subsequent biopsies showed an increase in the ratio of the areas of slow twitch to fast twitch fibers from 0.82 to 1.11 (p < 0.01). Oxidative capacity increased in both fiber types; anaerobic capacity increased only in the FT fibers. This study indicates the possibility of great enhancement of local muscle metabolic capability, particularly oxidative capacity, with endurance training, and strongly supports the notion of some degree of specificity of training.

Regarding the question of whether athletes are born or made, it appears that the genotype sets the rather wide limits, with the actual performance capability determined by the extent and type of training.

Further Studies on the Specificity of Training

Transferability is the converse of specificity of training. It is of considerable interest to anyone who must prescribe exercise programs to know to what extent training acquired under one set of circumstances transfers to performance under another set of circumstances. The DeLorme axiom states that "high-power (high-force), low-repetition exercises build strength; low-power, high-repetition exercises build endurance" and that "each of these types of exercise is wholly distinct and wholly incapable of producing the results obtained by the other."[14] In the extreme case, it seems clear that the DeLorme axiom must be correct, but there is also reason to think that there may be a rather large middle ground where, under certain conditions, the DeLorme axiom may not apply. De Lateur and co-

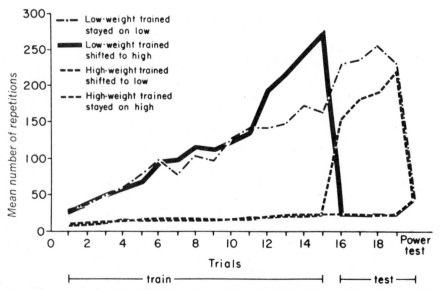

FIGURE 20–31. Mean scores for each of the four groups for each of 15 training trials and each of 4 test trials. The mean score for each of the four groups on the power test is also shown. (From de Lateur, B. J., Lehmann, J. F., and Fordyce, W. E.: A test of the DeLorme axiom. Arch. Phys. Med. Rehabil., 49:245–248, 1968.)

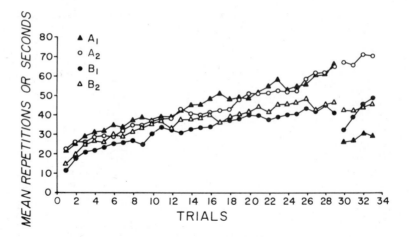

FIGURE 20–32. Results of the isotonic-isometric comparison. Groups A_1 and A_2 were isotonically trained. Groups B_1 and B_2 were isometrically trained. Group A_1 shifted to the isometric task on day 30. Group B_1 shifted to the isotonic task on day 30. (From de Lateur, B. J., Lehmann, J., Stonebridge, J., and Warren, C. G.: Isotonic vs. isometric exercises: A double-shift, transfer-of-training study. Arch. Phys. Med. Rehabil., 53:212–217, 1972.)

authors utilized a double-shift, transfer-of-training design to assess this axiom with the intensity range of 40 to 100 per cent of maximal.[11] Healthy young adult males were randomly assigned to one of four groups, two of which trained to fatigue on the high weight of 55 pounds and two of which trained on the relatively low weight of 26 pounds. The task was identical except for the amount of weight used. Subjects were seated in standard wooden chairs. To the metronome beat of 52/minute, the knee was extended on the count of one, held in full extension through the count of six, lowered on seven and raised again on one. Subjects were paid a small amount per repetition. Each session yielded a score. Thus training and testing were one and the same. At the completion of 15 sessions, one of the high-weight-trained groups shifted to the low-weight condition, and one of the low-weight-trained groups shifted to the high-weight condition and all continued for four more sessions. Results are shown in Figure 20–31. The transference was complete. In addition, when, in a fifth test session, all four groups were tested on a common power test (maximum work performed per unit time) the group averages were identical.

The task in the above-described study was qualitatively identical; only the amount of weight (and thus the repetitions needed to achieve fatigue) was different. The author carried out a subsequent study to assess the amount of transference of isotonic training to isometric performance and vice versa.[13] Healthy young adult males were randomly assigned to one of four groups, two isometric and two isotonic. The weight attached to the foot was the same for all, 50 pounds. The tasks were pure, i.e., no lifting or lowering for the isometric group and no holding of the knee in extension for the isotonic group. Subjects were again encouraged to go to the point of muscle fatigue by being paid per second of holding time for the isometric group and per repetition for the isotonic group (Fig. 20–32). At the completion of 29 sessions one isometric-trained group shifted to the isotonic condition and one isotonic-trained group shifted to the isometric condition, and all continued for five more sessions. In contrast to the DeLorme axiom study, there was very little transfer of training: subjects did much better on the task on which they had been trained.

Gollnick and co-workers used the biopsy technique to study the patterns of glycogen depletion in bicycling exercise of work intensities ranging from 30 to 150 per cent of $\dot{V}O_2$ max.[25] They found that the slow twitch, high oxidative (ST) fibers were the first to lose glycogen at all workloads below 100 per cent of $\dot{V}O_2$ max, but that as work continued the fast twitch (FT) fibers also became depleted of glycogen. At workloads exceeding maximal aerobic power, both fiber types lost glycogen. They concluded that there was primary reliance upon slow twitch fibers during submaximal endurance exercise, with recruitment of fast twitch fibers after slow twitch fibers were depleted of glycogen; during exertion requiring energy expenditure greater than maximal aerobic power, both fiber types were continuously involved in the task.

Gollnick et al. also studied glycogen depletion patterns in the vastus lateralis of six healthy males who carried out isometric contractions of various intensities related to

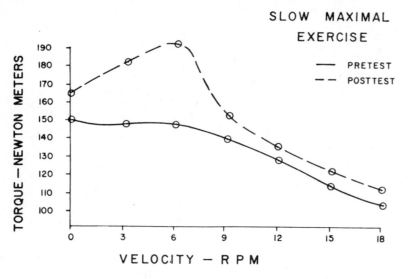

FIGURE 20-33. Peak torques of quadriceps plotted against velocity of contraction before (solid line) and after (dotted line) a maximal exercise regime at 6 RPM. (From Moffroid, M. T., and Whipple, R. H.: Specificity of speed of exercise. Phys. Ther., 50:1692–1700, 1970.)

their MVC.[24] In all experiments a selective glycogen depletion was observed. Instead of any gradation of depletion, there was a reversal of depletion patterns above and below the critical tension of 20 per cent of MVC. Below 20 per cent there was depletion of the slow twitch fibers; above 20 per cent the fast twitch fibers were depleted.

The above studies collectively suggest that for qualitatively identical tasks, comparable results from training in the range of 30 to 100 per cent MVC may be obtained as long as the task is carried to the point of fatigue (but it is much more difficult to reach true muscle fatigue with the lower weights; boredom is the more likely reason for cessation of the activity. For qualitatively different tasks, or for extreme quantitative differences, the best training is that task itself.

Newer dynamometric equipment has fa-

cilitated the study of the specificity of velocity of contraction in training, i.e., the extent to which it is possible to change the shape of the force-velocity curves by selective training. Moffroid and Whipple compared the results of six weeks of training on a slow (6 rpm) maximal task versus a fast (18 rpm) maximal task.[49] The outcome is shown in Figures 20–33 and 20–34. It may be said that training at the higher rpms transferred to the lowered velocities, but that training at the lower rpms had little or no transference to the higher velocities.

Having little or no positive transfer from training to a desired performance task is certainly inefficient and undesirable. It is possible, however, that an even more undesirable outcome may occur, i.e., negative transference or interference. Such an outcome was found by Kennedy and co-work-

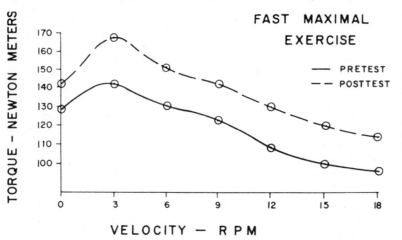

FIGURE 30-34. Peak torques of the quadriceps plotted against velocity of contraction before (solid line) and after (dotted line) a maximal exercise regime at 18 RPM. (From Moffroid, M. T., and Whipple, R. H.: Specificity of speed of exercise. Phys. Ther., 50:1692–1700, 1970.)

ers, who randomly assigned six distance runners to experimental and control groups whose training during running differed only in that the experimental subjects wore weighted wristlets, anklets, and belts. In pre- and post-training measurements it was found that the energy cost of a low-intensity run (9.7 km/hr at 0 per cent grade with weights removed) was *increased,* and an unexpected shift toward greater anaerobic metabolism was observed.[38]

Hickson carried out a study designed to determine how individuals respond to a combination of strength and endurance training as compared to the adaptations produced by either strength or endurance training separately. The endurance training referred to is not isolated muscle endurance but aerobic training. The strength training program (group S) consisted of lower extremity weight training 5 days per week for 10 weeks. The endurance training program (group E) consisted of 6 days per week for 10 weeks of cycle ergometer work or at least 30

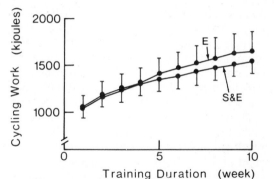

FIGURE 30–36. Increases in average total bicycle work per week during the 10 weeks of training in the endurance (E) and strength and endurance (S and E) groups. (From Hickson, R. C.: Interference of strength development by simultaneously training for strength and endurance. Eur. J. Appl. Physiol., 45:255–263, 1980.)

minutes of continuous running (cycle and running on alternate days). Groups S and E did both programs at the same intensities, and with at least two hours' rest between the two programs. Results are displayed in Figures 20–35 and 20–36. Based upon this outcome, Hickson suggests that at the upper limits in the development of strength, aerobic training inhibits or interferes with further increases in strength.[33] This again points out the importance of making the training as close to the performance task as possible.

Thus, one may say that for qualitatively identical or very similar exercises, there is a high degree of transfer of training for tasks ranging between 40 and 100 per cent of muscle contractile power (and perhaps as wide a range as 20 to 100 per cent) as long as the task (at whatever relative level) is carried to the point of fatigue, as previously operationally defined. In contrast, for qualitatively dissimilar tasks, or extreme quantitative differences, the best training for a task is that task itself.

Relative Roles of Mechanical Work Versus Fatigue

The results of the DeLorme axiom study showed no difference in ultimate performance ability between "low" (about 40 per cent MVC) and high (about 85 to 100 per cent MVC) weight-trained groups as long as all subjects worked to fatigue in training. However, the low-weight group required far more

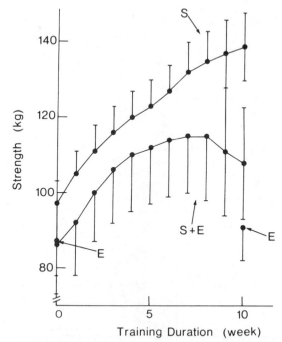

FIGURE 20–35. Strength changes in response to the three types of training. Measurements were made on a weekly basis in the strength (S) and strength and endurance (S and E) groups. The endurance (E) group was tested before and after 10 weeks of training. (From Hickson, R. C.: Interference of strength development by simultaneously training for strength and endurance. Eur. J. Appl. Physiol., 45:255–263, 1980.)

mechanical work and time to reach muscle fatigue. This suggested, but was not critically designed to show, that muscle fatigue was of greater importance in training than the amount of mechanical work performed. De Lateur et al.[12] carried out a two-phase, double-shift transfer-of-training study specifically designed to determine the relative importance of these two factors. In phase one, mechanical work was kept the same between right and left quadriceps, but one side, randomly determined, had more fatigue than the other. Subjects were paid for the number of repetitions (of complete cycles) performed by the fatigue side. The nonfatigue side had to match the number of repetitions on the fatigue side, but did so with one or more cycles of rest. Both sides lifted a 45-pound weight. The scheme for phase I and its five subsections is shown in Figure 20–37. The results are summarized in Figure 20–38. They may be interpreted as showing that more rest and less fatigue during training

result in poorer performance in the test period. In phase II with a new set of subjects, both sides exercised to fatigue during training, but one side, randomly determined, did so with a rest cycle between duty cycles and one side did so without a rest between duty cycles (see Fig. 20–37). Thus the side with a rest cycle did far more mechanical work than the side without in the process of going to fatigue bilaterally. The results are shown in Figure 20–39. The side that did more mechanical work did better in the test period, but not in proportion to the amount of time spent in training. For example, group one performed 91 per cent better than group two in the test period, in which both sides exercised to fatigue with a rest cycle between duty cycles, but spent 567 per cent more time in training. Comparing groups three and four in the test period, in which both sides exercised to fatigue without a rest cycle between duty cycles, one sees that group three, which trained with a rest cycle

	Seconds/Cycle	Nonrested Quad, Verbal Count	Rested Quad, Cycles Work/ Cycles Rest	Rested Quad, Verbal Count
Phase I	7	"up/2/3/4/5/6/down"	1/1	"up/2/3/4/5/6/down/rest/2/3/4/5/6/ready"
	6	"up/2/3/4/5/down"	1/2	"up/2/3/4/5/down/rest/2/3/4/5/6/7/8/9/10/11/ready"
	5	"up/2/3/4/down"	1/3	"up/2/3/4/down/rest/2/3/4/5/6/7/8/9/10/11/12/13/14/ready"
	4	"up/2/3/down"	1/4	"up/2/3/down/rest/2/3/4/5/6/7/8/9/10/11/12/13/14/15/ready"
	3	"up/2/down"	1/5	"up/2/down/rest/2/3/4/5/6/7/8/9/10/11/12/13/14/ready"
Phase II	7	"up/2/3/4/5/6/down"	1/1	"up/2/3/4/5/6/down/rest/2/3/4/5/6/ready"

FIGURE 20–37. The chart presents the number of seconds per cycle, the number of cycles of rest per cycle of work, and verbal counts for each leg under nonrested and rested conditions in Phase 1 and Phase 2. (From de Lateur, B. J., Lehmann, J. F., and Giaconi, R.: Mechanical work and fatigue: Their roles in the development of muscle work capacity. Arch. Phys. Med. Rehabil., 57:319–324, 1976.)

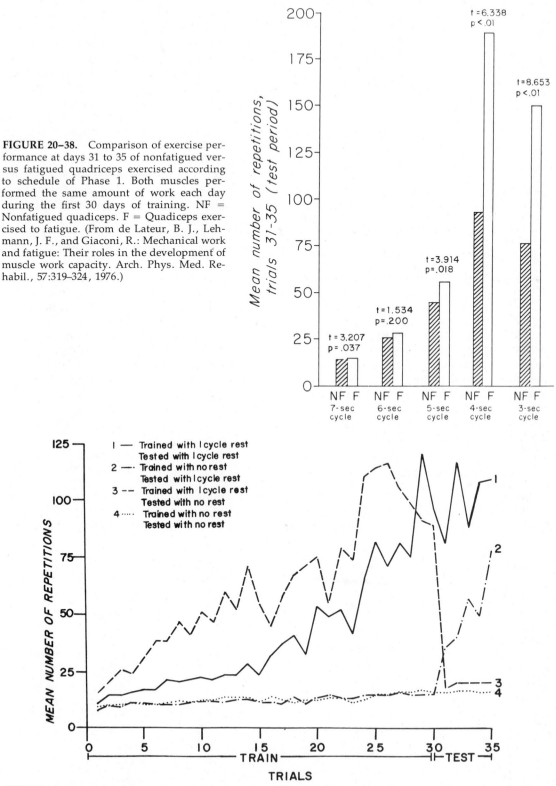

FIGURE 20–38. Comparison of exercise performance at days 31 to 35 of nonfatigued versus fatigued quadriceps exercised according to schedule of Phase 1. Both muscles performed the same amount of work each day during the first 30 days of training. NF = Nonfatigued quadiceps. F = Quadiceps exercised to fatigue. (From de Lateur, B. J., Lehmann, J. F., and Giaconi, R.: Mechanical work and fatigue: Their roles in the development of muscle work capacity. Arch. Phys. Med. Rehabil., 57:319–324, 1976.)

FIGURE 20–39. Comparison of exercise performance during training of quadriceps muscles with and without rest periods and during double-shift testing at days 31 to 35. Both rested and nonrested muscles were exercised to fatigue each day. (From de Lateur, B. J., Lehmann, J. F., and Giaconi, R.: Mechanical work and fatigue: Their roles in the development of muscle work capacity. Arch. Phys. Med. Rehabil., 57:319–324, 1976.)

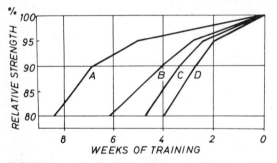

FIGURE 20–40. Weeks needed to reach limiting strength from an initial relative strength of 80 per cent: *A*, by submaximal training (one daily contraction at 65 per cent of maximum for one second); *B*, by standard training (one daily maximal contraction for one second); *C*, by one daily maximal contraction for 6 seconds; *D*, by multiple daily maximal contractions totaling 30 seconds in duration. (From Müller, E. A.: Influence of training and of inactivity on muscle strength. Arch. Phys. Med. Rehabil., 51:449–463, 1970.)

and thus had more mechanical work, did 21 per cent better than group four, which trained without a rest cycle but spent 917 per cent more time in training. Thus, it may be said that if time and willingness to spend it in training are not a limiting factor, pacing oneself to fatigue may be somewhat more *effective*, but going to fatigue without a rest cycle is much more *efficient*.[12]

Rate of Improvement and Rate of Loss

How much exercise provides optimal training and the fastest increases in strength and/or work capacity? The previously reported studies suggest that within wide limits, and provided there is no joint disease or tendinitis, the more exercise the better. Figure 20–40 shows that the time to reach the asymptote of "limiting strength" was less with heavier and more frequent isometric training.[52] Depending upon the previous state of training, Müller states that with maximal exercise the rate of increase may be 12 per cent/week. Rate of loss of strength, in the absence of any contraction of a muscle, is about 5 per cent/day (Fig. 20–41).

MacDougall et al. give somewhat different figures.[46] Following five to six months of heavy resistance training, increase of strength had averaged 5 per cent/week; after five to six weeks of immobilization in a cast, strength had decreased an average of 8 per cent/week. These apparent discrepancies between Müller and MacDougall can be reconciled if one recalls that the greatest increases with training and losses with immobilization occur early in the course, with subsequent leveling off. Moreover, isometric exercise within a cast against the resistance provided by the cast may retard the rate of loss of strength.

Isometric Programs

Brief isometric programs, as described by Hettinger and Müller[32] and others,[44, 58] have as advantages the fact that they can be done virtually anywhere, with no special equipment (using antagonistic muscles, for exam-

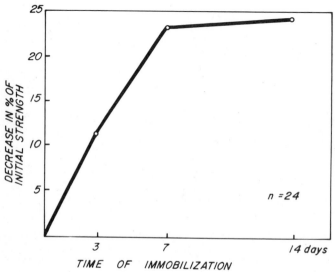

FIGURE 20–41. Observed decrease of strength per day of biceps of normal men when the arm was immobilized in a cast. (From Müller, E. A.: Influence of training and of inactivity on muscle strength. Arch. Phys. Med. Rehabil., 51:449–463, 1970.)

ple, as resistance), require very little time, and are highly effective in increasing isometric strength. However, since most activities in physical restoration and sport require some dynamic contractions (some of them quite rapid) it would be unwise to confine training only to isometric programs.

EQUIPMENT

Although exercise programs may be carried out with no special equipment at all, using only the force of gravity and the resistance of one's opposing muscles and/or ligaments, a wealth of equipment, ranging from simple to complex and from inexpensive to expensive, has become available.

In 1945 DeLorme described a technique of progressive resistive exercise that makes readily apparent use of the overload principle by literally increasing the load on the muscle.[14] (There are various ways to formulate the overload principle, some narrower and some broader. Very broadly, the overload principle holds that muscle performance cannot be improved unless the muscle is taxed beyond usual daily activity.) The distal part of the extremity moved by the muscle or muscle group to be trained is weighted in one of several ways. A typical method for the quadriceps involves the application of a quadriceps boot, sometimes called a DeLorme Boot, which is an iron "boot" (or full sole plate) with cross bar, iron weights of various sizes, collars and screws to hold weights on, and leather straps. Figure 20–42 shows a quadriceps

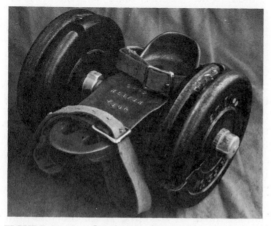

FIGURE 20–42. Quadriceps boot with crossbar and weights.

boot. At the beginning, and once a week thereafter, the 10 repetition maximum is determined. The daily program, then, consists of 10 repetitions (each repetition consisting of full extension of the knee of the seated subject) at each of several percentages of the 10 RM. A typical session would consist of 10 reps at 50 per cent, 10 at 75 per cent, and 10 at 100 per cent of the 10 RM. As strength increases, the 10 RM increases, and therefore the load is also increased.

It not infrequently happens that, because of the previous repetitions at 50 per cent and 75 per cent of the 10 RM, the subject is unable to carry out 10 reps at 100 per cent 10 RM. For this reason. Zinovieff et al. described a method which has been dubbed the "Oxford" technique.[76] All aspects are the same as the DeLorme technique except that during the exercise session, instead of starting with the lower weights and adding weight to reach 100 per cent of the 10 RM, the subject starts at 100 per cent and subsequently does 10 reps at 75 per cent and 10 reps at 50 per cent. In this way, the subject is less fatigued and is able to complete all of the prescribed repetitions. The results of the mechanical work versus fatigue study would suggest that the less fatigue is a training disadvantage rather than an advantage, but the critical transfer-of-training study of the "Oxford" technique versus the DeLorme technique remains to be done.

The Oxford and DeLorme techniques are highly effective, time-tested methods of strengthening muscle, but both have actual or potential disadvantages. One such disadvantage is that they are time-consuming, with the need to remove the collars from the bars or add or subtract weights and then replace the collars and tighten the screws. The problem of time consumption was even greater with earlier forms of the DeLorme technique, which involved 90 to 100 repetitions, 10 each at 10 per cent of the 10 RM, 30 per cent, 40 per cent, etc., to 100 per cent of the 10 RM.[15] This time-consumption is expensive in the use of therapist and patient time and is multiplied by the number of muscle groups studied. Another potential disadvantage of these techniques, applied to the seated subject attempting to strengthening his/her quadriceps, is that the force required to extend the knee in the early part of the range (e.g., between 90 and 80 degrees of flexion) is relatively small and becomes greater as the knee approaches full extension. (This illustrates the fact that most dynamic exercises are not correctly called isotonic.) This a purely mechanical factor and is quite distinct from the angle at which the muscle is *able* to exert maximal torque. To the extent that training is joint-angle specific, then the quadriceps will be undertrained in the early part of the range.

Several approaches have been made to the problems of time consumption and uniformity of training. One approach, used by the chapter author and others at the University of Washington hospitals, is to find a weight that the patient can lift three to five times and thereafter count repetitions to fatigue. So that the repetitions are a reliable measure of performance, they should be done to a metronome, raising the weighted limb on one beat and lowering it smoothly on the next. After the session when the patient reaches 30 repetitions, the weight is increased substantially, so that the patient reverts to the 3 to 5 RM range. Thus, the weight needs to be changed only once every several sessions instead of several times per session. Graph-

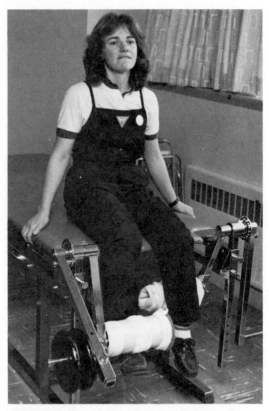

FIGURE 20–44. N-K table with the angle between load and lever arm set at 45 degrees.

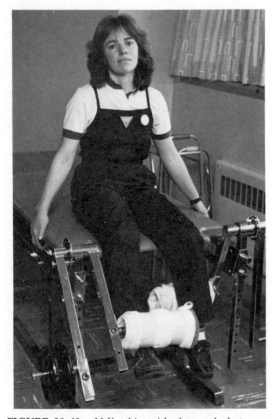

FIGURE 20–43. N-K table with the angle between load and lower arm set at 0 degrees.

ing repetitions is an easy way to record and reinforce progress in performance. This method helps reduce time consumption considerably, but does nothing about the problem of angle specificity during training.

Ankle and wrist cuff weights with Velcro closures can help with both problems to some extent. Whether used with the progressive resistive exercise (PRE) technique of DeLorme, with the Oxford technique, or with the author's technique, they will save time because of their rapidity of donning and doffing. They can help with the problem of undertraining of the early part of the range if the patient will add one set of repetitions in a different body position. For example, for the second set of quadriceps exercises, the patient could be supine, hip flexed 90 degrees, and take the weighted ankle from full knee flexion to full knee extension. This multiple-position exercise, however, increases the problem of time while helping with the problem of angle of training. Also, the maximal weight of the cuff is limited to about 20 lbs.

Another method to conserve time can be derived from the work of Hellebrandt, who

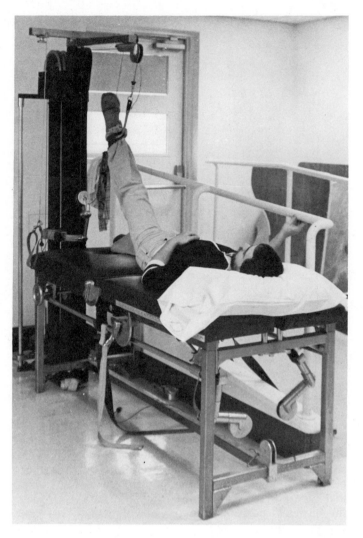

FIGURE 20–45. Exercising hip extension on an Elgin table.

showed that muscular performance could be improved by increasing the *rate* of training (rate of contraction) while keeping the load constant.[30] Thus, for example, a weight could be chosen which the patient can lift 10 to 20 times at the lowest metronome setting (raise on one beat; lower the weighted limb smoothly on the next beat). Thereafter, the load (weight) is kept the same, but each day the metronome setting is increased one notch. The patient carries out repetitions at this new *rate* to fatigue or 20, whichever is less. The problem of time is not only controlled but gets a bit better each day. To the author's knowledge, such a program is not widely used, but has much to recommend it, the chief drawback being possible annoyance of the tick-tock of the metronome.

The N-K table (Fig. 20–43) is a piece of equipment found in many physical therapy departments. It can help with the time and angle problems, to a limited extent. Weights can be added and removed rapidly, since a collar does not have to be used. Also, changing the angle between the load arm and lever arm (Fig. 20–44) will vary the angle of maximum load on the muscle. It will not, however, be a uniform load throughout the range.

The load *can* be kept uniform throughout the range by the use of pulleys or special cams. On the Elgin table, the load on the hip extensor (Fig. 20–45) or adductors (Fig. 20–46) is maintained nearly constant throughout their range. The single fixed pulley offers no mechanical (force) advantage, but does redirect the angle of pull. Thus, with a single fixed pulley, if a 10-pound weight is used, it requires a 10-pound force to lift or lower it at any point in the range.

At this point it should be recalled that the torque which can be exerted at any point throughout the range of motion is the net

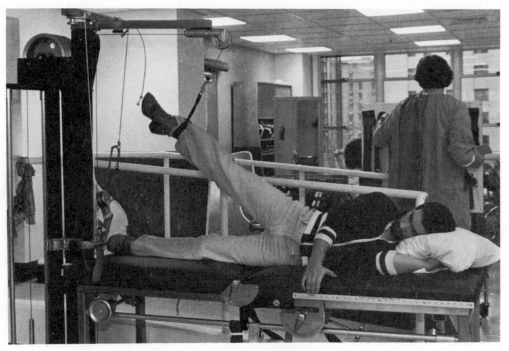

FIGURE 20–46. Exercising hip adduction on an Elgin table.

effect of the length-tension relationships and such mechanical factors as angle of application of the tendon of insertion, which vary independently. Figures 20–24 to 20–27 show variability of torque throughout the range for several muscle groups. Since the training effect upon a muscle depends not only upon load but upon the relationships of that load to the muscles' position of maximal voluntary contraction, a *constant* load will have a *variable* effect at different points in the range, having least effect where the muscle is capable of exerting the greatest torque. This complicates the angle-specificity problem further.

This angle-specificity problem is also addressed very well by the Cybex II isokinetic dynamometer, which limits the angular ve-

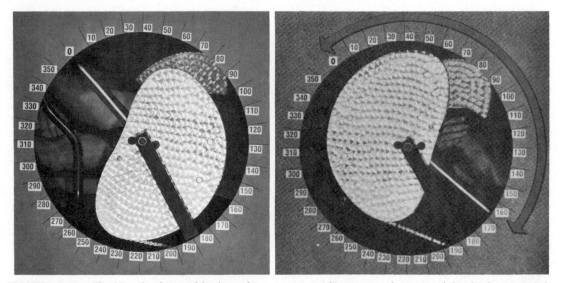

FIGURE 20–47. The Nautilus hip and back machine cam, providing range of motion of the thighs around the hips of about 160 degrees. (Photograph courtesy of Nautilus.)

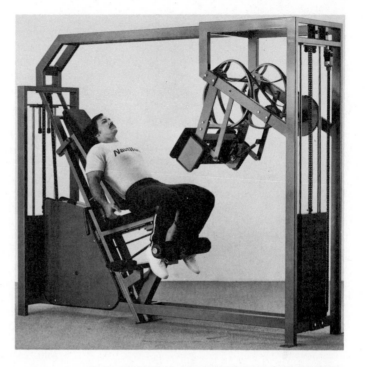

FIGURE 20–48. Nautilus compound leg machine, showing a subject performing a quadriceps extension. The upper portion of the apparatus is used to perform a compound leg press. (Photograph courtesy of Nautilus.)

locity of contraction (RPM; degrees/sec; radians/sec) to some preset rate that cannot be exceeded, no matter how forcefully the subject pushes against the lever arm. The device thus provides accommodating resistance that matches anything the muscle can produce (large or small) throughout the range.

The Nautilus system, so named because of somewhat fanciful resemblance of its special cam to a cross section of the sea creature of that name, thoughtfully addresses the problem of uniformity of load throughout the range (Figs. 20–47 and 20–48). Because of the variation of torque that the muscle can exert in various portions of the range, a constant load will not provide uniform stress to the muscle and therefore presumably not provide uniform training. The Nautilus equipment is responsive to this problem. The special cam varies the resistance to match the torque curve of each muscle group. Thus, variable resistance is used to provide uniformity of training throughout the range of motion. Because the resistance so closely matches the angle-specific torque capabilities of the muscle, the resistance subjectively feels uniform throughout the range. The Nautilus training program emphasizes slow, very forceful concentric and eccentric contractions, i.e., just to the right and to the left of isometrics on the force-velocity curve.

Cost of purchase and space required increase with the variety of Nautilus machines desired. At the time of this writing, the machines are more widely used in athletic departments or free-standing Nautilus programs than in hospital physical therapy departments.

The Cybex also addresses another problem, i.e., the specificity of rate of training. It was previously pointed out that force of contraction is dependent both upon muscular hypertrophy and upon "neural" factors, such as patterns of recruitment. Evidence was presented that the force-velocity curves can be altered to some extent and thus, if the task for which one is training requires quick movement, it would be wise to do at least some of the training at the higher RPM. The flexibility of this system allows the user to vary the program in many ways. He/she can, for example, begin training at slow RPM's and gradually increase the rate without the annoyance of the metronome accompanying Hellebrandt's and the author's systems. In contrast to any other system, the Cybex has the advantage that it automatically accommodates to any torque the muscle can produce at any rate of contraction. Also, the one system can be adapted to the various large muscle groups of the limbs. Immediate feedback and a permanent record of progress on moving graph paper may be obtained. At the time of this writing the price of the system, including recorder, but not including a work integrator, is about $17,000.

It may be noted that the proponents of the Nautilus and the Cybex systems use the same basis force-velocity curves to support the use of their respective systems, i.e., low-velocity, high-force versus high-velocity, lower-force training. Rather than viewing one system as superior to another, it may be wise to emphasize training specificity and to make the training as close as possible to the task for which one trains.

AEROBIC EQUIPMENT AND PHYSICAL DISABILITY

As has previously been mentioned, strength and local muscle endurance have been shown to be mathematically related over as large a range as 20 to 100 per cent of maximum contraction ability. However, improving the aerobic capacity of the individual requires prolonged low-level (left-hand portion of curve in Figure 20–16) reciprocal use of multiple muscle groups. There are many options (jogging, cycling, use of cycle ergometer, etc.) for able-bodied persons, but options for establishing a quantitative aerobic program for persons with lower-extremity physical disabilities, such as paraplegia, are more limited. A useful piece of equipment for persons with such disabilities is the Monark Rehab Trainer (Model No. 881, $810 as of this writing) (Fig. 20–49). This is a true ergometer, permitting quantification of work intensity (power) and total amount of external work accomplished and calories consumed. Programs with such equipment can be varied widely, but in order to improve aerobic capacity, a low enough intensity should be selected that the individual can continue for 20 to 30 minutes (less than 20 minutes may have insufficient training effect; greater than 30 minutes may be impractical owing to boredom and the expense of patient and therapist time). With improvement in training, the intensity can be increased.

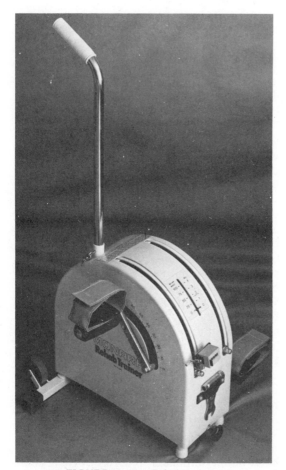

FIGURE 20–49. Rehab trainer.

REFERENCES

1. Abbott, B. C., Bigland, B., and Ritchie, J. M.: The physiological cost of negative work. J. Physiol., 117:380–390, 1952.
2. Arkin, A. M.: Absolute muscle power. The internal kinesiology of muscle. Research Seminar Notes, Dept. Orth. Surg., State U. of Iowa, 12D:123, 1938.
3. Asmussen, E., Hansen, O., and Lammert, O.: The relation between isometric and dynamic muscle strength in man. Comm. Dan. Natl. Assoc. Inf. Paral., 20:11, 1965.
4. Barnes, W. S.: The relationship between maximum isokinetic strength and isokinetic endurance. Res. Q., 51:714–717, 1980.
5. Bergström, J.: Muscle electrolytes in man. Scand. J. Clin. Invest., 14 (Suppl. 68):11–13, 1962.
6. Bethe, A., and Franke, F.: Beitrage zum Problem der willkurlich beweglichen Armprothesen. IV. Die Kraftkurven der indirekten naturlichen Energiequellen. Munch. Med. Wochenschr., 66:201–205, 1919.
7. Braune, W., and Fischer, O.: Die Rotationsmomente der Beugemuskeln am Ellbogengelenk des Menschen. Abh. Konigl. Sachs. Wissensch. Math. Phys. Klasse, Vol. 15, 1890.
8. Brunnstrom, S.: Clinical Kinesiology, 2nd Ed. Philadelphia, F. A. Davis, 1966.
9. Caiozzo, V. J., et al.: Training-induced alterations of *in vivo* force-velocity relationship of human muscle. J. Appl. Physiol., 51:750–754, 1981.

10. Close, R. I.: Dynamic properties of mammalian skeletal muscles. Physiol. Rev., 51:129–197, 1972.

11. de Lateur, B. J., Lehmann, J. F., and Fordyce, W. E.: A test of the DeLorme axiom. Arch. Phys. Med. Rehabil., 49:245–248, 1968.

12. de Lateur, B. J., Lehmann, J. F., and Giaconi, R.: Mechanical work and fatigue: Their roles in the development of muscle work capacity. Arch. Phys. Med. Rehabil., 57:319–324, 1976.

13. de Lateur, B. J., Lehmann, J., Stonebridge, J., and Warren, C. G.: Isotonic versus isometric exercises: A double-shift, transfer-of-training study. Arch. Phys. Med. Rehabil., 53:212–217, 1972.

14. DeLorme, T. L.: Restoration of muscle power by heavy resistance exercises. J. Bone Joint Surg., 27:645–667, 1945.

15. DeLorme, T. L., and Watkins, A. L.: Progressive Resistance Exercise. New York, Appleton-Century, Inc., 1951.

16. Desmedt, J. E., and Godaux, E.: Ballistic contractions in man: Characteristic recruitment pattern of single motor units of the tibialis anterior muscle. J. Physiol., 264:673–693, 1977.

17. Engel, W. K.: Selective and nonselective susceptibility of muscle fiber types. Arch. Neurol., 22:97–117, 1970.

18. Eriksson, O. N., Gollnick, P. D., and Saltin, B.: The effect of physical training on muscle enzyme activity and fiber composition in eleven-year-old boys. Acta Paed. Belg., 29 (Suppl):245–252, 1974.

19. Fick, R.: Anatomie und Mechanik der Gelenke. Teil III, Spezielle Gelenke und Muskelmechanik. Jena, Fischer, 1911.

20. Fugl-Meyer, A. R., Gustafsson, L., and Burstedt, Y.: Isokinetic and static plantar flexion characteristics. Eur. J. Appl. Physiol., 45:221–234, 1980.

21. Gollnick, P. D., Armstrong, R. B., Saltin, B., Saubert, C. W., IV, Sembrowich, W. L., and Shepherd, R. E.: Effect of training on enzyme activity and fiber composition of human skeletal muscle. J. Appl. Physiol., 34:107–111, 1973.

22. Gollnick, P. D., Armstrong, R. B., Saubert, C. W., IV, Piehl, K., and Saltin, B.: Enzyme activity and fiber composition in skeletal muscle of untrained and trained men. J. Appl. Physiol., 33:312–319, 1972.

23. Gollnick, P. D., Armstrong, R. B., Saubert, C. W., IV, Sembrowich, W. L., Shepherd, R. E., Saltin, B.: Glycogen depletion patterns in human skeletal muscle fibers during prolonged work. Pflügers Arch., 344:1–12, 1973.

24. Gollnick, P. D., Karlsson, J., Piehl, K., and Saltin, B.: Selective glycogen depletion in skeletal muscle fibers of man following sustained contractions. J. Physiol., 241:59–67, 1974.

25. Gollnick, P. D., Piehl, K., and Saltin, B.: Selective glycogen depletion pattern in human muscle fibers after exercise of varying intensity and at varying pedalling rates. J. Physiol., 241:45–57, 1974.

26. Gordon, E. E., Kowalski, K., and Fritts, M.: Protein changes in quadriceps muscle of rat with repetitive exercises. Arch. Phys. Med. Rehabil., 48:296–303, 1967.

27. Gregor, R. J., Edgerton, V. R., Perrine, J. J., Campion, D. S., and DeBus, C.: Torque-velocity relationships and muscle fiber composition in elite female athletes. J. Appl. Physiol., 47:388–392, 1979.

28. Guth, L.: "Trophic" influences of nerve on muscle. Physiol. Rev., 48:645–687, 1968.

29. Guth, L., Samaha, F. J., and Albers, R. W.: The neural regulation of some phenotypic differences between the fiber types of mammalian skeletal muscle. Exp. Neurol., 26:126–135, 1970.

30. Hellebrandt, F. A., and Houtz, S. J.: Methods of muscle training: The influence of pacing. Phys. Ther. Rev., 38:319–322, 1958.

31. Henneman, E.: Peripheral mechanisms involved in the control of muscle. In Mountcastle, V. B. (Ed.): Medical Physiology, 13th Ed. St. Louis, The C. V. Mosby Co., 1974, pp. 617–635.

32. Hettinger, T., and Müller, E. A.: Muskelleistung und Muskeltraining. Arbeitsphysiol., 15:111–126, 1970. Cited in Müller, E. A.: Influence of training and of inactivity on muscle strength. Arch. Phys. Med. Rehabil., 51:449–462, 1970.

33. Hickson, R. C.: Interference of strength development by simultaneously training for strength and endurance. Eur. J. Appl. Physiol., 45:255–263, 1980.

34. Hill, A. V.: Dynamic constants of human muscle, Proc. R. Soc. London, Series B, 128:263–274, 1940.

35. Hill, A. V.: The heat of shortening and dynamic constants of muscle. Proc. R. Soc. London, Series B, 126:136–195, 1938.

36. Ianuzzo, C. D.: The cellular composition of human skeletal muscle. In Knuttgen, H. G. (Ed.): Neuromuscular Mechanisms for Therapeutic and Conditioning Exercise. Baltimore, University Park Press, 1976, pp. 31–53.

37. Infante, A. A., Klaupiks, D., and Davies, R. E.: Length, tensions and metabolism during short isometric contraction of frog sartorius muscles. Biochim. Biophys. Acta, 88:215, 1964.

38. Kennedy, C., Van Huss, W. D., and Heusner, W. W.: Reversal of the energy metabolism responses to endurance training by weight loading. Percept. Motor Skills, 39:847–852, 1974.

39. Keul, J., Doll, E., and Keppler, D.: Energy Metabolism of Human Muscle. Medicine and Sport, Vol. 7. Baltimore, University Park Press, 1972.

40. Kidd, G., and Brodie, P.: The motor unit: A review. Physiotherapy, 66:146–152, 1980.

41. Knapik, J. J., and Ramos, M. U.: Isokinetic and isometric torque relationships in the human body. Arch. Phys. Med. Rehabil., 61:64–67, 1980.

42. Knuttgen, H. G.: Development of muscular strength and endurance. In Knuttgen, H. G. (Ed.): Neuromuscular Mechanisms for Therapeutic and Conditioning Exercises. Baltimore, University Park Press, 1976, pp. 97–118.

43. Kugelberg, E., and Edstrom, L.: Differential effects of muscle contractions on phosphorylase and glycogen types of fibers: Relation to fatigue. J. Neurol. Surg., Psychiatry, 31:415–423, 1968.

44. Liberson, W. T., and Asa, M. M.: Further studies of brief isometric exercises. Arch. Phys. Med. Rehabil., 40:330, 1959.

45. Lloyd, B. B.: World running records as maximal performances. Circ. Res., 20 and 21 (Suppl. I): I218–I226, 1967.

46. MacDougall, J. D., Elder, G. C. B., Sale, D. G., Moroz, J. R., and Sutton, J. R.: Effect of training and immobilization on human muscle fibers. Eur. J. Appl. Physiol., 43:25–34, 1980.

47. Maton, B.: Fast and slow motor units. Their recruitment for tonic and phasic contraction in man. Eur. J. Appl. Physiol., 43:45–55, 1980.

48. Milner-Brown, H. S., Stein, R. B., and Lee, R. G.: Synchronization of human motor units: Possible roles of exercise and supraspinal reflexes. E. E. G. Clin. Neurophysiol., 38:245–254, 1975.

49. Moffroid, M. T., and Whipple, R. H.: Specificity of speed of exercise. Phys. Ther., 50:1692–1700, 1970.

50. Monod, H., and Scherrer, J.: Capacité de travail statique d'un group musculaire synergique chez l'homme. CR soc. biol., 151:1358–1362, 1957. Cited in Simonson, E. (Ed.): Physiology of Work Capacity and Fatigue. Springfield, Ill., Charles C Thomas, Publisher, 1971, pp. 440–442.

51. Moritani, T., and de Vries, H. K.: Neural factors versus hypertrophy in the time course of muscle strength gain. Am. J. Phys. Med., 58:115–130, 1979.

52. Müller, E. A.: Influence of training and of inactivity on muscle strength. Arch. Phys. Med. Rehabil., 51:449–462, 1970.

53. Mundale, M. O.: The relationship of intermittent isometric exercise to fatigue of hand grip. Arch. Phys. Med. Rehabil., 51:532–539, 1970.

54. Mundale, M. O.: The relationship of isometric grip strength to isometric grip endurance. M. S. Thesis, University of Minnesota, Minneapolis, 1964.

55. Perrine, J. J., and Edgerton, V. R.: Muscle force-velocity relationships under isokinetic load. Med. Sci. Sports, 10:159–166, 1978.

56. Ramsey, R. W., and Street, S. F.: Isometric length-tension diagram of isolated skeletal muscle fibers in frog. J. Cell Comp. Physiol., 15:11–34, 1940.

57. Rohmert, W.: Ermittlung von Erholungspausen für statische Arbeit des Menschen. Int. Z. Angew. Physiol., 18:123–164, 1960. Cited in Simonson, E. (Ed.): Physiology of Work Capacity and Fatigue. Springfield, Ill., Charles C Thomas, Publisher, 1971.

58. Rose, D. L., Radzyminski, S. J., and Beatty, R. R.: Effect of brief maximal exercise on the strength of the quadriceps femoris. Arch. Phys. Med. Rehabil., 38:157–164, 1957.

59. Saltin, B., and Åstrand, P. O.: Maximal oxygen uptake in athletes. J. Appl. Physiol., 23:353–358, 1967.

60. Samaha, F. J., Guth, L., and Albers, R. W.: The neural regulation of gene expression in the muscle cell. Exp. Neurol., 27:276–282, 1970.

61. Samaha, F. J., Guth, L., and Albers, R. W.: Differences between slow and fast muscle myosin. J. Biol. Chem., 245:219–224, 1970.

62. Scherrer, J., and Bourguignon, A.: Changes in the electromyogram produced by fatigue in man. Am. J. Phys. Med., 38:148–158, 1959.

63. Schottelius, B. A., and Senay, L. C., Jr.: Effect of stimulation-length sequence on shape of length-tension diagram. Am. J. Physiol., 186:127–130, 1956.

64. Scudder, G. N.: Torque curves produced at the knee during isometric and isokinetic exercise. Arch. Phys. Med. Rehabil., 61:68–73, 1980.

65. Seliger, V., Dolejs, L., and Karas, V.: A dynamometric comparison of maximum eccentric, concentric and isometric contractions using EMG and energy expenditure measurements. Eur. J. Appl. Physiol., 45:235–244, 1980.

66. Shaver, L. G.: Maximum dynamic strength, relative dynamic endurance and their relationships. Res. Q., 42:460–465, 1971.

67. Simonson, E.: Recovery and fatigue. In Simonson, E. (Ed.): Physiology of Work Capacity and Fatigue. Springfield, Ill., Charles C Thomas, Publisher, 1971, pp. 440–458.

68. Smith, M. J., and Melton, P.: Isokinetic versus isotonic variable resistance training. Am. J. Sports Med., 9:275–279, 1981.

69. Soule, R. G.: Physiological response to physical exercise. In Knuttgen, H. G. (Ed.): Neuromuscular Mechanisms for Therapeutic and Conditioning Exercise. Baltimore, University Park Press, 1976, pp. 79–96.

70. Steindler, A.: Kinesiology of the Human Body. Springfield, Ill., Charles C Thomas, Publisher, 1955.

71. Thorstensson, A. G., Grimby, G., and Karlsson, J.: Force-velocity relations and fiber composition in human knee extensor muscle. J. Appl. Physiol., 40:12–16, 1976.

72. Tuttle, W. W., Janney, C. D., and Thompson, C. W.: Relationship of maximum grip strength to grip strength endurance. J. Appl. Physiol., 2:663–670, 1950.

73. Von Recklinghausen, H.: Gliedermechanik und Lahmungsprothesen. Berlin, J. Springer, 1920.

74. Wells, J. B.: Comparison of mechanical properties between slow and fast mammalian muscles. J. Physiol., 178:252–269, 1965.

75. Wilkie, D. V.: The relation between force and velocity in human muscle. J. Physiol., 110:249–280, 1950.

76. Zinovieff, A. N.: Heavy-resistance exercises; the "Oxford technique." Br. J. Phys. Med., 14:129–132, 1951.

21

BED POSITIONING

PAUL M. ELLWOOD, JR.

The prevention and treatment of contractures and decubiti through an effective bed positioning program is contingent upon proper equipment, a well-trained and well-motivated nursing staff, and appropriate physician's orders.

THE POSITIONING PRESCRIPTION

The positioning prescription should identify the equipment specifically needed for the positioning program, positions to be used, motions and positions to be avoided, and frequency of turning. In addition, it is important to recognize that the patient should assume increasing responsibility for his positioning program. If he is able, the patient should remind the staff when he needs to be turned, know where positioning equipment is kept, actually assist in changing positions, and ultimately assume full responsibility.

THE EQUIPMENT FOR EFFECTIVE BED POSITIONING

High-Low Bed. The use of beds that are adjustable to high (30 inches including the mattress) and low (20 inches including mattress) positions is recommended. With the bed in the high position, more comfortable and efficient nursing care and range of motion exercises can be carried out. In the low position, the bed can be set at the ideal height for wheelchair transfers or crutch walking.

Bed Boards. A ¾-inch plywood bed board equal in size to the spring frame is bolted between the spring and mattress (Fig. 21–1). Jointed (Gatch) features can be retained by breaking the continuity of the board at the hinge points. Some hospital beds now have a metal panel that substitutes for springs and provides excellent mattress support. Also available are slatted bed boards, which have the advantage of flexibility.

Mattresses. Firmness and durability are sought in mattress selection. Uniform firm support is obtained through a foam rubber mattress. A 4-inch foam rubber mattress made of 34 pound compression ratio material is the firmest available. Urethane foam of the same compression ratio is still undergoing evaluation for rehabilitation uses. The firm support provided by bed board and mattress is especially valuable in preventing hip flexion contractues.

Footboards. Heel cord contractures are prevented by the use of a footboard. It has been suggested, but not proved, that the footboard provides a valuable source of sensory input to the plantar surface of the feet so that the desirable extensor reflex dominance is maintained and the neuron networks normally involved in the standing position are activated. The board should be ½-inch thick and sufficiently high to keep the bed clothes from contact with the toes. To prevent decubiti over the posterior calcaneus and to facilitate prone positioning without knee flexion, the board is blocked 4 inches away from the end of the mattress (Fig. 21–2).

465

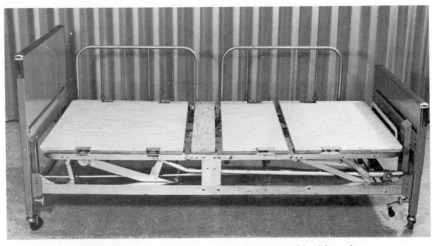

FIGURE 21–1. Three-quarter inch plywood bed board.

Short Side Rails. Side rails are used for safety, moving about, coming to a sitting position, and transferring in and out of bed (Fig. 21–3). Commercial short side rails are 33 inches long and should extend 11 inches above the level of the mattress. For most patients, the rails are attached only to the head end of the bed. If side rails are not required for protection, a single short rail is attached at the head end of the bed on the patient's stronger side to which he transfers.

Overhead Trapezes. Trapezes are rarely necessary to facilitate moving about in bed or for upper extremity exercise. In making unassisted transfers, they are not as useful as short side rails. They do simplify nursing care of very large patients or those in casts.

Positioning Frames (Foster, Stryker, and Others). When immobility of the spine is required, a bed consisting of canvas stretched on anterior and posterior frames that can be rotated along their long axes is used. Footboards for frames are often available and should be used. The narrow metal-rimmed canvas surface of the frame can be satisfactorily padded with 1 inch foam rubber covered with plastic. The foam rubber for the trunk section of the prone unit should be wider than the metal frame to protect the shoulders from pressure when the patient's

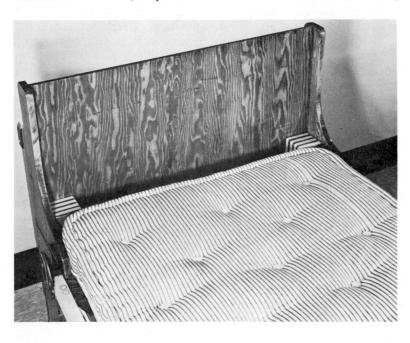

FIGURE 21–2. Foot board.

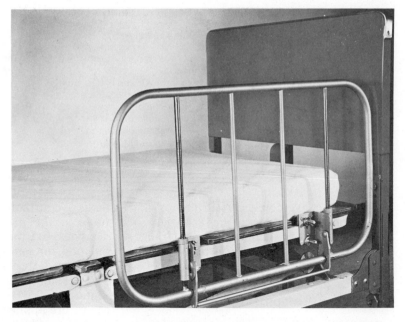

FIGURE 21–3. Short side rail.

arms are dropped downward for eating or reading. The foam rubber of the lower extremity section of the prone unit should be slightly longer than the canvas frame to protect the front of the patient's ankles. The foam rubber pieces of the supine section should cover the canvas to protect the patient's sacral area when using the bed pan. Arm boards are available for positioning the upper extremities of the quadriplegic patient.

Powered Rotating Frames. Electrically powered frames that rotate along their short axes can be used to substitute for both canvas frames and standing beds. They permit more comfortable positioning and changes in position by the patient or a single staff member by the operation of remote control switches. They are costly, however, and because of their complexity are more subject to mechanical failure.

Standing Beds. Electrically or manually controlled beds to elevate patients to the upright position are thought to aid in the reduction of osteoporosis and renal calculi, the maintenance of vascular tone (thus preventing postural hypotension), preservation of morale, and the shifting of weight-bearing to relieve pressure in other areas. Postural hypotension owing to pooling in splanchnic and lower extremity veins is prevented in part by the use of scultetus binders and by wrapping the legs with 6-inch elastic bandages. Blood pressure should be taken at frequent intervals by the attendant. No pa-

tient on a standing bed should be left unattended. Many patients cannot attain the upright position on the first occasion on the standing bed. A useful routine is to begin at 30 degrees for 30 minutes. When this is readily tolerated, increase by 5- to 10-degree increments. Binders and bandages are progressively eliminated after the patient attains 80 degrees.

Small Positioning Devices. Most quadriplegic patients will require two trochanter rolls, two shoulder rolls, three hand rolls, two small pillows, six large pillows, 6-inch-wide canvas straps and, in the presence of lower extremity abduction spasticity, a 6-inch-wide canvas strap lined with soft leather. The application of these devices is described later in this chapter.

THE POSITIONING PROGRAM

Positioning instructions and turning schedules are based on individual patient needs, but certain generalizations can be made about most disabilities that are associated with muscle weakness or joint deformity. In some institutions that serve large numbers of the chronically disabled, it has been found desirable to establish a set of positioning procedures for hemiplegia, quadriplegia, and paraplegia. The physician's order then may specify variations from the routine positioning procedure, positions to be avoided, and areas to be kept immobilized. Positions are

TABLE 21–1. SOME COMMON DEFORMING FORCES

Force	Resultant Deformity	Method of Prevention
Gravity	Sagging mattress and springs + gravity = hip flexion contractures	Firm mattress plus bed board, prone position, prone cart
Shape of the extremity surface	Configuration of the ankle and foot + gravity = external rotation of the lower extremity and a tight gastrocnemius	A trochanter roll and footboard
Muscular imbalance	High, above-knee, amputation + strong hip abductors = hip abduction contracture	Prone position with leg adducted and internally rotated
Spasticity	Paraplegia + flexor spasticity = hip and knee flexion contractures	Prone position, buttocks plus knees strapped in extension, prone cart, knee lockers during gait training

prescribed to overcome certain natural and pathologic forces, to provide a variety of joint positions for maintaining joint range, and to place the extremity in a more functional position (Table 21–1).

The Supine Position

Lower Extremities. The feet are positioned with the entire plantar surface firmly against the footboard. Contact with the posterior heel is avoided by placing it in the space between the mattress and the footboard which has been created by 4-inch-thick blocks. The legs are placed in a neutral position with the toes pointed toward the ceiling (Fig. 21–4). This position is maintained by friction of the feet against the footboard and a cloth roll placed under the greater trochanter (trochanter roll).

The knee and hips are positioned in extension (Fig. 21–5). Perhaps the most critical element of the lower extremity positioning program is the prevention of hip and knee flexion contractures. Hip flexion contractures in the presence of lower extremity weakness are the principal deterrents to ambulation for patients with hemiplegia, paraplegia, and above-knee amputations. Stance phase stability of the knee and hip joints requires full extension so that gravitational forces are applied against ligaments and the normal configuration of the joint rather than requiring muscle power.

Upper Extremities. Nurses should be cautioned to position only within the painless or nonresistive range of motion. Spasticity must, however, be differentiated from other forms of resistance to joint motion.

POSITION 1. The shoulder is abducted to 90 degrees and slightly internally rotated, the elbow is at 90 degrees, and the forearm is partially pronated (Fig. 21–6).

POSITION 2. The shoulder is abducted to 90 degrees or more and externally rotated to the greatest degree compatible with comfort. The elbow is flexed at 90 degrees and the forearm is pronated (Fig. 21–7).

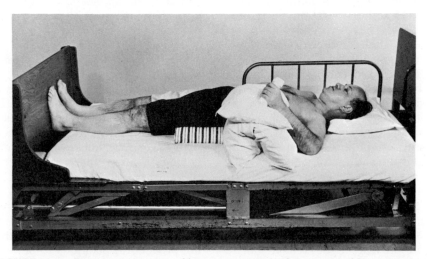

FIGURE 21–4. Routine positioning of lower extremities, plus one possible arm position.

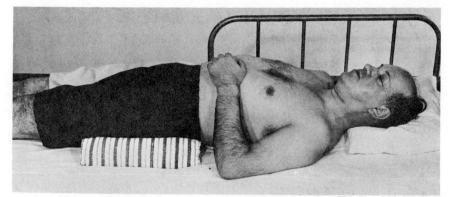

FIGURE 21–5. Use of trochanter roll in positioning of lower extremities.

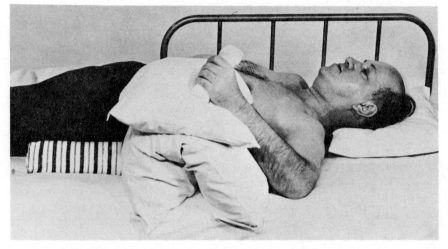

FIGURE 21–6. Positioning of the upper extremities, position 1.

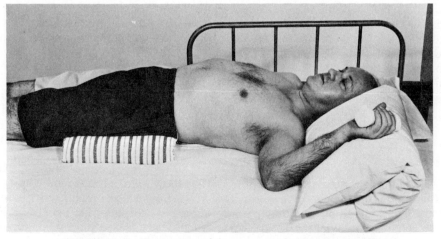

FIGURE 21–7. Positioning of the upper extremities, position 2.

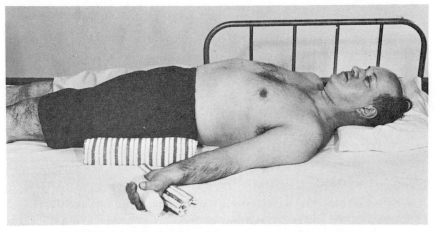

FIGURE 21–8. Positioning of the upper extremities, position 3.

POSITION 3. The shoulder is in slight abduction, the elbow extended, and the forearm supinated (Fig. 21–8).

Wrist and Hand

POSITION 1. The wrist is extended, the fingers are partially flexed at the interphalangeal and metacarpal phalangeal joints, and the thumb is abducted, opposed, and slightly flexed at the interphalangeal joint (Fig. 21–9). Maintenance of these positions is facilitated by the use of a hand roll (Fig. 21–10).

POSITION 2. This position is similar to position 1 except that the fingers are extended at the interphalangeal and metacarpal phalangeal joints. A palmar positioning splint can be used to maintain this position (Fig. 21–11). The positioning program for the wrist and fingers should be particularly directed to *maintenance of joint motion of the wrist* from neutral to a fully extended position, *a full range of motion in the metacarpal phalangeal joints*, flexion of the interphalangeal joints, and opposition of the thumb. To obtain tenodesis grasp in the quadriplegic patient who retains wrist extensor function, arthrodesis of thumb joints and interphalangeal joints to form a three-jawed chuck may be sought.

Side-Lying Position

Hemiplegic patients are most comfortable lying on their uninvolved side. Paraplegics and quadriplegics should be positioned on either side when they can tolerate it. The top leg is placed in a position of flexion at the hip

and knee. Through use of pillows, contact with the under leg is avoided. The inner (bottom) arm is externally rotated and partially extended. The outer (top) arm is kept away from the patient's chest (Fig. 21–12).

The Prone Position

The prone position is ordered when pulmonary, cardiac, and skeletal status permit. Many patients do not tolerate it well at first. It is highly advantageous in maintaining full extension of the hips and relieving pressure over vulnerable posterior bony prominences that so commonly are sites of decubiti. The prone position also has its vulnerable points such as the skin over the sternum, the iliac spines, the patella, and the dorsum of the foot. These areas should be inspected frequently. Foam rubber can be used above and below the contact points when pressure is producing focal ischemia. Synthetic fibers or sheepskin are also useful to protect the bony prominences. Narrow doughnut-shaped devices should *not* be used. They actually inhibit circulation to ischemic areas.

The prone position (Fig. 21–13) is simply one of good alignment with hips and knees extended. Toes should not be allowed to touch the footboard. The feet can be elevated slightly using a trochanter roll under the anterior ankle.

The arm is abducted slightly, extended at the elbow, and extended and supinated at the wrist. Finger flexion and wrist extension are achieved through the use of a hand roll. Shoulder rolls are placed lengthwise under each shoulder.

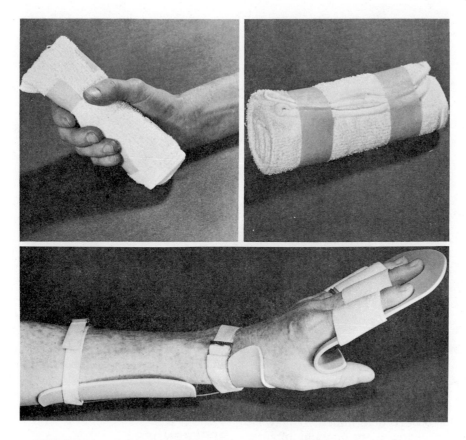

FIGURE 21–9. Positioning of the wrist and hand, position 1.

FIGURE 21–10. Hand roll for use in wrist and hand positioning.

FIGURE 21–11. Palmar positioning splint for use in wrist and hand positioning, position 2.

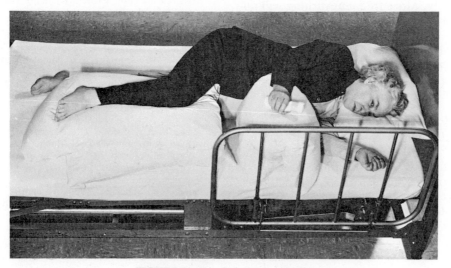

FIGURE 21–12. Side-lying position.

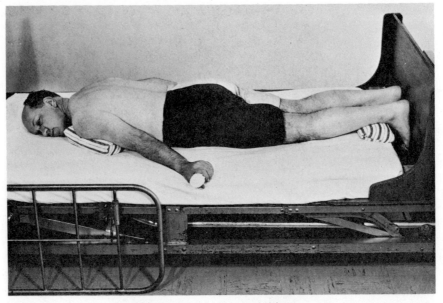

FIGURE 21–13.   Prone position.

FREQUENCY OF TURNING

Turning the patient every two hours is usually a safe routine to follow until the patient's skin sensitivity and tolerance of the positions have been determined. It may be necessary to decrease the amount of time spent in certain positions or it may be found that time in other positions can be increased to two and a half or three hours. Generally it is best to order the more prolonged positioning periods for the night hours, thus lessening the amount of turning at night and enabling the patient to sleep more satisfactorily. More frequent turning will automatically be needed during the day to allow for the desired positions for the patient's daily activities. Nursing staff should be encouraged to set up a definite schedule so that the patient will be in a proper position for activities (such as supine for physical therapy).

The physician should frequently check the skin in vulnerable areas to make certain that no decubiti are developing and to emphasize to the attending staff the importance of a proper turning schedule. Increased activities in the use of various appliances should call attention to new possible areas of ischemic ulceration. The patient who is spending a great deal of time in a wheelchair should have particularly close observation for possible ischemia in the region of the ischial tuberosities.

REFERENCES

1. Coles, C. H., and Bergstrom, D. A.: Bed Positioning Procedures. Minneapolis, American Rehabilitation Foundation, 1969.
2. Elson, R.: Practical Management of Spinal Injuries for Nurses. Baltimore, Williams & Wilkins Company, 1965.
3. Hicks, D., Scarlisi, S., Woody, F., and Skinner, B.: Increasing upper extremity function. Am. J. Nurs., 64:8:69–73, 1964.
4. Hirshberg, G., Lewis, L., and Thomas, D.: Rehabilitation: A Manual for the Care of the Disabled and Elderly. Philadelphia, J. B. Lippincott Co., 1964.
5. Kosiak, M.: Etiology and pathology of ischemic ulcers. Arch. Phys. Med., 40:1:62–69, 1959.
6. Kosiak, M.: Etiology of decubitus ulcers. Arch. Phys. Med., 42:1:19–29, 1961.
7. Larson, C., and Gould, M.: Orthopedic Nursing. St. Louis, the C. V. Mosby Co., 1970.
8. Strike Back at Stroke. U.S. Department of Health, Education and Welfare, Public Health Service Publication No. 596. U.S. Government Printing Office, Washington, D.C. 20201, 1960.
9. Sverdlik, S. S., and Chantraine, A.: A spongy cushion over hypersensitive areas of the skin to increase threshold to pain. Arch. Phys. Med., 45:1:430–432, 1964.

22

TRANSFERS — METHOD, EQUIPMENT, AND PREPARATION

PAUL M. ELLWOOD, JR.

A transfer is a pattern of movements by which the patient moves from one surface to another. This chapter is limited to a discussion of transfers to and from wheelchairs, since these are the earliest and most common types of transfer for the patient with neuromuscular disability. The ingredients of safe and efficient transfers are a combination of physical and perceptual capacities, proper equipment, and techniques that are suited to the patient's abilities. Firm, stable surfaces for the patient to move to and from are required for all transfers. It is also necessary that the patient have the ability to learn motor skills.

ASSISTED TRANSFERS

Techniques for assisted transfers are not demonstrated in this chapter. However, assistance by another person for physical support and reinforcement of learning may be required during early learning, or permanently for more severely disabled patients. In an assisted transfer, the same general techniques are used, with the assistant compensating for the patient's inabilities. Providing support at the waist with a transfer belt assures a good grip on the patient without restricting him from using his arms (Fig. 22–1).

STANDING TRANSFERS

Physical Requirements. The unassisted standing transfer requires good sitting balance without postural hypotension; the ability to maintain the hip and knee in a position of extension by means of voluntary muscle contraction, long leg braces, or extensor spasticity; reasonably strong shoulder depressors and adductors, elbow flexors and extensors; and, preferably, hand and wrist function on one side.

Preparing the Patient for Standing Transfers. Activities helpful in preparation for standing transfers are sitting on the edge of the bed without making a transfer; daily use of the standing bed, followed by actual standing at the parallel bar and practice in locking the knee; exercises designed to strengthen hip and knee extensors, shoulder depressors and adductors, and elbow and wrist extensors on the normal side; and mat work and bed activities to improve the ability to roll, balance, and shift weight.

The author is indebted to the staff of Sister Kenny Institute for the preparation of photographs and drawings used in this chapter.

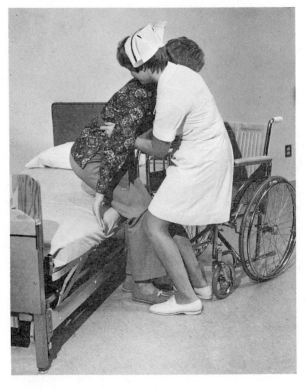

FIGURE 22–1. Using a belt around the patient's waist, the nurse assists her in a standing transfer.

Teaching Transfers. The process of teaching the patient to make a transfer with assistance is begun as soon as he is able to balance in the sitting position. Patients should be taught in short sequences and they should master each step before proceeding to the next. Even patients with no verbal language can be taught to transfer by repetition and demonstration. Visual motor-perceptual defects may prevent motor learning.

Technique. Most transfers are made toward the more normal or stronger side, regardless of the cause of the disability. This text uses as an example a hemiplegic patient, but the principles set forth apply to any patient who can attain a stable standing position during the course of his transfer.

BED TO WHEELCHAIR TRANSFER

Equipment. The necessary equipment includes a stable bed approximately the same height as the wheelchair (a short side rail attached at the head end of the bed is optional) and a wheelchair with brakes and detachable footrests. For the hemiplegic patient, the footrest on the normal side should be removed.

Layout. The wheelchair is on the patient's normal side; it is slightly angled toward the foot of the bed for the transfer out of bed (Fig. 22–2) and toward the head of the bed for the transfer into bed. The footrest adjacent to the bed is removed or swung aside.

Coming to a Sitting Position. The patient begins the sequence lying in the center of the bed. With her normal hand, she picks up her involved arm at the wrist and places the forearm across her abdomen (Fig. 22–3).

The patient places her normal foot under the knee of her involved leg and slides her foot down the leg to her ankle. She then partly flexes and lifts her involved leg with her normal foot and leg. Keeping the same foot-support position, she grasps the side rail with her normal hand and, rolling her legs toward her normal side, turns onto her side (Fig. 22–4).

Then, as she moves her legs over the edge of the bed, the patient grasps and pulls on the side rail and swings herself to a sitting position (Fig. 22–5). She makes full use of gravity and momentum by performing these motions in one unit. She then uncrosses her feet and places them firmly on the floor to maintain balance.

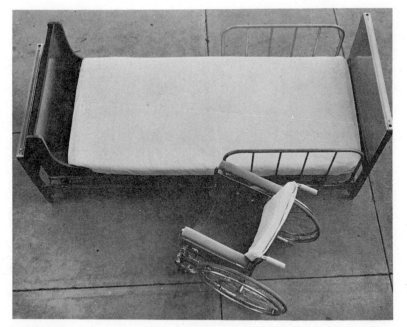

FIGURE 22–2. Position of the wheelchair for the standing transfer out of bed.

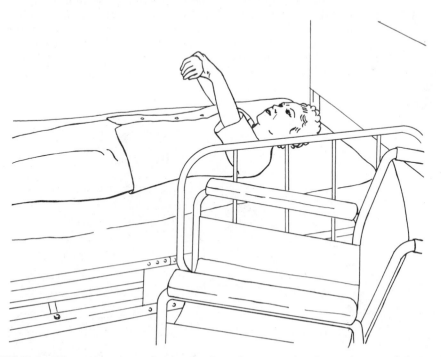

FIGURE 22–3. The patient moves her involved arm in preparation for coming to a sitting position.

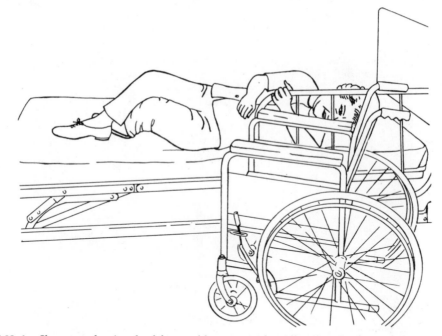

FIGURE 22–4. She moves her involved foot and leg, grasps the side rail, and turns onto her normal side.

Coming to a Standing Position and Completing the Transfer. From her sitting position at the edge of the bed, the patient locks the brakes on both sides of the wheelchair, locking the rear brake first. By leaning her trunk forward and pushing down at the same time with her normal hand and foot, she moves forward toward the edge of the bed. She then flexes her normal knee more than 90 degrees and moves her normal foot slightly behind the involved foot so that her feet will be free to pivot. Grasping the side rail (or the middle of the farther armrest of the wheelchair if balance is poor), the patient is now in a position for standing (Fig. 22–6).

She moves her trunk forward, pushes

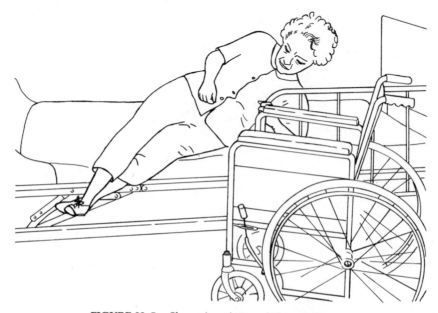

FIGURE 22–5. She swings into a sitting position.

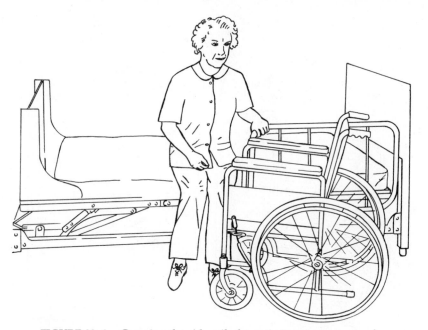

FIGURE 22–6. Grasping the side rail, the patient prepares to stand.

down with her normal arm, and, bearing most of her weight on the normal leg, comes to a standing position (Fig. 22–7).

She moves her hand to the middle of the far arm of the wheelchair and pivots on her feet, bringing herself into a position to sit down (Fig. 22–8). After sitting down in the chair, she adjusts her sitting position, unlocks the brakes, lifts her involved foot with her normal foot, and backs the wheelchair away from the bed. Finally the patient swings tne footrest into position and, lifting her involved leg with her normal hand, places her foot on the footrest.

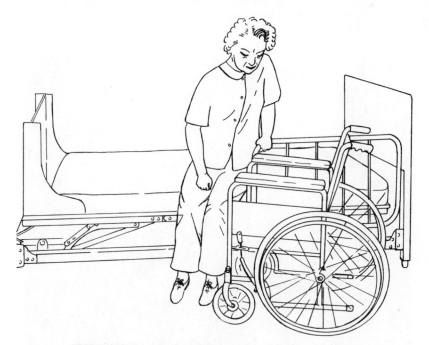

FIGURE 22–7. The patient comes to a standing position.

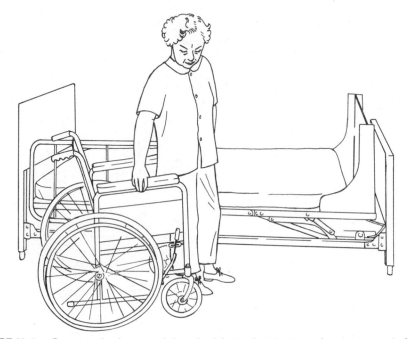

FIGURE 22–8. Grasping the far arm of the wheelchair, she pivots, and prepares to sit down.

The Standing Transfer from Wheelchair to Low Bed

Again, the transfer is made toward the normal side. The wheelchair faces the head of the bed (Fig. 22–9). After locking the brakes and taking her involved foot off the footrest, the patient swings the footrest out of the way. By leaning forward and pushing down, she moves forward toward the edge of the wheelchair until her feet are under her and her normal foot is slightly behind the involved foot. Holding onto the wheelchair armrest (or the side rail), the patient moves her trunk forward and, bearing her weight on her normal leg and arm, comes to a standing position. After standing erect, she moves her hand to the side rail and pivots on her feet,

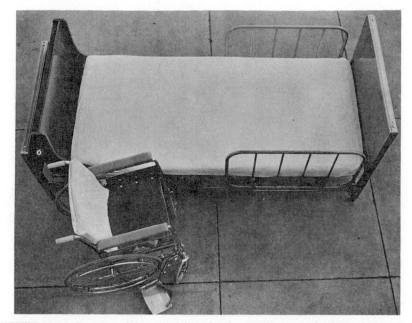

FIGURE 22–9. Position of the wheelchair for the standing transfer from chair to bed.

FIG. 22–10

FIG. 22–11

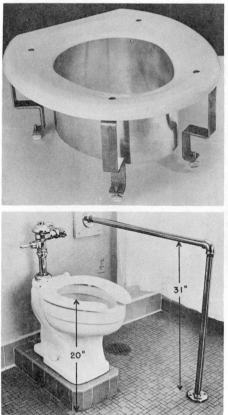

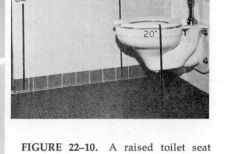

FIG. 22–12

FIGURE 22–10. A raised toilet seat attached to the toilet bowl facilitates transfer.

FIGURE 22–11. Position of the 45-degree angle handrail at the toilet for transfers.

FIGURE 22–12. Position of the right-angle handrail at the toilet.

bringing herself into a position to sit on the bed. Seated on the edge of the bed, she moves the wheelchair away so that she can swing her legs onto the bed and lie down.

Standing Transfer from Wheelchair to Toilet

A special requirement for an unassisted toilet transfer is that the patient be able to manage his clothing.

Equipment. Preferably, the toilet seat is mounted 20 inches from the floor. Raised seats that can be fastened securely to the toilet bowl are available from hospital supply companies (Fig. 22–10). The placement of a handrail generally depends on the position of the toilet in relationship to the side walls of the bathroom. The rail should be on the same side as the normal extremities when the patient is seated on the toilet. It is mounted on the wall at a 45-degree angle with the lower part of the bar placed 2 inches behind the leading edge of the toilet (Fig. 22–11). The length of the bar may vary from 15 to 35

inches. If for any reason the handrail cannot be attached to the wall beside the toilet, a right-angle rail may be bolted on the floor and wall (Fig. 22–12). The right-angle rail should extend 6 inches in front of the leading edge of the toilet.

Layout. The chair is angled with the patient's normal side adjacent to the toilet.

Transfer Procedure. After locking the brakes and removing her foot from the footrest, the patient swings the footrest out to the side (the clothing may be loosened at this time). Pushing down on the armrest with her normal hand, she moves forward in the chair, leans forward (Fig. 22–13), bearing most of her weight on her normal leg, and rises from the chair. Most of her lifting power should come from her normal leg. When standing, she uses the handrail to keep her balance and pivots on her feet until she is standing in front of the toilet (Fig. 22–14). Clothing is lowered and she sits down on the toilet.

To transfer from the toilet to the wheelchair, she reverses the procedure.

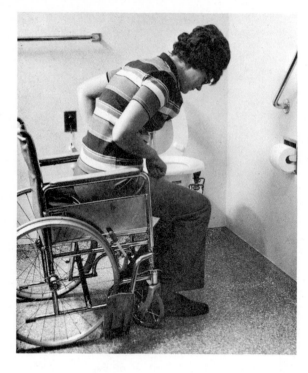

FIGURE 22–13. The patient has locked her wheelchair brakes, swung the footrest out of the way, and moved to the edge of the chair.

FIGURE 22–14. She pushes on the armrest to stand and reaches to the wall rail for support while turning and sitting down.

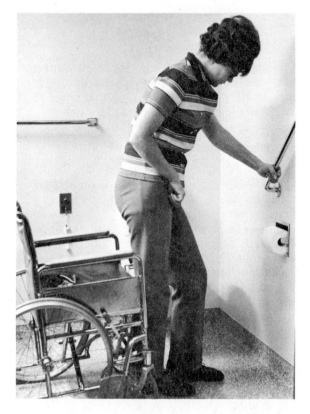

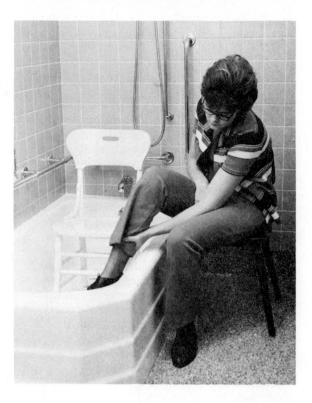

FIGURE 22–15. The patient places her involved leg in the tub.

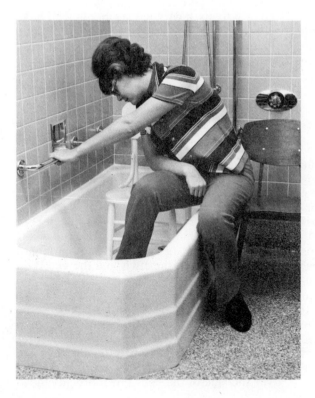

FIGURE 22–16. Using the wall rail for support, she slides onto the tub chair. She then moves her normal leg into the tub.

Bathtub Transfer

Getting in and out of the bathtub can be one of the most dangerous procedures for the patient and should always be supervised. Unlike most transfers, which should be made toward the patient's normal side, a tub transfer may be made toward either side, whichever is easiest for the patient.

Layout. A firm wooden chair should be placed beside the tub and another in the tub. These are used until the patient gains enough strength and confidence in his ability to transfer to a 9-inch or 5-inch stool or to the bottom of the tub. The legs of the chair placed in the tub should be shortened so that the seats of both chairs are the same height as the edge of the tub. Rubber tips attached to the bottom of the chair legs on the shorter chair protect the tub and prevent the chair from slipping. A shampoo hose is attached to the faucet. Safety tread tape is used in addition to a bath mat. The bath mat covers the rough surface of the tape and the tape keeps the mat from moving.

Transfer Technique. Pushing down on the chair seat with her normal hand, and on the floor with her normal leg, the patient moves to the edge of the chair and onto the edge of the tub. Then she picks up her involved leg with her normal hand and places it in the tub (Fig. 22–15).

Again pushing down with her normal arm and leg and using the wall handrail for support, she slides onto the chair in the tub (Fig. 22–16). She then lifts her normal leg into the tub.

SITTING TRANSFERS

There are three basic types of sitting transfers: a lateral sliding transfer requiring the use of a sliding board to bridge the space between the two surfaces; an anterior-posterior sliding transfer; and a lateral transfer without a sliding board.

In the sitting transfers described in this section, paraplegic patients are used as examples. The transfer techniques apply unmodified to patients with other lower extremity disabilities (e.g., double amputees). If upper extremity weakness is present, the assistance of another person may be required for the transfer. The type of transfer used depends upon the patient's ability and the specific situation.

Preparing the Patient for Sitting Transfers. The following activities are valuable in preparation for sliding and swinging transfers: daily use of the standing bed, leading to the ability to stand at 80 degrees without postural hypotension; training in coming to a sitting position and sitting on the edge of the bed without making a transfer (transfer training is begun when the patient can balance in sitting position); progressive resistive exercises designed to strengthen shoulder depressors and adductors, elbow flexors and extensors and wrist extensors and flexors; intensive mat work in the long sitting position to improve the ability to roll and balance and to elevate the hips; and hamstring stretching. For quadriplegic patients with weak triceps, training in locking the elbow is also included.

Bed to Wheelchair Lateral Transfer Using a Sliding Board

Physical Requirements. Good sitting balance and arms powerful enough to lift the hips from the bed (strong shoulder depressors and adductors and elbow and wrist extensors) are necessary. This transfer is seldom accomplished unassisted by patients with lesions above the seventh cervical vertebra. Unusual quadriplegics with lesions at the fifth to sixth cervical segments who have weak triceps can use their biceps to lock their elbows in hyperextension sufficiently well to accomplish a sliding board transfer without assistance.

Equipment. A stable bed approximately the same height as the seat of the wheelchair; a wheelchair equipped with brakes, swinging detachable footrests, and detachable armrests; and a sliding board are needed.

Layout. The wheelchair is placed next to the bed and facing the head or foot of the bed at a slight angle. The principle of transfer toward the stronger side applies here also. The armrest is removed from the side next to the bed and is hung on the back of the chair. After the patient is sitting, the sliding board is placed between the chair and the bed (Fig. 22–17).

Coming to a Sitting Position. Paraplegics in the early stages of training and some quadriplegics attain sitting positions in a manner similar to the hemiplegic; i.e., after the patient rolls onto his side, his legs are brought independently or with assistance over the side of the bed. For more advanced

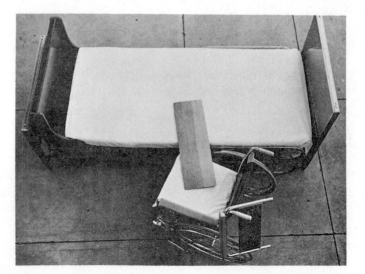

FIGURE 22–17. Position of the wheelchair and sliding board for a lateral sliding transfer.

FIG. 22–18

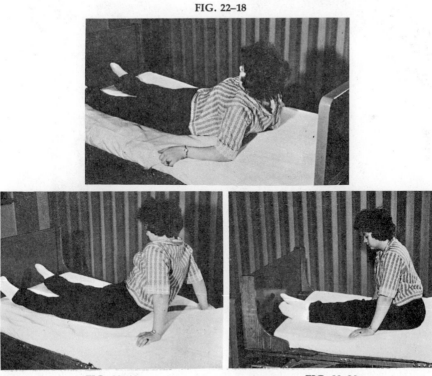

FIG. 22–19   FIG. 22–20

FIGURE 22–18. To come to a sitting position the patient raises her shoulders by pushing down on her forearms and gradually moving them backward.

FIGURE 22–19. She straightens her elbows, one at a time.

FIGURE 22–20. She "walks" her hands forward one at a time until her trunk is forward and she has reached an upright sitting position.

patients, particularly those with good sitting balance and loose hamstrings, the following procedure can be used in coming to a sitting position.

The patient raises her head and bends it forward, then places her hands on the bed beside her hips, palms down, elbows flexed. She raises her shoulders by pushing down on her forearms and gradually "walking" her forearms backward (Fig. 22–18).

She transmits her weight to her right forearm and flexes her head to the right as

FIG. 22–21   FIG. 22–22

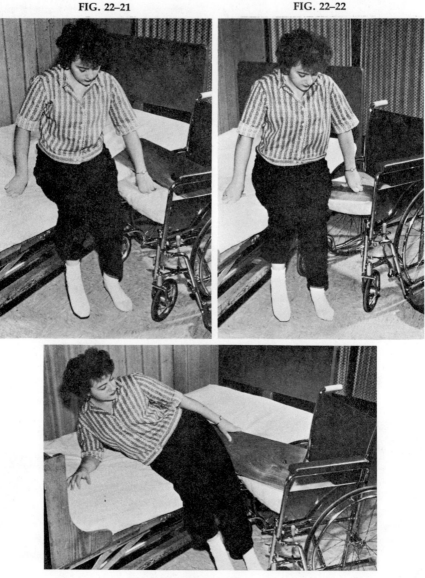

FIG. 22–23

FIGURE 22–21. She moves her legs over the side of the bed with her arms and slides to the edge of the bed in position for the sliding transfer to the wheelchair.

FIGURE 22–22. Leaning on her right forearm, the patient places one end of the sliding board under her.

FIGURE 22–23. She moves across the sliding board to the wheelchair.

she quickly straightens her left elbow. Keeping her left elbow in this locked position, she shifts her weight to her left arm and straightens her right elbow (Fig. 22–19).

To come to an upright sitting position, she must "walk" her hands forward one at a time until her trunk is forward. She must keep her head and shoulders slightly forward to maintain her balance and to keep from falling backward (Fig. 22–20). She performs lateral and anterior-posterior movements by using her upper extremities to push against the bed to raise her hips off the bed, moving in the desired direction while her hips are raised. She uses her fist rather than the palm of her hand for added height.

Transfer to the Chair. The patient reaches a sitting position on the side of the bed by moving her legs with her hands. She moves toward the edge of the bed, turning herself so that her knees are away from the wheelchair and her hips are toward the wheelchair (Fig. 22–21). As she turns, she must adjust her feet with her hands to bring them directly under her.

The patient leans over onto her right forearm, raising her left buttock off the bed enough to place one end of the sliding board under her (Fig. 22–22). Two corners of the board must rest securely on the bed and two corners must rest on the wheelchair seat or the board may slip or break.

Using her upper extremities for balance and movement, the patient carefully moves laterally across the sliding board into the wheelchair (Fig. 22–23). She then leans over onto her left forearm to raise her buttock off the board and removes the sliding board.

She replaces the armrest on the wheelchair and swings the left footrest into place. After placing her left foot on the footrest, she unlocks the brakes and moves away from the bed. Finally she swings the right footrest into place and places her right foot on the footrest. When the patient becomes adept at using the sliding board, she may be able to progress to transferring without it. The movement would then be performed by using her upper extremities to boost her hips short distances rather than by sliding.

Bed to Wheelchair: Anterior-Posterior Sliding Transfer

Physical Requirements. This transfer requires loose hamstrings and slightly more strength, particularly in the elbow extensors, and better balance than the lateral transfer.

Equipment. A bed that can be immobilized and set at approximately the same height as the wheelchair is needed.

Layout. The wheelchair is braked and placed with the front of the seat directly against the bed and the footrests are swung aside (Fig. 22–24).

Transfer Techniques. During the entire

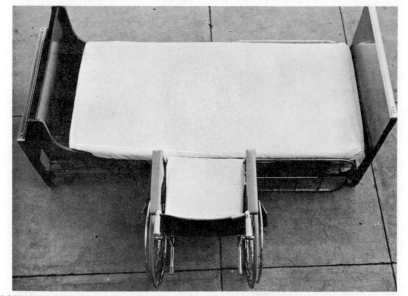

FIGURE 22–24. Position of the wheelchair for the anterior-posterior sliding transfer.

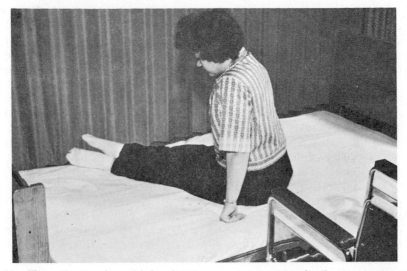

FIGURE 22–25. The patient pushes with her fists to move into position for the anterior-posterior transfer.

transfer, the patient keeps her head and shoulders slightly forward to maintain her balance and prevent her from falling backward. She moves her legs to the side of the bed away from the wheelchair by moving one leg at a time with her hands.

By pushing with her fists, the patient moves sideways and backward, moving each leg and hip alternately to bring her hips close to the wheelchair (Fig. 22–25).

When the patient is near the edge of the bed, she reaches behind her, places her hands on the middle of the wheelchair

armrests, and lifts herself gently back into the wheelchair (Fig. 22–26). It is for this stage of the maneuver that strength in the elbow extensors is essential.

She moves the chair away from the bed until only her heels are resting on the edge of the bed. She locks her brakes; then using the armrests for support, the patient leans to each side to swing the footrests into place (Fig. 22–27) and carefully places her feet on the footrests, watching to see that they are properly positioned. To get back into bed, she reverses the procedure.

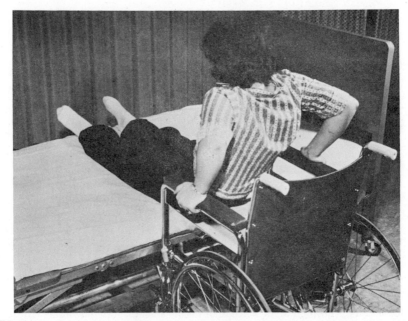

FIGURE 22–26. Grasping the middle of the wheelchair armrests, she lifts herself into the chair.

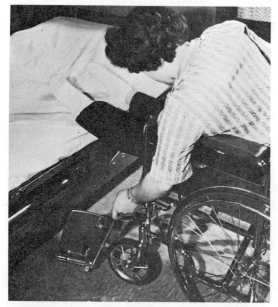

FIGURE 22–27.   The patient swings the footrests into place and positions her feet on them.

wheelchair as close as possible to the toilet. Then he relocks the brakes (Fig. 22–30). This final moving of the wheelchair is an important clue to a good transfer: it eliminates the space between the wheelchair seat and the toilet seat, thus reducing the distance the patient must cross. At this point, while he still has the support of the wheelchair armrests, the patient loosens his trousers and, by leaning from side to side, gradually works them under his buttocks to about midthigh.

Next he removes the armrest and places it on the back of the chair so that it will be within easy reach. He places one hand on the opposite side of the toilet seat and the other hand on the wheelchair seat. He uses his upper extremities to raise his hips and move toward the toilet (Fig. 22–31).

Several moves may be needed to complete the transfer. When the transfer procedure is completed, the patient must position his lower extremities.

Sitting Toilet Transfers

Equipment.   It is recommended that the toilet seat be approximately the same height as the wheelchair seat. In a rehabilitation center where many patients need a higher toilet, the fixture may be installed at a height of 20 inches. When a standard toilet seat 16 inches high is the only one available, a securely fastened raised toilet seat may be used (see Fig. 22–10).

Layout.   Depending upon the space in the bathroom, the patient should position the wheelchair parallel or at an angle to the toilet. If space does not permit the use of the wheelchair in the bathroom, an ordinary sturdy wooden straight-back chair with small casters or gliders may be used instead of the wheelchair, provided the patient has sufficient balance to manage a chair without the support of armrests.

Transfer Technique.   The patient lifts his feet off the footrests, places them on the floor one at a time, and swings the footrests out of the way. Next, he moves the chair until his knee is as close as possible to the toilet. He locks the wheelchair brakes (Fig. 22–28).

He shifts his hips so that he is sitting sideways on the chair and moves his legs so that his knees are away from the toilet (Fig. 22–29). He unlocks the brakes and moves the

Tub Transfers

Caution: When the patient has lost sensation to pain and temperature, the water temperature must be checked.

Equipment and Layout.   See the bath tub transfer on page 482.

Transfer Technique.   The patient transfers from a wheelchair to a straight chair next to the tub. Using his hands, he lifts each leg into the tub. He then straightens his knees and directs his feet toward the end of the tub so that his legs will move forward as he lowers himself into the tub. This is essential to a safe and efficient transfer. The patient positions his hands on the seat of the chair and on the handrail. Sometimes the edge of the tub may be used instead of a rail. Keeping his head and upper trunk forward, he gently lowers his body into the tub (Fig. 22–32). Gradual flexion of the elbows gives better control.

The Lateral Sitting Transfer Without Sliding Board — Bed to Wheelchair

Physical Requirements.   This transfer method can be used only by paraplegics with exceptionally good shoulder depressors and abductors as well as good balance. The patient must have the ability to lift his buttocks off the bed and move himself from the bed to the wheelchair in one motion. Male paraple-

FIG. 22–28

FIG. 22–29

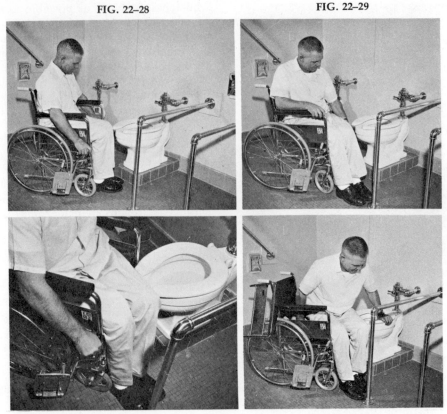

FIG. 22–30

FIG. 22–31

FIGURE 22–28. For the lateral transfer to the toilet the patient swings the footrests to the side, moves the wheelchair so that his knee is close to the toilet, and locks the brakes.

FIGURE 22–29. The patient moves so that he is sitting sideways on the wheelchair.

FIGURE 22–30. He unlocks the brakes and moves the wheelchair as close as possible to the toilet. Then he relocks the brakes.

FIGURE 22–31. Removing the armrest and placing one hand on the opposite side of the toilet seat, the patient lifts himself to the toilet seat.

gics who develop very strong upper extremities may even be able to transfer to different levels with ease.

Layout. The wheelchair is set at a 45-degree angle next to the bed. For close placement, the footrests are swung aside. Very strong patients find this maneuver unnecessary.

Transfer Techniques. The patient comes to a sitting position on the side of the bed. She turns so that her knees are away from the wheelchair and her hips are directed toward the wheelchair. She adjusts her legs to bring her feet directly under her. She moves her hand to the middle of the farther armrest. By pushing down with her upper extremities, she raises herself off the bed and swings in one motion to the wheelchair (Fig. 22–33). She turns her trunk as she lowers herself into the chair.

Car Transfers

Physical Requirements. This is an advanced transfer and can be accomplished unassisted only by patients with strong upper extremities.

Transfer Techniques. There are several methods by which patients can make a car transfer. If the patient wears long leg braces

FIGURE 22–32. After placing his feet in the bath-tub, the patient, using the handrail and the seat of the chair, lowers himself to a stool in the tub.

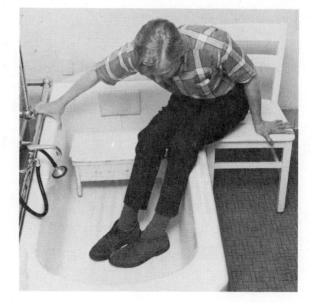

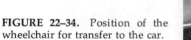

FIGURE 22–33. The patient pushes up on her arms to lift her buttocks from the bed to the wheelchair.

FIGURE 22–34. Position of the wheelchair for transfer to the car.

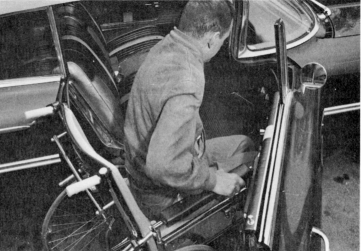

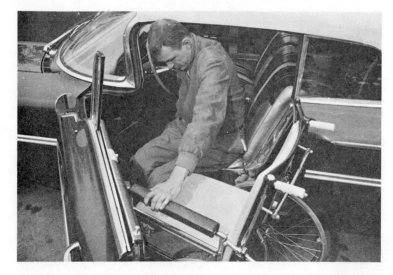

FIGURE 22–35. The patient performs a swinging transfer to the car seat.

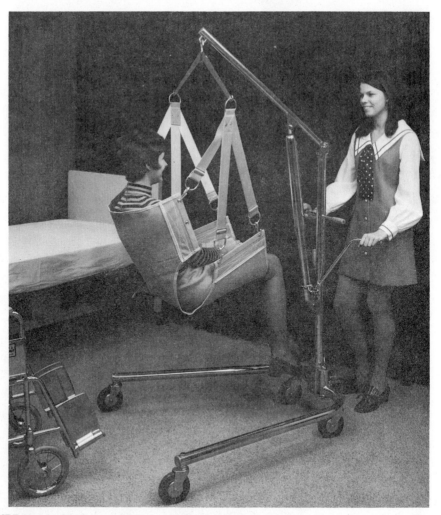

FIGURE 22–36. Mechanical lift for assistance in transfer. (Courtesy of Ted Hoyer & Company.)

or has sufficient extensor spasticity or one strong leg, he may be able to perform a standing transfer in which he stands, pivots, and sits on the edge of the car seat. If the windows are rolled down, he can grasp the window opening for support during the transfer.

If the car door opens wide enough, the wheelchair can be placed directly facing the seat of the car. The patient's legs can be placed on the seat of the car and the patient can then slide forward into the car. This method is exactly the same as the one described for the anterior-posterior transfer from the wheelchair to the bed. A wide sliding board facilitates this transfer, particularly for the bilateral lower extremity amputee with prostheses.

The wheelchair can be placed at an angle to the car and the patient may be able to perform a swinging transfer, moving to the side (Figs. 22–34 and 22–35). This again is the same procedure that is so frequently used for bed or chair transfers except that there is a wider space between the wheelchair seat and the car seat. If the patient does not have sufficient strength to bridge this gap, a sliding board 28 to 34 inches long may be used. A completely independent transfer includes the ability to bring the wheelchair into the car after the transfer has been made and to remove the wheelchair before transferring out of the car.

LIFTS

For patients who cannot accomplish a transfer without extensive assistance, the various hydraulic or mechanical lifts have been found to be very effective (Fig. 22–36). A properly trained small woman, using these devices, can successfully lift and transfer a man more than twice her size. Family members or attendants should be trained to use such equipment if excessive lifting is required to assist a transfer. The rehabilitation center should have lifts available for training demonstrations.

REFERENCES

1. Audiovisual Aids Utilized in Teaching Rehabilitation Nursing. New York, Educational Services Division, American Journal of Nursing Co., 1970.
2. Flaherty, P., and Jurkovich, S.: Transfers for Patients with Acute and Chronic Conditions. Minneapolis, American Rehabilitation Foundation, 1970.
3. Fowles, B. H.: Syllabus of Rehabilitation Methods and Techniques. Cleveland, Stratford Press Co., 1963.
4. Lawton, E. B.: Activities of Daily Living for Physical Rehabilitation. New York, McGraw-Hill Book Co., Inc., 1963, Chapter 3.
5. Narrow, B. W.: A hydraulic patient lifter. Am. J. Nurs., 60:1273–1275, 1960.
6. Rusk, H. A.: Rehabilitation Medicine, 2nd Ed. St. Louis, The C. V. Mosby Co., 1964, Chapter 6.

23

PRESCRIPTION OF WHEELCHAIRS

PAUL M. ELLWOOD, JR.

Whenever a person must spend much of his time in a wheelchair and whenever it is to be maneuvered by the patient rather than by other persons, a wheelchair prescription is a must. The prescription of wheelchairs by physicians is analogous to the prescription of drugs and requires attention to many of the same factors. The most important considerations include patient size, body weight, safety, diagnosis, prognosis, transfer technique, mode of propulsion, style of living, and cost. Wheelchair features can be selected to assist the patient in these individual matters. A rehabilitation nurse or physical therapist may be able to prescribe a wheelchair capably, but the physician should make sure that such persons are knowledgeable about both the patient and the types of basic chair variations available.

Since hundreds of possible combinations of wheelchair features are available, many extended-care facilities and rehabilitation units have found it essential to use a special form to ensure complete, rapid, and accurate wheelchair prescriptions (Fig. 23–1). Since a wheelchair is a costly item for the patient, it is imperative that his chair have only those features that are necessary to serve him optimally.

The major wheelchair manufacturers publish excellent catalogues that describe features and dimensions available on their chairs. Since wheelchairs are fitted to patients, not patients to wheelchairs, a rehabili-

tation facility should have available a group of sample chairs of different sizes with varied special features, such as detachable armrests and footrests and reclining backs. In this way, the patient and the staff can evaluate a wheelchair before actual purchase for an individual. If a variety of chairs are not available for trial, a wheelchair sales representative should be consulted about arranging to borrow or rent a chair for a brief period of time.

IMPORTANT FACTORS IN WHEELCHAIR SELECTION

Experience has shown that certain wheelchair features are virtually a requirement for a majority of handicapped persons. These include (1) a high degree of durability, (2) ease of folding, (3) easy propulsion, (4) brakes, (5) removable footrests, and (6) 8-inch front casters. These are not luxury but essential features for persons who use a wheelchair regularly. The following discussion considers the factors that must be taken into account for each individual.

The Patient's Size. Wheelchairs are available in three major sizes: a standard adult size, suitable for most adults; an intermediate or junior chair for small adults and older children; and a children's size, which is ideal for children up to the age of six years (Fig. 23–2). "Growing chairs" are available

492

WHEELCHAIR PRESCRIPTION

Name _____ Date Ordered _____

Address _____

To Whom Billed _____ Dealer _____

Brand Name _____ Model _____

Size:　Adult _____　　　　　　　　　Wheels – 24":　36 spokes _____
　　　　Junior _____
　　　　Large child _____　　　　　　Tires – 24":　Regular _____
　　　　Small child _____　　　　　　　　　　　Pneumatic _____
　　　　Special _____

Type:　Fixed back _____
　　　　　Added Height _____　　　　Axle:　Regular _____　Heavy duty _____
　　　　Semi-reclining _____
　　　　Full reclining _____　　　　　Handrims:
　　　　Amputee _____　　　　　　　Regular _____
　　　　　　　　　　　　　　　　　　　　Vertical projections – No. _____
Brakes:　Lever _____　　　　　　　　　Other _____
　　　　　Toggle _____
　　　　　　　　　　　　　　　　　　Front Casters:　8" regular _____
Detachable Footrests:　　　　　　　　　　　　　　8" semi-pneumatic _____
　　　　　Lift off _____
　　　　　Button _____　　　　　　　Cushion:　Seat:　2" _____　3" _____　4" _____
　　　　　Swinging _____
　　　　　Elevating _____　　　　　　　　Horseshoe _____
　　　　　　　　　　　　　　　　　　　　　Measurement _____
Footplates:　Regular _____　　　　　　　Protective Covering _____
　　　　　　Large _____　　　　　　　　Other _____

Heel Loops:　Right _____　Left _____　Back:　1" _____　2" _____

Armrests:　Padded _____
　　　　　Fixed _____　　　　　　　Measurement _____
　　　　　Removable _____　　　　　　　Protective Covering _____
　　　　　　Regular _____
　　　　　　Adjustable _____
　　　　　desk _____　　　　　　　　　Color of Upholstery: _____

Additional instructions:

Ordered By _____, M.D.

FIGURE 23–1. Wheelchair prescription form.

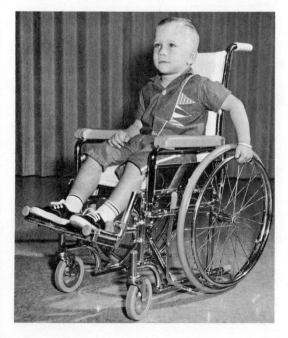

FIGURE 23–2. Child's wheelchair. (Courtesy of Sister Kenny Institute, Minneapolis.)

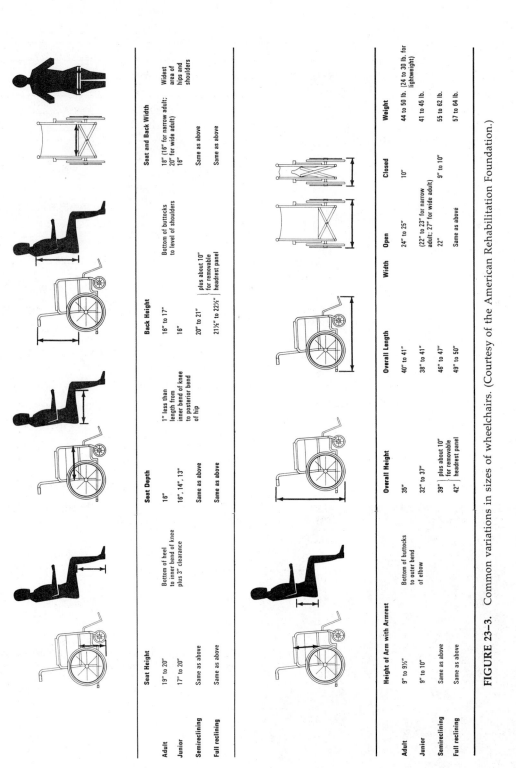

	Seat Height	Seat Depth	Back Height		Seat and Back Width
	Bottom of heel to inner bend of knee plus 3" clearance	1" less than length from inner bend of knee to posterior bend of hip	Bottom of buttocks to level of shoulders	plus about 10" for removable headrest panel	Widest area of hips and shoulders
Adult	19" to 20"	16"	16" to 17"		18" (16" for narrow adult; 20" for wide adult)
Junior	17" to 20"	16", 14", 13"	16"		16"
Semireclining	Same as above	Same as above	20" to 21"		Same as above
Full reclining	Same as above	Same as above	21½" to 22½"		Same as above

	Height of Arm with Armrest	Overall Height	Overall Length	Width Open	Width Closed	Weight
	Bottom of buttocks to outer bend of elbow					
Adult	9" to 9½"	35"	40" to 41"	24" to 25"	10"	44 to 50 lb. (24 to 30 lb. for lightweight)
Junior	9" to 10"	32" to 37"	38" to 41"	(22" to 23" for narrow adult; 27" for wide adult)		41 to 45 lb.
Semireclining	Same as above	39" plus about 10" for removable headrest panel	46" to 47"	22"	9" to 10"	55 to 62 lb.
Full reclining	Same as above	42"	49" to 50"	Same as above		57 to 64 lb.

FIGURE 23–3. Common variations in sizes of wheelchairs. (Courtesy of the American Rehabilitation Foundation.)

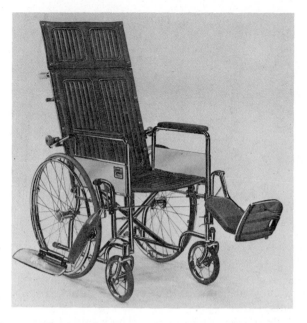

FIGURE 23–4. Wheelchair with semireclining back and headrest extension for trunk and neck weakness. (Courtesy of Everest & Jennings, Inc., Los Angeles, California.)

for those undergoing the period of rapid growth between ages 6 and 12 years. In determining wheelchair size, the critical dimensions are seat width and depth, the height of the seat from the floor, armrests of a height that allows the patient to rest his forearms comfortably without slumping or excessive shoulder abduction, and adjustable footrests set to provide an ideal distance from the popliteal fossa to the heel. (Figure 23–3 shows typical variations in wheelchair dimensions.) The patient's weight should be distributed over as great an area of skin surface as possible. In rare instances, custom sizes may be necessary.

Safety. For safety, particularly in making transfers, brakes are required on all chairs. It is essential that the bilateral lower extremity amputee with his higher center of gravity have a chair with more posteriorly placed rear wheels to prevent instability of the chair (see Fig. 23–12). The use of weights placed on the footrests of a regular chair will also compensate for this change in center of gravity. Another important safety measure is the seat belt, which can be attached at the hips, waist, or chest area.

Diagnosis and Prognosis. The patient's prognosis should be carefully considered in making the proper wheelchair selection. For instance, in progressive muscular dystrophy, future trunk weakness can be anticipated by selecting a chair with a semireclining back. Trunk weakness may be compensated for by

a semireclining or reclining back or perhaps by added back height. A head extension is attached to the back of the chair for patients with neck weakness (Fig. 23–4). Patients who have been bedridden for prolonged periods or those with postural hypotension may require a semireclining chair during the early stages of their rehabilitation program. Elevating foot and leg rests are available for situations in which incomplete knee flexion or dependent edema are problems (Fig. 23–5).

Most patients find that they are more comfortable using a cushion of some type. The presence of sensory loss from the fifth lumbar vertebra downward calls for the use of a foam rubber cushion, preferably 4 inches thick and horseshoe-shaped (Fig. 23–6). Cushions may also be filled with water, resin, gel, or air. Seat boards used under cushions can improve lower extremity posture (Fig. 23–7).

Transfer Techniques. Brakes are necessary for all transfers, and the transfer technique itself dictates the type of armrests and footrests chosen. For anterior sliding transfers, swinging detachable footrests permit placement of the chair closer to the surface to or from which the patient is moving. Lateral transfers (toward the arm of the wheelchair), with or without the use of a sliding board, require detachable arms plus a removable footrest (Fig. 23–8). For a standing transfer, footrests may not be a problem.

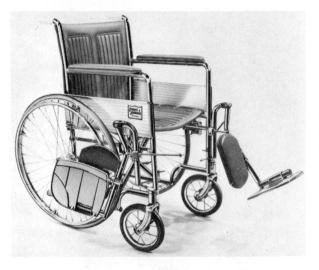

FIGURE 23–5. Elevating footrest and legrest. (Courtesy of Everest & Jennings, Inc., Los Angeles, California.)

If they are, a simple detachable footrest is adequate.

Propulsion Techniques. The mode of propulsion influences footrest and hand rim selection. Hemiplegic patients who propel the chair with their normal arm and leg require a detachable footrest on the uninvolved side. Chairs that are equipped with one-wheel drive are necessary only in triplegia, with weakness of both lower extremities and one upper, or in very unusual cases, such as a hemiplegic patient with a lower extremity amputation on the normal side.

For the patient with a poor grasp, as in quadriplegia or arthritis of the hands, vertical projections on the hand rim substantially assist propulsion (Fig. 23–9). Vertical projections (rather than horizontal) are preferred, since they do not widen the dimensions of the chair. Battery-powered wheelchairs are available for individuals with minimal arm power or control, who by one means or another can operate a small control stick that activates the wheels. These chairs weigh from 70 to 80 pounds without the batteries and cost $2000 and up.

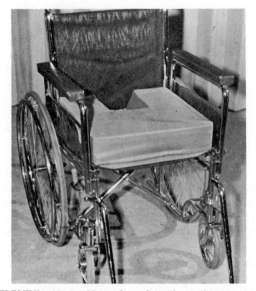

FIGURE 23–6. Horseshoe-shaped cushion used when there is sensory loss. (Courtesy of Sister Kenny Institute, Minneapolis.)

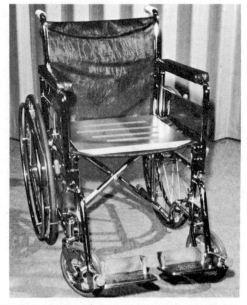

FIGURE 23–7. Seat board used under cushions. (Courtesy of Sister Kenny Institute, Minneapolis.)

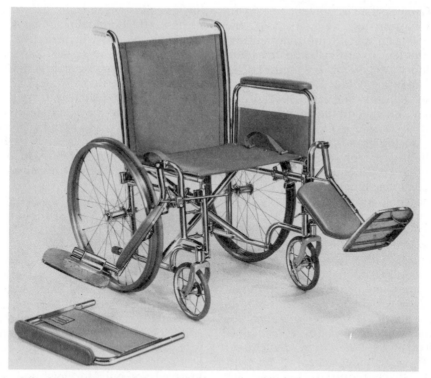

FIGURE 23–8. Wheelchair with detachable armrest removed and detachable legrest swung back. (Courtesy of Everest & Jennings, Inc., Los Angeles, California.)

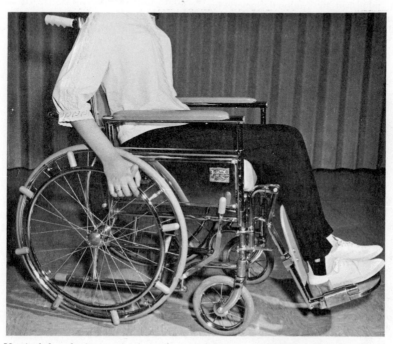

FIGURE 23–9. Vertical hand rim projections for weak grasp. (Courtesy of Sister Kenny Institute, Minneapolis.)

Style of Living. To circumvent certain architectural barriers of the household, the physician will need specific information from the family in order to prescribe chair modifications. Doorways should be measured to make sure they are wider than the overall open width of the open chair. Special narrowers can be attached to the chair to temporarily narrow its width by 2 to 4 inches (depending on the brand) to permit passage through slightly narrow doorways. Doorways can often be widened by 1 to 2 inches by simply removing inner moldings. In some instances an adult can be comfortably fitted with a junior chair, which is on the average 2 inches narrower than similar full-size models. Some brands of junior size wheelchairs, when equipped with removable arms, will often accommodate adults.

Several other important architectural dimensions for wheelchair living are found in the *American Standard Specifications for Making Building and Facilities Accessible to, and Usable by, the Physically Handicapped.** This document states, "The average turning space required (180 and 360 degrees) is 60 by 60 inches. . . . The average horizontal working (table) reach is 30.8

---

*American Standard Specifications for Making Buildings and Facilities Accessible to, and Usable by, the Physically Handicapped. New York, American Standards Association, published by National Society for Crippled Children and Adults, 2023 W. Ogden Avenue, Chicago, Ill. 60612, 1961.

inches, and ranges from 28½ inches to 33.2 inches. An individual reaching diagonally, as would be required in using a wall-mounted dial telephone or towel dispenser, would make the average reach (on the wall) 48 inches from the floor."

If ramps are installed for wheelchairs, a 5-degree incline may be lengthy but is most desirable. A recommended slope is not greater than a 1 foot rise in 12 feet. Guard rails are highly recommended on ramps to prevent the patient from slipping off the edge.

If the person's life takes him to areas where the ground is soft or uneven, pneumatic tires can be helpful in maneuvering such surfaces (Fig. 23–10).

Detachable desk arms are available for individuals who need to work closely at low desks and tables. The front 6 inches of the desk armrest are lowered to permit the wheelchair arms to pass under the table top (Fig. 23–11). These armrests can also be reversed. Another type of adjustable armrest is also available. These can be raised and lowered not only to clear under desks and tables but also to adjust for arm comfort and shoulder level of the individual.

It should be kept in mind that table legs or partitions also may inhibit the close approach to a work surface, unless the footrests can be swung aside or detached. A lap board can be placed over the arms of the chair when other adjustments are difficult.

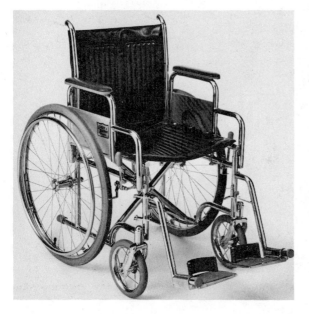

FIGURE 23–10. Wheelchair with pneumatic tires for use on soft or uneven surfaces. (Courtesy of Everest & Jennings, Inc., Los Angeles, California.)

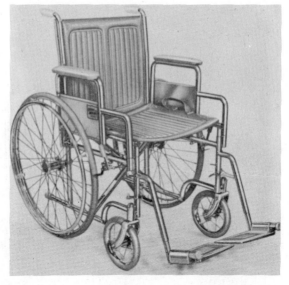

FIGURE 23–11. Wheelchair with desk arms positioned for close work at low tables. Arms can be reversed for comfort. (Courtesy of Everest & Jennings, Inc., Los Angeles, California.)

Persons who will give a chair rugged daily use with frequent moves in and out of cars and over curbs and other forms of abuse require either a heavy-duty chair or a regular chair with a heavy-duty axle. When a chair must be lifted up and down stairs frequently, or handled by a woman, consideration might be given to a lightweight but slightly less durable steel and aluminum chair, which weighs approximately 20 pounds less than comparable models.

Cost. Each special feature increases the cost of the chair. In most instances, quality is a function of price, but essential individual needs should never be sacrificed to economy.

SOME TYPICAL WHEELCHAIR PRESCRIPTIONS

Hemiplegia

PATIENT. The chair is for a 170-pound, 5-foot, 8-inch, right or left hemiplegic patient who is able to perform a standing transfer with assistance.

PRESCRIPTION. Adult chair, 8-inch front casters, 24-inch rear wheels, regular tires, brakes, button-detachable footrests with heel loops, padded armrests, fixed back, and 2-inch cushion for comfort.

Paraplegia

PATIENT. The chair is for a strong, 180-pound, 6-foot, paraplegic man who performs a sitting transfer. He expects to use his chair outside extensively on hard and soft surfaces.

PRESCRIPTION. Adult size wheelchair, 8-inch front casters with semipneumatic tires, 24-inch rear wheels, air cushion tires and heavy-duty axle (or a heavy-duty wheelchair), brakes, swinging detachable footrests with heel loops, padded removable armrests, fixed back, seat board, and a special horseshoe cushion (filled with air, gel, water, resin, or sponge rubber).

Quadriplegia

The chair is for a small quadriplegic female college student with a lesion at the sixth to seventh cranial segment who uses a sliding board to transfer.

PRESCRIPTION. Junior size, semireclining wheelchair, 8-inch front casters, 24-inch rear wheels, regular tires, hand rim with vertical projections, brakes, swinging detachable footrests with heel loops, adjustable detachable padded arms, seat board, and special 4-inch horseshoe cushion (filled with air, gel, resin, water, or sponge rubber), as shown in Figure 23–6).

Amputee

PATIENT. The chair is for a 5-foot, 10-inch, 145-pound, bilateral lower extremity amputee.

PRESCRIPTION. Narrow adult size amputee chair. Until an amputee chair (Fig. 23–12) is available, place sandbags on the footrests on a regular chair to prevent tipping of the

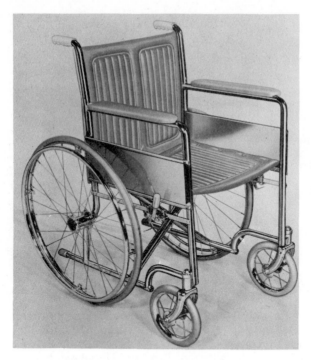

FIGURE 23–12. Amputee wheelchair. (Courtesy of Everest & Jennings, Inc., Los Angeles, California.)

chair due to the patient's altered center of gravity.

SUGGESTIONS FOR PURCHASE OF WHEELCHAIRS FOR INSTITUTIONS

Many institutions use chairs principally to transport non-disabled patients to and from such departments as admitting, x-ray, laboratory, physical therapy, and recreational therapy. A lightweight, folding, easy-to-push chair with brakes and a luggage rack and footrests is a good general-purpose chair that can be used by a majority of patients.

Once chairs for this requirement have been satisfied, an institution must look further into its needs to serve the kinds of patients who come for care. For a rehabilitation center or extended care facility where patients with a variety of disabilities are served, it is essential to have one or more chairs with brakes, removable armrests, and removable footrests. Such removable features permit exchange of parts and versatility within one chair. Certainly orthopedic areas and emergency areas require chairs with reclining back and elevating legrests. While a wheelchair must be individually prescribed for a handicapped person, careful thought must go also into the selection of chairs for an institution in order to prevent excessive expenditure on equipment that does not serve its particular patient population.

REFERENCES

1. Bergstrom, D. A.: Report on a Conference for Wheelchair Manufacturers Bulletin of Prosthetics Research, Spring, 1965, pp. 60–89.
2. Cicenia, E. F., et al.: Maintenance and minor repairs of the wheelchair. Am. J. Phys. Med., 35:206, 1956.
3. Fahland, B. B.: Wheelchair Selection — More than Choosing a Chair with Wheels. Minneapolis, Kenny Rehabilitation Institute, 1967.
4. Fowles, B. H.: Evaluation and selection of wheelchairs. Phys. Ther. Rev., 39:525–529, 1959.
5. Goldsmith, S.: Designing for the Disabled, 2nd ed. New York, McGraw-Hill Book Co., 1967.
6. Kamenetz, H. L.: The Wheelchair book. Springfield, Ill., Charles C Thomas, Publisher, 1969.
7. Lawton, E. B.: Wheelchair prescription. In Lowman, E. W.: Arthritis — General Principles, Physical Medicine, Rehabilitation. Boston, Little, Brown and Company, 1959.
8. Lee, M. H. M., et al.: Wheelchair Prescription. Public Health Service Publication No. 1666, undated. Superintendent of Documents, Washington, D.C. 20402.
9. Lowman, E. W., and Rusk, H. A.: Rehabilitation Monograph XXI: Self-Help Devices, Part 2. The Institute of Physical Medicine and Rehabilitation, New York University Medical Center, 1963.
10. Peizer, E., et al.: Bioengineering Methods of Wheelchair Evaluation. Bulletin of Prosthetics Research, Spring, 1964.

24

TRAINING FOR FUNCTIONAL INDEPENDENCE

LOREN R. LESLIE

The effectiveness of any program of medical intervention is determined by its therapeutic outcome. If possible, quantitative criteria should be used to measure outcome. Examples of rehabilitation outcome measurements are changes in muscle strength and endurance, degrees of range of motion, and levels of independence of physical function. The latter are referred to as self-care activities or activities of daily living, ADLs. This chapter presents a review of the basic principles involved in making a physically handicapped patient independent in the performance of those activities of daily living, as well as some of the systems utilized to measure ADL rehabilitation outcome.

The activities that must be performed to achieve functional independence may be classified as mobility activities, hygiene, eating, dressing, and bowel and bladder control. Mobility activities include bed position, transfers, wheelchair mobility, and ambulation. Most programs for training physically handicapped patients to become independent in the activities of daily living are adapted from the original work of George G. Deaver and Mary Eleanor Brown at the Institute for the Crippled and Disabled, New York City.[1]

Any activity that must be performed is analyzed by breaking it down into its simplest components, and exercises or therapies are selected that will increase the ability of the patients to perform each component motion until they can perform the total activity.[2, 3] In addition, many of the activities of daily living can be performed with a variety of mechanical aids and assistive devices.[4-7] It is often necessary for the patients to use assistive devices and aids early in the rehabilitation program; however, when they have developed some flexibility, strength, and endurance, less equipment may be required.

MOBILITY ACTIVITIES

Bed Mobility. The handicapped patient should be trained to shift about in bed, turn in both directions, sit erect in the long and short sitting positions, and reach objects on a bedside table. To facilitate bed mobility, the bed should have a ¾-inch plywood board under a firm flat mattress. A footboard should extend 4 inches from the lower end of the mattress, and the bed should have a half-length side rail to provide protection against falling and a handgrip for turning and positioning.

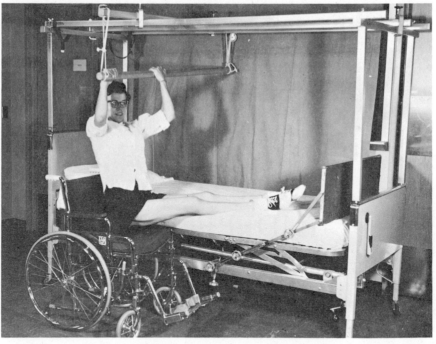

FIGURE 24–1. Transfer from bed to wheelchair by a paraplegic patient using a 4-foot trapeze bar. The long bar makes lateral transfers less difficult for any patient who has good strength in the upper extremities.

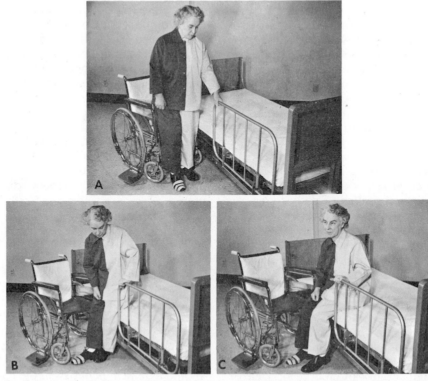

FIGURE 24–2. Sequence for independent transfer by a hemiplegic patient from a wheelchair to bed. The patient approaches the bed, locks the chair, and swings the footrest out of the way. She moves forward toward the edge of the chair seat and, grasping the arm rest, leans forward and pushes herself erect. After she is standing erect she grasps the side rail of the bed, pivots on her feet and lowers herself to sit on the bed. (From A Handbook of Rehabilitative Nursing Techniques in Hemiplegia. Minneapolis, Kenny Rehabilitation Institute, 1964.)

Patients with good arm strength may be able to push up to the erect sitting position. The side rail also may be used to pull themselves erect. Overhead trapeze bars enable patients to pull up to a sitting position and to transfer to a wheelchair beside the bed (Fig. 24–1).

Wheelchair Mobility. Wheelchair mobility includes transfers to and from the wheelchair, operation of the wheelchair, and sitting tolerance. The ability to transfer requires adequate strength to lift or shift the weight of the body, balance, and coordination. There are numerous methods of transfer.[8] The method of transfer selected should be the most convenient one in relation to the patient's residual abilities. To improve the ability to transfer, exercises are directed particularly to the muscles for shoulder depression, elbow extension, hand grip, hip extension, and knee extension.

For the patient with hemiplegia or generalized weakness who has head and trunk balance, the pivot transfer can be performed independently or with the assistance of one person with little effort (Fig. 24–2). This is probably the most frequently used transfer when assistance is available. The nurse or therapist prevents buckling of the patient's knees with his or her knee and, by supporting the hips, assists the patient to stand and balance. The patient may then be pivoted to change directions. This transfer is stable and safe. Its relatively low energy requirement permits the movement of a large patient and decreases the risk of a back injury by the attendant.

For the patient who has lower extremity paraplegia, transfer to and from the bed by use of a trapeze bar is convenient (Fig. 24–2). The bed should be at the same height as the seat of the wheelchair. If the arm of the wheelchair is removable, the patient can transfer horizontally without having to lift the body vertically. Wheelchairs with detachable footrests can be wheeled close to the bed so that the distance for transfer is minimal. The transfer method that requires the least strength utilizes a transfer board or sliding board along which the patient slides from the bed, toilet, or chair to the wheelchair.

Wheelchair mobility requires more than the ability of the patients to propel themselves with the upper extremities. It is imperative that they are able to lock both wheels and adjust the footrests. In addition, the patient should be able to remove and replace the removable armrests as applicable. Use of the uninvolved lower extremities may assist in propelling the chair in a straight line or in turning the chair in either direction.

The disabled person who has reduced sensation or lacks the ability to shift weight is in danger of developing tissue damage as a result of ischemic necrosis. Normally, people shift position frequently enough that ischemia is not a problem. If the pressure produced by the weight of the body on a given surface exceeds capillary pressure for more than 30 minutes, ischemic damage begins to occur in that area.[9] Usually this pressure is greatest beneath the bony prominences of the ischial tuberosities and the greater trochanters. In addition to shifting weight for a few seconds every 10 minutes, persons with sensory loss should have a seat cushion in the wheelchair to distribute the sitting pressure more evenly. Sitting time and wheelchair mobility may be limited to the time during which the patient can sit without evidence of injury to the skin.

Ambulation. Ambulation training is dealt with elsewhere in this text; however, it should be noted that successful ambulation as a functional mobility activity requires that the patient be able to transfer from sitting to standing independently and to utilize ambulation aids such as crutches, canes, or appliances with ease.

The degree of functional independence determines the extent of ambulatory proficiency required both in complexity and in endurance of effort. Ambulation for short distances on level, smooth surfaces may be entirely satisfactory for the patient who is homebound or limited to an institutional domicile. For most patients, however, ambulatory mobility must also include the ability to climb stairs, curbs, and inclines as well as to walk on uneven surfaces or textures. Training in walking in a variety of environmental conditions and in the use of private and public transportation is an integral part of achieving functional independence in mobility.

DRESSING

Patients should be evaluated for their ability to put on and take off the usual types of clothing. Most dressing ADLs can be accomplished using one-handed techniques, although limitations of range of motion may make it difficult to put the arms through sleeves or slip clothing of usual design over the feet. Impairment of hand and finger coordination may interfere with buttoning, lacing, tying, and other small motions. In those instances, the use of assistive devices such as button hooks, long-handled reachers, and shoe horns often enable patients to dress themselves independently. Frequently, minor adaptations in the design of clothing such as the relocation of buttons, hooks, or zippers or the substitution of elastic or Velcro closures make dressing easier.[10] Recently, specially designed clothing for the handicapped has become available commercially.

HYGIENE

The usual hygiene activities of washing, brushing teeth, shaving or applying make-up, combing hair, and using a handkerchief may require adapted equipment so that the patient can hold, control, or reach. Limitation of arm mobility or of grasp interferes with the performance of these activities. If the grasp is inadequate but the arm can be controlled, a holding device for such articles as a toothbrush, comb, or razor allows independence. Such a device may vary from a simple cuff to an elaborate splint or powered orthosis (Fig. 24–3). If the muscles of the shoulder or elbow are weak or incoordinated, a counterbalanced deltoid aid greatly increases the sphere of useful motion of the upper extremi-

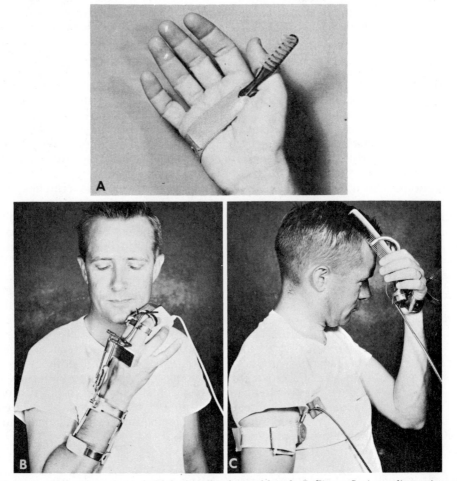

FIGURE 24–3. *A,* Cuff with pocket to hold the handle of a toothbrush. *B,* Finger flexion splint activated by wrist extension to hold a razor or other equipment for daily self-care. *C,* Robin-Aid splint hook attached to the hand for prehensile activities. The hook is closed by elastic bands and opened by abduction of the opposite arm.

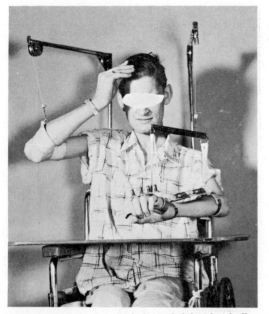

FIGURE 24–4. A counterbalanced deltoid aid allows flexion, abduction, and adduction of the shoulder with minimal muscular strength.

ty (Fig. 24–4). Motorized equipment such as electric razors or toothbrushes also make self-care easier for the patient with severe physical impairment. Bathing in a tub or shower requires the ability to transfer. A stool in the tub or shower may make independent transfers easier, and they should have nonskid mats or adhesive on the bottom for safety.

BOWEL AND BLADDER CONTROL

The establishment of bowel and bladder continence is needed to prevent perineal and sacral irritation. Urinary control may be achieved by an indwelling catheter; however, it is desirable to achieve a catheter-free status because of the multiple hazards of prolonged catheterization.[11] The use of condom catheter drainage or intermittent catheterization may be a part of the patient's self-care training. Bladder training is described in detail in Chapter 38.

Bowel control is somewhat easier to manage than bladder control. If normal bowel function cannot be restored, management of the bowel should prevent fecal incontinence, diarrhea, impaction, and irregularity.[12] Optimal function is established by developing regular bowel habits. The gastrocolic reflex may enable the patient to attempt a bowel movement on a toilet or commode. This reflex occurs 20 to 40 minutes after a meal. The same postprandial period should be used every day if the patient's schedule of activities permits. Adequate time without emotional stress must be allowed so that the patient can relax, adequate peristalsis can occur, and the bowel can be emptied.

Other stimulation of colonic peristalsis may be used. Stimulation of the anorectal reflex by gently dilating the anal sphincter with a gloved finger or by the use of a glycerin suppository is an effective means of initiating defecation. Irritation of the rectum by irritant suppositories, cathartics, or enemas should be avoided. Usually bulk-forming agents such as Colace or Senakot will suffice to maintain stool consistency and intestinal peristalsis. If an atonic bowel does require a stimulus, Dulcolox suppositories or tablets are preferred, although milk of magnesia, tap water, or Fleet enemas may be used to initiate peristalsis. The least irritating procedure that is effective should be used.

Fecal incontinence is controlled best by dietary management. In the absence of an infectious gastroenteritis, just decreasing condiments or roughage in food or adding such foods as cheese, apple sauce, or tea may be adequate to solve the problem. Pectin, kaolin, or Metamucil may decrease intestinal motility. On occasion, anticholinergic drugs may be necessary, but the use of opium preparations is unsatisfactory.

The optimal position for defecation is the squat; therefore, the use of a commode or toilet is preferable to the bedpan or chucks. In addition to increased comfort, the commode requires less energy than the bedpan.[13] Suitable handrails in the bathroom assist the patient in toilet transfers and in minimizing the danger of a fall.

EATING

The physically disabled patient may be unable to feed himself adequately because of loss of grasp, range of motion, or coordination. A holding device may be necessary for the knife, spoon, or cup. Adapted utensils are helpful (Fig. 24–5). If mobility or coordination of the upper extremities is limited,

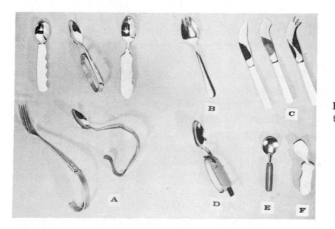

FIGURE 24–5. Adapted eating utensils for patients with impairment of grasp or reach.

devices such as a Warm Springs feeder (Fig. 24–6), rocker feeder, or balanced deltoid aid may be required.

Care should be taken in the placement of food on the plate or eating surface, especially if there is a visual field deficit. Difficulty in

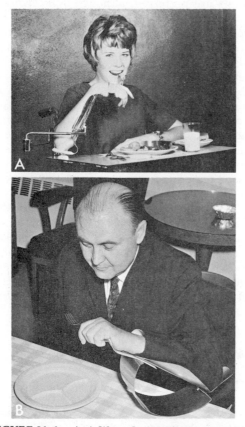

FIGURE 24–6. *A,* A Warm Springs feeder allows the patient to substitute shoulder depression to elevate the hand during eating. This device also assists the function of weak shoulder flexors, adductors and abductors, and weak elbow flexors. *B,* A forearm rocker feeder aids in the elevation of the hand during eating.

swallowing requires the appropriate selection of food consistency. Aspiration of liquid substances may occur in patients with bulbar paresis. Evaluation of the swallowing mechanisms should be a part of an ADL evaluation.

The oral ingestion of substances other than food, such as medications, is a part of functional independence training. Self-medication programs on the rehabilitation ward address the competence of the patient in the self-administration of prescribed drugs.

REHABILITATION ADL MEASUREMENT

Because self-care or ADL proficiency represent rehabilitation process outcomes and in addition are quantifiable, self-care rating systems are often used as indicators of rehabilitation effectiveness and program efficiency. Numerous assessment methods have appeared in rehabilitation literature, including the Barthel Index,[14] Pulses,[15] and Kenny Self Care Scale.[16] Combinations of these and other scales have been adapted to meet individual institution or program needs, or to form the basis for the functional component of a more comprehensive patient profile system.[17]

The importance of measuring functional outcome is emphasized by accreditation bodies such as the Commission on Accreditation of Rehabilitation Facilities, CARF, as a part of required program evaluation systems. Utilization review and third party payers such as Medicare often employ functional scales for documentation of rehabilitation effectiveness in the monitoring of health care services.

It is important to recognize, however, that rehabilitation for self-care and functional independence is more than an intrainstitutional exercise or a basis for documentation of rehabilitation program effectiveness. The ultimate outcome of training for functional independence is the use of this knowledge and techniques by patients in their home or post-discharge domicile. ADL training must be practical for daily use in order to be accepted by the patients and their families. For example, the time required by patients to dress or feed themselves may be excessive, resulting in family members or attendant staff providing assistance to expedite the process. If possible, these problems should be determined before the patient is discharged from the rehabilitation training program. Trial weekends at home or live-in facilities at the rehabilitation center should be utilized to assist families in learning to supervise the patient's self-care activities and to help determine the level of proficiency needed to function in the home environment. Home-bound health care or home nursing visits both before and after discharge are also useful to monitor self-care proficiency and to reinforce the patients and their families in accomplishing a level of optimal functional independence.

REFERENCES

1. Deaver, G. G., and Brown, M. E.: Physical Demands of Daily Life. New York, Institute for the Crippled and Disabled, 1945.
2. Lawton, E. B.: Activities of Daily Living for Physical Rehabilitation. New York, McGraw-Hill Book Co., 1963.
3. Rusk, H. A., and Taylor, E. J.: Living With a Disability. Garden City, New York, The Blakiston Co., 1953.
4. Self-Help Devices for Rehabilitation: Part I. New York University-Bellevue Medical Center Institute of Physical Medicine and Rehabilitation. Dubuque, Iowa, Wm. C. Brown Company, Publishers, 1958.
5. Self-Help Devices for Rehabilitation: Part II. New York University-Bellevue Medical Center Institute of Physical Medicine and Rehabilitation. Dubuque, Iowa, Wm. C. Brown Company, Publishers, 1965.
6. Goldsmith, S.: Designing for the Disabled, 2nd Ed. New York, McGraw-Hill Book Co., 1967.
7. Rosenberg, C.: Assistive Devices for the Handicapped. Minneapolis, American Rehabilitation Foundation, 1968.
8. A Handbook of Rehabilitative Nursing Techniques in Hemiplegia. Minneapolis, Kenny Rehabilitation Institute, 1964.
9. Kosiak, M.: Etiology of decubitus ulcers. Arch. Phys. Med., 42:19–29, 1961.
10. Kernaleguen, A.: Clothing for the handicapped. Physiother. Can., 30:135–138, 1978.
11. Price, M., Tobin, J. A., Reiser, M., Olson, M. E., Kubicek, W. G., Kottke, F. J., and Boen, J.: Renal function in patients with spinal cord injuries. Arch. Phys. Med., 47:406–411, 1966.
12. Mead, S.: A bowel training program in a rehabilitation center. Arch. Phys. Med., 37:210–213, 1956.
13. Benton, J. G., Brown, H., and Rusk, H. A.: Energy expended by patients on the bedpan and bedside commode. J.A.M.A., 144:1443–1447, 1950.
14. Mahoney, F. I., and Barthel, D. W.: Functional evaluation: Barthel index. Md. State Med. J., 14:61–65, 1965.
15. Moskowitz, E., and McCann, C. B.: Classification of disability in chronically ill and aging. J. Chronic Dis., 5:342–346, 1957.
16. Schoening, H. A., Anderegg, L., Bergstrom, D., Fonda, M., Steinkie, N., and Ulrich, P.: Numerical scoring of self-care status of patients. Arch. Phys. Med., 46:689–697, 1965.
17. Granger, C. V., Albrecht, G. L., and Hamilton, B. B.: Outcome of comprehensive medical rehabilitation: Measurement by PULSES profile and Barthel index. Arch. Phys. Med., 60:145–154, 1979.

25

TRAINING IN HOMEMAKING ACTIVITIES

LOREN R. LESLIE

Homemaking is probably the oldest vocation in history. In 1954 the Federal Rehabilitation Law was interpreted to include homemakers. Even earlier, in 1943, federal rehabilitation programs were included in the Social Security Law, and in 1946 homemaking was declared a vocation by the Vocational Rehabilitation Administration.[1]

Homemakers constitute the largest group among the disabled. One survey[2] pointed out that there were 1,875,000 women with arthritis, 4,000,000 women with cardiovascular disease, 175,000 women with active or arrested tuberculosis, 650,000 women with hemiplegia, and 800,000 women with orthopedic disabilities. The last group runs the gamut from tetraplegia to osteoarthritis of the hip. The total number of physically handicapped homemakers is now well over 10,000,000.

The disabled housewife is not the only one who can benefit from training in homemaking. Men with physical impairment often must assume homemaking roles in order to allow other members of the family to work outside the home (Fig. 25–1). Men and women with a chronic illness are often relegated to a condition of complete dependency. Their potential for independence through training has never been realized.

Children and young people with handicaps are certainly candidates for training. Development of homemaking skills may contribute to development of self-confidence and initiative.

It would be difficult to calculate the economic consequences of homemaking disability considering the diversity of tasks that a homemaker performs. Household management impacts not only on housekeeping but also on the emotional well-being of the individual and the family unit; therefore, the rehabilitation process must address much more than the development of work skills alone.

Homemaking activities — whether carried out by men, by women, or by children — contribute to the welfare of the family and to its economic productiveness and well-being. Homemaking itself is a composite of physical tasks, managerial functions, spirit, and emotional climate that holds the family or personality together and fosters development. The scope of activities related to homemaking include the following:

1. Care of self
2. Feeding the family
3. Marketing and shopping
4. Clothing the family
5. Housing and maintenance

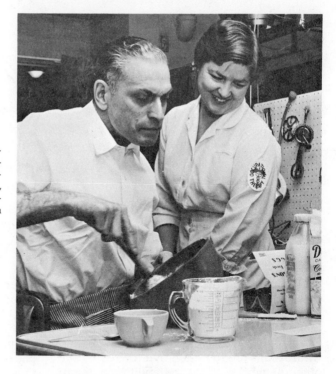

FIGURE 25–1. Men sometimes need homemaker training. (Connecticut Society for Crippled Children and Adults.) (From U.S. Department of Health, Education and Welfare, Vocational Rehabilitation Administration: Rehabilitation of the Physically Handicapped in Homemaking Activities, 1963.)

6. Family relations
7. Education and recreation
8. Community participation

ORGANIZATION OF A TRAINING PROGRAM

Training may be arranged as a community service, as part of a hospital service, or, when possible, as a combination of the two.[2]

There are many agencies and facilities in most communities with an interest in homemaking. In planning the program, one should consider the local medical society, physical and occupational therapists, visiting or public health nurses, social workers, voluntary agencies, such as the National Society for Crippled Children and Adults, homemaker services in welfare departments or family service groups, home economists, dietitians, architects, designers, builders, and industrial engineers. Physiatrists and other physicians, such as orthopedic surgeons, neurologists, and cardiologists, should be encouraged to help in the planning.

The ideal training program should be based in a rehabilitation center or in a hospital with a department of physical medicine and rehabilitation and should begin when the

homemaker is in the hospital.[3] Here the team concerned with the patient's rehabilitation can plan homemaking as an integral part of the general rehabilitation program. In addition, after discharge, the team can serve as a liaison to arrange continued training and follow-up. If the patient lives too far away from the rehabilitation facility, agencies in the patient's community can be alerted to his or her needs after return to the home.

The team may include all professional personnel in a department of physical medicine and rehabilitation. People most concerned are the physician (preferably a physiatrist), who directs training; the social worker, who acquaints the patient's family with the patient's particular needs and maintains the link with the physician, evaluates the possibilities for adaptations in the home, and helps in the purchase or procurement of special aids or devices; the physical therapist, who helps evaluate the patient's proficiency in activities of daily living and plans a conditioning program to maintain physical fitness; and the occupational therapist, who instructs in household management and the use of adaptive devices. Most often the actual home evaluation is carried out by a physical or occupational therapist who collaborates with the social worker. When the patient is a client of an outside agency,

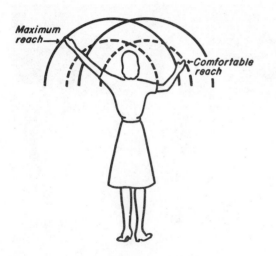

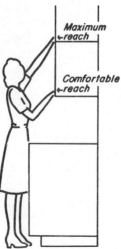

FIGURE 25–2. Determining vertical reaching areas. (From Rusk, H. A., et al.: A Manual for Training the Disabled Homemaker. Rehabilitation Monograph VIII, 2nd Ed. New York, The Institute of Physical Medicine and Rehabilitation, New York University Medical Center, 1961.)

coordination of the rehabilitative program may be directed by a rehabilitation counselor. A very useful addition to the team is the home consultant or home economist who is trained in many areas of homemaking and whose skills are too often overlooked by the other members of the rehabilitation team. Duties of team members should complement each other.

EVALUATION CONTENT

The goal of homemaker training is efficient resettlement of the patient in her place of work — the home. Evaluation should anticipate problems or difficulties that the patient will encounter in the home. Domestic activities involve consideration of the following:[4]

1. Range of Reach. One should consider the maximal reach required, both in a vertical and in a horizontal direction. Prescriptions of tools for reaching, allocation of equipment, and arrangement of working surfaces depend on these measurements (Figs. 25–2 and 25–3). Conditions that limit range of reach are those requiring that work be done sitting down, such as paraplegia, and those

severely limiting motion, such as crippling rheumatoid arthritis.

2. Movement from One Place to Another. A housewife may walk as much as 25 kilometers during her day's work. Cardiac patients, those limited to wheelchairs, and those requiring the use of canes, crutches, or leg braces are obviously limited.

3. Manual Activities. Patients with impaired use of hand or arm because of weakness, incoordination, or amputation may suffer limitations. It is this group that will call upon all the ingenuity the occupational therapist can muster.

4. Energy Consumption. Patients with cardiorespiratory diseases will usually find this the chief limiting factor. Bedmaking, ironing, or washing up requires the same rate of energy expenditure as housepainting, cabinetmaking, or plastering — 3 to 4.5 calories per minute. Passmore and Durnin[5] describe the energy costs of many common household activities.

5. Safety. Lack of coordination, of sensation, and of spatial orientation may prove dangerous when one handles hot or sharp objects. The danger of falling because of vertigo, loss of consciousness, syncopal at-

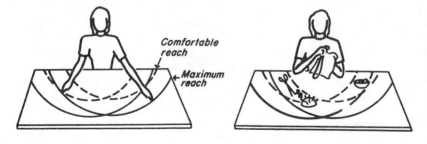

FIGURE 25–3. Determining horizontal reach areas. (From Rusk, H. A., et al.: A Manual for Training the Disabled Homemaker. Rehabilitation Monograph VIII, 2nd Ed. New York, The Institute of Physical Medicine and Rehabilitation, New York University Medical Center, 1961.)

tacks, or epilepsy must be guarded against. It is in this group that one should consider elimination of certain household tasks altogether.

6. Communication. Contact with the outside world through the telephone or directly in such activities as shopping is difficult for patients with language difficulty. The aphasic patient is an example of this problem.

Almost all rehabilitation centers and physical medicine and rehabilitation services in general hospitals have a training kitchen facility. In addition, bathroom and bed and sitting room training areas are often standard equipment. In such facilities, patients' skills in cleaning activities, meal preparation, meal service, laundry tasks, sewing, heavy household duties, marketing, child care, and special tasks may be thoroughly evaluated and plans made for adaptation in the home. Forms on which careful records are kept are an essential part of the training program. Accurate assessment of progress or changes in technique cannot be made any other way. Evaluation of skills in activities of daily living, such as bed-to-wheelchair transfer, walking, climbing, traveling, hand dressing, eating, and toilet activities, cannot be excluded from the program. Training in these areas must go on concomitantly with training in homemaking.

All members of the rehabilitation team try to help the homemaker to help herself. The primary therapeutic goal is work simplification — a scientific process of improving job method and adapting mechanical facilities to fit the physiologic capacity of the worker. We may add two more: improved physical fitness — increased capacity for work —and improvement in psychological motivation so that the patient is encouraged to become proficient.

PRINCIPLES OF WORK SIMPLIFICATION OR ECONOMY OF MOTION

Work simplification is of primary concern in homemaking training. The following outline is an excellent working guide.[2]

1. Whenever the condition allows, use both hands in opposite and symmetric motions while working.

2. Lay out work areas within normal reach. Arrange supplies in a semicircle.

3. Slide — do not lift and carry. Use a table with wheels when moving from one work area to another.

4. Use fixed work stations. Have a special place to do each job so that supplies and equipment may be kept ready for immediate use.

5. Use the smallest number of work elements. Select equipment that may be used for more than one job; eliminate unnecessary motions.

6. Avoid the work of holding. Use utensils that rest firmly and are secured by suction cups or clamps. This will free hands for work.

7. Let gravity work. Examples are a laundry chute, refuse chute, and gravity-feed flour bin.

8. Position tools in advance. Store them so that they are placed in position for immediate grasping and use. For example, hang measuring cup and spoons separately within sight.

9. Position machine controls and switches within easy reach. Household appliances should be chosen on the basis of ease of operation.

10. Sit to work whenever possible. Use a comfortable chair and adjust work-place height to the chair. Or use an adjustable stool or chair.

11. Use a correct work-place height. The height should be right for the homemaker and the job. There are no standard heights. Morant[6] points out that the dimensions of a work space suitable for persons of normal size may differ appreciably from the best that can be found to accommodate workers of all sizes and that in a work space, a change of even one-half inch may make an appreciable difference in the ease of operation and comfort of a considerable proportion of workers.

12. Good conditions are important —good light and ventilation, comfortable clothing, and ambient temperature.

Rules of work simplification are not enough. The patient must learn to manage herself and her needs before she can manage homemaking activities and her family. She must become proficient in her activities of daily living.[7] She must begin to think like an industrial engineer. Is her strength adequate for certain jobs? What is her need for rest periods? What is the best time of day for the performance of certain duties? Ought she to plan some jobs as a daily chore, a weekly

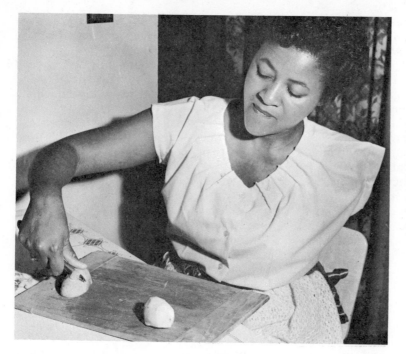

FIGURE 25–4. A spike on a board simplifies potato peeling. (J. A. Manter, University of Connecticut.) (From U.S. Department of Health, Education and Welfare, Vocational Rehabilitation Administration: Rehabilitation of the Physically Handicapped in Homemaking Activities, 1963.)

chore, or even a monthly chore? In what quantities ought food to be prepared? It is these and countless other questions that the homemaker tries to answer as she becomes more skillful in her job.

ASSISTIVE DEVICES, AND SELECTION AND ADAPTATION OF HOUSEHOLD EQUIPMENT

Tasks should be attempted without special aids. If it is decided that the homemaker will continue certain activities that require them, then plans can be made for the adaptation of a special aid or device. It would be unwise to plan for aids if the homemaker is not going to carry out activities for which the aids are designed.

Before planning to make a device, determine whether it is already available commercially. Often aids can be purchased more cheaply than they could be made. Basic considerations in the selection of devices are as follows:[8]

1. Use ordinary tools when they can be managed. Some homemakers hesitate to use tools that are obviously designed for the handicapped.

2. Homemakers are more likely to use assistive devices if they have a part in their selection.

3. Choose simple tools and, before their purchase or fabrication, consider the complications involved in taking them apart, keeping them clean, and finding a place to store them.

4. Consider an assistive device as temporary if that is possible. Change it as the homemaker acquires new skills.

Self-help devices or aids for the homemaker are used for stabilizing and holding objects (Figs. 25–4 and 25–5) or for extending reach and mobility (Fig. 25–6). In addition, one-handed aids (Fig. 25–7) and remote control devices (Fig. 25–8) may be useful in patients with limited upper extremity function.

Selection of proper appliances also can be of immense help to the homemaker. Care should be taken to see that all machines and

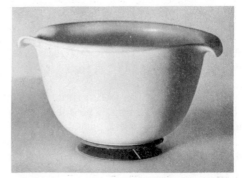

FIGURE 25–5. Suction bowel holder. (From Steinke, N., and Ericksson, P.: Homemaking Aids for the Disabled. Minneapolis, Kenny Rehabilitation Institute, 1963.)

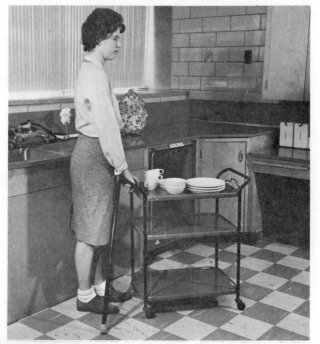

FIGURE 25–6. Wheeled utility table. The patient hangs her cane on the table rail and uses the table for support as she wheels it from place to place. (Courtesy of Kenny Rehabilitation Institute.)

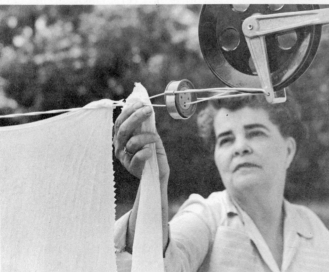

FIGURE 25–7. A twist line holds without pins. Just insert the edge of the garment between the lines and push the line ahead. It will twist and hold the garment. (From Zmola, G. M.: You Can Do Family Laundry with Hand Limitations. Storrs, Conn., University of Connecticut, School of Home Economics, 1959.)

FIGURE 25–8. Environmental control unit. By sipping or puffing into the mouthpiece the patient activates this device, which can remotely control appliances, lights, and communication aids.

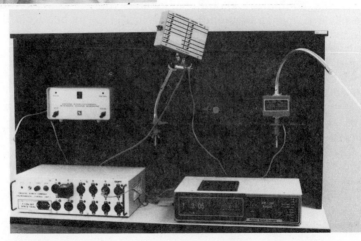

appliances have openings and controls that can be reached and operated easily. It is also important that such appliances are placed in a convenient location. The designs of small household appliances and their use are discussed by Klinger.[19] In general, it can be said that for the limited homemaker, front-opening equipment is better than top-opening equipment and that doors hinged on the side are best. A piece of equipment, such as a refrigerator, should not be purchased until the needs of the homemaker are clearly understood. Gas and electric utility companies can give very helpful advice.

REMODELING AND REARRANGEMENT OF HOME FACILITIES

In recent years there has been a great deal of emphasis on remodeling and rearrangement of home facilities, particularly kitchens. This work has emphasized space requirements for maneuvering a wheelchair, for vertical and horizontal reaches of the homemaker, for comfortable working heights, for necessary clearances of work areas, and for arrangement of the various centers such as sink center, range center, and mix center. Three basic kitchen arrangements, the U, the L, and the corridor, have been thoroughly worked out. There are advantages and disadvantages to each. Which one is best for a particular homemaker depends on her disability. However, the arrangement of the refrigerator, stove, and kitchen sink should form a work triangle. Most trips are made from the sink to the refrigerator and then to the stove.

The work center should have a definite and fixed place for all tools, utensils, and materials. This equipment should be located to permit a sequence of motion. Examples include the storage in the sink area of utensils that are first used with water, including all top-of-range utensils except skillets and pan covers. In the range area should be located utensils first used with heat, including covers to all utensils.

A logical extension of kitchen planning is the design of complete dwellings for the disabled. Obviously the limitations here are chiefly economic. In spite of these drawbacks, several approaches to housing for the disabled have been made. Design of dwellings for the disabled who require wheelchairs has been extensively discussed in two communications from the Testing and Observation Institute at Hellerup, Denmark,[9, 10] and in a recent publication by Laurie.[11]

At a conference of the International Society for Rehabilitation of the Disabled, the following criteria were stressed:[12]

1. The dwelling must allow the individual, whatever his handicap, to move about with maximal convenience and minimal effort.

2. The disabled person must be able to use all the facilities, not just the kitchen.

3. The dwelling must have maximal ease of communication with the outside world.

4. The house must have an adequate heating system.

5. Everything in the house must be planned for maximal serviceability and ease of maintenance.

6. The house must be usable regardless of the type of disability. It must never be planned for one disability only.

7. The price of every single component must be reduced to the absolute minimum.

Planning the home for a disabled person requires accurate information concerning the physical limitations imposed by the disability or illness and the actual space available in the house. A planning consultant can save time and money. Any new construction or remodeling of a home for the disabled should include the following dimensions:

1. Walkways and halls should be at least 3 feet wide.

2. Doorways should be a minimum of 32 inches in width to accommodate the average wheelchair or some motorized chairs, which may be 2 feet 5 inches in width.

3. Ramp slopes are recommended at no more than 8.3 per cent, or a one-foot rise in twelve feet.

4. Wall outlets should be no less than 16 inches from the floor.

5. Optimal table height for pull-out tables is 24 inches. If knee room is needed to accommodate a wheelchair, the height should be 30 inches, and for working while standing, 32 to 37 inches.

6. Sink heights should be 21 to 36 inches.

7. Toilet heights should be 15 to 23 inches.

8. An area of 15 square feet is required for wheelchair accommodation in a bathroom.

More detailed specifications are described

in the publication by Laurie,[11] which also includes references to other resource materials about adaptations, techniques, and remodeling plans.

CHILD CARE

Child care may be a particular problem for the disabled homemaker. It is important for her to develop a sense of discipline and responsibility in her children. Dressing the young child may be especially difficult for the handicapped mother. May et al.[8] have made some very practical suggestions concerning clothes for preschool children which make dressing much easier.

It may happen on occasion that a handicapped homemaker has handicapped children. In such cases good work habits and a sense of pride in accomplishment are invaluable. This is an excellent way to encourage independence.

All children, whether handicapped or not, work much better under established rules and regulation. Disciplinary problems arise more often when there are no standards and when the child is not made responsible. Wall[13] points out that the desire to be helpful and independent is often at its height when the child is four years old. Instead of making the child more dependent, the mother should give him the opportunity he needs to develop into a cooperative member of the family.

A mother who teaches her children to be independent early, whether they are handicapped or not, will make time available for her own needs — needs for rest, for cultural enrichment, and for other tasks not related to child care.

NUTRITION AND EXERCISE

During her training in the hospital or rehabilitation center the disabled homemaker should learn the principles of sound nutrition. This is of importance not only for herself but also for her family. Since mixes and canned and dehydrated foods may be sources of work simplification, it is imperative that the homemaker learn to incorporate them in a balanced diet. The hospital dietitian has a very helpful role to play here.

It is probably true, however, that the homemaker will suffer far more often from overnutrition than from malnutrition. Because disability may limit markedly the homemaker's opportunity to perform tasks that require intense, prolonged physical effort, she will tend to eat more than she needs. The result is obesity, which in turn will increase the cost of work.[14] An occasional patient, however, who is taking large doses of medication, or of several medications, may have little or no appetite. The goal in this instance is to control medications and encourage sound nutritional habits.

The recommendation for daily periods of cardiorespiratory and muscular exercise may appear contradictory after we have stressed work simplification and efficiency. On the contrary, short periods of relatively intense graded exercise are the basis of physical fitness and will increase the homemaker's ability to perform useful work. Some activity aside from the fixed duties of homemaking is also necessary to maintain flexibility and optimal range of motion of joints. An exercise program may be contraindicated in the case of a patient with severe cardiopulmonary disease.

PSYCHOLOGY OF DISABILITY AND FAMILY RELATIONSHIPS

The handicapped homemaker has fears and anxieties that those who are well can only dimly perceive. She must learn to accept the difference in her appearance and she must finally adjust her life to a central fact — disability is permanent and the most fervent wishing will not make it disappear. She is perturbed by doubts concerning her abilities, her role as a wife and sexual partner, and the way her children may respond to her altered appearance. Litman,[15] in a study of 100 patients undergoing treatment in rehabilitation centers, has emphasized the importance of family support in the rehabilitation process.

If we are to help the homemaker achieve successful resettlement in her home, the family must be encouraged to take an active part in the training. Frequent visits to the hospital by family members help the patient, but also allow them to see the patient at work, to discover what she can do, and to learn techniques of treatment that will be carried out at home.[16] Members of the rehabilitation team must learn to wait, to be patient, and to understand that the patient's adjustment is a dynamic, constantly changing process.[17]

Accounts of the trials and tribulations of disabled homemakers demonstrate that there are certain common factors in successful rehabilitation. They are courage, determination to succeed, family support, ability to change work habits and techniques, and intelligent use of available facilities.

The successful rehabilitation process is demonstrated in the words of a handicapped homemaker:

I am happy and thankful to do my own housework. I love to cook and wash and iron. It just is a thrill for me knowing I've done it myself, to see my clothes sparkling white and ironed smoothly, to see my family nicely dressed, and to see my husband's and son's eyes and hear their comments of pleasure as they enjoy their food.[11]

HOME CARE AND HOMEMAKER SERVICES

These subjects have some relation to training in homemaking and deserve definition. Home care is the provision of health care and supportive services to the sick or disabled person in his place of residence. It may be provided in a diversity of patterns or organization and service running the gamut from nursing service under a physician's direction to a program which is centrally administered and which, through coordinated planning, evaluation, and follow-up procedures, provides for physician-directed medical, nursing, social, and related services to selected patients at home. A logical link between the homemaker and the hospital would be a hospital extension service. Under titles XVIII and XIX of the Social Security Act (Medicare and Medicaid), home health care visits were included in a federal program of health insurance. Medicare benefits are limited to skilled nursing care or other therapeutic services prescribed by a physician and provided by an approved home health agency. This does not include homemaking services. Medicaid home health care benefits differ from Medicare in that eligibility for home health care for persons entitled to public assistance and Supplemental Security Income (SSI) is not related to the requirements for skilled care. Medicaid services may include home health aid services, medical equipment, and appliances. A new

title XX enacted in 1974 called for states to provide for health support services to meet the needs of children, the aged, the mentally retarded, the blind, the emotionally disturbed, and the physically handicapped. These services include those related to the management and maintenance of the home.[11]

Homemaker services are services offered to families disrupted by death, illness, or accident. A homemaker in this frame of reference is a trained housekeeper and cook who has skill in handling children. Such services are provided by many welfare and family agencies.[18] Home health aides have been added to homemaker services. Their function is to help improve the patient's level of independence by helping in the carrying out of instructions left by the occupational therapist, physical therapist, physician, or other supervisor. The nutritionist or dietitian may offer useful services through consultation to staffs of home health agencies, membership on a professional advisory committee, and teaching programs for home health aides. Such services may be extremely helpful to individuals whose disability is so severe that independent function will never be possible.

REFERENCES

1. Switzer, M. D.: Foreword. *In* Rehabilitation of the Physically Handicapped in Homemaking Activities. Proceedings of a Workshop. Highland Park, Ill., Jan. 27–30, 1963. U. S. Department of Health, Education and Welfare, Vocational Rehabilitation Administration.
2. Rusk, H. A., Kristeller, E. L., Judson, J. S., Hung, G. M., and Zimmerman, M. E.: Introductions. *In* A Manual for Training the Disabled Homemaker. Rehabilitation Monograph VIII, 2nd Ed. New York, The Institute of Physical Medicine and Rehabilitation, New York University Medical Center, 1961.
3. May, E. E.: Suggestions for the rehabilitation of the physically handicapped homemaker. Am. J. Occup. Ther., 8: Part I, 1962.
4. Petrie, A.: Rehabilitation of the housewife. Occup. Ther., 27:19, 1964.
5. Passmore, R., and Durnin, J. V. G. A.: Human energy expenditure. Phys. Rev., 35:801, 1955.
6. Morant, G. M.: Body sizes and work spaces. *In* Symposium on Human Factors in Equipment Design. The Ergonomics Research Society. Proceedings, Vol. 2, edited by W. F. Floyd and A. T. Welford. London, H. K. Lewis & Co., Ltd., 1954.
7. Mossman, P. L.: A Problem Oriented Approach to Stroke Rehabilitation. Springfield, Ill., Charles C Thomas, Publisher, 1976.
8. May, E. E., Waggoner, N. R., and Boettke, E. M.:

Homemaking for the Handicapped. New York, Dodd, Mead, and Company, 1966.

9. Leschly, V., Exner, I., and Exner, J.: General Lives in Designs of Dwellings for Handicapped Confined to Wheelchairs. Part I. Communications from the Testing and Observation Institute of the Danish National Association for Infantile Paralysis, No. 6. Hellerup, Denmark, 1960.

10. Leschly, V., Kjaer, A., and Kjaer, B.: General Lives in Designs of Dwellings for Handicapped Confined to Wheelchairs. Part 2. Communications from the Testing and Observation Institute of the Danish National Association for Infantile Paralysis, No. 6. Hellerup, Denmark, 1960.

11. Laurie, G.: Housing and Home Services for the Disabled. Hagerstown, Maryland, Harper and Row, 1977.

12. Planning of Dwellings. *In* ISRD Conference, The Physically Disabled and Their Environment, Stockholm, October 12–18, 1961. New York, International Society for the Rehabilitation of the Disabled, 1962.

13. Wall, J. S.: Play Experiences Handicapped Mothers May Share with Young Children. Storrs, Conn., University of Connecticut, School of Home Economics, 1961.

14. Gordon, E. E.: Development of the Applied Sciences to the Handicapped Homemaker. *In* Rehabilitation of the Physically Handicapped in Homemaking Activities. Proceedings of a workshop. Highland Park, Ill., January 27–30, 1963. U. S. Department of Health, Education and Welfare, Vocational Rehabilitation Administration.

15. Litman, T. J.: An analysis of the sociologic factors affecting the rehabilitation of the physically handicapped. Arch. Phys. Med. 45:9, 1964.

16. Peszczynski, M., Fowles, B., II, and Mohan, S. P.: Function of home evaluations in discharging rehabilitated severely disabled from the hospital. Arch. Phys. Med. Rehabil., 43:109, 1961.

17. Christopherson, V. A.: The patient and the family. Rehabil. Lit., 23:34, 1962.

18. Homemaker Services in Public Welfare. U. S. Department of Health, Education and Welfare, Welfare Administration, April, 1964.

19. Klinger, J. L.: Mealtime Manual for People with Disabilities and the Aging, 2nd Ed. New York, Institute of Physical Medicine, 1978.

20. Steinke, N., and Erickson, P.: Homemaking Aids for the Disabled. Minneapolis, Kenny Rehabilitation Institute, 1963.

21. Zmola, G. M.: You Can Do Family Laundry with Hand Limitations. Storrs, Conn., University of Connecticut, School of Home Economics, 1959.

26

UPPER EXTREMITY ORTHOTICS

LEONARD F. BENDER

FUNCTIONAL ANATOMY

The shoulder-elbow-wrist-hand unit is a remarkable evolutionary development modified as man arose and walked on his hind legs. The front legs developed the capacity for prehension and the mobility necessary to place the hand in an infinite number of positions.

The shoulder girdle is composed of seven joints: the costovertebral, costosternal, sternoclavicular, scapulocostal, acromioclavicular, suprahumeral, and glenohumeral.[1] Moving synchronously, these joints provide great mobility but only minimally essential stability. The glenohumeral joint is commonly referred to as the shoulder joint, in contrast to the group of joints that make up the shoulder girdle. Movements of the glenohumeral joint are controlled by two groups of muscles: (1) large muscles originating on the thorax and inserting on the humerus plus the deltoid and (2) smaller muscles that arise on the scapula and insert through the rotator cuff on the humeral head and neck. The combined action of the short rotator muscles (supraspinatus, infraspinatus, teres minor, and subscapularis) pulls the humeral head into the glenoid fossa and fixes it there, depresses and rotates the head of the hu-

merus, and, coupled with the deltoid muscle, assists in abduction of the arm through a rotatory force couple.[2] The short rotators receive their innervation primarily from the fifth and sixth cervical nerve roots through nerves that branch off the upper trunk and the posterior and lateral cords of the brachial plexus; they are spared in most cervical spinal cord injuries but are variously involved in injuries of the brachial plexus.

Elbow, forearm, and wrist motions combine to produce shortening and lengthening of the support system of the hand and rotation of the hand through 180 degrees from full pronation to extreme supination. Like a universal joint, these joints, in conjunction with the shoulder girdle, provide accurate and extensive positioning of the hand. Elbow flexor muscles are largely supplied by the fifth and sixth cervical nerve roots through the musculocutaneous nerve, while extensors are innervated by the sixth and seventh cervical nerve roots in the radial nerve.

The forearm anchors most of the muscles that flex, extend, and rotate the wrist and also provide power grip and metacarpophalangeal extension, while the muscles responsible for many fine functions of the fingers are located in the hand. The intrinsic muscles of the hand are supplied by the eighth cervi-

518

cal and the first thoracic nerve roots, while the muscles of the forearm receive innervation from all nerve roots of the brachial plexus.

Individual muscles for the thumb and little finger (fifth digit) makes these two digits uniquely mobile and useful. The first, second, and third digits are often used as a three-jaw chuck to grasp small objects. Napier has described this position as "precision grip."[3] It may be accomplished through fingertip, lateral, or palmar pinch. "Power grip" involves holding an object between flexed fingers and the opposed thumb. The same tool may be handled by either precision grip or power grip; it is the nature of the task, not the shape of the tool, that dictates which posture is employed. This difference must be carefully considered when prescribing orthoses or recommending surgery.

FORCES

Orthotic devices apply forces to the braced extremity. Therefore, it is important to recognize and attempt to understand the role of force in producing motion and desired activities.

A force can be described according to its magnitude, direction, and point of application.[4] All movement is either rotation, translation, or a combination of the two. Rotation is angular motion and translation is motion without change in angular orientation. Torque is the strength of a rotating tendency. The effectiveness of a force in causing joint motion depends both on its point of application or distance from the axis of rotation and on its magnitude. Moving the origin or insertion of a muscle to a different location may either decrease or increase the effectiveness of that muscle.

Levers can be used to amplify forces, and examples of all types of levers can be found in the musculoskeletal system. When applying force through orthoses, the principles of leverage and forces must be utilized to achieve optimal results.

PURPOSES OF ORTHOSES

Orthoses are used to (1) assist, (2) resist, (3) align, and (4) simulate function of part of the body. Orthoses that assist movement generally incorporate a method of storing energy and releasing it at a desired time; springs, rubber bands, compressed gas, and electricity may be used. They may also transfer muscle power from an accustomed use to a new one, as in balanced forearm orthoses or flexor hinge hand orthoses.

Occasionally, movements of the body need to be reduced; orthoses may restrict or resist movement by adding friction to orthotic joint movement or by using stops.

Alignment of joints damaged by arthritis or of a spine curved abnormally may be achieved through orthoses; such devices may reduce or possibly prevent deformity.

Certain surgical procedures may also achieve results similar to those produced by orthoses; in some instances an orthotic device may be used to simulate the result of proposed surgery.

CLASSIFICATION OF ORTHOSES

The confusing terminology used to describe braces, splints, calipers, appliances, and aids has included eponyms, descriptive phrases, and non-standardized terms. In 1971, the American Orthotic and Prosthetic Association urged the Committee on Prosthetic-Orthotic Education of the National Academy of Sciences to develop a standardized nomenclature. By mid-1972, a new terminology was developed and put into use;[5] in it all exoskeletal devices are called orthoses and they are described (1) by the joints they encompass, (2) by abbreviating each joint name to one letter, and (3) by using combinations of symbols to indicate the desired control of the designated function.

Orthoses may be made out of thin metal, heat-moldable plastic, epoxy resins, or plaster. The shorter the period of time one proposes using the device, the less durably it need be constructed. Thus, if one wishes to rest an inflamed joint for a few days, it is quite likely that a suitable orthosis can be constructed of plaster or heat-moldable plastic by the physician or by a therapist. But when use of the device for an extended period of time is anticipated, it will be cheaper and better to use metal, plastic, or epoxy resins and to have the device constructed by an orthotist.

TYPES OF ORTHOSES

A convenient way to describe orthoses is to divide them into static positioning devices and functional ones.

Static Orthoses

Shoulder Static Devices

The airplane splint is a classic example of a static positioning device applied to the shoulder. It holds the arm in approximately 90 degrees of abduction and permits no glenohumeral motion. It is held to the chest wall by straps or elastic bandages and is made of metal or plaster. Previously thought to be the best way to manage perinatal injury of the brachial plexus, it is no longer recommended for this purpose because it may contribute to the high-riding shoulder girdle frequently seen in Erb's palsy.[6] However, it is the orthosis of choice for burns of the axilla.

Elbow Static Devices

Static positioning orthoses are used at the elbow primarily to increase range of motion in either flexion or extension. They are contoured so that their straps exert force on the arm and forearm to gain the desired increase in range of motion. They may also be applied to prevent anticipated contractures after burns of the elbow region; turnbuckles may be used to increase the force applied to the area of contracture when one exists.

Wrist Static Devices

At the wrist, static orthoses are commonly used to provide immobilization. In a case of neurapraxia of the radial nerve with a good prognosis for quick recovery, a plaster cock-up splint which holds the hand in 15 degrees of dorsiflexion at the wrist and prevents wrist motion may suffice. If a long period of recovery is anticipated, a functional device would be more appropriate.

In rheumatoid arthritis, a plastic or metal orthosis can be applied to the volar surface of the forearm and the wrist and is held in place by three straps over the styloid processes of the radius and ulna, the metacarpals, and the mid-forearm.[7] When correctly applied, this device can help prevent or correct subluxation of the carpal bones volarly on the radius and ulnar deviation of the hand at the wrist.

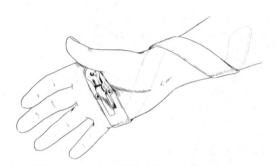

FIGURE 26–1. A spiral wrist orthosis with a spring-loaded clip on the palmar extension can be used to stabilize the wrist and to provide an attachment for writing and eating and other assistive devices.

Spiral orthoses also can stabilize the wrist by wrapping a metal or plastic strap from the palm to the mid-forearm in 1½ turns.

Static Hand Orthoses

Static hand orthoses vary considerably in design according to their purpose. They may be used to immobilize finger joints or to increase function by holding digits in a more favorable position.

Burns of the dorsum of the hand are appropriately splinted by holding the fingers on a platform with the IP joints extended, the MCP joints fully flexed, the thumb abducted, and the wrist slightly dorsiflexed.[8]

When the metacarpophalangeal joints are acutely inflamed, as in rheumatoid arthritis, these joints should be supported in a neutral position with a volar platform extending to the flexor crease of the proximal interphalangeal joint. This support is most easily provided through heat-moldable plastic splints that extend either to or across the wrist on the volar surface and have a lip on the ulnar border high enough to prevent ulnar deviation of the fingers and a dorsal strap just behind the head of the metacarpals to reduce volar subluxation of the phalanges.

As one considers different ways to increase function in a weak or partially paralyzed hand, there appear to be two basic classes of orthoses that may be used: the simple hand orthosis and some type of flexor-hinge hand orthosis.

The simple hand orthosis is a device that consists of a metal or plastic band that runs either over the dorsum of the hand from the thumb web to the volar surface of the fourth metacarpal or volarly from the dorsal surface of the second metacarpal across the palm to the dorsal surface of the fourth metacarpal. Each orthosis is held on the hand and pre-

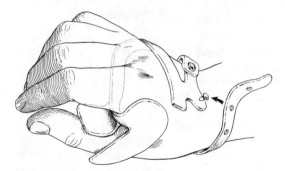

FIGURE 26–2. A simple or basic hand orthosis made from steel and held on by a plastisol strap. A large C bar is attached to hold the thumb abducted.

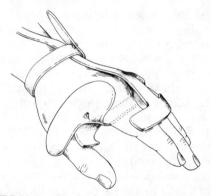

FIGURE 26–3. A wrist-hand orthosis with a metacarpophalangeal extension stop; this "lumbrical" bar can be used to enhance extension of the interphalangeal joints by the long finger extensor muscles in an ulnar nerve lesion.

vented from sliding off by a strap around the volar surface of the wrist. A small, rolled bar protrudes between the first and second metacarpals to prevent the orthosis from migrating proximally. If this bar is enlarged to form a letter C, it can be used to hold the thumb abducted from the palm. An extension of the basic orthosis over the first metacarpal will hold the thumb in a position of opposition. If the thumb is flail, it can be held in a pair of rings with a bar connecting them to the simple hand orthosis. A bar set dorsally over the proximal phalanges will prevent hyperextension of the metacarpophalangeal joints, yet this "lumbrical" bar will permit the long finger extensors to act to extend the interphalangeal joints.

Other units that may be added to a simple hand orthosis utilize springs or movable parts and will be considered under the heading of Functional Orthoses.

Static Finger Orthoses

Static finger orthoses can stabilize individual interphalangeal joints or combinations of interphalangeal joints. They are usually constructed of stainless steel in the form of complete or partial rings fastened together with narrow metal bars. They may also be spirals similar to those used across the wrist. An unstable interphalangeal joint can be prevented from hyperextending and can be made stable with one of these devices.

Functional Orthoses

Instead of immobilizing a joint or restraining its motion as static orthoses do, a functional orthosis improves function through the use of levers, pulleys, movable joints, and external power storage devices such as

springs, rubber bands, batteries, and tanks of compressed gas.

Functional Shoulder Orthoses

Functional orthoses to improve shoulder actions have not proven generally useful or successful. Several orthoses that were supported on the iliac crest and had uprights that extended to the axilla or laterally around the shoulder were designed and refined in the decades between 1950 and 1970.[9] They were relatively complex exoskeletal systems and have been discarded because they were cumbersome and difficult to fit and provided only limited additional function.

Functional Elbow Orthoses

Functional orthoses can be constructed for weakness or instability of the elbow. The

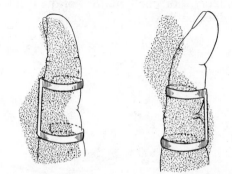

FIGURE 26–4. Static finger orthoses. The one on the left prevents fixed flexion of the proximal interphalangeal joint as is seen in a "boutonniere" deformity; the one to the right prevents hyperextension of the proximal interphalangeal joint, as may be seen in a "swan neck" deformity.

customary device has some type of pivot hinge aligned with the axis of the elbow joint, and stability is provided by cuffs above and below the elbow. Rubber bands, springs, or compressed gas may be used to assist either flexion or extension; generally, extension can be achieved through the pull of gravity and only flexion need be assisted. When elbow flexion muscle strength is less than antigravity and an elbow flexion assist is utilized, the orthosis must also incorporate a locking mechanism at the elbow to maintain a practical functional position for carrying loads. Elbow flexion assist may also be provided through a Bowden cable, which has the cable housing attached to a cuff around the arm while the cable extends through it from a figure eight harness around the shoulders to that portion of the orthosis that is below the elbow. Tension on the cable will flex the elbow and an elbow-locking mechanism operated by scapular elevation will permit a choice of several stable positions of the elbow.

Balanced Forearm Orthoses

Perhaps the most useful device to assist both elbow and shoulder function, in the presence of profound weakness in the upper extremity, is the balanced forearm orthosis. This can be mounted on a wheelchair, on a table or working surface, or occasionally on a belt around the person at the level of the iliac crest. It consists of a trough, in which the proximal portion of the forearm rests, a pivot and linkage system underneath the trough which can be adjusted and preset so that the patient can learn to produce motion at both the elbow and to a lesser extent the shoulder, with small motions of the trunk or shoulder girdle.

Functional Wrist Orthoses

Functional wrist orthoses are rarely used without hand orthoses. If it is necessary to assist wrist extension only, it can be done by a volar plastic or metal trough on the forearm attached with Velcro straps around the dorsum of the forearm. Pivot hinges at the side of the wrist must be attached to the forearm piece and to a palmar bar. Springs or rubber bands attached to short dorsal uprights on either side of the wrist hinge can be adjusted to give assistance to wrist extension.

A group of devices known as wrist-driven, flexor-hinge hand splints have been developed and will be discussed under "Functional Hand Orthoses," since they use wrist power to provide finger function, especially prehension.

Functional Hand Orthoses

Functional hand orthoses can be constructed by using a simple hand orthosis as a foundation and adding one or more special assistive devices.

A swivel thumb is a half-ring clip around the proximal phalanx of the thumb whose arm pivots from a point near the head of the second metacarpal to permit the thumb to swing in a fixed arc toward opposition from extension and abduction. The rigid pivot arm can be replaced with a spring wire and the thumb then not only can pivot but also can voluntarily be brought into adduction; abduction is assisted by the spring.

A first dorsal interosseus assist also attaches near the head of the second metacarpal and utilizes a spring wire and a plastic ring to pull the index finger into abduction; the plastic ring may be placed over either the proximal or the middle phalanx.

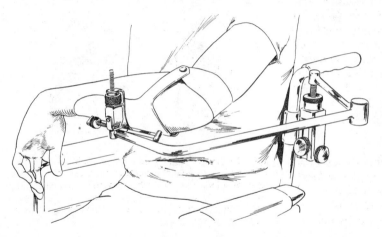

FIGURE 26–5. A balanced forearm orthosis mounted on a wheelchair. The patient's forearm rests in a trough. The pivot point of the trough and the position of the two movable arms must be carefully adjusted to achieve maximum range of hand placement in a patient with severe proximal weakness.

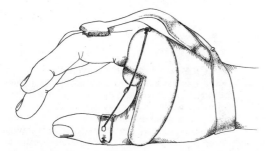

FIGURE 26–6. A spring swivel thumb assist has been added to a simple hand orthosis with a metacarpophalangeal extension stop. The thumb assist permits the thumb to be actively adducted and the spring will assist abduction. The thumb can also pivot across the palm toward the fifth digit.

A thumb interphalangeal joint extension assist is similar to a first dorsal interosseus assist but is attached near the head of the first metacarpal and exerts its pull on the distal phalanx of the thumb.

Interphalangeal extension assist in the absence of hand intrinsic muscles and long finger extensors can be achieved by mounting a "banjo"-shaped device on the hand orthosis and pulling on the distal phalanges through plastic rings attached to rubber bands that are fastened to the crossbar of the "banjo." Unfortunately, the device is cumbersome and the assisting force cannot be constant, since the rubber band tension increases with stretch.

Metacarpophalangeal extension assist no longer requires a "banjo." It can be accomplished by a bar similar in contour to a lumbrical bar but placed on the volar surface of the proximal phalanges with stiff coil springs holding each end of the bar to the hand orthosis. The springs must be placed to push the proximal phalanges into extension at the metacarpophalangeal joint and to permit full range of finger flexion.

Flexor-Hinge Hand Orthoses

Hand orthoses with various attachments described above work well in isolated and mild to moderate weaknesses or abnormal functions of the hand. However, when paralysis or weakness is widespread or severe, it may be advisable to use an orthosis built on the flexor-hinge hand principle. This principle permits only metacarpophalangeal motion, stabilizes the interphalangeal joints of digits two and three and both the interphalangeal and metacarpophalangeal joints of the thumb, creates a three-jaw chuck prehension, and may utilize several different power-assist sources. A hand with unstable metacarpophalangeal joints, such as is seen in rheumatoid arthritis, may need only the alignment provided by a finger-driven flexor-hinge hand orthosis. The intact muscles are used to flex and extend the metacarpophalangeal joints, and the orthosis guides the fingers in the desired path of movement.

In cervical spinal cord injuries where no muscles to flex or extend the fingers remain innervated, but the extensor carpi radialis muscle is intact, a wrist-driven flexor-hinge hand orthosis can be used. This device has a parallelogram of metal bars that transforms wrist extension and flexion into finger flexion and extension. Usually, the top bar of the parallelogram is adjustable in length so prehension can be accomplished in several different positions of wrist flexion or extension. Instead of being a hand orthosis, it is a wrist-hand orthosis with a cuff or trough on the forearm.

FIGURE 26–7. A wrist-hand orthosis with wrist extension assist and metacarpophalangeal extension assist. The wrist extension assist is provided by rubber bands dorsal to the axis of wrist motion, while metacarpophalangeal extension assist comes from coiled springs that support a volarly placed "lumbrical" bar. This orthosis is designed for use in radial nerve paralysis.

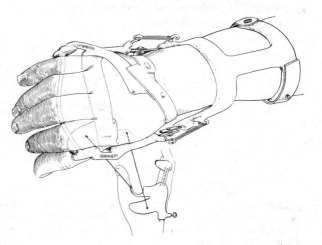

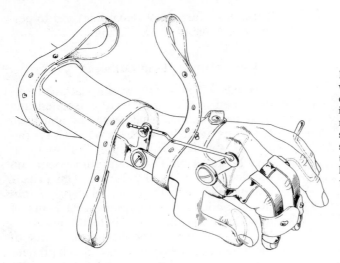

FIGURE 26–8. A wrist-driven flexor-hinge wrist-hand orthosis is operated by the power of wrist extension and is used in spinal cord injuries where no active finger function remains but wrist extension, elbow flexion, and shoulder motions are all at least antigravity strength. The top bar of the parallelogram at the wrist is adjustable in length so that prehension can be accomplished in different wrist positions.

A variation of the wrist-driven flexor-hinge hand orthosis has been developed. A one-piece molded dorsal cover for the three phalanges each of the second and third digits is adjustably attached by a cord to a wrist cuff. A hand orthosis with a thumb post holds the thumb in a stable position. Again, wrist extension causes finger flexion. The device is less bulky and somewhat less stable than the metal wrist-driven flexor-hinge hand orthosis with parallelogram bars.

Another newer variation of the wrist-driven flexor-hinge hand orthosis is the Key Grip or Lateral Pinch Orthosis. In this device, developed at Burke Rehabilitation Center, a wrist-driven orthosis holds the index fingers stabilized at the metacarpophalangeal and interphalangeal joints in a position of partial flexion and then pulls the thumb into flexion by a Bowden cable attached volarly at the wrist and to the plastic thumb post. This creates a lateral pinch type of grip that is preferred by some persons with severe paralysis of the hand.

When both the hand and the forearm muscles are paralyzed, a cable-driven or motor-driven flexor-hinge hand orthosis may be utilized. A Bowden cable can be attached to a figure eight harness similar to that used to operate the terminal device of an upper extremity prosthesis. Scapular abduction or humeral flexion will operate the orthosis. To provide prehension for an extended period of time without constant tension on the control cable, a clutch-locking device or spring-assisted prehension and a tension-relief control must be included. The development of small electric motors has made it possible to open and close a flexor-hinge hand orthosis electrically. Myoelectric control may be used, but the current state of the art leaves much to be desired. Reliable, implantable

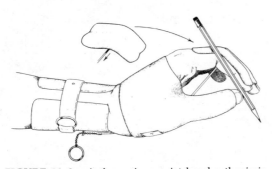

FIGURE 26–9. A three-piece wrist-hand orthosis is simpler, lighter, and less expensive than a wrist-driven flexor-hinge wrist-hand orthosis, yet it provides similar function.

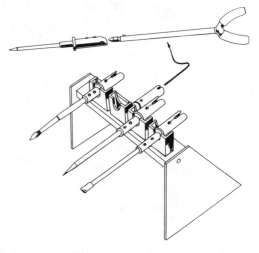

FIGURE 26–10. A mouthstick is grasped between the patient's teeth and can be inserted into a choice of several devices which hold a pencil, a paint brush, a pen, or a typing stick.

electrodes for controlled voltages are still in the developmental stage. Surface electrodes are not consistent or reliable from day to day; it is difficult to place them accurately daily, and varying skin impedance requires resetting the amplifier gain. Instead of myoelectric control, one can use on-off switches of many designs; generally, it is difficult to place them in a position where they can be utilized over extended periods of time. Often, these switches are attached to the wheelchair and operated by head motion or scapular motion; this correct relationship between the person and the switch is difficult to maintain.

Mouthsticks

A few devices have been developed which consist of a lightweight but strong metal tube or rod attached to a mouth piece and capable of holding simple tools like a pencil, pen, or paint brush. The rod is usually about 12 inches long, permitting the person to see what he or she is drawing or painting. The mouth piece should be carefully constructed by a dentist so that an accurate impression of the teeth or gums is made and the mouth piece constructed to the same contour. If simple half-rings or flat pieces are used, damage to the teeth is likely to result.

ENVIRONMENTAL CONTROL SYSTEMS

Electric devices are available which control a selection of a variety of outputs from one of a number of possible input mechanisms. They were developed to permit persons who have limited or no use of the extremities to turn on and off a small number of electric devices that can be plugged into the master control box. In one such device, 10 different electric appliances can be operated. The handicapped person can select

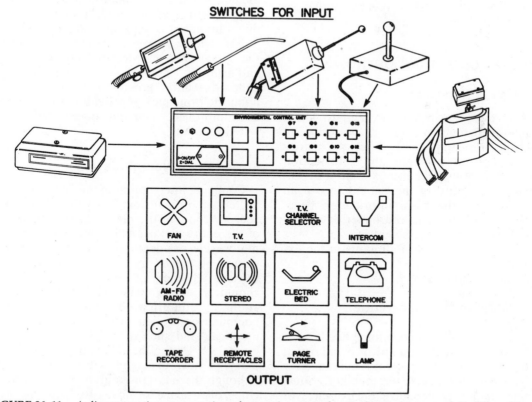

FIGURE 26–11. A diagrammatic representation of an environmental control unit. Any one of six different types of input switches can be used to control many different electrical applicances. The most appropriate switch is selected and attached to the control system. A small box contains scanning lights that move from the name or symbol of one device to the next at a controllable rate. Actuating the input switch starts the device scanning. When the desired appliance is reached by the scan, the input switch can be used to stop scanning and to actuate the appliance.

one of several control mechanisms: a sip-and-puff switch, a joy-stick switch, a manual rocker switch, and a toggle switch. Whichever switch works best for the person can be selected and attached to the control system. A small box on which scanning lights move from the name of one object to the next at a controllable rate is placed in a position where the handicapped person can see it. Each actuation of the control mechanism orders the scanning device to begin scanning or to stop at the desired point. When it stops at the desired point, a different mode of operation of the control switch turns on the device connected to that particular circuit; it may be a radio, an electric door controller, an electric window shade controller, a lamp, a television set, or a telephone. Any small device that can be operated electrically can be controlled by the environmental control system. In the case of a television set, there is a separate position on the scanning box for changing channels after the set is turned on. The telephone requires a special dialing device that performs the dialing function electronically and utilizes a speaker-phone so that no hands are needed.

EVALUATION FOR AN ORTHOSIS

Analysis of Handicap

What does the physician need to know about the patient in order to prescribe an orthosis for the upper limb? First, the history of the present problem and information about any other conditions that may influence the ability of the patient to use an orthosis form the basic information base. Evaluation of the impaired upper extremity includes accurate assessment of:

1. Range of motion of all joints in the extremity
2. Muscle strength
3. Sensation
4. Adequacy of skin coverage
5. Pain
6. Vocational and avocational needs

From a general standpoint, it is important to try to estimate the patient's tolerance for devices and his degree of mobility. Some people simply do not have the patience or motivation to use complicated devices, such as a myoelectrically controlled, motor-powered orthosis, and they would best be provided with a simpler device to achieve more limited function. Persons who are mobile in a wheelchair may need a different hand orthosis from those who walk because they must propel the wheelchair and the orthosis must not interfere with their mobility.

Prescription of Orthoses

The requirements of the patient must be established and the purpose of the device carefully delineated. The proposed device must be comfortable, provide adequate cosmesis, fill a real need, and be relatively inexpensive and lightweight. The many devices previously described are available, either through prefabricated kits or directly from an orthotist.

CONDITIONS REQUIRING ORTHOSES

The specific conditions that most frequently call for a prescription of orthotic devices include lower motor neuron lesions at any level from the spinal nerve root to the terminal branches of a peripheral nerve; upper motor neuron lesions, particularly those in the spinal cord and cerebral cortex; burns; and arthritis. The orthoses for these various conditions differ greatly, but all are based upon the principles of providing immobilization, improved alignment, or assisted or resisted function.

Lower Motor Neuron Lesions

Complete interruption of the brachial plexus, either by avulsion of all the motor and sensory roots of the plexus or by severance of the entire plexus, as is sometimes seen in motorcycle accidents and gunshot wounds, cannot be helped by currently available orthoses. Absence of motor power at the shoulder, elbow, wrist, and hand requires such a complicated, motor-powered, computer-controlled orthosis that it is impractical, and such a device is still experimental.[10] Upper brachial plexus (Erb's) palsy is now managed without splinting,[6] although there are probably still some advocates of airplane orthoses to hold the arm abducted and externally rotated.

Musculocutaneous nerve lesions may cause sufficient weakness of elbow flexion that an elbow flexion–assist orthosis is desired.

Ulnar nerve lesions in the distal forearm are best treated with a hand orthosis with "lumbrical bar." This permits the long finger-extensor muscles to extend the interphalangeal as well as the metacarpophalangeal joints. To enhance pinch, a first dorsal interosseus assist may be added. Ulnar nerve lesions above the elbow create an imbalance of wrist flexor pull but seldom require a wrist extension of the hand orthosis.

Median nerve lesions at the wrist create loss of active thumb abduction and opposition; they can be treated with a hand orthosis with spring-swivel thumb assist. Since the thumb adductor still functions, it is not advisable to use a swivel thumb with rigid post. Median nerve lesions above the elbow create a serious problem by paralyzing thumb flexion, abduction, and opposition as well as radial wrist flexion and all finger flexion, except for those fingers supplied by the ulnar innervated portion of the flexor digitorum profundus muscle. Precision grip is lost; power grip is weakened significantly. A wrist-driven flexor-hinge hand orthosis can be utilized, but the patient may prefer no device, since lateral prehension is still possible through muscles innervated by the ulnar nerve.

Radial nerve lesions above the elbow cause paralysis of the wrist, thumb, and finger extensors. The least cumbersome, most functional device is a wrist-hand orthosis with side wrist pivot hinges, wrist dorsiflexion assist, a spring-loaded "volar lumbrical bar" to assist metacarpophalangeal extension, and a thumb interphalangeal stabilizer.[11]

Lesions of two or more peripheral nerves simultaneously or partial lesions of one or more nerves require a careful evaluation of the functional loss so that the correct device can be prescribed.

Upper Motor Neuron Lesions

Transection of the cervical spinal cord with paralysis below the level of the damage creates a myotomal type of sparing. The upper extremity is supplied by cervical roots 4 through 8 and the first thoracic; since the interossei, lumbricals, and thenar and hypothenar muscles are largely supplied by the eighth cervical and first thoracic roots, they will be paralyzed in a lesion that spares the seventh cervical roots and above. Function may be improved in this case by a hand orthosis with "lumbrical bar" and thumb post, but most persons with this lesion seem to prefer to wear no device. Persons with sparing of the sixth cervical roots benefit from some type of wrist-driven flexor-hinge hand orthosis. Any of those previously described may be utilized. A spontaneous finger flexor tenodesis will usually develop if judicious physical therapy does not overstretch the long finger flexors, and the person will then be nearly as functional without a device as with it.

Sparing at the fifth cervical root level leaves the forearm and hand muscles paralyzed plus loss of elbow extension and weakened elbow flexion. Limited function can be obtained from a palmar band with clip, which can hold many small utensils or writing instruments. A spiral wrist orthosis can stabilize the wrist to enhance function of devices held in a palmar band. The spiral wrist orthosis may also be adapted to hold utensils and devices. A motor- or cable-driven flexor hinge hand orthosis can provide prehension and stability at the wrist. Since persons with this level of spinal cord injury usually have an electric wheelchair, a source of electricity is readily available and a motor-driven device becomes reasonably practical.

Cervical spinal cord injuries with sparing only of C4 and above leave the arm, forearm, and hand paralyzed, and there remains only weak shoulder function. A balanced forearm orthosis can usually provide hand placement and those devices used at the C5 level will provide hand function.

Environmental control systems that permit the handicapped person to operate a number of electrically powered devices are available with a variety of control switches that interface the handicapped person to the system. They may be very useful in high-level cervical spinal cord injuries.

Devices held in the mouth, either between the teeth or between the gums, can be used to operate devices such as an electric typewriter, control switches, and environmental control systems and may also be used for writing and drawing.

Burns

When burns damage the full-thickness of the skin, contractures can be expected to develop. The resultant deformities may be minimized by using static or functional orthoses early in the course of treatment.

Burns of the axilla are best treated by holding the arm abducted, especially after grafting. A padded metal or plastic orthosis that can be sterilized should be adjusted to hold the arm in maximum obtainable abduction. The orthosis may be needed for four weeks or more.

When the antecubital fossa is burned, the impending elbow flexion contracture can be minimized by using a padded metal trough to hold the elbow extended until the skin has healed.

Burns of the hands frequently involve the dorsum, since the hand may be used to shield the face. The resulting deformity of hyperextension of the metacarpophalangeal joints and flexion of the interphalangeal joints can be counteracted by a static, volar, wrist-hand orthosis that holds the wrist 10 degrees dorsiflexed, metacarpophalangeal joints fully flexed, and interphalangeal joints extended.[12] Later, a hand orthosis with rubber band metacarpophalangeal flexion assist and interphalangeal extension assist may be needed to improve motion. If the palm is burned, immobilization by a static dorsal orthosis will be needed for at least four weeks.

Arthritis

When rheumatoid arthritis involves the joints of the hand and wrist, various orthoses may be utilized. According to the theory of Smith et al.,[13] the pull of the flexor digitorum sublimis and profundus tendons at the metacarpophalangeal joint is largely responsible for the deformity of volar subluxation and ulnar drift and dislocation at the metacarpophalangeal joints. Based on this theory, immobilization of the metacarpophalangeal joints of the second through fifth digits, when those joints are acutely inflamed and swollen, has been instituted and a heat-moldable plastic orthosis that extends to the proximal IP joints of those digits on the volar surface and crosses the wrist to the mid-forearm has been designed. This orthosis must be carefully contoured to provide support at the base of the proximal phalanges and to create a shear force in the dorsal direction by pressing down upon the head of the metacarpals with a padded Dacron strap. Similarly, a strap over the styloid processes with pressure from the orthosis against the carpal bones from the volar aspect will reduce the

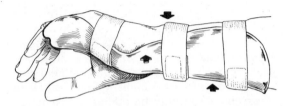

FIGURE 26–12. A plastic wrist-hand orthosis for use in rheumatoid arthritis. Carefully contoured, it extends to the proximal interphalangeal joints of the fingers to support the metacarpophalangeal joints and the wrist joints. It is designed to reduce deforming forces that contribute to ulnar deviation and volar subluxation at the wrist and fingers.

tendency to volar subluxation at that joint. By preventing ulnar deviation of the hand on the wrist and of the fifth digit on the hand, the tendency to ulnar dislocation will be reduced.

When only the wrist is acutely involved, the volar orthosis need extend only to the head of the metacarpals rather than to the proximal interphalangeal joint. A static wrist-hand orthosis then is carefully contoured to reduce the volar subluxation tendency of the carpal bones on the radius.

If only the proximal interphalangeal joints are acutely involved and are developing either "boutonniere" or "swan neck" deformities, the joint can be immobilized by using static interphalangeal joint orthoses.

When acute involvement of joints of the wrist and fingers is no longer present, but the collateral ligaments of the joints have stretched or deteriorated, it is possible to provide alignment to finger motion by using a finger-driven flexor hinge hand splint. Some persons may prefer to use no orthosis at this stage of the disease.

TRAINING THE PATIENT TO USE AN ORTHOSIS

The simpler positioning and functional splints require little or no training in their application and removal. However, modification of techniques of performing activities of daily living may be necessary and should be undertaken by the therapist most skilled in this area. The more complicated orthoses utilizing external power and the balanced forearm orthosis require hours of careful adjustment and training to maximize their usage.

PATIENT ACCEPTANCE OF ORTHOSES

It is essential that the orthosis be comfortable, cosmetic, complimentary, and cheap as well as being easy to put on and take off and to repair. Pre-prescription thought and discussion with the patient as well as the orthotist may save considerable time and effort. The patient must have the same goals and expectations for the orthosis that the physician and orthotist have. Effective communication among patient, physician, and orthotist will develop the best orthotic solution by specifying acceptable criteria to achieve their common goal.

An ugly but functional orthosis may be rejected by a patient who values appearance over function. A complicated orthosis may exceed the patient's gadget tolerance. If the device cannot easily be put on and removed, it may remain in the drawer. If the device provides improved function desired by the patient or decreased pain, the patient will ordinarily wear it as instructed. However, if the device impairs function and creates pain or discomfort, it may well be discarded. When patients with rheumatoid arthritis understand the necessity to protect joints, they, too, will wear the devices and they soon find that they are more comfortable. The extremely complicated devices with myoelectric controls must be carefully prescribed and must provide increased function without undue technical problems. They are the ones most likely to be rejected because the improved function they provide may be only marginal.

REFERENCES

1. Cailliet, R.: Shoulder Pain. Philadelphia, F. A. Davis Co., 1966.
2. Inman, V. T., Saunders, J. B. de C. M., and Abbott, L. C.: Observations on functions of shoulder joint. J. Bone Surg., 26A:1, 1944.
3. Napier, J.: The evolution of the hand. Sci. Am., 207:1–8, 1962.
4. Smith, E. M., and Juvinall, R. C.: Mechanics of bracing. In Licht, S. (Ed.): Orthotics, Etcetera. Baltimore, Waverly Press, 1966.
5. American Orthotics and Prosthetics Association Almanac, March, 1973, p. 11.
6. Johnson, E. W., Alexander, M. A., and Koenig, W. C.: Infantile Erb's palsy (Smellie's palsy). Arch. Phys. Med. Rehabil., 58:175, 1977.
7. Smith, E. M., Juvinall, R. C., Bender, L. F., and Pearson, J. R.: Flexor forces and rheumatoid metacarpophalangeal deformity. J.A.M.A., 198: 130–134, 1966.
8. Koepke, G. H., and Feller, I.: Physical measures for the prevention and treamtent of deformities following burns. J.A.M.A., 199:791–793, 1967.
9. Anderson, M.: Functional Bracing of the Extremities. Springfield, Ill., Charles C Thomas, Publisher, 1958.
10. Long, C.: Upper limb bracing. In Licht, S. (Ed.): Orthotics, Etcetera. Baltimore, Waverly Press, 1966.
11. Bender, L. F.: Prevention of deformities through orthotics. J.A.M.A., 183:946–948, 1963.
12. Koepke, G. H., Feallock, B., and Feller, I.: Splinting the severely burned hand. Am. J. Occup. Ther., 17:147–150, 1963.
13. Smith, E. M., Juvinall, R. C., Bender, L. F., and Pearson, J. R.: Role of the finger flexors in rheumatoid deformities of the metacarpophalangeal joints. Arth. Rheum., 7:467–480, 1964.

27

SPINAL ORTHOSES

STEVEN V. FISHER

As with any proper prescription, a spinal orthosis cannot be adequately prescribed without proper understanding of the anatomy, kinesiology, biomechanics, and pathophysiology of the disorder being treated.

The prescribing physician must be knowledgeable concerning the positive and negative effects of a spinal orthosis for a particular pathological condition. At times an accurate assessment of the pathophysiology and faulty biomechanics of the spine is difficult, making the proper prescription of an orthotic device an analytical problem. It is beyond the scope of this chapter to deal in sufficient detail with the anatomy, kinesiology, and disease conditions of the spine to allow a reader to become expert in the prescription of spinal orthoses. The basic principles of spinal bracing will be reviewed, and some of the common spinal orthoses will be discussed. The reader is referred to other sources for more detail.[1-4] Scoliosis bracing will not be considered.

Spinal bracing is used to decrease pain, to protect against further injury, to assist weak muscles, and to prevent or help correct a deformity.[4] These objectives are gained through the biomechanical effects of (1) trunk support, (2) motion control, and (3) spinal realignment.[3] When dealing with the cervical spine, an additional biomechanical effect is partial weight transfer of the head to the trunk when the patient is upright.

The negative effects of spinal orthoses must also be considered. Muscle atrophy and weakness may result from the use of spinal orthotics by reducing the amount of muscular activity needed to maintain trunk support. This problem can be partially avoided by an isometric exercise program. Control of the motion of an orthosis can promote contracture in the immobilized area. Psychological dependence on an orthosis[3] and increases in energy expenditure while ambulating with a spinal orthosis have been documented.[5]

Ralston found that when subjects walked at a comfortable speed while immobilized in a posterior plastic shell, a 10 per cent increase in oxygen consumption resulted. This factor must be taken into consideration when fitting a debilitated patient. Since axial rotation is necessary between the pelvis and shoulders during ambulation, not only is the energy consumption of ambulating increased, but there may be an increased motion at the unrestrained segments rostral and caudal to the orthosis.[3]

Nomenclature for spinal orthotics is confusing. Eponyms are commonly used for spinal orthotics and the standardized nomenclature given orthotic devices omits sufficient detail. Therefore a sketch of each orthosis discussed is shown. Orthotic devices are grouped according to level of the spine to which they are applied and the most common general types are shown. For further discussion of other spinal orthoses, detailed references are available.[2, 4]

530

CERVICAL ORTHOSES (C.O.)

General Considerations

The cervical spine provides the greatest range of motion of the entire spinal column in extent, direction, and variation of motion.[6] Cervical orthotic devices are often used in the treatment of neck disorders of both traumatic and non-traumatic etiology. Such orthoses are used to provide support and protection as well as limit range of motion. In general, cervical orthotic devices are most effective in limiting flexion and extension. With even the most effective cervical orthosis, lateral bending can only be limited to approximately 50 per cent of normal motion and rotation to 20 per cent of normal. Sagittal plane motion is better restricted, although the reported effect of the orthotic devices varies somewhat depending on the literature cited.[7-10]

Although the orthotic device must fit precisely, it should not be fitted so tightly that the pressure exerted by the orthotic device on the patient exceeds a capillary pressure of 20 to 30 mm Hg. If this does occur, the patient experiences ischemic pain. He will attempt to change his posture in the orthosis to provide comfort. If the orthosis is too tight, however, the patient will either loosen the orthotic device or reject it altogether. It has been shown that fitting a cervical orthotic device to within capillary pressure does not decrease the effectiveness of the orthosis as compared to the usual manner of fitting.[11]

Types of Orthoses

Collars

Cervical orthoses are of several basic design types. The first type to be considered is the collar made out of foam, which can be a firm plastizote material or a more rigid polyethylene. The foams may vary in their thickness or firmness. The hard collars (polyethylene) may have occipital and mandibular projections for added support. The collars are applied in a circular manner about the neck.

The effectiveness of the collars is limited. The soft cervical collar provides its restriction of motion more through a sensory feedback and a reminder to limit head and neck motion than through actual mechanical restriction of motion (Fig. 27-1).[7] A firmer cervical collar made out of a plastizote material with anterior and posterior plastic rigid supports (Philadelphia collar) limits the anterior-posterior cervical motion to approximately 30 per cent of normal (Fig. 27-2).[7, 8] This support allows 43 per cent of normal rotation and 67 per cent of lateral bending.[7] The firmer polyethylene collar with a mandibular and occipital piece demonstrates similar effectiveness in limiting anterior-posterior neck motion.[8] This collar, however,

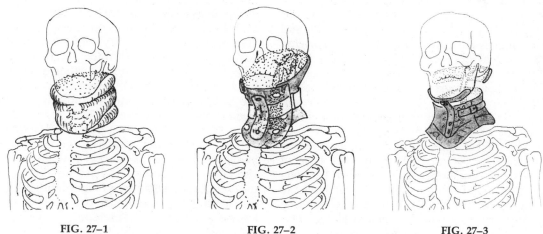

FIG. 27-1   FIG. 27-2   FIG. 27-3

FIGURE 27-1. Foam soft collar.

FIGURE 27-2. Firm Plastizote (Philadelphia) collar.

FIGURE 27-3. Polyethylene rigid collar with mandibular and occipital supports.

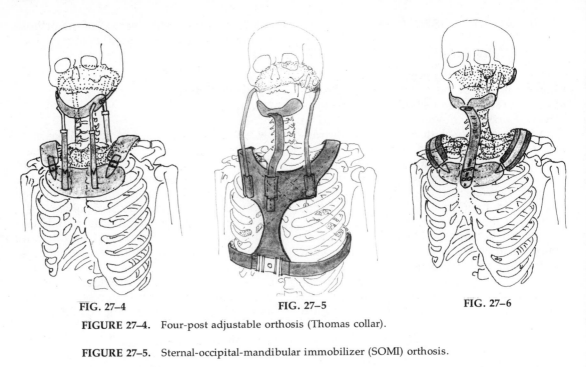

FIG. 27–4   FIG. 27–5   FIG. 27–6

FIGURE 27–4. Four-post adjustable orthosis (Thomas collar).

FIGURE 27–5. Sternal-occipital-mandibular immobilizer (SOMI) orthosis.

FIGURE 27–6. Two-post adjustable orthosis with mandibular and occipital supports.

can be quite uncomfortable because it rests over the clavicles (Fig. 27–3).

Rigid Supports

A more rigid type of orthosis fabricated with metal uprights can be classified as a "poster" appliance. The four-poster orthotic device (Fig. 27–4) consists of a chin and occipital piece connected with four uprights to a sternal and posterior thoracic plate.[4] The four posters are easily adjusted. This orthosis has been reported to allow sagittal motion of 5 per cent[8] to 21 per cent[7] of normal, rotation of 27 per cent of normal, and lateral bending of 46 per cent of normal.[7]

The SOMI (sternal occipital mandibular immobilizer) (Fig. 27–5) is another type of "poster" appliance. This support has one strip of metal running anteriorly to hold the chin piece and two rigid metal rods running posteriorly to hold the occipital piece.[5] The device is easily applied with the patient supine in the case of spinal cord injury and requires very little patient movement by the orthotist in its application and fitting. It is a comfortable orthosis and is very lightweight. The SOMI has been reported to allow 13 per cent[8] to 27 per cent[7] of normal sagittal motion, 34 per cent of rotation, and 66 per cent of lateral bending.[7] Both orthotic devices are quite effective in limiting cervical range of motion.

Other "poster" type appliances exist, for example, the two-poster (Fig. 27–6), and are probably as effective as the four-poster or the SOMI mentioned above, but they may provide less lateral stability. Johnson et al.[7] developed a cervicothoracic (CTO) four-poster brace that extended farther down the trunk and appeared to be more effective than the SOMI or four-poster in limiting overall sagittal plane movement. The Jewett J-21 brace (Fig. 27–7) is a two-poster CTO which extends well down the thorax, with rigid metal bands from the sternal pad across the shoulders and down the back to the lower thoracic band. This brace is more difficult for the orthotist to apply to the patient in a supine position. A "Peterson" is a similar cervicothoracic (CTO) two-poster but has enlarged mandibular and occipital supports and a forehead strap (Fig. 27–8). It is doubtful that the additional support offered, compared to the SOMI, warrants its prescription, especially in view of its difficulty in fitting

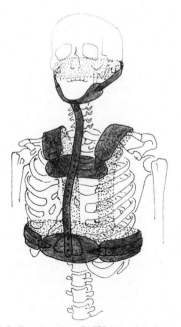

FIGURE 27–7. Jewett J-21 two-poster cervical orthosis with thoracic extension.

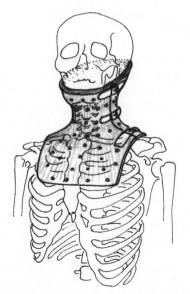

FIGURE 27–9. Molded "Minerva" cervical orthosis.

and pressure problems on the skin in the supine spinal cord injury patient.

Another type of cervical orthotic device could be classified as a custom-molded, total contact, chin-occipital-sternal-thoracic orthosis of the Minerva type (Fig. 27–9). This orthosis, if fabricated properly, would seem to control more lateral and rotatory move-

ment of the cervical spine than the "poster" type orthosis. A formal study of its effectiveness has not been published. As with any orthosis, the fabrication technique for this appliance is crucial to its success in limiting cervical range of motion. If more control of the cervical spine is required, rather than tightening an orthosis to unbearable limits, a rigid jacket made out of either plaster or polyethylene with a halo attached to the skull becomes necessary (Fig. 27–10).

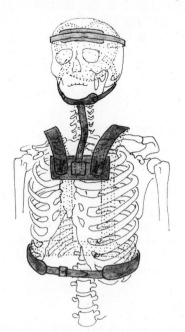

FIGURE 27–8. Peterson cervical orthosis with thoracic extension.

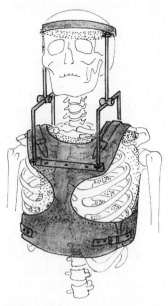

FIGURE 27–10. Halo-type cervical orthosis attached to a polyethylene jacket.

THORACOLUMBOSACRAL ORTHOSES

Lumbosacral and thoracolumbosacral orthoses are prescribed more frequently than cervical orthoses and there are more numerous variations of the designs for each type. This chapter will concentrate on the most commonly prescribed orthotic devices[12] and the representative types of design and material.

General Considerations

The work of Norton and Brown[13] was the first and still remains one of the most important articles dealing with the effectiveness of back braces. Some of the findings are pertinent to this discussion. Orthoses vary widely in their effectiveness in controlling the lower lumbar intervertebral levels. This variability of orthotic effectiveness probably relates to an individual's lumbar flexion pattern.

All spinal devices employ three-point pressure, and the effectiveness of each orthotic device in the production of controlling forces varies considerably. Orthotic devices that are well fixed to the chest but inadequately fixed to the pelvis produce a concentration of forces in the upper lumbar and thoracolumbar region as the trunk flexes. This leaves the lumbosacral segments unsupported. This was particularly noted in braces of the Taylor-type construction. In contrast, the chairback brace that has short supports tends to pull away from the body much less. In this way the supportive force offered by the orthotic device is maintained in the lumbosacral area.[13]

No brace actually immobilizes; it only tends to limit interspinous motion. No orthotic device can totally control the sagittal or axial lumbosacral motion.[13, 14] Therefore, if an orthotic device is to be effective, it must supply sufficient localized pressure over bony prominences to cause enough discomfort to remind the patient wearing the orthosis to change or maintain his posture in the orthotic device.

Increased abdominal pressure decreases the net force applied to the spine when attempting to lift a weight from the floor.[15] One of the major functions of a lumbar support, including corsets and rigid braces, is abdominal compression. The resultant increased intra-abdominal pressure thereby creates a semirigid cylinder surrounding the spinal column capable of relieving some of the imposed stresses on the vertebral column itself.[16] The lumbosacral support, when tightened within patient tolerance, decreases the intradiscal pressure at the lumbar spine by approximately 30 per cent.[17]

At rest both the chairback brace and the lumbosacral corset either decrease or have no effect on the electrical activity of back muscles in the majority of subjects. When the subjects walk at their comfortable walking speed, neither support has any effect on electrical muscular activity. However, when subjects wearing the chairback brace walk at a fast pace, the muscle activity increases in comparison with the activity of that muscle when no support is worn. It is thought that the greater electrical activity recorded in subjects walking rapidly while wearing the chairback brace reflects the increase in muscular exertion of the back muscles in attempting to overcome immobilization of the chairback brace.[18] Persons with back pain usually do not walk fast, and the significance of these electrical findings is limited.

It would seem that the biomechanical effect of trunk support is most importantly related to the increased abdominal cavity pressure created by the orthotic device. The motion control that is created by the orthotic devices might very well be more on the basis of painful stimuli to the subject wearing the brace, reminding him to correct his position, than by the actual three-point support system. Spinal realignment would be a very difficult task for an external support to perform passively. Active muscle realignment with the orthotic device seems necessary.

Types of Orthoses

These appliances can be classified as corsets, rigid braces, hyperextension braces, and jackets. All spinal orthoses with the exception of hyperextension braces give abdominal support. The ability of these devices to restrict motion has not been measured with as great detail as the cervical orthoses, so that the evaluation of effectiveness is more subjective.

Corsets

The most commonly prescribed lumbosacral support is the lumbosacral corset, which is prescribed approximately 44 per cent of the time.[12] In general a corset is made of canvas with rigid back steels. There is adjustable side or back lacing. A corset is a stock item and can be fitted by a corseteer without difficulty. The corset can be lumbosacral (LS) or thoracolumbosacral (TLS) in nature. The steels can be either rigid or semirigid. The corset's main purpose is to provide abdominal support. However, the steels serve to give a little support and to supply painful stimuli if the patient leans against the stays, especially the lateral ones. Therefore the corset not only gives some support but reminds the patient to maintain adequate posture.

Rigid Braces

Lumbosacral Orthoses (LSO). Of the rigid braces, the chairback brace is the most popular.[12] The chairback brace consists of two paraspinal uprights and two uprights in the mid-axillary line (Fig. 27–11). It may have an anterior corset or apron front with side lacing and is designed to control flexion-extension and lateral motion (Fig. 27–12).

Another lumbosacral orthosis commonly prescribed is the William's back brace, which is used primarily to control extension and lordosis, and to give some lateral control

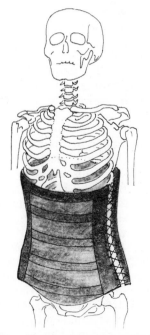

FIGURE 27–12. Chairback lumbosacral orthosis with side-lacing attachment of abdominal apron.

(Fig. 27–13). It is a specialized orthosis in that it allows free flexion but limits extension and uses a lever action and abdominal support to reduce lumbar lordosis.

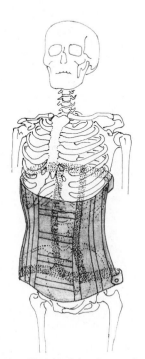

FIGURE 27–11. Chairback lumbosacral orthosis with attached abdominal apron closed by Velcro straps.

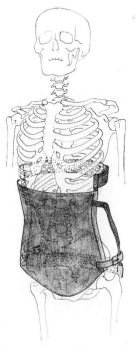

FIGURE 27–13. William's hyperextension lumbosacral orthosis.

Thoracolumbosacral Orthoses (TLSO).
There are two major types of thoracolumbosacral orthoses. The more common is the Taylor orthosis, which is constructed to restrict flexion and extension (Fig. 27–14). However, as mentioned earlier, this type of orthosis is ineffective for limiting the lumbar spine motion.[13] The Taylor orthosis limits thoracic motion only if the axillary straps are tightened to a point of discomfort. Therefore, when the patient loosens the straps because of discomfort, the orthosis becomes ineffective. This orthosis, therefore, seems to be a poor choice for thoracolumbosacral immobilization. The chairback brace with cowhorn or sternal pad attachments (Fig. 27–15), which transmits pressure through the sternum and ribs directly to the spine, provides better lumbosacral and thoracic immobilization than a brace by which force is transmitted through the pectoral girdle, which is attached to the spinal axis only by muscles and the sternoclavicular joints.

Molded jackets are made either of plaster of Paris or of a thermoplastic to conform to the contours of the body (Fig. 27–16). If made properly, they become a nearly total contact type of orthotic device. Therefore, the pressure distribution is more uniform and more support is afforded. These jackets are

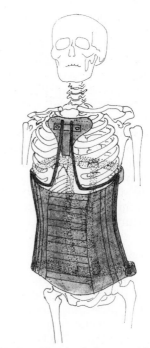

FIGURE 27–15. Chairback brace with sternal pad transmitting bony support to the thoracic spine.

used frequently for patients with spinal fractures or scoliosis to allow early mobilization and rehabilitation. They also may be of value when there are metastases in vertebrae to

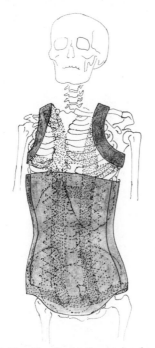

FIGURE 27–14. The Taylor thoracolumbosacral brace is too frequently prescribed and usually ineffective.

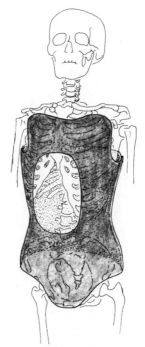

FIGURE 27–16. The molded jacket, when properly fitted, provides total contact support.

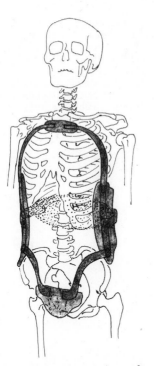

FIGURE 27-17. The hyperextension orthosis restricts spinal flexion by anterior pressure over the sternum and hypogastrium, and posterior pressure across the upper lumbar and lower thoracic region.

provide support and control pain. Donning and doffing the molded jacket is more difficult than with other orthoses.

The hyperextension orthosis differs from other devices because it does not have an abdominal apron and does not give abdominal support; it functions to give a hyperextension moment (Fig. 27-17). This hyperextension brace applies three-point pressure anteriorly across the upper lumbar or thoracolumbar spine. This orthosis is used to permit the upright position, especially to prevent flexion after a compression fracture of a vertebral body. It is not recommended, however, to manage compression fractures in osteoporotic elderly patients because it may place excessive hyperextension forces on lower lumbar vertebrae, which can induce posterior element fractures or exacerbate a degenerative arthritic condition.

It should be stressed that orthotic devices only partially limit rather than immobilize the spine. Spinal orthoses should be considered to be temporary devices. At the same time that the orthotic device is prescribed, a rehabilitation treatment plan should be outlined to attempt to rid the patient of the need for the device in the future.

REFERENCES

1. McCollough, N. C., III: Biomechanical analysis of the spine. *In* Atlas of Orthotics: Biomechanical Principles and Application. American Academy of Orthopedic Surgeons. St. Louis, The C. V., Mosby Co., 1975.
2. Berger, N., and Lusskin, R.: Orthotic components and systems. *In* Atlas of Orthotics: Biomechanical Principles and Application. American Academy of Orthopedic Surgeons. St. Louis, the C. V. Mosby Co., 1975.
3. Lusskin, R., and Berger, N.: Prescription principles. *In* Atlas of Orthotics: Biomechanical Principles and Application. American Academy of Orthopedic Surgeons. St. Louis, The C. V. Mosby Co., 1975.
4. Lucas, B. D.: Spinal bracing. *In* Licht, S. (Ed.): Orthotics, Etcetera. New Haven, Waverly Press, Inc., 1966, pp. 275–305.
5. Ralston, H. J.: Effects of immobilization of various body segments on energy cost of human locomotion. Proceedings of Second International Congress on Ergonomics, Dortmund, 1964. Suppl. to Ergonomics, 1965, pp. 53–60.
6. Caliet, R.: Neck and Arm Pain. Philadelphia, F. A. Davis Co., 1964.
7. Johnson, R. M., Hart, D., Simmons, E. F., Ramsby, G. R., and Southwick, N. O.: Cervical orthoses. J. Bone Joint Surg., 59A:332–339, 1977.
8. Fisher, S. V., Bowar, J. F., Awad, E. A., and Gullickson, G.: Cervical orthoses effect on cervical spine motion: roentgenographic and goniometric method of study. Arch. Phys. Med. Rehabil., 58:109–115, 1977.
9. Colachis, S. C., Jr., Strohm, B. R., and Ganter, E. L.: Cervical spine motion in normal women: Radiographic study of effect of cervical collars. Arch. Phys. Med. Rehabil., 46:753–760, 1965.
10. Hartman, J. T., Palumbo, F., and Hill, B. J.: Cineradiography of braced normal cervical spine: Comparative study of five commonly used cervical orthoses. Clin. Orthop., 109:97–102, 1975.
11. Fisher, S. V.: Proper fitting of the cervical orthoses. Arch. Phys. Med. Rehabil., 59:505–507, 1978.
12. Perry, J.: The use of external support in the treatment of low back pain. J. Bone Joint Surg., 52A:1440–1442, 1970.
13. Norton, P. L., and Brown, T.: The immobilization efficiency of back braces, their effect on the posture and motion of the lumbosacral spine. J. Bone Joint Surg., 39A:111–139, 1957.
14. Lumsden, R. M., and Morris, J. M.: An in vivo study of axial rotation and immobilization at the lumbosacral joint. J. Bone Joint Surg., 50A:1591–1602, 1968.
15. Morris, J. M., Lucas, D. B., and Bresler, B.: Role of the trunk in stability of the spine. J. Bone Joint Surg., 43A:327–351, 1961.
16. Morris, J. M.: Low back bracing. Clin. Orthop., 102:126–132, 1974.
17. Nachemson, A., and Morris, J. M.: In vivo measurements of intradiscal pressure: Discometry, a method for the determination of pressure in the lower lumbar discs. J. Bone Joint Surg., 46A:1077–1092, 1964.
18. Walters, R. L., and Morris, J. M.: Effect of spinal supports on the electrical activity of muscles of the trunk. J. Bone Joint Surg., 52A:51–60, 1970.

ADDITIONAL READINGS

Spinal Orthotics, New York University Post Graduate Medical School, Prosthetics and Orthotics, New York, 1973.

Kottke, F. J.: Evaluation and treatment of low back pain due to mechanical causes. Arch. Phys. Med. Rehabil., 42:426–440, 1961.

Bennett, R. L.: Orthotics for function. Part I: Prescription. Phys. Ther. Rev., 36:721–730, 1956.

Bloomberg, M. H.: Orthopedic Braces: Rationale, Classification and Prescription. Philadelphia, J. B. Lippincott Co., 1964.

Jordan, H. H.: Orthopedic Appliances, the Principle and Practice of Brace Construction. Springfield, Ill., Charles C Thomas, Publisher, 1963.

28

LOWER EXTREMITY ORTHOTICS

JUSTUS F. LEHMANN

Historically, design features for lower extremity orthotics have changed slowly. In recent years, however, two new factors have led to a rapid increase in the rate and number of changes, i.e., the application of engineering skills to orthotic design and the introduction and widespread availability of plastic materials suitable for use in these orthoses. As a result, not only are there many more designs from which to choose, but they are also constantly changing. Therefore, guidelines for evaluation of patients and selection of the appropriate orthosis assume an even greater importance than in the past. An understanding of the functional biomechanical principles used in orthotic design provides the foundation for these guidelines and simplifies the approach to the patient.[1]

ORTHOSES FOR SKELETAL AND JOINT INSUFFICIENCY

The design of these orthoses provides for adequate bone and joint alignment and allows quantifiable limits of lower extremity weight bearing through the skeletal system.

Ischial Weight Bearing Orthoses

Orthotic Components. These orthoses are designed to transmit force from the ischium to the orthosis and through the orthosis to the ground. The components consist of standard stainless steel bar stock for the uprights connected at the bottom by a stirrup, which is often riveted to a steel sole plate extending to the metatarsal head area. A rocker or patten bottom[2] may be added. The most common design of the weight bearing area used is a quadrilateral cuff of the same configuration as the quadrilateral socket of the prosthesis for an above-knee amputee.[3-7] The ischial (Thomas) ring[8] is no longer used as a standard design.

Biomechanical Function. The amount of reduction of force transmission through the skeletal system depends on several elements in the orthotic design such as the configuration of the ischial weight bearing area, the use of a locked or free knee joint, the design of the ankle joint, the sole plate, and the addition of a rocker or patten bottom. Training of the patient in the proper use of the orthosis also has a major effect on reliable weight bearing relief.

The use of the rigid quadrilateral cuff (Fig. 28–1) markedly improved the weight bearing function of the orthosis, which, in general, is maximal during heelstrike and drops off significantly during the pushoff phase. However, if the patient is trained to avoid active pushoff, which loads the skeletal system, weight bearing of the orthosis during the latter part of the stance is greatly improved. Also, the patient should be instructed in the appropriate utilization of the ischial seat of the orthosis, i.e., weight bearing with the ischium on the seat.[9, 10] In addition, the greater the clearance between heel and shoe

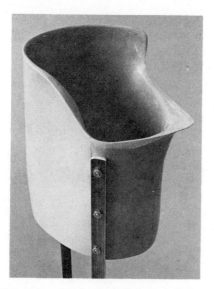

FIGURE 28–1. Rigid, quadrilateral cuff for ischial weight bearing orthoses. (From Lehrmann, J. F., Warren, C. G., de Lateur, B. J., Simons, B. C., and Kirkpatrick, G.: Biomechanical evaluation of axial loading in ischial weight bearing braces of various designs. Arch. Phys. Med. Rehabil., 51:331–337, 1970.)

provided during fitting, the greater the reliability of weight bearing through the orthosis. A minimum of 3/8 inch heel clearance as measured in mid-stance should be provided, and occasionally a greater amount may be desirable.

The ischial weight bearing orthosis with a quadrilateral cuff does not provide complete protection of the hip joint, since not all forces are transmitted through the ischial seat and, therefore, do not all bypass the hip joint. Actual measurements with an instrumental ischial seat show that only approximately 40 per cent of the force is transmitted through it,[10] the rest apparently passing from the quadrilateral cuff through the soft tissue mass of the thigh into the skeletal structure. Therefore, canes or crutches should be used to protect the hip joint.

The Thomas ring may be considered obsolete as a weight bearing orthosis. Because of the small contact area between the ischium and ring,[8] discomfort is frequently produced, causing patients to loosen the thigh lacer to obtain relief. The ischium then drops into the ring and the weight bearing function is lost.[10]

In general, the weight bearing function of an ischial weight bearing orthosis depends on design and training as follows:

1. The orthosis with fixed knee and patten bottom produces 100 per cent weight bearing through the orthosis.

2. The orthosis with locked knee, fixed ankle, rocker bottom, and training produces weight bearing through the orthosis at 90 per cent or more of body weight (Fig. 28–2).

3. The orthosis with locked knee and fixed

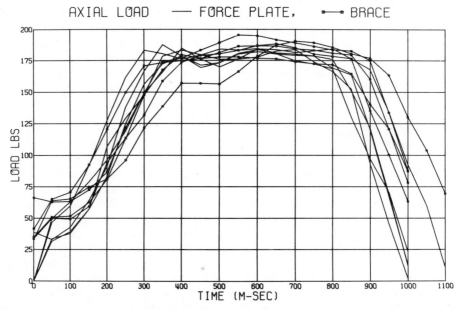

FIGURE 28–2. Axial loads developed on force plate and in uprights of a brace with fixed ankle, fixed knee, quadrilateral shell, and rocker bottom during five stance phases. (From Lehmann, J. F., Warren, C. G., de Lateur, B. J., Simons, B. C., and Kirkpatrick, G.: Biomechanical evaluation of axial loading in ischial weight bearing braces of various designs. Arch. Phys. Med. Rehabil., 51:331–337, 1970.)

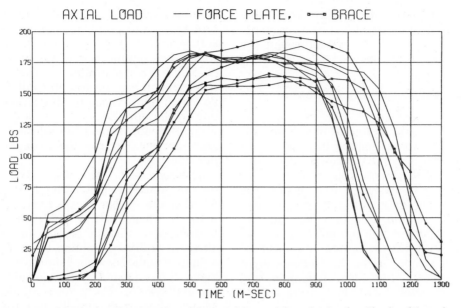

FIGURE 28–3. Axial loads developed on force plate and in uprights of a fixed ankle, fixed knee brace with a volunteer attempting active dorsiflexion to avoid pushoff during five stance phases. (From Lehmann, J. F., Warren, C. G., de Lateur, B. J., Simons, B. C., and Kirkpatrick, G.: Biomechanical evaluation of axial loading in ischial weight bearing braces of various designs. Arch. Phys. Med. Rehabil., 51:331–337, 1970.)

ankle, with training, produces weight bearing through the orthosis at approximately 86 per cent of body weight (Fig. 28–3).

4. The orthosis with locked knee and fixed ankle, without training, produces weight bearing through the orthosis at 50 per cent of body weight with little variation (Fig. 28–4).

5. The orthosis with a fixed knee, free ankle joint, with training, produces 50 per cent or more variable weight bearing through the orthosis throughout the stance phase.

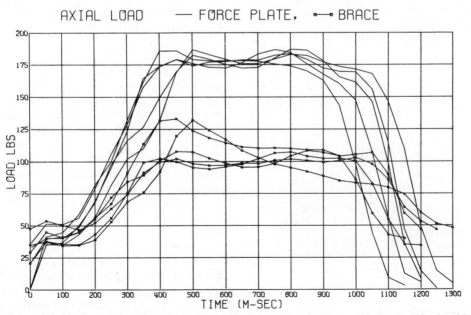

FIGURE 28–4. Axial loads developed on force plate and in uprights of a brace with fixed ankle, fixed knee, and quadrilateral shell during five stance phases. (From Lehmann, J. F., Warren, C. G., de Lateur, B. J., Simon, B. C., and Kirkpatrick, G.: Biomechanical evaluation of axial loading in ischial weight bearing braces of various designs. Arch. Phys. Med. Rehabil., 51:331–337, 1970.)

6. The orthosis with a fixed knee, free ankle joint, without training, produces 50 per cent or more weight bearing through the orthosis only during heelstrike.

Patellar Tendon Bearing Orthoses

Orthotic Components. The most important advance in the design of this orthosis is the use of a patellar tendon bearing cuff of the same design as the patellar tendon bearing socket of the below-knee prosthesis for amputees. It is designed to transmit the majority of the force from the knee through the patellar tendon area into the cuff and from there through the upright and shoe to the ground. A rocker bottom can also be fitted to the shoe, as in the ischial weight bearing orthosis. For ease of donning and doffing, the patellar tendon bearing cuff is

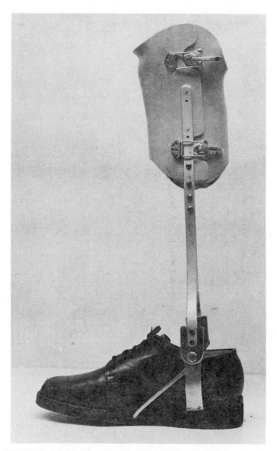

FIGURE 28–5. Patellar tendon bearing brace for limiting weight bearing, incorporating bivalved patellar tendon bearing cuff closed by skin boot buckles, standard uprights, double-stopped ankle joint, and sole plate extending to the metatarsal head area.

bivalved and must be closed by rigid ski boot type buckles to avoid the yielding found with soft leather or Velcro, which decreases the weight bearing function of the orthosis (Fig. 28–5).[11-14] To make effective use of the patellar tendon bearing area, the cuff should be flexed to approximately 10 degrees in relation to the uprights. If a fixed ankle joint is used, the stop should be adjusted to 7 degrees dorsiflexion from the 90-degree neutral position.[15]

Biomechanical Function. The weight bearing function of the orthosis depends on whether the design uses a fixed ankle joint with sole plate, a free ankle, or a rocker bottom as well as the amount of heel clearance. In addition, training has a significant influence, and the patient should be taught to avoid active pushoff, which would load the skeletal system. The patient should also be shown how to maximally use the weight bearing area of the patellar tendon bearing cuff.

The weight bearing function of the patellar tendon bearing orthoses of various designs can be summarized as:

1. If a free or cable ankle joint is used with 3/8 inch heel clearance, weight bearing function of the orthosis during the heelstrike phase is limited to approximately 42 to 44 per cent of the total force transmitted to the ground (Fig. 28–6). During the pushoff phase there is a marked drop-off to no weight bearing. However, with training the weight bearing function can be improved by avoiding active pushoff.

2. If a fixed ankle is used with heel clearance of 3/8 inch but no training is given, approximately 40 per cent of the total force transmitted to the ground is borne by the orthosis with a drop-off to approximately 30 per cent during the pushoff phase (Fig. 28–7).

3. In the same design using a fixed ankle and an increased heel clearance of 1 inch and training, more than 70 per cent of the weight is borne by the orthosis, with a drop of 50 to 60 per cent during the pushoff phase (Fig. 28–8).

4. With a fixed ankle and 1 inch heel clearance, the weight bearing during pushoff can be further improved by adding a rocker bottom. This makes the patient unstable in order to prevent active pushoff and also increases difficulty in ambulation. Weight bearing during the heelstrike phase is not

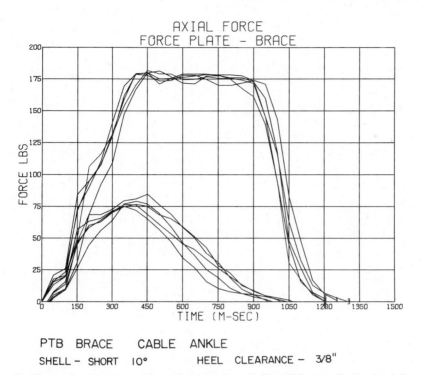

FIGURE 28–6. Patellar tendon bearing, cable ankle joint, short shell at 10 degrees flexion, heel clearance 3/8 inch. Upper curves force plate force, lower curves brace forces. (From Lehmann, J. F., Warren, C. G., Pemberton, D. R., Simons, B. C., and de Lateur, B. J.: Load bearing function of patellar tendon bearing braces of various designs. Arch. Phys. Med Rehabil., 52:367–370, 1971.)

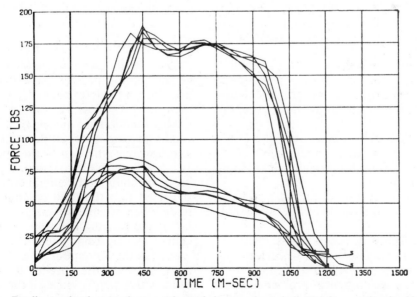

FIGURE 28–7. Patellar tendon bearing brace with rigid closure, short shell at 10 degrees, fixed ankle at 7 degrees, heel clearance 3/8 inch. Upper curves force plate force, lower curves brace forces. (From Lehmann, J. F., Warren, C. G., Pemberton, D. R., Simons, B. C., and de Lateur, B. J.: Load bearing function of patellar tendon bearing braces of various designs. Arch. Phys. Med. Rehabil., 52:367–370, 1971.)

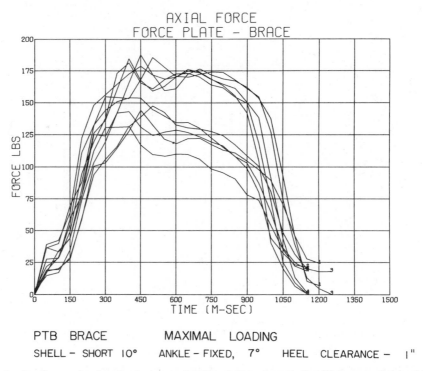

FIGURE 28–8. Patellar tendon bearing brace used with training, short shell at 10 degrees, fixed ankle at 7 degrees, flexion, heel clearance 1 inch. Upper curves force plate force, lower curves brace forces. (From Lehmann, J. F., Warren, C. G., Pemberton, D. R., Simons, B. C., and de Lateur, B. J.: Load bearing function of patellar tendon bearing braces of various designs. Arch. Phys. Med. Rehabil., 52:367–370, 1971.)

likely to be improved beyond the 70 per cent.

According to Davis and associates,[14] the indications for the use of patellar tendon bearing orthoses on a short-term basis are:

1. Healing of os calcis fractures
2. Postoperative fusions about the ankle
3. Painful conditions of the heel which have been refractory to conservative management and for which surgery is contraindicated.

The orthosis is recommended for long-term use in the following conditions:

1. Delayed unions or nonunions of fractures and fusions
2. Avascular necrosis of the talar body
3. Degenerative arthritis of the subtalar or ankle joint
4. Osteomyelitis of the os calcis
5. Sciatic nerve injury with secondary anesthesia involving the sole of the foot
6. Chronic dermatological problems, such as diabetic ulceration
7. Other chronic and painful conditions of the foot not amenable to surgery.

Davis identified as contraindications conditions of the skin and peripheral circulation such that pressure about the patellar tendon and popliteal regions cannot be tolerated.

Fracture Cast Bracing

Casts with patellar tendon or ischial weight bearing designs have been successfully used in the treatment of lower extremity fractures.[16] The biomechanics of the weight-bearing function are the same as those in the weight bearing orthoses described. In addition, however, the cast or the plastic materials used to encase the limb or a portion of it must maintain bony alignment. Sarmiento suggested that the fluid column of the soft tissue when completely encased may add to the weight bearing function.[17] This requires further investigation, since no significant difference in the amount of weight bearing was found between the patellar tendon bearing orthosis that tightly encased the entire leg to the ankle and an orthosis with a short patellar tendon bearing cuff.[16] The use of these orthoses in the management of fractures has been advantageous when compared to the traditional methods of treatment, since the period of immobilization is reduced, and even delayed union or nonunion fractures frequently heal well. Nickel et al. described 102 femoral fractures treated with ischial weight bearing fracture cast orthoses as healing after traction in an average of 12 weeks.[4-6] Similarly, Sarmiento used patellar tendon bearing orthoses in 382 patients with tibial fractures and reported an average healing time of 14.5 weeks.[18] No significant shortening of the limbs associated with this treatment was observed, and delayed and nonunion fractures responded well. It is likely that these orthoses are effective because they maintain bony alignment and limit weight bearing through the fracture site to a tolerable level, which promotes bone healing while simultaneously allowing early ambulation.

Weight Bearing Orthoses to Maintain and Correct Joint Alignment

In cases of joint disease such as rheumatoid arthritis, it may be desirable not only to limit weight bearing but also to support joint alignment. Orthoses used for this purpose are of the same design as the ischial and patellar tendon weight bearing orthoses; however, they are modified to maintain joint alignment and stability. They may also be used without the weight bearing features. Clinically, the major problems that can be treated with these types of orthoses occur at the level of the knee joint, as in rheumatoid arthritis where destruction and loosening of the medial collateral ligaments lead to valgus deformity. Orthoses can be designed to counteract the bending moment that forces the knee into valgus position. This is therapeutically significant, since the center of rotation for medial deviation of the knee is moved medial to the extension of the ground reactive force line, thus creating a moment arm that bends the knee further medially into valgus. Consequently, the more the knee is deformed, the greater the moment arm, and, therefore, the greater the deforming force. This is an accelerating process that can be prevented by the proper use of orthoses. The corrective force must be applied medial to the knee and countered by two forces, one applied to the limb above the knee and one below. The corrective force may be applied by a pressure pad to the medial side, but it is

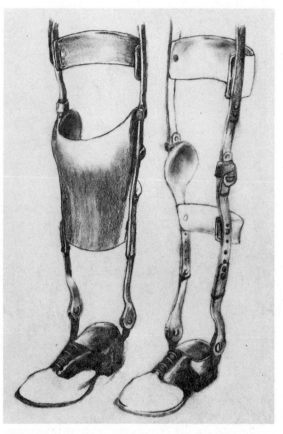

FIGURE 28–9. Braces with standard medial knee support (R) and pretibial shell (L).

better if a form-fitting plastic shell is added extending from below to just above the knee level (supracondylar extension). Thigh position can be better controlled by substituting a plastic, form-fitting shell for the standard thigh bands (Fig. 28–9).[19-21] The plastic shell, both above and below the knee, must be manufactured from an accurate plastic cast made when the limb is in its optimally correct position. When the orthosis allows free knee flexion and extension, it is important to align the center of rotation of the brace axis as accurately as possible to coincide with the location of the anatomical knee axis. Otherwise, the force generated by the relative motion of the orthosis and limb may further injure the diseased joint and make the wearing of the orthosis uncomfortable. Since only single axis knee joints are available for the orthoses and since the location of the instantaneous center of rotation of the anatomical knee changes with motion,[22] special attention must be given to optimal alignment. A

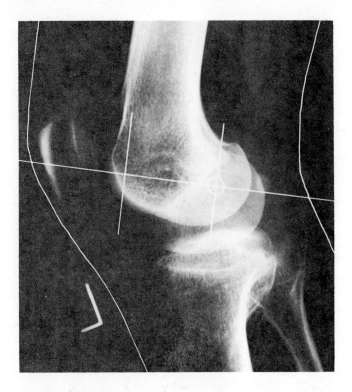

FIGURE 28–10. Location of knee axis.

commonly used method for aligning the orthotic knee joint with the anatomical joint axis is as follows:

1. Locate the maximum bony prominence of the medial femoral condyle.

2. Draw a line horizontally at the midpatella level and subdivide it into three equal parts.

3. The axis is located at the junction of the middle and posterior third (Fig. 28–10).

To check the alignment of the knee axis with the completed orthosis, the following points should be observed:

1. When the patient sits down, there should be no relative motion between the orthosis and the limb.

2. If the axis of the orthosis is too high, the lower thigh band will dig into the thigh.

3. If it is too low, the calf band will bite into the calf.[23]

In their evaluation of single and double upright orthoses for patients with rheumatoid arthritis and valgus deformity at the knee, Smith and Juvinall[20] found:

1. The use of a single upright is limited to conditions requiring a corrective force of 18 to 20 pounds.

2. Both the single and double upright orthoses could be worn only if flexion contracture at the knee was less than 15 and 20 degrees. They found that of 50 patients thus fitted, 38 patients wore their orthoses successfully for 7 to 48 months.

Knee extensor weakness or muscle imbalance, which may be caused by an absence of sensory feedback as in tabes dorsalis, may produce a genu recurvatum. In cases with muscle weakness, the patient stabilizes the knee against the posterior capsule and extension check ligaments by manipulating the ground reactive force line so that it falls in front of the knee, creating an extension moment. Thus, the knee is locked in extension. The posterior capsule is weak and will gradually yield. A "back knee" can be produced by a tight gastrocnemius, soleus, or other bony abnormalities fixing the foot in equinus, thereby creating an excessive extension moment at the knee, especially during the latter part of the stance. In addition to standard medical and/or surgical care and an appropriate physical therapy program, orthoses are prescribed for this condition. In mild genu recurvatum, often seen as a knee control problem in the early phase of recovery after the onset of hemiplegia, an ankle-foot orthosis with plantar and dorsiflexion stops and sole plate can be used as a training device. The ankle is set in some dorsiflexion. As the patient rocks over the heel from heelstrike to foot flat, the contact point with the ground is at the posterior edge of the heel, with the extension of the ground reactive force falling behind the knee joint, creating a bending moment, while during the pushoff phase, the adjustment of the ankle reduces the extension moment at the knee. It may be advisable in some cases to remove the dorsiflexion stop, but the patient must have enough voluntary control to keep from buckling during the heelstrike phase. The biomechanical details will be discussed in the section on ankle-foot orthoses for paralysis and paresis.

Most commonly, genu recurvatum is treated with a knee-ankle orthosis positioning the knee in slight flexion. The posterior capsule and check ligaments may tighten enough so that the patient might not have to wear the orthosis permanently. To achieve proper knee position, the upper thigh band should be relatively deep and the lower thigh bands relatively shallow. Thus, according to Bennett,[23] the knee is put in a flexion position. Better control can be achieved with a rigid plastic cuff instead of thigh bands, supplemented by a plastic posterior shell below the knee instead of a calf band.[24]

The knee cage is a relatively short orthosis extending from the area just above the knee to the area just below the knee. It has rigid cross-connections or bands between the orthotic uprights posteriorly and two counter forces applied by elastic straps just above and below the knee. More recently, plastics have been used to improve this design,[25]

although none of them has been totally satisfactory, some tending to slide off the leg. The hinged knee cage and the double anterior loop knee orthosis[25, 26] are some of the commonly used modifications of the knee cage. Also, plastic orthoses have been advocated.[25, 26]

The Toronto abduction orthosis for Legg-Perthes disease (Fig. 28–11) is a specialized orthosis for the hip joint.[27] This orthosis allows ambulation and knee and hip flexion while maintaining the hip at 45 degrees abduction and 18 degrees internal rotation. An angle of 90 degrees is maintained at all times between the legs. The treatment rationale is that the femoral head will re-form if weight bearing is allowed only in the abducted position.

ORTHOSES FOR WEAKNESS OF THE LOWER EXTREMITY

These orthoses are used in cases of paralysis and paresis from upper and lower motor neuron disease or in cases of weakness from muscle pathology. They also prevent the development of deformities.

Ankle Foot Orthoses

These are by far the most commonly used orthoses, and the most important reasons for prescribing them are that they provide (1)

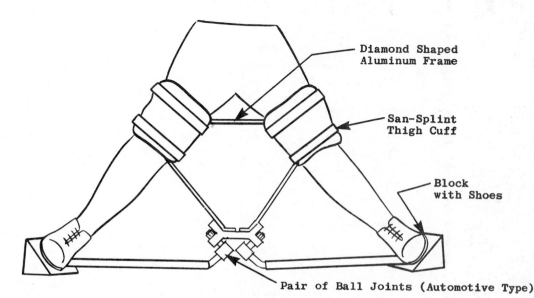

FIGURE 28–11. Toronto Legg-Perthes orthosis. (From Lehmann, J. F., de Lateur, B. J., Warren, C. G., and Simons, B. C.: Trends in lower extremity bracing. Arch. Phys. Med. Rehabil., 51:338–353, 1970.)

mediolateral stability at the ankle during the stance phase to prevent inadvertent twisting of the ankle; (2) toe pickup during the swing phase to prevent dragging of the toe, stumbling, and falling; and (3) pushoff stimulation during the latter part of the stance phase, thus approximating more normal gait and reducing energy expenditure.

All ankle-foot orthoses inevitably have a significant influence on knee stability. The criteria listed above take into consideration the fact that many patients may be able to ambulate without an orthosis; however they cannot do so safely because they may frequently fall, stumble, or twist an ankle. Thus the orthoses are prescribed in those cases to provide safety of ambulation.

The biomechanical function of different ankle-foot orthoses may be the same irrespective of materials and components used in their construction. This function can be demonstrated in the conventional metal double upright orthosis. This orthosis is attached to a firm Blücher[28] type shoe for ease of donning and doffing. Most commonly used is a stirrup, i.e., a steel plate bent in a U shape which is incorporated into the shoe. The upper ends form part of the ankle joints. A rigid steel sole plate is often riveted to the stirrup, extending into the sole of the shoe just short of the metatarsal head area. Designs such as the split stirrup with flat channels or stirrups that accommodate round calipers for attachments of the uprights allow the detachment of the uprights from the stirrup but have major disadvantages. The split stirrup sometimes inadvertently slips out of the channels or, because of dirt and corrosion in the channels, is difficult to remove. The round calipers eliminate the ankle joint and, therefore, the axis of motion is coincident with the instep rather than the anatomical ankle axis. Pistoning of the brace against the limb is thus inevitable, but this is less of a problem with children because of the short distance between the instep and ankle. The conventional ankle joint allows motion only on one plane, i.e., dorsiflexion or plantar flexion. The so-called free ankle does not significantly limit motion in either direction, and in order to prevent foot drop, a plantar flexion or posterior stop may be added (Fig. 28–12). A steel pin is inserted into the channel that rests against the posterior flange of the stirrup, stopping plantar flexion. The angle at which this occurs is determined by a set screw. A spring inserted into the same channel will also counteract plantar flexion somewhat and is called a "lift assist." A double-stopped ankle joint adds a similarly constructed dorsiflexion or anterior stop (Fig. 28–12) which, to be fully effective, is usually combined with a steel sole plate or a long flange stirrup extending to the metatarsal heads. The uprights consist of stainless steel bar stock or, for light weight, are made

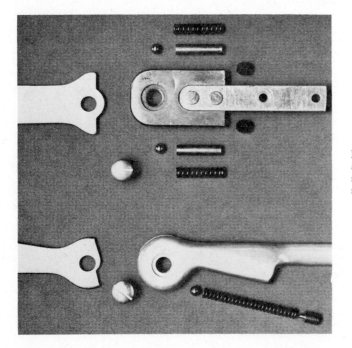

FIGURE 28–12. Double-stopped Becker ankle joint with pin and spring stops (top); single-stopped Klenzak ankle joint with spring assist (bottom).

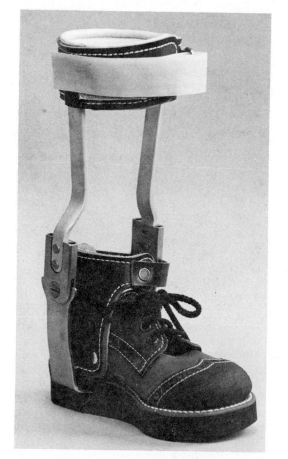

FIGURE 28–13. Inside T-strap correcting valgus position.

2. Ankle and knee stability: The plantar flexion stop at the ankle joint is a substitute for weak foot dorsiflexors, thus preventing toe drag and stumbling during the swing phase. In moderate to severe spasticity, a firm pin stop may be required to prevent a lapse into the equinus position; however, in flaccid paralysis or mild spasticity, a spring assist may be adequate.

Knee stability is also significantly influenced by the type of stop used. With a pin stop, the patient rocks over the posterior portion of his heel rather than letting the foot down slowly from heelstrike to foot flat through a contraction of the foot dorsiflexors. As a result, the ground reactive force is extended behind the knee joint (Fig. 28–14) with the moment arm (perpendicular distance from knee axis to force line) posterior to the knee, creating a bending moment at the knee greater than that produced by the normal lengthening contraction of the foot dorsiflexors. This bending moment must be overcome by knee extensor musculature. It is essential for the orthotic design to minimize this bending moment, since in many cases of significant weakness around the ankle, the muscles that extend to the knee are also affected. Therefore, during the swing phase, only the minimal force necessary to pick up the toe should be used. This would reduce the bending moment at the

of aluminum. They are posteriorly connected at the top of a rigid, padded calf band with an anterior soft closure.

The biomechanical function of the standard double-upright orthosis is as follows:

1. Mediolateral stability: This orthosis, when attached to a firm shoe, provides satisfactory mediolateral stability; however, in those patients with significant spasticity, such as stroke patients who tend to invert the foot, this is not the case. In such situations, a T-strap attached to the outside of the shoe covering the lateral malleolus and cinched around the middle upright can be added. When cinched, the lateral malleolus is pushed medially, thus correcting the varus (inversion) position. The valgus position, when there is a tendency toward eversion, can be corrected by attaching the T-strap to cover the medial malleolus and cinching it around the lateral upright (Fig. 28–13).

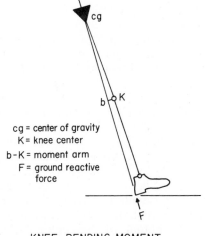

cg = center of gravity
K = knee center
b-K = moment arm
F = ground reactive force

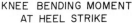

KNEE BENDING MOMENT
AT HEEL STRIKE

FIGURE 28–14. Knee bending moment at heelstrike (on photo). (From Lehmann, J. F.: The biomechanics of ankle foot orthoses: Prescription and design. Arch. Phys. Med. Rehabil., 60:200–207, 1979.)

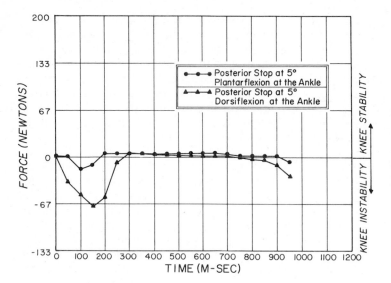

FIGURE 28–15. Force between leg and ankle foot orthosis at the calf band measured during stance, average of five consecutive steps. (From Lehmann, J. F.: The biomechanics of ankle foot orthoses: Prescription and design. Arch. Phys. Med. Rehabil., 60:200–207, 1979.)

knee because the resistance to plantar flexion is less. A spring assist, if adequate, should be used rather than the rigid pin stop.

The magnitude and duration of the bending moment at the knee is also influenced by the angle of the ankle at which the rigid plantar flexion stop is set. The bending moment is less if more plantar flexion is allowed than if the ankle is set in slight dorsiflexion (Fig. 28–15). There is a direct trade-off — the more dorsiflexion provided at the ankle, the better toe clearance during the swing phase but the greater the bending moment at the knee at heelstrike which the patient must overcome through voluntary muscle effort. Conversely, the more plantar flexion provided, the more toe drag during swing phase but the less bending moment at the knee at heelstrike. *Conclusion:* No more toe pickup than necessary should be provided by the posterior stop.

3. The anterior, dorsiflexion stop may be combined with a sole plate extending to the metatarsal head area. As the center of gravity of the body moves forward, the heel rises, the shoe pivots over the end of the sole plate, and pushoff is simulated. Consequently, the lowest point of the center of gravity pathway is elevated during the phase of double support; i.e., there is a reduction in the total amplitude of the center of gravity pathway. *Conclusion:* The dorsiflexion stop in combination with a sole plate is a substitute for the plantar flexion musculature, the gastrocnemius, and the soleus.

4. The dorsiflexion stop also has an effect

on knee stability (Fig. 28–16).[29] During the latter part of the stance phase, as the foot pivots over the metatarsal head area, a moment arm extending in front of the knee is created by the extension of the ground reactive force located at the ball of the foot. It is in the opposite direction of the moment arm during heelstrike and produces knee extension. The knee is locked in extension, since the posterior capsule and check ligaments prevent hyperextension. Since the posterior capsule and check ligaments are not particularly strong structures, repeated creation of too great an extension moment may result in

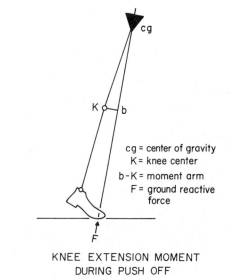

KNEE EXTENSION MOMENT
DURING PUSH OFF

FIGURE 28–16. Knee extension moment during pushoff (on photo). (From Lehmann, J. F.: The biomechanics of ankle foot orthoses: Prescription and design. Arch. Phys. Med. Rehabil., 60:200–207, 1979.)

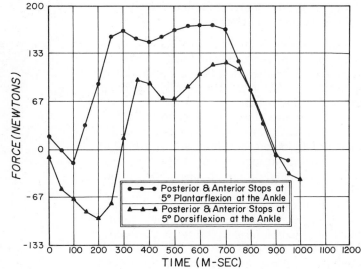

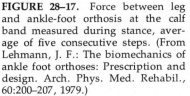

FIGURE 28–17. Force between leg and ankle-foot orthosis at the calf band measured during stance, average of five consecutive steps. (From Lehmann, J. F.: The biomechanics of ankle foot orthoses: Prescription and design. Arch. Phys. Med. Rehabil., 60:200–207, 1979.)

a genu recurvatum. This should be kept in mind when the patient is fitted with such an orthosis and, if needed, the stop should be adjusted. A spring plantar flexion assist is seldom used, as the forces needed to simulate pushoff easily overcome the spring and compress it, and as a result the foot remains flat on the ground.

The extension moment at the knee depends on the angle at which the dorsiflexion stop becomes effective (Fig. 28–17).[29] If the angle at the ankle is fixed at 5 degrees plantar flexion, the dorsiflexion stop increases knee stability over most of the latter part of the stance. The extension moment is of large magnitude, while the effect of the plantar flexion stop is of short duration and small magnitude. Thus, in this position, stability is gained during the latter part of the stance. Conversely, if the ankle is fixed at 5 degrees dorsiflexion by plantar and dorsiflexion stops, the bending moment at the knee during heelstrike is of long duration and large amplitude. Consequently, the stabilizing extension moment is of shorter duration and smaller magnitude. *Conclusion:* There is a trade-off between toe pickup and knee stability in that the more toe pickup or dorsiflexion of the ankle needed to clear the ground adequately during the swing phase, the more knee instability is produced by the plantar flexion stop during the heelstrike phase, and the less knee stability and pushoff simulation can be gained from the dorsiflexion stop, and vice versa.

If significant spasticity forces the foot into the equinus position during the swing phase, a solid posterior plantar flexion pin stop is needed to prevent the toe from dragging. If, at the same time, the adjustment of the stop, i.e., the angle at which it becomes effective, is such that the knee buckles during the heelstrike phase, the bending moment can be changed. This is accomplished by moving the location of the ground reactive force forward (Fig. 28–18),[29] either by cutting off part of the heel at a 45-degree angle or by inserting a cushion wedge into the heel.[30]

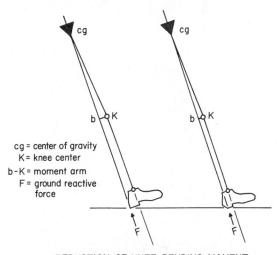

cg = center of gravity
K = knee center
b-K = moment arm
F = ground reactive force

REDUCTION OF KNEE BENDING MOMENT
DURING HEEL STRIKE PHASE BY HEEL CUTOFF

FIGURE 28–18. Reduction of knee bending moment during heelstrike by heel cutoff (on photo). (From Lehmann, J. F.: The biomechanics of ankle foot orthosis: Prescription and design. Arch. Phys. Med. Rehabil., 60:200–207, 1979.)

Use of Biomechanical Principles in Evaluation of Orthoses

With an understanding of the biomechanical function of the orthotic components, selection of the design that best corresponds to a patient's needs is greatly simplified. This is especially important in view of the many recent orthotic designs and modifications using new materials such as plastics, and it can be anticipated that there will continue to be a fairly rapid increase in modifications of existing designs, design changes, and materials used.

When prescribing an orthosis, it is of primary importance to determine the patient's need for mediolateral stability at the ankle, toe pickup, knee stability, and simulated pushoff. A gross assessment of the forces required, especially for toe pickup, is desirable. With this in mind, several examples of the application of biomechanical principles are as follows:

Orthosis with Single Metal Upright and Posterior Plantar Flexion Stop (Fig. 28–19). It is obvious that this orthosis does not provide as

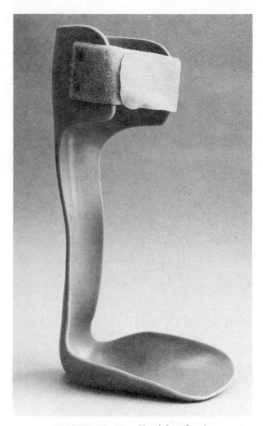

FIGURE 28–20. Teufel orthosis.

much mediolateral stability as a double upright orthosis, but the medial malleolus is less likely to be knocked by the opposite leg because of the absence of a medial upright. The plastic laminated shoe insert allows shoes to be changed, and, if an anterior dorsiflexion stop is added, the insert would also serve as a sole plate equivalent for pushoff. This design could be used as a toe pickup orthosis, but the patient using it should not have much spasticity driving the foot into an equinovarus position.

Teufel Orthosis (Fig. 28–20).[1, 31, 32] This orthosis is a stock item that is available in different sizes. As can be seen from its appearance, it provides limited mediolateral stability. It is effective in patients needing a moderate amount of force for toe pickup, but it provides little additional knee stability during the latter part of the stance. It is fairly rigid in resisting plantar flexion when stressed manually, but yields easily when the same amount of force is applied to push it into dorsiflexion. Because the orthosis acts as a posterior leaf spring allowing dorsiflexion, the center of rotation in the orthosis

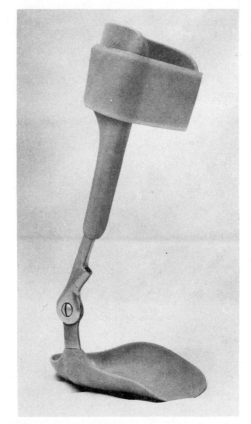

FIGURE 28–19. Orthosis with single upright and posterior plantar flexion stop.

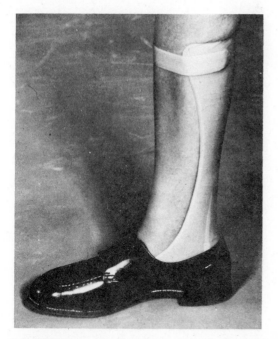

FIGURE 28–21. Seattle orthosis. (From Lehmann, J. F.: The biomechanics of ankle foot orthoses: Prescription and design. Arch. Phys. Med. Rehabil., 60:200–207, 1979.)

sign of this orthosis using plastics such as polypropylene (Fig. 28–22).[31] The cost of manufacture is thus reduced, since vacuum-forming techniques can be used with these plastics. The biomechanical function of this orthosis is basically the same as the Seattle orthosis; however, it is somewhat less rigid, depending on the thickness of the plastic used and the trim lines.

TIRR Orthosis (Engen) (Fig. 28–22). Polypropylene is used in the manufacture of this orthosis, which was designed by Engen.[31, 32] It is corrugated posteriorly for greater strength. The orthosis resists mild to moderate forces pushing it into plantar flexion, depending on thickness of plastic and trim line; however, there is very little resistance to being pushed into dorsiflexion. Depending on trim line, limited mediolateral stability is provided. Therefore, since the

differs from the location of the anatomical axis of the ankle, resulting in some relative motion between the orthosis and the limb, a problem in some patients.

Seattle Orthosis (Fig. 28–21). This orthosis is manufactured by lamination over a positive mold taken from a cast and was the first plastic orthosis described in the literature.[33, 34] The orthosis is rigid and encases the ankle, thereby providing the biomechanical equivalent to an anterior and posterior pin stop with a sole plate extending to the metatarsal head area. It provides maximal mediolateral stability, but since knee stability is dependent on the degree of plantar or dorsiflexion at which the foot is fixed, casting at the correct angle of the ankle is of critical importance, and heel and sole height of the shoe must be taken into consideration when casting. Consequently, shoes can be changed only if heel and sole height are the same as those of the shoes used for casting. A cushion wedge[34] or cutoff heel can be used to reduce the bending moment at the knee during heelstrike. The anterior portion of the orthosis can be slightly trimmed back to reduce the extension moment at the knee, if desired.

Lehneis in New York and the staff at Rancho Los Amigos have modified the de-

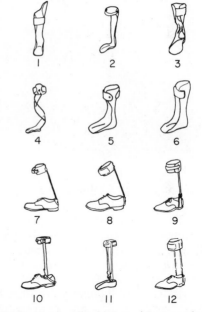

FIGURE 28–22. Small selection of recent orthotic designs:

1. Plastic solid ankle.
2. Teufel.
3. Texas Institute of Rehabilitation Research (Engen).
4. Institute of Rehabilitation Medicine Spiral.
5. Rancho Los Amigos.
6. Seattle.
7. Veterans Administration Prosthetics Center Shoe-Clasp.
8. Army Medical Branch Research Laboratory Posterior Bar.
9. VAPC Single Side Band.
10. University of California Biomechanics Laboratory Dual Axis.
11. New York University.
12. AMBRL — Double Upright.

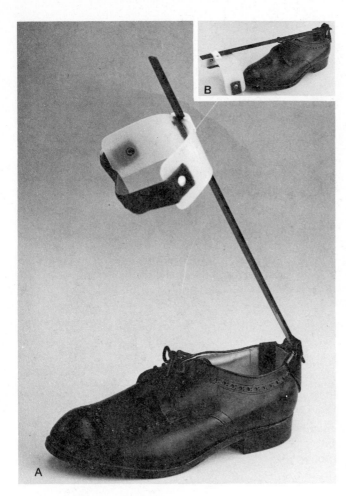

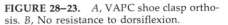

FIGURE 28–23. *A*, VAPC shoe clasp orthosis. *B*, No resistance to dorsiflexion.

orthosis gives little additional knee stability during pushoff or the latter part of the stance phase, its primary use is to provide toe pickup during the swing phase for patients with flaccid paralysis or mild spasticity.

VAPC Shoe Clasp Orthosis (Fig. 28–23).[1, 31, 35] This orthosis is a plastic leaf spring orthosis with its main advantage being that it is "ready made" and requires only a firm shoe for application. It can be attached to the heel counter of a shoe by a clasp and loosely to a calf band to absorb the relative motion of the orthosis against the limb. While the center of rotation of the ankle and the orthosis are in different locations, pistoning of the plastic bar within the calf band is possible. Although readily available and easily applied, this orthosis provides only moderate force for toe pickup and no significant mediolateral stability, and collapses readily into maximal dorsiflexion even in the absence of stress, thus contributing no additional knee stability (Fig. 28–23).

Spring Wire Orthosis.[36, 37] This orthosis provides only a moderate spring foot dorsiflexor assist for toe pickup. It resists dorsiflexion at pushoff in the same proportion, but the force is not strong enough to produce any significant pushoff stimulation. Mediolateral ankle stability is limited, and plastic orthoses are now frequently used instead of this orthosis.

University of California at Berkeley Dual Ankle Orthosis.[38] This is just one example of special orthoses designed for unusual conditions and, like the others in this group, is applicable to only a few patients. In developing this orthotic design, Inman and associates[39, 40] determined that the axis of inversion and eversion of the subtalar joint is 42 degrees from the horizontal plane and 23 degrees from the midline of the foot. With this information as the basis, an orthosis was designed with an axis for plantar and dorsiflexion and an axis located posteriorly at the heel of the shoe to allow inversion and eversion. A standard ankle joint is used which can be stopped or modified as in other orthoses. However, the use of this orthosis is limited, since it can seldom be used where there is weakness of the anterior leg musculature. The necessity for toe pickup requiring a stopped ankle joint implies that the foot dorsiflexors are either nonfunctioning or weak. Since these muscles are also part of the inversion and eversion group, most patients are unable to use this orthosis with its additional freedom to invert and evert, as they need mediolateral stability at the ankle.

Only a few of the available orthoses have been discussed or illustrated in Figure 28–22, but this relatively small number demonstrates the value of understanding and using the basic biomechanical principles when prescribing orthoses. This understanding not only allows more individualization but also eliminates the need for rote memorization of indications and contraindications.

In addition to the biomechanical principles discussed, another important consideration in prescription should be whether the orthotic design increases functional ambulation capability and decreases energy expenditure. A comparison between normal subjects and hemiplegic patients walking without an orthosis, with the Seattle orthosis, and with a double upright ankle-foot orthosis with anterior and posterior pin stops and sole plate showed the following:

1. Oxygen consumption was least in normal subjects for any given walking speed and highest in hemiplegics walking without an orthosis. When walking with an orthosis, oxygen consumption was reduced but was still considerably higher than that of normals.

2. There was no difference in oxygen consumption at various speeds with patients using the Seattle or the double upright ankle-foot orthosis.

3. The use of either the Seattle or double upright ankle-foot orthosis increased the comfortable walking speed, i.e., that walking speed at which the minimum amount of energy is required to cover a given distance. The use of either of these orthoses also increased the maximum walking speed when compared with the same patient walking without the orthosis. In these respects, there was no difference between the two types of orthoses used (Fig. 28–24).[41, 42]

4. Most importantly, however, while the patients walked safely with either of the orthoses, they had to be closely guarded

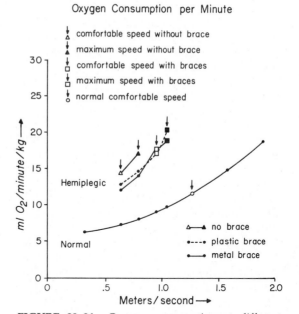

FIGURE 28–24. Oxygen consumption at different ambulation rates of a patient walking without orthosis and using a plastic laminated ankle-foot orthosis and an ankle-foot orthosis with double metal uprights, anterior and posterior stops, and sole plate extending to the metatarsal head area. (From Lehmann, J. F.: The biomechanics of ankle foot orthosis: Prescription and design. Arch. Phys. Med. Rehabil., 60:200–207, 1979. Redrawn from Corcoran.[41, 42])

against falls when walking without an orthosis.

In summary, proper bracing increases functional ambulation while decreasing energy consumption and provides a greater degree of safety for the patient. Second, even though the materials used and the appearance of orthoses are different, results are quantifiably similar, provided the same biomechanical design is used in the orthoses. Third, minor differences in the weight of the orthoses are not as important in determining energy consumption as biomechanical function and its influence on the center of gravity pathway.

Use of Biomechanical Principles in Checking Orthoses

After fitting to the patient, it is most important to check the orthosis to determine whether it fulfills its intended functions. This checking can be divided into several parts:

1. The simple fit of the orthosis should be checked in a static situation. There should be no pressure areas or areas where the orthosis may produce abrasions. With the metal dou-

ble upright orthosis, common problem areas include the impingement of the peroneal nerve as it passes around the fibular neck by the calf band and where the uprights touch the malleoli. The patient with a plastic orthosis should be managed in the same way as an amputee with a new prosthetic socket. Initially, frequent checks for pressure areas are necessary, and redness should fade after a short period of time. Skin intolerance must be built up by gradually increasing wear.

2. The dynamic checkout is very important. While the patient is standing, the sole and heel of the shoe should be flat on the floor. While walking, the patient should be closely observed for potential knee instability during the heelstrike phase from heelstrike to foot flat. This relates to the function of the plantar flexion or posterior stop of the orthosis or its equivalent. If, during the pushoff phase, a tendency toward back-knee is noted, this can be related to the anterior dorsiflexion stop and the length of the sole plate. During the entire swing phase, a determination should be made as to adequacy of toe clearance and, if a dorsiflexion spring assist is used, it should be observed for sufficient toe clearance.

3. The ankle should also be closely observed for possible movement. If the orthosis does allow movement, the axis of the ankle joint for plantar- and dorsiflexion should be aligned to coincide as closely as possible with the location of the anatomic joint axis. It was determined by Inman and associates[39] that this axis can be approximated by connecting the tips of the medial and lateral malleoli. This alignment prevents forces from developing between the orthosis and the limb. A special problem is present in plastic or posterior spring orthoses where the center of rotation in the orthosis differs from that of the ankle joint.

Knee-Ankle Orthoses

As in the ankle-foot orthoses, an understanding of the biomechanical function of these orthoses will allow their prescription and modification to meet the specific needs of a particular patient. New approaches to design have recently been introduced, and their advantages and disadvantages over the standard double upright metal orthosis can be best understood in terms of their biomechanical function. Knee-ankle orthoses are usually needed by patients who not only have weakness around the foot and ankle but also are unable to stabilize the knee securely during the weight bearing phase of the gait cycle. Weakness of this type may be caused by upper or lower motor neuron lesions. A severe disability commonly managed with these orthoses is spinal cord injury, including conus and cauda equina lesions. The orthoses may be used for functional ambulation or for ambulation as exercise. Patients with spinal cord injury usually use a swing-to or swing-through gait and become functional ambulators only at lesion levels below T10,[43, 44] their functional ambulation ability depending on age, strength, and coordination.

The knee-ankle orthosis should provide the following biomechanical functions during the stance phase:

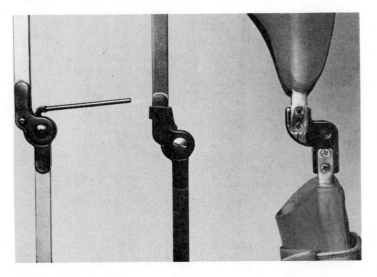

FIGURE 28-25. Swiss or bail lock, drop lock, and free knee.

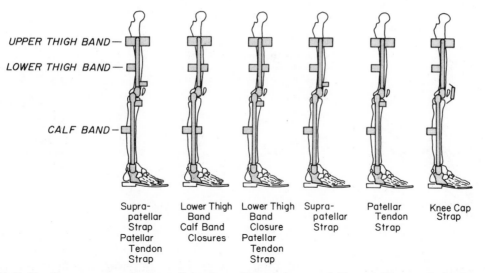

UPPER THIGH BAND —

LOWER THIGH BAND —

CALF BAND —

| Supra-patellar Strap Patellar Tendon Strap | Lower Thigh Band Calf Band Closures | Lower Thigh Band Closure Patellar Tendon Strap | Supra-patellar Strap | Patellar Tendon Strap | Knee Cap Strap |

FIGURE 28–26. Six common orthotic configurations. (From Lehmann, J. F., and Warren, C. G.: Restraining forces in various designs of knee ankle orthoses: Their placement and effect on anatomical knee joint. Arch. Phys. Med. Rehabil., 57:430–437, 1976.)

1. Mediolateral stability at the ankle.

2. Knee stability in cases where the ankle-foot orthosis is not adequate to control the knee.

3. Pushoff simulation during the latter part of the stance phase if equipped with an anterior dorsiflexion stop and a rigid sole plate extending to the metatarsal head area.

During the swing phase the posterior plantar-flexion stop should assure toe clearance.

Thus, the basic difference between the ankle-foot and knee-ankle orthoses is the stabilization of the knee by the knee-ankle orthosis. This is achieved by three force applications, one stabilizing force applied in front to keep the knee from buckling under load bearing, and two counterforces applied at the upper part posteriorly and at shoe level to keep the limb from moving. The components used to achieve such biomechanical function in the standard metal double upright orthosis, i.e., shoes, stirrups, ankle joints, calf bands, and uprights, are the same as those in the ankle-foot orthosis. Commonly available knee joint designs are a free knee, knee joint with a drop or ring lock, and a bail or Swiss lock (Fig. 28–25). At the top of the orthosis the two uprights are connected by a posterior, rigid, padded upper thigh band with anterior soft closure. This band should clear the ischium by approximately 1½ inches. Usually a lower thigh band with a soft front closure is also used. Knee stabilization is provided by a number of different devices, six common versions of which are shown in Figure 28–26.[45]

A pelvic band is sometimes used in conjunction with the knee-ankle orthosis.[46] The pelvic band is a padded, rigid steel band posteriorly and laterally which fits between the greater trochanter and the iliac crest. A soft front closure is used. The pelvic band is connected to the lateral uprights of the knee-ankle orthosis by a hip joint that may be locked, for instance, by a drop lock. Most hip joints of this type allow only flexion and extension movements.

Through an analysis of the function of this standard design, a determination can be made of the basic principles necessary for understanding the function of the orthosis. These principles are as follows:

1. Force applications should be well within tolerance limits, particularly in patients with anesthetic skin.

2. Forces should be distributed over tolerant areas of the tissues.

3. Unnecessary shear stresses liable to loosen ligaments of the knee should be avoided.

4. Energy consumption required for walking should be kept to a minimum.

5. The orthosis should allow ease of donning, doffing, and transfer activities.

In recent investigations,[45] the forces between the upper thigh band and thigh were measured, and no differences were found in the various designs applying the knee-stabilizing force. However, significant differ-

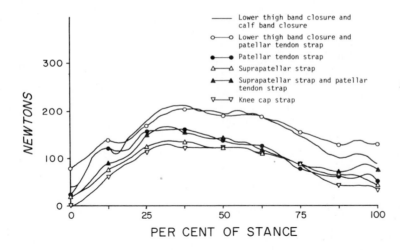

FIGURE 28–27. Total force required to stabilize the knee in the same patient using the six orthoses. (From Lehmann, J. F., and Warren, C. G.: Restraining forces in various designs of knee ankle orthoses: Their placement and effect on anatomical knee joint. Arch. Phys. Med. Rehabil, 57:430–437, 1976.)

ences were found in the amount of total stabilizing force required to counteract a given bending moment at the knee. The highest force was required when the lower thigh band and calf band were used together to stabilize the knee (Fig. 28–27). From these experiments it can be concluded that the knee-stabilizing force can be kept to a minimum if it is applied close to the knee center, since this provides a better leverage to counteract the bending moment at the knee. In addition, the more flexion allowed at the knee, the greater the bending moment during the weight bearing phase of the stance. Therefore it is essential that the orthosis be designed to keep the knee straight in the orthosis, thus reducing the required stabilizing force. It is equally important for an orthosis so designed to be correctly applied and the straps cinched evenly and tightly enough to prevent any bending during weight bearing (Fig. 28–28).

If one looks at the forces per strap that approximately represent the force per unit of

surface area of tissue, one finds very significant differences (Fig. 28–29). The lowest force per strap was found when the forces were applied close to the knee center and distributed over two straps such as the patellar tendon and suprapatellar straps. These straps also have the additional advantage of being applied to areas very tolerant of pressure, i.e., the patellar tendon and the musculature above the patella. Single straps can be safely used only if they are large enough to distribute the forces over a large area and especially if applied to tolerant areas such as the patellar tendon.

The forces required to counteract the knee bending moment by the application of stabilizing straps are biologically significant. The range of these forces was measured and found to be from 100 to 170 newtons during paraplegic ambulation using a swing-through gait. For the calculation of pressure, a variable contact area between tissue and the straps or bands was assumed. Depending on the width of the area of interaction between

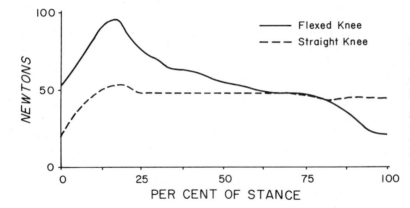

FIGURE 28–28. Comparison of total stabilizing force required with knee maintained as straight as possible and flexed at 12 degrees. (From Lehmann, J. F., and Warren, C. G.: Restraining forces in various designs of knee ankle orthoses: Their placement and effect on anatomical knee joint. Arch. Phys. Med. Rehabil., 57:430–437, 1976.)

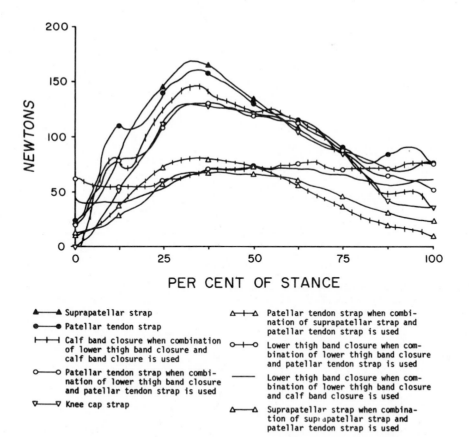

FIGURE 28–29. Forces on each of the individual strap closures stabilizing the knee in the same patient using the six orthoses. (From Lehmann, J. F., and Warren, C. G.: Restraining forces in various designs of knee ankle orthoses: Their placement and effect on anatomical knee joint. Arch. Phys. Med. Rehabil., 57:430–437, 1976.)

the band and the tissues, these pressures were on the order of magnitude of 10 newtons/sq cm or 750 mm mercury. In a poorly fitting orthosis the patient's ischium may be sitting on the edge of the upper posterior thigh band. The force interaction between the ischial area and the band was measured by determining the bending moment created in the orthosis uprights below the band. The forces in swing through ambulation ranged from 3 to 5 newtons. If one calculates the pressure for interaction between the tissue and various widths of the edge of the posterior thigh band, it is on the order of magnitude of 25 newtons/sq cm or 1875 mm mercury (Fig. 28–30). These are significant and potentially destructive forces and therefore should be kept to a minimum in an optimal orthotic design. Even then they occlude the blood flow; however, this occurs during ambulation only in the stance phase and, therefore, this temporary interruption of capillary flow is tolerated. However, toler-

ance may be exceeded if straps are used over less tolerant areas such as bony prominences.

Anatomically, knee shear varied greatly with the type of knee-stabilizing force applied (Fig. 28–31). In all cases, the initial shear during heel-strike was positive; i.e., the femur sheared forward on the tibia. During the latter part of the stance or pushoff, it sheared backward on the tibia; i.e., a negative shear was recorded. Two types of curves were obtained with the different orthotic designs, one with relatively even distribution of duration and amplitude between positive and negative shear, the other with a minimum positive shear during the heelstrike phase and a maximum amplitude and duration of negative shear during the latter part of the stance, with total shear amplitude negative and greater than in the other types of curves. It can be assumed that the latter distribution of shear would be destructive to knee ligaments, especially if the patients are

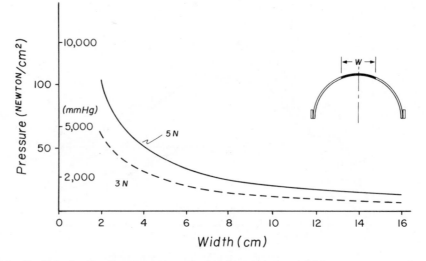

FIGURE 28–30. Possible distribution of pressure calculated assuming a variable contact area on the superior edge of the upper thigh band. (From Lehmann, J. F., and Warren, C. G.: Restraining forces in various designs of knee ankle orthoses: Their placement and effect on anatomical knee joint. Arch. Phys. Med. Rehabil., 57:430–437, 1976.)

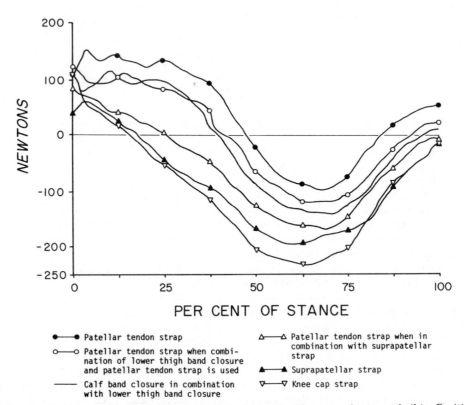

FIGURE 28–31. Anatomical knee shear showing force interaction between femur and tibia. Positive values indicate the femur shearing forward on the tibia; negative values indicate the femur shearing backward on the tibia. (From Lehmann, J. F., and Warren, C. G.: Restraining forces in various designs of knee ankle orthoses: Their placement and effect on anatomical knee joint. Arch. Phys. Med. Rehabil., 57:430–437, 1976.)

vigorous ambulators. The result is usually a back-knee or genu recurvatum. The explanation for this difference and the types of shear curves during the pushoff phase are shown in Figures 28–32 and 28–33.

If the force is applied by a patellar tendon strap (Fig. 28–32), the shear transmitted to the knee ligaments is reduced considerably, thereby decreasing the chance of loosening them. The explanation for this reduction in shear is as follows:

1. The shear measured in the orthosis is in an anterior direction, while the shear against the floor is in a posterior direction.

2. Shear transmitted through the skeletal system equals floor shear minus the shear measured in the orthosis.

3. Since these shear forces are vectors, the shear in the orthosis is added to the floor shear in the opposite direction. The shear in the skeletal system is therefore large and posterior.

4. This large amount of shear is transmitted up the skeletal leg column until another force is applied, in this case by the patellar tendon strap.

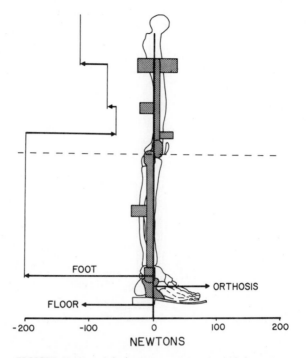

FIGURE 28–33. Schematic representation of shear in the limb and orthosis during pushoff, the stabilizing force above the knee. (From Lehmann, J. F., and Warren, C. G.: Restraining forces in various designs of knee ankle orthoses: Their placement and effect on anatomical knee joint. Arch. Phys. Med. Rehabil., 57:430–437, 1976.)

However, when the strap is applied above the knee, the total shear force is transmitted across the knee and might very well stretch the ligaments (Fig. 28–33). With this type application of force, the shear force generated in the leg column is not reduced until it meets another force about the knee.

If the strap is applied below the knee, the positive shear phase is enhanced, providing a more even distribution between positive and negative shear through the stance phase (Fig. 28–34). If, on the other hand, the stabilizing strap is applied above the knee, only a minimum amount of positive shear is transmitted through the knee during heelstrike, producing an even distribution between positive and negative shear (Fig. 28–35).

Efforts have been made to reduce the weight of the orthoses by eliminating unnecessary structural components, thus making them more functional and easier to don and doff. The Craig Scott orthosis[47-49] was specifically designed for this purpose for paraplegic patients. This orthosis eliminates the lower thigh band and calf bands, retains the bail lock at the knee, and applies a stabilizing

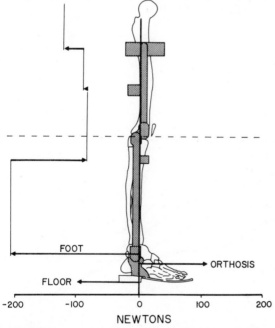

FIGURE 28–32. Schematic representation of shear in the limb and orthosis during pushoff, the stabilizing force below the knee. (From Lehmann, J. F., and Warren, C. G.: Restraining forces in various designs of knee ankle orthoses: Their placement and effect on anatomical knee joint. Arch. Phys. Med. Rehabil., 57:430–437, 1976.)

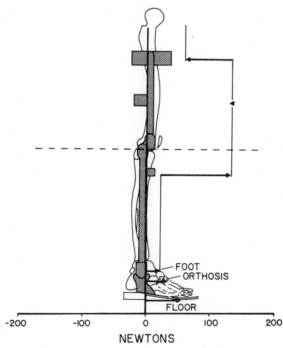

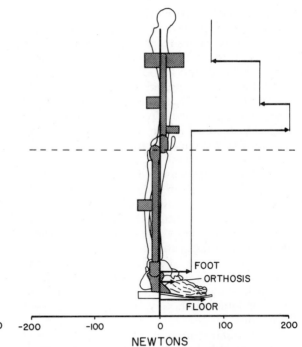

FIGURE 28–34. Schematic representation of shear distribution in limb and orthosis at heelstrike with stabilizing force below the knee. (From Lehmann, J. F., and Warren, C. G.: Restraining effects in various designs of knee ankle orthoses: Their placement and effect on anatomical knee joint. Arch. Phys. Med. Rehabil., 57:430–437, 1976.)

FIGURE 28–35. Schematic representation of shear distribution in limb and orthosis at heelstrike with stabilizing force about the knee. (From Lehmann, J. F., and Warren, C. G.: Restraining forces in various designs of knee ankle orthoses: Their placement and effect on anatomical knee joint. Arch. Phys. Med. Rehabil., 57:430–437, 1976.)

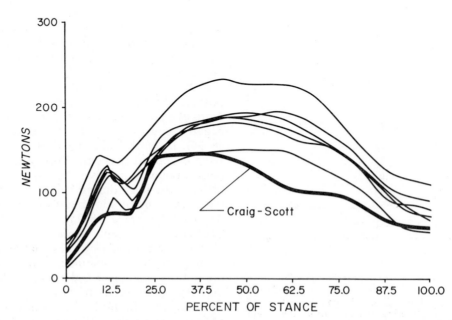

FIGURE 28–36. Total stabilizing force on knee as compared with six other configurations. (From Lehmann, J. F.: Lower limb orthotics. *In* Redford, J. B. (Ed.): Orthotics Etcetera, 2nd Ed. Baltimore, Williams & Wilkins Co., 1980, p. 320.)

force to the knee through an anterior pretibial rigid piece that may either be hinged and locked into position or permanently attached to the uprights. As in the conventional designs, a double pin–stopped ankle joint with a sole plate at the metatarsal head area is used. When this orthosis was evaluated (Fig. 28–36),[49] it was found that the total force required to stabilize the knee is small, since the force is applied near the knee center. If the forces applied by the pretibial piece are compared with forces applied by straps used in the other configurations, they are found to be relatively high, since only one strap is used for stabilization. In spite of careful fitting and padding, the original design of the shin piece applies too much force over the tibia so that functional ambulators suffer skin abrasions or unduly prolonged reddening after wearing the orthosis. This can be eliminated by widening the shin piece, manufacturing it from a plaster cast mold to make it form fitting, and extending the area of maximal pressure to the patellar tendon area. The shear forces were relatively small and well distributed in this orthosis, since the knee-stabilizing force was applied below the knee (Fig. 28–37). When the rigidity of the orthosis with reduction of rigid cross-connections between the uprights was tested, it was found that mediolateral displacement and rotation at the upper thigh band

level and posterior displacement at the knee level were minimal and temporary in the standard configuration of this orthosis. Only when all rigid cross-connections, including the bail, were removed between the upper thigh band and the stirrup below did the orthosis significantly deform under load conditions comparable to those measured in paraplegic ambulation. Thus, the Craig Scott orthosis with a bail for the knee lock and an anterior rigid pretibial shell should have adequate structural rigidity.

The ability to functionally ambulate, especially for paraplegic patients, depends largely on the amount of oxygen consumed.[50] With a knee-ankle orthosis, the amount of energy consumption during ambulation primarily depends on the influence of the design on the center of gravity pathway. The six conventional orthoses (see Fig. 28–26) share with the Craig Scott design the double pin–stopped ankle joint used in conjunction with a rigid steel sole plate extending to the metatarsal head area which provides a simulated pushoff. Another common design uses a single joint with a posterior plantar flexion stop to provide toe clearance during the swing phase, but allows free dorsiflexion. The difference in the center of gravity pathway curves is shown in Figure 28–38. As a paraplegic patient using a swing-through gait with crutches leans forward on the crutches, the

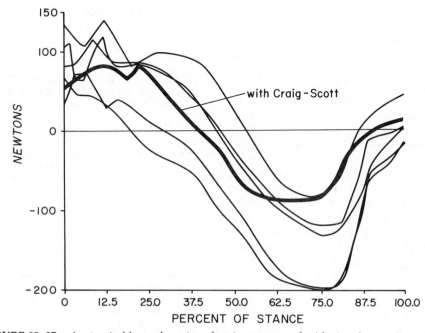

FIGURE 28–37. Anatomical knee shear (on photo) as compared with six other configurations.

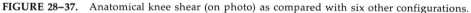

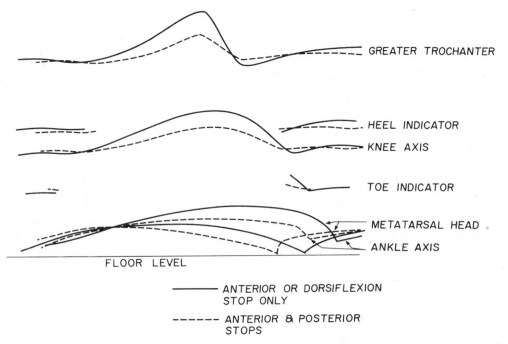

FIGURE 28–38. Difference in center of gravity pathway curves, first curve posterior stop only and second curve posterior stops.

heel rises and the center of gravity pathway is maintained at a relatively high elevation from the floor at the lowest point of the center of gravity pathway curve. This is the result of the dorsiflexion stop and the sole plate. The shoe and foot pivot over the end of the sole plate at this time. If the ankle joint allows free dorsiflexion, the sole of the shoe stays flat on the floor and the center of gravity at this point is at a lower elevation from the floor than in the orthosis equipped with a dorsiflexion stop and sole plate. As a result, the patient must lift more to clear the ground during the swing phase (Table 28–1). During the lift phase the actual difference in mechanical work between patients wearing these two designs of orthoses can be determined by multiplying the center of gravity displacement by the force exerted against the ground through the crutches. The latter can be measured through the use of a force plate. It was found[51] that the mechanical work was reduced by an average of 34 per cent. Since energy is also consumed when mechanical work is not done — i.e., for balance, shock absorption, deceleration — oxygen consumption was also measured (Table 28–2). The total energy consumption thus measured was reduced by the addition of the dorsiflexion stop and the sole plate. It is also inter-

esting to note that the greatest amount of energy consumed when the dorsiflexion stop and sole plate were used occurred during ambulation or in the first part of the rest period. However, with free ankle dorsiflexion this occurred late in the rest period, which suggests that these patients incurred an oxygen debt to a degree that would limit ambulation with this type of orthosis to walking for exercise purposes only. The same patients

TABLE 28–1. COMPARISON OF VERTICAL LIFT OF CENTER OF GRAVITY AREA

Patient No.	Sex	Level of Lesion	(n=10) Post. Stop	(n=10) Post. and Ant. Stop	t value (p*)
1	F	T12	13.2	9.0	5.998 (0.0001)
2	F	T7-8	12.0	6.85	6.414 (0.0006)
3	M	L2-3	21.6	13.3	5.534 (0.00002)

*p = probability

From Lehmann, J. F., de Lateur, B. J., Warren, C. G., Simons, B. C., and Guy, A. W.: Biomechanical evaluation of braces for paraplegics. Arch. Phys. Med. Rehabil., 50:179–188, 1969.

TABLE 28-2. COMPARISON OF ENERGY CONSUMPTION OF PATIENT AMBULATING WITH EACH BRACE

Intervals of O_2 Consumption	Post. Ankle Stop		Post. and Ant. Ankle Stop	
	Run 1	Run 3	Run 2	Run 4
Rest 1 min.	0.42 liter	0.44 liter	0.67 liter	0.66 liter
Ambulation 200 feet	2.48 liters	2.49 liters	2.56 liters	2.04 liters
Min. 1 and 2 rest	1.56 liters	1.58 liters	1.82 liters	2.22 liters
Min. 3 and 4 rest	3.35 liters	3.38 liters	1.01 liters	0.95 liters
Total O_2 consumed*	7.39 liters	7.45 liters	5.39 liters	5.21 liters
Total caloric* equivalent	36.95 Cal.	37.25 Cal.	26.95 Cal.	26.05 Cal.
Ambulation time	1 min., 11 sec.	1 min., 19 sec.	1 min., 13 sec.	1 min., 17 sec.

*Prerun rest not included in totals.
From Lehmann, J. F., de Lateur, B. J., Warren, C. G., Simons, B. C., and Guy, A. W.: Biomechanical evaluation of braces for paraplegics. Arch. Phys. Med. Rehabil., 50:179–188, 1969.

equipped with a dorsiflexion stop and sole plate could ambulate for greater distances and longer periods of time and would thus be more likely to become functional ambulators. Also, the double-stopped ankle joint with a sole plate provides a pla'form over which the patient can balance and, therefore, the standing balance without handholds or crutches was significantly increased with the use of this orthotic design.

Energy cost seems to be one of the major limitations on paraplegic ambulation. It is for this reason that Long and Lawton[43] believe that paraplegics at levels T10 and above would not become functional ambulators, a finding confirmed by Rosman and Spira.[52] They found that paraplegics at levels T1 through T6 did not use their orthoses. A few T7 to T11 paraplegics used their orthoses primarily for exercise purposes, while the functional ambulators usually had lesion levels at T12 or below. Patients with levels of lesion at L2 to L5 are especially likely to become functional ambulators. Clinkingbeard's[50, 53-55] group, in a study of paraplegics, found that the energy required for ambulation ranged from 2.32 to 9.05 kcal × 10^{-3}/m/kg. This represents a threefold increase when compared with normals.

Orthotic design features should make donning and doffing easy, and the time required for this was used as a measure of the difficulty encountered. When the Craig Scott orthosis was compared with the standard double upright orthosis using the patellar tendon–suprapatellar strap combination, the average donning time was 111 seconds for the Craig Scott and 153 seconds for the standard orthosis. The doffing time for the former was 28 seconds and for the latter 33 seconds. However, on evaluation of the Craig Scott, it was noted that it slid off the thigh when the patient sat because the posterior calf band normally restraining the orthosis was missing. This could be readily corrected by a posterior soft closure below the knee which, however, added four seconds to the doffing time.[49] It can therefore be concluded that one posterior connection between the uprights below the knee is essential to stabilize the orthosis on the limb when the patient sits. There was no difference between the standard orthosis and the Craig Scott design in transfer activities. Also, standing balance was identical, since these two types of orthoses are the same from the ankle joint down.

The necessity for a pelvic band is somewhat controversial. While a pelvic band designed with a lockable hip joint is frequently used for stabilizing the hips, patients can be quite stable when using a swing-through and swing-to gait without such a band. With crutches in front, the forces of gravity pull the hips into extension to provide stability, and hyperextension is checked by extremely strong ligaments. Following swing-through, the patient is stable with the crutches behind him. If the patient's trunk is arched, the center of gravity force line falls behind the hip joints into an area of support between the legs and crutches. The hips are again locked by the extension moment created by the force line falling behind the hip axis of flexion extension. In this manner patients can ambulate effectively without being encumbered by a pelvic band.

The literature suggests that excessive lumbar excursion is reduced by the use of a pelvic band and that it controls the forward

TABLE 28–3. LUMBAR EXCURSION, STRIDE LENGTH, AND CENTER OF GRAVITY AMPLITUDE WITH AND WITHOUT PELVIC BAND

	With Pelvic Band	Without Pelvic Band	Wilcoxon Test*
Mean maximum range of lumbar excursion (degrees)	29.0	26.8	$p < 0.05$
Mean stride length	0.96 m	1.03 m	$p < 0.05$
Mean center of gravity amplitude	10.8 cm	8.7 cm	$p < 0.05$

*Matched-pairs signed-ranks test.
From Warren, C. G., Lehmann, J. F., and de Lateur, B. J.: Pelvic band use in orthotics for adult paraplegic patients. Arch. Phys. Med. Rehabil., 56:221–223, 1975.

swing of the legs, especially in cases of uneven spasticity. An experiment was developed to test this suggestion by applying an electrogoniometer to the backs of paraplegic patients in order to estimate the maximal excursion of the lumbar spine throughout the gait cycle.[56] The results showed that while the hips were somewhat limited by the pelvic band, lumbar excursion was significantly increased as the lumbar spine compensated for lack of mobility at the hips. The use of the pelvic band resulted in a significant reduction of mean stride length and an increase in the center of gravity pathway amplitude (Table 28–3). Without the pelvic band, the patient walked with a lower center of gravity pathway amplitude (Table 28–3), and mobility at the hips allowed the patient to clear the ground more easily during the swing phase.

The assumption can be made from these measurements that energy consumption will be greater when the orthosis includes a pelvic band. Also, donning and doffing times were found to be longer. If the patient had some spasticity, it was found that standing balance was slightly improved. However, all patients tested learned to overcome their initial difficulties when using orthoses without pelvic bands and chose permanent orthoses without the band even though forward leg swing might be better controlled with the pelvic band. Therefore, in most cases of paraplegia, pelvic bands are probably unnecessary, although they may be useful in some exceptional cases of spasticity.[56]

In summary, the following biomechanical principles apply to the design and fitting of all knee-ankle orthoses:

1. Mediolateral stability of ankle and toe pickup during the swing phase is provided in the same fashion as in the ankle-foot orthosis. In addition, knee stability is provided during the stance phase and simulated pushoff.

2. To reduce the possibility of excessive forces being applied to the knee by bands or straps, the following should be observed:
   a. The orthosis should be designed and applied with the knee straight to reduce the bending moment at the knee.
   b. Any stabilizing straps should be applied close to the knee center to reduce the force required to counteract a bending moment at the knee.
   c. The straps or bands stabilizing the knee should distribute the required force over a large and also tolerant area such as the patellar tendon and suprapatellar areas.
   d. To reduce the shear on the knee ligaments, a major portion of the total knee stabilizing force should be applied below the knee.

3. An anterior dorsiflexion stop combined with a sole plate extending to the metatarsal head area simulates pushoff with a decreased center of gravity pathway and amplitude and a significant reduction of energy consumption.

4. The rigid platform provided by a double pin–stopped ankle joint combined with a sole plate provides better standing balance with the hands free.

5. Reduction of structural components in the standard double upright orthosis and its modifications (Craig Scott) is possible, but to maintain structural stability, at least one rigid cross-connection, which can be the bail at the knee lock, should be built into the orthosis between the rigid posterior upper thigh band and the stirrup

below. To restrain the orthosis from sliding off the leg when sitting, a strap or band applied posteriorly below the knee is necessary.

6. Pelvic bands are needed only in exceptional cases to control rotation or adduction of the legs in adults. The pelvic band combined with a hip lock reduces stride length, increases center of gravity amplitude, and makes donning, doffing, and transfers more difficult.

With the understanding of the basic principles of orthotic design, it is relatively easy to examine new designs and identify their functions. To illustrate this, the following can be determined by examining a design developed by Lehneis (Fig. 28–39):[57, 58]

1. Knee stabilizing force is applied in the suprapatellar and patellar tendon areas.

2. A rigid ankle is used which is functionally equivalent to an anterior and posterior stop with sole plate extending to the metatarsal head area.

3. The malleoli are encased to provide maximum mediolateral stability.

4. A posterior soft closure prevents the

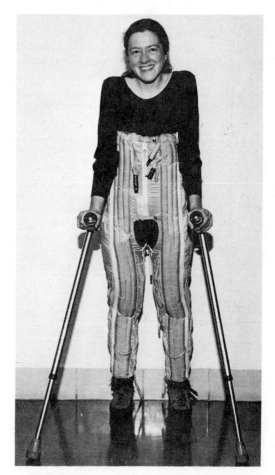

FIGURE 28–40.   Long pneumatic orthosis.

orthosis from sliding off the thigh when sitting.

5. The upper closure is equivalent to the posterior thigh band.

Pneumatic orthoses were introduced in this country for paraplegics by Silber and associates and were more recently tested by Ragnarsson.[59, 60] Inflatable tubes in front and back provide rigidity when properly inflated. Deflation allows bending at hips and knees for sitting. The long version of the orthosis covers the hips and a portion of the trunk (Fig. 28–40). This pneumatic orthosis has approximately the same length as a standard double upright metal orthosis. Toe pickup during the swing phase is provided by a pickup strap, and mediolateral stability at the ankle by wearing high-top boots. On evaluation of these orthoses, it was found:[61]

1. Much better mediolateral stability of the ankle and simulated pushoff could be produced by using the orthosis in combina-

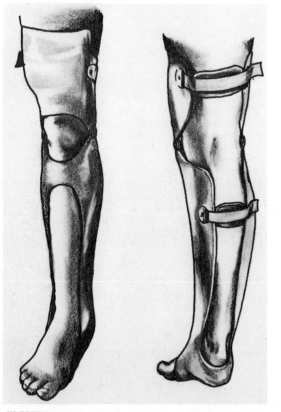

FIGURE 28–39.   Design developed by Lehneis. For further discussion, see references 57 and 58.

tion with a plastic ankle-foot orthosis of the Seattle or Rancho type as an insert. Only with this ankle-foot orthosis were our patients able to use the short orthosis effectively.

2. The center of gravity pathway amplitude was definitely greater when the patients used pneumatic orthoses rather than the standard double upright orthosis. The greatest amplitude was found with the short pneumatic orthosis even when used in combination with the ankle-foot orthosis. An equally large amplitude of the center of gravity pathway was observed when the patients wore the long pneumatic orthosis without the ankle-foot orthosis followed by the long pneumatic orthosis, using it in combination with the ankle-foot orthosis, and the least

amplitude was produced with the patients walking with the standard double upright orthosis with anterior and posterior stop and sole plate extending to the metatarsal head area. These larger amplitudes in the pneumatic orthosis were the result of the angular motion at the knee under the impact of heelstrike as well as some movement at the ankle even when used with the plastic ankle-foot orthosis. The ankle motion was maximal if the orthosis was used without the ankle-foot orthosis as an insert (Figs. 28–41 and 28–42).

3. When the metabolic requirements were measured, however, it was surprising that the long pneumatic orthosis required the least oxygen consumption in spite of the center of gravity amplitude being larger than

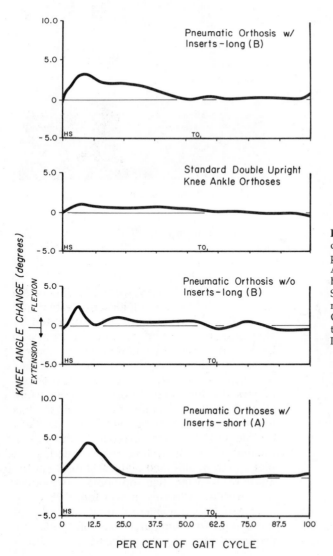

FIGURE 28–41. Measurement of angular changes produced at the knee while a T-12 paraplegic ambulates with different orthoses. Average of 10 runs with each orthosis. HS = heelstrike; TO = toe off. (From Lehmann, J. F., Stonebridge, J. B., and de Lateur, B. J.: Pneumatic and standard double upright orthoses: Comparison of their biomechanical function in three patients with spinal cord injuries. Arch. Phys. Med. Rehabil., 58:72–80, 1977.)

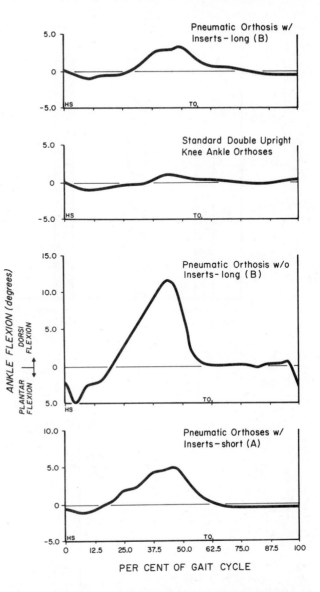

FIGURE 28–42. Measurement of angular changes produced at the ankle while a T-12 paraplegic ambulates with different orthoses. Average of 10 runs with each orthosis. HS = heelstrike; TO = toe off. (From Lehmann, J. F., Stonebridge, J. B., and de Lateur, B. J.: Pneumatic and standard double upright orthoses: Comparison of their biomechanical function in three patients with spinal cord injuries. Arch. Phys. Med. Rehabil., 58:72–80, 1977.)

that observed in the standard double upright orthosis. The difference was significant at the p≤0.05 level (Fig. 28–43), and the only explanation is the better stabilization of hip and trunk by the orthosis, resulting in less voluntary effort being required by the patient. Even when using the long pneumatic orthosis without the ankle-foot orthosis, which produced the largest center of gravity pathway amplitude, the oxygen consumption was equal to that of patients using the standard double upright orthosis.

4. Functional ambulation was evaluated by having the patients walk at a prescribed rate until they could no longer maintain that speed. Distances are plotted in Figure 28–44. At slow walking speeds, i.e., those below 70 meters per minute, patients wearing the long pneumatic orthosis with the ankle-foot orthosis as an insert could walk greater distances at the various speeds than those with other orthoses. This performance was closely followed by the use of the standard double upright metal orthosis. At higher speeds, the pneumatic orthoses were more likely to buckle at the knee with the increased impact of heelstrike. This increased the center of gravity amplitude significantly, rendering the pneumatic orthoses less efficient. The angular change at the knee increased from 4 degrees at 55 meters per minute to 10 degrees at 75 meters per minute. The center of gravity amplitude changed from 10.81 cm to 25.72 cm.

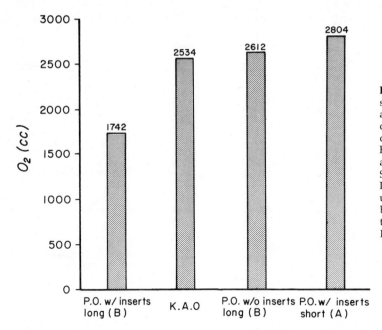

FIGURE 28–43. Total oxygen consumption while a T-12 paraplegic ambulated 300 meters with different orthoses. Average of 6 runs with each orthosis. PO = pneumatic orthosis, KAO = standard double upright knee ankle orthosis (From Lehmann, J. F., Stonebridge, J. B., and de Lateur, B. J.: Pneumatic and standard double upright orthoses: Comparison of their biomechanical function in three patients with spinal cord injuries. Arch. Phys. Med. Rehabil., 58:72–80, 1977.)

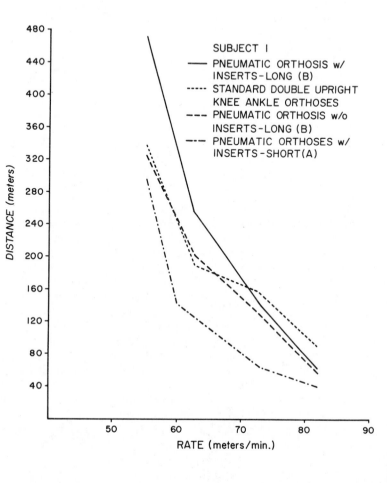

FIGURE 28–44. Maximum distance traveled by a T-12 paraplegic ambulating at various speeds while wearing different orthoses. (From Lehmann, J. F., Stonebridge, J. B., and de Lateur, B. J.: Pneumatic and standard double upright orthoses: Comparison of their biomechanical function in three patients with spinal cord injuries. Arch. Phys. Med. Rehabil., 58:72–80, 1977.)

5. For marginal ambulators and for ambulators who walk for exercise purposes only, the long pneumatic orthosis with the ankle-foot orthosis may be most effective. However, it was found that even paraplegic patients with good use of the arms had difficulties in correctly donning and doffing the garment. The inflation mechanism is, at the very least, cumbersome because it depends on availability of compressed gas cans or an electrical outlet for a pump.[61]

6. For early mobilization of recent paraplegics, the long pneumatic orthosis compresses the abdomen and legs, as pointed out by Silber, and reduces the likelihood of orthostatic hypotension.

7. The short pneumatic orthosis has none of the advantages of the long pneumatic orthosis, but most of its disadvantages.

Since the garment is available as a shelf item in different sizes and can be adjusted to individual patients, it may be used for the initial phase of mobilization of paraplegic patients. An additional benefit to the patient is the reduction of cost, as the orthosis can be reused by subsequent patients. For marginal ambulators or ambulators for exercise purposes only, the long pneumatic orthosis may be the choice in exceptional cases. For a functional ambulation, however, the standard double upright metal orthosis is preferred.

ORTHOSES USING ELECTRICAL STIMULATION

The concept of functional electrical stimulation was introduced by Liberson et al.,[62] and it is used primarily to control foot drop during the swing phase in hemiplegic patients. The theory upon which its use is based is the survival of the lower motor neuron, including the axon in upper motor neuron lesions; therefore, a contraction of the muscles innervated by the peripheral nerve can be induced by electrical stimulation of this nerve, although stimulation must be properly phased to obtain a functional result.[63]

There are two types of electrical stimulators available, one using external stimulation of the peroneal nerve through the skin, the other using an implanted electrode that is applied surgically to the nerve. Common to both applicators is a miniature electrical stimulator producing currents between 20 and 300 microseconds in duration per pulse, with a repetition of 30 to 100 cycles per second and a peak current below 90 milliamperes. The voltage requirements vary between 0 and 50 volts.[62-64]

In using an external stimulator, the power pack is worn on a waist belt, and the skin electrode is applied to the peroneal nerve below the fibular head, with the inactive electrode applied to the leg below. The stimulator is activated by a switch incorporated in the shoe which turns the stimulator on when the heel leaves the ground and off on heelstrike.[65]

When an implanted electrode is used, it must be surgically placed directly on the nerve with a flexible wire lead connected to a subcutaneously implanted receiver located over the anteromedial aspect of the thigh. The power pack for the stimulator and transmitter are worn at the waist, and the transmitter is connected to an antenna located on the surface of the skin over the implanted receiver. Phasing of the stimulation is controlled by a heel switch with a transmitter incorporated into the shoe, its signal being received by the receiver part of the stimulator-transmitter assembly at the waist (Fig. 28–45).[63]

According to Waters, conduction velocity of the nerve is not significantly affected by the stimulation.[66] Fuhrer found that repetitive stimulation slightly decreased skin impedance and slightly increased current levels.[67]

Both the external and implanted stimulators have been applied to hemiplegic patients with the ability to walk without an orthosis. However, certain criteria have been developed in various studies for the use of these types of functional orthoses. The following is a brief summary of the findings of these studies:

1. Waters et al. felt that it was necessary for the patient to be able to walk more rapidly than 25 m/min without an orthosis, that the patient should have good balance, and that the major gait problem should be foot drop, which could also be corrected by an ankle-foot orthosis.[68] Proprioception should also be intact, and, during the stance phase, the patient's ankle should not be plantar flexed more than 10 degrees.

2. In addition, Takebe et al. stated that the patient should be able to apply the electrodes

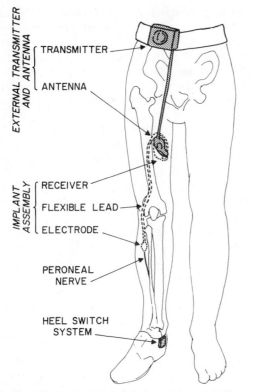

EXTERNAL TRANSMITTER AND ANTENNA
— TRANSMITTER
— ANTENNA

IMPLANT ASSEMBLY
— RECEIVER
— FLEXIBLE LEAD
— ELECTRODE

PERONEAL NERVE

HEEL SWITCH SYSTEM

FIGURE 28–45. Relative location of neuromuscular assist equipment on patient with right side hemiplegia. (From Lehmann, J. F.: Lower limb orthotics. *In* Redford, J. B. (Ed.): Orthotics Etcetera, 2nd Ed. Baltimore, Williams & Wilkins Co., 1980, pp. 320. Redrawn from Waters et al.[68])

manually without difficulty if the external stimulator is used and should also be able to tolerate the discomfort caused by stimulation.[65]

3. Liberson suggested that an increase in strength of foot dorsiflexors could be attributed to this therapy and that on a long-term basis it would be helpful in reeducating the patient's muscles, even without continued use of the electrophysiological orthosis.[62]

4. Rather than stimulating the peroneal nerve, Lee et al. applied a train of electrical pulses to a single skin area to induce a flexion reflex in order to effect an improvement in gait pattern during the swing phase.[69]

5. Dimitrijevic et al. claim that a reciprocal inhibition of the triceps surae results from stimulation of the foot dorsiflexors, and they therefore conclude that the electrophysiologic orthosis prevents undesirable ankle clonus.[70]

The principle upon which treatment with these electrophysiologic orthoses is based has also been applied, on an experimental basis, to major hip and thigh muscle groups of spinal cord–injured patients.[71] In addition, it has been used experimentally in the upper extremity in an effort to reduce wrist drop and improve functional grasp.[72, 73]

SUMMARY

An understanding of the biomechanical function of orthoses can markedly improve the prescribing physician's ability to select the most effective orthosis for each patient's needs. It has also led to better and more varied orthotic designs as well as to the development of new materials to be used in those designs. Patient acceptance has been enhanced because of the higher cosmetic value of many of the new orthoses, although patient acceptance through improved cosmesis should never be gained at the expense of psychologic treatment of the patient's problem. It should also be noted that prescription of an orthosis should always be an integral part of a comprehensive treatment program and should not be considered in isolation from other treatment strategies. The best results can be obtained only when other possibilities such as drugs or motor point blocks are also considered and a comprehensive treatment program developed that best suits the particular patient. If an orthosis is a part of the treatment program, then the biomechanical principles discussed in this chapter can be very helpful in the selection and ultimate effectiveness of that orthosis.

REFERENCES

1. Lehmann, J. F.: The biomechanics of ankle foot orthoses: Prescription and design. Arch. Phys. Med. Rehabil., 60:200–207, 1979.
2. Lehmann, J. F.: Lower limb orthotics. *In* Redford, J. B. (Ed.): Orthotics Etcetera, 2nd Ed. Baltimore, Williams & Wilkins Co., 1980, p. 320.
3. Russek, A., and Eschen, F.: Ischial weight bearing brace with quadrilateral wood top — preliminary report. Orthop. Prosthet. Appliance J., 12:31–35, 1958.
4. Nickel, V. L., and Mooney, V.: The application of lower extremity orthotics to weight bearing relief. Final narrative report. Rancho Los Amigos Hospital, Downey, California.
5. Lesin, B. E., Mooney, V., and Ashby, M. E.: Cast

bracing for fractures of the femur. J. Bone Joint Surg., 59A:917–923, 1977.

6. Mooney, V., Nickel, V. L., Harvey, J. P., and Snelson, R.: Cast brace treatment for fractures for the distal part of the femur. A prospective controlled study of one hundred and fifty three patients. J. Bone Joint Surg., 52A:1563–1578, 1970.

7. Grynbaum, B. B., Sokolow, J., and Fleischman, E. P.: An adjustable ischial weight bearing brace for early ambulation in lower extremity fractures. Arch. Phys. Med. Rehabil., 54:566–568, 1973.

8. American Academy of Orthopedic Surgeons: Orthopedic Appliances Atlas, Vol 1. Ann Arbor, Mich., J. Edwards, 1952, pp. 398–399.

9. Warren, C. G., and Lehmann, J. F.: Effect of training on the use of weight bearing orthoses. Phys. Ther., 55:487–492, 1975.

10. Lehmann, J. F., Warren, C. G., de Lateur, B. J., Simons, B. C., and Kirkpatrick, G.: Biomechanical evaluation of axial loading in ischial weight bearing braces of various designs. Arch. Phys. Med. Rehabil., 51:331–337, 1970.

11. McIlmurray, W. J., and Greenbaum, W.: A below knee weight bearing brace. Orthop. Prosthet. Appliance J., 12:81–82, 1958.

12. Nitschke, R. O., and Marschall, K.: The PTS knee brace. Orthop. Prosthet., 22:46–51, 1968.

13. Lehmann, J. F., de Lateur, B. J., Warren, C. G., and Simons, B. C.: Trends in lower extremity bracing. Arch. Phys. Med. Rehabil., 51:338–353, 1970.

14. Davis, F. J., Fry, L. R., Lippert, F. G., Simons, B. C., and Remington, J.: The patellar tendon bearing brace: Report of 16 patients. J. Trauma, 14:216–221, 1974.

15. Lehmann, J. F., Warren, C. G., Pemberton, D. R., Simons, B. C., and de Lateur, B. J.: Load bearing function of patellar tendon bearing braces of various designs. Arch. Phys. Med. Rehabil., 52:367–370, 1971.

16. Sarmiento, A., and Sinclair, W. F.: Application of prosthetics-orthotics principles to treatment of fractures. Artif. Limbs, 11:28–32, 1967.

17. Sarmiento, A.: A functional below-the-knee cast for tibial fractures. J. Bone Joint Surg., 49:855–875, 1967.

18. Sarmiento, A.: A functional below the knee brace for tibial fractures. A report of its use in 135 cases. J. Bone Joint Surg., 52:295–311, 1970.

19. American Academy of Orthopedic Surgeons: Atlas of Orthotics, 2nd Ed. St. Louis, The C. V. Mosby Co., 1975, p. 209.

20. Smith, E. M., Juvinall, R. C., Corell, E. B., and Nyboer, V. J.: Bracing the unstable arthritis knee. Arch. Phys. Med., 51:22–36, 1970.

21. Heizer, D.: Bracing design for knee joint instability. In Perry, J., and Hislop, H. (Eds.): Principles of Lower Extremity Bracing. New York, American Physical Therapy Association, 1967.

22. Frankel, V. H., and Burstein, A. H.: Orthopedic Biomechanics. Philadelphia, Lea & Febiger, 1970.

23. Bennett, R. J.: Orthotics for function. Part I: Prescription. Phys. Ther. Rev., 36:1–25, 1956.

24. Simons, B. C., C. P. O.: Personal communication.

25. Lehneis, H. R.: New developments in lower-limb orthotics through bioengineering. Arch. Phys. Med. Rehabil., 53:303–310, 1972.

26. American Academy of Orthopedic Surgeons: Atlas of Orthotics, 2nd Ed. St. Louis, The C. V. Mosby Co., 1975, pp. 216–219.

27. Fifth Workshop Panel on Lower Extremity Orthotics. Subcommittee on Design and Development, Committee on Prosthetics Research and Development. Division of Engineering, National Research Council, National Academy of Sciences, National Academy of Engineering. Atlanta Ga., April 3–4, 1968, p. 17.

28. Kamenetz, H. L.: Eponymic orthoses. In Redford, J. B. (Ed.): Orthotics Etcetera, 2nd Ed. Baltimore, Williams & Wilkins Co., 1980, pp. 705–706.

29. Lehmann, J. F., Warren, C. G., and de Lateur, B. J.: A biomechanical evaluation of knee stability in below knee braces. Arch. Phys. Med. Rehabil., 51:687–695, 1970.

30. McIlmurray, W., and Greenbaum, W.: The application of SACH foot principles to orthotics. Orthop. Prosthet. Appl. J., 13:37–40, 1959.

31. Rubin, G., and Dixon, M.: The modern ankle foot orthoses (AFO's). Bull. Prosthet. Res., Spring:20–40, 1973.

32. Stills, M.: Thermoformed ankle foot orthoses. Orthop Prosthet., 29:41–51, 1975.

33. Jebsen, R. H., Simons, B. C., and Corcoran, P. J.: Experimental short leg brace fabrication. Arch. Phys. Med. Rehabil., 49:108–109, 1968.

34. Simons, B. C., Jebsen, R. H., and Wildman, L. E.: Plastic short leg brace fabrication. Orthop. Prosthet. Appl. J., 21:215–218, 1967.

35. Siegel, I. M.: Plastic-molded knee-ankle-foot orthoses in the treatment of Duchenne muscular dystrophy. Arch. Phys. Med. Rehabil., 56:322, 1975.

36. Heizer, D.: Short-leg brace design for hemiplegia. In Perry, J., and Hislop, H. (Eds.): Principles of Lower Extremity Bracing. New York, American Physical Therapy Association, 1967.

37. American Academy of Orthopedic Surgeons: Atlas of Orthotics, 2nd Ed. St. Louis, The C. V. Mosby Co., 1975, p. 209.

38. LeBlanc. M.: A clinical evaluation of four lower limb orthoses. Orthop. Prosthet., 26:27–43, 1972.

39. Inman, V. T.: The Joints of the Ankle. Baltimore, Williams & Wilkins Co., 1976.

40. Inman, V. T.: UC-BL dual axis ankle control system and UC-BL shoe insert. Bull. Prosthet. Res., Spring:130–145, 1969.

41. Corcoran, P. J.: Evaluation of a plastic short leg brace. M. Sc. Thesis, University of Washington, Seattle, 1968.

42. Corcoran, P. J., Jebsen, R. H., Brengelmann, G. L., and Simons, B. C.: Effects of plastic and metal leg braces on speed and energy cost of hemiparetic ambulation. Arch. Phys. Med. Rehabil., 51:69, 1970.

43. Long, G., and Lawton, E. B.: Functional significance of spinal cord lesion level. Arch. Phys. Med., 36:249–255, 1955.

44. Stauffer, E. S.: Symposium on spinal cord injuries. Clin. Orthop., 112:1–165, 1975.

45. Lehmann, J. F., and Warren, C. G.: Restraining forces in various designs of knee ankle orthoses: Their placement and effect on anatomical knee joint. Arch. Phys. Med. Rehabil., 57:430–437, 1976.

46. American Academy of Orthopedic Surgeons: Atlas of Orthotics, 2nd Ed. St. Louis, The C. V. Mosby Co., 1975, p. 232.

47. Hahn, H.: Lower extremity bracing in paraplegics with usage followup. Paraplegia, 8:147–153, 1969.

48. Scott, B. A.: Engineering principles and fabrication techniques for Scott-Craig: Long leg brace for paraplegics. Orthop. Prosthet., 28:14–19, 1974.

49. Lehmann, J. F., Warren, C. G., Hertling, D., McGee, M., and Simons, B. C.: Craig Scott orthosis: A biomechanical and functional evaluation. Arch. Phys. Med. Rehabil., 57:438–442, 1976.

50. Fischer, S. D., and Gullickson, G.: Energy cost of ambulation in health and disability: A literature review. Arch. Phys. Med. Rehabil., 59:124–133, 1978.

51. Lehmann, J. F., de Lateur, B. J., Warren, C. G., Simons, B. C., and Guy, A. W.: Biomechanical evaluation of braces for paraplegics. Arch. Phys. Med. Rehabil., 50:179–188, 1969.

52. Rosman, N., and Spira, E.: Paraplegic use of walking braces: Survey. Arch. Phys. Med. Rehabil., 55:310–314, 1974.

53. Clinkingbeard, J. R., Gersten, J. W., and Hoehn, D.: Energy cost of ambulation in traumatic paraplegic. Am. J. Phys. Med., 43:157–165, 1964.

54. Gordon, E. E.: Physiological approach to ambulation in paraplegia. J.A.M.A., 161:686–688, 1956.

55. Gordon, E. E., and Vanderwalde, H.: Energy requirements in paraplegic ambulation. Arch. Phys. Med. Rehabil., 37:276–285, 1956.

56. Warren, C. G., Lehmann, J. F., and de Lateur, B. J.: Pelvic band use in orthotics for adult paraplegic patients. Arch. Phys. Med. Rehabil., 56:221–223, 1975.

57. American Academy of Orthopedic Surgeons: Atlas of Orthotics, 2nd Ed. St. Louis, The C. V. Mosby Co., 1975, p. 226.

58. Casson, J.: Advanced designs of plastic lower orthoses. Orthop. Prosthet., 26:24–30, 1972.

59. Silber, M., Chung, T. S., Varghese, G., Hinterbuchner, C., Bailey, M., and Hivry, N.: Pneumatic orthosis: Pilot study. Arch. Phys. Med. Rehabil., 56:27–32, 1975.

60. Ragnarsson, K. T., Sell, G. H., McGarrity, M., and Offir, R.: Pneumatic orthosis for paraplegic patients: Functional evaluation and prescription consideration. Arch. Phys. Med. Rehabil., 56:479–483, 1975.

61. Lehmann, J. F., Stonebridge, J. B., and de Lateur, B. J.: Pneumatic and standard double upright orthoses: comparison of their biomechanical function

62. Liberson, W. T., Homquest, H. F., Scott, D., and Dow, M.: Functional electrotherapy: Stimulation of the peroneal nerve synchronized with the swing phase of the gait of hemiplegic patients. Arch. Phys. Med. Rehabil., 41:101–105, 1960.

63. Gracanin, F., and Trnkoczy, A.: Optimal stimulus parameters for minimum pain in the chronic stimulation of innervated muscle. Arch. Phys. Med. Rehabil., 56:243–249, 1975.

64. Post, B. S., Foster, S., Rosner, H., and Benton, J. G.: Use of functional electrotherapy in neuromuscular diseases. N.Y. State J. Med., 63:1808–1811, 1963.

65. Takebe, K., Kukulka, C., Narayan, M. G., Milner, M., and Basmajian, J. V.: Peroneal nerve stimulator in rehabilitation of hemiplegic patients. Arch. Phys. Med. Rehabil., 56:237–240, 1975.

66. Waters, R. L., McNeal, D. R., and Tasto, J.: Peroneal nerve conduction velocity after chronic electrical stimulation. Arch. Phys. Med. Rehabil., 46:240–241, 1975.

67. Fuhrer, M. J., and Yegge, B.: Effects of skin impedance changes accompanying functional electrical stimulation of the peroneal nerve. Arch. Phys. Med. Rehabil., 53:276–281, 1972.

68. Waters, R. L., McNeal, D., and Perry, J.: Experimental correction of foot drop by electrical stimulation of the peroneal nerve. J. Bone Joint Surg., 57A:1047–1054, 1975.

69. Lee, K. H., and Johnston, R.: Electrically induced flexion reflex in gait training of hemiplegic patients: Induction of the reflex. Arch. Phys. Med. Rehabil., 57:311–314, 1976.

70. Dimitrijevic, M. R., Gracanin, F., Prevec, T., and Trontelj, J.: Electronic control of paralysed extremities. Bio. Med. Engineering, 3:8–14, 1968.

71. Varken, E., and Jeglic, A.: Application of an implantable stimulator in the rehabilitation of the paraplegic patient. Int. Surg., 61:335–339, 1976.

72. Burke, J. F., Pocock, G. S., and Wallis, W. D.: Electrophysiological bracing in peripheral nerve lesions. J. Am. Phys. Ther. Assoc., 43:501–504, 1963.

73. Merletti, R., Acimovic, R., Grobelnik, S., and Cvilak, G.: Electrophysiological orthosis for the upper extremity in hemiplegia: Feasibility study. Arch. Phys. Med. Rehabil., 56:507–513, 1975.

in three patients with spinal cord injuries. Arch. Phys. Med. Rehabil., 58:72–80, 1977.

29

PRESCRIBING PHYSICAL AND OCCUPATIONAL THERAPY

GORDON M. MARTIN

Well-written prescriptions for physical therapy and occupational therapy containing sufficient specific detail are essential to the effective use of these methods of treatment. Such written prescriptions provide the physician an opportunity to plan, specify, and correlate various techniques and procedures into a suitable program designed to improve or develop physical function to a realistic maximal goal. The prescription may be a simple one for short-term treatment, or it may provide a complex and changing program over a prolonged period for the severely and chronically handicapped patient. In any case, the prescription must be concise, clear, specific, and individualized. The suitability of the prescription and the effectiveness of the therapy are in large measure dependent on the physician's interest and knowledge of this field and his ability to work well with the therapists, at the same time keeping the patient interested, motivated, and cooperative.

Purposes. There are several important purposes of the detailed, specific written prescription. It provides the therapist with basic aims and specific procedures to be included in the treatment program and direc-

tions for carrying out specified evaluations. It is designed to ensure that the physician's orders will be followed and that misunderstandings between physician and therapist will not arise. It will provide a permanent record of the treatment prescribed and administered. Such records are valuable for use in the future care of a patient and in insurance or compensation cases. It will serve to protect both physician and therapist in case of medicolegal complications.

The Physician as Prescriber. Certain qualifications are expected of the person prescribing physical therapy, occupational therapy, or other rehabilitative procedures. Only a physician is licensed to prescribe. He need not be a physiatrist. He should, however, refer certain patients to, or consult with, a physiatrist when this would provide better service to the patient. The physician should have basic knowledge of the biophysical, physiologic, and psychologic effects of the various procedures used in physical and occupational therapy. He should know the indications for their use as well as the contraindications and limitations. He should have knowledge of the training, special abilities, and possible limitations of the therapists. He should be aware of equipment, facilities, and time available for physical treatment.

Preliminary Considerations. Before the physician turns the patient and the prescription over to the therapist, an adequate working diagnosis should be established based on history, physical findings, and laboratory tests as indicated. Only treatment and procedures that have been proven clinically to be beneficial should be prescribed. It should be ascertained that the prescription contains sufficient detail so that the therapist can proceed efficiently and with assurance. A summary of essential physical findings and diagnosis should accompany the prescription.

The type of treatment, the aims of treatment, and the result expected in the immediate future or in the long run should be explained to the patient. The costs of treatment should be evaluated and discussed with the patient; the need or availability of insurance or other aid may have to be determined if prolonged treatment is expected. The patient should be informed about the importance of home treatment procedures. The prescription should indicate instructions for treatment measures or procedures to be given the patient for use at home.

Common Errors

An awareness of common errors that are made in prescribing physical treatment can lead to more efficient and effective therapy.

Delay in starting treatments may unnecessarily prolong a period of disability and suffering. Often physicians err in assuming that stiffness or weakness following fractures or soft tissue trauma "will work itself out" with ordinary use or with some simple exercises merely described superficially to the patient in an office visit. The patient, too, may be reluctant to undertake treatments that will be time-consuming and expensive, and he may want to gamble on nature's tendency to bring about spontaneous improvement.

A "shotgun" type of prescription can be disadvantageous, as, for instance, in prescriptions for several types of heat in one therapy session, or for heat, massage, and exercise when only a concise prescription for therapeutic exercise is indicated. The type of treatment prescribed in the "shotgun" manner may detract from or miss the primary aim of the treatment. Such haphazard treatment is unnecessarily time-consuming for therapist and patient alike and hence is inefficient. The "shotgun" use of multiple procedures tends to be seen when a checklist order sheet is used. Although a checklist order sheet may be satisfactory for ordering laboratory tests, it does not permit an adequately detailed, individualized prescription for physical treatment.

Selection of Patients. If patients are not selected with some discrimination, the results are poor and the therapist's time and effort are exploited or wasted; under such circumstances patients may understandably become disillusioned or discouraged.

The severe psychoneurotic patient with multiple somatic complaints and lack of insight either will not benefit from therapy or will become overly dependent on both treatment and physical therapist. However, many patients with functional neuromuscular complaints who have tension anxiety states but possess some insight into their problems may be benefited greatly by physical and occupational therapy and by instructions in a program of home treatment and specified activities.

Patients having complaints of peripheral pains that are of thalamic or central nervous system origin do not benefit from physical therapy. Patients with progressive metastatic lesions are generally poor candidates for prolonged treatment. Patients with stroke or those with residual effects of cerebral trauma who remain semicomatose, confused, and stuporous, or who are unable or unwilling to cooperate, usually do not benefit significantly from prolonged physical therapy and rehabilitation.

The severely involved arthritic cripple can rarely be helped significantly by physical treatment alone. Frequently, an intensive program utilizing the combined efforts of a rheumatologist, orthopedic surgeon, and physiatrist will result in good progress.

Most patients who are hostile or uncooperative relative to treatment are poor candidates.

Other Errors. Vague, muddled, or inadequate prescriptions are of little use to a therapist. These may lack sufficient detail or specify treatment that cannot be carried out by the therapist or cannot be tolerated by the patient.

The therapist is sometimes expected or encouraged to select or prescribe the treatment. This is unethical, and it encourages the therapist to practice medicine without qualifications or license.

The patient should not be permitted to prescribe his own treatment, nor should the therapist be encouraged to "give him whatever he asks for."

Treatments that are given too infrequently may be a source of disappointing results. Generally, at first, daily or even twice-daily treatments are indicated. Later, the frequency may be decreased to two or three times weekly as progress is made and as the patient learns to carry on with treatment procedures at home. Treatment once weekly is essentially worthless except when it serves as a review and updating of a home treatment program.

The use of so-called "routine" orders results in a gross misuse of physical therapy. There is no such thing as the "arthritis routine," "hemiplegia routine," or "low-back routine." The prescription should be individualized and specific for each patient.

Telephoned or verbal orders should be considered only a temporary expedient and should be followed up by a properly written prescription.

Inadequate or delayed follow-up and recheck by the physician is a common pitfall that may unnecessarily prolong treatment. Generally, orders must be changed as response to treatment is observed and progress is made.

ESSENTIALS OF THE PRESCRIPTION

The essentials of the physical therapy or occupational therapy prescription should be recorded on a departmental record or order sheet, which should become a permanent part of the patient's office or hospital history and record file.

The diagnosis should be given, whether it is a final diagnosis or a tentative one. A brief summary of history and physical findings will provide pertinent information for the physical or occupational therapist and for the consulting physicians, residents, or interns who will be following the course of the patient. The patient's hospital, clinic, or office record is generally not available with the patient at the time of each treatment. Thus, the statement "see record" or "see history"

is useless to physicians and therapists who are treating or following the course of the patient in the department of physical medicine and rehabilitation. Measurements of range of motion and muscle strength that are recorded with the original prescription provide base lines for evaluation of progress.

The part or parts to be treated are to be determined by the physician and indicated on the order sheet. Procedures to be used with specifications as to apparatus, techniques, and time should have major prominence on the prescription sheet.

Special instructions or cautions should be clearly indicated. If a splint or bandage is to be removed during treatment, this should be recorded. The presence of diabetes, convulsive disorder, angina, or mental confusion should be clearly indicated so that the therapist can observe necessary precautions.

Home treatment instructions for the patient should be specifically ordered by the physician and the technical details of the instructions supplied by the therapist. Generally, instructions can best be given during the course of several treatment sessions. Printed or written instructions given to the patient serve as reminders of what to do, but "how to do it" can be learned properly only by actual *doing* it under close supervision of a competent instructor.

The number and frequency of treatments must be indicated and the date for the physician's recheck of the patient should appear on the prescription. In addition, the order sheet should include dates of treatment, names of therapists treating the patient, progress notes by physicians and therapists, and the patient's condition at time of dismissal as well as the final recommendations. See the sample prescriptions at the end of this chapter.

Physical Therapy

Thermotherapy. The essential elements of a prescription for thermotherapy are the following: the source of heat to be used — heat lamp, shortwave diathermy, warm tub bath, contrast bath, or others; the part to be treated, specifying local areas and the position of patient; the time or duration of application and number of daily applications; specifications regarding technique, listing of the type of applicator, such as coil, hinged drum, or vaginal electrode for shortwave diathermy, with electrode temperature specified for the last-named technique; and the intensity in terms of output or temperature measurement when possible. *Low intensity* must be indicated for anesthetic areas and in debilitated individuals or for those with a possible intolerance or sensitivity to heat. The temperature of the water should be indicated when hydrotherapy is prescribed.

Massage. In the prescription for therapeutic massage, the type or types must be specified. This may be the *stroking* or *kneading* types, which are usually combined, or *friction* massage, which may be specified for certain limited areas. Other types of manual massage or the use of mechanical massage devices are infrequently prescribed.

Specifications include indication of quality, that is, *deep* or *light* and *sedative* (most common) or *stimulating* massage. Avoidance of recent surgical incisions and varicosities should be noted.

The parts to be massaged should be specifically listed. Patients frequently attempt to have the therapist massage more extensive areas, which would prolong treatment time unreasonably. Therapeutic manual massage is time-consuming and should not be prescribed indiscriminately.

Electrical Stimulation. Prescription for electrical stimulation should be preceded by a manual muscle test, sensory test, and electrodiagnostic tests when indicated.

The types of current and apparatus used are interrupted galvanic or slow sinusoidal (6 to 40 cycles per second) for denervated muscle and faradic-like current or sine wave current of 30 to 1000 cycles per second for muscles when the lower motor neuron is intact.

Specifications should include the number of contractions or surges per minute, the approximate number of contractions at each session (generally 60 to 150), and the intensity of the current or the strength of contractions. Individual muscles, muscle groups, or nerves to be stimulated should be listed.

Transcutaneous electrical nerve stimulation (TENS) appears to be helpful for some patients with chronic pain syndromes in relatively localized areas but not with pain of extensive distribution.[1] Battery-operated stimulators producing impulses of 0.1 to 1 millisecond duration and generated at several frequencies and with controllable intensities are commercially available to patients on a rental or purchase basis. The use of such stimulators should be tested on a 2- or 3-day trial, and only if such a device is significantly effective should purchase or rental be prescribed. The prescription for TENS should indicate the specific area and the time of application, and it should request evaluation of the effectiveness of several frequencies and intensities.

Therapeutic Exercise. The prescription for therapeutic exercise is generally the most complex and difficult part of the prescription for physical therapy. It must be preceded by a complete evaluation of malfunction, including manual muscle tests, evaluation of range of motion, status of bones and joints, and noting of coordination problems. Frequently, several types of exercises should be prescribed for one or several different parts of the extremities or trunk. The prescription should indicate clearly just what exercise procedures the therapist is to employ. The type of therapeutic exercise is listed first.

PASSIVE. These are relaxed exercises without forcing or stretching. If stretching, forcing, or manipulation is desired, it must be clearly specified, since these are not true passive exercises.

ACTIVE ASSISTIVE. Exercises with assistance by the therapist or by an assistive apparatus are prescribed for parts with which the patient cannot carry out active exercise satisfactorily.

ACTIVE. These exercises are most frequently prescribed to maintain range of motion and increase strength and endurance.

RESISTIVE. Exercises against resistance are prescribed for strengthening muscles. Several satisfactory techniques and programs have been described for progressive resistive exercises. Indications are made regarding apparatus such as wall weights, sandbags, weighted boots, and manual resistance.

REEDUCATION. Reeducation exercises are prescribed for retraining in individual function and coordination of recovering paralyzed or paretic muscles or tendon transplants. They may be prescribed in any condition in which there are poor coordination and muscle imbalances.

COORDINATION. Exercises for coordination are of several types. Originally they were designed to utilize visual reflexes in replacing poor proprioceptive reflexes. Now they may be combined with reeducation exercises and with occupational therapy for any condition involving poor coordination and muscle imbalances.

RELAXATION. The principles of relaxation and the appropriate exercises are prescribed for patients with persistent muscle guarding and spasm and persistently hypertonic muscles as observed in patients with tension states.

Other specifications essential to the prescription for exercise include the specific parts to be exercised (joints, muscles, or an extremity), the number of exercise periods daily, the duration of each exercise period, indications as to grading or progression of the program, apparatus to be used, and exercises to be done by the patient at home on his or her own.

There are several reasons for failure of a prescribed exercise program. The prescribed program may be overwhelming to the patient. It may exceed the patient's capabilities and be overfatiguing or may aggravate pain or other symptoms; if so, it should be modified but not necessarily discontinued. There may be lack of cooperation, enthusiasm, or understanding on the part of the patient. Lack of care and attention to detail by the therapist administering the exercises may occur when the therapist has too many patients to treat and thus leaves the patient to exercise without adequate supervision.

Ambulation. Training and assistance with ambulation are often an important part of physical therapy. The decision as to the need for cane, German or axillary crutches, walker, braces, or other special assistive devices is the physician's prerogative.

Preliminary strengthening exercises may be needed and should be included in the prescription. Preparatory to crutch walking, progressive resistive exercises for latissimus dorsi, triceps, and biceps may be indicated along with those for quadriceps and hip extensors and abductors. Mat exercises, crawling, rolling, sitting, balance, transfers, or tilt-table procedures may precede ambulation for some patients (for example, paraplegics). Parallel bars may be prescribed for balance and security for patients learning correctly specified patterns of gait.

The type of crutch gait — four-point or three-point, with or without weight bearing, and the amount of weight bearing permitted; swing-to or swing-through; or walk-to or walk-through — should be specified.

Practice on curbs and steps is prescribed when the patient is competent in walking on level surfaces with cane or crutches. Getting in and out of chairs and bed correctly should be prescribed with the ambulation training. Crossing streets and getting in and out of cars are final steps in the ambulation prescription.

Occupational Therapy

The prescription for occupational therapy requires the same preliminary considerations and essentially the same evaluation and summary of history and physical status as are described for the physical therapy record. In some departments of physical medicine the prescription for occupational therapy is included on the same order sheet as that for physical therapy.

Certain factors are particularly important in the guidance of the occupational therapist. The diagnosis is again included. Present physical status and general condition of the patient should be given as well as the mental and emotional status and any significant psychologic factors. Indication should be made as to whether occupational therapy is to be done in bed or in the occupational therapy department, and the time to be devoted to these activities should be specified.

Specific aims and desired results should be indicated on the prescription. Functional or kinetic activities are prescribed for mobilizing, coordinating, or strengthening specific parts. Functional occupational therapy generally supplements physical therapy. Special sensory assessments and evaluation of motor function and coordination may be requested on the prescription form. The many therapeutic activities and special tests are described in Willard and Spackman's Occupational Therapy.[2]

Training in many of the activities of daily living is carried out by the occupational therapist. The physician should indicate whether the activities are to be done in bed or in a wheelchair, and what specific limitations will be encountered. Generally this work by the occupational therapist is correlated with certain phases of training in self-help, transfers, and daily living activities that are taught by the nursing staff and physical therapists. Special assistive devices may be designed and fashioned by the occupational therapist for the handicapped patient at the request of the physician. The prescription for functional occupational therapy can specify areas for special attention, i.e., dressing, grooming, eating, homemaking activities, fine coordination, increasing speed, or mobility.

Some occupational therapy departments can construct splints for preventing or controlling potential deformities of the hand of patients with rheumatoid arthritis or hemiplegia. Functional splints, such as a tenodesis splint for a tetraplegic, can be fitted in occupational therapy, and training and practice in their use may be prescribed.

Diversional, supportive, recreational, and avocational activities may be prescribed for the physically handicapped as well as for those with mental illness. Prevocational exploratory services are available on request or prescription in some occupational therapy departments.

The attitude the therapist is to take —

whether he or she should insist on productive work or merely invite or encourage the patient — should be indicated on the prescription. Suggestions or information as to the patient's likes, dislikes, attitudes, previous occupations, and hobbies may be of real value to the therapist in establishing good rapport and achieving an effective program of occupational therapy.

SAMPLE PRESCRIPTIONS

These sample prescriptions illustrate some of the principles that have been discussed. They are not to be considered as standard or routine prescriptions or necessarily ideal prescriptions for patients with the condition listed. Each prescription must be individualized and then modified as changing status indicates need for variations and progression.

DEGENERATIVE LUMBOSACRAL DISK WITH RADICULITIS, LEFT SIDE

Treatment	Time, Minutes	Specifications
Radiant heat	30	Lamp to low back and left hip (lying on right side)
Massage	10–15	Deep stroking and kneading, low back and left hip
Exercises		Abdominal strengthening exercises
		Non–weight bearing pelvic flexion
		Trunk flexion from sitting position
		Posture principles for low back and pelvis

Treat: Daily 3 times for instruction
Instruct: Heat lamp
         Exercises as listed above

ADHESIVE CAPSULITIS, RIGHT SHOULDER

Treatment	Time, Minutes	Specifications
Ultrasound	10	1.5 watts per sq. cm.
		Stroking technique, right shoulder
Massage	5–10	Deep stroking and kneading to right shoulder
Exercise	10–15	Active and assistive right shoulder
		Moderate stretch
		Wall ladder
		Overhead pulley
		Shoulder wheel
		Codman's exercise with 5 lb. sandbag

Treat daily. Physician's recheck after 5 treatments
Instruct: Infrared lamp 30 min. daily
         Active exercises and pulley and ladder assistive exercises, two times daily at home

LEFT HEMIPLEGIA (ONSET ON JANUARY 26)

Date	Treatment	Time, Minutes	Specifications
2–1	*Exercise* Passive	10	Left upper and lower extremities through normal range, 3-4 times each joint (remove footdrop splint for treatment)
2–7	Reeducation and coordination Active	20	Left upper and lower extremities Normal range, right upper and lower extremities (avoid fatigue; encourage use of normal extremities for activities of daily living)
2–16	Active and assistive Resistive		Left shoulder and elbow Left hip and knee Powder board with assistance for hip and knee flexion and extension, and hip abduction and adduction Right quadriceps 30 contractions daily — 10 each of $\frac{1}{2}$, $\frac{3}{4}$, and full 10 rep. max.*
2–18	*Gait training*	B.i.d.	Parallel bars with knee splint and foot support Sling left arm 1. Standing balance 2. Walking
2–22	Gait	B.i.d.	Start on glider cane with assistance (cane in right hand)
3–2	Gait	B.i.d.	Walk with regular cane and footdrop brace
3–6	Gait	B.i.d.	Climb stairs, ramp In and out of chairs In and out of car

2–1 Treat once daily in patient's room
   Physician check q. 3 days
2–7 Treat in physical medicine and rehabilitation department twice daily
2–8 Occupational therapy: Perceptual assessment. Activities to increase left upper extremity function. Activities of daily living.
3–4 Instruct in normal range of motion exercises for home use

*By "10 rep. max." (10 repetition maximum) is meant the number of pounds that can be moved through the full range 10 times.

RHEUMATOID ARTHRITIS (HANDS, ELBOWS, SHOULDERS, KNEES, AND FEET)

Treatment	Time, Minutes	Specifications
Radiant heat	30	Two bakers — patient supine (alternate with hydrotherapy)
Hydrotherapy	30, 3 times weekly	Hubbard tank — water temperature 102° F (38.9° C), with active assistive underwater exercise of shoulders, elbows, knees
	30	Contrast baths, hands and feet; once for instruction
Massage	20	Deep stroking and kneading to hands, shoulders, knees
Exercise	10	Active and assistive, work toward normal range in above joints Resistive isometric with 5 lb. sandbag, 10 contractions for each quadriceps. Later progressive resistive exercise program Posture correction and principles, stand, sit, lie
Gait	5	Supervise walking short distances In and out of chair Stair climbing
Treat daily for 2 weeks Occupational therapy:		Resting hand splints. Hand use and protection principles. Assessment of activities of daily living. Assistive devices.

Treat daily for 2 weeks
Instruct: Daily contrast baths at home, water temperature 110° F (43.3° C) and 65° F (18.3° C) for hands and feet
Warm tub bath twice a week, water temperature 102° F (38.9° C), 20 minutes
Home exercise program: active and progressive resistive

CHRONIC LEFT L5-S1 RADICULOPATHY (STATIC AND NIGHT PAIN, 2 YEARS AFTER LUMBAR LAMINECTOMY)

Trial of transcutaneous electrical nerve stimulation (TENS) for pain control or modification

Treatment	Time, minutes	Specifications
TENS	30	2 electrodes over left lumbar paraspinal area 2 electrodes over sciatic nerve, thigh, and popliteal area (place one on common peroneal, one at sciatic notch) Evaluate combinations of intensity and frequencies Have patient standing during trial

Treat 2 times daily, 2 or 3 days
Provide stimulator on loan for overnight if feasible
Physician recheck after 4 treatments

REFERENCES

1. Thorsteinsson, G., Stonnington, H. H., Stillwell, G. K., and Elveback, L. R.: Transcutaneous electrical stimulation: A double-blind trial of its efficacy for pain. Arch. Phys. Med. Rehabil., 58:8–13, 1977.

2. Hopkins, H. L., and Smith, H. D.: Willard and Spackman's Occupational Therapy, 5th ed. Philadelphia, J. B. Lippincott Company, 1978.

30

REHABILITATION OF PATIENTS WITH COMPLETED STROKE

THOMAS P. ANDERSON

Stroke is usually defined as a cerebral vascular accident. However, when the term is used in this broad sense, it also includes TIA's (transient ischemic attacks) which some writers believe comprise 60 to 75 per cent of all strokes.[24] Because these TIA's, by definition, result in complete recovery, they are not included in discussions about rehabilitation for stroke. This is the reason for using the term *completed stroke* when rehabilitation is discussed. In this chapter, when general references are made to completed stroke, it usually means the stereotypic completed stroke involving the middle cerebral artery. When it does not mean this, it will be so designated that the anterior cerebral artery or posterior cerebral artery or vertebral arteries are involved. Certainly not all completed strokes should be lumped together and considered to be the same, since they vary so widely in their manifestations (see Table 30–1) and hence in their evaluation and management. For example, brain stem strokes are significantly different in their manifestations and management from middle cerebral artery strokes.

Many of the principles in the rehabilitation of completed stroke apply to the hemiparesis resulting from traumatic brain damage, but there are sufficient differences so that gener-alizations for completed stroke should not be made for post-traumatic hemiplegia. Before a patient with completed stroke is evaluated for rehabilitation training, the professional should ask the question, "Is this stroke?" The differential diagnosis of completed stroke[25] is extensive, and with the new diagnostic procedures of various types of brain

TABLE 30–1. COMMON SYNDROMES OCCURRING AFTER CEREBRAL VASCULAR ACCIDENTS

Disturbance of consciousness
Mental confusion
Paralysis, paresis
  Motor
  Sensory
Spasticity
Incoordination
Dyspraxia
Anosognosia
Visual field deficits
Cognitive dysfunctions
Perseveration
Impaired judgment and planning
Impulsivity
Ataxia
Communication
  Language (aphasia)
  Speech production (dysarthria, dyspraxia, dysphonia)
Emotional lability

scans one may be able to determine not only whether this patient has a completed stroke but also the probable mechanism of the stroke, i.e., thrombosis, embolus, or hemorrhage. Furthermore, it is rare that one treats a patient with completed stroke as the only problem. There are usually concomitants such as hypertension, cardiac failure, angina, diabetes mellitus, peripheral vascular disease, and more.

Recovery

It should be kept in mind that there are two types of improvement that occur in completed stroke: neurologic recovery and improvements in functional abilities or performance. The neurologic recovery depends on the mechanism of the stroke and the location of the lesion, so that no one generalization about neurologic recovery is applicable to an individual case. However, it is generally agreed that 90 per cent of the neurologic recovery has occurred by the end of three months following onset of the stroke, with the exception of some hemorrhagic-type strokes that may continue to show some slow neurologic recovery for a longer period. The improvement in function depends upon the environment in which the patient with completed stroke is placed and how much training and motivation there is for him to learn to become independent again in self care and mobility. It is still not proved that the early initiation of rehabilitation treatment, particularly some of the facilitation techniques, can influence a greater return of neurologic function. However, there are other justifications for beginning rehabilitation early in the course of completed stroke, e.g., to prevent avoidable complications such as depression. Several studies[3, 20] or developing predictive factors to determine which patients are good candidates for stroke rehabilitation and which are not concluded that there is no single predictive finding in early evaluation of the stroke patient that is going to indicate what his long-term outcome is.

Should the Patient with Completed Stroke Have Rehabilitation?

The old myth that survival of patients with completed stroke is not sufficiently long to justify the great expense and effort of rehabilitation has been disproved by recent studies,[2, 4, 23] which show that at least 50 per cent of the survivors lived for 7 1/2 years or longer. A study has recently been completed comparing the long-term outcomes of those stroke patients who had rehabilitation with those who did not.[5] It showed that those who had rehabilitation had better long-term outcomes. There has also been some confusion about what rehabilitation is and where it should be done,[36] that is, in a nursing home versus a rehabilitation center. Stroke rehabilitation that is carried out in a comprehensive manner in a large rehabilitation center moves the stroke patient from a low level of functioning to a high level in a relatively short period of time, whereas the activities in physical therapy, occupational therapy, and other therapies in extended care facilities, community hospitals, and nursing homes could often be labeled maintenance rehabilitation, which is carried out to prevent the deterioration of function in the patient but does not actually rapidly progress him from a low level to a high level of function. Furthermore, studies are being considered that measure the cost benefits or the cost effectiveness* of stroke rehabilitation.[21] Many comprehensive rehabilitation centers have reported a reduction in the length of stay for stroke rehabilitation patients in recent years. Some outcome studies have shown that the gains during rehabilitation are maintained for as long as several years thereafter.[2, 4, 5] If the patient survives 22 months or longer after rehabilitation for completed stroke there is a lessening of costs.[21] There have appeared reports about the ineffectiveness of stroke rehabilitation in which there was no distinction made about the type of rehabilitation care provided in a small community hospital[36] and another in which patients were admitted to a large comprehensive rehabilitation center 40 days (on the average) after the onset of the stroke.[14] Most stroke rehabilitation programs are completed by patients before the end of 40 days after onset. In carrying out cost benefit studies of stroke rehabilitation, it has been recognized that not just financial benefits but all benefits should

---

*The term *cost benefits* usually refers to a comprehensive inclusion of all costs, direct and indirect, as well as all benefits, direct and indirect, whereas *cost effectiveness* usually refers only to the more direct costs and benefits. See Table 30–2 for examples.

TABLE 30–2. EXAMPLES OF DIRECT AND INDIRECT COSTS AND BENEFITS OF STROKE REHABILITATION

Direct Costs
  Hospital bills
  Doctors' bills

Indirect Costs
  Modification of home
  Special transportation
  Time lost from employment by family member

Direct Benefits
  Improved functions
  Improved performance
  Less dependency
  Employment

Indirect Benefits
  Improved quality of life
  Greater socializing
  Greater community involvement

be considered, such as those contributing to the quality of life of the patient.

Referral to a Rehabilitation Center?

Which patients with completed stroke should be referred to a rehabilitation center? Attitudes about this question have changed in recent years. It was formerly felt that there were such a great number of patients with completed stroke and so few comprehensive rehabilitation centers and such difficulty in transportation that the majority of stroke patients had no access to rehabilitation centers. However, now it is rare that any patient in southern Canada or the United States is more than a few hours' drive from a comprehensive rehabilitation center. Because there is such a wide variation in patients with completed stroke and their evaluations are so complex, the stroke patient should go to a rehabilitation center in order to have an individually designed rehabilitation program. After the principal aspects of stroke rehabilitation training have taken place in a rehabilitation center, some of the longer term aspects of rehabilitation training may be done in the home community, e.g., speech therapy.

When Should a Patient with Completed Stroke be Referred to a Rehabilitation Center?

Generally some principles of rehabilitation can be started on the first or second day after onset of stroke. Usually as soon as the stroke has stabilized, showing no further progression of neurologic deficits, it is desirable to move the patient to a rehabilitation service or ward, provided the patient can meet a few simple criteria such as having a level of consciousness that permits him to follow two-step or preferably three-step directions. Also, can the patient remember and apply today what he learned yesterday? If both of these criteria can be fulfilled, then it is not too early to transfer the patient with completed stroke for rehabilitation training.

In planning the organization of this chapter, it was decided that using the approach taken by each of the rehabilitation disciplines to the patient with completed stroke was not as appropriate as a problem-oriented approach to stroke rehabilitation. Instead of having one section of the chapter on evaluation of the stroke patient and another on management, the evaluation and management will be discussed for each problem that is taken up.

REHABILITATION DURING THE ACUTE PHASE OF STROKE

How soon after the onset of stroke should rehabilitation begin? Some rehabilitation procedures should begin on the first day, particularly those aimed at preventing the development of complications. How long does the acute stroke patient have to remain in bed or in a chair? In the past there has been a tendency to leave stroke patients in bed much too long for fear of making the stroke progress if the patient starts sitting up too soon. However, the practice of having stroke patients sit up early has proved this myth to be untrue. Most authorities agree that the stroke patient can start sitting up in bed, and even in a chair beside the bed, just as soon as the stroke has stabilized. There has been some difficulty in determining when the stroke has stabilized or has become completed. Some physicians feel that this stage has been reached when there has been no further evidence of progression of neurologic deficits for 48 hours.[6]

Enlightened rehabilitation practices applied early to the patient with completed stroke have made it apparent that many aspects of stroke that were formerly considered part of the natural history of completed stroke have, in reality, been complications that are preventable and avoidable.

Preventable Complications

Intellectual Regression. Probably the most common complication in completed stroke is intellectual regression due to sensory deprivation. Also some complications are enhanced by prolonged sensory deprivation, such as depression, short attention span, and poor motivation. There has been a tendency in the past to isolate the stroke patient during the acute phase to a quiet, dark room, disturbing him as infrequently as possible. He sometimes is placed in a bed so that he gets little, if any, stimulation from his environment: when he lies on his back he sees the ceiling and when he is lying on the one side to which he can turn he is able to see only a blank wall. While nursing personnel and physicians are briefly present on rounds, they sometimes have a tendency to speak of the patient in the third person, even in his presence. Without external stimulation from the environment, even the most well-integrated personality tends to deteriorate rapidly. For example, astronauts who were placed in dark, quiet tanks began to hallucinate within an average of 14 hours. It is true that some stroke patients at first have short attention spans and fatigue easily and quickly. Consequently the environmental stimulation has to be provided in brief intervals.

Depression. If sensory deprivation is prolonged, the patient soon develops depression along with the intellectual deterioration. There is then a tendency to blame depression on brain damage rather than on the environmental situation. More will be discussed about depression later in this chapter.

Physical Deterioration. With intellectual regression, depression, plus physical disability, the patient has an increasing dependency on the nursing personnel. Dependency frequently leads to resentment, and hence the patient becomes an increasing problem in nursing care. When this withdrawal, apathy, and depression are permitted to persist, it does not take long before a physical breakdown begins to develop. Decubitus ulcer occurs, particularly if the patient has some sensory deficits on the involved side or has been under the influence of heavy sedation or analgesia. Until the patient has learned to use the less affected side in changing his position in bed, it should be part of the standard nursing care procedures to change the patient's position frequently.

Contractures. Probably the second most common complication of completed stroke is the development of contractures, a complication that is generally avoidable. The presence of contractures has many effects on the stroke patient other than just his loss of motion. For example, when the contractures are permitted to progress, they soon become painful. The presence of contractures often enhances the amount of spasticity, and contractures can greatly interfere with ambulation. The two principal procedures that are used to prevent the development of contractures can both be accomplished by nursing personnel. These are (1) proper positioning of the more affected limbs in bed and when sitting, and (2) range of motion exercises to maintain full range of motion. There are excellent inexpensive monographs available for nursing personnel who are not familiar with proper positioning of the more affected limbs of the stroke patient.[27] The majority of nursing personnel in recent times have been well instructed in performing passive range of motion exercises to prevent contractures. It is the physician's duty to see that these exercises are ordered to be carried out routinely, daily, by nursing personnel, even though sometimes these exercises may also be carried out by a physical therapist who is involved. It should be pointed out that a distinction should be made between passive range of motion exercises that are performed by nursing personnel to *prevent* contractures and the stretching exercises for *correction* of contractures; the latter are usually performed by trained physical therapists.

Bladder Incontinence. After the onset of stroke the presence of urinary incontinence may be due to confusion, to communication disorder, or to the presence of a flaccid, distended bladder with dribbling overflow type of incontinence. If the involved extremities are quite flaccid and there is an altered level of consciousness, it is reasonable to assume that a situation has occurred in which catheter drainage is indicated. Later the neurologic effect on bladder function may change as peripheral reflexes return and perhaps some spasticity appears and the incontinence changes to an inability to inhibit the detrusor reflex. When the filling bladder begins to contract, the patient cannot postpone this urgency volitionally and incontinence results. In evaluating bladder dysfunction, three aspects of voiding have to be evaluated and considered;[26] namely, bladder filling, the detrusor activity for emptying the bladder, and the external sphincter relaxation that permits the flow of urine. In addition, there may be an impairment of urine flow by mechanical obstruction such as enlarged prostate or a scarred urethra. By asking the nursing service to initiate a total bladder training program, urinary dysfunction can often be accommodated without the demoralizing effect of incontinence on the patient and still avoiding the use of an indwelling catheter.

Urinary Sepsis. The period of urinary incontinence in many stroke patients does not last very long and in many male patients frequent changes of bed linen may be avoided by simply keeping a urinal in place, by using an external catheter to avoid bed wetting, or by simply arousing the patient at frequent intervals and offering the bedpan or urinal. Unfortunately, it is much easier to take care of the patient by using an indwelling catheter. The tendency is to leave the catheter in much too long. The longer the catheter, which acts as a foreign body, stays in the bladder, the greater the likelihood of urinary sepsis. It is rare to hear of a trial off catheter for the stroke patient being unsuccessful because it was tried too early.

Bowel Dysfunction. Even with severe brain damage intestinal peristalsis continues so that fecal material arrives at the rectum quite automatically without volition of the patient. When this happens, if the stroke patient is unable to inhibit the urge or reflex to defecate, fecal incontinence occurs. This type of incontinence often occurs along with urinary incontinence and is seen more commonly and more extensively in cases in which the brain damage is more extensive or even bilateral. However, even in those cases of bowel incontinence associated with severe brain damage, bowel incontinence can often be avoided by the initiation of a good bowel program by the nursing service. Such a program has to take many factors into consideration, such as the patient's previous habits of timing of bowel movements, diet, food intake, amount of physical activity, etc. Even though the patient may not be able to request a bedpan or commode, an individualized bowel program may take care of emptying

the rectum at a regular, natural time so that accidents are avoided at other times of the day. This training by the nursing service, sometimes called bowel training of the stroke patient, plays a large role in helping relieve depression by avoiding incontinence.

MOTOR ASPECTS

Paralysis and Weakness

Many people, when hearing the word *stroke*, think first of paralysis or weakness as the most outstanding characteristics of completed stroke. Hence, they tend to lose awareness that this process or weakness may not be the most disabling factor to the patient with completed stroke. In evaluating the extent and amount of paralysis and/or weakness, manual muscle testing is of limited value because the response of individual muscle groups to testing depends upon a wide variety of factors such as spasticity, incoordination, apraxia, uninhibited reflexes, relationship to gravity, and posture. It may take a considerable time before a full appreciation can be developed of how much motor function has been retained or regained. Often much more motor function can be demonstrated in the more affected lower extremity when the patient is supported in the standing position than when examined while lying supine.

Spasticity

During the recovery phase the limbs affected by the stroke progress from a state of flaccidity to increased stretch reflexes (spasticity) as manifested by increased deep tendon reflexes, clonus, and clasp-knife reaction to flexor and extensor synergies and finally to return of voluntary motor function. This general pattern of recovery may cease to progress at any phase. Hence spasticity cannot always be considered to herald return of voluntary motor function. For an excellent, yet brief, explanation of the neurophysiologic basis of spasticity, see Chapter 3 in Mossman's Problem Oriented Approach to Stroke Rehabilitation.[26] Some spasticity may be quite useful to the patient, particularly for standing and walking. In dealing with spasticity in the stroke patient, the professional should ask the question: "How disabling is it?"

There is a wide variety of pharmacologic and surgical approaches to spasticity. These tend to dominate consideration before these questions are asked: "Had the spasticity been about the same for a long period of time and only recently become sufficiently worse to produce an increase in disabling effects? If so, what has occurred that might be enhancing the spasticity?" Factors that are well known for enhancing spasticity include the presence of contractures, anxiety, extremes of heat or cold, or any ordinarily painful condition such as ingrown toenails, infection, or decubitus ulcer. An attempt should be made to eliminate or diminish these factors before any pharmacologic or surgical approach to treating the spasticity is tried. (See Chapter 11.)

The use of both heat and cold has been noted in some stroke patients to have some temporary effect on reducing the amount of spasticity. Sometimes this permits a brief period in which the patient can better practice certain exercises or neurophysiologic retraining. Probably the most well-publicized approach to spasticity is through drugs. There are several classes of these drugs that have different sites of action. Although some of them have proved to reduce measurably the amount of spasticity, when patients who have tried them are given the option of continuing or going without the antispasmodic, many give up the drug treatment and put up with the increased spasticity because they do not like the drug's side effects. Because most of the drugs used for spasticity also have some effect on the central nervous system functioning, particularly alertness, stroke patients tend to find these side effects more undesirable than the more pronounced spasticity. What is needed is a long-term follow-up study to determine how many patients continue taking drugs for spasticity over a long period of time.

The use of phenol blocks,[17] either for neurolysis of a main nerve trunk or for a few selective motor units intramuscularly, has been quite effective in reducing the amount of spasticity. These effects are not permanent but can be repeated when the spasticity increases again. Following such procedures some patients have had a complication of discomfort in the blocked muscle for two to three days. Surgical lengthening of tendons of the spastic muscles is rarely done anymore.

Incoordination

Incoordination in patients with completed stroke may be associated with spasticity, or it may be due to involvement of the cerebellum or cerebellar tracts. For evaluation and management of the latter, see the section on brain stem involvement. For incoordination associated with spasticity, see the section on management below.

Dyspraxia

In stroke patients dyspraxia is a disorder of voluntary movement wherein the individual cannot initiate a willed or planned purposeful movement or activity despite the presence of adequate strength, sensation, coordination, and comprehension. There is a wide variety of types of dyspraxia that are described in stroke patients, such as oral-verbal dyspraxia, constructional apraxia, dressing apraxia, ideational apraxia, and motor dyspraxia. It is the motor or kinetic dyspraxia that is most commonly encountered in stroke patients. A common example of motor dyspraxia is the patient who can perform a movement spontaneously quite accurately but when requested to perform this same act so that he has to plan the movement is then unable to initiate the movement. Once he is given some assistance to initiate the movement, he can then go ahead and complete it, often with good coordination or dexterity. This phenomenon has a definite neurologic basis, although it often resembles a problem in attitude, cooperation, comprehension, awareness, or motivation. Once it is recognized, it can be dealt with in rehabilitation training by giving the patient assistance for starting a complex performance which the patient completes successfully. The prognosis is good for overcoming most types of dyspraxia if consistent training is pursued. This is true even for oral dyspraxia and oral-verbal dyspraxia, which will be further discussed in the section on communication disorders.

Management of Motor Dysfunction

It is not difficult for the physician to write an adequate physical therapy prescription even for the paretic limb that continues to progress in neurologic recovery. The order can be written: "Re-education, including neurophysiologic techniques, for all muscle groups in the extremity; progressing each group as improvement occurs to active assistive, active, active against gravity, and finally resistive." This will permit the physical therapist to progress the patient along as neuromuscular functioning improves without having to have the physical therapy prescription rewritten at frequent intervals. The problem that is still quite controversial is the selection of neurophysiologic techniques to use for this returning function. Some people are under the incorrect impression that these neurophysiologic techniques are designed to overcome pathologic reflexes, but Kottke[19] points out that rather than there being pathologic reflexes, there are in stroke patients specific spinal and supraspinal reflexes that vary only in intensity or extent of response as the result of diminution or loss of inhibition because of damage to the higher centers. Kottke further points out that to train a normal adult to the peak of coordination in a specific activity, the activity must be performed with maximal skill for hundreds of thousands, possibly millions of repetitions. Just as coordination is developed by frequent and multiple repetitions, it is lost progressively over time with inactivity. Therefore, the therapeutic program should be adjusted to assure that coordination activities are repeated at frequent intervals throughout each day and continued until a functional level of activity is achieved. In the treatment of stroke, Kottke divides the neurophysiologic techniques into four phases, depending upon the state of neuromuscular function of the patient: (1) activation of nonresponsive muscles, (2) reinforcement of feedback, (3) inhibition of muscles not in a coordinated engram, and (4) improving performance of the engram. Instead of recommending any one of the many detailed techniques of treatment, he recommends that techniques be used that are appropriate for the state of neuromuscular function of the muscle group or limb in that individual patient which seem to be the most effective. One of the frustrations in using these neurophysiologic methods of treatment of stroke patients is that they have to be carried out over a long period of time, with many repetitions. In the short period of time that stroke rehabilitation usually takes place on an inpatient basis, there has been insufficient time to show much significant change with these methods.[34] Ideally those stroke patients who show a good early response to such training should have the opportunity of coming in as an outpatient for continuing the training over a long period of time.

SENSORY DEFICITS

Because the patient may not complain of sensory deficits, their importance in causing disability in the hemiplegic patient tends to be overlooked by rehabilitation professionals. This is particularly true in the upper extremity that has good return of voluntary motor functioning that is not utilized by the patient because of the persistent sensory deficits. This patient is accused of poor motivation or over-reaction emotionally for not using the upper extremity more. The types of sensory modalities involved in completed stroke in the order of importance of the disabilities they produce are proprioception, tactile sensation, vibration, pain, and temperature.

In some hemiplegics who have some sensory impairment but not complete sensory paralysis of the more involved limbs, there is a tendency to recognize all stimuli as pain. This is probably most pronounced in partial lesions in the thalamus. Such a situation makes carrying out range-of-motion exercises for prevention of contractures difficult because all light touch and movement of the involved extremities is recognized by the patient as pain. One of the ways this problem can be lessened is that the therapist, recognizing that the patient's sensation has the ability to adapt, does not change tactile sensations once she grasps the extremity for conducting the passive movements. After a few minutes, the patient's reaction of pain to the tactile sensation of having the limb held by the therapist will adapt. Then when the therapist performs the movements at the same rate of speed without sudden stops and starts, the amount of pain recognized by the patient from the movement will be lessened. In addition, the therapist needs to repeatedly reassure the patient that what is being done is not actually painful, but is just being misperceived.

The level of the lesion has considerable effect on the sensory deficit. Lesions of the ascending sensory tracts in the brain stem may produce sensory loss of the entire extremity, whereas higher lesions in the internal capsule or cortex tend to produce a loss of sensation greater distally than proximally. The ventral nucleus of the thalamus may be affected particularly following interruption of the posterior cerebral artery circulation. It is the level for the first appreciation of primary sensations of touch, temperature, pain, vibration, and some cruder aspects of proprioception. Projections from the ventral nucleus of the thalamus to the parietal cortex pass through the posterior limb of the internal capsule, which is a frequent site of damage with strokes involving the internal carotid or middle cerebral artery circulation. The sensory projections are commonly involved in conjunction with the descending motor tracts that pass more anteriorly in the internal capsule, giving rise to associated hemiplegia and sensory losses. It is the area of the parietal cortex where the crude sensations that were initially perceived by the thalamus undergo fine discrimination. Because the fibers within the internal capsule are more closely concentrated than the more diffused projections in the cortex, a lesion of equal size produces greater damage within the internal capsule than one in the cortex.

In the cortical sensory lesions impairing proprioception from about the knee down, the lower extremity can function adequately with a gross motor pattern for walking. Useful distal function in the upper extremity requires not only fine motor coordination for prehension but also sensory sophistication of a high order of complexity. Hence, when cortical proprioception is involved, there is a poorer prognosis for regaining useful function in the upper extremity than in the lower extremity. However, occupational therapists have found that teaching the patient visual monitoring of hand activity can help compensate for the impaired proprioception. Other cortical functions for sensation that can be tested are localization and discrimination of stimuli by tests of two-point discrimination, sensory extinction, stereognosis, and graphesthesia. After time is allowed for spontaneous recovery, the stroke patient who performs well on these tests of cortical functioning has a much better prognosis for use of the involved extremity in vocational rehabilitation.

Studies have shown that some stroke patients with impairment of sensation do recover some of the impaired sensation, usually within the first or second month.[35] The number experiencing recovery of sensory function varied depending on the types of sensation that were involved. Generally, one half to two thirds of the patients experienced some improvement in the sensory deficits. Those patients with no sensory deficits had a much shorter initial hospitalization. Those that made no recovery had still longer hospitalization than those with some recovery. It is still questionable whether retraining can help patients with impaired, but not absent, sensation to improve their recognition of these sensations for practical clinical purposes.

Anosognosia is a term coined by Babinski, but the meaning and cause of the condition are still not well understood. Generally the term applies to a condition in some patients with left hemiparesis or hemiplegia who do not recognize their left extremities as their own or who do not recognize the disabilities in those extremities. Friedlander[16] has pointed out that there are three theoretical mechanisms underlying anosognosia: (1) a defect in morphosynthesis, (2) a defect of body concept, or (3) a maladaptation to illness in a personality that premorbidly denied illness. Whatever the defect, the phenomenon of anosognosia significantly impedes rehabilitation training.

Visual Field Deficits

Vascular lesions of the brain can cause interference with vision if they occur anywhere along the visual pathways but occur more often in circulatory embarrassment in the middle cerebral artery territory and less commonly in the posterior cerebral artery distribution. The effect on vision may be complete ablation, so that it is referred to as a field cut (Fig. 30–1), or it may be partial. Since it is so difficult to distinguish between these two early after the onset of stroke, it is probably preferable to label such lesions as "visual field deficits." The pattern of involvement can vary from one quarter of a visual field, one half, or three quarters. It may involve the same amount of the visual field of each eye, which is the most common type of deficit. These deficits in visual field should not be called problems in perception nor perceptual deficits. The term *perceptual* relates to right hemisphere function.

Visual field impairments are often not rec-

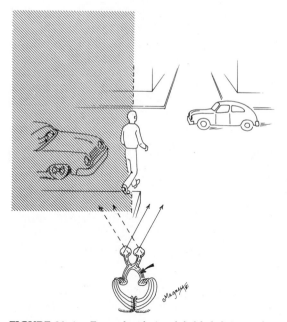

FIGURE 30–1. Example of visual field deficit on the left. The individual does not respond to the visual stimuli of the approaching auto on his left owing to a lesion in the optic radiation at the point of the arrow.

ognized and appreciated by the rehabilitation staff early after onset of stroke, but becoming aware of these problems allows the staff to help avoid a lot of frustration for the patient. For example, this is particularly true when the patient is learning to feed himself and the staff learns to place the food in his functioning field of vision, avoiding the side where the deficit is located. Some patients with these problems can learn to compensate for the visual field deficit. Some either learn to compensate very well so that the problem appears no longer to exist or perhaps actually make recovery and regain this visual functioning. One of the greatest problems in teaching such patients to compensate for the visual deficit is the patient's tendency to deny that such a visual impairment exists. This "denial" should not be confused with another condition called visual field neglect, in which the patient when tested by perimeter examination has full field of vision but clinically it is noted that the patient tends to ignore and neglect visual stimuli coming from the involved side. Often this type of extinction, or perceptual rivalry, is encountered in other areas of sensory perception such as double simultaneous stimulation and kinesthetic perception.

HEARING DEFICITS

Although there are not well-recognized specific deficits in hearing ability due to stroke, the impairment of hearing in stroke patients is quite common. It is usually assumed that the hearing loss was present prior to the stroke. It is well for the rehabilitation staff to suspect possible hearing difficulties in the older stroke patient. Audiometric examination is quite useful to the staff in knowing how to communicate with the stroke patient.

COGNITIVE AND OTHER DYSFUNCTIONS

Differences Between Right and Left Hemisphere Involvement

Generally it is recognized that the left hemisphere controls the right side of the body and is the dominant one for communication ability, while the right hemisphere controls the left side of the body and various integrative factors in cognition and intellectual functioning. However, it is erroneous to think that all stroke patients have only one side of the body involved. Even though the lesion may be in one side of the brain, the effects on the functioning are often bilateral so that we should say that one side is "the more involved" and the other side is "less involved," rather than saying left hemiparetic or right hemiparetic. It is also generally recognized that the intelligence quotient is made up of an average of the verbal IQ, which mainly represents left hemisphere function, and the performance IQ, which mainly represents right hemisphere function. The effects of left hemisphere lesions on communication will be dealt with under communication disorders later in this chapter.

Right Hemisphere Dysfunction

The right parietal lobe in the majority of people, including most left-handed people, provides the ability to correctly organize stimuli into concepts, the process termed *morphosynthesis*. Interference in this functioning is often termed *perceptual disorder*. However, because of the ambiguity of this term, such as applying it to visual field disorders, it is probably preferable to refer to dysfunctions of the right parietal lobe more specifically with terms such as *visual-spatial* and *visual-motor disorders*. These are seen in stroke patients most often as difficulties in performing activities of daily living where they seem impaired in making the right spatial analysis of problems they encounter. A classic example is the patient who easily verbally indicates there is something wrong with his shirt that interferes with his putting it on, yet he cannot recognize that it is one sleeve turned wrong side out that is interfering.

Some studies of rehabilitation of stroke patients have shown that patients with right hemisphere damage producing this type of deficit are slower in learning activities of daily living than those patients with left hemisphere involvement. However, other studies[3, 20] show that there is no difference between right and left involvement. Perhaps this variation may have occurred owing to differences in the number of nonverbal cues given in instructing the patient in his training in activities of daily living. There appears to be no correlation of visual spatial and visual motor dysfunctions with the amount of motor impairment in the left limb. Generally all patients who have had right hemisphere involvement should not be permitted to drive an automobile again until they have passed special testing for visual-spatial and visual-motor functioning as well as visual field neglect and other types of deficits.

Psychometric Testing

One of the most widely used tests of right parietal lobe functioning is the Bender-Gestalt Visual Motor Test. It consists of asking the patient to copy on paper meaningless geometric designs and dots. This is a cross-cultural type test that can detect spatial distortions, separations, and errors in orientation or rotation. It may also pick up unilateral visual field neglect. The Gram Kendall Memory for Design Test and Sequin Formboard require perception of visual-spatial relationships and discrimination of the test object by the patient. The Wechsler Adult Intelligence Scale has a variety of assembly and completion tasks involving varying levels of visual-spatial reasoning, analysis, and manipulation of relationships

as well as higher cognitive visual-spatial reasoning. It is the performance part of this test that is often low in patients with right hemisphere involvement, while their verbal IQ may remain quite high, similar to the premorbid level. These tests have not proved to be useful in their predictive value[3, 20] as had been hoped by an earlier study.

Other Dysfunctions

Perseveration is a repetitive and involuntary motor or verbal response that possibly was appropriate to a first stimulus but continues to be repeated even after the first stimulus has been removed and other new stimuli or instructions have been introduced. It is found in people with a wide variety of brain damage. It usually is associated with severity of involvement or indicative of recent involvement, since it often gradually subsides as neurologic recovery takes place.

Some patients with brain damage also exhibit a quality of behavior called impulsivity. This is most often encountered in patients who begin an action before they completely process what the full scope of the action will be. For example, they begin following instructions before the instructions have been completed. Patients exhibiting impulsivity seem to be unable to withhold response and make a judgment about which alternatives and course of action would be most appropriate. They come forth with a quick motor response without taking time for consideration of its appropriateness or its effects.

Another characteristic of brain damage that interferes with the rehabilitation process is impaired judgment and impaired planning and foresight. This can be easily tested and demonstrated by asking the patient to perform on Porteus mazes. Clinically it is manifested often when patients are undergoing homemaking evaluation in which they exhibit poor judgment or inability to plan or execute preparation of a meal. These dysfunctions tend to be most noticeable immediately after the onset of the stroke and gradually diminish with time. Often they completely disappear or reoccur only with marked fatigue. Since they tend to clear up spontaneously, either rapidly or gradually, it has been difficult to study training programs that might lead to eventual better resolution or more rapid resolution of the problem.

MOBILITY

During Acute Phase

Some patients with stroke view themselves at first as totally paralyzed instead of paralyzed on just one side of the body. They feel totally helpless. One of the first steps in overcoming this feeling is helping them learn to use the less involved arm and leg to move themselves in bed. Because the dangers of having the stroke patient sit up early have been exaggerated in the past, one should consider rolling up the head of the bed quite early, particularly while the patient is awake. When this is tolerated well, the patient can learn to come to a sitting position on the edge of the bed. The patient rolls to his less involved side and then uses the less involved lower extremity under the involved one to guide it over the edge of the bed and uses the less involved arm to push up to the sitting position. These techniques are well described and illustrated in a monograph on nursing procedures for stroke patients published by the Elizabeth Kenny Institute.[27]

Common to nearly all patients with completed stroke is the difficulty in maintaining sitting balance and, of course, standing balance. This problem seems to be not necessarily related to which hemisphere is involved but rather to learning to develop new reflexes for maintaining balance. There are three major determinants for maintaining balance in the normal individual: vision, proprioception, and labyrinthine function. Generally at least two of these three factors should be operating. If the patient has been left long in bed, transient hypotension due to the sudden change in posture may cause cerebral vascular insufficiency with transient vertigo. Undoubtedly visual spatial and visual motor dysfunctions could also interfere with maintenance of balance.

Another factor is the sense of verticality in the hemiplegic patient (Fig. 30–2). Special tests have been developed for measuring this, such as the Rod and Frame Test. Most studies[12] reveal that early after onset nearly all hemiplegic patients show some impairment of performance in ascertaining the vertical position of the test rod. Not all of the studies[10] agree that right hemiplegics perform this test better than left hemiplegics. Fortunately the sense of verticality and particularly the sense of balance can be re-

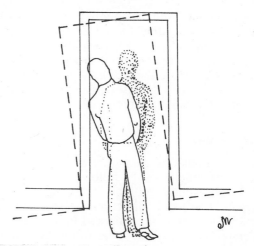

FIGURE 30–2. Illustration of the person with impaired sense of verticality.

learned. It is rare that these problems persist for a long period of time if the stroke patient has been given an adequate trial of relearning sitting balance while using visual input as well as proprioceptive input from the less involved upper extremity, and then relearning standing balance.

Transfers and Wheelchairs

Getting out of bed, particularly when he has learned to do so by himself, is probably more significant to the stroke patient than any other factor in overcoming the feeling that he is still a sick patient; it signifies that he is learning to become a person again instead of a patient. For the hemiplegic or hemiparetic there is a definite method to be used (see Chapter 18) even when the patient needs assistance or direction, so that eventually using this same procedure the patient can learn to perform the transfer without assistance. Detailed instructions of a step-by-step procedure of transfer training are well outlined in the Elizabeth Kenny Institute publication on stroke.[27] Each time a transfer is performed with assistance, training should be given so that eventually the patient will learn to do this independently.

For the stroke patient an important aspect of getting up in a wheelchair is to be able to propel the wheelchair independently. It is not necessary to have an expensive one-hand-drive wheelchair. If the patient has one good functioning upper extremity and lower extremity, he can quickly learn how to use that foot and hand together to propel forward and turn and guide the chair (see Chapter 23). Even patients with visual-spatial and visual-motor dysfunction associated with right hemisphere damage can learn by practicing to get themselves independently around the building.

Ambulation

For ambulation the patient with completed stroke should have the following:

1. The ability to follow instructions, preferably three-step directions. Even though the patient may have marked impairment in comprehension of verbal instructions he may be able to learn readily from nonverbal directions such as demonstrations.

2. Ability to maintain standing balance, which can be evaluated when the patient is transferring.

3. Absence of contractures in hip and knee flexors and heel cord.

4. Adequate return of voluntary motor function to stabilize the hip, knee, and ankle on the involved side. For the patient with completed stroke to learn to walk again, return of voluntary motor function is necessary in only one muscle group — the hip extensors. These muscles not only stabilize the hip in extension but also help stabilize the knee in extension by pulling backward on the femur. Lateral stabilization of the hip that is impaired by weakness or paralysis of the hip abductors can be compensated for by placing the opposite (less involved) hand on a stable object such as a cane. For paralysis or weakness of foot and ankle muscles, an ankle-foot orthosis (AFO) not only can help keep the forefoot up but also can aid medial and lateral stability of the ankle. If the AFO resists dorsiflexion beyond 90 degrees, it can also help add to stabilization of the knee to keep it from flexing during stance. It is rare that a patient with hemiparesis needs a long leg brace. In evaluating the patient to determine how much return of voluntary motor function is present, manual muscle testing while the patient is lying supine can be misleading. Often the stimulus of being in the upright standing position and attempting to bear weight on the more involved lower extremity brings out more voluntary motor function than is apparent when the patient is lying supine.

5. Intact position sense in the more involved lower extremity. This is not an absolute requisite because patients with impaired proprioception can learn to walk again using the sensory involved lower extremity.

Progression of Gait Training

For successful gait training of the patient with completed stroke, a well-trained physical therapist is most helpful, if not essential. The patient first learns balance holding onto a bar or other stable support standing. When the balance is beginning to be reliable, the patient learns to shift full weight onto the more affected lower extremity. Once this is feasible, the patient can begin performing gait drills standing in place, shifting the weight from one lower extremity to the other, back and forth. When this appears to be going well, with the hip, knee, and ankle well stabilized, actual walking at the bar can begin, with the aim of developing an optimal reciprocal pattern of gait. Once a good reciprocal pattern at the bar has been achieved, the patient progresses to using a four-point cane. A crutch at this point is not desirable because with a crutch the patient can easily develop a habit of leaning away from the more involved lower extremity, thereby not placing full weight on it, which will make progression later to a cane difficult. When the patient is doing well with a four-point cane and appears to have confidence, an attempt can be made to use a single-ended cane. The gait training is not completed, however, until the patient has learned to negotiate stairs and ramps. For the patient with right hemisphere involvement that has produced some spatial and visual motor impairment, the patient may have difficulty remembering which foot to use first when going up or down the stairs. However, this can sometimes be helped if the patient has good verbal functioning. He can learn verbally the little mnemonic device which goes, "up with the good foot, down with the bad."

Factors Interfering with Ambulation

1. *Paralysis and Weakness.* Since antigravity strength in the hip extensors on the more involved side is the only motor function required for walking, paralysis and weakness play little role in interference with gait training.

2. *Spasticity*. This is undoubtedly the most common disabling factor in gait training. When this occurs, first a search should be made for factors that may be enhancing the spasticity, such as pain, contracture, ataxia, fears, and anxiety. For many stroke patients spasticity that interferes with walking is most marked in the plantar flexors. This can often be adequately controlled by the use of an AFO. (See Chapter 28 on Lower Extremity Orthotics.) If the spasticity is rather marked, the Klenzak type brace seems to be more effective than the posterior molded plastic splint. It should be pointed out that there is no truth in the persistent old myth that spring action braces enhance spasticity.[22] An outside T-strap on a Klenzak brace may help lessen the problem of spastic invertors pulling the foot over laterally so that the patient has a tendency to walk on the outer edge of the foot. Intramuscular neurolysis may also be used to reduce the amount of spasticity.[17] A pharmacologic approach to spasticity in patients with completed stroke often adds a burden of having a central nervous system depressant effect. Drugs should be considered only when all the above measures have been tried and yet the spasticity is still interfering.

Common Pitfalls in Gait Training for Stroke Patients[7]

Some physical therapists who are eager to make the patient feel that progress is occurring in ambulation have a tendency to start the patient walking at a bar before he has learned adequately to shift his full weight onto the more involved lower extremity. This leads to the development of a pattern that will make it very difficult for the patient ever to progress to using a cane. There is also a tendency for both the therapist and the patient to want to graduate the patient away from the bar too soon before a good pattern is established and thereby create a situation of persistently poor gait pattern. Then once the patient has graduated from the bar and is walking well with a four-point cane, there is a tendency to move the patient to a single-ended cane too soon. In fact, the single-ended cane should not be used until the therapist notices no differences in the pattern whether the patient uses a four-point cane or a single-ended cane. For those patients with dyspraxia, a physical therapist has to learn to refrain from giving instructions for each movement in sequence but instead allow the patient to move ahead automatically as feasible.

ACTIVITIES OF DAILY LIVING

One-Handed Methods

The reader is referred to Chapter 24 on activities of daily living. For all those listed activities, methods have been worked out for one-handed performance. For specific written guides on stroke patients performing self care and other activities of daily living, the Sister Elizabeth Kenny publications[28] are excellent guides with good illustrations. For most patients with completed stroke the difficulties involved in learning activities of daily living are less commonly due to physical factors such as weakness and one handedness or to communication factors, but more often due to such problems as poor sitting balance, visual field defect, and visual-spatial and visual-motor dysfunctions.

Self Care

Training in self care by nursing personnel should begin early while the patient is still in bed. Even then he can begin learning to use his less involved extremities for turning himself in bed and feeding himself, and can start to perform some aspects of personal hygiene, to bathe himself, and eventually to learn to come to a sitting position on the edge of the bed without assistance. When sitting balance has been achieved, then the patient can start to learn to dress himself and also to transfer to a bedside commode or toilet. Finally when the patient has achieved standing balance and ability to transfer to and from a toilet independently, he needs still to learn to rearrange his clothing in a standing position before and after using the toilet.

Homemaking

It should not be assumed that it would be mainly female patients with completed stroke who are interested in evaluation and training in homemaking. Almost as many males are interested in including this in their rehabilitation training. Often this evaluation and training are postponed until shortly before discharge from the comprehensive inpatient rehabilitation period so that the patient may have attained his maximal potential in mobility and communication. Better recommendations for what the patient will be able and not able to do at home can then be made. Although most of this evaluation is done by the occupational therapist, the entire team contributes to determining some aspects of the evaluation. For example, the physical therapist reports on whether the patient should work from a wheelchair or a standing position, whether transfers are performed safely, and whether transfer to a stool in the kitchen is practical. The social worker reports on the family's general attitude toward the patient's return home and what their expectations are and if the patient will be expected to resume a full or limited homemaking role. The occupational therapist will report on such factors as the degree of function that remains in the more involved upper extremity, whether it can be used in a helping way or a stabilizing way, whether there is a visual field deficit, whether the patient has learned to compensate for it, and whether visual-spatial and visual-motor problems affect the patient's ability. The speech pathologist will recommend what communication methods should be used with the patient during the homemaker's evaluation, and the psychologist may be reporting from the psychometric testing about the patient's judgment and reliability. The homemaking evaluation itself gives a great deal of information about judgment, reliability, and ability to plan ahead.

When the final report of this evaluation is made, there are recommendations made about which activities will need no help, some help, much help, or complete help. Some of the other problems that affect the outcome of the homemaking evaluation are perseveration, impulsivity, ataxia, unreliability, and poor frustration tolerance. After the evaluation of homemaking abilities has been completed, the homemaking training often focuses on such factors as work simplification in the patient's home, organization of the work areas there, and determination of reaching ranges.

Other Activities

Consideration should be given to how the patient functions, not only in the home but also outside the home, and how the patient will be able to negotiate certain types of architectural barriers, use public transportation, go shopping, and drive an automobile. For driving an automobile special consideration should be given to such factors as slowed reaction time, visual field neglect, and visual-spatial dysfunction, which are usually not picked up in the average medical or driving evaluation for re-issue of a driver's license.

UPPER EXTREMITY PROBLEMS

Neurologic Recovery

In the typical middle cerebral artery stroke the upper extremity is usually more involved compared to the lower extremity and recovery is usually not as complete. With the exception of those patients whose stroke involved the anterior cerebral artery, the pattern of long-term return of motor function is usually more proximal, with the distal functioning in the fingers being the last to return. Stroke patients regaining full recovery of motor function in the upper extremity developed the onset of this return of function within the first two weeks of the onset of the stroke, and always within the first month.[8] Most subjects achieved full active movement within the first month and all of them by the third month. If the patient has gone six months beyond onset with no return of voluntary motor function in the hand, the prognosis for any return of useful function in that hand is poor. Carroll[13] found that if there was no return of voluntary motor function within the first week, it was unlikely the patient would regain "full use" of the hemiplegic upper extremity. There are other differences between the upper extremity and lower extremity on the involved side. For the lower extremity to be useful in ambulation it requires only minimal return of voluntary motor function, that is, the hip extensors, for that extremity to serve as a pillar for weight bearing. For the upper extremity to be useful there has to be almost complete return of voluntary motor and sensory function to provide fine coordination and finger dexterity. It is always difficult to know, even with knowledge of these statistical studies[8, 13] about return of function (Table 30–3), when to start training the premorbidly nondominant hand to become the dominant one. In the treatment of the upper extremity, therapists

TABLE 30–3. TIME AFTER ONSET UNTIL INITIAL VOLUNTARY MOTION IN UPPER EXTREMITY (MONTHS)

	1	2	3	4	>4
Patients recovering full motion	39	0	0	0	0
Patients recovering partial motion	17	5	5	1	0

Used with permission from Bard, G., and Hirschberg, G. G.: Recovery of voluntary motion in the upper extremity following hemiplegia. Arch. Phys. Med. Rehabil., 46:567–572, 1965.

often apply bilateral activities in the hope that movement might more readily return in the involved upper extremity. However, it has been pointed out[18] that the function thus occurring may be less efficient and inferior to the paretic hand's capability when it functions separately. There is still considerable question about whether specialized neurophysiologic techniques utilizing synergies and facilitation produce a significant improvement in the paretic hand. Stern et al.[33] indicated that the specialized facilitation techniques have no better results than a traditional approach in the stroke patient learning self care techniques. Others point out that for new patterns of motion to become effective and useful they have to be repeated many times over a long period of time. Hence, the short period of three to four weeks that a stroke patient is in traditional inpatient rehabilitation would not be long enough to show effective results. It would appear that before the value of these specialized neurophysiologic techniques can be determined in improving the function in the paretic hand, a group of patients would have to experience a long period of training as outpatients.

Painful Shoulder

In those patients with completed stroke who have a subluxation of the shoulder on the more involved side, there is a tendency always to blame the shoulder pain on the subluxation. However, many subluxed shoulders are not painful. What tends to be overlooked is a painful contracture of the shoulder that is also present. To give such a patient a sling without also adding stretching exercises to correct the contractures will fail to relieve the pain. Although no comparative studies are known to be reported, it is the clinical impression that the incidence of painful contractures is much less today than two or three decades ago when daily range-of-motion exercises were not as common and routine as they are at present. The number of patients with hemiparesis exhibiting a fully developed reflex sympathetic dystrophy involving the hand and shoulder also seems much less in recent years. When early signs of reflex dystrophy associated with vasoconstriction are detected, the vicious circle can usually be rapidly reversed by use of simple measures such as heat, gentle stretching exercises to regain full pain-free motions in the shoulder, oral analgesia, contrast baths for the hand and arm, and other similar measures to counteract the pain and vasoconstriction. If these are used frequently and vigorously before structural changes have had a chance to develop, it is seldom necessary to use more drastic measures for the reflex dystrophy such as stellate ganglion blocks.

The upper extremity with a subluxed shoulder can be supported by a sling. There are many types of slings (Fig. 30–3). The type most commonly used is the type that places most of the weight-bearing on the back of the neck. However, the other types of slings are more difficult to put on by the

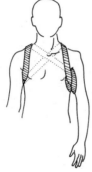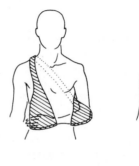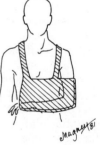

FIGURE 30–3. Some types of arm slings. From left to right: Bobath, common hemiplegic, Breuer-Kauper.

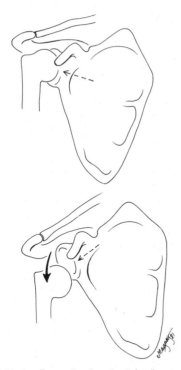

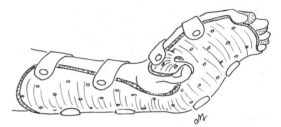

FIGURE 30–5. Pancake (resting) splint for hand and wrist.

FIGURE 30–4. Basmajian's principle. *Lower*, Drooping of the shoulder in some hemiplegics permits subluxation out of the downward tilted glenoid fossa (dotted arrow). *Upper*, Normally positioned shoulder prevents subluxation because the humeral head cannot displace laterally out of the upward tilted glenoid fossa (dotted arrow).

patients with visual-spatial and visual-motor difficulties. Basmajian[9] has pointed out that it is the downward droop of the glenoid fossa, which becomes less vertical, that enhances the subluxation of the shoulder (Fig. 30–4). Hence, he recommends retraining the upper trapezius to perform its function better in keeping the shoulder elevated in its normal position and thus preventing the downward droop and resulting subluxation.

Hand and Wrist

Probably the most common problem in the paralytic or paretic hand and wrist is the development of contracture, usually in the flexors. Some patients who have accepted the fact that the paralysis of the hand is going to be permanent wonder why they should bother with keeping up the range of motion exercises. Unfortunately, contractures can become painful, and even if they are not painful, the presence of a contracture enhances spasticity in the upper extremity and then indirectly also in the lower extremity, which may in turn interfere with walking. If

the patient and family understand this relationship, they do a better job of preventing contractures in the paralyzed, useless upper extremity.

The use of a pancake resting splint (Fig. 30–5) at night can be helpful in preventing the development of contractures of the finger flexors as well as the daily routine of stretching exercises. The patient who has some return of voluntary motor function in the upper extremity but spasticity in the more dominant flexors and thus tends to keep the hand and wrist in a flexed position would do well to use a dorsal cock-up splint for the hand to keep the hand and wrist in a better position of function and to prevent the spasticity in the flexors from dominating the posture of the hand (Fig. 30–6).

Dependent edema of the hand, sometimes extending up into the arm, occurs in hemiplegia, particularly when there is little, if any, voluntary motor function in the upper extremity. The pumping mechanism for helping the venous and lymphatic flow in the arm is impaired. When the dependent edema begins to accumulate, it is preferable to provide the patient with other means of keeping the extremity elevated rather than putting it in a sling against the patient's chest. It is more desirable to use a forearm tray on the patient's wheelchair with the hand end elevated. While the patient is lying down the involved upper extremity can be elevated on pillows. The use of the sling can be limited to times when the patient is walking.

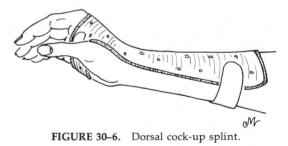

FIGURE 30–6. Dorsal cock-up splint.

COMMUNICATION DISORDERS

Confusion of Terms

Communication may be affected by either a language disorder, an impairment of speech production, or both. It is important to determine in which of these ways communication is affected, because impaired communication is very frustrating to the stroke patient and also because professionals dealing with the patient and the family will better understand how to communicate with the patient. There still tends to be an old persisting custom of referring to all communication disorders collectively as aphasia. Aphasia refers specifically to language problems and not to speech production problems.

Aphasia

Aphasia can be defined as an acquired impairment of verbal language behavior at the linguistic level caused by brain damage to the dominant cerebral hemisphere (usually the left).[29] It ordinarily affects to some degree all language areas such as understanding the speech of others, speaking, reading, writing, and arithmetic, but may involve principally verbal expression or principally comprehension. The term *aphasia* does not apply to language disorder associated with primary sensory deficits (for example, deafness), mental deficiency, psychiatric problems, or neuromuscular involvement of the speech mechanism. The majority of stroke patients with aphasic communication disorders have difficulty with both input (auditory comprehension and reading) and output (speaking and writing). Usually their impairment is more marked in one area than in another. Hence it is inappropriate to use specific labels such as *receptive aphasia, expressive aphasia,* and *mixed aphasia.* Terms sometimes used relating to impairment of verbal

expression are determined according to the classification used. Schuell and her colleagues[32] have designated five groups. Wepman and Jones[37] have a different type of classification: (1) syntactic aphasia, (2) semantic aphasia, (3) jargon aphasia, and (4) global aphasia. Aphasias can also be classified according to the anatomical localization of the lesion, such as Broca's aphasia and Wernicke's aphasia. Probably the most commonly used terms by speech pathologists are listed in Table 30–4, showing their distinguishing features in fluency, ability to repeat, and comprehension.

It is difficult to ascertain quickly what the patient's specific problems are in aphasia. Sometimes evaluation has to go on for many visits before the speech pathologist can adequately determine the types of aphasia and advise the other members of the rehabilitation team on how they should attempt to communicate with the patient. In a rehabilitation team most of the other members of the team may actually be performing more speech therapy than the speech pathologist, but the speech pathologist serves as the team's expert. The method used may vary considerably as the rehabilitation process progresses and the patient makes some improvement.

Because categorization of the type of aphasia is not easy and takes time, it is difficult for the speech pathologist to state early what the prognosis for regaining language function is, unless the patient happens to have severe global aphasia. If the patient is classified according to Schuell's groupings, the group that the patient is placed in has a hierarchy of prognosis, the poorest being for group five, i.e., irreversible aphasia syndrome, virtually complete loss of language skills. In patients with severely involved aphasia, the principal early benefits of speech therapy are the supportive care

TABLE 30–4. DISTINGUISHING FEATURES OF MAJOR FORMS OF APHASIA*

	Fluency	Ability to Repeat	Comprehension
Broca's aphasia	Nonfluent	↓	+
Transcortical motor aphasia	Nonfluent	+	+
Global aphasia	Nonfluent	↓	↓
Wernicke's aphasia	Fluent	↓	↓
Transcortical sensory aphasia	Fluent	+	↓
Conduction aphasia	Fluent	↓	+

* ↓ impaired
+ relatively intact

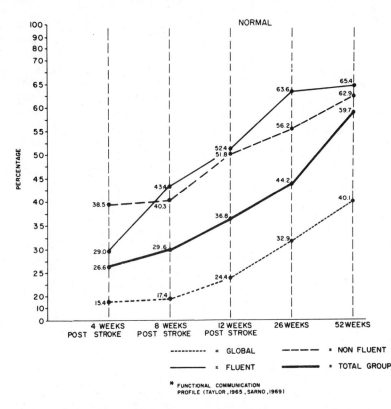

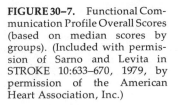

FIGURE 30–7. Functional Communication Profile Overall Scores (based on median scores by groups). (Included with permission of Sarno and Levita in STROKE 10:633–670, 1979, by permission of the American Heart Association, Inc.)

given to the patient by the speech pathologist.[30] Most speech pathologists agree that spontaneous recovery of speech is probably not finished until the end of the first three months. Following that time, as the patient reaches a plateau in his functional improvement with speech therapy and makes no progress for two or three weeks, speech therapy may be discontinued for a while or limited to a few drills that can be performed at home with a periodic follow-up. However, in most cases patients do show progress with speech therapy and it is feasible for the patient to continue speech therapy on an outpatient basis[31] (Fig. 30–7). This may continue for a long period of time, from 12 to 24 months. It is important to have evaluation by a speech pathologist for those patients with completed stroke who have a communication disorder.

Other Language Impairments in Stroke

Not all language impairments in stroke are due to involvement of specific speech areas in the left hemisphere. There may be confusion in language related to generalized reduced cognitive functioning. The patient with involvement of the right hemisphere may have impairment in language (particularly reading) due to visual-spatial and visual-motor impairment. In performing written arithmetic and reading he finds it difficult to follow the line across the page and to shift down from one line to the next. The speech pathologist can evaluate whether the patient is reliable in keeping his own checkbook and whether, even though he can read single words or sentences that are single lines, he cannot read an entire paragraph and control his eyes to read it in the proper sequence to get meaning. Even for these disorders there are some aspects of speech therapy that can be helpful, such as using a red line down the left margin of the page if the patient is having difficulty making his eyes track back far enough to the left. Also, if the patient has difficulty following a single line across the page in a paragraph, sometimes a piece of paper with a single line cut out, restricting visibility to one line at a time, will help.

Disorders of Speech Production

Dyspraxia. Dyspraxia in speech production is similar to dyspraxia in other kinds of motor function. It is an impairment of the ability of the patient to initiate simple voluntary motor acts. When the patient has difficulty in initiating voluntary motor function of the tongue and lips or cannot touch his tongue from one corner of the mouth to the other as directed or demonstrated, this condition is referred to as oral dyspraxia. On the other hand, some patients are able to move their tongue and lips on command or imitate tongue and lip movements of others but cannot initiate speech when asked to, even though they are capable of automatic speech that is quite clear and distinct. This is called oral verbal dyspraxia. Sometimes these patients need only a slight clue to get them started, such as making the first sound of a word. Unless the dyspraxia is severe, the prognosis is usually much better than the more severe forms of aphasia. However, it is not unusual for patients who have aphasia also to have some dyspraxia. It may take the speech pathologist working with the patient some time to be able to determine that both of these disorders are present. Hence, it is of great importance to have stroke patients with a confusing communication disorder evaluated by a speech pathologist who can advise others on the types of communication disorders present and on how to deal with the patient. For example, they can advise whether to try to guess the word that the patient is searching for, or to wait and give the patient time to find the word, or to give a clue by giving the first sound of the word that the patient is having difficulty initiating.

Dysarthria and Dysphonia. Other disorders of speech production are those associated with muscular weakness. Facial weakness on one side can be a cause of slurred speech referred to as dysarthria. Brain stem strokes may produce sufficient weakness in the laryngeal area to cause dysphonia or aphonia and render the patient speechless. Sometimes aphonic patients are mistakenly called aphasic and even assumed to have no auditory comprehension, when actually their only problem is difficulty in speech production. Of course, patients with dysarthria and dysphonia can communicate by writing, which is ordinarily unimpaired, but they have to perform this with their dominant hand.

EMOTIONAL RESPONSE AND PERSONALITY ASPECTS OF COMPLETED STROKE

In addition to the effects of brain damage on cognitive functioning and personality, the patient with recent onset of completed stroke reacts to the newly acquired disability in a manner similar to those with other types of new disability. These reactions can usually be categorized in order of occurrence and frequency as denial, depression, anxiety, and hostility.

There tends to be confusion regarding patients with brain damage who have the phenomenon of anosognosia, those who ignore the extremities on the involved side, and those who display the emotional response termed denial. Most feel that these are two separate phenomena, the anosognosia being neurological[16] and the denial being emotional.[15] They discourage the use of the term *anatomical denial* to substitute for the term anosognosia. Generally, denial is seen as a protective mechanism to allow the patient to get ready to accept the reality of the loss and thereby perhaps avoid a sudden profound depression.[26] Furthermore, most patients who experience completed stroke know of some stroke patients who had remarkable recovery. They like to cling to the idea that the neurologic deficits they have experienced may be only temporary.

Depression has been considered by some to be part of the natural history of stroke. They maintain that all patients with significant deficits in completed stroke are bound to experience considerable depression simply because brain damage itself causes depression. However, some of the depression may be preventable, particularly that associated with intellectual deterioration due to environmental deprivation due to isolation. Emotional lability associated with brain damage is sometimes confused with depression. The patient loses some of the inhibitory control over the expression of emotions, especially crying. This occurs with the slightest provocation but tends also to subside quickly. It often is much more easily tolerated by the patient and his family, particularly if the patient is male, if it is explained to them that this occurrence does not mean a weakness of character or that the patient is losing his mind and that usually it is not a permanent condition. Emotional lability gradually subsides, lasting rarely past the first year after onset of the stroke.

Nearly all patients with completed stroke have very easy fatigability. Some of these patients, when placed in an environment or situation in which they feel obligated to remain active for longer periods of time than they feel like doing, will experience cumulative fatigue that can sometimes give the impression of depression. During the early rehabilitation phase it is well for a patient to have rest periods in between appointments at various therapies. Generally for most stroke patients one of the most effective ways of counteracting depression is promoting a sense of progress and improvement. This can happen in rehabilitation, even when no further spontaneous return of neurologic function is occurring, if the therapist makes sure that the patient ends his daily periods of training with a performance he has learned to do well and provides positive verbal feedback to the patient for this successful performance.

It has been observed that premorbid personality traits of the patient appear to be exaggerated following completed stroke.[1] If the patient tended to be impulsive premorbidly, he tends to be even more impulsive after the stroke. For help in relieving both anxiety and depression reactions to stroke, counseling is certainly in order,[15] but nothing may be as helpful to the patient as seeing that he is making progress and improving his functional abilities and becoming less dependent. The professional staff working with the stroke patient who expresses hostility toward them should realize that sometimes this is a mechanism of the patient's saving himself from suffering acute guilt feelings and feeling responsible for his stroke. Rather, he puts the responsibility off onto the health care profession. This may be a way of having the stroke be less overwhelming to him.

Because there is a wide variation among people in all age groups in the amount of sexual activity they have, it cannot be assumed that sexuality is not important to the stroke patient; instead this subject should be explored.[11] For those patients who are concerned, specific counseling should be sought. The majority of stroke patients can continue to function sexually from a physical standpoint but need guidance and understanding from the health professionals and also their partners about readaptations that may need to be made.

BRAIN STEM INVOLVEMENT

One should be cautious in applying generalizations to an individual patient. Each patient should be evaluated and treated individually. This is certainly true for patients with involvement of the brain stem because it contains both the ascending and descending tracts as well as cranial nerve nuclei. Damage within this area can produce a wide variety of symptoms. An impairment of the vertebral vascular system in the brain stem can produce a crossed hemiplegia or quadriplegia as well as a variety of signs of cranial nerve, cerebellar, and sensory tract involvement. (See the section on dysarthria and dysphonia.) The patients with resulting ataxia may have normal motor strength but be quite disabled by their ataxia. There are specific types of coordination exercises for both upper and lower extremities that help the patient regain control of coordination and reduce the amount of ataxia. However, this type of training has to go on for a long period of time to produce significant clinical results observable in walking ability or in activities of daily living.

The speech pathologist can be of great help to patients who have brain stem involvement, not only to those who have difficulty in phonation but also to those who have difficulty in swallowing. Sometimes by experimentation the speech pathologist can find ways to enhance the swallowing mechanism so that the patient doesn't have to continue nasogastric tube feeding for a long period or have a gastrostomy performed.

VOCATIONAL ASPECTS

There has been a tendency in the past for patients who have completed stroke to be considered fit only for retirement, even though some of them may be considerably younger than retirement age. Part of this may be due to an attitude of the public of reluctance to hire or rehire a patient who has obvious hemiparesis. However, recent outcome studies[2, 4, 5] have made it clear that a larger percentage of patients with completed stroke are capable of some type of employment than had been assumed earlier. At the University of Minnesota a special long-term outcome study[4] of younger stroke patients was made because it was felt that vocational aspects may have been neglected. In these patients 54 per cent had returned to their usual daily activities, ranging from being employed full time or part time to being a full-time or part-time homemaker. In another study at the University of Minnesota,[2] only 53 per cent of post-rehabilitation stroke patients at all ages were unemployed at the time of follow-up. Hence the old attitude that most stroke patients are too old or too impaired to be able to get back into employment has been proved to be erroneous. Vocational rehabilitation replacement should be considered for all those patients with completed stroke who are under retirement age, if this is feasible.

REFERENCES

1. Allison, R.: The Senile Brain. London, Edw. Arnold, Ltd., 1962.
2. Anderson, E., Anderson, T. P., and Kottke, F. J.: Stroke rehabilitation: Maintenance of achieved gains. Arch. Phys. Med. Rehabil., 58:345–352, 1977.
3. Anderson, T. P., et al.: Predictive factors in stroke rehabilitation. Arch. Phys. Med. Rehabil., 55:545–553, 1974.
4. Anderson, T. P., et al.: Stroke rehabilitation: Evaluation of its quality by assessing patient outcomes. Arch. Phys. Med. Rehabil., 59:170–175, 1978.
5. Anderson, T. P., et al.: Quality of care of stroke without rehabilitation. Arch. Phys. Med. Rehabil., 60:103–107, 1979.
6. Anderson, T. P.: Management of completed stroke. J. Okla. State Med. Assoc., 63:403–411, 1970.
7. Anderson, T. P., and Kottke, F. J.: Stroke rehabilitation: A reconsideration of some common attitudes. Arch. Phys. Med. Rehabil., 58:175–181, 1978.
8. Bard, G., and Hirschberg, G. G.: Recovery of voluntary motion in upper extremity following hemiplegia. Arch. Phys. Med. Rehabil., 46:567–572, 1965.
9. Basmajian, J. V.: Muscles Alive: Their Functions Revealed by Electromyography. Baltimore, Williams & Wilkins, 1967.
10. Birch, H. G., et al.: Perception in hemiplegia: I. Judgement of vertical and horizontal. Arch. Phys. Med. Rehabil., 41:19–27, 1960.
11. Bray, G. P., et al.: Sexual functioning in stroke survivors. Arch. Phys. Med. Rehabil., 62:286–288, 1981.
12. Bruell, J. H., et al.: Perception of verticality in hemiplegia: Patients in relation to rehabilitation. Clin. Orthop., 12:124–130, 1958.
13. Carroll, D.: Hand function in hemiplegia. J. Chronic Dis., 18:493–500, 1965.
14. Feigenson, J. S., et al.: A comparison of outcome and cost for stroke patients treated in academic and community hospital centers. J.A.M.A., 240:1878–1880, 1978.
15. Fisher, S. H.: Psychiatric considerations of cerebral vascular disease. Am. J. Cardiol., 7:379–385, 1961.
16. Friedlander, W. J.: Anosognosia and perception. Am. J. Phys. Med., 46:1394–1408, 1967.
17. Halpern, D., and Meelhuysen, F. E.: Duration of relaxation after intramuscular neurolysis with phenol. J.A.M.A., 200:1152–1154, 1967.
18. Hausmanouva-Petrusewicz, I.: Interaction in simultaneous motor functions. A.M.A. Arch. Neurol. Psychiat., 81:173–181, 1959.
19. Kottke, F. J.: Neurophysiologic therapy for stroke. In Licht, S.: Stroke and Its Rehabilitation. New Haven, Conn., Elizabeth Licht, 1975.
20. Lehmann, J. F., et al.: Stroke rehabilitation: Outcome and prediction. Arch. Phys. Med. Rehabil., 56:383–389, 1975.
21. Lehmann, J. F., et al.: Stroke: Does rehabilitation affect outcome? Arch. Phys. Med. Rehabil., 56:375–382, 1975.
22. Machek, O.: Is elastic bracing contraindicated in spastics? Arch. Phys. Med. Rehabil., 39:245–246, 1958.
23. Matsumoto, N., et al.: Natural history of stroke in Rochester, Minnesota, 1955 through 1969: Extension of previous study 1945 through 1954. Stroke, 4:20–29, 1973.
24. McHenry, L. C., et al.: Essentials of stroke diagnosis and management. Philadelphia, Smith, Kline and French, 1973.
25. McHenry, L. C., and Jaffee, M. E.: Cerebrovascular disease, Part I. G.P., 37:88, 1968.
26. Mossman, P. L.: A Problem Oriented Approach to Stroke Rehabilitation. Springfield, Ill., Charles C Thomas, Publisher, 1976.
27. Rehabilitation Nursing Techniques—1: Bed Positioning and Transfer Procedures for the Hemiplegic. Minneapolis, Kenny Rehabilitation Institute, 1962.
28. Rehabilitation Nursing Techniques—4: Selfcare and Homemaking for the Hemiplegic. Minneapolis, Kenny Rehabilitation Institute, 1962.
29. Sarno, M. T.: Disorders of communication. In Licht, S.: Stroke and Its Rehabilitation. New Haven, Conn., Elizabeth Licht, 1975.
30. Sarno, M. T., Silverman, E., and Sands, E.: Speech therapy and language recovery in severe aphasia. J. Speech Hear. Res., 13:607, 1970.
31. Sarno, M. T., and Levita, E.: Recovery in treated aphasia in the first year post-stroke. Stroke, 10:663–670, 1979.
32. Schuell, H. M., et al.: Aphasia in Adults. Diagnosis, Prognosis and Treatment. New York, Hoeber, 1964.
33. Stern, P., et al.: Effects of facilitation exercise techniques in stroke rehabilitation. Arch. Phys. Med. Rehabil., 51:526–531, 1970.
34. Taylor, M., et al.: Perceptual training in patients with left hemiplegia. Arch. Phys. Med. Rehabil., 52:163–169, 1971.
35. Van Buskirk, C., and Webster, D.: Prognostic value of sensory defects in rehabilitation of hemiplegics. Neurology, 5:407–411, 1955.
36. Waylonis, G. W., et al.: Stroke rehabilitation in mid-western county. Arch. Phys. Med. Rehabil., 54:151–155, 1973.
37. Wepman, J. M., and Jones, L. V.: Five aphasias. A commentary on aphasia as a regressive linguistic phenomenon. In Rioch, D. M., and Weinstein, E. A.: Disorders of Communication. Baltimore, Williams & Wilkins Co., 1964.

31

REHABILITATION IN ARTHRITIS AND ALLIED CONDITIONS

ROBERT L. SWEZEY

The physiatrist is frequently called upon to assess and treat acute rheumatological and related musculoskeletal problems. He frequently serves as the primary diagnostician and manager to patients with degenerative joint disease and soft tissue rheumatism, as well as related discogenic disorders. He is therefore called upon to identify and distinguish systemic, inflammatory, and metabolic disorders that affect the joints and soft tissues, and the physiatrist may play a primary or adjunctive role in the management of these conditions. He must therefore be equipped to diagnose and/or understand the significance of various diagnostic categories of rheumatic diseases and to perceive when additional diagnostic clarification may be required in those patients referred for adjunctive therapies.

There are four major categories of rheumatological disorders to be considered. They include degenerative joint diseases, rheumatoid arthritis and related inflammatory processes, metabolic disorders affecting joints, and periarticular conditions. As is invariably the case in medical diagnosis, a careful history and physical examination are essential for an accurate diagnosis. A careful searching for clues of relevant systemic disease, such as a history of sun sensitivity, neuritis, urethritis, syphilis, exposure to hepatitis, and passage of a kidney stone, as well as

familial predispositions, may alert the clinician to select those diagnostic measures most likely to lead to a correct diagnosis.

From a musculoskeletal disease standpoint the clinician must first determine if the joint is indeed involved. Circumferential tenderness around the joint is highly indicative of an intra-articular process. In degenerative joint disease only one surface of the joint may be tender, but this is rarely the case in an inflammatory disorder. Restriction of joint motion, swelling, redness, and heat all point to intra-articular inflammatory disease. The clinician must then determine whether more than one joint is involved. Here again, careful palpation of all symptomatic joint margins may elicit evidence of more than one affected joint and lead to the appropriate polyarticular diagnostic category.

Table 31–1 outlines the major diagnostic considerations when one is confronted with a true monoarticular arthritis. In a monoarticular arthritis the most important decision to be made is whether or not infection is present. Synovial fluid aspiration is therefore essential; even if it is questionable whether synovial fluid has been obtained, a culture should be made from serum or blood from the aspirating needle.[1] Table 31–2 indicates various diagnoses that can be sorted out by an analysis of the synovial fluid. An elevated synovial fluid leukocyte count with a high

TABLE 31–1. DIAGNOSTIC CONSIDERATIONS IN MONOARTICULAR ARTHRITIS

Transient (< 2 Weeks)	Acute	Subacute-Chronic
Initial phase of polyarthritis	Infection – septic	Infection – granuloma, TB
Palindromic rheumatism	Gout/pseudogout	Gout/pseudogout
Intermittent hydroarthrosis	Rheumatoid and variants	Rheumatoid and variants
Acute periarthritis	Trauma	Osteoarthritis
		Tumor
		Neuropathic (Charcot)
		Chronic periarthritis

percentage of polymorphonuclear leukocytes suggests infection; an analysis for crystals using polarizing light with a red compensating filter is invaluable in identifying sodium urate or calcium pyrophosphate crystals. A low serum complement is suggestive of rheumatoid arthritis or lupus, and an elevated serum complement is suggestive of Reiter's syndrome. A depression of the synovial fluid sugar may be seen in a number of inflammatory disorders but is suggestive of infection. Less specific indicators of inflammation are an elevated synovial fluid protein and reduced synovial fluid mucin viscosity.

If the disorder is polyarticular, then a much wider range of diagnostic considerations must be entertained. Table 31–3 outlines many of those considerations and characterizes them further into the rheumatoid-like inflammatory disorders, the degenerative disorders, and acute and chronic metabolic disorders. In Table 31–4 the various diagnostic considerations that can be brought forward from the laboratory are outlined. Table 31–5 delineates those clues that can be obtained from x-ray of joints in addition to the affected joint or joints in question. Specific features of x-rays that are often diagnostic are outlined in Table 31–6, and Table 31–7 lists supplementary non-articular radiographic examinations that may be of great importance in establishing the final rheumatological diagnosis.

The various diagnostic laboratory and x-ray procedures accompanied by appropriate joint or other tissue biopsy will usually lead to the correct diagnosis, but only if the clinician has carefully performed his initial clinical evaluations. In making his assignment, there are *certain features that must be kept in mind if an accurate assessment of the clinical findings is to be made.* Whenever an apparent normal range of joint mobility is found where one has reason to suspect an abnormality, hypermobility on the *opposite side should be sought.* Bilateral *elbow joint contractures* are often telltale indicators of current or previous rheumatoid disease. They may, however, represent congenital abnormalities, and this can usually be established by asking the patient. Congenital flexion contractures of the proximal interphalangeal (PIP) joints of the fifth fingers are particularly common. Restricted flexion of the distal interphalangeal (DIP) joints to 45 degrees found in multiple joints or in symmetrical joints is usually a congenital variation. A normal PIP joint should flex beyond 90 degrees to approximately 110 to 120 degrees. A *subluxation of a small joint is detected by the sensation of a distinct ledge,* rather than an indented cleft (a bayonet configuration) at the adjacent joint margins. Most patients over age 50 have restriction of internal rotation of both hips. If restriction of mobility of the hip joints is asymmetrical or all planes of motion are restricted and painful, then hip joint involvement is highly suspect. Restrictions of joint mobility may be very difficult to assess in the presence of severe pain, and one should not assume a contracture where reflex muscle spasm may be restricting joint motion. Pain also alters the response on muscle testing. In the presence of joint disease, the joint should be placed and supported so as to minimize pain and then the muscle in question tested isometrically. If care is taken to avoid pain one will get a "normal" response to manual tests performed in the above manner unless true neuropathic or myopathic disease or muscle-tendon rupture is present.[2, 3]

DIAGNOSTIC AND THERAPEUTIC CONSIDERATIONS IN JOINT DISEASES

Just as certain features of various joint disorders help characterize them diagnosti-

TABLE 31–2. MAJOR CATEGORIZATIONS BY SYNOVIAL FLUID ANALYSIS

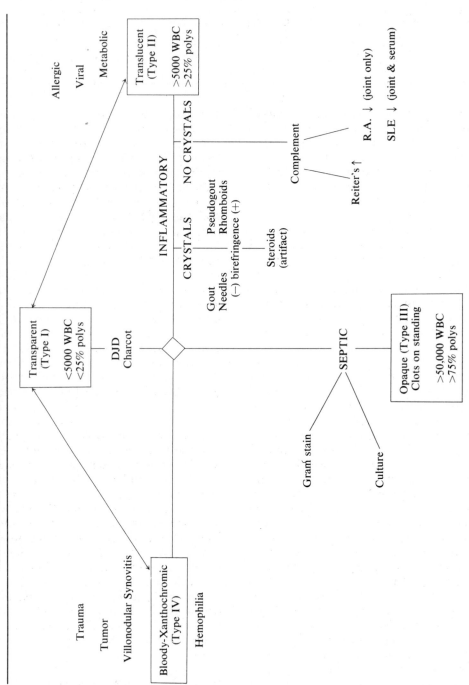

cally, the pathophysiology of the joint disorder, its natural history, the location of the joints that are affected, the severity of the joint involvements, and the customary response to treatment of the joint disorder in question will all help determine the ordering of specific therapeutic interventions.

Osteoarthritis (Degenerative Joint Disease)

Although osteoarthritis is relatively rare in young adults, it can be predictably diagnosed in association with the inevitable disc degeneration of the spine in all patients over the age of 50. The problem is whether or not roentgenographic confirmation of osteoarthritis can be correlated with clinical symptoms. Obviously this is not true in the case of spinal discogenic disease in the geriatric population, but *most patients with radiographic evidence of osteoarthritis in other axial or peripheral joints will either have or give a history of having had symptoms.*

Osteoarthritis is a disorder in which bony proliferation at the joint margins and subchondral bone is a consequence of deterioration in the articular cartilage. The earliest changes in osteoarthritis are a depolymerization of the glycoprotein ground substance surrounding the chondrocytes, and this is subsequently associated with fissuring of the overlying cartilage surface, wearing away of the cartilage surface, and bony proliferations that may lead to juxta-articular bony cyst formation with ultimate collapse of these cysts and derangements of joint surfaces.[4] The synovial fluid that nourishes the cartilage and lubricates the joint surfaces does not appear to be at fault as a lubricant, and the exact mechanism whereby the cartilage deteriorates cannot always be ascertained.[5-7]

In those disorders in which the osteoarthritis is secondary to a previous trauma or inflammation, the basis for the particular cartilage deterioration is apparent. In the so-called primary osteoarthritis a genetic factor is clearly operative, but the biochemical nature of the defect that renders the cartilage susceptible to deterioration has not yet been identified. Primary osteoarthritis is characterized by its dominant genetic inheritance pattern, which is fully expressed in females after the menopause and less often expressed in the male siblings. Characteristically it affects the distal interphalangeal joints and the carpometacarpal joint of the thumbs. The distal interphalangeal joint involvement creates bony prominences on the dorsal surface, originally described by Heberden, and similar subsequent involvement of the proximal interphalangeal joints is called Bouchard's nodes. Patients with severe primary generalized osteoarthritis may also have involvement of the knees, much less commonly the hips, and occasionally the small joints in the toes in addition to the first MTP joint.[7] Acromioclavicular joints may be affected, and only rarely are the glenohumeral joints involved. Generally the elbows and ankles are spared. The wrists, however, are occasionally involved in the joints between the navicular and lunate and navicular and greater multangular.

There are two distinctive features of primary osteoarthritis that merit comment. Although the typical development of Heberden's nodes is minimally symptomatic or asymptomatic, on occasion the onset can be fairly acute and accompanied by a cystic erythematous mass overlying the DIP joint, which is red and extremely tender. The mass, which may persist for months, consists of a mucinous cyst that communicates with the joint. Local steroid injections and rest or splinting will usually relieve the acute symptoms. Less commonly the distal interphalangeal and occasionally proximal interphalangeal joint involvement is characterized by an aggressive, erosive, destructive process that pathologically is manifested by an acute inflammatory reaction and that leads to marked destruction and derangement of the affected DIP and PIP joints, the so-called erosive osteoarthritis. Synovectomy and surgical stabilization of the affected joints may occasionally be necessary to preserve function in such cases.[8]

The *most disabling problem in the hand in association with primary osteoarthritis* is *the involvement of the first carpometacarpal joint.* Atrophy of the overlying thenar musculature and inhibition of normal joint use lead to an adductor contracture with impairment of grasp and pinch. Splinting to stabilize this joint in addition to occasional use of local steroid injections with gentle stretching of the adductor musculature between the thumb and index metacarpals can help preserve mobility (Fig. 31–1). Excision of the greater multangular or joint replacement and

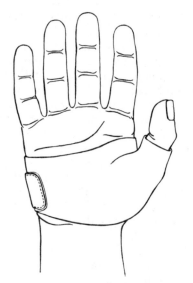

FIGURE 31–1. Plastic stabilizing splint to restrict motion of the carpometacarpal and metacarpophalangeal joints of the thumb. This splint allows full interphalangeal flexion. The distal palmar edge of the splint is proximal to the distal palmar crease so as not to restrict MCP flexion of the fingers. (From Swezey, R. L.: Arthritis: Rational Therapy in Rehabilitation. Philadelphia, W. B. Saunders Company, 1978.)

occasionally fusion of the carpometacarpal joint are occasionally necessary to relieve pain and preserve function. As is generally true in the management of osteoarthritis when avoidance of joint stress and/or stabilization and/or the use of occasional local steroid injections are insufficient, local heat, salicylates, and occasional use of other analgesics and/or nonsteroidal anti-inflammatory drugs may be helpful in management of the specific joint problem.

Osteoarthritis of the hip is an insidious problem of middle and late adult life that typically manifests itself with pain in the groin, as well as in the buttock and lateral thigh. Congenital shortening of the leg on the affected side, pathology of the opposite knee, a childhood slipped capital femoral epiphysis, and osteochondritis are common predisposing factors in addition to previous inflammatory arthritis or trauma.[7] Nevertheless, for most patients who develop osteoarthritis of the hip the cause is not easily ascertained. Pain in the buttock area is often attributed to the hip when in fact it may be due to lumbar discogenic disease. Pain in the upper lateral thigh may be due to trochanteric bursitis, which is commonly seen in

association with osteoarthritis of the hip, but it may also be an unrelated problem. In addition to pharmacological measures, which again include salicylates, mild analgesics, nonsteroidal anti-inflammatory drugs, and a trial of local steroid injections, the rehabilitative management consists of relief of weight-bearing stresses by the use of a cane or crutches, early stretching of the tight hip musculature to maintain good mobility and joint surface apposition for optimal joint nutrition, and strengthening of the hip musculature.[9] Activities that cause undue stress, including jogging and hiking, are best avoided. In all overweight patients with arthritis in weight-bearing joints, weight reduction is an important factor. Bicycling may be tolerated if there is little inflammatory reaction in the hip. Swimming is the optimal overall exercise, both for mobilizing the hip and strengthening the musculature and for its general conditioning effect on patients whose athletic activities are otherwise circumscribed. When pain cannot be well controlled with the above regimens and particularly when pain consistently disturbs rest at night and/or functional activities are greatly limited, surgical therapy is indicated.[10, 11]

Osteoarthritis of the knee is frequently a result of damage secondary to meniscal injury and other trauma. Patellofemoral compartment degeneration (chondromalacia of the patella) is a disorder that affects young people and is the exception to the usual pattern of medial tibiofemoral joint disease with narrowing of the tibiofemoral compartment and early proliferation of osteophytes on the opposing medial tibial and femoral borders.[12] People with genu varus deformities carry the bulk of their weight-bearing stresses in the medial compartment and are predisposed to osteoarthritis in that area, as opposed to those with valgus angulation of the knee joint, who are predisposed to lateral tibiofemoral joint disease.

The treatment of osteoarthritis of the knee includes the same drug and local steroid considerations previously described for the hip, as well as the recommendations for avoidance of weight-bearing stress. In all disorders of joints, as is particularly obvious in the knee, atrophy of the related musculature occurs as a consequence of the reduction in active use of the affected joint. Quadriceps strengthening and instruction in body mechanics to avoid unnecessary knee stress

TABLE 31–3. DIFFERENTIAL DIAGNOSIS OF POLYARTHRITIS

POLYARTHRITIS

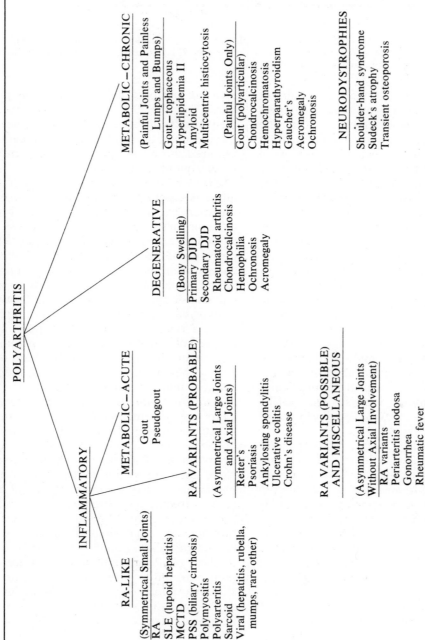

INFLAMMATORY

RA-LIKE

(Symmetrical Small Joints)
RA
SLE (lupoid hepatitis)
MCTD
PSS (biliary cirrhosis)
Polymyositis
Polyarteritis
Sarcoid
Viral (hepatitis, rubella, mumps, rare other)

METABOLIC–ACUTE

Gout
Pseudogout

RA VARIANTS (PROBABLE)

(Asymmetrical Large Joints and Axial Joints)
Reiter's
Psoriasis
Ankylosing spondylitis
Ulcerative colitis
Crohn's disease

RA VARIANTS (POSSIBLE) AND MISCELLANEOUS

(Asymmetrical Large Joints Without Axial Involvement)
RA variants
Periarteritis nodosa
Gonorrhea
Rheumatic fever
Pulmonary osteoarthropathy
Serum sickness (drug reactions)
Sickle cell disorders
Relapsing polychondritis
Periodic disorders (FMF)
Henoch-Schönlein's
Behçet's

DEGENERATIVE

(Bony Swelling)
Primary DJD
Secondary DJD
Rheumatoid arthritis
Chondrocalcinosis
Hemophilia
Ochronosis
Acromegaly

METABOLIC–CHRONIC

(Painful Joints and Painless Lumps and Bumps)
Gout–tophaceous
Hyperlipidemia II
Amyloid
Multicentric histiocytosis

(Painful Joints Only)
Gout (polyarticular)
Chondrocalcinosis
Hemochromatosis
Hyperparathyroidism
Gaucher's
Acromegaly
Ochronosis

NEURODYSTROPHIES

Shoulder-hand syndrome
Sudeck's atrophy
Transient osteoporosis

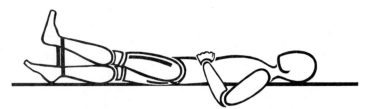

FIGURE 31-2. Isometric counter-resistance exercise of quadriceps vs. contralateral gluteal and hamstring muscles using an elastic band or belt looped over both ankles. (From Swezey, R. L.: Arthritis: Rational Therapy in Rehabilitation. Philadelphia, W. B. Saunders Company, 1978.)

that may occur when arising from chairs or toilet stools that are too low are key features in successful management. Isometric strengthening of the quadriceps musculature should be initiated in a regimen consisting of 6 seconds of quadriceps strengthening twice daily (Fig. 31-2). The exercise should be performed in a position of maximum comfort, which is usually in extension for the patient with osteoarthritis of the knee, and particularly for those patients with patello-femoral compartment disease. There is no established basis for the additional use of iso-tonic or isokinetic exercise, although these may be added if desired, but only when pain permits (see discussion of exercise in arthritis).[13]

Flexion contractures in osteoarthritic knees are usually minimal, and apparent contractures in more advanced cases may be a consequence of bony obstruction; therefore, range of motion exercises may not be required in many cases of osteoarthritis of the knee.

Attention to leg length discrepancies should be given, and at least a 50 per cent compensation in the height of the shortened extremity should be made. For both the hip and the knee, good supporting footwear is essential to minimize joint stress. A shock-absorbing sole is useful; however, the sole should not be made of a crepe so soft that it creates an unstable gait because of excessive yielding at heel strike. A maximum heel height of one inch is recommended for any patient with osteoarthritis of the knee, and this is particularly important in patients with patellofemoral joint compartment disease, for which a negative heel may actually be preferred.

When conservative measures have failed to provide sufficient pain relief or restoration of function, surgical procedures must be considered. The success rate of the numerous variations on total knee replacement does not approach that of the total hip procedures.[10, 11, 14, 15] The postoperative management is difficult because of pain and because more cooperation on the part of the patient is required during the postoperative period to restore mobility and function.

Osteoarthritis of the foot and ankle. The ankle is essentially spared by osteoarthritic disorders except as a consequence of trauma or secondary to another disease process such as rheumatoid arthritis. The management of these problems includes the usual pharmacological and local steroid therapy considerations, avoidance of weight-bearing stresses, and use of appropriate supporting footwear. Supportive footwear may include a high-top shoe, a rigid shank, a cushion heel, and a rocker sole. In those patients in whom distress is not being controlled by these measures, a below-knee weight-bearing brace or surgical therapy must be considered.[16] *Osteoarthritic changes in the proximal tarsal joints* are not uncommon; the bony prominences protruding from the dorsal surfaces of these joints are common and sometimes symptomatic. Therapeutic considerations include good supporting footwear with multiple lacings to give a supporting corset effect to the proximal tarsal joints.

The most common problems in the forefoot are those that affect the great toe. Hallux valgus and secondary osteoarthritis of the first MTP joint and/or IP joint are common disabling disorders. Appropriate shoewear with adequate room in the forefoot and a rigid sole with the roll-over or rocker feature or an orthosis providing similar features to minimize stress in the joints is helpful.[16] Local steroid injections are occasionally of value in relieving acute symptomatology. Surgical therapy to improve cosmesis is useful and can be helpful in relieving pain in refractory cases. The status of prosthetic arthroplasties of the MTP joint is not established, but this may hold promise to achieve not only improved cosmesis and pain relief, but also improved toe-off function during ambulation.

Soft Tissue Rheumatism (Bursitis and Fibrositis)

If until the recent advent of reconstructive surgery osteoarthritis has been the step-child of rheumatology, then the soft tissue disorders have been the orphans. Musculoskeletal complaints attributable to soft tissue rheumatism probably account for the vast majority of rheumatological disorders. Because the complaints are often mild and accepted as part of the natural course of events and because many of the problems are self-limited and the justification for surgical intervention almost nil, there has been relatively little interest in defining the nature of these problems and in developing rational approaches to their management. Perhaps the major deterrent to careful assessment of these disorders is the lack of "objective" findings such as laboratory or x-ray confirmation of a diagnosis. Calcium deposits in tendons and bursae may be found on occasion, and they may or may not correlate with the clinical condition in question. The clinician is left with his fingertips and thumbs and his knowledge of anatomy and kinesiology to locate the source of the patient's complaint. Having done so, he must presume more knowledge than he can confirm in establishing the diagnosis, e.g., is the painful shoulder due to a rotator cuff tendinitis, a bicipital tendinitis, a subacromial bursitis, a referred cervical myalgia, an idiopathic adhesive capsulitis, or a true arthritis? The examiner's knowledge, hands, and the lack of supporting evidence for other conditions allow him to make his diagnosis — i.e., bicipital tendinitis. Who can refute him?

There are, in fact, a number of disorders that are commonly seen and for which either definitive or presumptive diagnoses of soft tissue rheumatism can be made.[17] In general, one can say that *the management of soft tissue disorders* will depend on their severity and chronicity. Treatments will consist variably of the use of cold applications in acute processes; warm compresses in more chronic processes; diathermy for diffuse chronic processes, and ultrasound for focal chronic processes; rest of the part, which may include immobilization by sling or splint in the more acute disorders and functional splinting in more quiescent disorders; and adjunctive therapy consisting of analgesics and nonsteroidal anti-inflammatory drugs, depending on the severity of the process.[18] By and large *those focal disorders* of ligaments, tendons, or bursae (see muscle trigger areas) *that are either very severe* or *very persistent, e.g.,* lasting more than three or four weeks, are most expeditiously treated by the use of a local steroid injection consisting of approximately 5 mg of triamcinolone in 1 to 2 ml of 1 per cent lidocaine, followed by range-of-motion exercises to increase mobility if mobility of the affected joint area has been lost and then isometric exercises of the affected related musculature. Isometric exercises are first performed in a restricted range and, when tolerated, at the extremes of joint range with or without the addition of isokinetic exercise. Instruction in body mechanics is essential to help avoid the stresses that predispose to the problem.

Fibrositis Syndrome. The most elusive disorder of the various conditions that can be categorized under soft tissue rheumatism is the fibrositis syndrome. It consists of local and focal areas of muscle tenderness (*trigger areas*) usually limited to the region of the axial skeleton extending over the shoulder and hip areas and out onto the trunk. Occasionally ramifications of this disorder will be felt in so-called trigger areas as far as the ankle, and not uncommonly in the posterior calf in either of the heads of the gastrocnemius muscle or at the musculotendinous juncture of the soleus muscle.[19-21] The term *fibrositis* is undoubtedly a misnomer, because true inflammation has not been observed.[22] The basic pathology appears to be the development of hyperirritable and usually anatomically predictable so-called "trigger" areas of muscle spasm, usually as a consequence of pain referral from axial skeletal or, less commonly, large proximal joint derangements.[19-22] Pathologically whereas inflammation is lacking, an increased intracellular amorphous deposit with increased numbers of mast cells, platelets, and giant intracellular myofilaments has been observed.[22] Electromyographic abnormalities have been inconsistent, but short duration high-pitched motor unit potentials have been noted by several observers when a needle electrode is inserted into the trigger point. There has been no evidence of consistent motor unit firing nor evidence of muscle spasm per se by electromyographic criteria.[21, 23] A recent report indicates a disturbance of normal delta wave sleep patterns in patients with the fibrositis syndrome with reduction in symptoms as a consequence of chlorpromazine therapy used to induce normal sleep patterns.[19] From a clinical standpoint a fibrositic syndrome may therefore occur as a primary disorder, perhaps related to sleep disturbance, and as a secondary disorder related to a variety of focal or general inflammatory and degenerative joint disorders. The recognition of the primary fibrositic syndrome is important in that many of these patients who are tense, worried, and particularly fearful that they are developing a severe arthritic disease are greatly benefited by the reassurance that this is not the case. These patients are susceptible to cold and drafts. Fatigue and nervous tension aggravate their symptoms. They should be cautioned against exposing themselves to these stresses, but at the same time it should be pointed out that the only danger is temporarily increased pain and discomfort, and not a progressive crippling joint problem.

Mechanical stresses from inappropriate body mechanics during activities or during sedentary occupations should be avoided. Typically, it is suggested to the patient that he obtain a firm mattress or place a board under the mattress and that he obtain proper seating and lighting as well as needed spectacles for reading purposes or television viewing. Instructions are given in general warm-up and conditioning exercises to maintain body mobility and conditioning so that unaccustomed activities are less apt to precipitate fibrositic stresses. When symptoms are persistent, the local trigger areas can be treated with ice massage, fluorimethane spray and stretch techniques, kneading massage, local heat, local electrical stimulation, and local ultrasound, in addition to mild analgesics such as aspirin or acetaminophen.[21, 24, 26] Local 1 per cent lidocaine injections are often helpful in the management of severe or refractory "trigger" areas. Note that since the trigger areas are apparently areas of reflex muscular irritability rather than inflammation, the addition of local steroids to injection therapy offers no additional advantage and may produce unneeded local irritation at the injection site.

The fact that tension, fatigue, and psychological stresses exacerbate this problem does not make it a psychogenic rheumatism per se, but psychological and social counseling may be of additional benefit in many of these patients. When the fibrositic nodules occur secondary to other pathology such as lumbar or cervical discogenic disease, appropriate therapy directed to these problems, in addition to the local therapy to the reflex trigger areas, may facilitate the total management.

Some of the *common locations for trigger areas* in muscles are the origins and insertion of the upper trapezii at the base of the skull and just superior to the superior medial angle of the scapulae along the lower third of the medial angle of the scapulae and the rhomboid, in the paracervical musculature, at the lateral edge of the quadratus lumborum, at the origin of the erector spinae just medial to the posterior superior iliac spine, in the gluteus medius origin just below the iliac crest, and in the areas overlying the sciatic outlet, the subgluteus medius, and subgluteus maximus bursae.[20, 21, 25, 26] Less commonly they can be found in the scalenes, infraspinati, anterior tibials, gastrocnemii, and soleus muscles.[20, 21, 25, 26]

Often confused with these focal trigger areas are fibrofatty nodules that may range in number from one to many and that are typically located in the region of the posterior superior iliac spines.[27] These are benign and in this author's experience never a cause of symptoms. Severe and diffuse stiffness, aching, and "fibrositic" symptoms are characteristic of polymyalgia rheumatica and accompany rheumatoid arthritis, ankylosing spondylitis, hypothyroidism, and viral infections.

Focal Syndromes

Tendinitis and bursitis occur as a consequence of repeated low grade irritation due to unaccustomed or excessively strenuous activity in otherwise normal structures or as a result of such activity that is poorly tolerated in abnormal structures. Typical examples are trochanteric bursitis associated with hip joint disease or anserine bursitis in association with osteoarthritis of the knees. Calcific deposits (calcium hydroxyapatite crystals) in tendinous areas, most notably the rotator cuff tendon, may be extruded into adjacent bursae and produce an acute crystal-induced bursitis.[28] This is often an extremely painful disorder, such that the patient suffers agonizing pain even at rest and will not accept the best intended examination. X-ray documentation of this diagnosis may or may not be made because of the edema associated with the inflammatory reaction and the diffusion of the extruded calcium hydroxyapatite crystals into the swollen bursal area. Calcium hydroxyapatite crystals associated with tendinitis may also occasionally be seen in the region of the trochanteric bursa and rarely in the region of the short thumb extensor tendon in association with De Quervain's disease.

There is a disorder, acute calcific periarthritis, in which calcific deposits recur variously, most commonly in the region of the extensor carpi ulnaris at the wrist and in and around the small joints of the hands.[29] Although usually idiopathic, it may rarely be seen in association with either hyperparathyroidism or as a complication of chronic kidney disease, in particular, renal dialysis.[30]

Acute bursitis, with or without local crystal extrusions, is treated with analgesic medication, cold or ice applications, immobilization, and nonsteroidal anti-inflammatory agents.[28] If a prompt response is not seen, short-term oral steroids (if not otherwise contraindicated) such as prednisone in a dose of 0.5 mg/kg for three or four days will usually provide relief. Local steroid injections are equally beneficial, but when the pain is extremely severe, the patient may not accept this procedure. When symptoms have abated sufficiently, first gentle range of motion exercises followed later by active stretching to restore loss of mobility and finally isometric exercises to regain strength should be instituted.

A *rule of thumb in the management of all painful joint disorders* is to *restore mobility as a first priority* rather than risk exacerbation of symptoms in a strengthening regimen that might lead ultimately to aggravation of the joint problem and loss of motion and function. It should also be mentioned that local corticosteroid injections into tendons can cause collagen necrosis, and a steroid should never be forced from the syringe but rather should flow freely into the tendon sheath or bursal space during the injection. Excessive use of a damaged tendon made possible by pain relief from steroid injection may predispose a tendon to rupture. The patient should be instructed to avoid excessive use of tendinous structures following injections for a period of four weeks.

There are several bursal areas in addition to the subacromial bursa that merit comment. The *olecranon bursa* may swell as a consequence of rheumatoid arthritis, often with associated subcutaneous nodule formation, and it may also become swollen without severe pain in patients with gout. Where there is no adequate explanation for the olecranon bursal swelling, the bursa should be aspirated and a synovial fluid analysis made. There are two bursae that are consistently present around the hip: the *subgluteus medius bursa,* which lies deep to the insertion of the gluteus medius muscle at the superior angle of the greater trochanter, and the *subgluteus maximus bursa,* which lies beneath the latter muscle at the inferior lateral edge of the greater trochanter near the insertion of the gluteus maximus into the fascia lata. These bursae become irritated in association with mechanical stresses about the hip joint secondary to arthritis of the hip, leg length discrepancies assoicated with contractures of the muscles attaching to the fascia lata (the fascia lata syndrome), or static or dynamic postural stresses in association with low back pain.[31] In many instances in which lumbar discogenic disease is present and pain is referred, trochanteric bursal irritation can be confused with radiculitis because of its referral into the lateral thigh. It is difficult, if not impossible, to determine whether or not the focal tenderness found in the trochanteric bursal locations is secondary to muscle trigger areas or to bursal involvement per se, but in this author's experience, in contrast with muscle trigger areas, local steroid injections have proved to be far more effective than any other therapeutic intervention regardless of whether the hip joint or a lumbar disc disease was the inciting factor.

When the bursitis is severe, cold compresses are useful; when the bursitis has largely subsided, gentle mobilizing exercises are performed, initially with the patient supine with the knees flexed and feet flat, and then both legs rotated to the side opposite that of the affected bursa in a manner to cause a mild stretch but to avoid exacerbating pain. When the contralateral knee can be rotated to touch the floor, then a more advanced pelvis and hip rotation exercise can be instituted (Fig. 31–3).

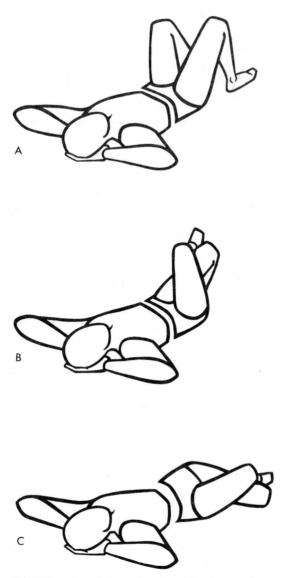

FIGURE 31–3. Active assisted stretch of external rotary components of hip and lumbosacral fascia. (From Swezey, R. L.: Arthritis: Rational Therapy in Rehabilitation. Philadelphia, W. B. Saunders Company, 1978.)

The *anserine bursa* lies on the anterior medial surface of the tibia about 2 to 3 cm below the tibial plateau. It separates the junction of the sartorius, gracilis, and semitendinosus muscles from the tibia. Irritation of this bursa occurs in association with osteoarthritis of the knee and the mechanical stresses that accompany varus deformity.[32] Treatment directed toward relieving irritation in the knee, improving the quadriceps function, and stabilizing the knee with an elastic knee support, and the use of a cane or crutches all may be beneficial. Local steroid injections are very useful in obtaining prompt relief and may obviate the need for more aggressive therapy to the knee joint per se. As in all chronic conditions, analgesics and nonsteroidal anti-inflammatory drugs may be of additional benefit. In addition to the anserine bursa, there are bursae located between the skin and the patella — the so-called prepatellar bursa, the suprapatellar bursa or pouch, which is actually a part of the knee joint itself, and the small bursae lying between the medial or lateral collateral ligaments and the joint margins.[33] These small bursae can become highly irritated in patients with osteoarthritis of the knee and will respond to measures outlined for the anserine bursa.

There are several other bursae that much less commonly cause symptoms. The ischiogluteal bursa, when irritated, can be a source of pain on sitting (Weaver's bottom). Hyperflexion of the thigh performed with the knee flexed to eliminate sciatic stretch will cause exquisite tenderness over the ischial tuberosity. Modification of patients' activities and the use of padded seating, as well as the general therapeutic principles previously described, are recommended. There are bursae lying superficial to and deep to the Achilles tendon that can be irritated. These may be affected in association with ankylosing spondylitis, and indeed this disorder would be suspected when bursitis in this area is observed. In addition to the usual therapeutic consideration, the use of a cushioned and raised heel to minimize stretch on the Achilles tendon may increase comfort and minimize recurrences.

Tendinitis

The hypermobility of the glenohumeral joint may predispose it to the stresses that make tendinitis and bursitis so common in this joint area. Except in those cases in which aspiration of the subacromial-deltoid bursa reveals synovial fluid and calcium hydroxyapatite crystals, there is really no sure way to distinguish between subacromial bursitis, rotator cuff tendinitis, and biceps tendinitis. Calcification in the rotator cuff tendon may suggest that a tendinitis exists, but does not prove its etiology in the patient's shoulder complaint. The clinician can palpate the anterior capsule of the glenohumeral

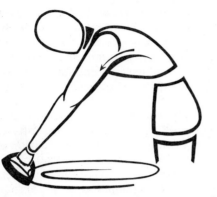

FIGURE 31–4. Gravity-assisted active pendular shoulder exercise to increase range of motion. There is better relaxation if the patient lies prone with the arm hanging over the side of the plinth and a 5-pound weight is suspended from the wrist. (From Swezey, R. L.: Arthritis: Rational Therapy in Rehabilitation. Philadelphia, W. B. Saunders Company, 1978.)

FIGURE 31–5. Shoulder mobility exercises using a wand to provide active assistance from the opposite upper extremity. (From Swezey, R. L.: Arthritis: Rational Therapy in Rehabilitation. Philadelphia, W. B. Saunders Company, 1978.)

joint just lateral to the coracoid process, and the findings of an accentuation of tenderness in this area suggest intra-articular glenohumeral joint disease. By the same token, palpation over the acromioclavicular joint may localize a diagnosis to that area. One is left with palpation in most instances to arbitrarily distinguish between biceps tendinitis and rotator cuff tendinitis. With the arm in the anatomical position, the biceps tendon passes anteriorly over the humerus, and local tenderness in that area as opposed to tenderness over the greater tuberosity is the usual basis for distinguishing these two disorders. A positive Yergason's sign — shoulder pain elicited by resisting supination and external rotation of the forearm while the upper arm is kept adducted and fixed alongside the trunk — adds strong support to the diagnosis of biceps tendinitis.[28] As a practical matter one uses palpation to attempt to localize the seat of the pathology and then is guided clinically by what is found. If rotator cuff tendinitis or biceps tendinitis is suspected, local measures depending on the severity of the problem are used for pain relief, and stress of the affected area is avoided. By and large the use of diathermy and ultrasound or other modalities is not as effective as local steroid injections in obtaining prompt subsidence of pain. The use of local cold or heat and occasionally transcutaneous nerve stimulation may facilitate joint mobilization. Because of the propensity of the glenohumeral joint to undergo

contracture, early and prompt attention is directed toward mobilizing exercises beginning with pendulum (Codman) exercises (Fig. 31–4) in the more acute cases, and progressing through reciprocal pulleys and wand exercises to attempt to restore full mobility if possible when pain has subsided (Figs. 31–5 and 31–6). When pain is under sufficient control that resistive exercises can

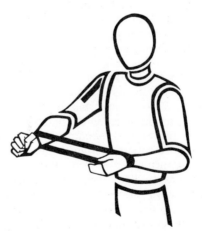

FIGURE 31–6. Isometric bilateral shoulder abduction and external rotation resistance exercise using a belt around the wrists. (From Swezey, R. L.: Arthritis: Rational Therapy in Rehabilitation. Philadelphia, W. B. Saunders Company, 1978.)

be commenced, isometric exercises first to the deltoid and then to the external and internal rotators are taught. These should be performed in the comfortable range of motion of the shoulder in order to obtain forceful contractions and to avoid exacerbating the painful shoulder disorder itself. Exercises to increase mobility of the shoulder should focus first on restoration of flexion and then on external and internal rotation.[34] When these are restored, abduction is usually restored as well, and, if not, can be more easily accomplished at the time that the other motions have returned toward normal and pain has abated. To attempt to achieve abduction, particularly with the hand pronated, is to risk impingement of the greater tuberosity on the coracoacromial ligament and exacerbation of pain and prolongation rather than amelioration of the shoulder problem.

Lateral and Medial Epicondylitis ("Tennis" and "Golfer's" Elbows). Epicondylitis is a strain of the tendinous insertions of the finger and wrist extensors (lateral epicondylitis) or flexors (medial epicondylitis) and occurs as a consequence of repetitive and/or forceful actions by these muscle groups either in work or in recreational activities. "Tennis elbow" can occur in various hand activities such as wood chopping, hammering, and nut grinding, and the same applies to medial epicondylitis. Management of these problems consists of rest of the affected extremity, avoidance of stress (handshaking by politicians and ministers is a notorious offender), use of mild analgesics and cold or warm compresses, depending on the severity of the disorder and the effectiveness of these modalities.[35, 36] Local ultrasound can be tried, but this has not often proved to be effective in this author's experience, and local steroid injections are generally the most effective way to restore pain-free functional activities.[37] To insure that function can be restored, reconditioning of the affected musculature by graded isometric and isotonic exercises is recommended when pain permits.[34] Wearing a forearm strap measuring approximately one and one-half inches in diameter over the bulky muscular area approximately 4 to 5 cm distal to the cubital fossa helps minimize stress at the insertion of the muscle groups on the epicondyles. Caution should be taken in injecting steroids in the region of the medial epicondyle to assure that the ulnar nerve is avoided.

Flexor Tenosynovitis (Trigger Fingers). Tenosynovitis can affect any of the fingers and thumb and cause irritation and/or crepitation. Most commonly and dramatically the patient's attention is drawn to this problem by a tendency for a finger or fingers to become "stuck" after forceful flexion and for them to become "unstuck," "triggered," in a jerking and often very painful fashion by forcible extension of the affected joint. Tenosynovitis can occur as a manifestation of a systemic disorder, but most often it is idiopathic or a consequence of unusual hand stress. Palpation of the tendon area at the MCP joint will usually elicit tenderness and creptitation and often a sense of a nodular thickening under the examining finger. Similar findings are less commonly observed at the IP joint on its palmar surface. Specific therapeutic interventions for these problems include modification of tools with built-up handles to avoid joint stress and other work modification measures. The use of a simple elastic splint designed to permit partial but not full flexion of the finger may relieve symptoms and expedite subsidence of these problems.[38] In persistent or very painful cases, local steroid injections into the tendon sheath are usually beneficial. Rarely surgical release of tendinous constraints or synovectomy is required.

De Quervain's Disease (Stenosing Tenosynovitis of the Long Thumb Adductor and Short Thumb Extensor Tendons). Pain in the region of the thumb may be difficult to localize. Osteoarthritis of the first MCP joint or carpometacarpal joint is commonly a cause of thumb pain in the older age group in the absence of other associated arthritic disorders. IP joint involvement is also a possible source of thumb pain, as is the carpal tunnel syndrome and flexor tenosynovitis. As common as any of these disorders is De Quervain's disease. Careful examination will usually reveal tenderness along the lateral aspect of the radial styloid, frequently extending into the area just volar to the anatomical snuff box. There may be mild swelling over the radial styloid extending somewhat proximally and dorsally. On occasion evidence of calcification in the tendon or tendon sheath can be noted on x-ray. The tenderness along the radial styloid as opposed to articular or other tendon areas is crucial to the diagnosis. Finkelstein's test (sign) consists of putting the affected tendons on stretch by placing the thumb across the palm of the hand, grasping it with the fingers, and then ulnar-cocking the hand.[39] This can cause exquisite pain in the region of the radial styloid at the point of stenosis of the affected tendons. Care must be taken to first test the unaffected side because this test can cause mild to moderate discomfort in apparently normal patients. Therapy consists of avoidance of stress, mild analgesics, and local steroid injections. The use of a splint to stabilize the base of the thumb while permitting full flexion of the IP joint is very useful in restoring function and relieving pain (see Fig. 31–1). Surgical release of the stenosed tendon sheath is rarely necessary.[39, 40]

Peroneal Tenosynovitis. Tenosynovitis affecting these tendons as they pass behind the lateral malleolus is usually seen in association with other foot pathology, most notably marked pes planus or spasticity of the foot secondary to upper motor neuron lesions. Tenderness, swelling, and heat are frequently noted. Correction of the predisposing factors, ice or heat, analgesics, nonsteroidal anti-inflammatory drugs, and local injections are used depending on the severity and persistence of the problem.

Morton's Neuroma. Although not properly a tendinitis or bursitis or even an arthritis, pain in the ball of the foot which may be burning and quite disabling is so commonly confused with an arthritic or related disorder that a Morton's neuroma is appropriate to consider here. The junction of the medial and lateral plantar nerves of the foot in the area underlying or plantar to the intermetatarsal ligament between the third and fourth distal metatarsal heads places the thickened nerve in jeopardy from compression due to tight shoes or high heels.[41] This is particularly true in the foot that is beginning to spread with increased age or in disorders associated with edema formation. The diagnosis is suspected by palpation of the exquisite tenderness between the third and fourth metatarsal heads and usually occurs in the absence of local callus formation and/or marked tenderness in the adjacent joints. A local injection of 1 per cent lidocaine into the tender area will usually cause a prompt subsidence of tenderness. Symptoms can be relieved by wearing appropriate footwear with restricted heel height, metatarsal pads, and ample room for the forefoot structures. Local steroid injections into the irritated area will often give lasting

relief; however, the problem tends to recur if appropriate shoe modifications cannot be made, and surgical excision is sometimes necessary.[41] Following surgery the patient should be advised and encouraged to continue to wear appropriate footwear to avoid recurrences.

Morton's neuroma is a true nerve entrapment syndrome but one that is *not* diagnosable by nerve conduction studies. The most common disorder in the latter category is the carpal tunnel syndrome. This, along with the relatively infrequent tarsal tunnel syndrome, lateral femoral cutaneous nerve entrapment, and others as well, are discussed in Chapter 4.

Ganglions. Related to tendon degeneration, these mucus-containing cystic masses may occur in a number of locations, most commonly around the wrist and less commonly about the fingers, over the dorsum of the foot, and around the ankle. They may be associated with a localized tenosynovitis or may be asymptomatic and present merely as a very firm mass that moves with tendon motion and sometimes disappears in certain positions of the wrist or hand, only to reappear when the position is changed. If the margins of the suspected ganglion on the dorsal surface of the wrist are not well defined and rather tend to blur, a tenosynovitis related to a systemic process should be seriously considered, most notably rheumatoid arthritis and its related disorders. Avoidance of stressful activities or movements in painful cases is helpful, as is splinting. Ganglia may subside spontaneously and when they are asymptomatic usually do not require treatment. Those that are painful will usually respond to local steroid injections. Surgical excision may be required in some instances, but again there is a tendency for the lesions to recur after apparently successful surgery.[42]

Dupuytren's Contracture. This consists of a painless nodular thickening of the palmar fascia, which usually originates in the region overlying the palmar surface of the third or fourth metacarpophalangeal joints. A progressive proliferation of this fascial tissue may lead to a gradual contracture of all of the fingers into the palm.[43] The plantar fascia is similarly affected in some cases.[43] This process is frequently seen in association with the late stages of the shoulder-hand syndrome.[28] Attempts to prevent progression of the con-

TABLE 31–4. LABORATORY DETERMINATIONS OF DIAGNOSTIC HELP

Laboratory Test	Helpful in Following Conditions
INITIAL SURVEY	
Antinuclear factor (ANF or ANA)	JRA (chronic iritis), MCTD, PSS, SLE
Complete blood count	Anemia, infection, leukemia, leukopenia (Felty's syndrome), sickle cell disorders, SLE
Culture, blood	Sepsis, SBE
Culture, special site (mouth, anus)	Gonorrhea, sepsis
Rheumatoid factor (latex)	RA (falsely positive in chronic inflammation, leprosy, liver disease, SBE, syphilis)
Sedimentation rate	Inflammatory disorders, PMR (high)
SMA 12	
Alkaline phosphatase	Acromegaly, biliary cirrhosis, fracture, Paget's disease
Calcium, inorganic phosphorus	Hyperparathyroidism, sarcoidosis, vitamin D intoxication
Cholesterol	Type II hyperlipidemia
Glucose	Charcot joint disease, diabetes mellitus
Lactic acid dehydrogenase (LDH), SGOT	Hepatitis with arthritis, polymyositis
Total bilirubin	Biliary cirrhosis, hepatitis
Urea nitrogen	Vasculitis with renal disease
Uric acid	Gout
Urinalysis, routine	Amyloidosis, metabolic disease, renal calculus, systemic vasculitis
AUGMENTED SURVEY	
Anti-streptolysin-O (ASO) titer	Rheumatic fever
Creatinine phosphokinase, aldolase	Polymyositis
Deoxyribonucleic acid (DNA), extractable nuclear antigen (ENA)	SLE, MCTD
Hemoglobin electrophoresis	Sickle cell disorders
Heterophile agglutinins	Infectious mononucleosis
HLA B27	Ankylosing spondylitis, RA-variants, Reiter's syndrome
Protein electrophoresis	Agammaglobulinemia, multiple myeloma, sarcoidosis, Sjögren's syndrome, SLE
Serum amylase, lipase	Arthritis in pancreatic disease
Serum complement	Polyarteritis, serum sickness, SLE (reduced)
Triiodothyronine (T-3), thyroxine (T-4)	Arthralgia, hyper- or hypothyroidism, myopathy
VDRL (Venereal Disease Research Laboratories)	Charcot joint disease, secondary syphilis, SLE (biologic false positive)
SUPPLEMENTAL SURVEY	
Coagulation profile	Clotting disorders
Cryoglobulin, immunoglobulins	Lymphomatous disorders, serum protein abnormalities
LE test (LE prep)	SLE (when anti-DNA or antibody against acidic nuclear glycoprotein cannot be obtained)
Serum iron (transferrin)	Hemochromatosis, iron deficiency

Abbreviations: JRA—juvenile rheumatoid arthritis; LE—lupus erythematosus; MCTD—mixed connective tissue disease; PMR—polymyalgia rheumatica; PSS—progressive systemic sclerosis; RA—rheumatoid arthritis; SBE—subacute bacterial endocarditis; SGOT—serum glutamic oxaloacetic transaminase; SLE—systemic lupus erythematosus; SMA 12—sequential multiple analysis (12 tests).

Table adapted from Rehabilitation in joint and connective tissue disorders. *In* Medical Knowledge Self-Assessment Program in Physical Medicine and Rehabilitation Syllabus. Chicago, American Academy of Physical Medicine and Rehabilitation, 1977, p. G6. Reprinted with permission from the publisher.

tracture by daily metacarpophalangeal stretching exercise or splinting can be tried. There is no established treatment to arrest the process, but surgical release of the tissue causing the contracture can restore function. Postsurgical recurrences are common.[43]

Rheumatoid Arthritis

The most dramatic and usually the most devastating of the arthritides is rheumatoid arthritis. Unlike the descriptive "ovia" in synovia, which alludes to the egg white–like mucinous characteristic of synovial fluid, the "oid" in rheumatoid deliberately obfuscates all those disorders that are similar to, but can be separated from, rheumatic fever. It follows, therefore, that under the umbrella of the term *rheumatoid arthritis* one can find a wide variety of joint and systemic manifestations, a wide variety of clinical presentations, a wide variety of clinical courses, a wide variety of numbers and locations of joints affected, and a wide variety of responses to therapy or indeed to the absence of therapy. Therefore it is clearly beyond the scope of this chapter to attempt to delineate all of the clinical, pathological, and therapeutic ramifications that might occur under the diagnostic rubric of rheumatoid arthritis. One has only to witness the recent fragmentation of juvenile rheumatoid arthritis (JRA) into at least three subgroups — systemic onset disease (Still's disease), polyarticular disease, and pauciarticular disease — and its further differentiation into subsets of rheumatoid factor–positive and rheumatoid factor–negative polyarthritis and pauciarticular arthritis associated with chronic iridocyclitis with and without sacroiliitis.[44] These types of JRA are further distinguished from rheumatic fever, juvenile ankylosing spondylitis, lupus erythematosus, rheumatoid variants, and dermatomyositis.[44] Advances in the techniques for tissue typing play a major role in ability to distinguish a number of apparently similar disorders that are currently classified as rheumatoid arthritis.[45] It is too early to determine whether or not most of these disorders are indeed similar in etiology (witness the broad spectrum of manifestations of syphilis) or whether indeed genetic factors primarily affecting the immune control mechanisms are the determinants of individual responses to a variety of pathogenetic factors.[46, 47] An example of the latter is the susceptibility of those persons who carry the HLA B27 tissue antigen to the development of Reiter's syndrome as a consequence of infections with Salmonella, Shigella, and Yersinia organisms.[45]

At the time of this writing the explosion of information relating to the immunological aspects of rheumatoid arthritis and related disorders still permits only a glimpse at the basic mechanisms and only a hint as to how different immunologic responses in clinically similar disorders come about and how they operate. The recent association of HLA Dw-4 with rheumatoid arthritis caused a reexamination of genetic factors in rheumatoid disease.[47] It is now known that rheumatoid factors may exist not only in the IgM class, but are also found in the IgG and IgA immunoglobulin classes and create complexes of various affinities and sizes, and therefore sensitivities to detection by classic rheumatoid factor analyses.[48] The importance of rheumatoid factor complex binding with syn-ovial fluid complement in the genesis of the inflammatory reaction of a rheumatoid joint is well documented, and the association with circulating immune complexes and the more virulent systemic complications of rheumatoid arthritis and vasculitis has also been demonstrated.[48] The demonstration of synovial plasma cell production of IgG rheumatoid factors and their relationship to synovial fluid IgG rheumatoid factor complexes has also been established.[48] The role of the T cell, which is the predominant cell in both the synovial fluid and peripheral blood, as a significant factor in the pathogenesis of rheumatoid arthritis is dramatically illustrated by the remissions in rheumatoid arthritis demonstrated through thoracic duct drainage of circulating T lymphocytes. The interactions between local tissue antigens (including collagen), T lymphocytes, B lymphocytes, plasma cells, rheumatoid factor production, immune complex formation, and release of lymphokines from activated T cells and lysosomal enzymes from activated leukocytes and macrophages are all significant parts of a complex web of events. These events, partially determined by genetic susceptibilities and to an indeterminant degree by environmental factors, coalesce in the ultimate manifestations of rheumatoid joint disease and determine the presence or absence of systemic complications.[48]

Whatever the mechanisms, the ultimate effect is that rheumatoid arthritis is usually manifested as a disorder that symmetrically involves the small joints of the hands and feet. Characteristically, to the exclusion of most noninflammatory disorders, it affects the MCP joints, and almost as frequently the PIP joints, wrists, elbows, shoulders, knees, ankles, and proximal tarsal and metatarsal phalangeal joints. Less commonly, the temporomandibular joints, the cervical spine, and the hips are affected. The joint pathology consists of a chronic granulomatous process that is associated with proliferation of the synovial lining, overgrowth of articular surfaces by a pannus of this proliferating granulomatous synovial tissue, an undermining of the joint margins, and a destruction of the overlying cartilage. Penetration of the proliferating synovia into the subchondral bone leads to cyst formation and, in more severe cases, to complete destruction of the articular surfaces with fibrous or, more rarely, bony ankylosis.[48]

As in all things in nature, the symmetry of

the joint involvement is never perfect, nor is the intensity of the inflammatory reaction consistent in the various joints that may be affected. The disorder may be monocyclic, characterized by a generalized flare, which may be either insidious or acute in onset and which may last a period of months and then remit. It may be cyclical, with one to several joints involved for durations as short as a few days to as long as years and with joints variously involved such that one PIP joint may undergo severe destructive changes and an indolent inflammation may persist in a knee, while other joints may be variously affected acutely or not affected at all. The lack of predictability of the course of the disease makes generalizations about its treatment extremely complex and assessment of the results of therapy equally confusing. In general, those patients who develop early destructive changes manifested by x-ray examination require more aggressive therapy in order to control and contain the disease. The presence of high titer rheumatoid factor, rheumatoid nodules, and/or antinuclear antibodies in patients with rheumatoid arthritis is usually associated with more severe arthritic disease than in those cases in which these serological manifestations are lacking.[49]

Patients with rheumatoid arthritis and rheumatoid factor (usually high titer) commonly develop subcutaneous granulomatous nodules at points of pressure, most notably in the region of the olecranon bursa; similar granulomatous lesions can be seen in the lung, heart, sclerae, and even the meninges. The presence of severe necrotizing vasculitis, which is a rare complication of rheumatoid arthritis, may be manifest by small or large areas of gangrene and peripheral neuropathies, the most characteristic pattern of which is the so-called mononeuritis multiplex — a series or cluster of unrelated sensory or motor neuropathies secondary to vasculitis. These complications are related to circulating immune complex formation and their deposition into the endothelia of small and large arteries. The use of high dosages of steroids and immunosuppressive therapy may be life-saving in such cases.[48]

The systemic nature of rheumatoid arthritis is typically more subtle and associated with weight loss, low grade fever, severe generalized stiffness, depression, and less commonly generalized lymphadenopathy, pleuritis, pericarditis, and sicca (Sjögren's) syndrome. This latter syndrome is characterized by lacrimal and salivary involvement with dry eyes and dry mouth, as well as, in severe cases, dryness of other mucus-secreting tissue surfaces.[50] Gamma globulins, antinuclear antibodies, and rheumatoid factor are commonly found in high titers. Sjögren's syndrome can occur in association with other connective tissue diseases and as a primary disease. It may be associated with the development of lymphomas.[50] Felty's syndrome is another rare complication of severe rheumatoid arthritis associated with neutropenia, anemia, hepatosplenomegaly, and in many cases susceptibility to infection. Disturbances in hematopoiesis and antileukocyte antibodies leading to impaired phagocytosis and enhanced removal of polymorphonuclear leukocytes in the circulation by margination and splenic sequestration are important factors in this disorder. In Felty's syndrome the indications for splenectomy are still not firmly established; the role of gold therapy has some credibility; the status of lithium carbonate in stimulating granulopoietic activity is currently being investigated.[48]

It is important to recognize in the management of rheumatoid arthritis the role of a number of drugs which, among other things, inhibit prostaglandin synthetase activity. These include aspirin in the dose of approximately four grams daily and a rapidly expanding number of nonsteroidal anti-inflammatory drugs that have superseded phenylbutazone, because of its various toxicities, and indomethacin, because of its poor tolerance and requirement for high-dosage therapy for suppression of rheumatoid arthritis.[51] These now include ibuprofen, naproxen, and phenoprofen in the phenylalkanoic acid group; tolmetin sodium, which is related to indomethacin, in the pyrrole group; and clinoril, a fluoridated indole, or sulfone.[51, 52] These drugs have in common a prostaglandin synthetase–inhibiting effect and share to a greater or lesser extent the side-effects of gastrointestinal irritation, central nervous system disturbance, dermatitis, tendency to salt retention, and, according to occasional reports, bone marrow suppression.[51] In general they are all as effective as high-dose salicylates and have fewer side effects, and in particular cause less gastrointestinal bleeding than aspirin. There are many potential hazards when two or more drugs are prescribed simultaneously, and this is true of many antirheumatic drug combinations.[53, 54] At this time it is not possible to predict which of these drugs will be effective or tolerated in any given patient. A trial of each in turn in full dosages for a period of at least two weeks is recommended in the event that a month's trial of full-dose salicylates has already proved ineffective in controlling inflammatory manifestations of rheumatoid arthritis and its related and variant disorders.[51, 52]

When nonsteroidal anti-inflammatory drugs have proved inadequate or where the aggressive and destructive nature of the ongoing rheumatoid disease is of sufficient severity, an agent that will better control the basic disease process is required. The three agents most widely used for this purpose are gold compounds (gold thiomalate and gold thiosulfate), D-penicillamine, and antimalarials (hydroxychloroquine). The mechanism of action of these agents has not been established, but the efficacy of both gold and penicillamine has been confirmed.[55, 56] Both gold and penicillamine have serious side effects, most notably bone marrow suppression and renal insufficiency, and require close observation of the patient for these as well as other manifestations of drug toxicity. Both agents require two to six months for an effect to be determined and require long-term maintenance therapy. The role of hydroxychloroquine is more controversial; both because its efficacy is less firmly established and because of the potential for an irreversible retinopathy, many clinicians have been reluctant to use the agent.[57] Nonetheless, hydroxychloroquine, which also requires two to four months for its effect to be established, continues to have a role in the management of rheumatoid arthritis. Two agents currently under investigation are levamisole, an agent capable of stimulating cell-mediated immunity, and azathioprine, an agent capable of causing immune suppression.[48] Both of these drugs have demonstrated their capability of suppressing rheumatoid arthritis. Both drugs have a wide spectrum of toxic side effects with a thus-far reversible agranulocytosis, the most severe for levamisole, and the emergence of carcinoma in patients treated with azathioprine as the most alarming of these.[48]

Systemic steroid therapy is occasionally required for suppression of symptoms in patients with otherwise uncontrollable rheumatoid arthritis. The prednisone dosage should be kept below 7.5 mg to minimize (but certainly not avoid) the disastrous consequences of iatrogenic Cushing's disease.[58] Local steroid injection into affected joints and tendon sheaths is a major adjunctive therapy in the management of rheumatoid arthritis and related disorders.[59, 60] Large joint injections of approximately 20 mg of prednisone or its equivalent and small joint injections of dosages ranging variously from 2.5 mg for an interphalangeal joint to 10 to 15 mg for an intercarpal or wrist injection and 5 to 10 mg for a tendon sheath injection are efficacious.[59, 60] The risk of tendon rupture and joint destruction from repeated injections or excessive use of recently injected joints is recognized; however, one must weigh the risk of the destructive rheumatoid process versus its amelioration and suppression by steroids against the inherent joint- and tendon-damaging properties of the local steroids per se.[61, 62] At this time it is very difficult to determine with precision exactly what that trade-off is in any given case. The usual recommendation of not more than three or four injections per joint per year would certainly avoid any serious problems; however, more frequent injections, particularly in non–weight-bearing joints such as the shoulder, may be required to assist in maintaining mobility and compliance in an exercise regimen designed to prevent progression of contracture or reverse joint contracture.[63] In the author's experience, injections given as frequently as every two weeks for a series of three injections into a shoulder may safely be administered during a concomitant course of intensive therapy designed to overcome contracture. One must bear in mind that there are individual cases in which the risk of the destructive effects of repeated intrasynovial injections administered to maintain joint function is justified when weighed against the equally destructive surgical alternative — which may not be accepted by the patient.

Basic Principles of Joint Therapy in Inflammatory Joint Disease

Repetitive joint movement and in fact any joint activity not specifically performed in a therapeutic context will create undesirable joint stress and tend to aggravate an inflammatory joint disorder. In addition to the

TABLE 31–5. X-RAY SURVEY

1. HANDS (posterior-anterior)	Osteoarthritis, rheumatoid arthritis, sarcoid, chondrocalcinosis (calcification of the triangular cartilage in wrist)
2. CHEST (posterior-anterior and lateral)	Tuberculosis, sarcoid and other granulomata, pneumonitis and pleuritis with collagen vascular disease, malignancy, erythema nodosum, osteoporosis, compression fractures
3. CERVICAL SPINE (lateral in mild flexion)	C1-C2, subluxation in rheumatoid arthritis. C2-C3, fusion in juvenile rheumatoid arthritis. C4-C7, fusion in ankylosing spondylitis, osteophytes in degenerative joint disease of cervical spine.
4. PELVIS (posterior-anterior)	Sacroiliac joint disease in ankylosing spondylitis, hip joint disease, and calcification of symphysis in chondrocalcinosis.
5. KNEE (standing anterior-posterior)	Degenerative joint disease, rheumatoid arthritis, Charcot (or neuropathic) arthritis, and chondrocalcinosis of menisci.

pharmacological efforts to suppress joint inflammation, patients should be cautioned to avoid both physical and mental exhaustion, and rest should be prescribed sufficient to insure that both general fatigue and local joint fatigue and discomfort are kept at a minimum. This usually requires eight hours of bedrest at night and at least an hour nap in the day for patients with very active generalized rheumatoid and related joint diseases.

Splinting of affected joints during the acute phase of the disorder should be designed to maintain optimum functional position and insofar as possible permit functional activities to take place.[64] Although immobilization of arthritic joints for three to four weeks has been shown to ameliorate the inflammatory process in the splinted joints without significant risk of contracture, this degree of immobilization is warranted only for short periods of time in patients with a very severe acute form of inflammatory joint disease prior to control by pharmacological means.[64] There are two splints of particular value in this regard: one is a static working wrist splint designed to stabilize the inflamed wrist (which can be extended to include partial stabilization of the MP joints), and the other is a posterior molded leg splint to stabilize the knee and/or ankle.[64]

The patients should be carefully instructed in body mechanics and joint protection and pacing of their activities to minimize joint stress and maximize postural patterns that will best preserve joint function.[65] A firm mattress, the use of built-up handles for grasp, avoidance of a pillow under the knee to prevent hip and knee and ankle contractures, and prone positioning during rest to minimize hip flexion contracture are some of the basic considerations in this regard. The use of raised toilet seats, raised chairs, and raised beds to facilitate transfer are protective of lower extremity joints and also minimize stress on upper extremities — in particular the hands, which might be required to assist in transfer.[65]

The use of modalities as specific curative treatments for joint diseases has no established value. Generally moist heat administered as a compress or by tub, shower, or pool is most effective in providing pain relief, and this is particularly useful just prior to any exercise therapy.[66]

Patients with rheumatoid arthritis and related diseases suffer not only from painful joints but also from the indignities that loss of function and the visible alterations in their bodies impose. "Psychic rest" may require social counseling, psychological counseling, sexual counseling, psychiatric counseling, and/or pharmacological intervention, as well as patient and family education. Patients and their families must learn the nature of the disease, the specifics of the regimens for drugs, exercise, and other therapeutic modalities, and the optimal ways for compliance with these regimens.[67]

The coordination of the health professionals and integration of their effort into a team-like configuration to optimize the potential beneficial effects to the patient and his or her family require that each health professional be highly skilled in his profession and both trained and experienced in the management of the various rheumatic diseases. The various disciplines must cooperate and collaborate and must often, therefore, subordinate some of their own areas of interest or expertise in the conduct of the patient's treatment program. Unfortunately the ideal configuration of such highly experienced health care professionals working with arthritis patients in a smooth and efficient manner is rarely achieved because of the lack of such trained personnel and because of the bureaucratic barriers that exist or are all too often created to interfere with coordinated rehabilitative team therapies.[68, 69]

Exercise Therapy

Strengthening. Since repeated and stressful joint motion will aggravate an inflammatory joint disorder, it is essential that these movements be kept to a minimum during therapeutic exercise. From the standpoint of strengthening the musculature that activates an affected arthritic joint (a task that is essential if sufficient strength is to be available for the joint to perform its essential functional tasks in a smooth and coordinated fashion), one must design the exercises to strengthen those muscles in a manner that minimizes joint irritation and pain. If one provokes pain, forceful muscular contractions will be inhibited and the stimulus required for muscle strengthening may not be achieved.[70]

What is required of the musculature related to an arthritic joint is that it perform brief dynamic or static holding activities essential to basic functions such as lifting a cup of tea, arising from or sitting down onto a chair, walking across the room, dressing, etc. These are basically "weight-lifting" functions associated with Type II (glycolytic, anaerobic) muscle fiber activity that is capable of brief, forceful, resistive contractions.[71] These fibers are strengthened preferentially by isometric contractions. This is fortunate because one can position the affected arthritic joint in the least painful posture (usually in midjoint range, with all aspects of the joint capsule under minimal stretch) and then a brief maximum contraction can be performed isometrically.[70] The basic principles of brief isometric exercises are discussed elsewhere, but their efficacy in the face of inflammatory joint disease has also been shown.[70, 72-74] A six second maximum contraction twice daily (with the patient instructed to count out loud while forcibly exhaling to avoid a Valsalva stress) is prescribed for each muscle group unless contraindicated by cardiovascular considerations.[70] The use of an elastic belt or rubber loop made of dental dam or tire inner tube or of a partially inflated beach ball is a practical way to provide proprioceptive feedback as the extremity is "isometrically" contracting against a barely yielding resistance[70] (see Figs. 31–2 and 31–7).

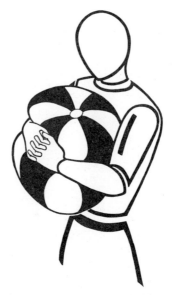

FIGURE 31–7. Isometric exercise to strengthen biceps brachii bilaterally using beachball resistance. (From Swezey, R. L.: Arthritis: Rational Therapy in Rehabilitation. Philadelphia, W. B. Saunders Company, 1978.)

The isometric exercise regimen can help to provide useful coordinated functional movements with joints protected from adverse stress during the exercise program. With subsidence in the joint disease, isotonic activities and exercise can be incorporated into the overall patient management program. However, whereas isotonic *functional activities* may not be avoidable (e.g., the secretary may have to type), isotonic and isokinetic *exercise* has not been shown to have any specific added value in the management of inflammatory joint disease. Nonetheless, when the patient's general condition improves, a desire for overall physical exercise beyond that which is incurred in daily activities is frequently expressed. Swimming is usually the most suitable exercise for such purposes because the buoyancy (and warmth) of water minimize joint stress.

Stretching. The basic principles of avoidance of joint irritation by repeated movement or stressful actions apply to stretching as well as to strengthening exercise.[70] In general, the nature of the exercise will depend on the acuteness of the joint process. When joint inflammation is severe and pain is great, the goal of therapy is to minimize further loss of joint movement. As the severity of the inflammation decreases, restoration of joint mobility and/or preservation of joint movement becomes the objective. Once a joint has

TABLE 31–6. DISORDERS FOR WHICH X-RAY IS OFTEN DIAGNOSTIC

Bone and Joint	Osteophyte	Sclerosis	Free Joint Ossicles	Joint Narrowing	Bone Proliferation	Periosteal Proliferation	Bone Resorption	Joint Margin Erosion	Bony Cysts	Osteoporosis	Cartilage Calcification	Extra-Articular Calcification	Subluxation	Bony Ankylosis	
Osteoarthritis (DJD)	x	x	x	x	x				x						Asymmetric joint narrowing. Findings of DJD are common in gout, chondrocalcinosis, trauma, osteochondromatosis.
Neuropathic (Charcot)	x	x	x		x	x	x		x		x		x		Highly variable findings with large effusions characteristically observed.
Ochronosis	x	x	x	x	x		x	x	x		x				Disk calcifications and severe generalized DJD.
Acromegaly	x	x			x										Tufting of terminal phalanges due to bone growth. Widening of joint spaces due to cartilage growth.
Rheumatoid (RA)				x	x		x	x	x	x			x	x	Diffuse cartilage loss (joint narrowing), marginal erosions of MCP & MTP joints.
Juvenile RA				x	x	x	x	x	x	x			x	x	Hypoplastic mandible, irregular epiphyseal closures. Fusion of C2-C3 or C3-C4.
Psoriasis				x	x	x	x	x	x	x			x	x	Destructive widening of DIP joints.
Septic arthritis				x		x	x	x	x	x					Soft tissue changes only are seen for 2 to 3 weeks.
Hyperparathyroidism							x		x	x		x			Resorption of radial aspect of middle phalanges and of distal clavicles.

Disorder	Comments
Paget's	Secondary DJD is common.
Aseptic necrosis	Cartilage loss and secondary DJD come late.
Tophaceous gout	Calcification of tophus.
Chondrocalcinosis	May occur coincidentally in other diseases.
Calcific periarthritis	Calcifications may be transient.
Scleroderma (P.S.S.)	Subcutaneous calcifications. Resorption of distal phalanges is typical.
Reiter's	When periosteal thickening or bone proliferation on the anterior calcaneus is present.
Pulmonary osteoarthritis	Distal ends of long bone ± clubbing.
Sarcoid	Usually x-ray is of no assistance.
Ankylosing spondylitis (A.S.)	These findings apply to sacroiliac joints and axial joints.
Osteochondromatosis	Single to multiple.

DISORDERS FOR WHICH X-RAY OFTEN SUGGESTS THE DIAGNOSIS

Amyloidosis	Large soft tissue shoulder masses are rare but distinctive.
Chronic SLE	MCP and PIP subluxations without erosions are suggestive.
Hemochromatosis	Erosions of index and middle MCP joints.
Lymphomas	
Multicentric reticulohistiocytosis	Can be confused with RA, psoriasis, gout.

become subluxed or dislocated no exercise will restore alignment, but if the malalignment is due to contracture alone then there is a reasonable expectation of restoration of joint mobility, provided the articular surfaces are not excessively damaged or deranged. Therapeutic exercise in all patients with inflammatory joint disease should be performed when the patient is at his best. This usually means sometime in the mid morning when the characteristic morning stiffness has subsided. The use of moist heat or cold (as preferred by the patient) to minimize joint discomfort and, if need be, supplementary analgesics may be prescribed so as to be effective at the time of the exercise regimen.[70]

In the very acute phase of joint inflammation, active and gently assisted exercises with one to three gentle repetitions once or twice daily is usually all that will be tolerated in the effort to preserve joint mobility. At this state splinting and posture-corrective measures are used to maintain functional position of joints.[64, 65] As inflammation subsides and the goal is increase of joint motion, the patient is instructed to repeat the specific exercise three to five times with the initial repetitions being in essence a "warm-up" and the final two or three repetitions the actual stretching exercise just into the range of pain. The rule of thumb is that no exercise, strengthening or stretching, should cause severe pain at the time the exercise is performed, nor should it cause pain lasting more than two hours, nor should it be associated with either increased joint inflammation or excessive pain on the day following the exercise regimen.[70]

When inflammation is only moderate, the exercise regimen to increase mobility where contractures have occurred can be performed three to four times daily. In those joints for which the goal is maintenance of motion, once-daily exercise should suffice. It should be borne in mind that the patient's compliance with an exercise regimen that is painful, time consuming, and fatiguing and that requires repetitive performances will be markedly attenuated as the complexity, frequency, and pain of these regimens are increased. The goals of exercise therapy should be precisely defined and once they are achieved they should be revised so that either a new goal requiring additional exercise is prescribed and the previous exercise is discontinued or the regimen is altered according to the newly perceived needs and realities. It must be remembered that patients with inflammatory joint disease tend to have a variable course in terms of the overall disease and in terms of the problems relating to any given joint at any given time. This is particularly true as new medical treatments are implemented during the course of the joint disorder.

Key Joint Problems in Rheumatoid and Related Arthritides

Temporomandibular Joint. The temporomandibular (TM) joint is occasionally the source of significant trouble to patients with rheumatoid arthritis. Transient pain is not uncommon, but on occasion a destructive process involving one or both of the temporomandibular joints can cause severe disability. Mandibular contracture, loss of interincisor separation or lateral translation in mastication, and even mandibular resorption may be noted; however, the chief problem is pain on mastication. Persistent transient inflammatory reactions not ameliorated by a soft diet and local heat can often be relieved by local steroid injections into the TM joint with due care that the facial nerve is avoided. Arthroplasties and joint replacement are occasionally necessitated by severe TM joint pain and malfunction.[75] Mandibular hypoplasia is a sequela in some cases of JRA and may require mandibular reconstruction.

Cervical Spine. Subluxation of C1 on C2 may rarely lead to severe upper and lower neuron complications and death. Painful C1-C2 subluxations without neurological deficit are best treated with a soft or plastic collar fitted to minimize hyperflexion of the cervical spine.[76] All patients with cervical spine involvement should be cautioned to avoid excessive neck manipulation in a dental chair, under anesthesia, during x-ray procedures, or in therapy.[77] Even in cases where neurological manifestations have occurred, the use of these collars and instruction in appropriate body mechanics may suffice.[76] When the atlas is sufficiently eroded to allow penetration of the odontoid process into the foramen magnum, the risk of catastrophic neurological damage due to spinal cord compression is great, and surgical intervention may be mandatory. Mid or lower cervical instability and subluxation secondary to rheumatoid disease is also a common complication and may lead to spinal cord compression.[76] All of these complications tend to be more prevalent in patients on long-term steroid therapy, which may reflect both a complication of steroid therapy and a selection of more severely involved patients. When neurological signs and symptoms cannot be stabilized with the use of cervical immobilization, which in the case of the lower cervical spine is best effected by a Philadelphia collar or SOMI brace, surgical stabilization may be required.[64, 76] Unfortunately, the poor quality of bone in patients with these complications may militate against a successful stabilization procedure.

Shoulders. Both the acromioclavicular joint and the glenohumeral joint are commonly involved. Swelling of the glenohumeral joint is often difficult to detect. Contractures of the glenohumeral joint capsule occur early, should be avoided when possible, and an attempt to reduce them should be made as soon as they are detected. A progressive exercise program may commence, with pendulum (Codman's) exercises, progress to reciprocal pulleys, finger-wall "walking," and "wand" exercises, accompanied in the last instance by isometric exercises to the deltoid and internal and external rotators (see Fig. 31–5 and 31–6).[34] Local steroid injections may permit more rapid restoration of shoulder motion. Patients should be instructed to avoid excessive reaching, repetitive overhead activities, and movements such as mopping, sweeping, etc. When these are unavoidable, the use of long-handled, light-weight tools or power tools, and an arrangement of household supplies to avoid unnecessary stretching or the use of reachers where appropriate should be instituted. The status of total shoulder arthroplasties remains to be determined.[78]

Elbow. Elbow contractures are common in rheumatoid arthritis and occur with pain and/or minimal effusions in the elbow joint. The use of local steroids to minimize swelling and inflammation while accompanied by extension exercises tends to minimize the problem and help reverse early contractures. Fixed contractures in extension are extremely difficult to overcome, and attention should be directed at preventing loss of flexion because of the severe functional embarrassment in self-care activities that this loss of range of motion can impose — particularly in patients with rheumatoid arthritis, whose shoulder and wrist mobility are often impaired as well. Flexion exercises, active and assisted, should be designed to maintain mobility and increase mobility where loss of range is detected. Pronation and supination of the elbow and wrist, particularly the latter, require range-of-motion exercise to preserve mobility.[79] Platform crutches facilitate crutch walking in patients with wrist and elbow involvement. Synovectomy combined with radial head resection is a useful procedure for pain relief but creates difficulties for some crutch users.[80, 81] Considerable experimentation in total elbow prostheses is being done, but no entirely satisfactory resolution of the problems has been forthcoming as yet.[82]

Wrist. In contrast to most other joints affected in rheumatoid arthritis, the intercarpal joints have a tendency to undergo bony fusion. This may bridge the radiocarpal joint space or be associated with subluxations in that same area. When the wrist is affected, a static working wrist splint may be employed to minimize joint irritation during function (Fig. 31–8). This should be accompanied by twice-daily wrist range-of-motion exercises to minimize loss of mobility. Chronic wrist

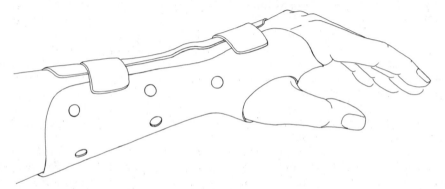

FIGURE 31–8. Static wrist stabilizing (working) splint. This splint is a custom-molded thermo-labile plastic splint. It extends from distally just proximal to the distal palmar crease to the proximal one third of the forearm. There is a wide aperture for thumb clearance. It is useful in arthritis of the wrist and to prevent hyperflexion and hyperextension of the wrist in the carpal tunnel syndrome. (From Swezey, R. L.: Arthritis: Rational Therapy in Rehabilitation. Philadelphia, W. B. Saunders Company, 1978.)

pain may require surgical intervention. Wrist synovectomy with removal of severely eroded ulnar styloids (the Darrach procedure) may permit restoration of useful function. Temporary fixation to permit a fibrous ankylosis or a bony fusion may be necessary to stabilize the wrist. Replacement arthroplasties are gaining acceptance as a method to preserve mobility and stability and relieve wrist pain.[83]

Communication with the intercarpal and radiocarpal joints and the overlying extensor and underlying flexor tendons is common in rheumatoid arthritis and can be associated with tenosynovitis. Rupture of the extensor tendons is very commonly associated with tenosynovitis and a prominent dorsally subluxed distal ulnar head and ulnar styloid erosions. Prompt surgical intervention when a tendon rupture is detected should be made in order to minimize the extent of surgery and further loss of function in adjacent fingers.

Hands. The selection of the metacarpophalangeal joint as a primary locus of rheumatoid arthritis leads to a weakening of the joint-supporting structures, contractures of the interosseous musculature, and, as a consequence of the stresses imposed by normal hand activities, the characteristic ulnar deviation and swan neck deformities.[84] Splinting to stabilize the MCP joints accompanied with exercises designed to stretch the interossei may help prevent these deformities, but this has not been established.[64]

Subluxation of the lateral slips of the extensor tendons volarly in association with attenuation or rupture of the central slip at its attachment on the dorsum of the base of the middle phalanx leads to PIP contracture and the boutonnière deformity.[84] The intact extensor tendon attachment to the dorsum of the base of the distal phalanx tends to maintain the DIP joint in hyperextension.[84] This can lead to a loss of effective apposition during pinch unless range of motion to the DIP joint is prescribed for maintenance of the DIP joint's mobility or to overcome an incipient contracture. It is doubtful that any exercise can prevent the PIP contractures that occur with the boutonnière deformity; however, the use of local steroid injection into the joint may minimize the inflammatory process and the progression of the PIP lesions, particuarly when systemic antirheumatic disease therapy can be anticipated to ultimately control the disease. Splinting to stabilize the thumb CMC, MCP, and IP joints can reduce pain and improve function.[64]

The role of synovectomy, either chemical or surgical, in the management of rheumatoid joints in the hand or elsewhere remains controversial.[85-87, 89] Joint arthroplasties of the MCP joints have been shown to improve cosmesis and relieve pain, but cannot be relied upon to improve function.[88] Surgical treatment of the PIP joints is less predictable in its outcome with the exceptions of stabilizing procedures designed to improve function. Arthroplasties to stabilize the CMC joint in the thumb, replacement of the trapezium or stabilization of the thumb IP joint, and replacement of the MCP joint in the thumb are useful in selected cases.[85, 89]

Hip. Progressive destructive changes in the hip are not uncommon in rheumatoid arthritis and are even more common in rheumatoid variant disease. Exercises to maintain mobility, posture corrections to minimize hip flexion contractures, and strengthening by isometric contractions of the hip musculature can be helpful in preventing progressive weakness and irreversible deformity.[90] Swimming and pool therapy are very useful. Relief of weight-bearing stresses by crutch or cane is often required. Raised toilet seats and elevated seating minimize stress during transfer. Reachers and special dressing devices, such as stocking putter-on-ers and long-handled shoe horns, can facilitate function.

Fortunately, when satisfactory control cannot be achieved by conservative means, a total hip prosthesis offers an excellent functional solution to the pain of progressive inflammatory hip disease.[91] Long-term experience is lacking in the use of these prostheses in young patients, but their use in middle-aged and older patients appears safe and represents a major achievement in the management of arthritic disorders.[91] The rheumatoid arthritis patient has the advantage of being generally less active than the patient who has osteoarthritis and hip involvement and hence tends to have less risk of abusing the replaced joint and stressing the prosthesis.

Knee. The knee is commonly involved in rheumatoid arthritis. Inflammation of the knee leads to rapid quadriceps atrophy and weakness, which minimize the joint protective action of the key muscle for this crucial weight-bearing joint. Possibly as a result of the quadriceps inhibition, pain, and resultant weakness, patients with rheumatoid arthritis tend to externally rotate the hip, pronate the foot, and stabilize the knee by leaning into the medial collateral ligament rather than relying on the quadriceps to support the knee in its unstable flexed position during weight bearing. Whatever the mechanism, medial collateral ligament overstretching and valgus deformity are the usual late manifestations of rheumatoid knee involvement. Effusions of the knee, unless accompanied by a lax or overstretched capsule, restrict knee movement particularly in extension and predispose the knee to flexion contractures. The use of a pillow under the knee for support and comfort tends to further aggravate this problem and must be avoided. Stabilization of the knees with a posterior removable splint to maintain position at rest during the acute phases is therefore extremely important and should be combined with aspiration and/or local steroid injections when knee effusions preclude full extension.

Relief of weight-bearing stresses by crutches or canes is useful. In patients with very unstable knees a long-leg, plastic-metal orthosis can provide stability and pain relief, but long-leg orthoses are not well accepted by most patients. The use of an elastic knee support with or without metal side hinges is sometimes helpful in relieving pain even though it provides little actual stabilization for the knee.

Quadriceps isometric exercises with the knee in partial flexion can be initiated as soon as pain permits. Range-of-motion exercises should be performed with assistance twice daily in acute stages, and more frequently if a contracture persists and exercise is tolerated. Traction and serial casting can be helpful in overcoming contractures.[18, 64] Synovectomy of the knee may buy time and pain relief if performed at a time before severe destructive changes have occurred.[85-87] In those patients with marked loss of joint cartilage and destructive changes with uncontrolled active painful synovitis, a joint replacement prosthesis will be required.[92] It should be noted, however, that in those patients in whom the disease can be well controlled by antirheumatic drugs, the x-ray appearance alone should not dictate the decision for surgical treatment.

A complication of rheumatoid arthritis and variant disease in the knee is the rupture of a popliteal cyst that may form as a posterior extension of the knee joint in the presence of inflammatory joint disease. This can result in pain in the calf and swelling in the leg, and is frequently confused with thrombophlebitis.[93] Ultrasound studies can detect posterior effusions, and arthrography can document synovial rupture. A local steroid injection into the knee will usually cause a rapid subsidence of the inflammatory reaction in the calf, and this should be followed with one to three days of elevation and warm compresses to reduce the swelling and irritation in the leg.

Ankle and Hindfoot. The ankle is commonly involved in rheumatoid arthritis and in variant disease. With or without destructive changes in the articular surface, significant problems with ambulation are common. Relief of weight-bearing forces with crutches or a cane should be attempted. Stress on the foot itself during gait can be partially relieved by the use of a Sach heel and rocker sole, and in more severe cases this shoe modification can be attached to a below-knee weight-bearing brace to partially relieve some of the load on the ankle joint.[16] Local steroid injections are often beneficial.

Synovectomy is rarely useful in recalcitrant cases where severe destructive changes have not yet occurred, and the role of total ankle replacement is gaining acceptance over arthrodesis in severe chronic ankle problems.[85] Caution in making a recommendation for ankle surgery should be exercised because very often both the ankle and the proximal tarsal joints are involved. The latter may be a source of more discomfort than the ankle, in which case the results of ankle surgery may be disappointing indeed.

Rheumatoid involvement of the *proximal tarsal joints* may affect any or all of these joints and is occasionally associated with bony ankylosis similar to that seen in the wrist. Selected local steroid injections can be helpful. The use of shoe modifications and bracing as described under the ankle are also of value. The shoe selected for the patient with proximal tarsal involvement should be a Blucher model with a steel shank and multiple lacings such that, when it is properly laced, a corset-like effect can be achieved to help stabilize the proximal tarsal joints.

The *subtalar joint* is commonly involved in

rheumatoid arthritis. Inflammation of the bursae surrounding the insertion of the *Achilles tendon* with or without associated rheumatoid nodule formation is not uncommon. Pain at the insertion of the plantar fascia on the anterior surface of the calcaneus as well as at the insertion of the Achilles tendon posteriorly is commonly seen in rheumatoid variant diseases. The use of a Sach heel, as well as a cushioned inner heel, is helpful in relieving stress on the hindfoot structures during heel-strike and weight bearing. Occasionally undermining and filling the heel with soft foam for further relief is of value. A raised heel can reduce stress in cases of Achilles tendinitis. Cane, crutches, and below-knee weight-bearing braces may be required. Again, local steroid injections may be useful in relieving persistent symptoms.

The Forefoot. Characteristic rheumatoid involvement of the metatarsophalangeal joints leads to secondary muscle contractures and a kaleidoscope of deformities that most commonly include hallux valgus, hyperextension of the MTP joints with hyperflexion of the PIP joints, and a bunionette deformity of the fifth toe. Compounding these so-called hammer toe and bunion deformities are the hard callosities that occur on the dorsal surface of the PIP joints, on the lateral surfaces of the first and fifth toes, and under the depressed metatarsal heads. The metatarsophalangeal joints can be further traumatized as their protective fat pads are pulled distally by the toe contractures.

The use of a shoe with a rigid shank to provide stability, a metatarsal pad to relieve the weight-bearing stress on the metatarsophalangeal joints with ample width to allow room for the splayed toes medially and laterally, and ample depth of the toe box to allow for the cocked-up deformities of the PIP joints will help minimize pain on walking. The soles should be cushioned, and a crepe or rippled sole is helpful; however, a sole that is too soft can create instability beneath the foot during ambulation. Metatarsal bars can be placed on the outside of the shoe and perform the same service as a metatarsal pad. They have the advantage of not altering the volume on the inside of the shoe in which the foot must be contained, but they have the disadvantage that they may cause the patient to trip over slight defects in the pavement. The rheumatoid foot generally tends to undergo pronation due to stretching of lax proximal tarsal and subtalar ligaments. Good supporting footwear, therefore, is essential to minimize these deforming forces, and a molded insole should be provided to maintain the foot such that the longitudinal arch is held stable in its most comfortable position. Attempts to correct the depressed longitudinal arch usually result in pain on ambulation, and there is no evidence that they are successful. When attempts to relieve pain by shoe correction and pharmacological therapy fail or when the patient rejects on cosmetic grounds shoes designed to accommodate and support the arthritic foot, then surgical treatment is advisable. Resection of metatarsal heads and/or the bases of the phalanges can be anticipated to provide excellent pain relief as a consequence of functional gait and a more varied choice of footwear to the patient.[92] The status of prosthetic implants in the first MTP joint as well as other joints in the forefoot is not yet clear.[92]

Rheumatoid Arthritis Variants

Ankylosing Spondylitis. Ninety per cent of patients with ankylosing spondylitis are HLA B27 positive.[94] This disorder characteristically affects young men with variable pain in the low back and buttocks, and often progresses to involve the dorsal and cervical spine and may originate initially in any of these areas. Sacroiliitis is the hallmark of this disorder, and varying progression of bony proliferation leading to fusion between the vertebral bodies and loss of spinal mobility is a distinctive feature.[95] It has recently been shown that whereas the clinical manifestations of the full-blown picture of ankylosing spondylitis are relatively rarely seen in women, the disorder in a mild form probably occurs as often in women as in men when assessed on the basis of HLA B27 antigen positivity, back complaints, and sacroiliitis.[96]

The joints that are characteristically affected are those of the axial skeleton, which include the temporomandibular, the acromioclavicular, and the sternoclavicular joints, as well as the rib articulations. A loss of chest expansion is a characteristic clinical sign, as is early loss of lumbar flexion and atrophy of the lumbar paraspinal musculature. Iritis can lead to loss of vision, aortitis can necessitate aortic valve replacement, apical pulmonary infiltration may be associated with loss of pulmonary function, and amyloidosis, a rare complication, may lead to renal failure.

The characteristic pathological feature of this disorder is enthesitis (an inflammation of ligamentous and tendinous insertions).[97] Focal areas of pain in these locations may be very troublesome, and this is particularly true of the insertion of the Achilles tendon into the plantar fascia with the accompanying heel pain that may be a severe disabling complication of this disorder.

Hip joint involvement occurs in about 20 per cent of patients and may lead to severe disability because of the concomitant loss of motion in the spine. Further, surgical procedures such as total hip operations have a higher incidence of failure than does surgery for other disorders because of the tendency for heterotopic bone deposition and ankylosis to occur following hip surgery.[91, 98]

Pharmacological treatment consists of the use of nonsteroidal anti-inflammatory drugs. Patients with ankylosing spondylitis often will respond to lower dosages than are usually effective in other conditions (e.g., indomethacin, 25 mg two to three times daily may suffice to ameliorate severe spondylitic back and neck pain).

Rehabilitative Therapy. *Exercise* to maintain position and pulmonary expansion, as well as postural corrective measures, is the mainstay of rehabilitation therapy. Bracing to prevent kyphosis is of doubtful value. The patient should be instructed to use a firm mattress and a minimal pillow (or a Jackson pillow, which allows for lateral cervical support in the side lying position but does not cause cervical flexion in the supine position). *Prone positioning* for periods of at least one hour daily during the active phase of the disease and in patients with hip joint involvement is stressed.

EXERCISES. Early morning warm-ups should be prescribed to facilitate daily activities. This consists of having the patient assume the "all-fours" position (on the hands and knees in bed), rock back onto the heels, rock forward onto the shoulders, alternately stretch one arm and the opposite leg and indeed to crawl when necessary to facilitate mobility. Neck and back extension exercises can be initiated from the "all-fours" position. Both upper extremities and the upper

back and neck are then extended against gravity as far as possible and this stretch is held for a count of three. This exercise can be repeated three to five times and the holding phase continued to the point of fatigue to encourage strengthening of the erector spinae musculature. The patient can be more vigorously exercised in the prone position with a pillow placed under the upper abdomen and lower thorax. Alternating arm and leg extension is then followed by simultaneous upper extremity extension and simultaneous lower extremity extension, and then both upper and lower extremity and neck extension stretches with isometric holding at the extreme of the stretch to increase strength in the extensor muscles. Range of motion of the cervical spine consists of gentle flexion-extension, rotation, and lateral flexion movements in a series of three to five repetitions.[70] Neck extension and posture can be reinforced by having the patient attempt to place the occiput against a wall or door and slide up and down doing partial knee bends.[70] Rotation of the thoracic spine is best performed with the patient straddling a chair and twisting, first to one side and then to the other. This is done at least once daily for maintenance, and two to three times daily during the early phase of the disease, where evidence for loss of mobility is found. If patients with ankylosing spondylitis are kept under observation, the need for continuing exercise in each area can be assessed and the exercise regimen reduced to its essentials. Progress can be gauged by the ability of the patient to touch the floor, by measurements of chest expansion, by measurements of the occiput-to-wall distance while standing, and by the Schober test, a measurement of the lumbosacral vertebral interspinous lengthening during lumbar flexion.

In those patients in whom a relentless deformity and pain are not responsive to nonsteroidal anti-inflammatory drugs, the use of x-ray therapy should be considered; however, the late complications of acute myelogenous leukemia following x-ray therapy should be heavily weighed in considering this modality. A vertebral osteotomy can be performed to correct spinal alignment when severe flexion deformity has not been preventable or has already occurred. The failed total hip operation in patients with ankylosing spondylitis may be salvaged to the extent that mobility at the expense of instability can be restored by a Girdlestone procedure that consists of amputation of the femoral head and neck.[99]

The peripheral joints most commonly involved outside of the axial skeleton are the knees and ankles. The small joints in the hands and feet as well as wrists and elbows may also be involved, but generally the synovitis that occurs is less damaging to peripheral joints than to the axial and spinal joints, and is less destructive in the majority of cases than that seen in rheumatoid arthritis.[95] Treatment of peripheral joint involvement from a physiatric standpoint is essentially that of rheumatoid arthritis. From a pharmacological standpoint local steroid therapy and systemic nonsteroidal anti-inflammatory drugs are the only agents effective in this disorder, and drugs such as antimalarials, D-penicillamine, and gold compounds are not indicated.

Reiter's Syndrome

Reiter's syndrome is another disorder in which the HLA B27 antigen occurs in 90 per cent of cases.[94] This is also typically a disease of young males characterized by arthritis, usually asymmetrical and typically in weight-bearing joints, conjunctivitis or iritis, and a nonspecific urethritis.[100] Balanitis, a painless stomatitis, diarrhea, and an acute pustular psoriasis are very commonly associated.[100] About one third of the patients develop features of ankylosing spondylitis. Synovial fluid analysis typically reveals an elevated synovial fluid complement.[100]

Patients are managed with nonsteroidal anti-inflammatory drugs, although the response is usually incomplete. The attacks tend to be self-limiting, lasting two to four months with a recurrence rate of 15 per cent per year.[100] In some patients the development of a severe generalized psoriasis, ankylosing spondylitis, persistent hindfoot and heel pain, or systemic complications may result in considerable disability.[100] The physiatric management is as described under ankylosing spondylitis and rheumatoid arthritis.

Psoriatic Arthritis

Psoriatic arthritis in the majority of cases is essentially indistinguishable from rheumatoid arthritis except that rheumatoid factor and nodules are not present.[101] Skin lesions usually antedate the arthritis, and exacerbations and remissions of psoriatic arthritis are poorly correlated with the course of the skin lesions.[101] The presence of HLA B27 antigen is highly correlated with the development of spondylitic manifestations in those patients with psoriasis. The HLA B13 and B17 antigens have been associated with HLA B27–negative patients with psoriasis and peripheral arthritis.[102] Distinctive features of psoriatic arthritis include the seronegativity, distal interphalangeal joint involvement, periosteal proliferation, and the association of nail fissuring, pitting, or undermining keratosis. Occasionally (as in Reiter's syndrome as well) the arthritis may affect predominantly one digit, causing an inflammatory dactylitis with considerable overlying soft tissue inflammation — the so-called "sausage" digit. Severe osteolysis at the opposing articular surfaces may occur in peripheral and occasionally in proximal joints. A tendency to bony fusion may typically be seen in severe cases of psoriatic arthritis. These latter manifestations are more likely to occur in patients with generalized psoriatic erythroderma. The severe resorptive arthropathy in which the loss of bone-stock and joint surface is so extensive that the skin overlying the fingers or wrists may fold upon itself — the so-called main-en-lorgnette syndrome — may occur in a variety of arthritic conditions but most typically occurs in psoriatic and rheumatoid arthritis.[103]

The physiatric treatment of psoriasis is that of rheumatoid arthritis. The pharmacological therapy at this time does not include penicillamine or hydroxychloroquine. Hydroxychloroquine has been shown to exacerbate psoriasis.[101] Gold therapy is being re-evaluated at this time, and in severe cases immunosuppressive therapy, particularly methotrexate, may be required for control of the disease.[104] Steroids are occasionally necessary for control of the joint disease and they also ameliorate the skin manifestations. Local skin therapy, including topical steroids and various modifications of the Goeckerman regimen, may alleviate the skin manifestations but do not seem to alter the course of the joint disease.[105]

Arthritis and Colitis

The HLA B27 antigen has again helped us to understand the association between chronic inflammatory disorders of the gastrointestinal tract and ankylosing spondylitis.[94] Patients with ulcerative colitis or Crohn's disease may develop erythema nodosum with transient arthritis; episodes of usually symmetrical, nondestructive large joint synovitis, which may persist for weeks or months and subside; and localized sacroiliac disease and/or full blown ankylosing spondylitis.[106] The course of the ankylosing spondylitis, once initiated, is independent of the activity of the bowel disease.[106] The use of nonsteroidal anti-inflammatory drugs in these patients requires some caution because of the possibility of exacerbating the diarrheal disorder.

Systemic Lupus Erythematosus (SLE) and Related Disorders

There are several rheumatic diseases that in some instances resemble each other so closely that they cannot be distinguished with confidence. Some of these disorders may on occasion so closely resemble rheumatoid arthritis in their articular manifestations that terms such as *cross-over disease* or *overlap syndromes* are applied. As refinements in immunological, pathological, and clinical observations multiply, the criteria for distinctions between the various entities included in this section tend to wax and wane in their ability to distinguish the specific disorders sufficiently that a practical therapeutic strategy can be made for a given case.[107] Systemic lupus erythematosus (SLE) has many evidences of an autoimmune disturbance affecting almost every tissue and organ structure at various times in various individuals. Several drugs, including hydralazine, procainamide, isoniazid, chlorpromazine, and anticonvulsants, have been associated with a lupus-like syndrome, but in the majority of cases the inciting antigen remains unknown.[107] In both the NZB-NZW mouse and in man evidence for a viral etiology of a lupus-like disorder is compelling, but a viral etiology has not been established.[107, 108] A characteristic double-stranded DNA and IgG anti-DNA complex is a hallmark of SLE and is expressed in the LE cell test. The interaction of these complexes with complement probably accounts for the severe renal disease and many of the other manifestations of this disorder. Almost all patients with SLE have significant titers of antinuclear antibodies, and particularly anti-DNA and anti-Sm antibodies.[107] A depression of serum complement is commonly found in SLE, particularly in those patients with active nephritis. An hereditary complement deficiency (C2) has been associated with the HLA 10 and HLA 18 tissue types in a typical lupus syndrome in two families.[107] Elevation of gamma globulin is frequently seen and may be associated with a biologically false-positive serological test for syphilis.

Medical management of systemic lupus will depend on the nature and severity of the problems. Steroid therapy is a mainstay in those patients with severe systemic manifestations and may be used in conjunction with immunosuppressive therapy. Patients with mild manifestations and particularly dermatological manifestations may respond to antimalarial therapy, salicylates, or nonsteroidal anti-inflammatory drugs.[107, 109]

From a physiatric standpoint there are several problems that may require attention. The arthritis may be extremely painful without objective findings other than joint margin tenderness. It may, on the other hand, be associated with a severe and destructive arthritis — a "rheumatoid cross-over." Polymyositis or myopathy secondary to steroid therapy is frequently seen in association with lupus and is treated as discussed under polymyositis. The severe central nervous system manifestations including coma and hemiparesis or paraparesis are treated initially with high dose steroids, and ultimately their rehabilitative management will be that required by the persisting neurological deficit. The arthritis per se is managed symptomatically along the lines outlined for rheumatoid arthritis.

Progressive Systemic Sclerosis (PSS) or Scleroderma

All of the disorders in this section on systemic vasculitis are associated with Raynaud's phenomenon, and this is particularly true of PSS. Progressive tightening of the skin of the hands, often later progressing onto the forearms, face, trunk, and legs, is characteristic. The onset may be associated with a generalized edematous phase that may subside, leaving minimal skin-fascia adherence or severe progressive sclerodermatous changes. Hyper- and hypopigmentation in the affected areas of the skin are commonly seen; scarring of the fingertips associated with ischemic changes and Raynaud's phenomenon may be painful.[110] Subcutaneous calcification may on occasion be diffuse, and extrusions of calcification through the skin may occur associated with pain and disability, particularly when these occur in the palmar and digital areas. Systemic complications include pulmonary fibrosis, dysphagia secondary to esophageal hypomotility, and malabsorption syndrome.[110] A rare fulminant renal failure with hypertension is usually lethal. The so-called CREST syndrome is an acronym for calcinosis, Raynaud's phenomenon, esophageal hypomotility, sclerodactyly, and telangiectasia, all of which may be seen in any given case of PSS.[110]

A useful clinical sign for the diagnosis of scleroderma is an inability to pinch a fold of skin overlying the dorsum of the middle phalanges. The sign, when found bilaterally in the absence of previous traumata or generalized edema, is very suggestive of skin-periosteal tethering secondary to scleroderma. The biopsy of the skin tends to be helpful only in those cases in which the clinical diagnosis is obvious and tends to be equivocal when the clinician has the greatest need for pathological confirmation. The laboratory is usually not helpful, although antinuclear antibodies with a speckled or nucleolar fluorescence are commonly seen. Rheumatoid factor may be present in about 25 per cent of cases.[110]

The treatment medically is supportive with the use of steroids in those patients with associated myositis. The physiatric treatment consists of exercise and night splinting to prevent contractures and maintain mobility and strength. There is no evidence that the severe deforming contractures can be overcome by any physiatric measure, and in this author's experience, except in those patients in whom the edematous phase of scleroderma has subsided leaving relatively little residua, the results of aggressive exercise and splinting have been disappointing. Raynaud's phenomenon is treated by encouraging the use of gloves, avoidance of cold exposure, and meticulous skin hygiene. Some patients have been reported to respond to control of skin temperature by biofeedback techniques.[111]

Polymyositis (Dermatomyositis)

Polymyositis may accompany SLE, PSS, polyarteritis, or mixed connective tissue disease, and it may occur in association with malignancy or as an idiopathic process in its own right.[112] When the characteristic lavender (heliotrope) discoloration appears about the eyes and scaling erythematous lesions appear over the extensor surfaces of the knuckles and on the chest in association with proximal muscle weakness, a diagnosis of dermatomyositis can usually be established. Muscle tenderness and a mild symmetrical polyarthritis may be seen in association with this disorder. In children a vasculitis is commonly found, and secondary calcinosis and contractures are frequently seen.[112] The prognosis is generally better in children than in adults.[113] Evidence points to an autoimmune T cell stimulation by muscle tissue as a significant mechanism in the pathogenesis of polymyositis.[114] Clinically in addition to proximal muscle weakness, the elevation of serum muscle enzymes, particularly creatine phosphokinase (CPK), is most helpful in establishing the diagnosis.[114] Other enzymes that are frequently elevated include lactic dehydrogenase (LDH), aldolase, serum glutamic oxaloacetic transaminase (SGOT), and serum glutamic pyruvic transaminase (SGPT). Monitoring of one or two of these elevated enzymes during therapy is extremely useful because they will often revert toward normal or away from normal prior to the clinical remission or exacerbation of muscle weakness. Supporting electromyographic evidence suggesting muscle disease can be helpful, and a muscle biopsy is usually confirmatory.

Medical treatment consists of steroids in an initial dosage of at least 1 mg/kg daily until symptoms are controlled and then gradual tapering to a maintenance dose — usually 20 mg of prednisone daily or greater.[114] If after several months the disease is poorly controlled, immunosuppressive drugs may be required.[114]

The rehabilitative treatment consists of maintenance or restoration of joint mobility and posture, avoidance of contractures, and facilitation of functional activities with the use of assistive devices as required by the degree of muscle weakness. Strengthening exercises in the face of active myositis should be undertaken with caution because the effects of resistive exercises on the existing muscle inflammatory disease have not been adequately assessed.[70] Patients are usually encouraged to increase their activity commensurate with their increasing strength until enzymes are either stabilized or return to normal, at which time resistive exercises can be employed in an effort to obtain maximal muscle strength. It should be remembered that steroid therapy per se may be responsible for a proximal myopathy and that full restoration of strength in patients with polymyositis is rarely achieved.[114]

Mixed Connective Tissue Disease (MCTD)

This disorder, which closely resembles SLE and PSS and myositis, has been clinically characterized by the presence of tightly swollen fingers with sclerodermatous changes, Raynaud's phenomenon, hypergammaglobulinemia, and the presence of high titers of an RNAse-sensitive extractable nuclear antigen.[107, 115] These patients in general less frequently manifest severe chronic renal or CNS disease, but in the aggregate may manifest essentially any and all of the serological or clinical features of SLE, PSS, or polymyositis.[107, 115] The myositis and arthralgias can be controlled by steroids, and the management is essentially that of lupus, scleroderma, or myositis, depending on which symptoms are manifested.[115]

Polyarteritis

There are a number of distinctive disorders associated with autoimmune disturbances that in addition to the above described entities may be associated with necrotizing lesions in blood vessels ranging from venules to large arteries. The disorders can manifest variously transient skin rashes and include catastrophic multi-system diseases affecting literally every tissue in the body.[116] Joint manifestations are a common accompaniment of many of these disorders, and the arthritis is typically painful but not progressive or destructive.[116] The association of hepatitis B and an immune complex vasculitis that may be transient or chronic has recently been described.[116] Diagnosis is established by muscle or testicular biopsy, and in patients with large vessel vasculitis a celiac angiography may demonstrate arterial aneurysmal lesions in the mesenteric and renal vessels.[116]

Medical treatment consists of steroids and/or immunosuppressive therapy. The physiatrist will be called upon to treat patients with residual neurological deficit, myositis, and post-gangrene complications.

Polymyalgia Rheumatica (PRM)

This disorder affects patients usually after age 50 and is more commonly seen in women than in men. Fatigue, severe stiffness, and aching, particularly over the shoulder girdles and pelvic girdle, in association with weight loss, depression, low-grade fever, and a markedly elevated sedimentation rate, are the hallmarks of this disorder. Mild joint manifestations may be distinguished from the generalized stiffness, and the associated giant cell arteritis affecting the temporal and other medium-sized arteries, supplied particularly by the carotid arterial tree, may lead to blindness and stroke.[117, 118] In this age group the presence of low titer rheumatoid factor and/or antinuclear antibodies is not uncommonly found and has no diagnostic significance. The muscle enzymes are normal. Diagnosis is usually made on the basis of the clinical features and a very high sedimentation rate.

A therapeutic trial of low-dose steroids, 7.5 to 10 mg of prednisone daily, may produce a marked remission within a few days. Temporal artery biopsy can be performed when the diagnosis remains in doubt, but as the arteritis tends to skip areas, a negative biopsy does not exclude the diagnosis.[117] When temporal or CNS arteritis is suspected, prednisone in a dose of 40 mg daily is administered for six weeks and then reduced to 10 mg or less for maintenance therapy.[117]

Physiatric management consists of range-of-motion and general reconditioning exercises.

Metabolic Arthropathies

Gout. This is typically an acute monarticular arthritis that will commonly involve the great toe. Rarely it can be chronic and polyarticular and involve small joints in the upper extremities in a manner that closely mimics rheumatoid arthritis.[119] Tophaceous deposits usually occur late and typically occur in the olecranon bursae. Attacks tend to be abrupt in onset, often occurring during the early morning hours and reaching peak intensity within a period of 24 hours. The acute attacks are self-limiting and usually pass off within a matter of one to four weeks. Between attacks the patients are generally symptom free. An elevated serum uric acid is the hallmark of this disorder, and the diagnosis is confirmed by demonstration in the synovial fluid of negatively birefringent crystals of monosodium urate.[120] Crystals may be aspirated from bursae, particularly the olecranon bursae, or scraped from accessible tophaceous deposits, most notably the subcutaneous tophi overlying the ear cartilage. In advanced cases severe destructive arthritis associated with tophaceous deposits can be seen.

Medical management consists of the use of uricosuric agents, typically probenecid in a dose of one half gram twice to three times daily. This drug should not be used in the presence of renal disease, and is usually not effective when the serum uric acid is consistently above 10 mg per 100 ml.[120] In these cases allopurinol is administered in a once-daily dose of 300 mg. This agent may be required prophylactically when intensive immunosuppressive therapy is used in the treatment of malignancy.[120] Many patients with mild hyperuricemia (less than 10 mg per 100 ml) may never develop gout and do not require treatment.[120] Conversely, an occasional patient with a "normal" serum uric acid may develop a severe gouty diathesis.[119] Colchicine in a dose of 1 mg stat and 0.5 mg every hour either until symptoms begin to abate; nausea, vomiting, and diarrhea occur; or approximately 10 tablets have been administered can be used as a therapeutic test when the diagnosis cannot be otherwise confirmed. Pseudogout, discussed below, may occasionally respond to this regimen as well. Maintenance dosages of colchicine of two to four tablets daily may help prevent attacks during the first few months of administration of either uricosuric or allopurinol therapy.

The physiatric management of gout is essentially no treatment in the acute attacks because in general the modalities tend to do nothing to relieve the discomfort, and the attacks respond promptly to nonsteroidal anti-inflammatory drug therapy. The use of canes or crutches as a joint protective measure, however, may facilitate ambulatory activities. Patients with chronic generalized gout may require additional functional retraining and the use of assistive devices and a reconditioning regimen.

Pseudogout (Chondrocalcinosis). Pseudogout consists of a gout-like attack occurring in patients who have either radiographically evident, or sometimes undetectable, chondrocalcinosis.[121, 122] This is a disorder characterized by the deposition of calcium pyrophosphate dihydrate crystals in the articular cartilages.[122] These crystals are weakly positively birefringent and tend to be rhomboid or needle-shaped when observed in the synovial fluid under polarized light.[122] Extrusion of these crystals from the adjacent cartilage precipitates the inflammatory response. X-rays of the wrists, knees, and symphyses may reveal calcifications on the triangular cartilage, menisci, and symphysis, respectively.[121, 122] Chondrocalcinosis and pseudogout may be associated with hyperparathyroidism, hemochromatosis, and Wilson's disease and may be seen as a familial disorder as well.[122] Most often it is idiopathic in origin and in contrast to gout it may occur in conjunction with diverse rheumatological conditions, including rheumatoid arthritis, gout, osteoarthritis, and Charcot joints.[122] The acute attacks may respond to local steroid injections or nonsteroidal anti-inflammatory drugs. Chondrocalcinosis may be manifested as a chronic smoldering arthritis often accompanying a severe osteoarthritis. Maintenance therapy may require ongoing nonsteroidal anti-inflammatory drugs, and the use of colchicine may be of value in suppressing the recurrent attacks in some cases.[122] Rehabilitative treatment is symptomatic and supportive.

Miscellaneous Arthritic Disorders

Neuropathic Joint Disease (Charcot Joint). Patients with a loss of sensory innervation and/or pain sensation, typically in association with tabes dorsalis, diabetes mellitus, or syringomyelia, may develop a disorder of joints that is characteristically marked by a relative lack of pain as compared to the amount of swelling and inflammation manifested. A Charcot joint may rarely present as an inflamed, rapidly destructive process or typically as an indolent, relatively painless, markedly swollen, unstable crepitant joint.[123] Radiographically loose bodies, cartilage destruction, and irregular repair with large osteophytes and indeed fractured osteophytes are seen.[123] The association of chondrocalcinosis and pseudogout has been recently noted and may be an aggravating factor.[122] Treatment is sympto-

TABLE 31–7. X-RAYS OFTEN HELPFUL IN DIAGNOSING EXTRA-ARTICULAR MANIFESTATIONS

1. Barium swallow	Polymyositis and progressive systemic sclerosis (PSS)
2. Dental x-rays	Resorption of lamina dura in hyperparathyroidism and PSS
3. Upper GI	Duodenal widening in progressive systemic sclerosis
4. Small bowel follow-through	Crohn's disease
5. Barium enema	Ulcerative colitis, wide-mouth diverticuli in PSS
6. Chest x-ray	Granuloma, infection, TB, sarcoid, Wegener's granulomatosis, rheumatoid arthritis, progressive systemic sclerosis. SLE, periarteritis nodosa, malignancy
7. Abdominal arteriogram	Polyarteritis (aneurysms)
8. Bone scan	Malignant disorders or osteomyelitis

matic. The use of stabilizing braces or splints and/or canes or crutches is frequently helpful in improving function and relieving discomfort. Surgical stabilization and wound healing in general in patients with Charcot joints are fraught with failure, and the status of joint replacement in such cases remains to be determined.[123]

Reflex Sympathetic Dystrophies (Shoulder-Hand Syndrome and Sudeck's Atrophy). A diffuse, usually severe tenderness, swelling, and pain affecting a hand, foot, or entire extremity, causing marked restriction of motion, characterizes these disorders. Typically in the early phases there is edema and there may be some erythema that over a period of weeks evolves into a condition characterized by a cool, clammy, atrophic, and contractured hand, foot, or extremity. This disorder is attributed to a sympathetic or autonomic instability and has been associated with angina pectoris, myocardial infarction, stroke, thoracic surgery, cervical disc disease, fracture, and/or minor and sometimes inapparent trauma.[124, 125] In the case of the *shoulder-hand syndrome,* typically the hand is involved early and the shoulder later; however, only the shoulder or only the hand may be affected. The elbow is characteristically spared. Dupuytren's contractures are commonly seen in the later stages. Technetium scans have demonstrated diffuse articular involvement and often symmetrical involvement where clinically the disorder is unilater-al.[125] X-rays typically show a severe demineralization with a characteristic patchy, blotchy appearance, and marginal bony erosions may be noted. Synovial biopsy has demonstrated proliferation and increased vascularity of the synovium but minimal inflammation.[125] A peculiar *regional migratory transient osteoporosis* has been shown in one case to be associated with evidence of lower motor neuron denervation by electromyographic studies.[124, 126]

Medical treatment of these disorders includes the use of sympathetic ganglion blocks in the early phases, which may be repeated serially once or twice a week if symptoms are well controlled, and alternatively or subsequently the use of prednisone. Prednisone administered in a dose of approximately 1 mg/kg for a period of one week, tapered rapidly over the subsequent two or three weeks, appears to suppress the pain and discomfort in both the localized and migrating varieties of this disorder.[124, 126] Analgesics are used as needed, with all due caution to avoid addiction.

Rehabilitative therapy to prevent contractures and deformities in the acute phases consists of appropriate splinting and positioning followed by active assisted to active range-of-motion exercises as soon as they can be tolerated. Functional activities for upper extremity involvement include the use of built-up handles and adapted equipment and activities to encourage joint mobilization and function. In lower extremity cases partial relief of weight-bearing by crutches and/or canes and the use of wading tanks or pools to permit weight-bearing stresses as early as possible is helpful in restoring ambulation. A pool provides a particularly comfortable medium for exercise therapies generally in these cases. With foot involvement the use of below-knee weight-bearing braces may facilitate ambulation. Transcutaneous nerve stimulation may also relieve pain sufficiently to permit earlier participation in functional and exercise activities. Local steroid injections into the shoulder and manual manipulation of the glenohumeral joint as well as in the distal joints (at a time when the disease is controlled and relatively quiescent and such maneuvers can be tolerated) may help facilitate restoration of mobility and function.

Hypertrophic Pulmonary Osteoarthropathy. This disorder is characterized by painful joint swelling and typically by clubbing of the fingers and toes. Periosteal elevation is usually seen, particularly in the distal radius, ulna, tibia, and fibula, and may be detected by Tc-labeled diphosphate.[127] Painful swelling of the knees, ankles, wrists, and occasionally the finger joints can easily confuse this disorder with rheumatoid arthritis. The synovial fluid findings are noninflammatory. Although this condition may occur as a familial male sex-linked dominant trait, it typically is associated with an underlying systemic disease, most notably primary pulmonary carcinomata.[127, 128] Other disorders that have been associated with pulmonary osteoarthritis include chronic suppurative pulmonary disease, subacute bacterial endocarditis, biliary cirrhosis, ulcerative colitis, regional enteritis, and congenital heart disease. Eradication of the underlying disease can result in remission of the associated pulmonary osteoarthropathy.[128]

In addition to treatment of the underlying disease the use of analgesics, nonsteroidal anti-inflammatory drugs, and in some cases moderate dosages of steroids are given for symptomatic relief. The physiatric treatment per se is also symptomatic.

Infectious Arthritis. Septic arthritis may result in a variety of bacterial infections and is typically an acute monarticular process. Synovial fluid analysis, including Gram stain and culture, is the key to the establishment of the diagnosis.[129] Some of the common organisms in acute septic arthritis include streptococci, staphylococci, gonococci, *Hemophilus influenzae*, and Pseudomonas organisms.[129] The latter organism is particularly seen in patients who are either drug users or have immunosuppression from any cause, and may produce an acute or indolent arthritis. The chronic infections include tuberculosis, brucellosis, coccidioidomycosis, and other fungal infections. Identification of the organism and prompt systemic antibiotic therapy are essential to control the infection.[130] Antibiotics should be accompanied by daily or twice-daily aspirations if necessary to relieve distention and to remove as much debris and infectious material as possible in acute infections.[130] When this cannot be accomplished or when the infection is poorly controlled, surgical drainage may be indicated, and this is particularly true when the hip joint is affected in children.[131] The joints are splinted during the acute phase, and mobilization is commenced as soon as tolerated by pain. The use of ice or cold compresses for control of pain in the early phase is helpful, and subsequently warm compresses or submersion of the affected extremity in a tank or tub can be helpful in restoring mobility. Splinting should be performed in a manner to preserve function and the splint should be removed once or twice daily for gentle assisted range-of-motion exercises during the acute phases and more frequently as symptoms abate. More vigorous active or resistive exercises and/or weight-bearing are best deferred until the signs of infection have been largely brought under control and are stabilized and cultures are no longer positive.

A number of viruses can produce a transient nondestructive arthritis.[132] The only exception to this is smallpox, and at this time it would appear that this disease has been eradicated.[132]

Summation

The rheumatological disorders mentioned here (and numerous others that are either rare or insignificant in their effects on joints) are clearly a highly diverse group of conditions that may at one extreme be associated with lethal complications or severe joint destruction and disability and at the other an insignificant, almost subliminal, arthralgia. Further, any specific arthritic disease in any given individual, or any given joint in an individual with multiple joints involved may be highly capricious in its effects. One may see, therefore, severe joint destruction in erosive osteoarthritis, or a minimal, transient PIP joint effusion in one finger in a patient with psoriatic arthritis. An appreciation of the nature of the specific diseases and their spectra of presentations and variable courses is essential to appropriate management. The resources available to the clinician include judicious use of pharmacological therapy, selected use of therapeutic modalities, meticulous attention to joint protective measures, rationally prescribed selective exercise therapy, timely referral for surgical treatment, and a concern with the patient's total psychological, physiological, and socioeconomic functioning. There is clearly a great need to develop in health professionals the skills to meet these enormous challenges.

REFERENCES

1. Clarke, J. T.: The antibiotic therapy of septic arthritis. In Schmid, F. R. (Ed.): Clin. Rheum. Dis., 4:63, 1978.
2. Hines, T. F.: Manual muscle examination. In Licht, S. (Ed.): Therapeutic Exercise, 2nd ed. New Haven, E. Licht, 1965, p. 163.
3. Kendall, H. O., Kendall, F. P., and Wadsworth, G. E.: Muscle Testing and Function, 2nd Ed. Baltimore, Williams and Wilkins Co., 1971, p. 3.
4. Howell, D. S., Sapolsky, A. I., Pita, J. C., and Woessner, J. F.: The pathogenesis of osteoarthritis. Semin. Arthritis Rheum., 5:365–383, 1976.
5. Sokoloff, L.: The Biology of Degenerative Joint Disease. Chicago, University of Chicago Press, 1969, p. 81.
6. Bennett, J. C. (Ed.): Twenty-third rheumatism review. Arthritis Rheum., 21:R105, 1978.
7. Lee, P., Rooney, P. J., Sturrock, R. D., Kennedy, A. C., and Dick, W. C.: The etiology and pathogenesis of osteoarthritis: A review seminar. Arthritis Rheum., 3:189–218, 1974.
8. Peter, J. B., Pearson, C. M., and Marmor, L.: Erosive osteoarthritis of the hands. Arthritis Rheum., 9:365, 1966.
9. Swezey, R. L.: Arthritis: Rational Therapy and Rehabilitation. Philadelphia, W. B. Saunders Company, 1978, p. 182.
10. Bodyns, J. H. (Ed.): Symposium on total joint replacement: Achievements and expectations, Part I. Geriatrics, 31:45–93, 1976.
11. Dobyns, J. H. (Ed.): Symposium on total joint replacement: Achievements and expectations, Part II. Geriatrics, 31:47–85, 1976.
12. Smillie, I. S.: Diseases of the Knee Joint. London, Churchill Livingstone, 1974, p. 75.
13. Swezey, R. L.: Arthritis: Rational Therapy and

Rehabilitation. Philadelphia, W. B. Saunders Company, 1978, p. 184.
14. Peterson, L. F. A., Bryan, R. S., and Combs, J. J.: Surgery for arthritis of the knee. Bull. Rheum. Dis., 25:794–797, 1974-75.
15. Lotke, P. A., Ecker, M. L., McCoskey, J., and Steinberg, M. E.: Early experience with total knee arthroplasty. J.A.M.A., 32:2403–2406, 1976.
16. Swezey, R. L.: Arthritis: Rational Therapy and Rehabilitation. Philadelphia, W. B. Saunders Company, 1978, pp. 113–118.
17. Bennett, J. C. (Ed.): Twenty-third rheumatism review. Arthritis Rheum., 21:R121–R123, 1978.
18. Swezey, R. L.: Arthritis: Rational Therapy and Rehabilitation. Philadelphia, W. B. Saunders Company, 1978, pp. 133–147.
19. Smythe, H. A., and Moldofsky, H.: Two contributions to understanding the fibrositis syndrome. Bull. Rheum. Dis., 28:928–931, 1977-78.
20. Simons, D. G.: Muscle pain syndromes — Part I. Am. J. Phys. Med., 54:289–211, 1975.
21. Simons, D. G.: Muscle pain syndromes — Part II. Am. J. Phys. Med., 55:15–42, 1976.
22. Awad, E. A.: Interstitial myofibrositis: Hypothesis of the mechanism. Arch. Phys. Med. Rehabil., 54:449–453, 1973.
23. Kraft, G. H., Johnson, E. W., and LaBan, M. M.: The fibrositis syndrome. Arch. Phys. Med. Rehabil., 49:155, 1968.
24. Swezey, R. L., and Spiegel, R. M.: Evaluation and treatment of local musculoskeletal disorders in elderly patients. Geriatrics, 34:56–75, 1979.
25. Travell, J.: Symposium on mechanism and management of pain syndromes. Proc. Rudolf Virchow Med. Soc., 16:1, 1957.
26. Bonica, J. J.: Management of myofascial pain syndromes in general practice. J.A.M.A., 164:732–738, 1957.
27. Copeman, W. S. C.: Fibro-fatty tissue and its relationship to certain "rheumatic" syndromes. Br. Med. J., 2:191–192, 1949.
28. Bland, J. H., Merrit, J. A., and Boushey, D. R.: The painful shoulder. Semin. Arthritis Rheum., 7:21–47, 1977.
29. Carroll, R. E., Sinton, W., and Garcia, A.: Acute calcium deposits in the hand. J.A.M.A., 157:422–426, 1955.
30. Bluestone, R.: Calcific periarthritis and hemodialysis. J.A.M.A., 223:548, 1973.
31. Swezey, R. L.: Pseudo-radiculopathy in subacute trochanteric bursitis of the subgluteus maximus bursa. Arch. Phys. Med. Rehabil., 57:387–390, 1976.
32. Brookler, M. I., and Mongan, E. S.: Anserine bursitis. Calif. Med., 119:8–10, 1973.
33. Smillie, I. S.: Diseases of the Knee Joint. London, Churchill Livingstone, 1974, p. 140.
34. Swezey, R. L.: Arthritis: Rational Therapy and Rehabilitation. Philadelphia, W. B. Saunders Company, 1978, p. 186.
35. Nirschl, R. P.: Tennis elbow. Primary Care, 4:367–382, 1976.
36. Goldie, I.: Epicondylitis lateralis humeri (epicondylalgia or tennis elbow): A pathogenetical study. Acta Chir. Scand. Suppl., 339, 1964, pp. 1–189.
37. Clark, A. K., and Woodland, J.: Comparison of

two steroid preparations used to treat tennis elbow using the hypo spray. Rheumatol. Rehabil., 14:47–49, 1975.

38. Swezey, R. L.: Arthritis: Rational Therapy and Rehabilitation. Philadelphia, W. B. Saunders Company, 1978, p. 86.

39. Turek, S. L.: Orthopaedic Principles and Their Application, 3rd Ed. Philadelphia, J. B. Lippincott Co., 1977, p. 906.

40. Boyes, J. H.: Bunnell's Surgery of the Hand, 5th Ed. Philadelphia, J. B. Lippincott Co., 1970, p. 445.

41. Kelikian, H.: Hallux Valgus, Allied Deformities of the Forefoot and Metatarsalgia. Philadelphia, W. B. Saunders Company, 1965, p. 359.

42. Boyes, J. H.: Bunnell's Surgery of the Hand, 5th Ed. Philadelphia, J. B. Lippincott Co., 1970, pp. 666–670.

43. Boyes, J. H.: Bunnell's Surgery of the Hand, 5th Ed. Philadelphia, J. B. Lippincott Co., 1970, pp. 225–239.

44. Bennett, J. C. (Ed.): Twenty-third rheumatism review: Juvenile rheumatoid arthritis. Arthritis Rheum., 21:R34–R36, 1978.

45. Brewerton, D. A. (Ed.): Symposium on histocompatibility and rheumatic disease. Ann. Rheum. Dis., 34(Suppl. 1):1–65, 1975.

46. Brewerton, D. A.: HLA-B27 and the inheritance of susceptibility to rheumatic disease (Joseph J. Bunim Memorial Lecture). Arthritis Rheum., 19:656–668, 1976.

47. Bennett, J. C.: Future research directions: The infectious etiology of rheumatoid arthritis: New considerations. Arthritis Rheum., 21:531–538, 1978.

48. Bennett, J. C. (Ed.): Twenty-third rheumatism review: Rheumatoid arthritis. Arthritis Rheum., 21:R17–R33, 1978.

49. Linn, J. E., Hardin, J. G., and Halla, J. T.: A controlled study of ANA+ RF− arthritis. Arthritis Rheum., 21:645–651, 1978.

50. Bennett, J. C. (Ed.): Twenty-third rheumatism review: Sjögren's syndrome. Arthritis Rheum., 21:R72, 1978.

51. Huskisson, E. C.: Antiinflammatory drugs. Semin. Arthritis Rheum., 7:1–20, 1977.

52. Willkens, R. F.: The use of nonsteroidal antiinflammatory agents. J.A.M.A., 240:1632–1635, 1978.

53. Buckingham, R. B.: Interactions involving antirheumatic agents. Part I. Bull. Rheum. Dis., 28:960–965, 1977-78.

54. Buckingham, R. B.: Interactions involving antirheumatic agents. Part II. Bull. Rheum. Dis., 28:966–971, 1977-78.

55. Bluhm, G. B.: The treatment of rheumatoid arthritis with gold. Semin. Arthritis Rheum., 5:147–165, 1975.

56. Mowat, A. G., and Huskisson, E. C.: D-penicillamine in rheumatoid arthritis. Clin. Rheum. Dis., 1:319–333, 1975.

57. Popert, A. J.: Chloroquine: A review. Rheumatol. Rehabil., 15:235–238, 1976.

58. Jasani, M. K.: The importance of ACTH and glucocorticoids in rheumatoid arthritis. Clin. Rheum. Dis., 1:335–365, 1975.

59. Fitzgerald, R. H.: Intrasynovial injection of steroids, uses and abuses. Mayo Clin. Proc., 51:655–659, 1976.

60. Balch, H. W., Gibson, J. M. C., El-Ghobarey, A. F., Bain, L. S., and Lynch, M. P.: Repeated corticosteroid injections into knee joints. Rheumatol. Rehabil., 16:137–140, 1977.

61. Halpern, A. A., Horowitz, B. G., and Nagel, D. A.: Tendon ruptures associated with corticosteroid therapy. West. J. Med., 127:378–382, 1977.

62. Gibson, T., Burry, H. C., Poswillo, D., and Glass, J.: Effect of intra-articular corticosteroid injections on primate cartilage. Ann. Rheum. Dis., 36:74–79, 1976.

63. Steinbrocker, O., and Argyros, T. G.: Frozen shoulder: Treatment by local injections of depot corticosteroids. Arch. Phys. Med. Rehabil., 55:209–213, 1974.

64. Swezey, R. L.: Arthritis: Rational Therapy and Rehabilitation. Philadelphia, W. B. Saunders Company, 1978, pp. 103–124.

65. Swezey, R. L.: Arthritis: Rational Therapy and Rehabilitation. Philadelphia, W. B. Saunders Company, 1978, pp. 97–102.

66. Swezey, R. L.: Arthritis: Rational Therapy and Rehabilitation. Philadelphia, W. B. Saunders Company, 1978, pp. 133–148.

67. Swezey, R. L.: Arthritis: Rational Therapy and Rehabilitation. Philadelphia, W. B. Saunders Company, 1978, pp. 149–154.

68. Halstead, L. S.: Team care in chronic illness. A critical review of the literature of the past twenty-five years. Arch. Phys. Med. Rehabil., 57:507–511, 1976.

69. National attack on arthritis. Congressional Record, Vol. 120, No. 155 (Part II, S-19129), October 11, 1974, pp. 1–10.

70. Swezey, R. L.: Arthritis: Rational Therapy and Rehabilitation. Philadelphia, W. B. Saunders Company, 1978, pp. 21–45.

71. Edington, D. W., and Edgerton, V. R.: The Biology of Physical Activity. Boston, Houghton Mifflin Co., 1976, p. 57.

72. Muller, E. A.: Influence of training and of inactivity on muscle strength. Arch. Phys. Med. Rehabil., 51:449, 1970.

73. Machover, S., and Sapecky, A. J.: Effect of isometric exercises on the quadriceps muscle in patients with rheumatoid arthritis. Arch. Phys. Med. Rehabil., 47:737, 1966.

74. Ekblom, B., Lovgren, O., Alderin, M., Fridstrom, M., and Satterstrom, G.: Effect of short-term physical training on patients with rheumatoid arthritis, II. Scand. J. Rheum., 4(2):87, 1975.

75. Marbach, J. J.: Arthritis of the teporomandibular joints and facial pain. Bull. Rheum. Dis., 27:918–921, 1976.

76. Bland, J. H.: Rheumatoid arthritis of the cervical spine. J. Rheum., 1:319–342, 1974.

77. Ornilla, E., Ansell, B. M., and Swannell, A. J.: Cervical spine involvement in patients with chronic arthritis undergoing orthopaedic surgery. Ann. Rheum. Dis., 31:364–368, 1972.

78. Linscheid, R. L., and Beckenbaugh, R. D.: Total shoulder arthroplasty: Experimental but promising. Geriatrics, 31:64–69, 1976.

79. Swezey, R. L.: Arthritis: Rational Therapy and Rehabilitation. Philadelphia, W. B. Saunders Company, 1978, p. 37.

80. Dickson, R. A., Stein, H., and Bentley, G.: Excision arthroplasty of the elbows in rheumatoid disease. J. Bone Joint Surg., 58B:227–229, 1976.

81. Brattstrom, H., and Khudairy, H. A.: Synovectomy of the elbow in rheumatoid arthritis. Acta Orthop. Scand., 46:744–750, 1975.

82. Dobyns, J. H., Bryan, R. S., Linscheid, R. L., et al.: The special problems of total elbow arthroplasty. Geriatrics, 31:57–61, 1976.

83. Jackson, I. T.: Surgery of the hand in rheumatoid arthritis. Clin. Rheum. Dis., 1:401–428, 1975.

84. Swezey, R. L.: Dynamic factors in deformity of the rheumatoid hand. Bull. Rheum. Dis., 22(Nos. 1, 2):649–656, 1971.

85. Goldie, I. F.: Synovectomy in rheumatoid arthritis: A general review and an eight year follow-up of synovectomy in fifty rheumatoid patients. Semin. Arthritis Rheum., 3:219–251, 1974.

86. Arthritis and Rheumatism Council and British Orthopaedic Association: Controlled trial of synovectomy of the knee and metacarpophalangeal joint in rheumatoid arthritis. Ann. Rheum. Dis., 35:437–442, 1976.

87. Arthritis Foundation Committee on Evaluation of Synovectomy: Multicenter evaluation of synovectomy in the treatment of rheumatoid arthritis. Arthritis Rheum., 20:765–771, 1977.

88. Robinson, H. S., Kokan, P. J., MacBain, K. P., and Patterson, F. P.: Functional results of excisional arthroplasty for the rheumatoid hand. Can. Med. J., 108:1495–1499, 1978.

89. Brown, P. W.: Hand surgery in rheumatoid arthritis. Semin. Arthritis Rheum., 4:327–363, 1976.

90. Swezey, R. L.: Arthritis: Rational Therapy and Rehabilitation. Philadelphia, W. B. Saunders Company, 1978, p. 182.

91. Haberman, E. T., and Feinstein, P. A.: Total hip replacement arthroplasty in arthritic conditions of the hip joint. Semin. Arthritis Rheum., 7:189–231, 1978.

92. Cracchiolo, A.: Surgery of the knee and foot in rheumatoid arthritis. Clin. Rheum. Dis., 1:383–400, 1975.

93. Williams, R. C.: Rheumatoid Arthritis as a Systemic Disease. Philadelphia, W. B. Saunders Company, 1974, p. 210.

94. Bluestone, R.: HL-A antigens in clinical medicine. Disease-a-Month, 23:1–27, 1976.

95. Romanus, R., and Yden, S.: Pelvo-Spondylitis Ossificans. Chicago, Year Book Publishers, Inc., 1955, p. 63.

96. Calin, A., and Fries, J. F.: Striking prevalence of ankylosing spondylitis in "healthy" W27 positive males and females. N. Engl. J. Med., 293:835–839, 1975.

97. Ball, J.: Enthesopathy of rheumatoid and ankylosing spondylitis. Ann. Rheum. Dis., 30:213–223, 1971.

98. Dwosh, I. L.: Reankylosis high in hip patients. Orthop. Rev., 5:77–78, 1976.

99. Vatopoulos, P. K., Diacomopoulos, G. J., Demiris, C. S., et al.: Girdlestones operation — Follow-up study. Acta Orthop. Scand., 47:324–328, 1976.

100. Good, A. E.: Reiter's disease: A review with special attention to cardiovascular and neurological sequelae. Semin. Arthritis Rheum., 3:253–286, 1974.

101. Roberts, M. E. T., Wright, V., Hill, A. G. S., and Mehra, A. C.: Psoriatic arthritis. Ann. Rheum. Dis., 35:206–212, 1976.

102. Roux, H., Mercier, P., Maestracci, G., et al.: Psoriatic arthritis and HLA antigens. J. Rheumatol. (Suppl.) 3:64–65, 1977.

103. Swezey, R. L., Bjarnason, D. M., Alexander, S. J., and Forrester, D. B.: Resorptive arthropathy and the opera-glass hand syndrome. Semin. Arthritis Rheum., 2:191–244, 1972.

104. Dorwart, B. B., Gall, P., Schumacher, H. R., and Krauser, R. E.: Chrysotherapy in psoriatic arthritis. Arthritis Rheum., 21:513–515, 1978.

105. Harber, L. C.: Photochemotherapy of psoriasis. N. Engl. J. Med., 291:1251–1252, 1974.

106. Haslock, I., and Wright, V.: The arthritis associated with intestinal disease. Bull. Rheum. Dis., 24:750–755, 1973.

107. Bennett, J. C. (Ed.): Twenty-third rheumatism review. Systemic lupus erythematosus. Arthritis Rheum., 21:R51–R70, 1978.

108. Wigley, R. D.: Models of rheumatic disease occurring spontaneously in mice. Semin. Arthritis Rheum., 7:81–95, 1977.

109. Dubois, E. L.: Antimalarials in the management of discoid and systemic lupus erythematosus. Semin. Arthritis Rheum., 8:33–51, 1978.

110. Campbell, P., and LeRoy, E. C.: Pathogenesis of systemic sclerosis: A vascular hypothesis. Semin. Arthritis Rheum., 4:351–368, 1975.

111. Emery, H., Schaller, J. G., and Fowler, R. S., Jr.: Biofeedback in the management of primary and secondary Raynaud's. American Rheumatism Association, 40th Annual Meeting, Chicago, June, 1976, p. 77.

112. Talbott, J. H.: Acute dermatomyositis-polymyositis and malignancy. Semin. Arthritis Rheum., 6:305–360, 1977.

113. Carpenter, S., Karpat, G., Rothman, S., et al.: The childhood type of dermatomyositis. Neurology, 26:952–962, 1976.

114. Bennett, J. C. (Ed.): Twenty-third rheumatism review. Polymyositis and dermatomyositis. Arthritis Rheum., 21:R83–R89, 1978.

115. Sharp, G. C., Irvin, W. S., May, C. M., et al.: Association of antibodies to ribonucleoprotein and Sm antigens with mixed connective-tissue disease, systemic lupus erythematosus and other rheumatic diseases. N. Engl. J. Med., 295:1149–1154, 1976.

116. Fauci, A. S., Haynes, B. F., and Katz, P.: The spectrum of vasculitis. Ann. Intern. Med., 89:660–676, 1978.

117. Fernandez-Herlihy, L.: Polymyalgia rheumatica. Semin. Arthritis Rheum., 1:236–245, 1971.

118. Huston, K. A., Aunder, G. G., Lie, J. T., et al.: Temporal arteritis. Ann. Intern. Med., 88:162–167, 1978.

119. Talbott, J. A., Altman, R. D., and Yu, T. S.: Gouty arthritis masquerading as rheumatoid arthritis or vice versa. Semin. Arthritis Rheum., 8:77–114, 1978.

120. Klinenberg, J. R. (Ed.): Proceedings of second conference on gout and purine metabolism. Arthritis Rheum., 18:659–894, 1975.

121. Rubinstein, H. M., and Shab, D. M.: Pseudogout. Semin. Arthritis Rheum., 2:259–280, 1972.

122. McCarty, D. J.: Diagnostic mimicry in arthritis — patterns of joint involvement associated with calcium pyrophosphate dihydrate crystal deposits. Bull. Rheum. Dis., 25:804–808, 1974.

123. Bruckner, F. E., and Howell, A.: Neuropathic joints. Semin. Arthritis Rheum., 2:47–69, 1972.

124. Swezey, R. L.: Transient osteoporosis of the hip, foot and knee. Arthritis Rheum., 13:858–868, 1970.
125. Kozin, F., McCarty, D. J., Sims, J., and Genant, H.: The reflex sympathetic dystrophy syndrome. Am. J. Med., 60:321–331, 1976.
126. McCord, W. C., Nies, K. M., Campion, D. S., and Louie, J. S.: Regional migratory osteoporosis: A denervation disease. Arthritis Rheum., 21:834–838, 1978.
127. Lokich, J. J.: Pulmonary osteoarthropathy. J.A.M.A., 238:37–39, 1977.
128. Fischer, D. S., Singer, D. H., and Feldman, S. M.:

129. Sommers, H. M.: The microbiology laboratory in the diagnosis of infectious arthritis. Clin. Rheum. Dis., 4:63–82, 1978.
130. Parker, R. H., and Schmid, F. R.: Antibacterial activity of synovial fluid during therapy of septic arthritis. Arthritis Rheum., 14:96–104, 1971.
131. Sledge, C. B.: Surgery in infectious arthritis. Clin. Rheum. Dis., 4:159–168, 1978.
132. Sauter, S. V. H., and Utsinger, P. D.: Viral arthritis. Clin. Rheum. Dis., 4:225–240, 1978.

Clubbing, a review with emphasis on hereditary acropachy. Medicine, 43:459–479, 1964.

32

TRAUMATIC AND CONGENITAL LESIONS OF THE SPINAL CORD

MURRAY M. FREED

During the past four decades our understanding of the care of individuals with spinal cord injury has developed and improved more than during the previous 50 centuries. Yet it remains, because of its multisystem involvement, one of the most catastrophic injuries — socially, economically, and physically — which can occur to the young adult.

The earliest available documentary on spinal cord injury is found in the Edwin Smith surgical papyrus, estimated to have been written between 2500 and 3000 B.C., with certain commentaries added 1000 years later.[1] Legend has it that the author was Imhotep, physician to the Pharoah. He described a man with a broken neck who was paralyzed in all his extremities, whose excretory function was characterized by constant dribbling, and whose muscles were wasting away. Under medical treatment was noted, "an ailment not to be treated." This dictum, because the injury's complications were poorly understood, was followed for millennia.

The century prior to World War I saw such advances in surgical procedures for spinal cord injury as laminectomy, nerve section, cordotomy, rhizotomy, and sympathectomy. During the Balkan wars of 1912–1913 there was a mortality rate of 95 per cent within a few weeks.[2] Thompson Walker, commenting in 1917, noted that of approxmately 450 British soldiers with spinal cord injuries who had survived evacuation from World War I battlefields and been brought to the Star and Garter and King George hospitals, 179 died of urinary tract infection during a period of two years.[3] Among American troops during World War I, 80 per cent of the 2324 men who had received injury to the spinal cord died before they could be returned from overseas.[4] Of the remainder, who were successfully evacuated to this country, 10 per cent survived the first year; in 1946 it was estimated that less than 1 per cent of those

Portions of this chapter are taken from Tedeschi, C. G., Eckert, W. G., and Tedeschi, L. G.: Forensic Medicine: A Study in Trauma and Environmental Hazards. Chapter 3, Murray M. Freed: Long-term disability from spinal cord injury. Philadelphia, W. B. Saunders Company, 1977, pp. 76–87.

who survived the first year were still alive. Two decades after the end of World War I, Hinman wrote that most fatalities among patients with spinal cord injuries were still due to urinary tract infections and bedsores, and the failure to prevent or control these complications accounted for over 80 per cent of deaths.[5]

Improved understanding of the management of the bladder dysfunction secondary to transverse myelopathy and improved nursing care for the prevention of bedsores accounted for significant changes in survival rates just prior to and during World War II. In the United States it was the work of the late Dr. Donald Munro, and in Great Britain of Sir Ludwig Guttmann, that made them prophets in the management of the spinal cord injury and the decrease in its complications.

In 1943, Munro reported a mortality rate of 0.575 in 40 patients during the previous nine-and-one-half-year period.[6] Sepsis of the genitourinary tract and bedsores accounted for 30.4 per cent of the deaths. In 1946, Kirk stated that there were at that time 1400 paraplegic patients in service hospitals and that the results constituted a tribute to the professional competence of the Army doctors in the war.[7] In 1958, a Veterans Administration study of 5743 patients with spinal cord injuries who survived the immediate handling and the potential early complications in service hospitals and who were subsequently treated, between 1946 and 1955, for their traumatic paraplegia or quadriplegia disclosed an overall mortality rate of 0.139.[8]

As the incidence of urinary tract complications declines with progressively better methods of bladder management and with "prompt adequate care,"[9] the potential longevity of the spinal cord–injured individual will approach normal.

SCOPE OF THE PROBLEM

Spinal cord injury occurs most frequently in younger age groups: 80 per cent are under age 40. The median age is 23, the mean 29, and the most common age 20 years. Fifty per cent of the injuries occur in the 15- to 25-year-old group. Fifty-three per cent of the spinal cord injured have an impairment of quadriplegia, and 82 per cent are male.[9]

In 1957, Michaelis estimated, there were approximately 10 new cases of spinal injury per million of the population of a country.[10] In a study during the years 1960 to 1967 in Switzerland, Gehrig and Michaelis concluded that the annual incidence was 15 per million population, with an annual increase of 1.7 per cent.[11] A 1967 Canadian estimate was 12 to 15 per million.[12] In 1969, Young reported estimates that the number of persons experiencing spinal injury in the United States ranged between 3,500 and 10,000 annually, an incidence of between 20 and 50 per million population.[13] Owens and Sharman found an incidence of 12.3 per million in New England in 1970 and predicted an annual increase to 15.6 by 1980 and 17.1 by 1990.[14] Brown gave an incidence of 20 to 30 per million population annually in the 14- to 50-year age group.[15] The National Spinal Cord Injury Data Research Center in a 1979 report describes an annual incidence of 30 to 35 per million based on individuals who do not succumb prior to hospital admission. The overall incidence may well be on the order of 50 per million.[16]

Young noted that of the roughly 200 million population in the United States in 1969 it was estimated that the spinal cord injury population constituted approximately 500 per million or a total of 100,000 at that time.[13] Sharman and Owens estimated a prevalence of 46,700 in 1970 and predicted 75,200 by 1980 and 108,300 by 1990.[14] In the 14- to 50-year age group the prevalence was 161 per million for Hawaii in 1971, 121 per million for Nevada in 1970, and 119 per million for Maine and 121 per million for Massachusetts in 1972.[17, 18]

The Gehrig and Michaelis Swiss study disclosed that 36 per cent of spinal cord injuries occurred on the road and in traffic; 35 per cent occurred at work, and 29 per cent occurred at home and in sports.[11] The Nevada study showed 52 per cent resulting from automobile accidents; in Maine the percentage was 51.6,[15] while in Hawaii it was 21.[17, 18] A Canadian study of 1737 cases in 1967–1968 revealed that 37 per cent were due to motor vehicle accidents, 37 per cent to industrial accidents, and 7 per cent to diving.[19] The National SCI Data Research Center reported in 1979 that 46 per cent were due to vehicular accidents, 16 per cent to falls, and 10.6 per cent to diving accidents. Regional differences in etiology occur; in the National Pool penetrating wounds (gunshot and stabbing) accounted for 12 per cent, in the South Florida Regional System for 30 per cent, and in the New England Regional System for 6.1 per cent.[16]

Mechanisms of Injury

By definition, paraplegia is paralysis of the lower extremities and all or a portion of the trunk. When the arms are also involved, the term *quadriplegia* is used to describe the impairment.

Fracture-dislocation of the cervical spine is a consequence of sudden and violent flexion or, less frequently, of extension and rotational or horizontal forces. The vertebral fracture-dislocation may result from a direct blow or from acceleration injuries. Motor vehicle accidents are the leading cause of cervical cord trauma, with diving accidents the leading cause in sports injuries. Thoracic spine fractures may result from a direct blow such as occurs in a cave-in from violent flexion in the seated position or from a penetrating missile. Thoracolumbar fracture-dislocations are most common at the T12-L1 site and follow violent flexion such as occurs in a fall from a height. In such an occurrence the initial force may strike the calcanei, with the likelihood of fracturing these bony segments, following which the remaining force causes a sufficient degree of flexion at the thoracolumbar junction to produce a fracture-dislocation. The most common sites of fracture-dislocation injuries are the C5-6, C6-7, and T12-L1 junctions. Certain parts of the spine are relatively protected from injury, namely, the upper thoracic and lower lumbar regions.[21]

Those instances in which radiologic examination shows no fracture or dislocation but in which there is substantial cord damage prove to be hyperextension injuries to the cervical spine in persons with spondylosis.[22] The spinal cord, already compromised by a narrow canal, is compressed by the further narrowing caused by hyperextension of the cervical spine. In addition, Hughes points out, vertebral artery obstruction may occur in the absence of radiologic evidence of fracture and produce a central region of ischemia or infarction in the cervical cord.[22]

In the case of a fracture-dislocation with damage to the entire thickness of the cord, all function at and distal to the site of injury is lost. Thus, there is total sensorimotor loss in the area of the body supplied from the site of injury and below.

Following injury to the cord, vascular and biochemical changes lead to complete infarction and necrosis of the injured segment. The actual mechanism for reduction of spinal cord blood flow after trauma is poorly understood. According to Tator it may be a direct mechanical effect on the blood vessels or there may be a biochemical explanation.[23] There is not only a direct injury to the axons and blood vessels at the time of injury but also a secondary chain of events resulting in hypoxia, edema, and ultimate infarction. Osterholm and his co-workers were of the opinion that norepinephrine release at the site of injury causes severe vasoconstriction that leads to ischemia and hemorrhagic necrosis of the cord.[24]

Early Care

The acute care of the spinal cord–injured individual is directed to stabilization of the medical condition, treatment of associated injuries when present, and appropriate immobilization.

Although steroid therapy is almost universally used for resolution of edema of the injured spinal cord, proof of its beneficial effects is lacking. The use of hyperbaric oxygen in the reduction of permanent cord damage after trauma remains in the realm of the mythical and currently serves only to raise false hopes for the patient.[26]

In the cervical fracture patient, in lieu of skeletal traction, prolonged bed immobilization may be avoided by posterior fusion, anterior interbody fusion, or halo immobilization in appropriate instances. In the case of thoracic spine fractures, immobilization in recumbency is indicated until the acute period is over, for a period of rest in bed is all that is required before application of bracing. In those instances of thoracolumbar fracture for which fusion is indicated, Harrington rod application may be the treatment of choice.

Laminectomy is no longer the routine procedure that it was a decade ago. Any decision for surgical intervention is made after careful consideration of what may be accomplished; when complete paralysis has lasted more than one to two days there is usually no useful recovery.[27, 28]

Surgery is considered when the paralysis

shows a spread of neurologic involvement without obvious cause or in the instance of anterior cord syndrome with incomplete paralysis and the finding of anterior compression by radiographic study.

For a clearer understanding of the signs and symptoms resulting from spinal cord damage, it is germane to describe the scheme of segmental distribution.[25] The surface regions of the body supplied by the sensory (dorsal) roots of a spinal cord segment through the spinal nerves are called dermatomes. These have been determined by clinical studies and documented (Fig. 32–1). The segmental innervation of voluntary muscles has also been recorded; most muscle groups are innervated from two or more spinal cord segments as shown in Table 32–1.

For better understanding of the complications of spinal cord injury and the prognosis, the description of the impairment is based on the functional level of motor and sensory loss rather than on the anatomical location of the spinal column injury. Thus, "a complete level below C5" or "a C5 sensorimotor quadriplegia" denotes that C5 is the last functioning segment of the spinal cord. This is the terminology in use in the leading spinal cord injury centers and is the one propounded by Michaelis.[10] For the pathologist additional information including the site of bony injury is described so that he may correlate the neurologic or orthopedic findings with the histologic findings, since the level of spinal cord involvement may be at variance with the bony injury.

Motor Loss

It is a rare individual who survives complete injury to the third or fourth cervical cord segments, since respiratory difficulties secondary to loss of function ensue. Damage below the fourth cervical segment spares the diaphragm for breathing; the only other significant musculoskeletal functions remaining are neck muscle function and the ability to shrug the shoulders.

Statistically there exist critical levels of spinal cord function (Table 32–2). The described levels of remaining musculoskeletal function are consistent with intact function at the specific spinal cord segment and all those proximal to it, with loss of function to a

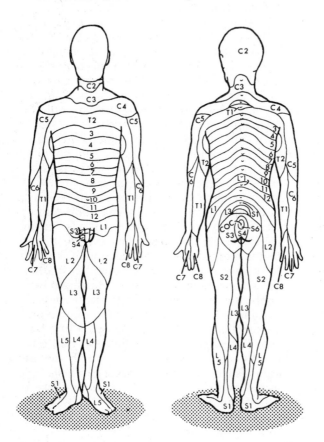

FIGURE 32–1. Spinal nerve dermatomes. (From Tedeschi, C. G., Eckert, W. G., and Tedeschi, L. G.: A Study in Trauma and Environmental Hazards. Philadelphia, W. B. Saunders Company, 1977, p. 78.)

TABLE 32–1. SEGMENTAL INNERVATION OF MUSCLES

Neck	Flexion	
	Extension	C1,2,3,4
	Rotation	
Shoulder	Flexion	C5,6
	Abduction	C5,6
	Adduction	C5,6,7,8
	Extension	C5,6,7,8
Elbow	Flexion	C5,6
	Extension	C7,8
Forearm	Pronation	C6,7
	Supination	C5,6,7
Wrist	Extension	C6,7
	Flexion	C6,7,T1
Hand	Gross extension of fingers	C6,7,8,
	Gross flexion of fingers	C7,8,T1
	Fine digital motion	C8,T1
Back	Extension	C4 to L1
Chest muscles for breathing		T2 to T12
Diaphragm		C2,3,4
Abdominal muscles		T6 to L1
Hip	Flexion	L2,3,4
	Abduction	L4,5,S1
	Adduction	L2,3,4
	Extension	L4,5,S1
	Rotation	L4,5,S1,2
Knee	Extension	L2,3,4
	Flexion	L4,5,S1
Ankle		L4,5,S1,2
Foot		L5,S1,2
Bladder		S2,3,4
Bowel	Rectum and anal sphincter	S2,3,4
Generative system		
Erection	Sacral cord	S2,3,4
Ejaculation	Lumbar cord	L1,2,3

TABLE 32–2. CRITICAL LEVELS OF SPINAL CORD FUNCTION

C4	Diaphragm, midcervical extensors and flexors.
C5	Partial strength of all shoulder motions and elbow flexion.
C6	Normal power of all shoulder motions and elbow flexion; wrist extension, with indirectly permits gross grasping by the fingers.
C7	Elbow extension, flexion, and extension of fingers.
T1	Completely normal arms and hands.
T6	Upper back extensors, upper intercostal muscles.
T12	All muscles of thorax, abdomen, and back.
L4	Hip flexion, knee extension.
L5	Partial strength of all hip motions with normal flexion, partial strength of knee flexion, partial strength of ankle and foot motion.

particular levels of the spinal cord, it is possible to categorize the performance to be expected of patients injured at and between these levels (Table 32–2; Figs. 32–2 to 32–10). The understanding of critical levels makes possible the prediction of ultimate function in the absence of complications in the well-trained, well-motivated spinal cord–injured person (Table 32–3).

greater or lesser degree in all distal segments.

The sensory sparing may be determined from the dermatome diagram (see Fig. 32–1).

FUNCTIONAL SIGNIFICANCE OF SPINAL CORD LESION LEVEL

Although general principles can be mentioned for the management of patients with spinal cord injuries, the specific program for an individual patient must be modified according to the level of the lesion. The lower the level of the injury, the greater the amounts of muscle power available to the patient for his rehabilitation. Because certain functional groups of muscles are activated at

Fourth Cervical Level

The quadriplegic in whom the fourth cervical segment is spared has good use of the sternomastoids and the trapezius and upper cervical paraspinal muscles. He is incapable of voluntary function in the arms, trunk, or lower extremities. The completely paralyzed arms may be supported on balanced forearm orthoses (mobile arm supports; feeders). The patient then uses ''body English'' and changes in head position to raise and lower the hand. A mouthstick may be useful in typing, writing, dialing, and turning pages.

The most practical method of replacing lost function is by use of ''sip and puff'' pneumatic control for operation of the wheelchair, including the reclining back. It is also appropriate for operation of an environmental control unit (ECU) to manage telephone, radio, television, and cassette tape recorder operation; page turning; and door locking. For those with insufficient ventilatory strength to manage the pneumatic control, tongue pressure and humidity switches are being developed. Voice activating mechanisms bode well for the future.[31]

TABLE 32–3. FUNCTIONAL SIGNIFICANCE OF SPINAL CORD LESION LEVEL

Activities	C4	C5	C6	C7	T1	T6	T12	L4
Self Care								
Eating	−	+	+	+	+	+	+	+
Dressing	−	−	±	+	+	+	+	+
Toileting	−	±	±	+	+	+	+	+
Bed Independence								
Rolling, sitting up supine	−	−	±	+	+	+	+	+
Moving about, sitting	−	−	±	+	+	+	+	+
Wheelchair Independence								
Transfer to and from	−	−	±	+	+	+	+	+
Mobility	*+	+	+	+	+	+	+	+
Ambulation								
Functional	−	−	−	−	−	±	±	+
Attendant								
Lifting	+	+	±	−	−	−	−	−
Assisting	+	+	±	−	−	−	−	−
Homebound Work	+	+	+	+	+	+	+	+
Outside Job	+	+	+	+	+	+	+	+
Private Car	−	+	+	+	+	+	+	+
Public Transportation	±	±	±	±	±	±	±	+
Braces or Devices	+ EC	+ Hand	+ Hand	−	+ LL	+ LL	+ LL	+ SH
Communication Skills								
Writing	*+	+	+	+	+	+	+	+
Typing	*+	+	+	+	+	+	+	+
Dictating machine	*+	+	+	+	+	+	+	+
Telephone	*+	+	+	+	+	+	+	+

*Requires pneumatically operated equipment or adaptive devices controlled by mouth.
EC = Environmental control; Hand =hand devices; LL = long leg brace; SH = short leg brace.

Fifth Cervical Level

The patient with a functioning fifth cervical segment can use the deltoid and biceps muscles to accomplish activities of daily living. Partial continued weakness of the deltoid and biceps may make it necessary to use a balanced forearm orthosis for support of the elbow and shoulder, especially in the early stages of the rehabilitation program. Overhead sling suspension may be used as an interim measure if it appears that permanent orthoses will not be necessary; the patient needs a substitute for nonfunctioning hand and wrist musculature. Fixed support of the wrist and fingers is used, and adapted devices are then applied to the patient's hand by another individual and kept in place until a new activity is started. Skillful use of these devices requires much training and practice.

The quadriplegic whose lesion is below the fifth cervical segment can be expected to feed himself, perform some grooming activi-

ties, help a little with upper extremity dressing, help apply bracing, push his wheelchair for short distances (with special projections on the wheelchair rims), turn pages, and use the electric typewriter.

Patients with lesions at the fourth and fifth cervical levels require help for lifting and assisting. A hydraulic lift may be necessary to help the family move the patient from bed to wheelchair. Beds for all patients with spinal cord injuries should be adjusted to wheelchair height. Removable armrests are essential components of all wheelchairs for the spinal cord injured.

Sixth Cervical Level

At the sixth cervical level of involvement, the individual has virtually fully innervated shoulder musculature, elbow flexion, and radial wrist extension; the last permits graded control of the wrist, with gravity performing the flexion movements. Wrist extension

Text continued on page 653

C4

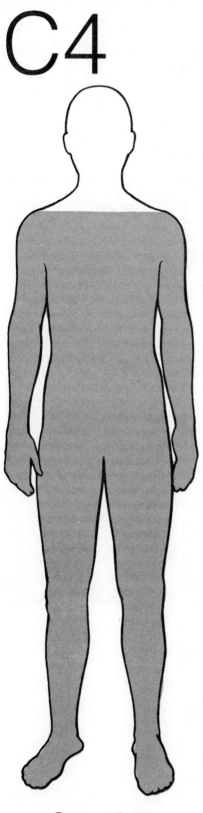

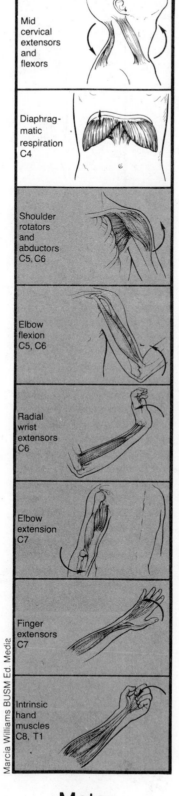

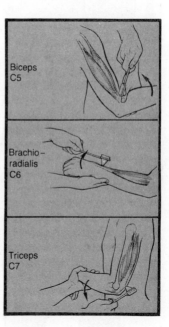

Sensation   Motor   Reflex

FIGURE 32–2. Effects of injury with sparing at the fourth cervical level.

C5

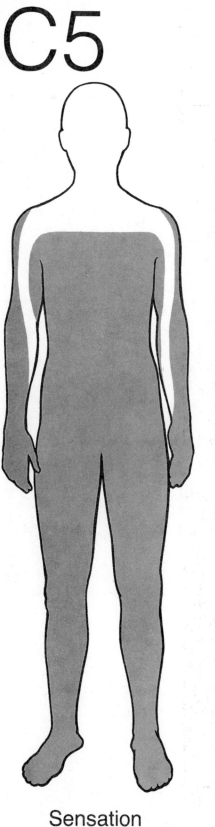

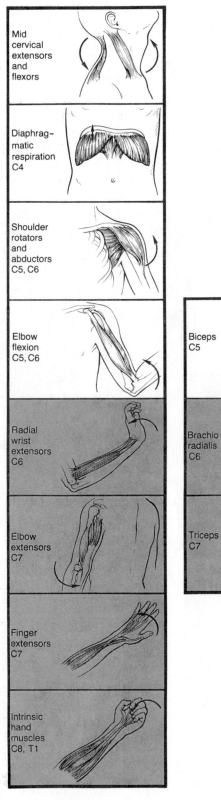

Sensation Motor Reflex

FIGURE 32–3. Effects·of injury with sparing at the fifth cervical level.

C6

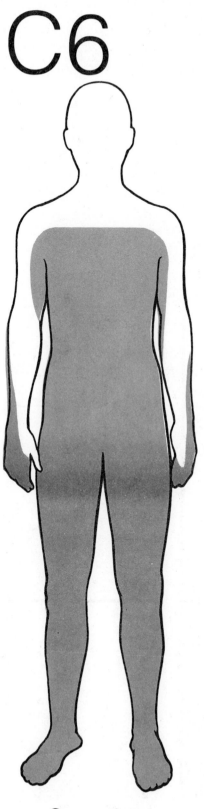

Sensation

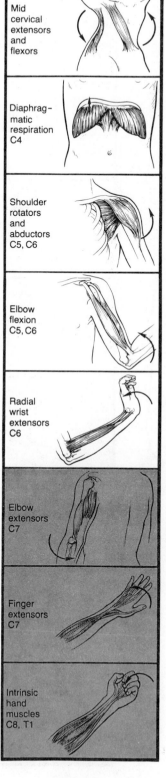

Mid cervical extensors and flexors

Diaphragmatic respiration C4

Shoulder rotators and abductors C5, C6

Elbow flexion C5, C6

Radial wrist extensors C6

Elbow extensors C7

Finger extensors C7

Intrinsic hand muscles C8, T1

Motor

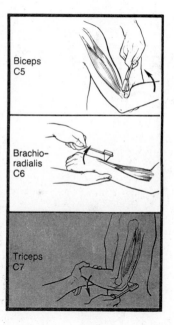

Biceps C5

Brachioradialis C6

Triceps C7

Reflex

FIGURE 32–4. Effects of injury with sparing at the sixth cervical level.

C7

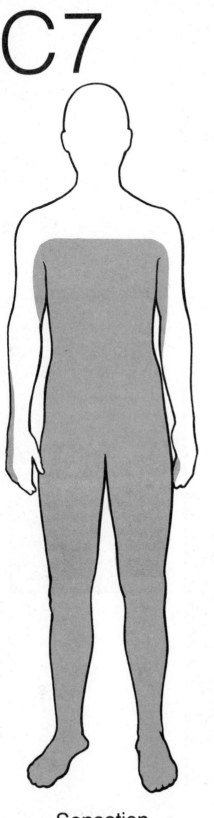

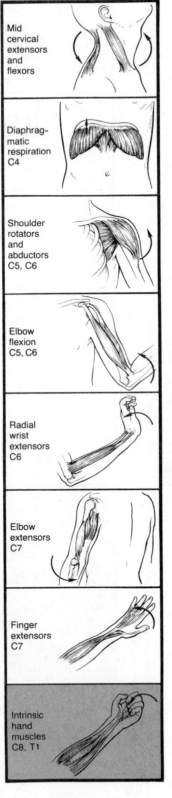

Mid cervical extensors and flexors

Diaphrag-matic respiration C4

Shoulder rotators and abductors C5, C6

Elbow flexion C5, C6

Radial wrist extensors C6

Elbow extensors C7

Finger extensors C7

Intrinsic hand muscles C8, T1

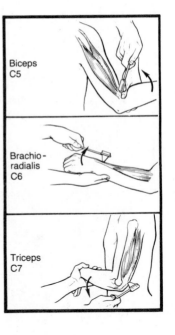

Biceps C5

Brachio-radialis C6

Triceps C7

Sensation   Motor   Reflex

FIGURE 32–5. Effects of injury with sparing at the seventh cervical level.

can be harnessed through special "tenodesis" spints to drive the fingers into flexion; sometimes a surgical finger flexor tenodesis can be performed for the same purpose. Many patients prefer simply to use leather cuffs strapped to their hands, into which such implements as tooth brushes, forks, and spoons can be inserted.

The patient injured below the sixth cervical segment can perform all the activities of patients with higher level lesions and in addition can be more helpful in dressing himself, often doing it completely, can propel his wheelchair long distances, and usually can transfer himself from bed to chair using the overhead trapeze or a modified push-up with elbow stabilization by shoulder adduction. Beginning at this level, individuals should be able to drive an automobile with manual controls and additional adaptive equipment.[32] A van with hydraulic lift makes the entire procedure easier, in that transfers are eliminated.

Seventh Cervical Level

The major functional additions at the seventh cervical segment are the use of the triceps and the extrinsic finger flexors and extensors. This patient is able to do push-ups in the sitting position and therefore can transfer himself from bed to chair. He can grasp and release and is usually able to operate his hands without splints.

This patient is independent at the wheelchair level.

As the patient grows older, less functional independence should be expected from him; reductions in capability vary with the individual, his physiologic age, and his physical abilities.

First Thoracic Level

This individual has normal upper extremities with a strong chain of stabilization to the thorax but lacks trunk musculature for full sitting balance and intercostal and abdominal musculature to supplement diaphragmatic breathing.

However, this person should be completely independent from a wheelchair in that he can dress and feed, manage toileting needs, accomplish transfers, drive a car with manual controls, and hold a job away from home requiring self-transportation as can the low-level quadriplegic.

Sixth Thoracic Level

The paraplegic at this level has upper intercostal function and upper back control and thus has an added increment of respiratory reserve. There should be wheelchair independence for activities of daily living.

This individual may be provided with orthoses for standing but should not be expected to walk because of the unusually increased energy demands of such ambulation.

Twelfth Thoracic Level

At this level the individual has full abdominal and virtually full back control as well as intact respiratory reserve. There should be complete independence in activities of daily living. Functional ambulation continues to be a problem, since the energy demands make it highly impractical for the vast majority. Nevertheless, orthoses should be considered for physiologic standing and walking.

Fourth Lumbar Level

This person has the use of the hip flexors and knee extensors and can stand without orthoses and walk without external support. However, because of severe weakness of the glutei coupled with loss of ankle power, there is a laborious waddling gait. Ambulation is assisted by use of ankle-foot orthoses and by crutches. Failure to use such support will result in genu recurvatum and abnormal lumbar spine strain.

This is a virtually completely independent individual. There is difficulty in stair climbing and in those activities requiring repetitive changing from seated to standing positions.

Thus, the individual with a T1 level has complete innervation of all portions of the upper extremities, but lacks trunk and breathing musculature except for the diaphragm. The individual with a T12 level has normal upper extremities with a chain of strong fixators in the normal trunk to give virtually unlimited function of the upper extremities in the seated position.

Text continued on page 659

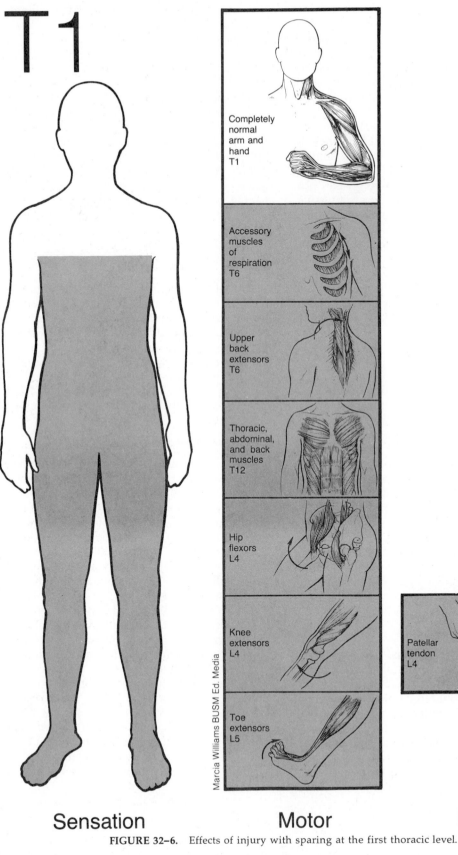

Sensation   Motor   Reflex

FIGURE 32–6. Effects of injury with sparing at the first thoracic level.

T6

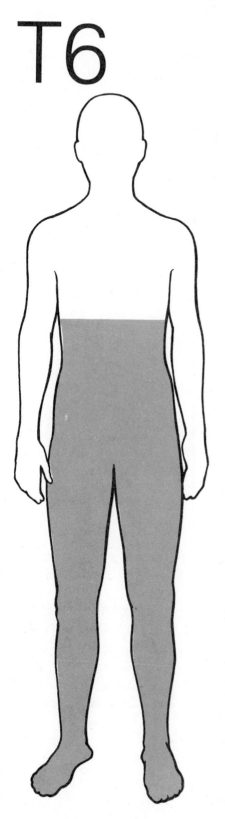

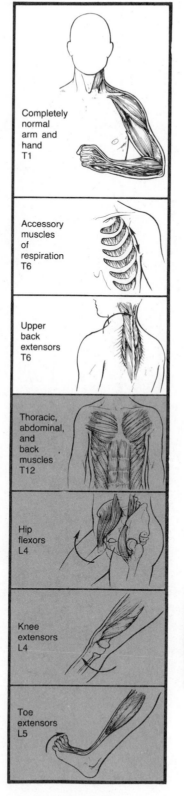

Completely normal arm and hand T1

Accessory muscles of respiration T6

Upper back extensors T6

Thoracic, abdominal, and back muscles T12

Hip flexors L4

Knee extensors L4

Toe extensors L5

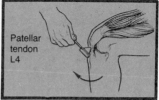

Patellar tendon L4

Sensation   Motor   Reflex

FIGURE 32–7. Effects of injury with sparing at the sixth thoracic level.

T12

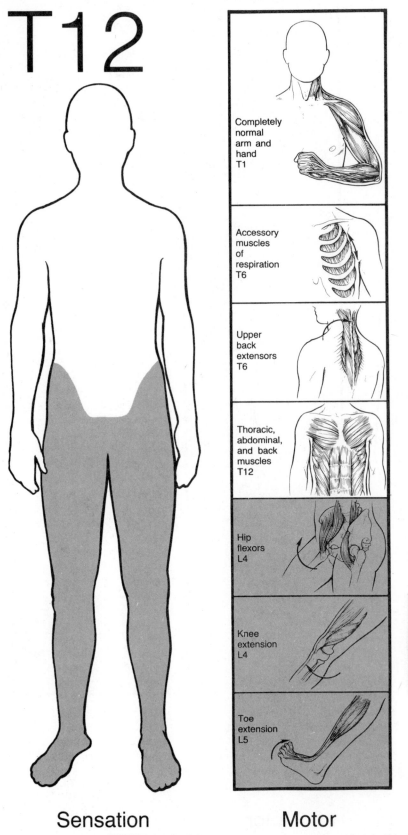

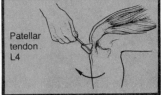

Sensation   Motor   Reflex

FIGURE 32–8. Effects of injury with sparing at the twelfth thoracic level.

L4

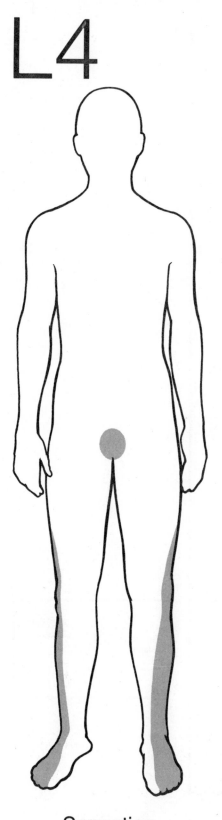

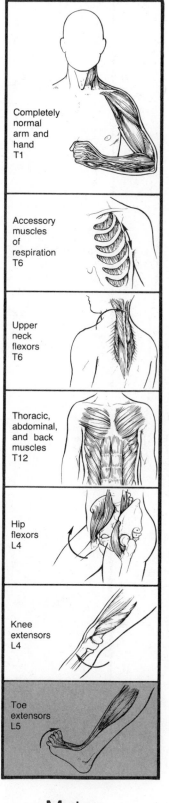

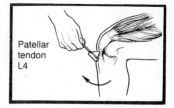

Sensation   Motor   Reflex

FIGURE 32–9. Effects of injury with sparing at the fourth lumbar level.

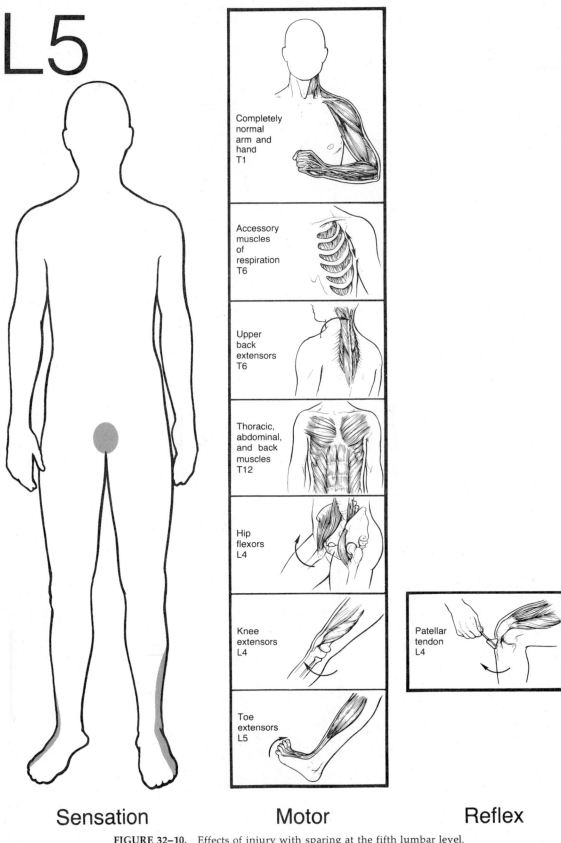

L5

Completely normal arm and hand T1

Accessory muscles of respiration T6

Upper back extensors T6

Thoracic, abdominal, and back muscles T12

Hip flexors L4

Knee extensors L4

Patellar tendon L4

Toe extensors L5

Sensation   Motor   Reflex

FIGURE 32–10. Effects of injury with sparing at the fifth lumbar level.

Congenital Spinal Cord Lesions

The most common group of spinal cord lesions are those resulting from incomplete closure of the vertebral canal. This is commonly seen as posterior spina bifida, in which there is a defect of the laminae; although it may occur at any level, it is most common in the lumbosacral region.[33] When only the laminar defect is present, it is designated spina bifida occulta. Spina bifida denotes an external sac of meninges. When there are adhesions between the cord and connective tissue, cord gliosis, and cavitation, these result in neurologic impairments. Meningocele exists when there is a bulging subcutaneous sac containing mainly meninges and fluid; it also may contain nerve roots. In myelomeningocele, the sac contains central nervous tissue which represents damaged spinal cord with nerve roots; frequently there is a mass of fibrous gliosis with no evidence of intact neurons. In meningomyelocystocele, the meningeal sac contains badly malformed spinal cord. Usually only the anterior half has a semblance of normal anatomy. The central nervous tissue is mainly glial.

Ames and Schut note that 80 per cent of those with meningomyelocele have hydrocephalus and bowel and bladder incontinence.[34] Stark comments that upper motor neuron involvement occurs and that this is the fundamental neurologic problem;[35] unexplained by myelodysplasia, it is "probably acquired before, during or shortly after birth."

To develop the potential of those who survive, a well-organized program is required. The contribution of the neurosurgeon is the management of local surgery and the hydrocephalus and that of the orthopedist the lower extremity deformities. The urologist deals with studies of the urinary tract and corrective reconstructive measures when indicated and the pediatrician and physiatrist with the child's physical and emotional growth and development.[35a] These are joined by a host of coprofessional persons to take advantage of the improved life span. This life span has resulted from the slowing of renal damage, by *judicious* use of antibiotics, uterovesicle junction surgical alteration, bladder neck resection, and urinary diversion.

The functional significance of the level of neurologic sparing is similar to that of the traumatically spinal cord injured. The child with spina bifida can usually become ambulatory. Orthoses are prescribed consistent with neurologic impairment. Hip and knee deformities may respond to conservative measures, including flexibility exercises and plaster cast wedging; in the former, family members become major participants. Orthopedic surgical correction may be necessary with incomplete results from conservative measures.

Psychological Reaction

On the premise that the spinal cord–injured individual has suffered one of the most physically and socially catastrophic injuries and appreciating that this person has been physically driven back to infancy in terms of requiring assistance for bathing, dressing, feeding, body elimination, and mobility — there are staggering adjustments to make over the coming weeks, months, and years (see also Chapters 21 to 24 and 38).

Much is accomplished through psychological support therapy and social casework. However, as the length of hospitalization decreases to an average length of stay of 80 to 130 days, the emotional adjustment no doubt will occur after discharge. Treischmann notes that psychological adjustment usually requires 18 to 24 months.[29]

Since the physical rehabilitation aspect is carried out over a shorter inpatient stay, the patient's depression and denial may make it difficult for him to adequately participate in the program. One of the essential tasks of the physician is to facilitate the process by carefully explaining the realities of the injury to the patient and the family. The physician as well as other coprofessional personnel need to be sensitive to how the patient and the family respond to the prognosis. They may not be able to "hear" the prognosis until they can handle the anxiety. Involvement of family and friends is important lest they undermine the treatment and reinforce the denial.

It has been suggested that the "stage theory of adjustment" may no longer be valid.[30] Each new crisis, such as getting out of bed for the first time, the first visit outside the hospital, and the first weekend therapeutic home leave, requires adjustment and coping. The patient may go through all of the stages several times a week or even in a day.

Because depression may manifest itself as self-neglect, attention will need to be directed to ensuring that the spinal cord–injured person is assuming responsibility for scrupulous self-care and for required medical attention.

Bladder Dysfunction

The bladder does not exist as an independent structure but is part of a highly complex reflex mechanism. In normal micturition there is a balance between the expulsive and retentive forces so that after timely bladder emptying there is no postvoiding residual bladder urine. An understanding of this function clarifies the role of the reflex mechanisms in the neurogenic bladder.[36] Bors classified neurogenic bladders into two types on the basis of the neuronal involvement: upper motor neuron and lower motor neuron.[37] The presence of reflex activity in a neurogenic bladder is consistent with an upper motor neuron lesion, and the absence of reflex activity denotes lower motor neuron involvement. He suggested that the bulbocavernosus reflex be used to test the integrity of the spinal sacral reflex arc, thus ruling out trauma to the conus medullaris or cauda equina. Stimulation of the glans penis, of the vesical and urethral mucosa, or of the detrusor produces contraction of the pelvic floor musculature and the anal sphincter. Traction on an indwelling catheter also serves as a stimulus to this reflex. Bors and Comarr note that micturition starts as a purely spinal reflex in infancy and childhood, with the sacral segments of the cord as the only link for transmission of impulses to and from the target structures.[38] Thereafter this develops into a willed process; the spinal activity of smooth and striated muscle becoming integrated with brain function so that the sacral segments, later in life, are the sites for "transmission and modulation" of afferent and efferent impulses between the higher parts of the central nervous system and the so-called target organs.

The upper motor neuron reflex bladder functions without a catheter when there is reciprocation between action of the detrusor and the sphincter. Inability to empty occurs when there is lack of reciprocal action between these two or when voiding reflexes are aborted prior to completion of bladder emptying.

In the lower motor neuron bladder there is lack of reflex detrusor function, and the individual voids by vigorous abdominal straining (see also Chapter 38).

Bowel Dysfunction

The innervation for release of the anal sphincter tone is the same as that for bladder evacuation, the sensory innervation for appreciation of terminal bowel distention, the same as for bladder distention. The stimulus to bowel emptying is distention. Thus the individual with spinal cord injury prior to regulation training experiences alternating phases of constipation and uncontrolled defecation, since the voluntary muscle component inhibits bowel emptying.

Respiratory Dysfunction

The three major motors for breathing are the diaphragm innervated from C2 through C4, the intercostal muscles innervated from T2 through T12, and the abdominal muscles from T6 through L1. The individual with quadriplegia has been spared only the diaphragm. According to Bergofsky, this type of breathing is adequate at rest but requires abnormally large energy expenditure when large tidal volumes are needed to satisfy increased metabolic demands.[39] Thus, the acute and chronic respiratory failure observed in quadriplegic patients arises from two sources: the inefficiency resulting from instability of the costal insertions of the diaphragm and the increased work of breathing due to increased intra-abdominal pressure caused by unusually large excursions of the diaphragm.

Additionally, the lack of abdominal muscle also results in a cough that is feeble at best, with consequent difficulty in clearing secretions in respiratory infections. This same problem with cough is encountered in lower-level injuries down to the point at which there is significant intact function in the lower thoracic cord. Impaired respiratory function, including the inability to cough effectively, is especially hazardous in the patient with high-level spinal cord injury who develops respiratory tract infection; with pooling of secretions, airway obstruction leads to atelectasis.

In those patients whose level of injury is at the C4 segment or above, there is the likelihood of denervation of the phrenic nerve, resulting in some degree of diaphragmatic paralysis. In addition, there may well be associated thoracic cage injuries. For the newly injured patient, measures are instituted to prevent pulmonary atelectasis, infection, and edema. Ventilator assistance and tracheostomy may be required.

When diagnosis of diaphragmatic paralysis is confirmed, further study is undertaken to assess the state of phrenic nerve transmission so that consideration may be given to phrenic nerve "pacing" after an appropriate trial interval to establish use of accessory muscles and glossopharyngeal breathing.[40-42]

Sexual Dysfunction

Talbot points out that much of the misinformation that has "pervaded society and eventually the medical profession about spinal cord injury patients and their impotence is derived not from medical sources but from a literary source."[43] This source, *Lady Chatterly's Lover,* tells of a World War I paraplegic whom D. H. Lawrence deemed impotent. As Talbot notes, D. H. Lawrence, who was a considerable poet and novelist, was not a physiologist.

Trieschmann states that we must recognize that the onset of a physical disability does not eliminate sexual feelings any more than it eliminates hunger or thirst; that there are many different kinds of sex acts available for satisfaction and a disability may interfere with only a certain number of these; and that the sexuality of the disabled individual must be evaluated in terms of his particular pattern of relating to others.[44] Therapeutic efforts must include the disabled individual's partner, since both must learn new patterns of behavior.[45] Hohmann adds that the patient wants to develop attitudes so that he is free to engage in whatever sexual behavior is organically possible and psychologically acceptable to him and his partner.[46] Cole asks about the paraplegic or quadriplegic man with complete transection, then continues: "His penis may become erect; his nipples may erect. His muscles may develop spasms; his blood pressure, pulse and respiration may increase. The skin of his scrotum may tense. He may develop a skin flush. Emission or ejaculation is unusual." Thus, "the spinal cord patient is capable of most of the sexual responses of the able-bodied."[47]

Corresponding responses in the spinal cord–injured female have also been suggested.[45]

The sexual act in the male consists of erection, ejaculation, and orgasm. Erection may be induced by either of two stimuli, central or somesthetic and local tactile, and depends on the integrity of the second, third, and fourth spinal sacral segments for parasympathetic innervation and to a much lesser extent on the segments from T11 to L1 for sympathetic innervation.[48] Hyperemia results, through vasodilatation and patency of the arteriovenous shunts, from activity of the sacral innervation transmitted through the cauda equina and pelvic nerves (nervi erigentes).

In the spinally injured man, local tactile stimulation provides the mechanism for erection. The success in achieving erection by this method is dependent on the level of the spinal cord injury. In one collected series, the overall success rate has been stated to be 77 per cent.[48] In the Bors and Comarr study of 529 cases the success rate for erection in complete upper motor neuron lesions was 93 per cent, while that in incomplete lesions was 99 per cent.[49] Miller claims that erections occur in 80 per cent of patients with cervical cord lesions.[50] Much remains to be learned about this function in the man with spinal cord injury — certainly with understanding and communicating partners the success rate will be higher.

Ejaculation includes seminal emission and the ejaculation proper.[48] The first, dependent on the peristaltic action of the vasa deferentia, seminal vesicles, and prostate, is mediated through the sympathetic nervous system. The second results from contractions of the pelvic floor muscles and the bulbospongiosus and ischiocavernosus muscles.

Tarabulcy, in his collected series, stated that though 35 per cent had coitus, only 10 per cent achieved ejaculation.[48] The Bors and Comarr study described ejaculation in 5 per cent of those with complete lesions and 32 per cent of those with incomplete lesions.[49]

Orgasm has been described as a sensation resulting from contraction of the smooth muscles of the genitalia and the striated muscles of the pelvic floor coinciding with the ejaculation.[48] Because of the absence of peripheral sensory appreciation, the experience of orgasm is perforce altered in the man with spinal cord injury. Significant numbers of individuals, however, report pleasurable sensations in the genital region and also in an area of intact body surface innervation above the level of injury, particularly the nipple area (T5) when this is spared.

The estimates of the number of men with spinal cord injuries who have sired children has been on the order of 1 to 5 per cent.[48, 49] To date this has been ascribed to the lesser frequency of successful coitus (35 per cent), to loss of ejaculation and impaired spermatogenesis due to nutritional or hormonal or neurogenic causes or chronic urinary tract infection, and finally to occlusion of seminal passages due to infection.[48]

Recent studies have demonstrated that electric massage of the genitalia has tripled the overall incidence of ejaculation.[51] Use of intrathecal injections of prostigmin has produced specimens for study as well as for artificial insemination in individuals incapable of ejaculation.[51] These techniques are not without danger, since ejaculations may be accompanied by symptoms of severe autonomic dysreflexia, including hypertension and cardiac arrhythmia.[52]

The male with a cauda equina injury with consequent striated muscle paralysis has a dribbling ejaculation rather than the projectile type. Erection is achieved by some 25 per cent of such men, ejaculation by a lesser number, and progeny by 5 per cent.[49]

In certain instances, with the benefit of careful assessment of the psychological needs and with counseling, there may be indication for a penile endoprosthesis.[53-56]

Less information is available concerning sexual function in the female because fewer women suffer spinal cord trauma. In our clinic the percentage has been under 15. The sequence of events in the sexual act corresponds to that in the male.[48] The tumescence of the clitoris and labia minora is the equivalent of erection. The seminal emission equivalent is contraction of the smooth muscle of the uterus, and the equivalent of ejaculation is the rhythmic contraction of the vaginal sphincter, the ischiocavernosus, and the pelvic floor musculature. Orgasm may be experienced as a pleasurable sensation at the level of demarcation between intact and lost sensation rather than vaginally; in some instances this sensation is vaginal in location.

Following injury, the woman with spinal cord injury may have an interval with loss of menstrual periods or irregularity with eventual return to regularity. The likelihood of pregnancy after spinal cord injury is unchanged, since fertility is unimpaired, and pregnancy and labor may proceed without complications. During labor in persons with a lesion at or above the T4-T5 level, the manifestations of autonomic dysreflexia may develop and should be distinguished from eclampsia.[57] It may be difficult to know when labor is beginning in patients with injuries above T10 because of lack of appreciation of uterine contractions.[58]

If the fetus has not been harmed in the accident in which the pregnant woman received the spinal cord injury and if the woman remains free of renal infection, there is all likelihood that a normal child will result.

Pregnancy complicated by paraplegia is threatened more than in normal circumstances by the trauma itself, the immediate post-traumatic situation of the patient and by chronic infections and anemia in pregnancies, following cord injury.[59]

Orthostatic Hypotension

A frequent and dismaying problem encountered by patients with spinal cord injury, particularly those with quadriplegia, is the inability to tolerate the upright position because of orthostatic hypotension. This is characterized by nausea, lightheadedness, and even syncope. For most, this is of a temporary nature and passes with increasing periods in the upright position. For a small number, it persists and requires mechanical or pharmaceutical control. Deprived of the sympathetic response that prevents pooling of blood in dependent parts and with poor tissue turgor, which allows extravasation of fluid, orthostatic hypotension occurs.

Vallbona and his colleagues have suggested that in cases of complete transection of the cervical spinal cord and sympathetic denervation below the lesion, there is insufficient release of catecholamines in response to sudden positional changes.[60] Slow release of antidiuretic hormone, cortisol, and aldosterone may also play a role.

Temperature Adjustment

Maintenance of body temperature results from a balance of heat production and heat dissipation. Temperature-sensitive structures in the superficial and deep regions of the body act as a warning system to the central temperature-sensitive receptors in the anterior preoptic region of the hypothalamus.[61] A rise in central temperature results in vasodilatation and sweating in the periphery, while central cooling results in vasoconstriction and shivering. Downey states that the central receptors probably play a dominant role in the thermoregulation, with skin responses functioning mainly in short-term regulation.[62]

According to Guttmann and his colleagues, T8 is the highest level at which a patient can maintain rectal temperature at 37° C in an environmental temperature from 18° to 40° C.[61] Patients with higher levels are poikilothermic in response to heating or cooling. In patients with spinal injury shivering occurs only in muscles innervated above the level of the lesion.[63] Miller comments on the presence of rudimentary thermoregulation at the cord level.[50]

Although the mechanism is not fully understood, the person with spinal cord injury does have difficulty adjusting to extremes of ambient temperature, and the higher the level the greater the difficulty.[64]

Metabolic Alterations

Bone

Prolonged bed rest is known to produce not only muscle atrophy but demineralization of bone as well. In the paralyzed individual this tendency is compounded, particularly in the bony structures below the level of the spinal cord lesion. The development of osteoporosis in the proximal femur makes the individual vulnerable to minimal trauma to the extent that even the ordinary activity of turning in bed may result in a hip fracture.

Serum Protein

In quadriplegics the median value of the total protein in both the immediate and late postinjury states is at the lower limits of normal.[65] In the later stages there is a gradual increase in the gamma globulin fraction. Once the serum protein changes have occurred, there is rarely return to normal.[66] Attempts to alter this situation in preparation for decubitus ulcer reconstructive surgery have proved fruitless both by nutritional supplement and intravenous albumin infusion. An adequate hemoglobin level has been the most promising preoperative achievement.

Hypercalcemia

Maynard and Imai report immobilization hypercalcemia in growing adolescent quadriplegics.[67] The mechanism is described as an imbalance of osteoblastic and osteoclastic activity in growing adolescents wherein osteoclastic activity with bone resorption is increased and the high increased calcium load is inadequately excreted by the kidneys, with resultant hypercalcemia. This phenomenon must be distinguished from primary hyperparathyroidism. The clinical manifestations of anorexia, nausea, malaise, headache, polydipsia, polyuria, and lethargy are noted most commonly four to eight weeks after injury when the condition occurs in the adolescent spinal cord–injured person. Recommendations for long-term control have been courses of corticosteroids or oral phosphates.[67]

Gynecomastia

Breast enlargement, either unilateral or bilateral, is not uncommon in the patient with spinal cord injury. In our own experience the incidence has been up to 5 per cent. The enlargement has been ascribed to an increase of circulatory estrogens resulting from hepatic dysfunction. Cooper and his colleagues commented that the liver impairment resolves within 8 to 10 weeks.[68] An understanding of this phenomenon will avoid the decision to perform breast biopsy.

Cooper and Hoen described temporary elevation of urinary 17-ketosteroid levels during the first 48 hours after spinal injury.[70] Thereafter 50 per cent of paraplegic males showed a decrease for a period of 10 weeks to 7 years. Kaplan and his co-workers noted that, in their study of 60 patients, 63.3 per cent showed little or no 17-ketosteroid response to ACTH and 58.3 per cent showed little or no 17-hydroxysteroid response.[69] Further, testicular atrophy and impaired spermatogenesis have been ascribed to disturbance of pituitary gonadal feedback.[71]

Autonomic Dysreflexia

Autonomic dysreflexia is characterized by elevation of blood pressure on the order of 100 to 200 mm of mercury systolic and 50 to 100 mm of mercury diastolic, headache, slowing of the pulse, flushing and sweating of the face, and nasal congestion. The possibility of convulsions and cerebral hemorrhage with death exists.[72]

Based on reflex activity, either viscerovascular or somatovascular, the syndrome occurs because of impaired vascular segmental activity resulting from spinal cord damage above the splanchnic outflow, that is, above levels between T4 and T6. Young comments that the autonomic systems (sympathetic and sacral parasympathetic) remain without control from higher regulatory centers. Thus the reflex mechanisms function in "unrestricted reflex revelry with disastrous consequences to the patient."[73]

Afferent impulses from the offending site enter the posterior gray matter, where they may initiate segmental reflexes and, as well, ascend in the cord to synapse with neurons in the intermediolateral columns of the thoracic cord, initiating autonomic vasoconstrictor reflexes.[74-76] In the able-bodied, inhibitory impulses from higher brain centers regulate the vasoconstriction reflexes. In the high-level spinal cord injured, the descending inhibitory impulses are blocked at the level of the cord injury, allowing the autonomic reflexes to go uncontrolled. The sole response to the uncontrolled blood pressure elevation is the bradycardia initiated by the baroreceptors in the aorta and carotid sinus and mediated through the medullary vasomotor centers.

Elicited by noxious stimuli to the body parts below the level of injury, the reflex most frequently occurs in response to distention of bladder and bowel. Rossier and his co-workers note that during labor in patients with high thoracic or cervical levels of injury, the manifestations of autonomic dysreflexia should not be confused with preeclampsia.[77]

Bladder calculi, urinary tract infection, and decubitus ulcers have also been implicated.[76] When none of the aforementioned conditions is the cause, presence of an ingrown infected toenail should be sought as the stimulus. Autonomic dysreflexia has already been well documented in patients with high-level spinal cord injuries during cystoscopy.[78] Bors and Comarr note that autonomic dysreflexia may reach a peak after a lapse of time following the spinal cord injury and then subside, but may recur after many years of quiescence.[38]

While seeking a not easily detectable source of the difficulty, chlorpromazine hydrochloride (Thorazine) may be of great assistance. When removal of the noxious stimulus does not result in resolution of the dysreflexia, treatment with amyl nitrite or nitroglycerin should be used initially. Although treatment with guanethidine (Ismelin) has been found useful, concomitant orthostatic hypotension may be a problem. In the instance that blood pressure levels rise above 160 mm systolic and/or 120 diastolic, intravenous therapy with hydralazide hydrochloride (Apresoline) or trimethaphan camsylate (Arfonad) may be indicated. In desperate situations spinal anesthesia or peripheral (pudendal or sacral) nerve blocks may be considered.

Ramos, Freed, and Marek demonstrated the basis for the transient mild sweating, cutis anserina, coldness, chills, and at times headache that occur at the time of bladder emptying, in high-level spinal cord–injured persons with acceptable reflex bladder emptying.[79] Although physical examination, including blood pressure measurement, revealed no abnormal findings, urodynamic studies with concurrent blood pressure and electrocardiographic measurements revealed a drop in heart rate, a rise in blood pressure from $115\pm12/70\pm11$ to $173\pm20/101\pm15$ at peak filling ($p < 0.001$). In a small number there was lengthening of the PR interval. In the paraplegic patient the heart rate increased from 72 to 82, while the blood pressure rose from $131\pm14/77\pm10$ to $131\pm24/84\pm4$ ($p = 0.05$). They have termed this phenomenon *subclinical autonomic dysreflexia*.

POTENTIAL COMPLICATIONS

Infection and Calculus Formation

The normal urinary tract is bacteria-free except adjacent to the distal portion of the urethra, and ordinarily the urine is sterile. The neurogenic bladder with large postvoiding residual urine volumes due to obstructive uropathy or impaired expulsive force provides the milieu for bacteria growth. Further, the indwelling catheter, when this is required, provides an entrance mechanism for bacteria from the external environment into the bladder.

The normal bladder mucosa is ordinarily resistant to bacterial entrance; the neurogenic bladder mucosa does not have this protective mechanism.

The person with spinal cord injury is also prone to kidney bacterial infection, since obstruction to urine flow makes the kidney more liable to infection; the neurogenic bladder dysfunction results in bladder infection, which in turn results in kidney infection. The spread of infection is, in a significant number of instances, fostered by the presence of vesicoureteral reflux due to involvement of the intramural portion of the ureters and of the ureteral orifice that is sufficient to interfere with normal function. In the absence of reflux, however, bacteria can reach the kidney by the ascending route.

Urinary stasis favors precipitation of salts resulting in calculus formation. Stones in spinal cord–injured patients consists mainly of phosphates and carbonates of calcium, magnesium, and ammonium. Also, the presence of infection as well as a foreign body in the bladder sets the stage for formation of stones in the bladder and kidney and less commonly in the prostate and seminal vesicles. The presence of calculus also concurrently fosters the infection.

The incidence of urinary tract calculi had been acknowledged to be from 22.5 to 68.7 per cent until after World War II.[80] The most important measure in decreasing calculosis, prevention of infection, has best been achieved by the wide acceptance of intermittent catheterization. Guttmann and Frankel demonstrated an overall incidence of 0.43 per cent in 476 patients treated with intermittent catheterization who were admitted to a spinal cord injury center within 14 days of injury.[81]

Ischemic Ulceration

Decubitus ulcers or ischemic ulcerations are one of the major problems confronting any patient who remains in one position, either sitting or recumbent, for prolonged periods of time.[82] The most frequently involved areas are the sacrum, the trochanters of the hip, the ischial rami, and the malleoli and heels. These are sites with relatively little tissue interposed between the skin and bony prominences. Thus, the person with spinal cord injury, who may be unable to move or turn himself frequently and who has no sensation of pressure, is especially prone to ulceration because he lacks perception of

pressure and because circulation to denervated areas is inadequate.

Munro wrote that the propensity for development of ulcers was based on interruption of the autonomic reflex arcs that controlled circulation to the skin; therefore, there was no response to pressure in the normal protective manner.[82] Later Kosiak demonstrated that decubitus ulcers were ischemic in nature and resulted from prolonged tissue ischemia when pressure applied exceeded capillary pressure at sites overlying bony prominences.[83, 84]

Because hydrostatic pressures in capillaries are low and because cessation of flow occurs even in the presence of positive arterial pressure it seems logical that complete tissue ischemia may be present when pressures on the order of capillary pressure are applied.[85]

Thus an ischemic destructive process occurs with application of high pressure of short duration or prolonged low pressure. According to Kosiak these are localized areas of cellular necrosis; the microscopic changes are characterized by edema, loss of cross-striations and myofibrils, hyalinization of fibers, neutrophilic infiltration, and phagocytosis by neutrophils and macrophages.[84, 85] In animal studies these changes were produced by pressure of 50 mm of mercury for one hour in animals with a ligated femoral artery, but did not occur with pressure of 100 mm of mercury for two hours in the normal animal.

Deep Vein Thrombosis

Among the complications to which the spinal cord injured person is subject is deep vein thrombosis. Steinberg[86] points out that more than 100 years after Virchow postulated that "three factors had to cause venous thrombosis: a change in rate of blood flow, vessel wall changes, and a change in blood coagulability, the precise role of each of these factors is poorly understood." Further, "there is no clear-cut evidence at this point in time that prolonged rest by itself, without other contributing factors, predisposes to the development of venous thrombosis."

Although Guttmann and others opined that the most important factor is stagnation of blood flow,[87-89] Wessler's demonstration that it took eight hours before blood trapped between two ligatures of dog's vein fully coagulated indicated that other factors certainly play a role.[90] Clagett and Salzman note that there are elevations in plasma procoagulants and fibrinogen and an increase in platelet number and reactivity following surgery and injuries.[91]

Deep vein thrombosis and its consequence, pulmonary embolism, represent a serious complication in traumatic spinal cord injury, most commonly within the first month after injury.[92, 93] Deep vein thrombosis develops more frequently in complete than in incomplete lesions and with greater frequency in thoracic and cervical injuries.[87, 91] The incidence of deep vein thrombosis has been estimated to be from 12.5 to 58 per cent in the spinal cord injured[89, 91, 93, 94] and pulmonary embolism on the order of 5 to 10 per cent.[89, 92, 95] Subclinical episodes of pulmonary embolization may occur more frequently than is commonly recognized.[96]

With the generally accepted emphasis on prevention, at least once daily thigh and calf girth measurements at indelibly marked levels are indicated to detect swelling. Proper application of full leg elastic bandages has proved more valuable than stockings, since the rapid onset of thigh atrophy negates the effectiveness of commercially available full length elastic stockings. The prophylactic administration of low dose heparin in the amount of 5000 units twice daily is low in risk and is becoming acceptable although not fully substantiated as a preventive measure. This regimen has been recommended for the first month, followed by Coumadin for the next two months.[97, 98] Aspirin and full anticoagulation carry the risk of increased bleeding at the spinal cord injury site, particularly early after the injury or after spinal surgery and, in the quadriplegic, increase the likelihood of gastric bleeding where the incidence is already appreciable.

Heterotopic Bone Formation

Heterotopic bone formation is a not uncommon complication of spinal cord injury but one not possible to predict in a given patient. It has an incidence of 16 to 53 per cent.[99, 100] Heterotopic bone formation is in most instances noted as an incidental finding during the course of x-ray examination. It forms periarticularly below the level of le-

sion and is associated with hips, knees, shoulders, elbows, and the lumbar paravertebral areas. The most common time for development is in the period from one to four months after injury, with rare occurrence after one year.

The findings may be of the "acute" type, presenting as an inflammatory reaction including local heat, swelling, and redness, or only swelling or induration. To be considered in the differential diagnosis are deep vein thrombosis, cellulitis, joint sepsis, hematoma formation, and fracture. The important consideration is to rule out deep vein thrombosis, for the onset of both thrombosis and heterotopic bone formation is most common in the first months after injury.

The finding of elevated serum alkaline phosphatase is only suggestive early in the course of heterotopic bone formation. X-ray examination may not reveal positive findings during the first two weeks; a bone scan is the most reliable diagnostic measure and more importantly in late stages as the determinant in deciding on maturity of the process.

It has been accepted that heteroptic bone formation following spinal cord injury requires aggressive passive range of motion[100, 101] for prevention of the ankylosis that severely limits activities of daily living; rest may well increase the joint motion limitations. Disodium etridonate (diphosphonate) has been proposed for the treatment and prevention of heterotopic bone formation. In the therapeutic dosage of 5 mg per kg per day for 12 weeks, it does not retard healing of any fractures but will prevent further ossification of the process of heterotopic bone formation. In those instances, when there is insufficient response to physical therapeutic measures, surgical intervention is indicated, but only after the bone formation has been demonstrated to be mature.

Spasticity

Every individual who suffers a spinal cord injury develops spasticity to a greater or lesser degree following an interval that may be as short as hours or as long as months. More commonly it occurs within the first two to three weeks following the injury. The development of this phenomenon is an indication that the muscle stretch reflex has become isolated from its supraspinal inhibitory-modulation system so that the alpha and dynamic fusimotor neurons are abnormally excitable.[102] The extensor mechanisms recover first, usually in the lower extremities, with a posture of extension that is difficult to overcome.[102, 103]

Spasticity may have a salubrious effect on activities of daily living in that it provides knee stability in the upright position on a reflex basis, by its effect in expulsion of urinary bladder contents, and by its torque force on bone to maintain bone density. It may, on the other hand, interfere by preventing comfortable wheelchair sitting, by hampering transfer activities and other activities of daily living, and by preventing the bladder from becoming a useful reservoir of urine. Finally, there is the probability of heel cord shortening, pronation deformity at the ankles, and adductor tightness at the hips.

When the spasticity interferes with activities to a sufficient degree and is not overcome by daily routine flexibility exercises, medication should be considered. The most commonly used pharmacologic agents are diazepam (Valium), dantrolene sodium (Dantrium), and baclofen (Lioresal). Although diazepam is probably the most widely used and is a polysynaptic inhibitor, it has a short duration.[103] It has been noted that in many instances a part of its effect may be due to its less specific psychotherapeutic properties.[103] Dantrolene sodium requires careful follow-up of liver function because of its side effects, which are dose related and more common in younger patients. Dantrolene sodium acts on skeletal muscle with a primary effect on extrafusal fibers affecting excitation contraction, coupled with possible effect on intrafusal fibers as well.[104-106]

According to Pedersen, "classification of drugs according to their site of action is often difficult because of incomplete knowledge of the pathophysiology of spasticity and because the agents may have more than one site of action."[103] Further, the site may vary with dosage.

In animal studies, baclofen has shown an inhibitory effect on both monosynaptic and polysynaptic activities.[103] Studies have shown that baclofen's site of action is the Ia fibers, including the alpha motor neurons in the area of presynaptic inhibition.[107] In the past barbiturates had been used for spasticity. However, the effective intake for relief of the spasticity produced concomitant drowsiness.

Baclofen in four divided doses to the recommended maximum of 80 mg daily is indicated initially for troubling spasticity. When required, small doses of diazepam or dantrolene sodium may be given for obtaining an adjuvant effect, thus avoiding the side effects of larger doses. Thus several effective preparations are available for spasticity which have proved to be beneficial in improving activities of daily living.

Invasive procedures such as intrathecal alcohol instillation or phenol instillation may resolve the problem of spasticity, but they also damage ventral and dorsal roots and thus preclude development of a reflex bladder and reflexogenic penile erection.[108] Peripheral nerve blocks with phenol, although effective, have demonstrated a side effect of painful paresthesias.[109-111] Awad has proposed the use of an electrical stimulator to localize a motor nerve. The use of an injection needle as the stimulating probe enables the localization of the nerve fibers and simultaneous blockage of these fibers.[111] He feels that phenol has withstood the test of time and is accepted as a local blocking agent, since it is free of local irritation and systemic toxicity in the amounts used. Moreover, its immediate onset of action makes it possible to determine the results of the blocks instantaneously. Further, he adds that phenol has the advantages of a reasonably long duration of action, of being easily sterilized without loss of activity, and of ready availability at low cost. When phenol is injected in or around the motor nerve to a spastic muscle, it abolishes the spasticity by interruption of the pathway of the increased activity of the stretch reflex. It does this by blocking the afferent proprioceptive and efferent fibers.[112]

Surgical measures have included obturator neurectomy for adductor spasticity which interferes with nursing care and ambulation, sciatic neurectomy for spastic knee flexors and plantar flexors, and tendon lengthening, particularly for the Achilles' tendon and knee flexors.

Malignant Disease

Melzak noted that since infection of the urinary tract is still very common in the patient with spinal cord injury, it would be appropriate to study the incidence of bladder cancer in these individuals.[113] In Great Britain's National Spinal Injuries Centre, his 20-year study beginning in 1944 of 3800 persons with spinal cord injury resulted in the finding of 11 cases of bladder cancer, an incidence of 0.28 per cent. The earliest was diagnosed after 13 years, the latest after 42 years. The youngest patient was 37 years old. Because the vast majority of his patients smoked he hesitated to accuse smoking as the cause; it is, however, recognized that smokers have a greater incidence of bladder carcinoma. The only common factors proved to be long-standing chronic urinary infection and cystitis, and long-standing catheter drainage. Bors and Comarr found malignant genitourinary tract disease in 0.64 per cent of 2322 patients.[30] The diagnosis was made 10 to 22 years following injury.

Hypertension

In his postmortem study of 122 paraplegics between 1945 and 1962 Tribe found a surprisingly large incidence of hypertension. "Critical assessment of both clinical and pathologic evidence revealed 41 cases of definite hypertension amongst the 122 paraplegics."[114] He concluded that the hypertension was associated with chronic pyelonephritis. Hypertension was an infrequent finding in other studies.[115-119]

Amyloid Disease

Chronic suppurative infection in the urinary tract, in bedsores, and in underlying bone resulting in disturbance of protein metabolism may be responsible for amyloid disease of the secondary type in patients with spinal cord injury. The amyloidosis is widespread, with the most serious involvement in the kidney.

Pain

Many patients with injuries to the spinal cord or cauda equina experience pain at some time in early or late course of their illness.[120]

Persistent intractable pain is a problem in a limited number of individuals with spinal cord injury. Gooddy suggests that the pain experienced below the level of the spinal cord lesion may be transmitted through the sympathetic nervous system.[121]

Krueger believed that in most instances the pain originates from lesions of the intraspinal contents, either from intact or partially intact nerve roots or from neuroma formation in severed roots or at the proximal stump of the severed spinal cord, or in the transitional zone immediately above the lesion in cases of nontransecting spinal cord injuries.[120]

Another type of pain has been labeled "visceral pain" and follows distention by enemas or distention of the urinary bladder.[28] This discomfort is abdominal in nature. Visceral abnormality such as peptic ulcer or cholecystitis may also produce vague nonlocalizing abdominal discomfort.

Gastrointestinal Function

The transport of products of digestion through the intestine results from peristaltic action that arises from the autonomic plexuses within the bowel wall. Quadriplegic individuals are known to have a high rate of incidence of peptic ulcer that may well be of the stress type. Miller points out that this ulcer phenomenon may be due to unopposed vagal action, as are the ileus and hypermotility.[122]

Superior mesenteric artery syndrome is a complication occurring in the high-level spinal cord injured, which although infrequent, is of great importance.[123, 124] The occlusion of the third portion of the duodenum by the superior mesenteric artery in its downward course is produced by traction on this artery on its mesentery or by any downward displacement of the small intestine. This duodenal obstruction results in sudden onset of persistent vomiting of large amounts of fluid. The upper abdomen is distended and tympanitic. Recommended is conservative care, including avoidance of the supine posture after meals, upward manual displacement of the abdominal viscera, and adequate support of the abdominal wall; when these preventive conservative measures are of no avail, then surgical correction becomes necessary.[123]

SPECIALIZED HOSPITAL UNITS FOR CARE OF THE PATIENT WITH SPINAL CORD INJURY

The great advantage of using a categorically oriented system of care for the patient with spinal cord injury was first proved by Dr. Donald Munro in the 1930's in his unit in the Boston City Hospital. That a significant number of such patients could not only survive but could also return to a productive and functional life status was later confirmed by Guttmann in England, Weiss in Poland, Cheshire in Australia, Michaelis and Rossier in Switzerland, Bors and Talbot in the United States Veterans Administration, Gregg in Ireland, Meinecke in Germany, and Young and Freed in the United States.[125-135]

The complex nature of the manifestations of spinal cord injury and the potential for life-threatening complications, as well as for complications whose avoidance could decrease the hospital stay and minimize the psychologic trauma, makes mandatory the provision of care in a facility especially organized for providing holistic care for this injury.

A lifetime of care begins after discharge from the hospital. The ongoing goals include refinement of physical gains already achieved, maintenance of achieved functional ability and adjustment, and identification of potential or already developed problems. This care includes regular outpatient re-evaluation as well as periodic inpatient study at intervals of 6 to 18 months.

Upon departure from the hospital, the person with spinal cord injury will, when possible, be discharged to his home, which will have been physically altered. His family will have become familiar with his total needs, and ideally his schooling, retraining, and vocational placement will have been arranged.

SPECIAL CONSIDERATIONS

Provided with adapted devices to exploit the full potential of his physical functioning and with removal of architectural barriers in the home and community, the individual with spinal cord injury, no matter what the level, can leave his home, make his way by wheelchair (the most essential equipment for mobility) and hand-control–operated motor vehicle, and participate in educational, vocational, recreational, and even social welfare pursuits in behalf of others.

These accomplishments require doors sufficiently wide to permit wheelchair entrance and egress; replacement of entrance stairs by ramps with grades of no greater than 8 per cent; widening of corridors to allow maneuverability of wheelchairs; construction of

bathrooms both in public buildings and at home to allow maneuverability in the chair and transfer from the chair onto the toilet and return; and adjustment of public telephones, electric light switches, plugs, elevator operating buttons, and door latches to the height of the person seated in the wheelchair. Internal environmental temperature adjustment is also important in view of the intolerance of the person with spinal cord injury to extremes of heat and cold. Elevator accessibility in multistoried school buildings will permit him to attend regular classroom instruction with his peers.

Prejudice by potential employers and real estate managers remains a problem, as does that of transportation companies. The potential of the person with spinal cord injury, in the absence of medical and psychologic complications but even in the presence of multiple physical impairment, is unmeasurable.

Rusk avers:

You don't get fine china by putting clay in the sun. You have to put the clay through the white heat of the kiln if you want to make porcelain. Heat breaks some pieces. Disability breaks some people. But once the clay goes through the white-hot fire and comes out whole, it can never be clay again; once a person overcomes a disability through his own courage, determination and hard work, he has a depth of spirit you and I know little about.[136]

REFERENCES

1. Elsberg, C. A.: The Edwin Smith surgical papyrus and the diagnosis and treatment of injuries to the skull and spine 5000 years ago. Ann. Med. Hist., 3:271, 1931.
2. Poer, D. H.: Newer concepts in the treatment of the paralyzed patient due to war-time injuries of the spinal cord. Ann. Surg., 123:510, 1946.
3. Thompson Walker, J. W.: Hunterian Lecture on the bladder in gunshot and other injuries of the spinal cord. Lancet, 1:173, 1917.
4. Kuhn, W. G.: The care and rehabilitation of patients with injuries of the spinal cord. J. Neurosurg., 4:40, 1947.
5. Hinman, F.: The treatment of paralytic bladder in cases of spinal cord injury. Surgery, 4:649, 1938.
6. Munro, D.: Thoracic and lumbosacral cord injuries. J.A.M.A., 122:1055, 1943.
7. Kirk, N. T.: Wartime activities of the Army Medical Department. N. Engl. J. Med., 235:182, 1946.
8. Controller, Department of Medicine and Surgery: Mortality Report on Spinal Cord Injury. Reports and Statistics Service, Veterans Administration, (Nov. 13), 1958.
9. Young, J. S., and Northrup, N. E.: Statistical

Information Pertaining to Some of the Most Commonly Asked Questions About SCI. Phoenix, Arizona, National Spinal Cord Injury Research Center, 1979.

10. Michaelis, L. S.: Discussion of papers read at the 1967 Scientific Meeting of the International Medical Society of Paraplegia. Paraplegia, 5:180, 1967.

11. Gehrig, R., and Michaelis, L. S.: Statistics of acute paraplegia and tetraplegia on a national scale. Paraplegia, 6:93, 1968.

12. Canadian Neurosurgical Society: Report of a Sub-Committee. Paraplegic Care in Canada, 1969.

13. Young, J. S.: The Southwest Regional System for Treatment of Spinal Injury. Proposal to U.S. Department of Health, Education, and Welfare, April 25, 1969.

14. Sharman, G. J., and Owens, K. A., Jr.: Spinal Cord Injury. Report to the National Paraplegia Foundation, Boston, September, 1970.

15. Brown, L. M.: Maine's Spinal Cord Injured. Study Report to Bureau of Rehabilitation, Department of Health and Welfare, Augusta, Maine, August, 1972.

16. Unpublished data of the National Spinal Cord Injury Model Systems Project, sponsored in part by the National Institute for Handicapped Research and received from the following projects: University of Alabama Spinal Cord Injury System, University of Alabama in Birmingham, Birmingham, Alabama; Southwest Regional System for Treatment of Spinal Injury, Good Samaritan Hospital–St. Joseph's Hospital, Phoenix, Arizona; Northern California Regional Spinal Injury System, Santa Clara Valley Medical Center, San Jose, California; Southern California Regional Spinal Injury System, Rancho Los Amigos Hospital, Downey, California; Rocky Mountain Regional Spinal Cord Injury System, Craig Hospital, Englewood, Colorado; South Florida Regional Spinal Cord Injury System, University of Miami School of Medicine, Miami, Florida; Midwest Regional Spinal Cord Injury Care System, Northwestern Memorial Hospital, Rehabilitation Institute of Chicago, Northwestern University, McGaw Medical Center, Chicago, Illinois; New England Regional Spinal Cord Injury System of University Hospital, Boston University Medical Center, Boston, Massachusetts; Missouri Regional Spinal Cord Injury System, University of Missouri School of Medicine, Columbia, Missouri; New York Regional Spinal Cord Injury System, Institute of Rehabilitation Medicine, New York University, New York, New York; Regional Spinal Cord Injury System of the Delaware Valley, Thomas Jefferson University, Philadelphia, Pennsylvania; Texas Regional Spinal Cord Injury System, The Institute for Rehabilitation and Research, Houston, Texas; Virginia Regional Spinal Cord Injury System, Woodrow Wilson Rehabilitation Center, Fishersville–University of Virginia, Charlottesville, Virginia; Northwest Regional Spinal Cord Injury System, University of Washington, Seattle, Washington.

17. Wilcox, E., Kuwamoto, H., and Shauffer, E. S.: Statewide census of spinal cord injured persons. Hawaii. December, 1971. (Cited in 13).

18. Wilcox, E.: Statewide census of spinal injured persons. Nevada, 1970. (Cited in 14.)

19. Canadian Paraplegic Association: Paraplegic Survey, 1967–68.

20. Lipschitz, R.: Associated injuries and complications of stab wounds of the spinal cord. Paraplegia, 5:75, 1967.

21. Griffiths, H. J.: The radiology of spinal cord injury; a review article. Proceedings 18th U.S. Veterans Administration Spinal Cord Injury Conference, October, 1971. Washington, U.S. Government Printing Office, 1972, p. 43.

22. Hughes, J. T.: Vertebral artery insufficiency in acute cervical spine trauma. Paraplegia, 3:2, 1964.

23. Tator, C. H.: Acute spinal cord injury. A review of recent studies of treatment and pathophysiology. Can. Med. Assoc. J., 107:142, 1972.

24. Osterholm, J. L., Mathews, G. J., Irvin, J. D., and Evangelakos, E. T.: A review of altered norepinephrine metabolism attending severe spinal injury. Proceedings 18th U.S. Veterans Administration Spinal Cord Injury Conference, October, 1971. Washington, U.S. Government Printing Office, 1972, p. 17.

25. Freed, M. M.: Teaching Syllabus; Rehabilitation Medicine. Boston University School of Medicine, 1972.

26. Helme, W. B.: The Soviet's cruel hoax. Model Systems' SCI Digest, 1:9, 1979.

27. Hardy, A. G., and Rossier, A. B.: Spinal Cord Injuries, Orthopedic and Neurologic Aspects. Stuttgart, Thieme, 1975.

28. Guttmann, L.: Spinal Cord Injuries: Comprehensive Management and Research. Oxford, Blackwell, 1973.

29. Trieschmann, R. B.: The Psychological, Social and Vocational Adjustments to Spinal Cord Injury: A Strategy for Future Research. Washington, D.C., RSA-HEW Monograph, 1978, p. 11.

30. Dunn, D.: Adjustment to Spinal Cord Injury in the Rehabilitation Hospital Setting. Doctoral Dissertation, University of Maryland, 1969.

31. Youden, M., Dickey, R. E., Sell, G. H., and Stratford, C. D.: Instrumentation for the severely disabled: An update. Model Systems' SCI Digest, 2:16, 1980.

32. Hofkosh, J. M., Sipaljo, J., and Brody, L.: Driver education for physically disabled: Evaluation, selection and training methods. Med. Clin. North Am., 53:685, 1969.

33. Hughes, J. T.: Pathology of the Spinal Cord. Philadelphia, W. B. Saunders Company, 1978.

34. Ames, M. D., and Schut, L.: Results of treatment of 171 consecutive meningoceles — 1963 to 1968. Pediatrics, 50:466, 1972.

35. Stark, G. D.: The nature and cause of paraplegia in myelomeningocele. Paraplegia, 9:219, 1971.

35a. Halpern, D., et al.: Pediatric Rehabilitation. Syllabus MKSAP in Physical Medicine and Rehabilitation. C1-30. Chicago, Am. Acad. Phys. Med. Rehabil., 1977.

36. Abramson, A. S.: The neurogenic bladder. Arch. Phys. Med. Rehabil., 48:480, 1967.

37. Bors, E.: Neurogenic bladder. Urol. Survey, 7:177, 1957.

38. Bors, E., and Comarr, A. E.: Neurologic Urology. Baltimore, University Park Press, 1971.

39. Bergofsky, E. J.: Quantitation of function of respiratory muscles in normal individuals and quadriplegic patients. Arch. Phys. Med. Rehabil., 45:575, 1964.
40. Glenn, W. W. L.: Diaphragm pacing: Present Status. Pace, 1:357, 1978.
41. Farmer, W. C., Glenn, W. W. L., and Gee, J. B. L.: Alveolar hypoventilation syndrome, studies of ventilatory control in patients selected for diaphragm pacing. Am. J. Med., 64:39, 1978.
42. Glenn, W. W. L., Holcomb, W. G., Shaw, R. K., Hogan, J. F., and Holschuh, K. R.: Long term ventilatory support by diaphragm pacing in quadriplegia. Am. J. Surg., 183:566, 1976.
43. Talbot, H.: Discussion of papers read at the meeting of the International Medical Society of Paraplegia. Paraplegia, 9:63, 1971.
44. Trieschmann, R. B.: Sex, sex acts and sexuality. Arch. Phys. Med. Rehabil., 56:8, 1975.
45. Griffith, E. R., and Trieschmann, R. B.: Sexual functioning in women with spinal cord injury. Arch. Phys. Med. Rehabil., 56:18, 1975.
46. Hohmann, G. W.: Reactions of the individual with a disability complicated by a sexual problem. Arch. Phys. Med. Rehabil., 56:9, 1975.
47. Cole, T. M.: Spinal cord injury patients and sexual dysfunction. Arch. Phys. Med. Rehabil., 56:11, 1975.
48. Tarabulcy, E.: Sexual function in the normal and in paraplegia. Paraplegia, 10:201, 1972.
49. Bors, E., and Comarr, A. E.: Neurological disturbances of sexual function with special reference to 529 patients with spinal cord injury. Urol. Survey, 10:191, 1960.
50. Miller, J. M., III: Autonomic function in the isolated spinal cord. In Downey, J. A., and Darling, R. C. (eds.): Physiological Basis of Rehabilitation Medicine. Philadelphia, W. B. Saunders Company, 1971.
51. Guttmann, L., and Walsh, J. J.: Prostigmin assessment test of fertility in spinal man. Paraplegia 9:39, 1971.
52. Rossier, A. B., Ziegler, W. H., Duchosal, P. W., and Meylan, J.: Sexual function and dysreflexia. Paraplegia, 9:51, 1971.
53. Morales, P. A., Suarez, J. B., Delgado, J., and Whitehead, E. D.: Penile implant for erectile impotence. J. Urol., 109:641, 1973.
54. Gee, W. F., McRoberts, J. W., Raney, J. O., and Amsell, J. S.: Impotent patient: Surgical treatment with penile prosthesis and psychiatric evaluation. J. Urol., 111:41, 1974.
55. Scott, F. B., Bradley, W. E., and Timm, G. W.: Management of erectile impotence: Use of implantable inflatable prosthesis. Urology, 2:80, 1973.
56. Furlow, W. L.: Therapy of impotence. In Krane, R. J., and Siroky, M. B. (eds.): Clinical Neuro-Urology. Boston, Little, Brown and Co., 1979.
57. Rossier, A. B., Ruffieux, M., and Ziegler, W. H.: Pregnancy and labour in high traumatic spinal cord lesions. Paraplegia, 7:210, 1970.
58. Robertson, D. N. S.: Pregnancy and labour in the paraplegic. Paraplegia, 10:209, 1972.
59. Guller, H., and Paeslack, V.: Pregnancy damage and birth complications in the children of paraplegic women. Paraplegia 10:213, 1972.
60. Vallbona, C., Lipscomb, H. S., and Carter, R. E.: Endocrine response to orthostatic hypotension in quadriplegia. Arch. Phys. Med. Rehabil., 47:412, 1966.
61. Guttmann, L., Silva, J., and Wyndham, C. H.: Thermoregulation in spinal man. J. Physiol. (Lond.), 142:406, 1958.
62. Downey, J. A.: Physiology of temperature regulations in man. In Downey, J. A., and Darling, R. C. (eds.): Physiological Basis of Rehabilitation Medicine. Philadelphia, W. B. Saunders Company, 1971.
63. Sherrington, C. S.: Notes on temperature after spinal transection, with some observations on shivering. J. Physiol. (Lond.), 58:405, 1924.
64. Johnson, R. H.: Temperature regulation in paraplegia. Paraplegia, 9:137, 1971.
65. Arieff, A. J., Pyzik, S. W., Tigay, E. L., and Bersohn, J.: Some metabolic studies in quadriplegia following spinal cord injury, Ill. Med. J., 117:219, 1960.
66. Robinson, R.: Serum protein changes following spinal cord injuries. Proc. R. Soc. Med. 47:1109, 1954.
67. Maynard, F. M., and Imai, K.: Immobilization hypercalcemia in spinal cord injury. Arch. Phys. Med. Rehabil., 58:16, 1977.
68. Cooper, I. S., Rynearson, E. H., MacCarty, C. S., and Power, M. H.: Metabolic consequences in spinal cord injury. J. Clin. Endocrinol., 10:858, 1950.
69. Kaplan, L., Powell, B. R., Grynbaum, B. B., and Rusk, H. A.: Comprehensive Follow-up Study of Spinal Cord Dysfunction and its Resultant Disabilities. Chap. V., New York, Institution of Rehabilitation Medicine, 1966.
70. Cooper, I. S., and Hoen, T. T.: Metabolic disorders in paraplegics. Neurology (Minneap.) 2:332, 1952.
71. Naftchi, N. E., Viau, A. T., Sell, G. H., and Lowman, E. W.: Pituitary gonadal axis dysfunction in spinal cord injury. Arch. Phys. Med. Rehabil., 57:552, 1976.
72. Thompson, C. E., and Witham, A.: Paroxysmal hypertension in spinal cord injuries. N. Engl. J. Med., 239:291, 1948.
73. Young, J. S.: Use of guanethidine in control of sympathetic hyperreflexia in persons with cervical and thoracic cord lesions. Arch. Phys. Med. Rehabil., 44:204, 1963.
74. Kurnick, N. B.: Autonomic hyperreflexia and its control in patients with spinal cord lesions. Ann. Intern. Med., 44:678, 1956.
75. Cole, T. M., Kottke, F. J., Olson, M., Stadal, L., and Neiderloh, J.: Alterations of cardiovascular control in high spinal myelomalacia. Arch. Phys. Med. Rehabil., 48:259, 1967.
76. Kewalramani, L. S.: Autonomic dysreflexia in traumatic myelopathy. Am. J. Phys. Med., 59:1, 1980.
77. Rossier, A. B., Ruffieux, M., and Ziegler, W. H.: Pregnancy and labour in high traumatic spinal cord lesions. Paraplegia, 7:210, 1970.
78. Snow, J. C., Sideropoulos, H. P., Kripke, B. J., Freed, M. M., Shah, N. K., and Schlesinger, R. M.: Autonomic hyperreflexia during cystoscopy in patients with high spinal cord injuries. Paraplegia, 15:327, 1978.
79. Ramos, M. U., Freed, M. M., and Marek, R. J.:

Simultaneous cardiovascular, electromyographic and urodynamic evaluation of patients with spinal cord injury. Model Systems' SCI Digest, 2:31, 1980.

80. Guttmann, L.: Official Medical History of Second World War. Vol. Surgery: Intermittent Catheterization, p. 465. London, H. M. Stationery Office, 1953.

81. Guttmann, L., and Frankel, H.: The value of intermittent catheterization in the early management of traumatic paraplegia and tetraplegia. Paraplegia, 4:63, 1966.

82. Munro, D.: Care of the back following spinal cord injuries. N. Engl. J. Med. 233:391, 1940.

83. Kosiak, M.: Etiology of decubitus ulcers. Arch. Phys. Med. Rehabil., 42:19, 1961.

84. Kosiak, M.: An effective method of preventing decubitus ulcers. Arch. Phys. Med. Rehabil., 47:724, 1966.

85. Kosiak, M.: Etiology and pathology of ischemic ulcerations. Arch. Phys. Med. Rehabil., 40:62, 1959.

86. Steinberg, F. U.: The effects of immobilization on circulation and respiration. In Steinberg, F. U.: The Immobilized Patient: Functional Pathology and Management. New York City, Plenum Medical Book Co., 1980.

87. Guttmann, L.: Venous thrombosis and pulmonary embolism. In Guttmann, L.: Spinal Cord Injuries: Comprehensive Management and Research, 2nd Ed. Oxford, Blackwell Scientific Publications, 1976.

88. Naso, F.: Pulmonary embolism in acute spinal cord injury. Arch. Phys. Med. Rehabil., 55:275, 1974.

89. Shull, J. R., and Rose, D. L.: Pulmonary embolism in patients with spinal cord injuries. Arch. Phys. Med. Rehabil., 47:444, 1976.

90. Wessler, S.: Studies in intravascular coagulation. I. Coagulation in isolated venous segments. J. Clin. Invest., 31:1011, 1952.

91. Clagett, G. P., and Salzman, E. W.: Prevention of venous thromboembolism in surgical patients. N. Engl. J. Med., 290:93, 1974.

92. Watson, N.: Venous thrombosis and pulmonary embolism in spinal cord injury. Paraplegia, 6:113, 1969.

93. Perkash, A., Prakash, V., and Perkash, I.: Experience with management of thromboembolism in patients with spinal cord injury: Part I. Incidence, diagnosis and role of some risk factors. Paraplegia, 16:322, 1978–79.

94. Bors, E., Conrad, C. A., and Massell, T. B.: Venous occlusion of lower extremities in paraplegia patients. Surg. Gynecol. Obstet., 99:451, 1954.

95. Walsh, J. J., and Tribe, C.: Phlebothrombosis and pulmonary embolism in paraplegia. Paraplegia, 3:209, 1965.

96. Wessler, S., Cohen, S., and Fleischman, F. G.: The temporary thrombotic state. N. Engl. J. Med., 254:413, 1956.

97. Watson, N.: Anti-coagulant therapy in the prevention of venous thrombosis and pulmonary embolism in the spinal cord injury. Paraplegia, 16:265, 1978–79.

98. Hachen, H. J.: Anti-coagulant therapy in patients with spinal cord injury. Paraplegia, 12:176, 1974.

99. Venier, L. H., and Ditunno, J. F., Jr.: Heterotopic ossification in the paraplegic patient. Arch. Phys. Med. Rehabil., 52:475, 1971.

100. Stover, S. L., Hataway, C. J., and Zeiger, H. E.: Heterotopic ossification in spinal cord injured patients. Arch. Phys. Med. Rehabil., 56:199, 1975.

101. Wharton, G. W., and Morgan, T. H.: Ankylosis in the paralyzed patient. J. Bone Joint Surg., 52(A):105, 1970.

102. Lance, J. S., and Buchi, D.: Mechanisms of spasticity. Arch. Phys. Med. Rehabil., 55:332, 1974.

103. Pedersen, E.: Clinical assessment and pharmacologic therapy of spasticity. Arch. Phys. Med. Rehabil., 55:344, 1974.

104. Joynt, R. L.: Dantrolene sodium: Long term effects in patients with muscle spasticity. Arch. Phys. Med. Rehabil., 57:212, 1976.

105. Zorychta, E., Esplin, D. W., Capek, R., et al.: Actions of dantrolene in extrafusal and intrafusal striated muscle. Fed. Proc., 30:669, 1971.

106. Monstea, A. W., Herman, R., and Meeks, S., et al.: Cooperative study for assessing effects of pharmacologic agents on spasticity. Am. J. Phys. Med., 52:163, 1973.

107. Curtis, D. R., and Felix, D.: GABA and prolonged spinal inhibition. Nature New Biol., 231:187, 1971.

108. Sheldon, C. H., and Bors, E.: Subarachnoid alcohol block in paraplegia. J. Neurosurg., 5:389, 1948.

109. Khalili, A. A., Hammel, M. H., Forster, S., and Benton, J. G.: Management of spasticity by selective nerve block with dilute phenol solutions in clinical rehabilitation. Arch. Phys. Med. Rehabil., 45:513, 1964.

110. Moritz, M. H.: Phenol block of peripheral nerves. Scand. J. Rehabil. Med., 5:160, 1973.

111. Awad, E. A.: Phenol block for control of hip flexor and adductor spasticity. Arch. Phys. Med. Rehabil., 53:554, 1972.

112. Meelhuysen, F. E., Halpern, D., and Quast, J.: Treatment of flexor spasticity of hip by paravertebral lumbar spinal nerve block. Arch. Phys. Med. Rehabil., 49:717, 1968.

113. Melzak, J.: The incidence of bladder cancer in paraplegia. Paraplegia, 4:85, 1966.

114. Tribe, C. R.: Causes of death in early and late stages of paraplegia. Paraplegia, 1:19, 1963.

115. Freed, M. M., Bakst, H. J., and Barrie, D. L.: Life expectancy, survival rates and causes of death in civilian patients with spinal cord trauma. Arch. Phys. Med. Rehabil., 47:457, 1966.

116. Ebel, A.: Discussion of the pathology in selected cases of spinal cord injury. Proceedings: 9th Annual Clinical Spinal Cord Injury Conference, October, 1960. Washington, U.S. Government Printing Office, 1961.

117. Finkle, J. R.: Discussion of the pathology in selected cases of spinal cord injury. Proceedings: 9th Annual Clinical Spinal Cord Injury Conference, Ocober 1960. Washington, U.S. Government Printing Office, 1961.

118. Halladay, L. W.: Discussion of the pathology in selected cases of spinal cord injury. Proceedings: 9th Annual Clinical Spinal Cord Injury Conference, October, 1960. Washington, U.S. Government Printing Office, 1961.

119. Lowry, R.: Discussion of the pathology in selected cases of spinal cord injury. Proceedings: 9th Annual Clinical Spinal Cord Injury Conference, October, 1960. Washington, U.S. Government Printing Office, 1961.

120. Krueger, E. G.: Management of painful states in injuries of the spinal cord and cauda equina. Am. J. Phys. Med., 39:103, 1960.

121. Gooddy, Y.: On the nature of pain. Brain 80:118, 1957.

122. Miller, J. M., III.: Autonomic function in the isolated spinal cord. *In* Downey, J. A., and Darling, R. C. (eds.): Physiological Basis of Rehabilitation Medicine. Philadelphia, W. B. Saunders Company, 1971.

123. Ramos, M. U.: Recurrent superior mesenteric artery syndrome in a quadriplegic patient. Arch. Phys. Med. Rehabil., 56:86, 1975.

124. Raptou, A. D., LaBan, M. M., and Johnson, E. W.: Intermittent arteriomesenteric occlusion of duodenum in quadriplegic patient. Arch. Phys. Med. Rehabil., 45:418, 1964.

125. Guttmann, L.: History of the National Spinal Injuries Centre, Stoke Mandeville Hospital, Aylesbury. Paraplegia, 5:115, 1967.

126. Weiss, M.: Fifteen years' experience on rehabilitation of paraplegics at the Rehabilitation Institute of Warsaw University. Paraplegia, 5:158, 1967.

127. Chesire, D. J. E.: The complete and centralised treatment of paraplegia. Paraplegia, 6:59, 1969.

128. Michaelis, L.: Opening of the Swiss Paraplegic Centre in Basle. Paraplegia, 5:158, 1967.

129. Rossier, A. B.: Organization and function of the French Swiss Paraplegic Centre. Paraplegia, 5:166, 1968.

130. Bors, E.: The Spinal Cord Injury Center of the Veterans Administration Hospital, Long Beach, California. Paraplegia, 5:126, 1967.

131. Talbot, H. S.: Rehabilitation in a changing world. Paraplegia, 7:146, 1969.

132. Gregg, T. M.: Organization of a Spinal Injury Unit within a Rehabilitation Centre. Paraplegia, 5:163, 1967.

133. Meinecke, F. W.: Opening of the Centre For Spinal Injuries and other severely disabled persons at the Orthopaedic Clinic of Heidelberg University. Paraplegia, 5:104, 1967.

134. Young, J. S.: Development of systems of spinal injury management with a correlation to the development of other esoteric health care systems. Ariz. Med., 27:1, 1970.

135. Freed, M. M.: The Spinal Cord Injury Center, Scope. B.U.M.C., 1:16, 1968.

136. Rusk, H. A.: A World to Care For. New York, Random House, 1972.

33

AFTERCARE OF FRACTURES

MILAND E. KNAPP

Problems in the aftercare of fractures may arise from bony causes, soft tissue injuries, and edema. Bony causes, such as malunion, delayed union, or nonunion, will not be discussed in this chapter, since they do not properly come under the heading of physical medicine. Soft tissue injuries, including lacerations of nerves, tears of ligaments and joint capsules, and injuries to tendons and muscles, also will not be discussed in this chapter, since they require definitive treatment, often surgical in nature, and although physical measures are commonly useful in their treatment, most of these measures will be discussed under other headings. Persistent edema, in my opinion, is the most common cause of disability following fractures. This problem will be discussed in detail.

Traumatic edema fluid is produced either by the original injury or by mechanical factors following the injury. Extravasation of blood into the soft tissues is a constant accompaniment of fracture. In addition to this, extravasation of edema fluid into the soft tissues may result in so much swelling and interference with normal blood supply that extensive blisters may form, covering sometimes the entire extremity. The extravasated blood and edema fluid must be removed by one of two methods. If return flow circulation is restored adequately and early, both the blood and edema fluid may be

removed by absorption into the general body circulation with no undesirable residual effects.

If, on the other hand, the swelling persists longer than a week or two, the swelling may be removed by organization instead of absorption, with the eventual production of fibrous scar tissue. This process is similar to and proceeds at the same time as the organization which results in the production of fibrous callus in the process of normal bone healing. It is desirable that fibrous tissue develop between the bone ends, since this is the first stage of fixation of the fracture. However, it is not desirable for fibrosis to occur in muscles or between such solid structures as tendon, joint capsule, bone, and strong fascial layers, since these parts are normally movable and the fibrosis limits movement.

"*Oedema is glue,*" says Watson-Jones. Since the fibrous tissue produced between the bone ends and within the soft tissues is developed at exactly the same time, it is obvious one cannot wait for the bone to heal before treating the soft tissue damage. There are two apparently antagonistic objectives to be obtained simultaneously. First, the bone ends must be held immobile and in constant apposition until healing occurs. Second, the soft tissues must be kept moving to prevent fibrosis and subsequent limited painful mo-

674

tion. However, the objectives are really not as antagonistic as it might appear, since pressure tends to promote bone healing and activity increases circulation to the part and this, too, aids in bone healing. It is necessary at the time of reduction to ascertain that the apparatus that maintains immobility of the bone ends is so arranged that maximal activity of soft tissues can be obtained starting immediately after the reduction of the fracture.

The aftercare of fractures may be divided into early and late stages.

TREATMENT IN THE EARLY STAGE

Active Motion. The most effective, as well as the most available and the least expensive, method of removing edema fluid is active motion. However, in order that this may be accomplished the surgeon must trim the cast to allow function or apply the retaining apparatus in such a manner that maximal function is possible. For instance, if function of the metacarpophalangeal joints of the hand is to be retained, it is necessary that the immobilizing apparatus not extend distal to the flexion crease of the palm.

Active motion is effective in removing edema fluid because it assists return flow circulation. Normal return flow circulation is carried on to a large degree by muscle activity. The veins are provided with valves that will not allow the blood to flow distally so that when the muscle squeezes down on the vein, blood is forced proximally. The blood cannot return through the valve so the area fills up from below and blood is again ready to be forced back toward the heart. This same mechanism is present in the lymphatics.

Elevation. If it is not feasible to remove the edema fluid by active motion, the next best method is elevation. However, it must be remembered that for elevation to be effective the distal part of the extremity must be above the proximal and the proximal part above the heart. This is a practical method in fractures of the lower extremity when the patient is in bed. Under these circumstances, elevation can be accomplished fairly easily. In the upper extremity, however, elevation is not usually practical because the hand would have to be up in a position above the elbow and the elbow above the shoulder. In frac-

tures of the upper extremity the patient is not ordinarily put to bed, so this method is not available. The use of a sling is not elevation because the hand and forearm in a sling are below the shoulder by the length of the arm.

Physical Therapy. If neither of these methods is feasible or effective, treatment must be given by what is ordinarily designated as physical therapy. The usual procedures are heat, massage, and motion.

HEAT. The physiologic effects of heat may be summarized briefly as relief of pain, increase in the arterial blood supply, increased edema because of the increased capillary pressure produced, and softening of fibrous tissue.

The type of heat used is not usually important. Hot packs or hot soaks are quite convenient, as is infrared radiation. In a department of physical medicine, whirlpool baths or similar methods of heat application are usually used. Diathermy is not advisable in the early stages following fractures because, as a result of its greater effectiveness, it often causes increased pain by increasing edema. Heat should always be followed by massage or exercise.

MASSAGE. The physiologic effects of massage are relief of pain if the massage is given efficiently and expertly, increase of venous circulation because the stroke of the massage is toward the heart, reduction of swelling as a result of the enhanced return flow circulation, and stretching of fibrous tissue (see Chapter 17).

The massage should be mild so that pain is relieved instead of increased, but it should be firm enough to give good edema reduction. Violent manipulation or painful types of massage should be avoided because of the possibility of displacing fragments before healing has occurred.

EXERCISE. If possible, massage should be followed by active exercise. If it is necessary to remove the supporting apparatus for exercise, the therapist should assist the patient in carrying out the exercise motion, either by overcoming gravity for him or by supporting a part of his body while the exercise is being performed. Passive motion should never be used in the early stage after fracture because fear of pain may cause the patient to resist any passive motion and the so-called passive motion is transformed into resistive motion with the patient doing the resisting. Assisted active exercise is the exercise of choice in early fractures.

To summarize, during the period of immobilization of the fracture, physical treatment is used to reduce swelling as soon as possible and to maintain range of joint motion, muscular strength, and dexterity.

TREATMENT IN THE LATE STAGE

If the removal of edema fluid is delayed until the bone is healed, soft tissue adhesions will have become firmly established and may be solid enough to limit motion as well as cause pain. Unfortunately it is common practice to refer patients for physical therapy two months or more after the original injury, when fibrosis and contractures, painful motion, muscle atrophy and weakness, and persistent brawny edema make the danger of permanent impairment of function obvious. Treatment at this time is entirely different from treatment in the early stage. Now the objectives of treatment are to remove whatever edema is still present, to soften and stretch fibrous tissue, to increase the range of joint motion, to restore circulatory efficiency, to increase muscular strength, and to retrain muscular dexterity.

HEAT. Heat may be used for sedation, to increase circulation and to soften fibrous adhesions. The type of heat used is not extremely important and depends more upon the availability of the modality and the pathologic conditions present in the patient than on any specific properties of the various methods of heat application. In my experience, relaxation is best obtained by the use of moist heat. The whirlpool bath is valuable because heat, massage, and active motion are possible simultaneously in it. Hot packs are often useful, particularly for areas that cannot be treated easily in the whirlpool. Diathermy and short-wave diathermy may be used. Infrared radiation is not as effective in the late stage as it is during the early stages.

MASSAGE. Again, the heat is followed by massage with emphasis upon deep stroking and compression movements in order to stretch the fibrous adhesions as well as to get rid of any edema that may still be present. This treatment may be considerably more vigorous than that used during the early stage. Tender areas are made less tender by

massage. The intramuscular movement produced by the kneading and friction motions helps to stretch adhesions so that a greater range of motion is possible.

EXERCISE. Heat and massage should always be followed by exercise. The most effective regimen begins with assisted active exercise followed by free motion and then resistive exercise as the patient improves. Forced stretching of fibrous bands may be necessary in order to obtain maximal range of motion. It may be done manually or by prolonged stretch using a weight over a period of a half hour or more (Chapter 18).

Manipulation under anesthesia should be used only if no other method is effective and then should be considered very carefully because of the danger of increasing the disability. If this method is used, it must be followed immediately by physical measures designed to overcome the pain and maintain the range of motion obtained by the manipulation. As the patient gains in range of motion and strength and as pain is decreased, occupational therapy becomes particularly useful because the patient's interest in the object he is making encourages prolonged effort (see Chapter 29). Projects may be chosen to increase range of motion, strength or coordination, and manual dexterity. When the exercise is to be continued for months, the projects should be suitable for home use after discharge from the hospital.

SPECIAL PROBLEMS

A few special problems seem worth discussing in some detail because physical treatment may prevent serious complications if the condition is recognized before irreversible changes have occurred.

Myositis Ossificans

During the healing process, calcification may occur in the soft tissues as well as around the bone. Frequently it follows hemorrhage into the muscle or a hematoma in the tissue spaces. The patient usually complains of pain and limited motion. Examination shows palpable localized induration, which may be deep in the tissues. X-ray examination reveals calcification diffusely in the muscle or localized to fascial planes. Continuous hyperemia will assist absorption into the circulation, and the calcification will often disappear without surgical removal.

I have used the following technique: The involved part is wrapped in a bath blanket or other insulating material to prevent heat loss. Gauze bandage holds it in place. Short-wave diathermy is then applied to the part as frequently as is convenient. The insulating padding remains in place between treatments to maintain the hyperemia. The diathermy may be applied for a half hour every two hours, all day, if the patient is hospitalized. If he is an outpatient, it should be repeated at least twice daily for an hour at a time. This treatment must be continued consistently for at least a month. A follow-up x-ray may show beginning absorption at that time, but two or more months of treatment is usually needed. During the treatment period, unusual exercise and stretching of the contracted muscle is prohibited because trauma may further injure the muscle and increase the calcification. When the calcium has nearly disappeared from the muscle itself and the range of motion is approaching normal, treatment may be discontinued. Calcification remaining in the fascial planes is of no clinical significance.

Atrophy

Atrophy of Disuse. This form of atrophy follows any prolonged immobilization and involves not only the bone but the muscle as well. X-ray examination may show marked loss of bone density. Heat is often useful in relieving pain and in softening tissues to overcome contractures, but active exercise is the essential treatment. Roentgenograms should not be used to gauge improvement, because recalcification is extremely slow and the patient will be clinically normal long before the x-ray becomes normal.

Reflex Sympathetic Dystrophy. This may follow minor fractures. Sudeck's acute posttraumatic bone atrophy, the shoulder-hand syndrome, and causalgia are common examples of reflex sympathetic dystrophy. X-rays often show marked bone atrophy with a patchy distribution. It is important to recognize these causes of pain and disability because relief may be greatly accelerated by blocking, with local anesthetics, the sympathetic ganglia supplying the area. Such blocking should be done in addition to the usual physical treatment, as early as the diagnosis can be made, because results improve with early treatment. In these dystrophies hyperemia is present, as evidenced by swelling, redness of the skin, and bone atrophy. Therefore, heat is not usually beneficial. If heat is desired to relieve pain, it should be used cautiously and if the pain is not relieved or is increased, as is common, the heat should be discontinued. The essential part of the physical treatment is active exercise. Increase in strength and decrease in atrophy result, even though active motion may be painful at first.

Volkmann's Contracture

Volkmann's ischemic contracture requires immediate recognition and treatment to prevent severe disability. It usually follows a supracondylar fracture of the humerus but may also follow fracture of both bones of the forearm. Arteriospasm or rupture of blood vessels causes swelling, which compresses the muscles and nerves within the fascial sheath. Necrosis of muscles, of nerves, or even of bone and cartilage may result. The fibrosis produced during healing shortens the muscles on the flexor surface of the forearm, so the fingers contract down into the palm and become nonfunctional. Immediate emergency treatment to relieve pressure or repair arterial injury is imperative. This is a real emergency because even a few hours of delay may result in irreparable damage. When a patient with a forearm or elbow injury complains of pain, sedatives should not be given until the physician has examined the extremity to be sure that this condition is not developing.

If adequate treatment is delayed too long, developing contractures may be prevented or reduced by physical treatment started as early as possible and continued intensively until maximal improvement is obtained. Whirlpool bath followed by massage plus interrupted direct current stimulation to the paralyzed muscles should be started at once. A pancake splint with a malleable wrist section may be adjusted to maintain the length of the flexor muscles as it increases with intensive treatment. The treatment should continue for at least six months to a year. In some cases where severe damage has occurred, reparative or cosmetic surgery may be needed.

Shoulder Dislocation

Following shoulder dislocation, even though the dislocation is satisfactorily reduced, disability may result.

1. Scapulo-humeral contracture may limit motion. Treatment consists of heat, massage, and scapulo-humeral motion.

2. The axillary nerve may be injured by pressure of the humeral head as it slips into the axilla. Its motor fibers supply the deltoid and teres minor muscles only, while its sensory distribution is to a variable but small area near and slightly posterior to the deltoid insertion. Nerve damage is often unrecognized because the symptoms are masked by a Velpeau bandage or similar retaining apparatus. Removal of the bandage a month or so later reveals that the patient cannot abduct his arm. Then physical therapy is prescribed. The true nature of the injury can be identified by merely stimulating the deltoid muscle with a tetanizing current. If the tetanizing current produces muscle contraction, the nerve is intact. If the muscle does not respond to the tetanizing current, even though some voluntary motion may be present, nerve damage has occurred and the muscle should be treated to prevent fibrosis and limitation of motion.

Treatment consists of interrupted negative direct current stimulation in addition to heat, massage, and scapulo-humeral motion. When good voluntary function has returned, the electric stimulation can be discontinued and active exercise prescribed to develop maximal strength.

3. Loss of function at the shoulder joint may also result from rupture of the short rotator tendons. In this case, the head of the humerus, which is normally held in place by the short rotator cuff during abduction, rides upward and strikes the acromion, which limits abduction. In complete rupture, the only effective treatment is surgical suture. In partial rupture, immobilization in an abducted position and cautious maintenance of range of motion may be adequate to maintain function while the tendon heals.

Hip Fracture

Hip fractures present special problems requiring careful treatment. Intertrochanteric fractures usually heal satisfactorily in about four months because the blood supply is adequate. Open operation with internal fixation secures accurate reduction and maintains contact. However, one must realize that the internal fixation is not intended to support weight bearing. Many older persons will not walk between parallel bars or on crutches without putting the injured foot to the ground. The plate may break or screws may loosen with weight bearing. Therefore, if the patient cannot be taught to walk without bearing weight on the fractured extremity, he should not be allowed to try independent ambulation until the bone has healed sufficiently to support his weight.

In intracapsular fractures, non-union is frequent because the major portion of the blood supply comes through the neck of the femur. Since this is broken, the femoral neck and head may not receive an adequate blood supply. Non-union is common and aseptic necrosis may supervene even when union is solid. Again, weight bearing should not be allowed until healing has occurred, and this may take six months. Therefore, the patient must be taught to walk with crutches or a walkerette with a three-point type of gait. It is important to maintain range of motion and strength in both types of fracture. Treatment by whirlpool bath or Hubbard tank, followed by range of motion exercise, is helpful and active exercise should be started as early as possible. Gait training in the parallel bars and graduating to underarm crutches should start as soon as the patient can be trusted to keep his weight off the injured extremity.

REFERENCES

1. Knapp, M. E.: Treatment of fracture sequelae. Lancet, 79:106–112, 1959.
2. Knapp, M. E.: Physical medicine in the treatment of fractures. (Panel Discussion, American Medical Association, Atlantic City, N.J., June 12, 1947.) JAMA, 137:136–139, 1948.
3. Knapp, M. E.: Physical therapy in fractures about elbow joint. (Read at Annual Session at Cleveland, Ohio, Sept. 3, 1940.) Arch. Phys. Ther., 21:709–715, 1940.
4. Knapp, M. E.: Role of physical therapy in fractures. (Read at American Congress of Physical Therapy. New York, Sept. 8, 1939.) Arch. Phys. Ther., 21:401–407, 1940.
5. Watson-Jones, R.: Fractures and Other Bone and Joint Injuries, 2nd ed. Baltimore, Williams and Wilkins Co., 1941, p. 48.

34

MANAGEMENT OF MOTOR UNIT DISEASES

ERNEST W. JOHNSON
MICHAEL A. ALEXANDER

DEFINITIONS

Motor unit diseases include those conditions affecting the anterior horn cell, its axon, the myoneural junction, and muscle fibers.

Anterior Horn Cell. Examples of diseases that affect the anterior horn cell include acute anterior poliomyelitis, amyotrophic lateral sclerosis (progressive spinomuscular atrophy), Kugelberg-Welander disease, Werdnig-Hoffmann disease, and myelitis.

Axon. Conditions that affect the axon are peripheral nerve injuries, Guillain-Barré syndrome (idiopathic polyneuritis), toxic neuropathies, diabetic neuropathy, Charcot-Marie-Tooth disease, and other heredofamilial peripheral neuropathies.

Myoneural Junction. Myasthenia gravis and myasthenic syndrome in small cell carcinoma of the lungs affect the myoneural junction.

Muscle Fiber (and Cell Membrane). Diseases that affect muscle fibers include progressive muscular dystrophy (Duchenne type), restrictive muscular dystrophy (fascio-scapulohumeral), myotonic dystrophy, polymyositis (dermatomyositis), metabolic myopathy (e.g., thyrotoxic), hypokalemic and hyperkalemic myopathies, congenital myopathies (e.g., nemaline, central core), and others.

MANAGEMENT

In a majority of motor unit diseases there is no specific treatment to effect a cure. The ideal approach would be prevention — vaccination for virus diseases, education to prevent toxic polyneuropathies, genetic counseling for hereditary diseases, and such measures as desensitization for allergic diseases. Therefore, the management is directed largely toward symptoms that appear during the course of the disease.[31] This management should be divided into (1) prospective care and (2) expectant care. Prospective care includes all those measures that should be used irrespective of the chronic disease, that is, all the usual techniques that are given to healthy children and adults. Expectant care includes anticipation of deformities and other complications that may be expected during the course of a progressive or chronic condition and using aggressive measures to prevent or minimize these. An example is tightness in muscular dystrophy that may lead to premature loss of ambulation. Another example is the ventila-

679

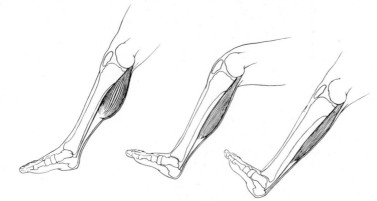

FIGURE 34–1. Tightness of two joint muscles is likely to occur in motor unit diseases. Proper stretch requires application of kinesiologic principles.

TABLE 34–1. FREQUENT AREAS OF SOFT TISSUE TIGHTNESS

Neck flexors	M-P extensors
Shoulder adductors	Rectus femoris
Elbow flexors	Hip flexor
Pronation	Tensor fascia lata
Web space	Knee flexor
	Gastrocnemius-soleus

tory insufficiency that accompanies many of the advanced motor unit diseases. This can be managed by early mechanical ventilatory devices.

Pain. In acute poliomyelitis, polyneuritis, and polymyositis, pain may be a significant symptom.[22] Control of pain may require both pharmacologic and physical treatment. Salicylates and codeine are often adequate, but narcotics should be used sparingly as they can produce respiratory depression. Physical treatment used with or without mild analgesics adequately controls pain in most cases.

Tightness. Soft tissue shortening may be present at all stages in motor unit disease. Two-joint muscle tightness often appears in the first week (Table 34–1). Physical treatment includes passive, active, and active assistive stretching, usually after the application of heat. If a heated pool is available both can be combined. Positioning can facilitate prolonged stretch and prevent deformity.[24] Bracing effective in the prevention of contractures requires careful attention to kinesiology when used to correct deformity (Fig. 34–1).

Deformity. Malalignment of body segments represents a negative aspect of general management. Care must be taken that prescribed equipment is not, in fact, causing progressive deformity. Children are fre-

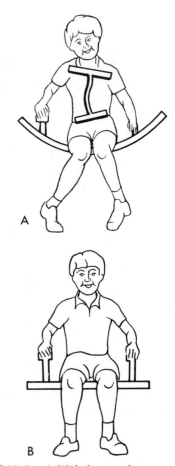

FIGURE 34–2. *A*, Wide hammock seat promotes deformity. *B*, Proper positioning includes a firm seat and correct arm height.

quently placed in large wheelchairs to allow for growth, often sitting on a sling with one hip higher, legs internally rotated and adducted, and leaning on one elbow (Fig. 34–2*A*). Progression from postural asymmetry to structural deformity becomes inevitable. A minimal chair prescription should include a

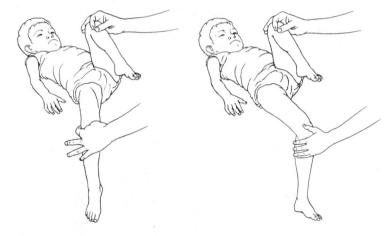

FIGURE 34–3. Iliotibial band—examination for tightness in abduction with hip fully extended.

firm seat, lumbar support, and adequate arm support (Fig. 34–2*B*). Malalignments can usually be prevented by positioning, selective stretching, and bracing (Fig. 34–3). If fixed or advancing rapidly they may be corrected or decelerated by surgical procedures or occasionally by mechanical stretching with serial casts and dynamic bracing. At the knee wedging casts are contraindicated, as they may produce tibial subluxations or supracondylar femoral fractures. Careful continuing observation, particularly during growth spurts, is essential to identify early deformities.

Weakness.   Weakness, while present in all motor unit disease, varies in its presentation and effect on rehabilitation. Proximal weakness interferes with gait, transfers, and gross movement, while distal weakness interferes with fine motor skills. Physical treatment can begin with kinesiologic and biofeedback techniques and may progress to strengthening exercises in some instances. Conventional wisdom dictates caution in the use of progressive resistive exercises in progressive motor unit diseases in spite of suggestive evidence to the contrary.[9] Bracing may provide benefits both in the post-surgical phase and in functional abilities. The anterior stop on an ankle-foot orthosis can provide knee stability for the Duchenne muscular dystrophy patient after iliotibial band releases. Polypropylene orthotic devices are both light weight and cosmetically superior to metal braces.

Ventilation.   With decreasing ventilatory sufficiency there is a need for mechanical assistance.[1] Appropriately prescribed extrathoracic ventilative aids may eliminate the need for tracheostomy and intratracheal volume respiratory support (Fig. 34–4). As signs of hypoxia and hypercapnea appear, the cuirass or plastic wrap (Fig. 34–5) will enhance gas exchange in the recumbent position. In late stages of motor unit disease, oral positive pressure, pneumobelt, or cuirass ventilators can be used throughout the day energized from the wheelchair battery.

Functional Ability.   Translation of specific motor and sensory residuals into complicated and practical function is the essence of physical treatment. This ability is often more limited by intelligence and motivation than by actual impairments. Examples of functional training include locomotion, dressing,

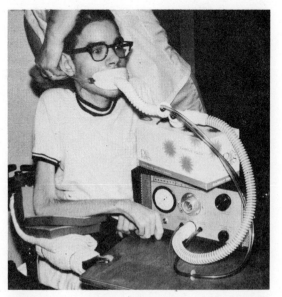

Figure 34–4.   Home use of intermittent positive pressure device in a far-advanced case of Duchenne dystrophy. (Note shield to compensate for facial muscle weakness.)

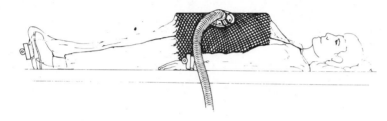

FIGURE 34–5. Plastic wrap (raincoat) respirator uses negative extrathoracic pressure.

eating, and other activities of daily living. Assistive devices (Fig. 34–6), substitutive training, and selective surgical procedures, e.g., tendon transfer, releases and arthrodeses, all represent medical (generic) management techniques.

PROGNOSTIC CATEGORIES

Symptomatic management is modified to relate to the expected prognosis. Motor unit diseases may be divided into four categories with respect to prognosis.

Progressive Conditions. In progressive conditions the primary pathologic lesions worsen at various rates. Amyotrophic lateral sclerosis, which may be fatal in three to five years, is rapidly progressive. Werdnig-Hoffmann disease appearing in the first few days also falls in this category. Kugelberg-Welander syndrome falls in a more intermediate progression, as does Duchenne muscular dystrophy. Charcot-Marie-Tooth disease (not fatal) progresses slowly.

Transient Conditions. Conditions whose effects regress with complete, or nearly com-

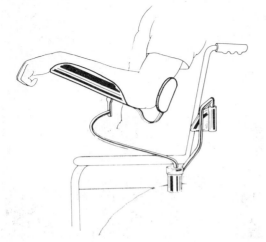

FIGURE 34–6. Balanced forearm orthosis. (From Chyatte, S. B., Long, C., II, and Vignos, P. J.: The balanced forearm orthosis in muscular dystrophy. Arch. Phys. Med., 46:633–636, 1965.)

plete, recovery after specific tissue injury or disease or for which specific treatment may be available for control or alleviation may be categorized as transient. Examples are Guillain-Barré syndrome (acute idiopathic polyneuritis), thyrotoxic myopathy, and, occasionally, myasthenia gravis.

Static Conditions. Static conditions are those in which a specific pathologic lesion occurs, usually as a single insult, leaving permanent deficits. Acute anterior paralytic poliomyelitis, cauda equina injuries, and severe peripheral nerve injury are examples.

Miscellaneous Conditions. There are some motor unit diseases, e.g., polymyositis, whose course is highly variable. Polymyositis (dermatomyositis) may regress with almost complete disappearance; it may become arrested at any stage, leaving residuals; or it may be progressively fatal.

A distinction must be made between truly progressive diseases and those that apparently progress, by the onset or worsening of secondary deformities, as growth occurs. Individuals may lose functional abilities by becoming overweight, or children may lose functional abilities as they grow larger or reach a plateau in motor development. Motor unit disease in growing children is more likely to produce deformities whether the condition is progressive or static.

Deformities resulting from asymmetric tightness of an iliotibial band[21] (tensor fasciae latae) are scoliosis (type I according to Bennett's classification); pelvic tilt; subluxation of the opposite hip; flexion contracture, internal rotation deformity, and abduction contracture of the hip; abduction and external torsion of the tibia; and supination deformity of the foot.

Adverse reactions to physical treatment in motor unit diseases may include burns from hot packs or other heating agents, soft tissue tearing with calcification, fractures of osteoporotic bones, or weakness from overwork. Early unsupervised activities and substitutive movement may result in incoordination.

Asymmetric strengthening or ill-advised ambulation may aggravate deformities. Over-bracing may cause retardation or limitation of functional ability. Adverse psychologic reactions may occur; for example, depression when unreachable goals are presented to the patient or his family.

PROGRESSIVE MUSCULAR DYSTROPHY

This disease is characterized by an insidious onset of weakness and tightness.[2, 17-19, 30]

Physical Treatment. Vigorous flexibility exercises should be begun early.[16] These must be taught to the parents for effective home stretching. Suspension and adjustment of the therapeutic exercise program should be determined by periodic rechecks—at least every three months.[20]

Contractures occur early and are severe, probably because the muscle itself is the site of the pathologic lesion. Tightness occurs early in two-joint muscle groups, e.g., gastrocnemius-soleus groups, tensor fascia lata, hip flexors, and hamstrings in the lower extremities (Fig. 34–7). Weakness occurs first in the gluteus maximus, then in the abdominal muscles, foot dorsiflexors, neck flexors, and lower pectorals, and finally in the quadriceps and deltoids.

Each patient should be examined for tight-

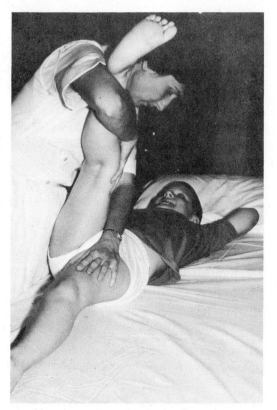

FIGURE 34–8. Stretching the hamstring muscles in a patient with Duchenne muscular dystrophy.

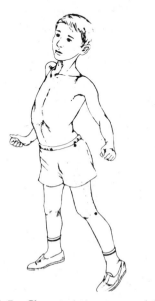

FIGURE 34–7. Characteristic stance of Duchenne dystrophy: increased lordosis, widened stance, and equinus of the feet.

ness and an individual home program should be prescribed. It is desirable to have a rather intensive and repeated home instruction period with the parents doing the exercises under the supervision of the therapist (Fig. 34–8). In the upper extremity the forearm pronators and wrist and finger flexors often are tight areas.

The collapsing spine needs careful attention to positioning and support.[14] Lateral support and a level seat coupled with built-in extension support of the lumbar spine (Fig. 34–9) helps to immobilize the facets (Fig. 34–10), providing further stability. Exercises to stretch tight spine extensors are counterproductive, as optimally these children's spines should be tight in slight hyperextension.

Strengthening exercises are of unproven value, and clinical impressions suggest acceleration of the weakness may result. Functional training is often helpful, particularly as the patient moves from independent ambulation to assisted ambulation and then to wheelchair ambulation.

Bracing and ambulation aids should be

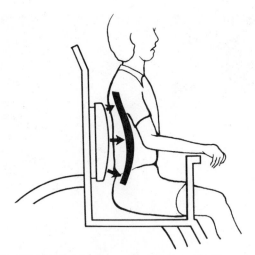

FIGURE 34–9. Lumbar support is provided to maintain extension of the lumbar spine.

minimal, since this is a generalized disease with the individual performing at his maximal energy expenditure. Gowers[15] in 1902 pointed out that deformities are the principal reason for early loss of ambulation in muscular dystrophy. If the patient is falling several times each day, long leg braces to stabilize the knees may prolong limited but functional ambulation for several years.

Surgical Management. Selective surgical release of tightness that resists conservative management may prolong and facilitate functional abilities.[12] Rapid convalescence is imperative, i.e., immediate postoperative ambulation in long leg casts after lower extremity surgery and using plastic jackets after spinal fusion to facilitate immediate sitting.[25]

For early inversion instability of the foot, transplantation of the posterior tibial tendon

to the lateral dorsum of the foot may be indicated. Another solution is an ankle-foot orthosis. If lengthening of the gastrocnemius-soleus tendon is needed to accommodate the orthosis, it may be necessary to stabilize the knee. If the deformity is unilateral, lengthening of one side and not the other may result in pelvic obliquity. Achilles tendon lengthening can be disastrous if one does not anticipate the loss of knee stability, which has been maintained by the fixed equinus of the foot. One should have the patient measured preoperatively so that he can go directly from plaster to orthoses.

Surgical release of the iliotibial tract is often quite helpful in prolonging ambulation and often is not performed as early as it should be. The tight tensor fosters knee instability as the patient increases his lumbar lordosis to stabilize his weight line behind his flexed hips, increasing torque to flex the knee.

In the past, surgical correction of spinal deformity with its surgical risk and prolonged immobilization resulted in excessive morbidity and mortality.[34] Improvement in surgical technique and the advent of Harrington and Dwyer instrumentation, permitting internal fixation, have improved the risk as well as the surgical outcome. Internal fixation and polypropylene bracing still allow these children to continue to be mobile. The physician can balance the progression of disease and the accelerating deformity and in many cases allow the child to continue to sit and preserve respiratory function that could have been lost through chest wall distortion.

The surgical connection of equinovarus foot deformity in a nonambulatory patient is

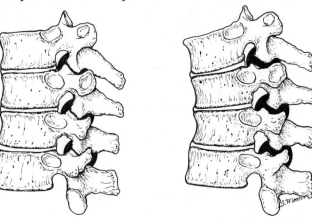

FIGURE 34–10. Extension of spine (left) stabilizes facets.

largely for cosmetic reasons and ease of footwear applications.

Surgery in this group of patients carries the additional risk of malignant hyperthermia, and the operative team should be prepared to monitor and intervene rapidly. It is the authors' opinion that surgery in these children, when elective, should be performed at regional pediatric surgical centers.

General Management. In Duchenne muscular dystrophy, an X-linked recessive genetic pattern, counseling the parents is a necessity.[8, 33] Fewer than one half of the patients will have a family history of progressive muscular dystrophy, since this gene has an extremely high rate of mutation. Estimates suggest one mutation per 10,000 genes per year. When the mother has been identified as a possible carrier by the appearance of an affected son, her daughters are suspected of being carriers (one half may be). As there is definite association between decreased mental function and muscular dystrophy in specific pedigrees, care should be taken to place reasonable expectations on their intellectual skills. All parents of patients are urged to have their names put on the mailing list of the Muscular Dystrophy Association so that the newsletter will provide a means for keeping up with the latest facts. This contact with a reliable source of information is often a deterrent to "doctor shopping" and frustrating trips for "miracle cures" at the urging of well-meaning friends and relatives.

Empathetic attitudes and forthright advice may lessen the fears and frustrations that are inevitable. Periodic checks by a physician conversant with physical management should be done as needed, usually every three to four months. Attendance at regular school as long as possible is recommended.

Spinal Muscular Atrophy

This disease offers such a broad spectrum of presentations and survival that great care should be taken to avoid considering this a short-term survival disease. Age of onset, family presentation, and progression of symptoms can be compatible with long-term survival. Recent literature has pointed out the chronicity in some cases.[26]

Physical Treatment. Again the hallmark of management is maintenance of mobility and flexibility. Vigorous attention must be given to the potential for tightness in two-joint muscles. Bracing plays some role, but this is often later in the course of the disease. There is a high probability for development of scoliosis, and meticulous care must be taken to identify curves and asymmetric tightness and precursors to scoliosis at the earliest possible moment. These paralytic curves do poorly in Milwaukee braces and do much better in bivalved polypropylene body jackets. Close attention to seating and positioning is indicated, as in the child with Duchenne dystrophy.

Medical Treatment. The same close attention to preventive medicine is warranted as in previous entities. Patients with these syndromes are also subject to the dilemmas of adolescence, as these children often retain mobility and encounter the same crises as peers. They should all have instruction in human sexuality and in addition genetic counseling. This will avoid misunderstanding and obviate some stress.

Surgical Treatment. These children for spinal surgery. Preoperative evaluation of respiratory function allows anticipation of pulmonary problems. Those with a vital capacity of 40 per cent or greater rarely require tracheostomy. Internal fixation and fusion to the sacrum are usually required. Rapid postoperative mobilization is accomplished with a bivalved polypropylene body jacket.

General Management. Common sense and cautious optimism are warranted in the older child, and the key phrase is anticipation for prevention.

AMYOTROPHIC LATERAL SCLEROSIS

Physical Treatment. Treatment measures should anticipate progression. Minimal bracing and ambulation aids are helpful for prolonged and safe ambulation. To prolong ambulation efforts, the patient should be taught how to fall safely. Positioning and therapeutic exercise are prescribed to prevent deformities. Early in the course of the disease this will maintain ambulation and functional ability, and later it will facilitate nursing care.

Medical Treatment. When there are bulbar symptoms and a prognosis of continuation for more than several months, a gastrostomy and tracheostomy may be helpful. If there is a short-term prognosis, intramuscular injection of Prostigmin (1 cc. of a 1:1000 dilution) 30 minutes before eating may temporarily facilitate swallowing. Fasciculations will be intensified, however.

A home suctioning device is often necessary. Mechanical ventilatory aid may be needed in later stages. Home management is very possible even in the terminal stages with an understanding family. It is important to keep an optimistic attitude in dealing with the patient and his family.

GUILLAIN-BARRÉ SYNDROME (ACUTE IDIOPATHIC POLYNEURITIS)

Full recovery is expected, although some patients die because of respiratory failure and a few have residual weakness. In the authors' experience this permanent weakness may have resulted from prolonged periods of hypoxia during the acute phase.

Pain is treated as in poliomyelitis. Tightness is prevented and corrected by positioning and early stretching. Weakness is usually reversible over a period of two months to as long as two years. If the onset is acute, ordinarily the recovery is more rapid. An insidious onset may foretell delayed recovery, perhaps over a period of a year or more, and some patients may never regain full strength. Strengthening exercises and exhaustive activities may aggravate the weakness or result in a relapse.

Temporary ambulation aids include wrapping the foot early with an elasticized bandage for dorsiflexion support, temporary splints at the knee, and a light spring wire brace later for footdrop if needed. Ambulation is begun in the parallel bars, proceeding to underarm crutches, forearm crutches, canes, and then to only occasional aid as progress continues. Temporary upper extremity aids include the mobile arm support, hand splints, and other adaptive devices.

Pressure ulcerations are frequent complications in this condition, especially if the patient is in the respirator. Ventilation insufficiency should receive early mechanical aid, as in muscular dystrophy. In acute motor unit illness that affects ventilation, mechanical assistance should usually be started when the vital capacity begins to fall and should be employed in all instances when it reaches 50 per cent. Myasthenia gravis, metabolic myopathy, and similar reversible conditions ordinarily do not need physical treatment except for ambulation aids during the period of weakness and functional training in safe ambulation.

STATIC MOTOR UNIT DISEASES

Acute Anterior Paralytic Poliomyelitis

The literature is replete with excellent descriptions of the proper management of this entity.[3-6, 22, 23] Prevention was by the Salk vaccine (formalin-killed virus) in the past and is now by the Sabin vaccine (attenuated live virus).

PHYSICAL MANAGEMENT

Early Stage. Management is based on the three clinical manifestations in the early phase (the first six weeks) of the disease. For muscle pain hot moist packs (Kenny) are applied three or four times daily in mild to moderate cases or continuously in severely involved patients.

Muscle tightness in the early stage may represent altered physiology at the internuncial pool; later soft tissue tightness probably involves fascial tightness. Early proper positioning and passive exercises following applications of hot packs are indicated.

Asymmetric muscle weakness is the cardinal sign of poliomyelitis. In the early stage, weakened segments are protected by positioning; later, selective reeducation and strengthening exercises are begun while protection is continued with bracing and limited activity.

Intermediate Stage. Various authorities support different views about management in the intermediate stage (six weeks to six months). The authors prefer to differentiate the growing child from the adult at this stage.

In the growing child the muscles are selectively reeducated and stretched to ensure maximal function of weakened body segments and minimize deformity. Limited activities, especially in the upright position, and limited ambulation are necessary. Precise support with bracing and careful observation are essential. Substitutive patterns are allowed in the child after six months if they do not appear to contribute to deformity.

In adults substitutive patterns are permitted early as a compromise for increasing functional ability.

Late Stage. Beyond six months of ideal management a clear estimation of the probable functional ability and potential sources of deformity is usually possible. The spine of the growing child should be checked radiographically at least yearly and more often during periods of rapid growth. Adults need periodic observation for orthotic adjustment and for detection of possible loss of function due to overwork.

There are several general rules of physical treatment. Active exercise should be deferred until the pain is relieved, and selective strengthening should be deferred if there is a significant tightness of the muscle group. Progressive resistive exercises and functional training unavoidably encourage substitutive patterns. Development of substitutive patterns usually inhibits activation of the prime movers; for example, the anterior tibial may drop out of the pattern of dorsiflexion (peroneal flip) if walking is initiated before this muscle is able to carry out its action. Asymmetric strengthening should be avoided because it may aggravate or initiate scoliosis. Overwork can cause further weakness in specific muscle groups. Tightness should be retained if it is symmetric and if weakness is present; for example, back extension tightness in the presence of severe weakness of back extensors.

Orthotic devices are used to prevent deformity (e.g., Hoke corset), to provide support (e.g., long leg brace), to protect a weakened muscle group (e.g., opponens splint), or to increase function (e.g., mobile arm support).

MEDICAL MANAGEMENT

In the respiratory system it is important to recognize and treat reduced ventilation early.[32] Having the patient count slowly and loudly will permit an adequate clinical estimation of the ventilation reserve. The number of counts is multiped by 100 cc. to estimate the vital capacity. The patient should have mechanical respiratory aid if the vital capacity drops below 50 per cent or if it is dropping rapidly even if above 50 per cent. While the patient is in the respirator, cough-ing and periodic deep breathing will reduce the episodes of atelectasis and pneumonitis.

Swallowing difficulties require meticulous nursing care, especially in the acute stage. If the patient is in a respirator a tracheostomy is usually indicated if there is pharyngeal muscle weakness. Tracheostomy is also indicated in vocal cord abductor muscle paralysis, since the airway is compromised.

Early urinary retention is common; an indwelling catheter should be avoided. Adequate urinary output is 1.5 liters per square meter of body surface per 24 hours. This will minimize urinary calculi and infection.[28]

In the acute stage with encephalitis it is important to observe carefully for possible Cushing's ulcer with gastrointestinal bleeding. In the convalescent stage constipation is often a problem. Severe muscle weakness and atrophy result in a loss of potassium stores, which predisposes to episodes of paralytic ileus. This is a most common reason for an ''acute'' distention of the abdomen in severely involved polio patients.

Hypertension in the acute phase is usually secondary to hypoxia, but it may be due to bulbar involvement. Bulbar involvement may also result in hypotension.

Surgical Management. In the acute stage tracheostomy may be necessary. In the intermediate stage surgical procedures are used for the release of soft tissue or urinary calculi removal. Tendon transfers and arthrodesis to improve function or correct deformity are done in the late stage.

General Management. Attendance at regular school is recommended whenever possible for children. A conference with the teacher to discuss positioning and modification of activities is usually necessary. A forthright but encouraging attitude on the part of the attending physician is essential for both the parents' and the child's well-being. Adult patients' questions regarding prognosis should be answered honestly with encouragement. Early vocational planning is imperative, and the patient's emotional needs should be identified and met at appropriate stages of his rehabilitation.

Congenital Myopathies

These myopathies, in the past lumped under benign congenital hypotonia, are usually nonprogressive.[33] Like muscular dystrophy

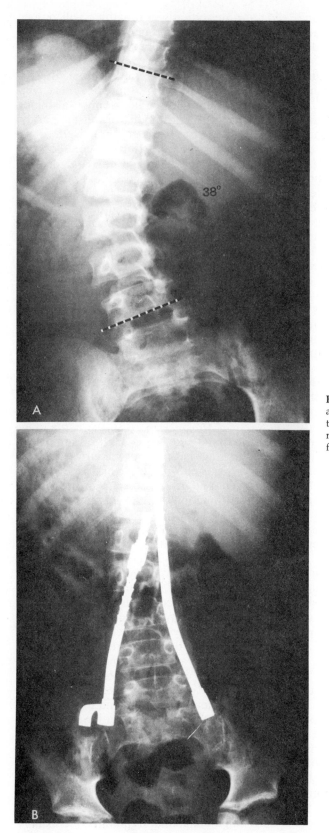

FIGURE 34–11. *A*, Rapidly progressing curve in a patient with fiber type disproportion. *B*, To retain ambulation, early fusion with Harrington rods and plastic jacket prevented loss of function from immobilization.

they require rapid postoperative mobilization and attention to tightness. With their good prognosis, vigorous efforts should be made to maintain good alignment of the spine (Fig. 34–11). One may lose ambulation after fusion owing to loss of spine mobility, but the potential hazard of the collapsing spine usually outweighs this risk.

Arthrogryposis

The syndrome of arthrogryposis multiplex congenita is believed to arise from an absence of fetal movement.[10] Experimental immobilization of the fetus by several techniques has led to this syndrome of soft tissue "ankylosis" and "clubbing" of multiple joints with the articular surfaces remaining intact.

Physical Management. These children often require early surgical intervention to facilitate standing. The parapodium (Fig. 34–12) is suitable as an initial standing device. Several observers should be evaluating upper extremity function to anticipate problems in ADL. An upper extremity orthosis may be needed to correct deformity as well as enhance motor function.[11, 13]

Surgical Management. As these children usually have normal intelligence and sensory function, they do well with transplants, such as substitution of the pectoral for the biceps function. A unilateral triceps transfer will substitute for elbow flexion, and this will leave one arm with active extension to accomplish toileting.

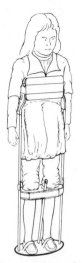

FIGURE 34–12. A static parapodium supports the extended joints against gravity to aid standing.

Medical Management. The electromyogram in these children usually shows large motor unit action potentials (MUAP) with a reduction in the number of MUAP. Such findings are considered "neuropathic" disease. These cases are static and do not progress. Both autosomal dominant and recessive patterns of inheritance have been reported.[29] Counseling of family and the child at the appropriate age is indicated.

MISCELLANEOUS MOTOR UNIT DISEASES

Included in this category are motor unit diseases that may progress, become arrested, or improve. Polymyositis (dermatomyositis) is a classic example. It appears to be a primary inflammatory disease of the muscle fiber.[27]

Physical treatment is based on the following three principles: maintaining flexibility, minimizing pain by application of heat (hot tub baths or home baker), and use of minimal bracing or ambulation aids if needed.

In medical managemement, some authorities feel that high doses of steroids are helpful during an exacerbation or an acute onset.

SUMMARY

The aim in management of progressive motor unit diseases is to prolong functional abilities; in static diseases, to protect from deformity and increase functional ability; and in transient diseases, to maintain flexibility and facilitate return of function.

The key to management of motor unit diseases is the maintenance of the patient's flexibility, especially of the multi-joint muscles, and careful, regular follow-up.

REFERENCES

1. Alexander, M. A., Johnson, E. W., Petty, J., and Stauch, D.: Mechanical ventilation of patients with late stage Duchenne muscular dystrophy: Management in the home. Arch. Phys. Med., 60:289, 1979.
2. Archibald, K. C., and Vignos, P. J.: A study of contractures in muscular dystrophy. Arch. Phys. Med., 40:150–157, 1959.

3. Bennett, R. L.: Evaluation of end results of acute anterior poliomyelitis. J.A.M.A., 162:851–854, 1956.
4. Bennett, R. L.: Evaluation and treatment of lower motor unit lesions involving the shoulder, arm, forearm and hand. Arch. Phys. Med., 41:54–61, 1960.
5. Bennett, R. L.: Use and abuse of certain tools of physical medicine. Arch. Phys. Med., 41:485–496, 1960.
6. Bosma, J. F.: Significance of the pharynx in rehabilitation of poliomyelitis disabilities in cervical area. Arch. Phys. Med., 38:363–368, 1957.
7. Chyatte, S. B., Long, C., II, and Vignos, P. J.: The balanced forearm orthosis in muscular dystrophy. Arch. Phys. Med., 46:633–636, 1965.
8. Cohen, H. J., Molnar, G. E., and Taft, L. T.: The genetic relationship of progressive muscular dystrophy (Duchenne type) and mental retardation. Develop. Med. Child. Neurol., 10:754–765, 1968.
9. De Lateur, B. J., and Giaconi, R. M.: Effect on maximal strength of submaximal exercise in Duchenne muscular dystrophy. Am. J. Phys. Med., 58:26–36, 1979.
10. Drachman, D. B.: The syndrome of arthrogryposis multiplex congenita. Birth Defects: Original Article Series, Vol. VII, No. 2, pp. 90–97, Feb., 1971.
11. Drumond, D. S., Siller, T. S., and Cruess, R. L.: Management of arthrogryposis multiplex congenita. Chapter 5, Instructional Course Lectures, Am. Acad. Orthopaed. Surg., 23:79–95, 1974.
12. Eyring, E. J., Johnson, E. W., and Burnett, C.: Surgery in muscular dystrophy. J.A.M.A., 58:4–7, 1977.
13. Friedlander, H. L., Westin, G. W., and Wood, W. L.: Arthrogryposis multiplex congenita — A review of forty-five cases. J. Bone Joint Surg., 50A:89–112, 1968.
14. Gibson, D. A., and Wilkins, K. E.: The management of spinal deformities in Duchenne muscular dystrophy. Clin. Orthop. Related Res., 108:41–51, 1975.
15. Gowers, W. R.: Myopathy and a distal form. Br. Med. J., 2:89–92, 1902.
16. Hoberman, M.: Physical medicine and rehabilitation: Its value and limitations in progressive muscular dystrophy. Am. J. Phys. Med., 34:109–117, 1955.
17. Jebsen, R. H., Johnson, E. W., Knobloch, H., and Grant, D. K.: Differential diagnosis of infantile hypotonia. J. Dis. Child., 101:8–17, 1961.
18. Johnson, E. W.: Examination for muscle weakness in infants and small children. J.A.M.A., 168:1306–1313, 1958.
19. Johnson, E. W.: Pathokinesiology of Duchenne muscular dystrophy: Implications for management. Arch. Phys. Med., 58:4–7, 1977.
20. Johnson, E., and Braddom, R.: Overwork weakness in fascioscapulohumeral muscular dystrophy. Arch. Phys. Med., 52:333–336, 1971.
21. Johnson, E. W., Weingarden, H., and Alexander, M.: Asymmetric iliotibial band contracture following muscle biopsy: Case report. Arch. Phys. Med., 58:28–29, 1977.
22. Knapp, M. E.: The contribution of Sister Elizabeth Kenny to treatment of poliomyelitis. Arch. Phys. Med., 36:510–517, 1955.
23. Knowlton, G. C.: Physiologic background for neuromuscular reeducation and coordination. Arch. Phys. Med., 35:635–638, 1954.
24. Lowenthal, M., and Tobis, J. S.: Contractures in chronic neurologic disease. Arch. Phys. Med., 38:640–645, 1957.
25. Moe, J. H., Winter, R. B., Bradford, D. S., and Lonstein, J. E.: Neuromuscular deformities. In Scoliosis and Other Spinal Deformities. Philadelphia, W. B. Saunders Co., 1978.
26. Pearn, J. H., Gardner-Medwen, D., and Wilson, J.: A clinical study of chronic childhood spinal muscular atrophy. J. Neurol. Sci., 38:23–37, 1978.
27. Pearson, C. M.: Serum enzymes in muscular dystrophy and certain other muscular and neuromuscular diseases. N. Engl. J. Med., 256:1069–1075, 1957.
28. Plum, F.: Prevention of urinary calculi after paralytic poliomyelitis. J.A.M.A., 168:1302–1306, 1958.
29. Rosenmann, A., and Arad, I.: Arthrogryposis multiplex congenita: Neurogenic type with autosomal recessive inheritance. J. Med. Genet., 2:91–94, 1974.
30. Stevenson, A. C.: Muscular dystrophy in Northern Ireland. Ann. Eugenics, 18:50–93, 1953.
31. Swinyard, C. A., et al.: Gradients of functional ability of importance in rehabilitation of patients with progressive muscular and neuromuscular diseases. Arch. Phys. Med., 38:574–579, 1957.
32. Vallbona, C., and Spencer, W. A.: Systematic classification of the chronic sequelae of poliomyelitis. Arch. Phys. Med., 42:114–121, 1961.
33. Walton, J. N., and Nattrass, F. J.: On the classification, natural history and treatment of myopathies. Brain, 77:169–231, 1954.
34. Wolfe, J. S., and Bagenstore, J. E.: Malignant hyperthermia: A complication of orthopaedic surgery. Orthopaedics, 3:211–214, 1978.

35

CRANIAL NERVE PALSIES AND BRAIN STEM SYNDROMES

BERNARD SANDLER

This discussion will include only those affections which commonly fall within the purview of the physiatrist. For a more complete picture the reader is referred to neurologic texts.[1-4] We shall also include those conditions which do not properly involve *only* the cranial nerves or brain stem. For example, amyotrophic lateral sclerosis involves cortical neurons, the corticobulbar tracts, cranial nerve nuclei, the corticospinal tracts, and the anterior horn cells. In these cases we shall emphasize diagnosis and treatment as they relate to the cranial nerves and brain stem.

DEFINITIONS

The term *brain stem* refers to the medulla oblongata, pons, and the midbrain; their cranial nerve nuclei; and the ascending and descending tracts passing through them.

Lesions affecting pathways between the cerebral cortex and brain stem are called *supranuclear;* lesions in the brain stem nuclei are *nuclear;* and lesions of the cranial nerves are *infranuclear.* A fourth category involves lesions of the ascending and descending tracts connecting the spinal cord and supranuclear structures.

THE CRANIAL NERVES

Cranial nerves I and II, the olfactory and the optic, respectively, are from an embryologic point of view not nerves at all but extensions of the brain. Occasionally the physiatrist will see a case of anosmia produced by an olfactory groove meningioma. Multiple sclerosis is the chief cause of optic nerve involvement. At times the physiatrist may see patients with optic nerve involvement caused by leukemia, syphilis, arteriosclerosis of the brain, gliomas, meningiomas, pituitary tumors, metastatic carcinoma, aneurysms, or trauma.

The oculomotor, trochlear, and abducens nerves and their nuclei may be involved as a result of trauma, multiple sclerosis, encephalitides, tumors, aneurysms, alcohol poisoning, syringobulbia, diphtheria, diabetes, meningitides, venous sinus thrombosis, poliomyelitis, vascular accidents in the brain stem, and heavy metal poisoning. Because of its long course the abducens is especially subject to damage from increased intracranial pressure.

The trigeminal nerve may be affected by neoplasms, trauma, aneurysms, meningitides, and polyneuritides. The sensory and motor nuclei are damaged by tumors, vascu-

691

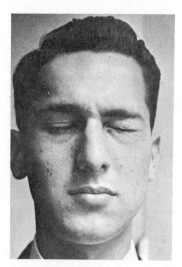

FIGURE 35–1. Right peripheral facial palsy (incomplete). (Courtesy of Dr. A. Ornsteen, Philadelphia.)

lar lesions, syringobulbia, multiple slcerosis, encephalitides, and amyotrophic lateral sclerosis.

The facial nerve may be injured by neoplasms, meningitides, Paget's disease, osteomyelitis, herpes zoster, ear infections, polyneuritides, diphtheria, tetanus, and leprosy. Trauma from gunshot or knife wounds and forceps delivery is not uncommon. Neuromas growing from the acoustic nerve may frequently involve the facial nerve. Bilateral facial palsies are most frequently seen in the Guillain-Barré syndrome, leprosy, leukemia, syphilis, and meningococcal meningitis. The facial nucleus is involved in poliomyelitis, amyotrophic lateral sclerosis, vascular accidents, and multiple sclerosis.

Bell's palsy is an infranuclear affection of the seventh nerve which is frequently seen by the physiatrist. It commonly follows exposure to cold. Presumably the paralysis is caused by edema of the nerve, which results in compression against the hard walls of the facial canal and ischemia. The eye cannot be made to close, nor the forehead to wrinkle. This paralysis of the upper facial musculature distinguishes the condition from central facial palsy seen in hemiplegic patients (Fig. 35–1). Alter[5] believes there is a tendency for Bell's palsy to occur in family members because of inherited traits such as a narrow facial canal or a small stylomastoid foramen.

A conservative regimen of treatment consists of superficial heat and sympatholytic agents to increase blood supply, reduction of edema by use of steroids, maintenance of muscle tone by massage and electrical stimulation, and muscle reeducation through exercise when voluntary function returns.[6] Taverner et al.[17] claim a marked decrease in severe denervation of the facial nerve in patients treated with ACTH gel intramuscularly when oral corticosteroids fail.

Surgical intervention is a subject of controversy. Kettel[7] has suggested the following as criteria for intervention: (1) Palsy accompanied by severe pain from the onset behind the homolateral ear. (2) No sign of return of function in two months. (3) Cases of incomplete spontaneous recovery. (4) Relapsing palsies. The value of surgery is predicated on the hope that some nerve fibers not yet undergoing degeneration may be preserved.[18] If this is true, then prompt decompression on evidence of beginning degeneration seems indicated.

Anastomosis of the facial nerve with the phrenic, spinal accessory, or hypoglossal nerves has been proposed in those cases in which there is little or no return of function in one year. Cosmetic procedures for support of sagging facial musculature by means of muscle slings or fascial strips have been helpful. Lagophthalmos has been improved by tarsorrhaphy.[6] Edgerton[19] believes that dynamic muscle transfers have great advantages over nerve anastomoses or static support with fascia lata, tendons, or synthetic material.

Prognosis can be made more accurate through the use of electromyographic techniques. If fibrillation potentials are discovered two to three weeks after onset, one may infer that axonal degeneration has taken place and that recovery will be delayed. On the other hand, absence of such potentials points to a simple neurapraxia with a good prognosis. Langworth and Taverner[8] point out that a loss of response to electrical simulation of the nerve is a grave sign and that conduction latency above 4 milliseconds signifies partial denervation. More recent electrodiagnostic tests such as electrogustometry[20] and the facial nerve excitability measurement[21] give information concerning impending degeneration of nerve fibers earlier than is possible with electromyography, and may help decide whether surgical intervention is warranted.

Annoying complications and sequelae of Bell's palsy are associated movements, contractures, lacrimation during eating (crocodile tears), gustatory sweating, parageusia, and hemispasm.

Herpetic palsy (Hunt's syndrome) is characterized by severe pain in and behind the ear and a herpetic eruption on the tympanum and in the external auditory canal.

The acoustic nerve may be injured by salicylates, streptomycin, quinine, and many other drugs. It is also involved by meningitides, cerebellopontine angle tumors, and degenerative processes in the middle and inner ear. The nuclei are damaged by tumors, demyelinating disease, vascular lesions, and inflammatory processes.

The glossopharyngeal nerve and its nucleus are rarely damaged by isolated lesions. Neoplasms and vascular lesions will usually involve neighboring nerves as well.

The vagus nerve is damaged by various neuritides, particularly the diphtheritic and "infectious" types. It may also be compressed by tumors or aneurysms. Lesions of the pharyngeal branch result in swallowing difficulty. Involvement of the recurrent laryngeal branch produces hoarseness and dysphonia. Superior laryngeal involvement is reflected in a weak voice. The nuclei of the vagus are damaged by poliomyelitis, tumors,

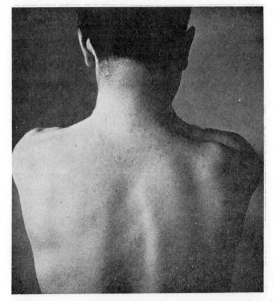

FIGURE 35–3. Trapezius palsy, right. Elevation of the arms in the forward plane of the body, i.e., flexion, causes lateral displacement of the scapula. Note atrophy of the superior third of the trapezius muscle and the firm approximation of the inferior angle of the scapula to the chest wall. (From Haymaker, W., and Woodhall, B.: Peripheral Nerve Injuries, 2nd Ed., 1953.)

syringobulbia, vascular lesions, multiple sclerosis, and amyotrophic lateral sclerosis.

The spinal accessory nerve is involved by neuritides, meningitides, extramedullary tumors, and neck trauma. The nucleus is damaged by the same conditions that involve the vagus. It is important for diagnostic reasons to distinguish between trapezius palsy and palsy of the serratus anterior (Figs. 35–2 to 35–4).

The hypoglossal nerve may be affected by all the processes that involve the vagus and spinal accessory nerves. Injury to the nerve causes the tongue to deviate to the paralyzed side when it is protruded (Fig. 35–5). When the tongue lies in the mouth, however, it may deviate slightly toward the uninvolved side. Fasciculations are noted in amyotrophic lateral sclerosis and syringobulbia. In supranuclear lesions the tongue is little affected. It may deviate slightly to the paretic side on protrusion.

Guillain-Barré Syndrome

This polyradiculoneuropathy is described in another portion of the handbook. The condition is of concern to the physiatrist because it may require prolonged medical

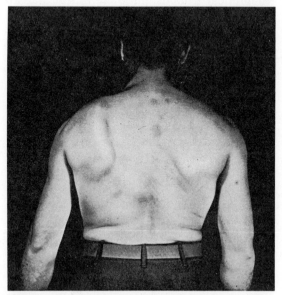

FIGURE 35–2. Trapezius palsy, left. The posterior triangle of the neck was penetrated by a bullet. Subsequently the patient became unable to shrug the left shoulder or to raise the left arm above the horizontal plane. The upper one half of the trapezius is atrophic. An attempt to abduct the arm leads to flaring of the vertebral border and to lateral displacement of the scapula. (From Haymaker, W., and Woodhall, B.: Peripheral Nerve Injuries, 2nd Ed., 1953.)

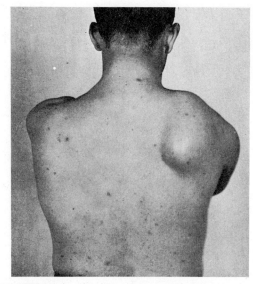

FIGURE 35–4. Winging of the scapula in serratus anterior palsy. When elevation of the arm is attempted the scapula becomes winged and moves upward and laterally. Abduction of the arm was not impaired. (From Haymaker, W., and Woodhall, B.: Peripheral Nerve Injuries, 2nd Ed., 1953.)

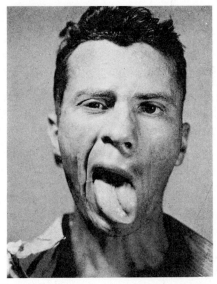

FIGURE 35–5. Atrophy and paralysis of the left side of the tongue due to missile wound of the left side of the neck, with missile entrance in the region of the mastoid process. The tip of the tongue deviates toward the paralyzed side. (From Haymaker, W.: Bing's Local Diagnosis in Neurological Diseases. St. Louis, The C. V. Mosby Co., 1956.)

management. It has been said that it involves proximal muscles chiefly. However, Wiederholt et al.[9] point out that the distal musculature in arms and legs may be severely involved. The musculature supplied by the cranial nerves is also more often involved than is usually thought (Table 35–1).

Nerve conduction studies when done serially may accurately chart the recovery of the patient. Artificial respiration after elec-

tive tracheostomy should be considered immediately on development of bulbar signs. Steroids in the acute phase may be of help on theoretical grounds, but there is little statistical support for their use.[10] Postural hypotension is also seen.[11] It is postulated that there is involvement of the intermediolateral cell column and consequently damage to autonomic function. It is important to remember that positive pressure respiration may pro-

TABLE 35–1. DISTRIBUTION OF MUSCLE WEAKNESS ON INITIAL EXAMINATION: 97 PATIENTS*

Distribution		Instances
Weakness		
Both upper and lower extremity		88
Proximal and distal parts of both extremities affected	66	
Other combinations	16	
Neck		44
Facial muscles (subsequently 6 more)		28
Lower extremity (proximal and distal in 7, distal in 1)		8
Extraocular muscles		5
Upper extremity		2
Anal sphincter		2
Palate		1
Tongue		1
No weakness of upper or lower extremity		5

*From Wiederholt, W. C., Mulder, D. W., and Lambert, E. H.: The Landry-Guillain-Barré-Strohl syndrome or polyradiculoneuropathy: Historical review, report in 97 patients, and present concepts. Proc. Mayo Clin., 39:427–451, 1964.

duce marked peripheral pooling in the absence of reflex venous constriction and thus aggravate the tendency toward hypotension.

Poliomyelitis

Poliomyelitis is no longer the scourge of former years but still merits our attention as a cause of profound weakness. It has been estimated that approximately 15 per cent of the cases have involvement of the brain stem nuclei. The facial, palatal, and pharyngeal muscles are most often involved, but ocular and glossal muscles are also affected. Muscles of mastication are involved less often.[4]

Infantile Spinal Muscular Atrophy

This disease is one of several which affects infants and young children. It falls into the "floppy" infant category and may on occasion be confused with muscular dystrophy. Walton[12] discussed the infantile hypotonias under the headings of infantile spinal muscular atrophy, symptomatic hypotonia (which includes cerebral palsy and a host of metabolic disorders), and benign congenital hypotonia. The last category is far from clear at the present time. Such cases may on the one hand be formes frustes of Werdnig-Hoffmann disease, and on the other perhaps examples of universal muscular hypoplasia.[13]

Since some patients with infantile spinal muscular atrophy may reach adulthood,[14] it is important to be constantly vigilant against upper respiratory infection, the development of scoliosis and pulmonary insufficiency, and the development of contractures. The disease is genetically determined and may afflict one in four children in any sibship.

Tetanus

The cephalic form of tetanus may cause severe involvement of cranial nerves. The cause has not been clearly elucidated, but it is thought that the toxin may act on both the neuromuscular junctions and cell bodies in the anterior horns and cranial nerve nuclei.[15] Trismus, spasm of the pharyngeal muscles and glottis, and stiffness of the facial muscles are common findings. Cranial nerve palsies may develop. Aside from treatment with anti-tetanus serum, maintenance on artificial respiration is important. Muscle relaxation has been approached in various ways; curare, chlorpromazine, and barbiturates are most commonly used.

Diphtheria

Diphtheritic neuropathy has some interesting characteristics. It tends to come on slowly — perhaps three weeks after infection — and involves many cranial nerves. Palatal weakness and faulty accommodation due to involvement of the ciliary muscle usually are seen first. This is followed by paralysis of the pharyngeal, facial, and external ocular muscles. Palatal and ciliary involvement distinguish it from Guillain-Barré syndrome.

Multiple Sclerosis

All sorts of combinations of brain stem involvement are possible in this disease. The clinical picture depends on the random location of the plaques. In the terminal stage bulbar palsy may be total.

Amyotrophic Lateral Sclerosis

This disease has a so-called bulbar form that may involve chiefly the bulbar nuclei. It is usually fatal in three to five years and in the terminal stages requires respiratory support and nursing care.

BRAIN STEM SYNDROMES

Basilar Artery Syndromes. The basilar artery supplies the medulla, pons, midbrain, and cerebellum by way of the paramedian, short, and long circumferential branches. There are various clinical pictures involving the cranial nerves and long tracts. Most common findings are hemiplegia, tetraplegia, various cranial nerve palsies, pseudobulbar palsy, and respiratory disturbances. In thrombosis of the main trunk the outcome is almost invariably fatal.

Vascular Lesions of the Brain Stem. Each side of the brain stem has an independent blood supply. Syndromes may be divided into paramedian (area supplied by short vessels from the vertebral and basilar arteries) and lateral (area supplied by vessels with a long course before they enter the brain stem) (Fig. 35–6).

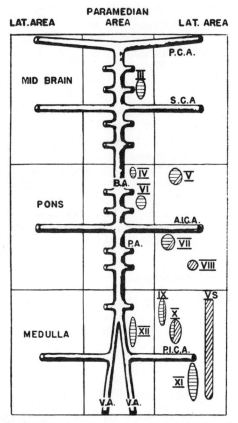

FIGURE 35–6. Brain stem nuclei and their blood supply. Roman numerals refer to cranial nerve nuclei. Horizontal lines in the nuclei indicate motor nuclei; diagonal lines indicate sensory nuclei. (From Holtzman, M., Panin, N., and Ebel, A.: Anatomical localization of common vascular brain syndromes. Am. J. Phys. Med., 38:133–135, 1959.)

THE PARAMEDIAN AREA. This area contains the motor nuclei of the third, fourth, sixth, and twelfth cranial nerves, the corticobulbar and corticospinal tract, and the medial lemniscus. Vascular accidents produce syndromes characterized by paralysis of one or more cranial nerves on the homolateral side and paralysis or paresis on the opposite side.

Weber's syndrome is produced by damage to the third nerve and cerebral peduncle. There is ophthalmoplegia on the ipsilateral side and paralysis of the arm or leg on the opposite side.

The Millard-Gubler syndrome involves the sixth and seventh nerves on the ipsilateral side and the corticospinal tract on the opposite side (Fig. 35–7).

Foville's syndrome consists of paralysis of conjugate gaze to the side of the lesion in addition to the findings in the Millard-Gubler syndrome.

Another lesion lower in the stem produces twelfth nerve palsy with contralateral hemianesthesia and hemiplegia.

THE LATERAL BRAIN STEM AREA. Vessels supplying this area also supply the cerebellum. In addition to cerebellar dysfunction there may be involvement of the fifth, seventh, and tenth motor nuclei, the fifth and eighth sensory nuclei, the spinal lemniscus, and the sympathetic pathways.

Wallenberg's syndrome (posterior inferior cerebellar artery) produces dysphagia, dysarthria, impairment of pain and temperature sensation in the face, Horner's syndrome, nystagmus, and cerebellar signs on the ipsilateral side. Contralaterally there is impairment of pain and temperature sensation of the body (Fig. 35–8).

Thrombosis of the anterior cerebellar artery produces homolateral deafness, facial paralysis, Horner's syndrome, and loss of sensation of touch in the face. On the opposite side there is impairment of pain and temperature sensation. Homolateral cerebellar signs are also present.

Superior cerebellae artery thrombosis produces homolateral involuntary movements, loss of hearing, and facial paralysis. Contralaterally there is loss of pain and temperature sensation over the entire half of the body.

Pseudobulbar Palsy. Theoretically this condition may be produced by bilateral lesions in the brain stem. The term implies,

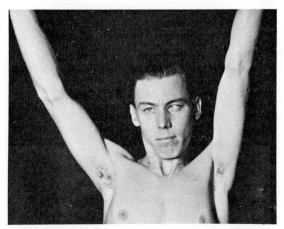

FIGURE 35–7. Patient with left abducens palsy and right hemiparesis. Seventh nerve palsy is not evident in this picture. (Courtesy of Dr. A. Ornsteen, Philadelphia.)

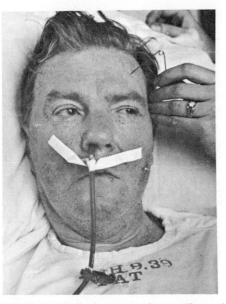

FIGURE 35–8. Wallenberg's syndrome. The patient has hypesthesia of the left side of the face and left Horner's syndrome. Difficulty in swallowing necessitates the nasogastric tube. (Courtesy of Dr. A. Ornsteen, Philadelphia.)

however, interruption of the corticobulbar pathway. The chief cause is multiple arteriosclerotic lesions in both hemispheres. There may be emotional outbursts, personality changes, aphasia, loss of memory, deterioration of intellective function, and moderate difficulty in speaking, chewing, and swallowing. Psychiatric evaluation and support may be necessary.

GENERAL MEDICAL MANAGEMENT

It is obvious that patients with brain stem involvement may be desperately ill and require long-term medical management. Attention must be given to nutrition and electrolyte balance, and care must be taken to prevent urinary tract and respiratory infections and thrombophlebitis.

Respiratory Management. Many of the problems discussed have in common the need for management of respiratory difficulty. Beaver[16] cites the most common causes of admission to a respiratory unit as the following: injuries to brain or brain stem, Guillain-Barré syndrome, poliomyelitis, tetraplegia, prolonged coma, virus encephalomyelitis, myasthenia gravis, myopathies, and bulbar palsy. Respiratory failure has

many causes. From a physiologic point of view, they can be classified as atmospheric, ventilatory, circulatory, hematologic, and cytologic.

Tracheostomy should be considered early for many reasons: (1) it enables secretions to be removed by suction; (2) it provides an obstruction-free airway; (3) it reduces the dead space by 70 cc., which may prove lifesaving; (4) it allows immediate employment of mechanical assistance; (5) it makes humidification and endobronchial medication easy; (6) in some cases, especially postoperative, it may serve as insurance against respiratory complications.

The merits of positive pressure ventilation as compared with the tank respirator have been argued. The advantages of positive pressure are definite: the patient is less restricted psychologically and physically, nursing and physical therapy procedures are performed more easily, transport is easy, and there is no difficulty with the neck seal and handling the tracheostomy. On the other hand, these machines are more delicate and there is less margin for error. There is interference with cardiovascular activity by reversal of the thoracic pump mechanism, direct tamponage of the heart, and inhibition of alveolar capillary circulation when intraalveolar tension exceeds 8 mm Hg.

There are conditions in which the mechanical support of respiration may be contraindicated. A patient literally dying from amyotrophic lateral sclerosis can only be made uncomfortable and unhappy if life is prolonged in a senseless way. The author remembers well a young woman kept alive for a year at great cost to her family in terms of money and anxiety. This woman was far from grateful. She had not been allowed to die simply and comfortably. Tracheostomy and oxygen given through a catheter would have permitted a far more comfortable and dignified death.

REFERENCES

1. Haymaker, W.: Bing's Local Diagnosis in Neurological Diseases. Translated, revised and enlarged from the 14th German edition. St. Louis, The C. V. Mosby Co., 1956, pp. 118–224, 241–253.
2. Grinker, R. R., Bucy, P. C., and Sahs, A. L.: Neurology, 5th Ed. Springfield, Ill., Charles C Thomas, Publisher, 1960, pp. 402–463.
3. Ford, F. R.: Diseases of the Nervous System in Infancy, Childhood, and Adolescence, 4th Ed.

Springfield, Ill., Charles C Thomas, Publisher, 1960, pp 20–43.

4. Merritt, H. H.: A Textbook of Neurology. Philadelphia, Lea and Febiger, 1955.

5. Alter, M.: Familial aggregation of Bell's palsy. Arch. Neurol. 8:55, 1963.

6. Ghiora, A., and Winter, S. T.: The conservative treatment of Bell's palsy. A review of the literature, 1939–1960. Am. J. Phys. Med. 41:213, 1962.

7. Kettel, K.: Surgical treatment in atraumatic facial palsies. J. Laryngol., 73:491, 1959.

8. Langworth, E. P., and Taverner, D.: The prognosis in facial palsy. Brain, 86:465, 1963.

9. Wiederholt, W. C., Mulder, D. W., and Lambert, E. H.: The Landry-Guillain-Barré-Strohl syndrome or polyradiculoneuropathy: Historical review, report on 97 patients, and present concepts. Proc. Mayo Clin., 39:427, 1964.

10. Marshall, J.: The Landry-Guillain-Barré syndrome. Brain, 86:55, 1963.

11. Birchfield, R. I., and Shaw, C.: Postural hypotension in the Guillain-Barré syndrome. Arch. Neurol., 10:149, 1964.

12. Walton, J. N.: The "floppy" infant, Cereb. Palsy Bull., 2:10, 1960.

13. Krabbe, K. H.: Congenital generalized muscular atrophies. Acta Psychiatr. Scand. 33:94, 1958.

14. Brandt, S.: Werdnig-Hoffmann's infantile progressive muscular atrophy, Copenhagen, Munksgard, 1950.

15. Abel, J. J., Hampil, B., and Jonas, A. F., Jr.: Researches on tetanus: Further experiments to prove that tetanus toxin is not carried in the peripheral nerves to the central nervous system. Bull. Johns Hopkins Hosp., 56:317, 1935.

16. Beaver, R.: The Management of Respiratory Failure. In Modern Trends in Neurology — 3. Ed. D. Williams, Washington, Butterworth, Inc., 1962.

17. Taverner, D., Kemble, F., and Cohen, S. B.: Prognosis and treatment of idiopathic facial (Bell's) palsy. Br. Med. J., 4:581, 1967.

18. Alford, B. R., Weber, S. C., and Sessions, R. B.: Neurodiagnostic studies in facial paralysis. Ann. Otol., 79:227, 1970.

19. Edgerton, M. T.: Surgical correction of facial paralysis: A plea for better reconstructions. Ann. Surg., 165:985, 1967.

20. Peiris, O. A., and Miles, D. W.: Galvanic stimulation of the tongue as a prognostic index in Bell's palsy. Br. Med. J. 2:1162, 1965.

21. Campbell, E. D. R., Hickey, R. P., Nixon, K. H., and Richardson, A. T.: Value of nerve-excitability measurements in prognosis of facial palsy. Br. Med. J. 2:7, 1962.

36

REHABILITATION FOR DEGENERATIVE DISEASES OF THE CENTRAL NERVOUS SYSTEM

JEROME W. GERSTEN

During the past few decades acute disease has been managed with much more success than previously. This has been the result primarily of advances in surgical techniques and antibiotic medication. There has therefore been a progressive shift in attention toward chronic diseases, and especially those classified as degenerative. Degenerative diseases have been characterized by a progressive course and occurrence in older age groups. Defining degeneration as deterioration adds little to understanding. The term *abiotrophy*, the inability of tissue to survive, has often been used to define the degenerative process, but it too says little concerning etiology. Some diseases initially categorized as degenerative are now known to be viral in etiology. Creutzfeldt-Jakob disease is an example of this. This is cortical atrophy, mainly frontal, with neuronal loss in cerebral cortex, basal ganglia, thalamus, brain stem, and spinal cord. There is rapidly progressive dementia, with motor abnormalities. The disease is, however, transmissible, and is now classified among the slow virus diseases. The physiatrist often is responsible for the management of patients with degener-

ative disease and attempts to improve or maintain functional capacity. The more common of these diseases will be examined in the following discussion.

Dementias

The major characteristic of the dementias is decrease in intellectual capacity, with memory deficit — recent worse than remote, confusion, disorientation in time and space, and difficulty in learning and in recognition. There may be behavioral problems and alteration in personality. These patients must be differentiated from those with mental retardation, depression, or primary language disorder. The dementias may be primary, with no other associated pathology, or secondary. Among the latter are those due to drugs, severe sensory deficit (especially auditory or visual), metabolic defect (folic acid deficiency), tumor, trauma, infection, or circulatory disorder (multi-infarct dementia).

The primary dementias are the more frequent, and have, in the past, been divided into the presenile (Alzheimer's disease), with onset before age 65, and the senile, with onset after that age. This distinction is now considered arbitrary and of no significance. Approximately 4 to 5 per cent of people over 65 show moderate to severe senile dementia, and 65 per cent of these have Alzheimer's disease. The prevalence rate of the advanced cases is 3/1000 of the whole population. The senile form of Alzheimer's disease may rank fourth or fifth as a cause of death in the United States. Eleven per cent of those over 65 have at least a mild form of dementia. The cause of premature neuronal degeneration — presumably due to biochemical defect — is unknown, although genetic elements have been implicated.

Age of onset of Alzheimer's disease is generally between 50 and 60, with females affected more often than males. Occurrence is generally sporadic. Onset is slow, with cognitive deficits noted above, but relentlessly progressive, with a course under five years. Myoclonus may occasionally be a prominent symptom. Movement later becomes slow and apraxic, with difficulty in ambulation, and the patient is eventually confined to bed.

The brain weight is decreased and there is gross atrophy of gyri. Sulci are wider and there is ventricular dilatation. Degeneration and neuronal loss are general, although especially marked in the hippocampus and association areas. Cells show granulovacuolar changes. Neurofibrillary tangles are prominent on microscopic examination. These are bundles of microtubules that twist in helical fashion, with a period of 800 Å. Senile plaques contain a core of amyloid (extracellular) surrounded by enlarged neurites. The degree of dementia has been correlated positively with the number of plaques and tangles.

Cerebral blood flow, O_2 consumption, respiratory rate, and phosphokinase content are reduced in the dementias, with decrease in cerebral metabolism occurring early with neuronal atrophy, and diminished blood flow appearing early in arteriosclerotic dementia. There is a positive correlation between mean hemisphere flow and the degree of dementia in multi-infarct patients, but no such relation in primary dementia.

Choline acetyl transferase, an enzyme involved in the synthesis of acetylcholine, is decreased in Alzheimer's disease, especially in the hippocampus. This parallels the degree of neuropathologic change and may be related to memory defect. Other biochemical changes include brain decrease in homovanillic acid (HVA), 1-dopa, dopamine, and noradrenaline, and cerebrospinal fluid decrease in HVA, gamma aminobutyric acid, and 5-hydroxyindole acetic acid. In one study, the level of HVA was inversely related to the degree of motor deficit.

The major aspects of care are preventive, designed to keep an individual as active and independent as possible in either home or institution. Physical activity must be encouraged, to whatever degree possible (maintain strength, ROM, alertness); stimuli must be maintained — visual, auditory, and social; safety must be enhanced (familiar objects, adequate lighting, avoidance of throw rugs and slippery surfaces, grab bars, etc.); and diet must be kept at an optimum level. Depression may be managed with tricyclic antidepressants, but the response is usually not satisfactory. Abnormal behavior may be treated with major tranquilizers. Specific treatment is not yet available. Vasodilators and hyperbaric oxygen have not been of value. In recent studies hydergine (dihydroergotamine) has been given in doses of 6 to 12 mg daily, with beneficial effect on mental alertness, sociability, and memory. Hydergine inhibits phosphodiesterase, and its presumed beneficial effect in dementia has been offered as evidence for a metabolic etiology. Much more evidence is required to determine the precise role of hydergine in the management of the dementias.

Parkinson's Disease

Parkinson's disease is the most common degenerative disease involving the basal ganglia. Although idiopathic disease (paralysis agitans) is the most common type observed at the present time, postencephalitic, arteriosclerotic, postanoxic, traumatic, or drug (reserpine, phenothiazine, α-methyldopa) etiologies also may occur. It is not likely that a single mutant gene can be involved as a cause of Parkinson's disease. More likely causation is a combination of many genetic and nongenetic factors. A more likely etiology for the idiopathic type would thus seem to be the multifactorial. A single major cause is therefore not likely to be found.

Prior to 1918, most cases of Parkinson's disease were of the idiopathic type. Following the epidemic of encephalitis lethargica (von Economo's disease) from 1918 to 1926, the pattern was altered for a period. From 1920 to 1943 there were two peaks of onset of Parkinson's disease, a small secondary peak in the third decade, representing postencephalitic cases, and a larger peak in the sixth, or sixth and seventh decades, representing the idiopathic type. Incidence of the postencephalitic type is now decreasing, and the curve representing age of onset is again unimodal, with the late peak. In the United States there are approximately 40,000 to 50,000 new cases per year. The incidence under the age of 50 is approximately 5 to 8/100,000, rising to 35/100,000 at age 50 to 59, and 100/100,000 at age 60 to 69. Over 1 per cent of the population over 50 may be involved, with a prevalence of approximately 350,000 to 400,000.

The most consistent neuropathological findings are those noted in the melanin-containing cells of the brain stem — the substantia nigra and locus ceruleus. There is loss of nerve cells with reactive gliosis, especially in the substantia nigra. In idiopathic parkinsonism eosinophilic intracytoplasmic inclusions (Lewy bodies) are present. Degeneration of dopaminergic neurons in the zona compacta of the substantia nigra, with degeneration of an unmyelinated nigrostriatal pathway, results in decreased dopaminergic activity at striatal dopamine receptors. These changes are related to the motor abnormalities in parkinsonism.

Dopamine (DA), an inhibitory neurotransmitter (membrane stabilizer), is present in highest concentration in the caudate and putamen. Eighty per cent of the brain content of DA is localized at these two sites. In parkinsonism there is a decrease in melanin content of substantia nigra cells, a selective decrease of DA in caudate and putamen, and a decrease in homovanillic acid (HVA) (a monoamine catabolite). There is a decreased urinary excretion of free DA in Parkinson's disease. The lower the level of free urinary DA, the greater the functional deficit, and the more severe the akinesia and rigidity. Most patients with parkinsonism have decreased DA release, a presynaptic DA deficiency, and a decrease in cerebrospinal fluid HVA levels. Parkinsonian symptoms may represent an imbalance between inhibitory dopaminergic stimuli and excitatory cholinergic stimuli in the striatum.

Dopaminergic inhibition can be demonstrated by the effect of iontophoretically applied DA, via micropipette, on spontaneous electrical activity of caudate nucleus cells. In 50 to 60 per cent of these cells the firing rate is decreased. In addition, electrical stimulation of the substantia nigra markedly depresses the firing rate of a large number of caudate neurons. In Parkinson's disease, the decrease in inhibition may be related to an imbalance in activity of the α and γ motor systems, with an increase in α activity and a decrease in γ activity. Increase in excitability of the α motoneuron pool has been demonstrated in examination of the H-reflex, of maximal H/M ratio, and of the recovery curve of the H response. Excitability of the α motoneuron pool is decreased following L-dopa administration. With microelectrodes in Ia afferents in man, increased static fusimotor activity has been demonstrated in parkinsonian patients. Although overactivity of the fusimotor system is an important part of parkinsonian rigidity, there is no primary defect in this system.

Onset of idiopathic parkinsonism usually occurs after the age of 50 (mean of 57.1 in one study). Common early symptoms and important in diagnosis are tremor, rigidity, and bradykinesia. Tremor, at a rate of 3 to 6/sec, is a frequent initial symptom, is manifest in distal parts of the extremity, is present at rest, and is often inhibited by the initiation of voluntary movement. Tremor may be initiated on attempting to maintain the upper extremity abducted in an unsupported position. It is increased by emotional stress and may disappear during sleep. Tremor probably results from increased activation of the α motoneuron system, with rhythmic discharge through the VL nucleus of the thalamus.

Rigidity, an early parkinsonian symptom, does not respect the concept of reciprocal innervation, and increased electrical activity and tone may be present in flexor and extensor muscles simultaneously. This disorder of reciprocal inhibition may also be demonstrated by low intensity stimulation of the tibial nerve. In the normal subject tibialis anticus and soleus respond simultaneously in only a small number of instances. In parkinsonian patients simultaneous response in these two muscles occurs in 77 per cent. Electrical activity in parkinsonism may be present in muscles at rest and is not affected by the velocity of motion. There may be, however, excessive reflex response to muscle stretch. Alternating tightening and releasing may produce cogwheeling. Bradykinesia, the slow and difficult initiation of voluntary movements, is independent of rigidity, although the two are often associated. It is noted especially on initiation of voluntary, repetitive acts and may be related to increased central inhibition of the γ neuron, via the VL nucleus of the thalamus. Slow movement is the result mainly of a motorial defect, although the role of arousal or alerting is not clear.

Control of posture is an important function of the basal ganglia, and postural disturbance is frequent in parkinsonism. The classic posture in parkinsonism is one of head flexion, thoracic kyphosis, shoulder protraction and abduction, and arm flexion. Gait is slow and shuffling, with difficulty in starting to walk, and loss of associated movements. Additional symptoms include weakness and easy fatigue, muscle pain — which may on occasion be severe, flexion contracture and decreased ROM, speech disturbance (decrease in articulation clarity, loss of vocal intensity, and loss of modulation of speech), and autonomic disturbance (salivation and oily skin). There may be intellectual deterioration, with memory impairment and perceptual deficit. On the WAIS, scores are much lower in performance than in verbal areas, especially so in perceptual organization, digit symbol, block design, and object assembly.

Treatment of parkinsonism may be pharmacologic, physical, or surgical — the last playing a much less important role at the present time. The basis for major pharmacologic therapy is the DA depletion in the striatum in parkinsonism and the restoration of DA toward normal levels. DA does not cross the blood-brain barrier. The precursor, L-dihydroxyphenylalanine (L-dopa), which does cross the barrier, must be administered orally and is then converted to DA in the striatum. Unfortunately, L-dopa is also converted to DA peripherally, through action of dopa-decarboxylase. Dopa-decarboxylase inhibitors block extracerebral conversion of L-dopa to DA, and lower doses of L-dopa are thus therapeutically effective. Unfortunately, 30 per cent of parkinsonian patients fail to respond to L-dopa. In addition, there are disturbing side effects, such as hypotension; uncontrolled movements of tongue, oral or buccal muscles, and jaw; and depression. There may be a role for ergot alkaloids that selectively inhibit prolactin secretion — bromocriptine and lergotrile. These drugs penetrate the blood-brain barrier more readily than L-dopa, and act directly on DA receptors in the striatum, probably with both presynaptic and postsynaptic effects. Other drugs that may be of value are the anticholinergics, and the antihistamines and β-adrenergic blockers for tremor.

Drug therapy alone is not sufficient and must be combined with a physical therapeutic program. The program is designed to correct faulty posture or maintain good posture, maintain or increase ROM, and maintain ambulation and hand function. With regard to posture, attention must be focused on the tendency toward neck flexion, thoracic kyphosis, hip flexion, and knee flexion. Prevention of contracture is an important element in maintenance of good posture. Gait training will be enhanced by successful attempts to improve posture. Ambulation is improved when there is a slightly broader base, when steps are longer, when there is conscious dorsiflexion of toes on beginning the swing phase, and when associated movements of the upper extremities are encouraged. Speech training should emphasize deep breathing and attention to rhythm and articulation. Singing may be of considerable benefit.

Huntington's Disease

Huntington's disease (HD) affects approximately 12,000 to 14,000 people in the U.S (6.5/100,000). It is transmitted as an autosomal dominant degenerative disease and is characterized primarily by severe degeneration and atrophy in the striatum, with lesser involvement of the neocortex and diencephalic-limbic structures. Vascular etiology has been suggested in one study. There is marked atrophy and loss of small neurons in the basal ganglia, caudate nucleus, and putamen, and more diffuse loss of neurons in the cerebral cortex, especially in frontal lobes. Although the basal ganglia show the major involvement, there also is damage to fine structure of cerebral cortical neurons. There is intense gliosis in regions of neuron loss, with accumulation of lipofuscin in neurons and glia. The caudate nucleus may show severe loss of choline acetyltransferase activity. Functionally there is dopaminergic hyperactivity, associated with decreased GABA inhibition. The concentration of GABA and the activity of glutamic acid decarboxylase are reduced in the basal ganglia. Symptoms are decreased by reserpine, which depletes striatum of DA (destroying storage sites), and by haloperidol, which blocks DA receptors (and blocks action of DA). In the normal subject the H reflex is elicited readily in quadriceps, hamstrings, and gastrocnemius-soleus, and with difficulty and infrequently elsewhere. In Huntington's disease the H reflex was elicited in the anterior tibial muscle in 8 of 9 patients and in 5 of 8 subjects at risk. In the same study the reflex could be elicited in only 1 of 30 normal subjects, in the anterior tibial muscle. Lymphocytes from HD patients respond to the presence of brain tissue from HD patients by producing migration inhibition factor. The significance of this observation is not known.

Huntington's disease is characterized by intellectual deterioration and involuntary choreiform movements. Symptoms usually begin after the age of 30, initially with abrupt, clumsy, and jerky movements. These movements are increased by emotional or physical stress and disappear during sleep. Later there are choreiform movements (jerking of fingers and wrists) and proximal dystonic movements. Ultimately there are slurred speech, dementia, and functional motor impairment, with death 10 to 15 years from onset. In patients with early involvement, the major neuropsychological deficit is severe impairment in memory function with relative preservation of IQ scores. There is difficulty in learning new material. In later stages there is nonfocal deficit, with poor performance on all tests except picture-naming. This differentiates HD from the presenile dementias, in which naming disorders and aphasia are common. Phenothiazine, reserpine, and haloperidol may be used to decrease adventitious movements.

Olivopontocerebellar Degeneration

Olivopontocerebellar atrophy is one of a group of genetic disorders with autosomal dominant or recessive inheritance. It is one of the spinocerebellar degenerations that occurs in adult or late middle life. The abiotrophic process is associated with premature degeneration of neurons and axons, possibly due to enzymatic deficits. There is involvement of cerebellum, with loss of Purkinje cells and cells in molecular and granular layers, pontine nuclei, and olives. Ataxia of trunk and extremities, dysarthria, tremor of head and trunk, and gait impairment progress steadily and result in incapacity within 5 to 10 years. Dementia, cranial nerve deficit (with speech disorder, ptosis, facial muscle atrophy, dysphagia), and extrapyramidal signs may also be present.

Friedreich's Ataxia

Friedreich's ataxia, the most common of the spinocerebellar degenerations, occurs at an earlier age (5 to 15), and involves the cerebellum to some degree (Purkinje cells and dentate nuclei). There is major involvement, however, in the dorsal half of the spinal cord, with atrophy predominantly in the dorsal columns, but also in the lateral corticospinal tract and dorsal and ventral spinocerebellar tracts. The disease is slightly more frequent in males than in females, with autosomal dominant or recessive inheritance. Ataxic gait is an early symptom, due to cerebellar and proprioceptive deficits. Awkward movements, intention tremor, slurred speech, and pes cavus occur later. Cavus is especially common in those with corticospinal tract involvement since childhood. In the presence of distal atrophy in the lower extremities, short leg braces may be helpful in prolonging the ability to ambulate.

Amyotrophic Lateral Sclerosis

Amyotrophic lateral sclerosis (ALS) (motor neuron disease) involves selective neuronal degenerative loss in the frontal cortex (Betz cells of motor cortex), the motor cranial nerve nuclei, and anterior horn cells in the ventral gray matter of the spinal cord, associated with degeneration of corticospinal tracts. Variants include progressive bulbar palsy, progressive muscular atrophy, and primary lateral sclerosis. In 20 to 25 per cent the disease does not fit any of the above patterns. Neurofibrillary changes (tangles) in cerebrum and brain stem have been found especially in ALS on Guam. Such tangles are rare in the classic sporadic case of ALS.

Among the suggested etiologic factors have been slow virus infection of motor neurons, toxin, autoimmune mechanism with antibody destruction of motoneurons, and abiotrophy. Serum from patients with ALS has been demonstrated to be toxic to anterior horn cells of the mouse. Some link has been suggested between poliomyelitis and ALS. The majority of the cases are sporadic. In 5 to 10 per cent, the disease is familial, with autosomal recessive inheritance.

ALS is more common than one might expect, and is responsible for 0.1 per cent of deaths in the world. It affects males twice as often as females and usually begins in the fourth decade, with a peak in the fourth and fifth decades. The age of onset seems to be earlier in hereditary than in sporadic ALS. Atrophy, weakness, fasciculations, and paralysis are characteristic symptoms. Atrophy is most often apparent in the hand, either unilateral or bilateral, and is accompanied by weakness, dysarthria, fasciculations, muscle pain, and spasticity. Weakness in the lower extremities usually involves the dorsiflexors before the plantar flexors and results in progressive foot drop. When intercostal muscles weaken, respiration is impaired and secretions may accumulate in the respiratory tract with fatal outcome. Bulbar muscle involvement leads to difficulty in swallowing (pharyngeal weakness), chewing, and coughing. Fifty per cent of patients die within three years, 80 per cent in 5 years, and 90 per cent in 10 years. Patients with bulbar involvement die sooner.

The diagnosis is essentially a clinical one, but electrodiagnostic studies may be of assistance. These show fibrillations and fasciculations, with normal nerve conduction velocity. Recruitment is impaired, with large, longer duration and polyphasic motor unit action potentials. There is motor unit loss, with suggestion that transsynaptic degeneration contributes to this process, and enlargement of some of the remaining motor units. Terminal reinnervation by collateral sprouting may result in large motor units. Abnormalities of muscle innervation have been reported. There may be decremental response to repetitive nerve stimulation.

Treatment of the primary problem is not yet possible. Guanidine and neostigmine may slow the progress of the disease for a short period, presumably by release of quantal packets of acetylcholine at the motor end plates. From the earliest phase of the disease, and for as long as possible, attempts must be made to keep ROM normal and avoid contracture. Initially this is achieved by active exercises, later by passive ones. Exercises to maintain or increase strength should be directed at least toward those muscles that are unaffected. Involved muscles should be approached more cautiously, fatigue should be avoided, and exercise periods should be short. It is possible that excessive exercise of involved muscles may increase weakness.

As weakness progresses, and functional impairment ensues, appropriate assistive devices may enable the patient to perform adequately in the community, or at home, for a longer period. These include short or long opponens hand orthosis and foot-ankle orthosis for foot drop. At a later stage, devices to assist in rising from a chair or a wheelchair may be necessary. Neck stability may be maintained by collar or brace.

Excessive salivation may be a problem. Transtympanic neurectomy has been suggested as a solution. Medication, such as methantheline, amitriptyline, methylphenidate, and clonidine may decrease secretions. Suction devices may be necessary to prevent aspiration and pneumonia. Involvement of bulbar musculature may result in difficulty in swallowing. This may be managed by preparing foods that can be swallowed more easily (blender use), by cricopharyngeal myotomy, or by esophagostomy (more rarely, gastrostomy). When respiratory function becomes severely impaired (with MBC less than 30 liters/minute), the use of assistive respiratory devices, or tracheostomy, should be considered.

REFERENCES

General

1. Gilroy, J., and Meyer, J. S.: Medical Neurology, 2nd Ed. New York, Macmillan Publishing Company, 1975, pp. 165–223.
2. Merritt, H. H.: A Textbook of Neurology, 5th Ed. Philadelphia, Lea and Febiger, 1973, pp. 431–571.
3. Nicholi, A. M., Jr. (Ed.): The Harvard Guide to Modern Psychiatry. Cambridge, Mass., Harvard University Press, 1973, pp. 297–318.

Dementias

4. Manuelidis, E. E., Gorgacz, E. J., and Manuelidis, L.: Viremia in experimental Creutzfeldt-Jakob disease. Science, 200:1069–1071, 1978.
5. Kahana, E., Alter, M., Braham, J., and Sofer, D.: Creutzfeldt-Jakob disease: Focus among Libyan Jews in Israel. Science, 183:90–91, 1974.
6. Heston, L. L.: Alzheimer's disease, trisomy 21, and myeloproliferative disorders: Associations suggesting a genetic diathesis. Science, 196:322–323, 1977.
7. Freemon, F. R.: Evaluation of patients with progressive intellectual deterioration. Arch. Neurol., 33:658–659, 1976.
8. Faden, A. I., and Townsend, J. J.: Myoclonus in Alzheimer disease. Arch. Neurol., 33:278–280, 1976.
9. Crapper, D. R., Dalton, A J., Skopitz, M., Scott, J. W., and Hachinski, V. C.: Alzheimer degeneration in Down syndrome: Electrophysiologic alterations and histopathologic findings. Arch. Neurol., 32:618–623, 1975.
10. Terry, R. D.: Dementia. Arch. Neurol., 33:1–3, 1976.
11. Katzman, R.: The prevalence and malignancy of Alzheimer disease. Arch. Neurol., 33:217–218, 1976.
12. Hachinski, V. C., Iliff, L. D., Zilhka, E., Du Boulay, G. H., McAllister, V. L., Marshall, J., Russell, R. W., and Symon, L.: Cerebral blood flow in dementia. Arch. Neurol., 32:632–637, 1975.

Parkinson's Disease

13. Kondo, K., Kurland, L. T., and Schull, W. J.: Parkinson's disease — Genetic analysis and evidence of a multifactorial etiology. Mayo Clin. Proc., 48:465–475, 1973.
14. Hoehn, M. M.: Age distribution of patients with parkinsonism. J. Am. Geriatrics Soc., 24:79–85, 1976.
15. Hull, J. T.: The prevalence and incidence of Parkinson's disease. Geriatrics, 25:128–133, 1970.
16. Hoehn, M. M., Crowley, T. J., and Rutledge, C. O.: Dopamine correlates of neurological and psychological status in untreated parkinsonism. J. Neurol. Neurosurg. Psychiatry, 39:941–951, 1976.
17. Klawans, H. L., et al.: Calcification of the basal ganglia as a cause of levodopa-resistant parkinsonism. Neurology 26:221–225, 1976.
18. Lloyd, K., and Hornykiewicz, O.: Parkinson's disease: Activity of L-dopa decarboxylase in discrete brain regions. Science, 170:1212–1213, 1970.
19. Connor, J. D.: Caudate unit responses to nigral stimuli: Evidence for a possible nigro-neostriatal pathway. Science, 160:899–900, 1968.
20. Herbison, G. J.: H-reflex in patients with parkinsonism: Effect of levodopa. Arch. Phys. Med. Rehabil., 54:291–295, 1973.
21. Fujita, S., and Cooper, I. S.: Effects of L-dopa on the H-reflex in parkinsonism. J. Am. Geriatrics Soc., 19:289–295, 1971.
22. McLeod, J. G., and Walsh, J. C.: H-Reflex studies in patients with Parkinson's disease. J. Neurol. Neurosurg. Psychiatry, 35:77–80, 1972.
23. Cherington, M.: Parkinson's disease, L-dopa, and the H-reflex. In Walton, J. N., Canal, N., and Scarlato, G. (Eds.): Muscle Diseases. Proceedings of an International Congress. Milan, May 19–21, 1969. Amsterdam, Excerpta Medica, 1970, pp. 197–200.
24. Landau, W. M., Struppler, A., and Mehls, O.: A comparative electromyographic study of the reactions to passive movement in parkinsonism and in normal subjects. Neurology 16:34–48, 1966.
25. Burke, D., Hagbarth, K.-E., and Wallin, B. G.: Reflex mechanisms in parkinsonian rigidity. Scand. J. Rehabil. Med., 9:15–23, 1977.
26. Delwaide, P. J., et al.: Polysynaptic spinal reflexes in Parkinson's disease. Neurology, 24:820–827, 1974.
27. Heilman, K. M., Bowers, D., Watson, R., and Greer, M.: Reaction times in Parkinson disease. Arch. Neurol., 33:139–140, 1976.
28. Klawans, H. L., and Topel, J. L.: Parkinsonism as a falling sickness. J.A.M.A., 230:1555–1557, 1974.
29. Delong, M. R.: Activity of pallidal neurons during movement. J. Neurophysiol., 34:414–427, 1971.
30. Rigrodsky, S., and Morrison, E. B.: Speech changes in parkinsonism during L-dopa therapy: Preliminary findings. J. Am. Geriatrics Soc., 18:142–151, 1970.
31. Gersten, J. W., Marshall, C., Dillon, T., Schneck, S., Orr, W., and Nelson, C.: External work of walking and functional capacity in parkinsonian patients treated with L-dopa. Arch. Phys. Med. Rehabil., 53:547–554, 1972.
32. Loranger, A. W., et al.: Intellectual impairment in Parkinson's syndrome. Brain, 95:405–412, 1972.
33. Bianchine, J. R., Shaw, G. M., Greenwald, J. E., and Dandalides, S. M.: Clinical aspects of dopamine agonists and antagonists. Fed. Proc., 37:2434–2439, 1978.
34. Coyle, J. T., and Snyder, S. H.: Antiparkinsonian drugs: Inhibition of dopamine uptake in the corpus striatum as a possible mechanism of action. Science, 166:899–901, 1969.
35. Chase, T., and Watanabe, A. M.: Methyldopahydrazine as an adjunct to L-dopa therapy in parkinsonism. Neurology, 22:384–391, 1972.
36. Wener, J., Rosenberg, G., Grad, B., and Wener, S.: Cardiovascular effects of levodopa in aged versus younger patients with Parkinson's disease. J. Am. Geriatrics Soc., 24:185–188, 1976.
37. Weiner, W. J., and Klawans, H. L., Jr.: Lingual-facial-buccal movements in the elderly. I. Pathophysiology and treatment. J. Am. Geriatrics Soc., 21:314–320, 1973.
38. Cherington, M.: Parkinsonism, L-dopa and mental depression. J. Am. Geriatrics Soc., 18:513–516, 1970.
39. Lees, A. J., Haddad, S., Shaw, K. M., Kohout, L. J., and Stern, G. M.: Bromocriptine in parkinsonism. Arch. Neurol., 35:503–505, 1978.
40. Lieberman, A., Estey, E., Kupersmith, M., Gopinanthan, G., and Goldstein, M.: Treatment of Parkinson's disease with lergotrile mesylate. J.A.M.A., 238:2380–2382, 1977.
41. Boshes, L. D., and Doshay, L. J.: Practical man-

agement of Parkinson's disease. Geriatrics, 19:644–653, 1964.

42. Mier, M.: Mechanisms leading to hypoventilation in extrapyramidal disorders, with special reference to Parkinson's disease. J. Am. Geriatrics Soc., 15:230–238, 1967.

Huntington's Disease

43. Mason, S. T., Sanberg, P. R., and Fibiger, H. C.: Kainic acid lesions of the striatum dissociate amphetamine and apomorphine stereotypy: Similarities to Huntington's chorea. Science, 201:352–355, 1978.

44. Barkley, D. S., Hardiwidjaja, S., and Menkes, J. H.: Huntington's disease: Delayed hypersensitivity in vitro to human central nervous system antigens. Science, 195:314–316, 1977.

45. Butters, N., Sax, D., Montgomery, K., and Tarlow, S.: Comparison of the neuropsychological deficits associated with early and advanced Huntington's disease. Arch. Neurol., 35:585–589, 1978.

46. Walsh, A. C., and Melaney, C.: Huntington's disease: Improvement with an anticoagulant-psychotherapy regimen. J. Am. Geriatrics Soc., 26:127–129, 1978.

47. Chase, T. N., Watanabe, A. M., Brodie, K. H., and Donnelly, E. F.: Huntington's chorea. Arch. Neurol., 26:282–284, 1972.

48. Johnson, E. W., Radecki, P. L., and Paulson, G. W.: Huntington disease: Early identification by H reflex testing. Arch. Phys. Med. Rehabil., 58:162–166, 1977.

49. Norton, W. T., Kahlid, I., Tiffany, C., and Tellez-Nagel, I.: Huntington disease: Normal lipid composition of purified neuronal perikarya and whole cortex. Neurology 28:812–816, 1978.

Olivopontocerebellar Degeneration

50. Landis, D. M. D., Rosenberg, R. N., Landis, S. C., Schut, L., and Nyhan, W. L.: Olivopontocere-bellar degeneration. Arch. Neurol., 31:295–307, 1974.

Amyotrophic Lateral Sclerosis

51. Meyers, K. R., Dorencamp, D. G., and Suzuki, K.: Amyotrophic lateral sclerosis with diffuse neurofibrillary changes. Arch. Neurol., 30:84–89, 1974.

52. Bjornskov, E. K., Dekker, N. P., Norris, F. H., and Stuart, M. E.: End-plate morphology in amyotrophic lateral sclerosis. Arch. Neurol., 32:711–712, 1975.

53. Wolfgram, F., and Myers, L.: Amyotrophic lateral sclerosis: Effect of serum on anterior horn cells in tissue cultures. Science, 179:579–580, 1973.

54. Brody, J. A., Edgar, A. H., and Gillespie, M. M.: Amyotrophic lateral sclerosis: No increase among U.S. construction workers in Guam. J.A.M.A., 240:551–552, 1978.

55. McKhann, G. M., and Johnson, R. T.: Amyotrophic lateral sclerosis: Summary of a conference. Science, 180:221–222, 1973.

56. Giménez-Roldán, S., and Esteban, A.: Prognosis in hereditary amyotrophic lateral sclerosis. Arch. Neurol., 34:706–708, 1977.

57. Mulder, D. W., and Howard, F. M., Jr.: Patient resistance and prognosis in amyotrophic lateral sclerosis. Mayo Clin. Proc., 51:537–541, 1976.

58. Mulder, D. W., Rosenbaum, R. A., and Layton, D. D., Jr.: Late progression of poliomyelitis or forme fruste amyotrophic lateral sclerosis? Mayo Clin. Proc., 47:756–761, 1972.

59. Brown, W. F., and Jaatoul, N.: Amyotrophic lateral sclerosis: Electrophysiologic study. Arch. Neurol., 30:242–248, 1974.

60. Smith, R. A., and Norris, F. H., Jr.: Symptomatic care of patients with amyotrophic lateral sclerosis. J.A.M.A., 234:715–717, 1975.

61. Sinaki, M., and Mulder, D. W.: Rehabilitation techniques for patients with amyotrophic lateral sclerosis. Mayo Clin. Proc., 53:173–178, 1978.

37

SPINE: DISORDERS AND DEFORMITIES

RENE CAILLIET

Spine disorders and deformities causing pain and disability have many varying etiologies, but all have a common denominator of pain and impairment. The diagnosis, as in all musculoskeletal problems, demands knowledge of normal functional anatomy, knowledge of tissue sites capable of causing pain or dysfunction, skill in a meaningful examination, and an awareness of necessary confirmation tests and their interpretation. Only then can a specific diagnosis result and meaningful treatment ensue.

The spine is a flexible rod composed of superincumbent functional units supported in equilibrium upon the sacral base. The upright position, held in a balanced equilibrium with minimum muscular effort, is possibly only because the line of the center of gravity falls through the major weight-bearing joints. These are through the first thoracic, twelfth thoracic and fifth lumbar vertebrae, in front of the knees, and through the hip joints. In a "locked" knee stance, the center of gravity falls further in front of all of these joints (Fig. 37–1).

The individual functional unit consists of two vertebral bodies separated by the intervertebral disc designed to bear weight; neural arches that surround and protect the neural tissues; posterior articulations that guide specific movement and prevent other movements; and bony processes that provide mechanical sites for musculature attachment (Figs. 37–2 and 37–3).

The spine's mechanical function is the basis of the structure and action of these functional units, and pain and disability result from injury, inflammation, disease, and infection of elements of the functional unit.

The intervertebral discs have a fibrous outer layer (annulus) enclosing a central gelatinous nucleus pulposus. The fibers attach and insert around the circumference of the vertebral end plates and intertwine to permit movement, maintain intradiscal pressure, and keep the vertebral bodies together against distracting forces. They also limit the extent of rotation of one vertebra upon its immediate subjacent vertebra.

The disc is a mucopolysaccharide gelatinous avascular aneural tissue that acts mechanically to keep the vertebral bodies separated. The annular fibers keep the vertebral bodies together. As the bodies are kept apart, the facet joints posteriorly are also kept apart and the intervertebral foramina are kept open. The posterior joints (the zygapophyseal joints, or facets) are non–weight-bearing but are in opposition and determine the amplitude and direction of the movement of each intervertebral segment (Fig. 37–4).

The vertebral column, composed of superimposed functional units, must be viewed from the erect position, which is posture, and the functional kinesthetic basis of daily activities. Both in their normal state are asymptomatic; in the abnormal state they are painful and disabling.

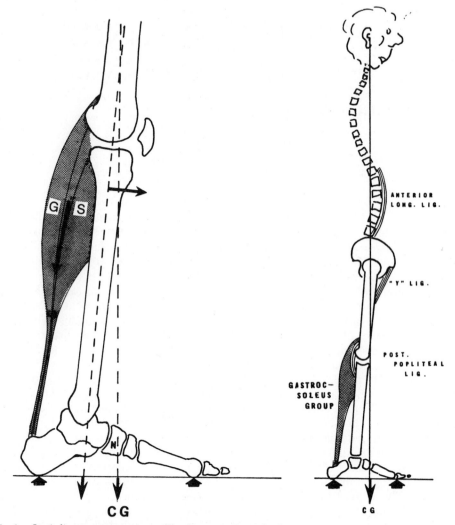

FIGURE 37—1. Static ligamentous posture. The figure on the right shows erect man leaning on his anterior longitudinal ligament (also upon his facets) with his knees locked in extension and leaning upon his anterior hip ligaments ("Y" ligament of Bigelow). Only the ankle cannot be locked, but mere gastroc tonus will balance the leg that leans forward 2 to 3 degrees. The gastroc soleus group pulls the leg back over the foot that is fixed upon the floor as shown in the figure to the left. (From Cailliet, R.: Low Back Pain Syndrome, 2nd Ed. Philadelphia, F. A. Davis Co., 1968, p. 27.)

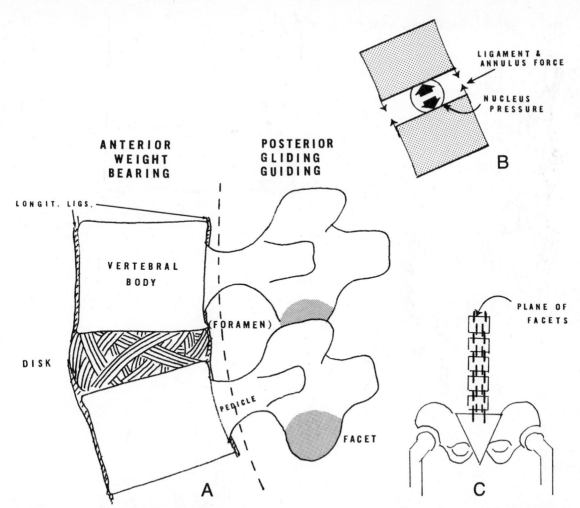

FIGURE 37–2. Functional unit. The anterior weight-bearing portion consists of two adjacent vertebrae separated by the disc. This portion is reinforced by longitudinal ligaments. The posterior portion contains the facets (articulations) that oppose each other in the sagittal plane. The foramina through which emerge the spinal nerves are depicted. The intradiscal pressure within the nucleus separates the vertebrae. This pressure is opposed by the annulus and the longitudinal ligaments. (From Cailliet, R.: Low Back Pain Syndrome, 3rd Ed. Philadelphia, F. A. Davis Co., 1981, p. 3.)

FIGURE 37–3. Functional unit: dorsal view. Lumbar vertebral functional unit viewed from above. (From Cailliet, R.: Low Back Pain Syndrome, 2nd Ed. Philadelphia, F. A. Davis Co., 1968, p. 6.)

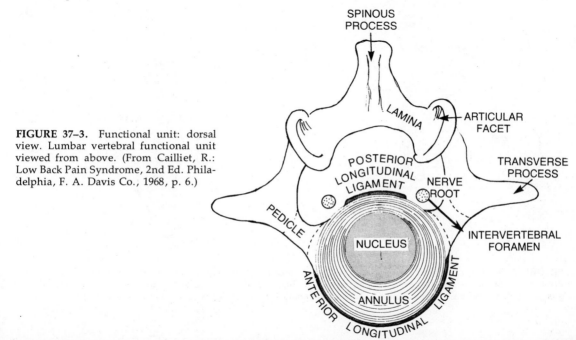

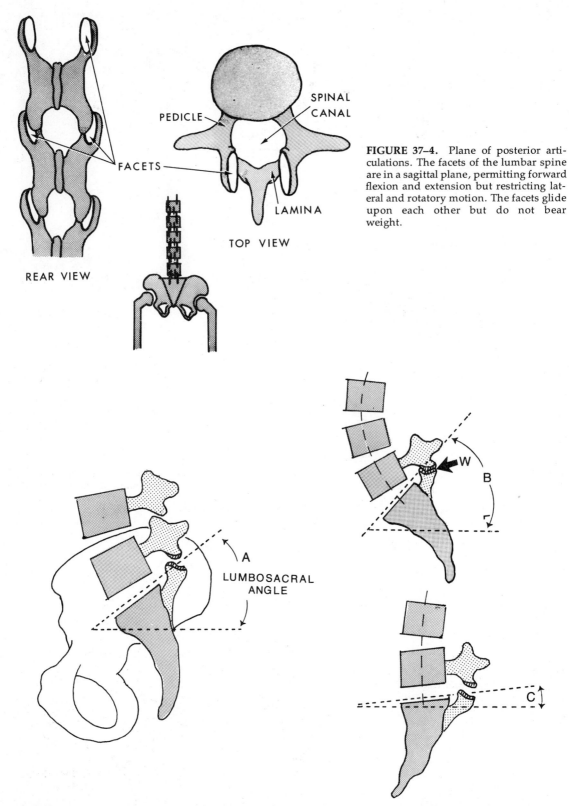

FACETS

PEDICLE

SPINAL
CANAL

LAMINA

TOP VIEW

REAR VIEW

FIGURE 37–4. Plane of posterior articulations. The facets of the lumbar spine are in a sagittal plane, permitting forward flexion and extension but restricting lateral and rotatory motion. The facets glide upon each other but do not bear weight.

A
LUMBOSACRAL
ANGLE

W
B

C

FIGURE 37–5. Facet weight-bearing due to increased lordosis. *A,* reveals the normal lumbosacral angle in which the facet surfaces are not abnormally compressed. *B,* Because of the increased sacral angle, the facets become weight-bearing and pain may result. *C,* shows the separation of the facets as the sacral angle decreases.

Erect stance is maintained by ligamentous support and intermittent muscular contraction. The angle of the pelvis maintains the balance of the superincumbent lumbar, thoracic, and cervical lordotic and kyphotic curves (Fig. 37–5). The equality of leg length and horizontality of the pelvis determine the erectness of the vertebral column.

LOW BACK PAIN

The most common of musculoskeletal pains that confront the physiatrist is the low back pain syndrome. There are numerous etiologies and theoretical mechanisms that require careful history, precise clinical examination, and specific laboratory confirmation.

Organic disease, such as multiple myeloma, Paget's disease, metastatic invasion, spondylitis, compression fractures, vascular lesions, etc., must always be considered and ruled out by appropriate studies. Low back pain referred from other sites must also be ruled out, e.g., sacroiliac pain referred from the thoracolumbar junction (T12).

The mechanical low back etiologies can be classified as static (postural) or kinetic (faulty biomechanics). Of the static type etiology, the most prevalent is excessive lordosis (Fig. 37–6). The mechanism is weight-bearing assumed by the facet joints, posterior compression of the disc causing posterior compression upon the posterior longitudinal ligament, and closure of the intervertebral foramina.

The diagnosis is based on the history and, during the examination, re-creation of the hyperextension of the lumbar lordosis which reproduces the patient's pain symptoms.

X-ray examination frequently reveals increase in the lumbosacral angle with approximation of posterior facets, but this cannot be quantitated with normal values. Narrowing of intervertebral disc space between L4-L5 and L5-S1 is increasingly more prevalent with age and can be elicited in 50 to 60 per cent of adults past the age of 50 years. Treatment is that of decreasing lordosis and developing good abdominal wall strength: in essence, improving posture and modifying working and standing positions.

Spondylolisthesis and Spondylolysis

These are structural abnormalities of the spine that can give rise to low back pain.

Spondylolisthesis

Spondylolisthesis, which is a forward slipping of the superior upon the immediately inferior vertebra (e.g., L4 upon L5 or L5 upon S1), has numerous etiologies. Normally, L5 is prevented from slipping forward

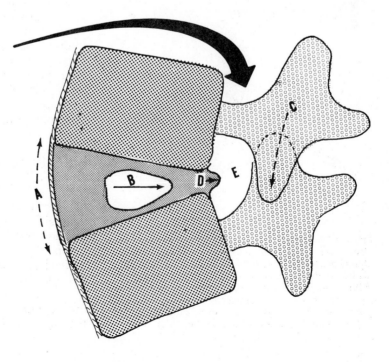

FIGURE 37–6. Static low back pain. Increased lumbar lordosis fully extends anterior longitudinal ligament (A), compresses nucleus (B), which then bulges posteriorly (D) and presses upon sensitized posterior longitudinal ligament. Neural arch approximates (E), compressing facets (C) and narrowing intervertebral foramina (E). (From Cailliet, R.: Low Back Pain Syndrome, 3rd Ed. Philadelphia, F. A. Davis Co., 1981, p. 59.)

upon S1 by the annular fibers of the intervertebral disc, mechanical block of the posterior facets, and an intact neural arch and pedicles. Defects of any of these structures can permit listhesis.

Spondylolysis

A defect in the pars interarticularis, termed spondylolysis, may be evidenced in listhesis (Fig. 37–7). There is some controversy as to whether this is a congenital defect, a neonatal fracture, or a condition acquired in adult life. There is incomplete agreement as to whether the listhesis follows or causes the defect. The pars interarticularis may merely be elongated without a break in continuity.

When there is a deficiency of normal mechanics that prevent excessive shear, only

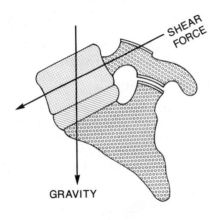

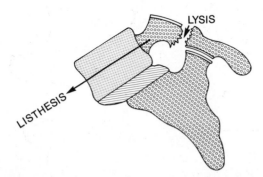

FIGURE 37–7. Mechanism of spondylolisthesis. Gravity compression combined with shear stress of the oblique vertebral angle does not cause forward sliding (listhesis) due to mechanical action of neural arch. With defect in the arch, facet, or pars interarticularis, the shear stress is unopposed, allowing listhesis. (From Cailliet, R.: Low Back Pain Syndrome, 3rd Ed. Philadelphia, F. A. Davis Co., 1981, p. 188.)

the annular fibers of the disc prevent listhesis. In the elderly and the excessively lordotic, disc degeneration may permit listhesis, with secondary facet and isthmus changes.

Diagnosis of this condition is the finding of excessive segmental lordosis and often a palpable bony prominence of the lumbosacral segment. Specific diagnosis is by A-P, lateral, and bilateral oblique x-rays of the lumbosacral articulation.

Attenuation of the pars interarticularis with or without a break in continuity occurs early in life, at 14 years in girls and 16 years in boys, and becomes symptomatic. There may be gradual slipping, but onset of pain may be sudden and violent. Neurologic involvement, including hamstring spasm, occurs as a result of compression of the cauda equina.

The usual conservative management is reduction of excessive lordosis to decrease the sacral angle. This requires an exercise program, weight reduction, and occasionally bracing or corsetting. The following exercises are recommended:

1. Instructions in pelvic tilting, in both the prone and the erect position, to decrease lordosis.

2. Low back stretching exercises.

3. Abdominal isometric strengthening exercises.

4. Posture and functional daily activities performed with decreased lordosis.

Severe progression of pain and neurological impairment are indications to consider surgical intervention. Merely finding a pars interarticularis defect is not an indication for surgery, as many patients with x-ray defects have no symptoms because their defect is held securely by fibrous binding. Other sources of low back pain in the presence of this condition must be considered.

KINETIC LOW BACK PAIN

The spine moves in a specific integrated manner as dictated by the facet alignments, ligamentous limitations, and neuromuscular mechanisms. To permit pain-free movements, daily activities must not exceed these limitations. The normal spine articulates in the following coordinated manner:

1. The lumbar spine flexes and extends in a sagittal plane as directed by the plane of the facets. In forward flexion the sacrospinal

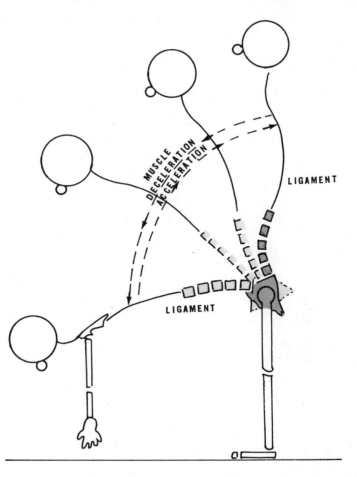

FIGURE 37–8. Muscular deceleration and acceleration of the forward flexing spine from the erect ligamentous support to the fully flexed ligamentous restriction. Muscle eccentric and concentric contraction permits forward flexion and re-extension. (From Cailliet, R.: Low Back Pain Syndrome, 3rd Ed. Philadelphia, F. A. Davis Co., 1981, p. 46.)

muscles actively elongate until full flexion has been reached, at which point the muscles cease to contract, probably by inhibitory impulses arising from the vertebral ligaments. This has been termed the "critical point" (Fig. 37–8).

2. Forward flexion occurs to the point of reversing the lumbar lordosis; it is limited by the supraspinous ligaments posteriorly and the posterior fibers of the annulus fibrosus.

3. Pelvic rotation occurs about the hip joints to change the sacral angle.

4. The erector spinae muscles elongate to gradually decelerate the forward flexion and smoothly contract to regain the erect lordotic posture.

5. Forward flexion and re-extension physiologically conform to "lumbar-pelvic rhythm" and must adhere to the direction dictated by the facet joints (Fig. 37–9).

Violation of the above can result in low back pain with or without nerve root entrapment causing local and, ultimately, radicular pain.

The lumbar spine facets, by their alignment, prevent lateral and rotatory movement of the functional unit in the erect or hyperextended position, but in flexion the facets separate and thus place all the rotatory torque stress upon the annular fibers. The rotatory movement in the flexed posture is a major factor in disc herniation and degeneration.

Sites and Causation of Pain

Most anatomic structures of the functional units are capable of eliciting pain. Some tissues are more sensitive as nociceptive sites and can be postulated as the major sites of local or referred pain (Fig. 37–10).

In the functional unit the following conclusions have been substantiated:

1. The posterior longitudinal ligament is innervated by the posterior recurrent meningeal nerve and has clinically been confirmed as a source and site of pain.[1]

2. The nucleus pulposus of the interver-

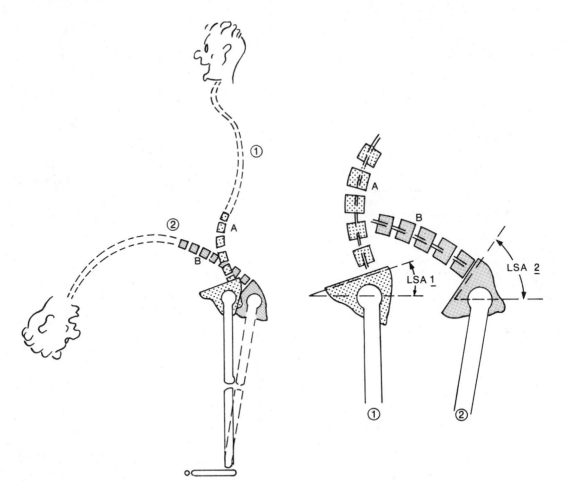

FIGURE 37–9. Lumbar pelvic rhythm. As the lumbar lordosis reverses there is a simultaneous synchronous pelvic rotation as depicted in LSA_1 to LSA_2.

tebral disc normally is avascular and aneural and remains controversial as a source of pain.[2-4] Intradiscal injections of irritating substances have been found to cause low back pain,[5] especially when there has been some herniation of the nucleus into the surrounding annulus.

Mechanisms of Pain

Poor conditioning and faulty biomechanical action probably cause most kinetic low back pain. Weak abdominal muscles impose a great stress upon the discs and allow increased lordosis.[6, 7] Improving the strength of back muscles has not proved to be beneficial except in patients who perform excessively strenuous work and have become debilitated from their usual occupation by an intercurrent illness or injury.

Faulty bending, stooping, and lifting cause

the vast majority of low back injuries. In the flexed position the facets separate and place all the rotatory torque forces upon the annular fibers when flexion is accompanied by rotation. These fibers have limited extensibility and will rupture, pull away from the endplate, and ultimately permit the normally enclosed nucleus pulposus to escape[8] into the surrounding annulus. In reextending from the flexed position, if reextension of the lumbar lordosis occurs before the pelvis is derotated, the facets can "lock" or the annular fibers of the disc can become torn. Back pain with or without radiculitis can result (Fig. 37–11).

Clinical Manifestations

Careful history elicits the exact manner in which pain was produced. Distraction of the

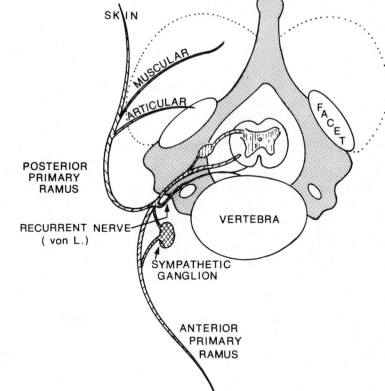

FIGURE 37–10. Innervation of the cervical and lumbar roots: The posterior primary ramus divides into skin, muscular, and articular branches; the anterior primary ramus, with a sympathetic innervation, proceeds to the dermatome and myotome areas. The recurrent nerve supplies the posterior longitudinal ligament and the dura.

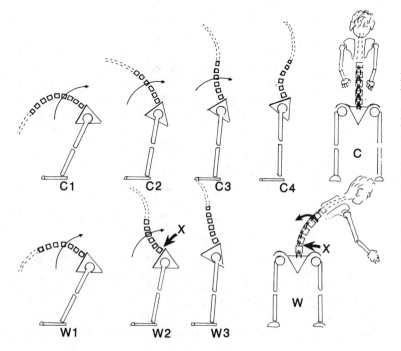

FIGURE 37–11. Proper and improper flexion reextension. Upper figure depicts proper reextension with simultaneous derotation of the pelvis and return of the lumbar lordosis. Bottom figure shows premature return of the lordosis before adequate derotation of the pelvis. Pain occurs from this forward cantilevered excessive lordosis. Faulty reextension to the erect posture is further aggravated by rotating the lumbar spine, thus causing the facets to become asymmetrically aligned and the disc to be subjected to rotating torque forces. (From Cailliet, R.: Low Back Pain Syndrome, 3rd Ed. Philadelphia, F. A. Davis Co., 1981, p. 77.)

patient by anxiety, depression, anger, haste, etc., may cause faulty biomechanical function.

Clinical Findings

1. Erector spinae spasm causes the antalgic posture and limited flexion. The exact muscles that are involved are not clearly delineated.
2. Functional scoliosis is usually away from the side of the radicular pain but not necessarily always present in that direction.
3. "Positive S.L.R.": straight-leg raising may be limited due to its effect on rotating the pelvis, protective hamstring spasm, or stretch pain of the irritated sciatic nerve. Pain from simultaneous nuchal flexion, or ankle dorsiflexion, while performing the test, corroborates the "positive" straight-leg raising to be a nerve pain.
4. Neurological deficit: objective findings such as sensory or motor impairment of a root(s), or subjective paresthesias or hypesthesia in dermatome areas.

Treatment of Acute Low Back Pain

1. Rest in antigravity position: semiflexion usually best tolerated.
2. Medication for pain.

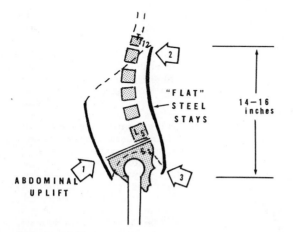

FIGURE 37–12. Corset principle for "flat lumbar spine." The three-point principle of the corset shows the long stays with contact at T₁₂ and low point at sacrum. The stays are flattened. The forward position of the corset presses up against the abdomen and also presses the back against the stays. (From Cailliet, R.: Low Back Pain Syndrome, 3rd Ed. Philadelphia, F. A. Davis Co., 1981, p. 127.)

3. Explanation and reassurances to the patient.
4. Frequent local applications of ice to decrease painful muscle spasm.

After the acute condition subsides, gradual ambulation with carefully outlined manner of bending, stooping, and lifting is taught and initiated. If an acute episode has been one of a number of frequent episodes, or if pain remains to significant degree after a period of bed rest, a back brace or corset may be of value. The brace (1) must be fitted for a specified *limited* time in conjunction with a gradual exercise program and instruction in proper posture and functional habits; (2) must assist by its contour in decreasing lumbar lordosis;[12] (3) must have an uplift abdominal support; (4) must be long enough posteriorly to contact the sacrum and limit thoracolumbar function (Fig. 37–12).

CHRONIC LOW BACK PAIN

Persistence of disabling pain with equivocal physical findings requires (1) psychological evaluation; (2) consideration of intra-articular facet steroid anesthetic injection; (3) posterior primary division chemical rhizotomy; (4) transcutaneous electrical stimulation; (5) biofeedback for relaxation training; (6) epidural steroid injection.[11, 12]

Indications for Surgical Referral

The primary indication for surgery is progressive neurological deficit(s) in spite of a period of adequate conservative treatment. Persistence of incapacitating pain after a prolonged conservative treatment program that causes economic duress to the patient is an indication for surgical consideration. This must follow psychological as well as physiological evaluation of the patient.

Presence of urinary retention, indicating a "neurogenic" bladder, is not a surgical emergency. Urinary retention may be treated conservatively and usually responds well without surgical intervention.

Myelography is usually required by most surgeons before surgery to give a differential diagnosis and confirm the level of the lesion. The dye currently used in contrast studies is of potential danger as a possible cause of arachnoiditis. Careful clinical evaluation and electromyographic localization are useful to avoid Pantopaque studies. Air myelography and new dyes may some day replace current techniques.

DEGENERATIVE DISC DISEASE: "OSTEOARTHRITIS"

Dehydration and fragmentation of the intervertebral disc with consequent effects upon the functional unit constitute the entity of degenerative disc disease. Over the years, trauma and possibly inherited vulnerability gradually dehydrate the disc, decreasing its hydromatic effectiveness. The vertebral bodies approximate, causing laxity of the longitudinal ligaments. The intradiscal pressure forces disc matrix between the bodies and ligaments, which gradually forms the nidus for osteophytes (Fig. 37–13).

Anterior compression of the functional unit causes posterior approximation, narrowing the intervertebral foramina and approximating the zygapophyseal joints. Owing to compression the facet joints undergo degenerative hypertrophic changes. All the tissues capable of pain are made more vulnerable, and the stability and flexibility of the functional unit are impaired. These changes may remain asymptomatic until the back is used in a faulty manner[13] or exposed to severe external forces.

SPINAL STENOSIS

Narrowing of the spinal canal (Fig. 37–13) can cause a specific clinical entity termed "pseudoclaudication." The patient afflicted with spinal stenosis complains of pain in the distribution of a nerve root (so-called "sciatica") after a period of walking or prolonged standing. Pain coming on after a period of walking, were it true claudication (on a vascular basis), would subside or disappear when the walking stopped. In spinal stenosis the patient must sit or assume a flexed posture to decrease the lumbar lordosis. The pain subsides and the patient can resume walking.

Pseudoclaudication after prolonged standing also can be relieved by a flexion posture to decrease the lumbar lordosis. This may be accomplished by squatting or sitting.

Conservative management is possible by "flat back exercises" to decrease the lordo-

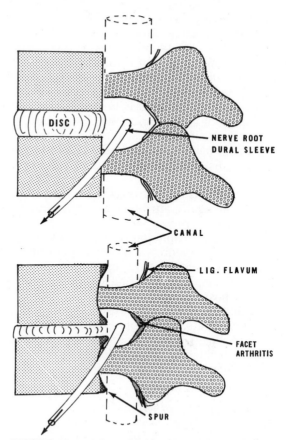

FIGURE 37–13. Spondylosis. Upper figure depicts normal functional unit, lower figure spondylosis. With disc narrowing, spurs form on the vertebrae, narrowing the foramen and compressing the facets. Facet degenerative arthritis results, bulging the ligamentum flavum into the spinal canal. Spinal stenosis results. (From Cailliet, R.: Low Back Pain Syndrome, 3rd Ed. Philadelphia, F. A. Davis Co., 1981, p. 181.)

sis and/or by wearing a lumbar brace. The specific diagnosis is made clinically and verified by x-ray, CAT scan, or myelography. Surgical decompression may be required when disability persists in spite of conservative management or disability increases to an unacceptable level.

CERVICAL PAIN

Pain in the neck, or from the neck, constitutes the second most prevalent musculoskeletal disability confronting the physiatrist. The functional unit in most ways is identical to the lumbar spine segment, except that it glides in an anterior-posterior direction. Flexion separates the neural arches and extension approximates them. Flexion opens the intervertebral foramina and extension closes them.[14] Rotation opens the intervertebral foramina and extension closes them.[14] Rotation opens the foramina on the side from which the head is turned and closes those toward which the head is turned.[15] This fact is important in evaluating the clinical history and the physical findings and explains mechanisms of pain in the neck and pain referred in the distribution of the cervical nerve roots.[16]

Pain and disability from the cervical spine can be generally attributed to either trauma or arthritis. Trauma includes (1) hyperflexion-hyperextension injury with soft tissue trauma; (2) posture in which hyperlordosis causes foraminal closure, nerve entrapment, and facet impingement; and (3) chronic "tension," postural or emotional, in which the unit and all its tissues, especially the muscular elements, are compressed, resulting in pain. Arthritis is usually of the degenerative type, in which all of the changes described in the lumbar spine are in evidence.

Cervical Pain or Cervical Referred Pain

The history reveals whether the pain is acute or chronic and describes the mechanism considered to cause the pain, and the physical examination reveals which tissues are involved and the degree of injury. Reproduction of symptoms by positions and movements of the head and neck clarify the mechanism and give indication for meaningful treatment. Muscle testing of the upper extremity plays a valuable part in the neurologic examination to determine the site and extent of nerve root entrapment.[17]

Treatment

The acute condition requires rest, relaxation of tissues, and decrease of inflammation. Rest by reclining is the best method. A collar that is comfortable and custom fitted is of value but does not significantly immobilize the cervical spine. Modalities such as icing, massage, heat, ultrasound, and manipulation have their indications and are beneficial when properly applied. Modifications of posture and daily activities are usually mandatory. Cervical traction essentially decreases lordosis, opens the foramina, and elongates the erector spine. This is of clinical value if it is applied to cause slight flexion of the cervical spine. All other modalities listed for the low back, as well as indications for surgical interventions, apply to the cervical spine.

In rheumatoid arthritis there is definite atlantoaxial instability due to decrease and resultant laxity of the supporting ligamentous tissues that encircle the odontoid process. Subluxation of the atlas upon the axis can occur from trauma, and treatment of a moderate severity can similarly cause disruption of the joint. As the contents of the spinal canal are the cord and its roots, subluxation can result in a high level quadriplegia. The rheumatoid arthritic patient must be protected from such a stress by avoidance of specific activities and excessive treatment and should be guarded by a collar or brace.

SCOLIOSIS

Scoliosis is the most deforming orthopedic problem confronting children. It is a potentially progressive condition that affects children during their active growth phase. Ultimate structural changes can only be corrected surgically; thus, early recognition and aggressive treatment are necessary.[18-20]

Scoliosis is unphysiological lateral curving from the midline. Owing to vertebral alignment, the mechanical alignment of the posterior articulations, and the ligamentous muscular constraints of the vertebral column, lateral curving is gradually accompanied by simultaneous rotation of the vertebral bodies toward the convex side of the curve. The curvature at first is functional in that it is reversible and disappears in the recumbent posture, but gradually it undergoes structural changes. A structural scoliosis is a fixed curve that does not correct on lateral bending or in the supine position. The lumbar rotation is mild in its cosmetic appearance but by virtue of the ribs being firmly attached to the thoracic vertebrae, the ribs undergo rotatory structural deformities in thoracic rotation. Lumbar scoliosis is more apt to cause low back pain.

The symptoms of scoliosis are primarily those of undesirable appearance. The cosmetic sequelae are significant in that scoliosis is more frequent in girls by a ratio of 9:1. Another sequela that justifies treatment is

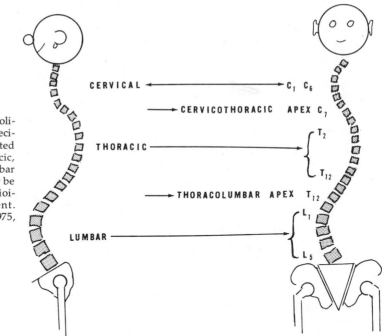

FIGURE 37–14. Spinal level of scoliosis curvatures. The scoliosis is specified to exist at the spinal level related to either the cervical, cervicothoracic, thoracic, thoracolumbar, or lumbar vertebrae. More than one level may be involved. (From Cailliet, R.: Scoliosis: Diagnosis and Management. Philadelphia, F. A. Davis Co., 1975, p. 22.)

the prevalence of cardiopulmonary complications secondary to rib cage deformity with impairment of vital capacity, pulmonary hypertension, and cor pulmonale. Pain is considered to be the third sequela, but there is controversy regarding the incidence of pain in this entity as compared to that in a comparable population of nonscoliotic patients.

Scoliosis is specified as to its site in the vertebral column of its apex: a cervical curve has its apex from C1 to C6, thoracic curve between T2 and T12, lumbar curve between L1 to L4, and the thoracolumbar curve at T12 to L1 (Fig. 37–14). Curves are also designated as primary or compensatory (secondary). They are also termed major or minor depending on their prominence and significance. By standardization of the Scoliosis Research Society, all curves are now measured by the Cobb method (Fig. 37–15). Recordable measurement of rotation remains unstandardized.

Early examination is best done by the examiner sighting horizontally along the spine of the patient, who stands with hips flexed at 90 degrees and legs fully extended. Early minimal curves are frequently seen only in this type of examination (Fig. 37–16).

Curving may progress until epiphyseal closure is completed and the end of growth has been reached. This end point is estimated by

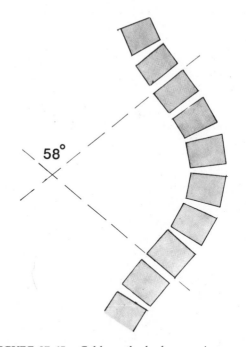

FIGURE 37–15. Cobb method of measuring curvature. A line is drawn along the upper margin of the vertebra that inclines most toward the concavity. A line is also drawn on the inferior border of the lower vertebra with greatest angulation toward the concavity. The angle of these transecting lines is noted and recorded. The apical vertebra is noted but does not enter into the measurement. (From Cailliet, R.: Scoliosis: Diagnosis and Management. Philadelphia, F. A. Davis Co., 1975, p. 29.)

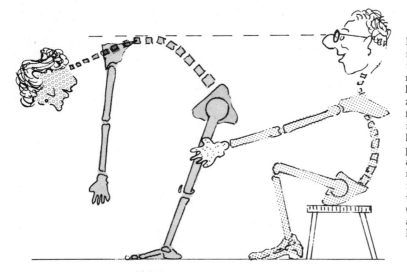

FIGURE 37–16. Clinical examination method for scoliosis. With the patient bent forward at a right angle (90 degrees) at the hips, the examiner sights horizontally down the entire spine from behind. The patient's legs must be fully extended at the knees, his arms dangling with palms facing, and his feet preferably bare. This method of examination will disclose early minimal scoliosis not easily seen when the child is erect. (From Cailliet, R.: Scoliosis: Diagnosis and Management. Philadelphia, F. A. Davis Co., 1975, p. 33.)

viewing the iliac crest apophysis (Fig. 37–17). When the iliac apophysis has completely crested the ilium and has fused, all vertebral growth is considered terminated.[21] Curves of 50 degrees or more are capable of progression even after apophyseal closure by virtue of disc compression on the concave side of the curve.

Treatment

In a young child with definite potential for growth, a curve of 10 to 15 degrees can be evaluated at three-month intervals with standing standardized x-rays during standing. If there is beginning rotation, even with merely 10 to 15 degrees of lateral deviation, a Milwaukee brace is indicated. An unbalanced curve that deviates laterally to the center of gravity is a poor prognostic sign (Fig. 37–18). These curves tend to progress rapidly. The principal aim of treatment is to realign the spine directly above the sacrum (Fig. 37–19).

A 20-degree curve is indication for bracing. A 50-degree curve is difficult to brace and should be considered for correction and internal fixation with a Harrington rod and surgical fusion. Curves of 50 degrees or

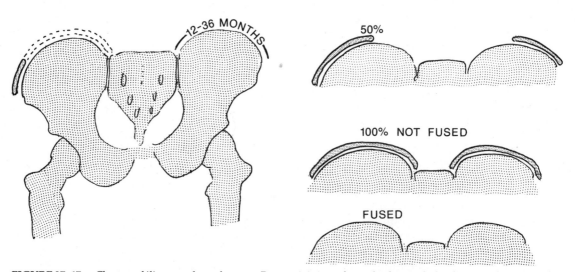

FIGURE 37–17. Closure of iliac apophyseal center. By termination of vertebral growth the iliac apophyses are also considered to be fused and spinal growth ended. (From Cailliet, R.: Scoliosis: Diagnosis and Management. Philadelphia, F. A. Davis Co., 1975, p. 37.)

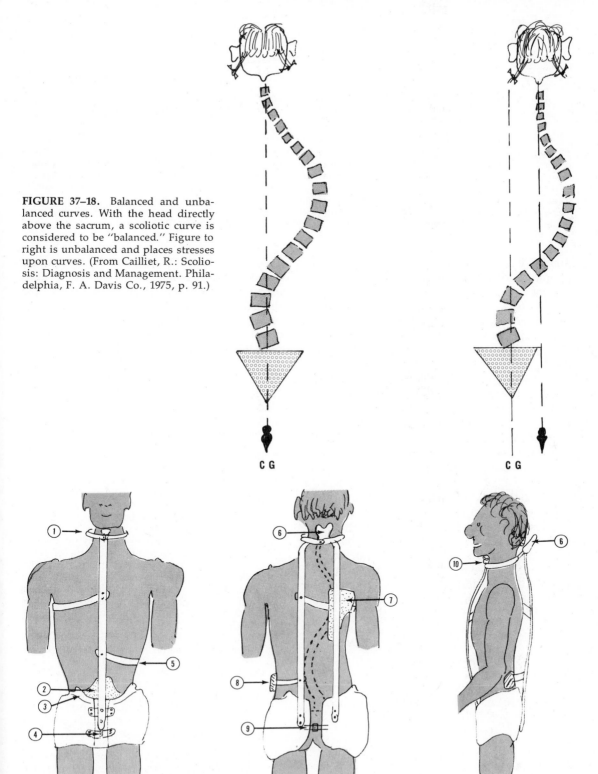

FIGURE 37–18. Balanced and unbalanced curves. With the head directly above the sacrum, a scoliotic curve is considered to be "balanced." Figure to right is unbalanced and places stresses upon curves. (From Cailliet, R.: Scoliosis: Diagnosis and Management. Philadelphia, F. A. Davis Co., 1975, p. 91.)

FIGURE 37–19. Milwaukee Brace. 1, Cervical ring. 2, Abdominal pad. 3, Iliac crest band. 4, Closure of iliac band for removal of brace. 5, Lateral band. 6, Occipital pad. 7, Lateral and posterior thoracic pad. 8, Lateral lumbar pad. 9, Posterior fringe. 10, Mandibular pad. (From Cailliet, R.: Scoliosis: Diagnosis and Management. Philadelphia, F. A. Davis Co., 1975, p. 68.)

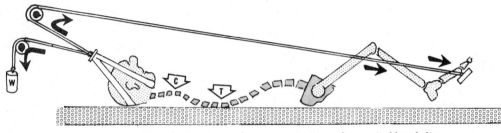

FIGURE 37–20. Cotrel traction. With the patient in the supine position, the cervical head sling passes over a pulley that permits traction by extending the legs against the crossbar attached to the rope. The duration and strength of the traction are graded to the tolerance of the patient under the physician's supervision. When the leg traction force is released, the weight (W) exerts the traction. Cotrel traction (personal observation) distracts the cervical spine (C) with diminution of traction in the thoracic spine (T) and no traction in the lumbar spine. This caudal decrease in traction is undoubtedly due to friction forces of the body on the surface of the bed or plinth. (From Cailliet, R.: Scoliosis: Diagnosis and Management. Philadelphia, F. A. Davis Co., 1975, p. 83.)

greater have been shown to progress *after* apophyseal closure and to predispose the patient to cardiopulmonary complications.

Exercises per se will not deter a curvature that is progressing in a growing child but will maintain flexibility and improve posture. Children placed in a Milwaukee brace or its equivalent must be given exercises to perform within the brace and while out of the brace.[22] The Milwaukee brace, or its equivalent, is a kinetic, not a static, brace. The lateral pads hold the lateral curves from going further but *do not* passively correct. The exercises of "pulling away" from the pads are considered to be the corrective forces.

The pelvic band fits the pelvis and decreases the lordosis. The collar head band applies distracting forces which elongate the spine, thus decreasing the cervical, thoracic, and lumbar curves. The lateral or posterolateral pads prevent further lateral rotatory deformity and indicate to the patient the direction from which to distract in the exercises. In children with "round back," an increased dorsal kyphosis, either idiopathic or from Scheuermann's disease, a Milwaukee brace with specific exercises is effective. Traction, specified by Cotrel, has strong European advocacy. This is applied for inpatient, clinic, or home use and supplemented with exercises (Fig. 37–20).

Conclusion

Early detection of scoliosis or round back and energetic treatment with proper conserv-ative methods prevent the inevitable cosmetic and disabling conditions in later life. These are some of the challenges presented to the physiatrist. Treatment, after careful clinical evaluation of painful disabling and deforming spinal disorders, must be based on precise knowledge of functional anatomy.

REFERENCES

1. Smyth, M. J., and Wright, W.: Sciatica and the intervertebral disc, an experimental study. J. Bone Joint Surg., 40A:1401–1418, 1958.
2. Holt, E. P.: The question of lumbar discography. J. Bone Joint Surg., 50A:720–726, 1968.
3. Hirsch, C.: Etiology and pathogenesis of low back pain. Isr. J. Med. Sci., 2:362–370, 1966.
4. Hirsch, C., Ingelmark, B. E., and Miller, M.: The anatomical basis for low back pain. Acta Orthop. Scand., 33:1–17, 1963.
5. Cloward, R. B.: Cervical diskography: A contribution to the etiology of mechanism of neck, shoulder and arm pain. Ann. Surg., 150:1052–1064, 1959.
6. Bartelink, D. L.: The role of abdominal pressure in relieving the pressure on the lumbar intervertebral discs. J. Bone Joint Surg., 39B:718–725, 1957.
7. Davis, P. R., and Traup, J. D. G.: Effects on the trunk of erecting pit props at different working heights. Ergonomics, 9:475–484, 1966.
8. Cailliet, R.: Soft Tissue Pain and Disability. Philadelphia, F. A. Davis, 1977.
9. Mennell, J. M.: The therapeutic use of cold. J. Am. Osteopath. Assoc., 74:1146–1158, 1975.
10. Morris, J. M., and Lucas, D. B.: Physiological considerations in bracing of the spine. Orthop. Prosthet. Appl. J., 17:37–44, 1963.
11. Delke, T. F. W., Burry, H. C., and Grahame, R.: Extradural corticosteroid injection in the management of lumbar nerve root compression. Br. Med., 2:635–637, 1973.
12. Burn, J. M. B., and Langdon, L.: Lumbar epidural

injection for treatment of chronic sciatica. Rheumatol. Phys. Med., 10:368–374, 1970.

13. Epstein, J. A., Epstein, B. S., Rosenthal, A. D., Carras, R., and Lavine, L. S.: Sciatica caused by nerve root entrapment in the lateral recess — the superior facet syndrome. J. Neurosurg., 36:5:584–589, 1972.

14. Cailliet, R.: Neck and Arm Pain. Philadelphia, F. A. Davis, 1964.

15. Fielding, J. W.: Cineroentgenography (dentgenography) of the normal cervical spine. J. Bone Joint Surg., 39A:1280–1281, 1957.

16. Jackson, R.: The Cervical Syndrome, 2nd Ed. Springfield, Ill., Charles C Thomas, Publisher.

17. Cailliet, R.: Scoliosis: Diagnosis and Management. Philadelphia, F. A. Davis, 1975.

18. Rabin, G. C. (Ed.): Scoliosis. New York, Academic Press, 1973.

19. Hoppenfeld, S.: Scoliosis: A Manual of Concept and Treatment. Philadelphia, J. B. Lippincott, 1967.

20. Roaf, R.: Vertebral growth and its mechanical control. J. Bone Joint Surg., 42B:40–59, 1960.

21. Blount, W. P., and Bolinski, J.: Physical therapy in the nonoperative treatment of scoliosis. Phys. Ther., 47:919–925, 1967.

22. Cailliet, R.: Exercises for scoliosis. In Basmajian, J. (ed.): Therapeutic Exercise, 3rd Ed. Baltimore, The Williams and Wilkins Co., 1978, pp. 430–449.

SUPPLEMENTAL BIBLIOGRAPHY

American Academy of Orthopedic Surgeons: Symposium on the Spine. November, 1967, pp. 188–240.

Badgley, C. E., and Arbor, A.: The articular facets in relation to low back pain and sciatic radiation. J. Bone Joint Surg., 23:481–496.

Bennett, R. L.: Recognition and care of elderly scoliosis. Arch. Phys. Med., 42:211–225, 1961.

Bergquist-Ullman, M., and Larsson, U.: Acute low back pain in industry: A controlled study with specific reference to therapy and confounding factors. Acta Orthop. Scand., Suppl. 170, 1977.

Blount, W. P.: The Principles of Treatment, According to Curve Patterns of Scoliosis and Round Back with the Milwaukee Brace. Postgraduate Course in the Management and Care of the Scoliosis Patient. New York Orthopedic Hospital, 1969.

Bourdillon, J. F.: Spinal Manipulation. New York, Appleton-Century Crofts, 1970.

Cailliet, R.: Low Back Pain Syndrome. Philadelphia, F. A. Davis, 1962.

Chrisman, O. D., et al.: A study of the results following rotatory manipulation of the lumbar intervertebral disc syndrome. J. Bone Joint Surg., 46A:517–526, 1964.

Cobb, J. R.: Outline for study of scoliosis. Instruct. Lect. Am. Acad. Orthop. Surg., 5:261–275, 1948.

De Palma, A. F., and Rothman, R. H.: The Intervertebral Disc. Philadelphia, W. B. Saunders Co., 1970.

Falconer, M. A., McGeorge, M., and Begg, A. C.: Observations on the course and mechanism of symptom-production in sciatica and low back pain. J. Neurol. Neurosurg. Psychiatry, 2:13, 1948.

Farfan, H. F.: Mechanical Disorders of the Low Back. Philadelphia, Lea and Febiger, 1973.

Harrington, P. R.: Treatment of scoliosis —Correction and internal fixation by spine instrumentation. J. Bone Joint Surg., 44A:591–610, 1962.

Hirsch, C.: Studies on the mechanism of low back pain. Acta Orthop. Scand., 24:261, 1951.

Holt, L.: Cervical, dorsal and lumbar spinal syndromes. Acta Orthop. Scand., Suppl. 17, 1954.

Kraus, H.: Clinical Treatment of Back and Neck Pain. New York, McGraw-Hill Book Co., 1970.

Lewin, T.: Osteoarthritis in lumbar synovial joints. Acta Orthop. Scand., Suppl. 73, 1964.

Magora, A.: Investigation of the relationship between low back pain and occupation, age, sex, community, education and other factors. Industr. Med. Surg., 39:465–471, 1971.

Moe, J. H.: Management of idiopathic scoliosis. Clin. Orthop., 20:169–184, 1957.

Morris, J. M., Lucas, D. B., and Bresler, B.: The role of the trunk in the stability of the spine. J. Bone Joint Surg., 43A:327, 1961.

Nachemson, A. L.: Lumbar intradiscal pressure. Acta Orthop. Scand., Suppl. 43, 1960.

Nachemson, A. L.: The lumbar spine: An orthopedic challenge. Spine, 1:59–71, 1976.

Nachemson, A.: Physiotherapy for low back pain patients. Scand. J. Rehab. Med., 1:85–90, 1969.

Norton, P. L., and Brown, T.: The immobilizing efficacy of back braces: Their effect on the posture and motion of the lumbosacral joint. J. Bone Joint Surg., 39A:111, 1957.

Sarno, J. E.: Therapeutic exercise for back pain. In Basmajian, J. (ed.): Therapeutic Exercises, 3rd Ed., Baltimore, The Williams & Wilkins Co., 1978.

Schmorl, G. H., and Junghanns, H.: The Human Spine in Health and Disease. New York, Grune and Stratton, 1959.

Stern, R. A., Wolf, J. R., Murphy, R. W., and Akeson, W. H.: Aspects of chronic low back pain. Psychosomatics, 14:52–56, 1973.

Turek, S. L.: Orthopaedics. Philadelphia, J. B. Lippincott, 1959.

Williams, P. C.: Conservation management of lesions of the lumbosacral spine. Instruct. Lect., Am. Acad. Orthop. Surg., 10:90–121, 1953.

38

MANAGEMENT OF NEUROGENIC DYSFUNCTION OF THE BLADDER AND BOWEL

INDER PERKASH

THE BLADDER

The management of neurogenic bladder dysfunction is too important to be left as a matter for occasional consultation. The urologist should be an active member of the team that follows the patient day by day. By the same token, any physician charged with the overall care of patients with this disorder, whatever his own specialty, must have an understanding of the urinary tract dysfunction and the methods available for treatment according to the needs of the individual patient. Improvement of patient care in the clinical problems of voiding dysfunction lies in a better understanding of neurophysiology and pharmacology of micturition and the ability to apply these principles in the study of micturition (urodynamic evaluation) in such patients.

Neuroanatomy and Neuropharmacology

The essential peripheral components of voiding and continence are the bladder musculature (detrusor), bladder neck mechan-

ism, posterior urethral smooth muscle, and striated pelvic and periurethral muscles. The smooth muscle fibers of the bladder body are described as being composed of three layers — the external and internal longitudinal layers and the middle layer, which is the thickest and is composed of circularly running muscle fibers. All layers intermingle and the muscular wall of the bladder is to be considered as a continuum of smooth musculature, the vesical detrusor.[1] However, as the detrusor muscles converge on the internal orifice of the bladder, they tend to become oriented into three layers.[2] The most caudal of the middle circular fibers are thickened and prominent and they form the true bladder neck. This concentric ring of "middle circular layer" fibers is complete anteriorly, while posteriorly it fuses with the trigone. This structure was first described by Heiss in 1915,[3] but later Hutch[4] demonstrated that anatomically and functionally the "fundus ring" or "Heiss ring" fuses with the deep trigone to form a structure that he called the "base plate." A considerable amount of smooth muscle from the bladder extends into the posterior urethra. The striat-

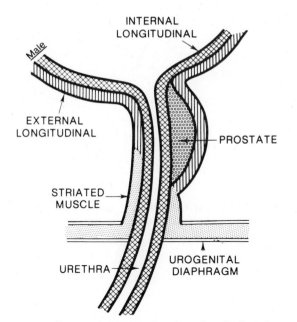

FIGURE 38–1. Schematic drawing of sagittal section showing relationship and extent of striated and plain muscles in the male posterior urethra. (After Hutch.)

ed muscle component of the urethra consists of pelvic floor musculature and periurethral extension. In male subjects the periurethral striated muscle extends between the urogenital diaphragm and the apex of the prostate. This is illustrated in the schematic drawings (after Hutch) in Figures 38–1 and 38–2.

The female urethra and the posterior urethra in the male essentially resemble each other except for the presence of the prostate in the male urethra, which partly displaces the homogeneous anatomic configuration seen in the female urethra. Recent histochemical and electron microscopic studies[5] show a well-developed circular smooth muscle extension from the bladder to the entrance of the ejaculatory ducts in males and a rather less developed extension in females. Furthermore, the distribution of sympathetic nerve fibers in the smooth muscle coat is sparse by comparison with the male bladder neck region. This finding goes along with the necessity for prevention of retrograde ejaculation in the male.

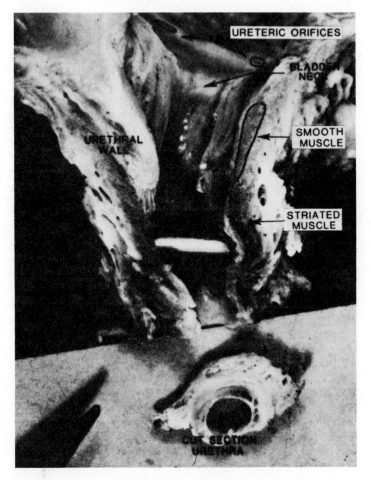

FIGURE 38–2. Musculature and interior bladder neck and cross section of male urethra.

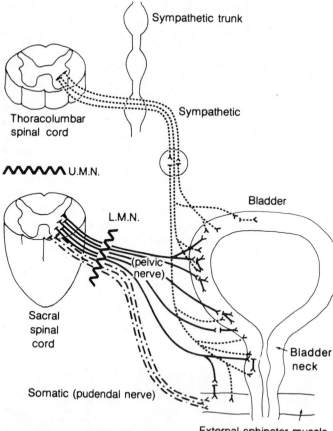

FIGURE 38–3. Innervation of the bladder. (U.M.N. = Upper motor neuron, L.M.N. = lower motor neuron.)

Parasympathetic Nerve Supply. The detrusor muscle is richly supplied by parasympathetic fibers originating from the anterior gray columns of the second, third, and fourth sacral segments of the spinal cord. Figure 38–3 illustrates the innervation of the bladder. It passes through pelvic splanchnic nerves to synapse in the intramural and extramural bladder ganglia. From these ganglia, postganglionic fibers travel to the detrusor muscle. In view of the peripheral location (mostly in the bladder wall) of the parasympathetic postganglionic cell bodies, damage to the pelvic nerves results largely in decentralization rather than denervation of the bladder (autonomous bladder). The parasympathetic nerves secrete acetylcholine at the motor nerve endings and are therefore called cholinergic nerves. This innervation to the bladder is so profuse that nearly every smooth muscle cell is individually supplied by one or more cholinergic nerves. Thus it indicates the importance of the parasympathetic supply initiating and sustaining bladder contraction at micturition.

Sympathetic Nerves. The sympathetic nerve supply originates in cells in the lateral gray column of the spinal cord from the level of T11 to L2. When the sympathetic nerves are stimulated, the nerve endings produce noradrenalin; the muscles that possess alpha-adrenergic receptors contract when noradrenalin is present. Those muscles that possess beta-adrenergic receptors relax, however, in the presence of noradrenalin. The bladder of man[5] shows a predominance of alpha-adrenergic receptors in the muscles of the bladder neck and the proximal urethra and beta-adrenergic receptors in the detrusor muscle of the bladder. Figure 38–4 diagrammatically illustrates the distribution of autonomic receptors of bladder and urethra. Thus, the effect of sympathetic stimulation is to contract the bladder neck and relax the detrusor muscle. The noradrenalin that is produced by the sympathetic nerve endings also acts as an inhibitor of the acetylcholine produced by the parasympathetic nerve endings. When the sympathetic nerves are stimulated, the smooth muscle of the prostate,

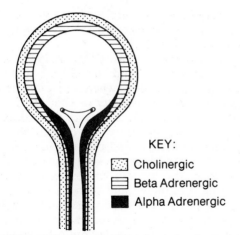

KEY:

▨ Cholinergic

▤ Beta Adrenergic

■ Alpha Adrenergic

FIGURE 38–4. Distribution of autonomic receptors of the bladder and urethra.

seminal vesicles, and ejaculatory ducts contract, resulting in ejaculation. The muscles of the bladder neck simultaneously contract, thereby preventing semen from entering the bladder. A disturbance of this function may result in sterility.

Striated External Urethral Sphincter. There are two components of striated sphincter muscle around the posterior urethra. The circularly arranged fibers surrounding the membranous urethra are usually referred to as external sphincter, and the striated fibers around the prostatic urethra are designated periurethral muscles (see Fig. 38–1). The periurethral striated sphincter is innervated mostly through the pudendal nerve, with fibers originating from the anterior gray columns of the second, third, and fourth sacral segments of the cord. The striated sphincter (external sphincter) fibers around the membranous urethra are considered to be slow twitch muscle fibers and are vital for the maintenance of continence. It has also been demonstrated histochemically[7] that the external urethral sphincter (also called a rhabdosphincter by Gil-Vernet[8] and Winkler[1]) receives triple sympathetic-parasympathetic-somatic innervation. This important study gives a morphologic basis to the observation that the action of the external sphincter is normally coordinated with the bladder smooth muscle.[9-11]

Recent neuropharmacologic studies indicate antagonistic roles of prostaglandins (PGE$_2$ and PGF$_2$) in a variety of organ systems, including bladder.[12-14] PGE$_2$ decreases norepinephrine (NEN) output as well as end-organ responsiveness to NEN and thus is a potent vasodilator and as such antisympathetic. On the other hand, PGF$_2$ increases NEN output at the synaptic terminals and usually causes vasoconstriction. In relation with coordinated activity of bladder, bladder neck, and posterior urethra, prostaglandins may play an important role in the synergistic activity of sympathetic and parasympathetic fibers.

The Central Innervation. Sensory receptors that primarily detect changes in length and tension have also been found in laboratory animals. They connect directly to the brain stem in the pons where the central micturition center is located.[15-17] A variety of positive and negative feedback loops have been uncovered which are believed important in sustaining and then terminating micturition.[18] Although a local reflex arc originating in the bladder, with a sacral micturition center in the conus, produces bladder contractions, the coordination of micturition is known to be influenced by several suprasegmental centers.[19] The cortical centers provide for adequate volitional control of micturition, inhibit uninhibited contractions, and maintain adequate bladder capacity and minimal residual urine. Thus, normal bladder and bladder outlet function is maintained by suprasegmental centers through both autonomic and voluntary nervous control, where the urine keeps collecting in the bladder with gradually increasing feedback through autonomic nerves, maintaining control through cortical awareness and initiating micturition through voluntary effort and the somatic system. Normal micturition is, therefore, entirely a voluntary act secondary to voluntary active contraction of the bladder. Simultaneously, also, contraction of abdominal musculature and diaphragm takes place to raise intra-abdominal pressure, which is not essential for normal micturition. On the other hand, a patient with a cauda equina lesion and an areflexic (noncontractile) bladder may be able to void only after raising his intra-abdominal pressure by suprapubic compression or by bearing down (Credé/Valsalva maneuver).

Normal Voiding

Normal persons can feel when the bladder contains approximately 100 ml of urine. The normal person will also feel a desire to pass urine when the bladder contains 300 to 400 ml of urine. As the bladder fills, the striated muscle sphincter remains contracted; the contraction is mediated through a primitive reflex known as the holding reflex. Normal people do not, however, contract their bladders until they voluntarily trigger the voiding mechanism. The urethral sphincter first relaxes, and then the bladder contracts. A few seconds are required to initiate the voiding process, during which the person must voluntarily get the system working. Thus, if the person feels inhibited or embarrassed (as for example when the patient must void in front of the doctor), the entire process may be slow in starting or may not take place at all.

The first action to take place is the overcoming of the holding reflex. The periurethral striated sphincter is relaxed. At the same time, the bladder neck will relax; immediately thereafter the detrusor muscle of the dome of the bladder contracts, and voiding takes place through a completely open bladder neck and urethra. Voiding will normally continue until the bladder is empty, but voiding can voluntarily be stopped at any point in the process. This extraordinarily well-coordinated process requires perfect synergy between the sympathetic, parasympathetic, and somatic nerve supply. Any dyssynergia in any of these three nerve supplies will lead to difficulties in voiding.

Study of Micturition (Urodynamic Evaluation)

Urodynamic studies in the broad sense of the term include the urine flow rate, the cystometrogram, the urethral pressure profile, and the voiding cystourethrogram. Neuropharmacologic testing with drugs before and after these tests is also being used increasingly to determine the efficacy of a therapeutic drug. Measurement of urine flow rate is done by asking the patient to void into an instrument that can simultaneously record the peak urine flow and also graphically record the pattern of voiding. The total volume divided by the time will give the flow rate per second. Reduced peak flow and increased voiding time could be due to the obstructing effects of the prostatic urethra, to neurogenic bladder dysfunction, or to an overdistended areflexic bladder. To resolve whether decrease in flow is due to bladder or urethral factors, a cystometrogram, along with simultaneous electromyography of the periurethral sphincter and the urethral pressure profile, is helpful.

The cystometrogram (CMG) helps assess bladder function and provides volume-pressure relationship when the bladder is gradually filled with water or CO_2. This test evaluates the contractability of the detrusor muscle, its adjustability to volume, and its capacity to stretch, and the patient's sensation of fullness, desire to void, and pain. The pressure in the bladder can be measured by inserting a catheter and using a water manometer or by a pressure sensor and a multiple channel recorder. A rectal balloon inserted at the same time can discriminate between intravesical and intra-abdominal pressure. The methodology is illustrated in Figure 38–5.

We perform such studies only on patients whose urine is sterile or whose urinary infection is covered adequately with a suitable antibiotic. It is helpful to have the rectum empty. Spinal cord injury patients should have their bowels emptied on the evening before the studies. The patient is asked to void immediately prior to the study to estimate the amount of the residual urine. The cystometrogram is performed by introducing the catheter into the bladder and emptying it completely. Carbon dioxide or sterile water (at 37°C) is introduced as the bladder pressure is simultaneously recorded. Patients must inform the physician or nurse as soon as they notice any sensation of fullness in the bladder and must also announce when they feel the desire to void. Patients are then instructed to void, and during voiding, patients are asked to cease voiding.

The urethral pressure profile is intended to provide an index of urethral resistance to bladder output, enable an assessment of urinary continence, provide distinction between a distensible and fibrotic sphincter urethral segment, and contribute information to enable characterization of detrusor-sphincter dysynergia. However, the intraurethral pressure is a function of the catheter size, the hole size through which fluid is perfused, the fluid perfusion rate, and the distensibility of the urethral sphincter segment; for want of standardization, it is difficult to interpret functionally the value of the peak urethral pressure taken with a certain catheter at a given perfusion rate. A mechanical puller is attached to the catheter to pull it

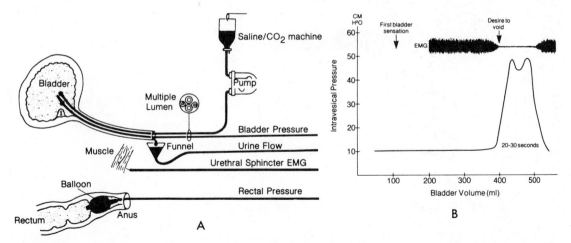

FIGURE 38–5. *A,* Schematic diagram showing method of urodynamic recording of urethral pressure profile, intra-abdominal pressure, and EMG of extenal urethral sphincter. *B,* Recording of simultaneous normal cystometrogram and EMG of external urethral sphincter.

through the urethra at a known rate while carbon dioxide is introduced. The urethral pressure is simultaneously recorded. The methodology is illustrated in Figure 38–6.

When the normal bladder is filled with increasing volumes of fluid, the intravesical pressure usually rises 10 to 15 cm water. Figure 38–5*B* illustrates normal CMG and simultaneous EMG of external urethral sphincter. Any sudden rise in bladder pressure during filling beyond 15 to 20 cm water is indicative of an unstable bladder. Most incontinent females show this instability with no other associated neurogenic bladder dysfunction. Any long tract disease in the spinal cord leads to increased instability, which

manifests itself as uninhibited bladder contractions over which the patient has no control. Normal people do not show uninhibited contractions. Complete lesions above the bladder center in the conus lead to a reflex bladder (Fig. 38–7). Lesions in the conus or lesions involving the cauda equina usually lead to a lower motor neuron (areflexic) bladder.

Simultaneous sphincter electromyography and CMG are helpful to diagnose complex neurogenic bladder dysfunctions such as detrusor sphincter dyssynergia. This is illustrated in Figure 38–8. Notice that the urethral EMG activity increases with each detrusor contraction (upper tracing). The

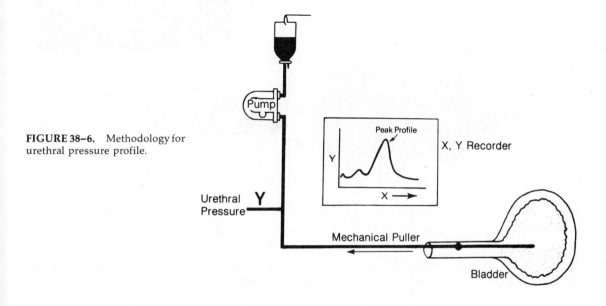

FIGURE 38–6. Methodology for urethral pressure profile.

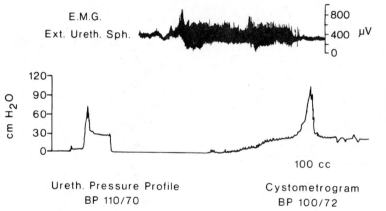

FIGURE 38–7. Reflex bladder contraction when the bladder was fillled with 200 cc.

bladder neck and urethra do not open at all during voiding cystourethrography.

Interprettation of Urodynamic Findings. When normal people are asked to hold their urine, the EMG activity of their periurethral striated sphincter increases significantly. On attempts to bear down and pass urine, activity decreases markedly; in fact, normal people can usually abolish the external urethral sphincter EMG activity. A sustained voiding pressure on the CMG in excess of 100 cm of water can eventually produce vesicoureteral reflux; this indicates the need for medication with alpha-adrenergic blocking agents or anticholinergic drugs or for sphincterotomy. The beneficial effects of these drugs are easily proved by demonstrating that the urethral pressure falls significantly after the administration of phentolamine (Fig. 38–9).

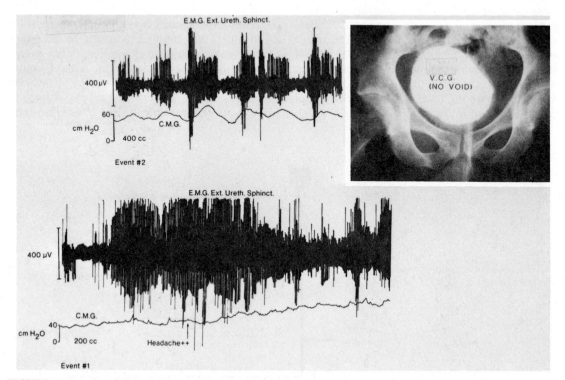

FIGURE 38–8. Simultaneous cystometrogram and external urethral sphincter EMG show detrusor-sphincter dyssynergia. Event #2 (upper CMG tracing) shows increased EMG activity corresponding to each detrusor contraction. Voiding cystourethrogram shows lack of bladder neck funnelling and no dye in the urethra.

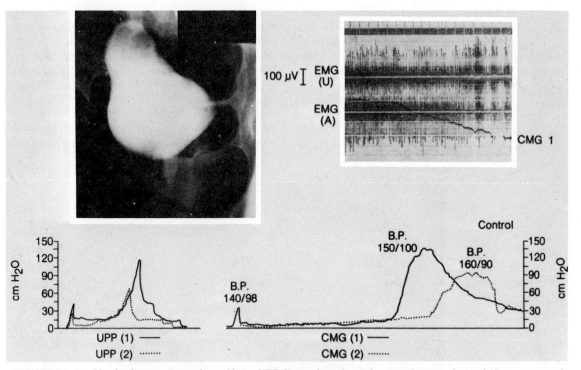

FIGURE 38–9. Urethral pressure peak profile — UPP(2) — after phentolamine shows a drop of 45 per cent and CMG(2) after phentolamine shows a drop of about 35 per cent in maximum voiding pressure. Voiding cystourethrogram shows opened bladder neck but inadequately opened external urethal sphincter. Simultaneous CMG and EMG of external sphincter (U) and anal sphincter (A), and CMG (1) show detrusor-sphincter dyssynergia.

During a cystometrogram, normal people will feel full after 100 ml of gas/water has been introduced into the bladder. Normal people will want to void when the bladder contains 400 to 500 ml (see Fig. 38–5B). At no time during bladder filling should the bladder pressure rise above 15 to 20 cm water in normal people. Patients with hyperreflexia, however, will void spontaneously when the bladder contains about 100 ml of gas or fluid. Hyperreflexia is common in patients with upper motor neuron lesions during or shortly after an episode of acute cystitis.

When normal people are instructed to void, electrical activity ceases first in the periurethral striated sphincter. Then the bladder pressure increases and the person voids. At this point, bladder and urethral pressures approximate each other. In patients with detrusor sphincter dyssynergia, the striated periurethral sphincter contracts during voiding instead of relaxing, as noted on the EMG.[20] This in turn generates high pressures in the bladder, bladder neck, and urethra. Urodynamic studies performed be-fore and after administration of alpha blockers, when demonstrating significant drops both in UPP and voiding pressures, can help determine therapeutic usefulness of these drugs in individual patients.[21]

Types of Neuromuscular Dysfunction of the Bladder

A patient with a neuromuscular dysfunction of the bladder may have either a contractile bladder or a noncontractile bladder. Two main types of contractile bladder are known to exist. The first is called the uninhibited bladder. In this condition, after the bladder has attained a certain volume, which is usually less than normal, the voiding reflex is triggered so that the patient voids and is essentially incontinent. The patient can, however, also void voluntarily. Such patients may be able to avoid incontinence by voiding before the bladder is full enough to trigger the voiding response.

The second type of contractile bladder is called the reflex bladder (Fig. 38–7). In this condition there is no voluntary control; voiding occurs through the spinal cord reflex and is completely involuntary. Bladder volumes required to initiate voiding are also less than normal. This type of bladder has also been called the automatic bladder, because it contracts automatically when it has reached a given volume.

The noncontractile bladder may be of three varieties. The first occurs when there is a lower motor neuron lesion, which involves both the sensory and the motor limbs of the reflex arc (Fig. 38–10). Such bladders are cut off entirely from outside control and are therefore autonomous or self-governing. Hence the name for this condition: the autonomous bladder. The second variety of noncontractile bladder is that which occurs in a patient who has an upper motor neuron lesion but has developed overdistention of

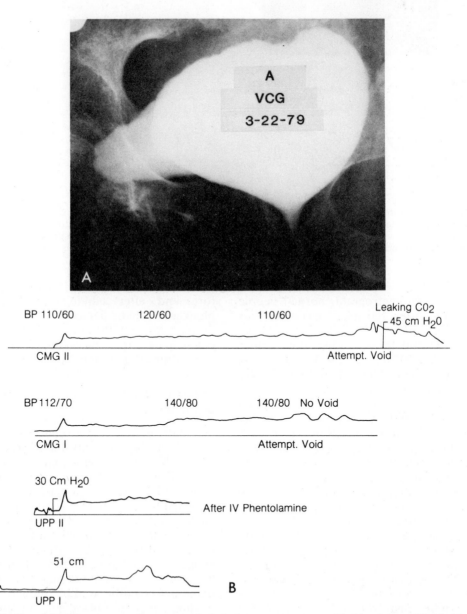

FIGURE 38–10. *A*, Voiding cystourethrogram typical of a lower motor neuron bladder shows a big bladder with a smooth wall which seems to be sinking into the pelvis due to a lax pelvic floor (compare with Fig. 38–8 — reflex upper motor neuron bladder). *B*, CMG I and CMG II before and after phentolamine show noncontractile bladder. UPP II after phentolamine shows drop of peak profile pressure from 51 cm to 30 cm H_2O.

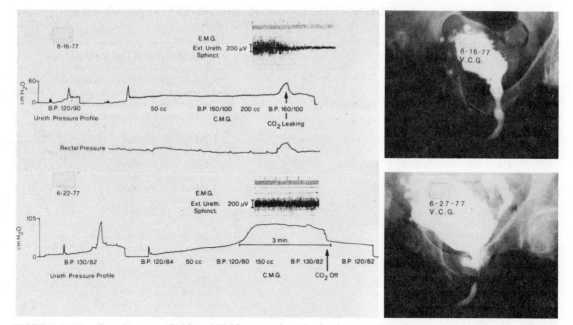

FIGURE 38–11. Simultaneous CMG and EMG external urethral sphincter show (lower tracing) detrusor-sphincter dyssynergia and voiding study shows non-opened external urethral sphincter and reflux. After transurethral sphincterotomy (upper tracing) bladder is noncontractile. Arrow points at the rise in CMG pressure which is simultaneous with an increase in rectal pressure, indicating that this was due to the rise in intra-abdominal pressure.

the bladder (Fig. 38–11). The third variety is due to a loss of the sensory pathway, either the posterior nerve roots or the sensory pathway in the spinal cord.

Noncontractile bladders are also called areflexic bladders. If a small amount of contractility is still present, they are called hyporeflexic bladders.

Common Causes of Neuromuscular Disorders of the Bladder

Neuromuscular disorders of the bladder are either congenital or acquired. Myelodysplasia is the common congenital cause.

Acquired lesions can affect any part of the central or peripheral nervous system. Common neurologic disorders leading into bladder dysfunction are shown in Table 38–1.

Intracranial Lesions. Intracranial lesions affect either the cortical centers or the suprasegmental pathway. Milder lesions usually cause an uninhibited bladder; more advanced lesions usually cause a reflex bladder. Common causes for such disorders are vascular lesions, such as cerebrovascular accidents, ischemia due to arteriosclerosis, intracranial neoplasms, multiple sclerosis, and Parkinson's disease.

Spinal Lesions Affecting the Suprasegmental Pathway. Spinal cord lesions above the detrusor center in the cord will result in an uninhibited bladder when the suprasegmental pathways are only slightly involved or a reflex neurogenic bladder when the lesion has destroyed all spinal cord pathways to the spinal cord detrusor center. The most common lesions involving the spinal cord are spinal cord injury, spinal cord neoplasm, intervertebral disc disease, and multiple sclerosis.

Cauda Equina Lesions. When the cauda equina is involved, the resultant bladder dysfunction is usually a noncontractile bladder. Common causes are trauma and neoplasms.

Lesions of the Posterior Nerve Roots and Sensory Pathways in the Spinal Cord. These lesions usually cause either a hyporeflexic or an areflexic bladder. The bladder is generally very large in such cases. The most common cause now is diabetes mellitus. All patients with diabetes mellitus who have this lesion also have peripheral neuropathy. In some diabetic patients, the metabolic disturbance leading to neuropathy also involves a deficiency of Vitamin B_{12} and folic acid. This lesion may also be due to tabes dorsalis, which is currently rare.

TABLE 38–1. COMMON NEUROLOGIC DISORDERS LEADING TO BLADDER DYSFUNCTION

Neurologic Disorder	Usual Type of Dysfunction
Suprapontine lesions	Detrusor hyperreflexia with absent detrusor-sphincter dyssynergy
Delayed CNS maturation (childhood)	Persistence of uninhibited bladder beyond age 2-3. Enuresis later on.
Cerebral atherosclerosis (old age)	Uninhibited bladder
Early multiple sclerosis	Uninhibited bladder
Brain neoplasm	Uninhibited bladder
Pernicious anemia	Uninhibited bladder
Lesions below pons	Usually associated with detrusor-sphincter dyssynergy
Spinal cord injuries	Reflex bladder
Spinal cord neoplasms—primary or secondary	Reflex bladder
Syringomyelia	Reflex bladder
Advanced multiple sclerosis	Reflex bladder
Extensive brain neoplasms	Reflex bladder
Extensive brain trauma	Reflex bladder
Conus lesion	Absent detrusor-sphincter dyssynergy
Cauda equina injuries or neoplasms	Areflexic bladder (autonomous bladder)
Acute transverse myelitis	Areflexic bladder (autonomous bladder)
Extensive rectal carcinoma	Areflexic bladder (autonomous bladder)
Following abdominoperineal resection of rectal carcinoma	Areflexic bladder (autonomous bladder)
Perivesical fibrosis following extensive pelvic surgery or trauma	Areflexic bladder (autonomous bladder)
Herniated intervertebral disc	Areflexic bladder (autonomous bladder)
Myelodysplasia and spina bifida	Areflexic bladder (autonomous bladder)
Poliomyelitis	Areflexic bladder (motor-paralytic, sensory intact)
Injury, neoplasms and herniated disc involving motor nerves to the bladder	Areflexic bladder (motor-paralytic, sensory intact)
Diabetes mellitus	Areflexic bladder (sensory-paralytic bladder, areflexic due to overdistention)
Tabes dorsalis	Areflexic bladder (sensory-paralytic bladder, areflexic due to overdistention)
Guillain-Barré syndrome	Areflexic bladder

TABLE 38–2. DRUGS HAVING A PHARMACOLOGIC ACTION ON THE BLADDER, PRIMARILY THROUGH THE PERIPHERAL AUTONOMIC INNERVATION

Drugs	Mode of Action	Alteration in Bladder Function
Cholinergic drugs Acetylcholine	Physiologic neurotransmitter for bladder contractions	Increases intravesical pressure and facilitates voiding
Muscarinic Bethanechol Methacholine	Physiologic neurotransmitter for bladder contractions	Increases intravesical pressure and facilitates voiding
Nicotinic Nicotine	Nicotine-like response resembles sympathetic stimulation mediated through release of norepinephrine	
Anticholinergics	Blockage of endogenous transmitter at postsynaptic receptor	Reduces bladder contractility and may lead to urinary retention
Atropine Propantheline d-Tubocurarine	Atropine blocks muscarinic action and d-tubocurarine blocks nicotinic action of acetylcholine. Propantheline blocks muscarinic action and also has a ganglion-blocking action.	
Reserpine Guanethidine	Essentially adrenergic neuron blocker	
Phenothiazines Antihistaminics	Mild anticholinergic action	
Adrenergic Alpha adrenergic response Phenylephrine Ephedrine Imipramine	Sympathomimetic response (response mostly on alpha adrenergic receptors) Action similar to alpha adrenergic stimulation	Increases bladder outlet and urethral pressure
Alpha blockers Phenoxybenzamine Phentolamine Prazosin HCl	Sympatholytic response	Lower bladder outlet and urethral pressures
Beta stimulants Isoproterenol Progesterone	Sympathomimetic	Lower urethral pressure
Beta blockers Propranolol	Sympatholytic	Increases urethral pressure

Lesions of the Anterior Horn Cells. These lesions will also lead to the development of noncontractile bladders. An isolated lesion of the anterior horn cells is usually due to poliomyelitis, which is now rare.

Adverse Drug Effects. Many different drugs that variously affect the autonomic nervous system may cause or prevent bladder dysfunction (see Table 38–2). Tricyclic antidepressants, antihistaminics, and phenytoin can all cause incomplete bladder emptying. Clinically significant adverse and unwanted pharmacologic effects on voiding function usually appear in patients whose voiding status already borders on being pathologic.

Evaluation and Management of the Spinal Cord Injury Bladder

Inadequate voiding in spinal injury patients could be caused by several factors, including an areflexic bladder, detrusor–external urethral sphincter dyssynergia, fixed scarred bladder neck, and enlargement of the prostate. There may also be excess alpha-adrenergic activity demonstrable at the bladder neck leading to bladder–bladder neck dyssynergia and autonomic dysreflexia.

Neurourologic Evaluation. A systematic approach to define bladder dysfunction problems during rehabilitation of the spinal cord injury patient is of utmost importance, since early recognition and management will prevent urologic complications and permanent renal damage. Neurologic examination should include testing perianal sensations to find out any sacral sparing. Presence of anal tone, anal reflex, and bulbocavernosus reflex only indicate intact conus and local reflex arc. However, detection of voluntary contraction of anal sphincter (determined with a finger in the anal canal) indicates intact voluntary control and in the presence of quadriplegia it indicates central cord type incomplete lesion. Combined studies such as CMG with EMG of external urethral sphincter should help determine the neurogenic dysfunction and also find out the presence of

significant detrusor-sphincter dyssynergia. A drop in urethral pressure profile (about 20 per cent or more) after intravenous phentolamine (5 to 7.5 mg) defines the role of alpha blockers such as phenoxybenzamine for therapeutic use to improve voiding (see Figs. 38–9 and 38–10B). Radiologic examination should include initial intravenous urography and voiding cystourethrograms to assess upper tracts and to rule out vesicoureteral reflux. Voiding radiologic studies with ciné control are also useful for the diagnosis of bladder neck problems and detrusor-sphincter dyssynergy.

Immediately following injury for a period of one day to usually three to four weeks, all deep reflexes below the level of injury are absent; this is usually referred to as the "shock phase." The bladder is areflexic during this period and needs a careful periodic or continuous drainage, and provocative testing such as introduction of 4 ounces of sterile cold water at 4°C does not evoke bladder reflex activity. The ice water test is positive when introduction of cold water is almost immediately followed by rapid rejection of water and catheter out of the bladder. Carefully planned bladder decompression during the shock phase can prevent the areflexic bladder from developing overdistention and atony:

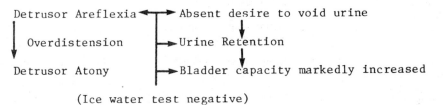

(Ice water test negative)

FIGURE 38–12. Bladder overdistention during spinal shock phase.

Intermittent catheterization (I.C.), rather than leaving a continuous indwelling catheter for drainage of the bladder, when used from the onset reduces incidence of infection and stone disease.[22] If done with regularity, it allows decompression of bladder and helps monitor the residual urine. It also allows detection of return of spontaneous voiding on the part of the patient and heralds recovery from the shock phase. Both aseptic and "clean" techniques have been advocated; however, the author prefers an aseptic

technique in acute spinal injury patients, particularly when it is desired to avoid bacteremia in patients prior to or immediately following spinal surgery and also in patients whose condition is complicated by thromboembolism due to deep vein thrombosis. In acute spinal injury patients with deep vein thrombosis, unsterile I.C. technique may lead to disseminated intravascular clotting.[23]

Intermittent Catheterization Technique. Intermittent catheterization using a size 12 or

TABLE 38–3. INTERMITTENT CATHETERIZATION RECORD

Date	Time	Intake	Reflex Voiding Spontaneous	Stimulation (ml)	Residual Urine (ml)	Total Urine (ml)	pH
10-7-75	11:00a	...	...	80	20	100	7.5
10-15-75	10:30a	...	...	500	180	680	6.5
10-17-75	1:30p	...	...	500	250	750	5.0
10-21-75				300	500	800	5.5

14 catheter is started every 4 hours. The patient's fluid intake is restricted to about 2 liters in 24 hours. Monitoring is done on a special sheet (Table 38–3). Intake and output are recorded synchronously with the catheterization every day. Table 38–3 shows only pertinent data; therefore information from several days has been omitted.

Catheterization intervals are extended to 6 and 8 hours with increasing spontaneous voiding between the periods of catheterization. It is preferred not to allow more than 400 to 500 ml of residuals, since this may lead to overdistention. Intermittent catheterization is stopped when balanced bladder is achieved. The bladder is considered "balanced" when (1) the patient can pass adequate urine on reflex or easily with the Credé/Valsalva maneuver; (2) residual urine is approximately 150 ml or less; and (3) there are no pathologic changes in the genitourinary tract.

An areflexic bladder may retain a fair amount of urine. Therefore, during catheterization when urine flow ceases, the bladder is gently aspirated through the catheter, preferably with a bulb syringe or with suprapubic pressure applied while the catheter is still in the bladder, to empty the bladder completely. After each catheterization, the bladder is irrigated with about 50 ml of normal saline containing 120 µg/ml neosporin and 60 µg/ml polymyxin B. Irrigation is continued while the catheter is being pulled through the urethra. The patient is instructed in bladder retraining using the Credé/Valsalva maneuver and stimulation of the suprapubic region (e.g., by tapping or pulling hairs) between the catheterizations and also prior to intermittent catheterization to trigger voiding. Urine pH is recorded after each catheterization; pH values over 7.0 may invariably be associated with infection due to urea-splitting organisms.

Transient high or low residuals may be noticed with infection.[24] Residuals of less than 50 ml are invariably associated with some degree of bladder infection. True volumes of residuals are seen after eradication of infection. An anecdotal example (see Table 38–3) is a T3 paraplegic patient admitted 21 years after injury with repeated urinary tract infections. Previous transurethral resection of the prostate (TURP) was carried out in 1969. On admission residual urine was 20 ml and urinary pH was 7.5; urine culture was positive ($> 10^5$) for *Proteus rettgeri*. After control of infection, residual urine was 180 ml one week later. Two weeks after admission urine culture showed no growth and residual urine was 500 ml. Transurethral sphincterotomy was performed three weeks after admission. At discharge one month after admission, residual urine was less than 100 ml and no infection was noted.

Patients with spinal cord lesions above the conus on intermittent catheterization for 8 to 10 weeks following injury usually show adequate spontaneous voiding if overdistention of the bladder is prevented and they do not have an enlarged prostate, stricture of the urethra, detrusor–bladder neck or detrusor-sphincter dyssynergia.

Prolonged intermittent catheterization with limitation on fluid intake is frustrating for spinal cord–injured patients with complete lesions and is even a hindrance to their complete rehabilitation. Therefore, the early recognition of patients in whom I.C. may not be successful is important, and such patients need careful urologic intervention to establish an early catheter-free status. Studies of micturition, including simultaneous cystomanometry and periurethral striated EMG and voiding cystourethrography, are therefore needed to define the dysfunctional neurogenic bladder problems. Trial with alpha-adrenergic blockers and/or striated

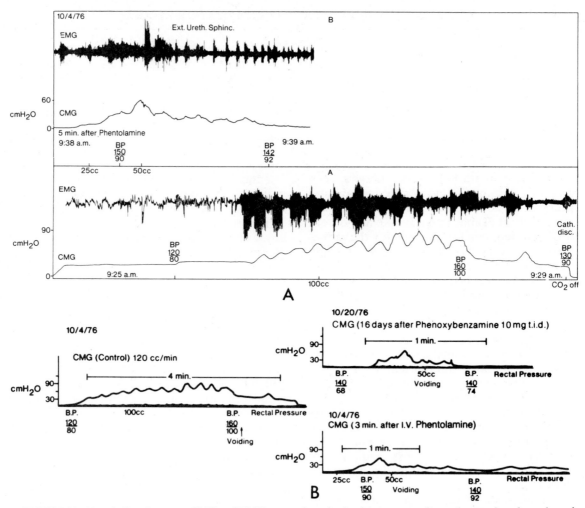

FIGURE 38–14. *A,* Simultaneous CMG and EMG external urethral sphincter recordings show reduced number of bladder contractions and less dyssynergia after phentolamine. Similar result was obtained 16 days later (*B*) with oral phenoxybenzamine when patient voided more adequately in less time.

muscle relaxants may help improve voiding in some patients with minimal sphincter dyssynergia. Therapeutic efficacy of these drugs can be evaluated by repeating the urodynamic study.

An illustration is shown in Figure 38–13. Cystomanometry before phentolamine testing (control), after phentolamine, and then 16 days after oral phenoxybenzamine shows marked improvement in voiding. The control study shows sustained detrusor contractions for over 4 minutes to empty his bladder, as against 1 minute after I.V. phentolamine; also, after oral therapy with phenoxybenzamine, detrusor contractions were less sustained and the voiding phase lasted just over a minute. The study shows the usefulness of phentolamine testing in such patients.

Autonomic Dysreflexia and Detrusor-Sphincter Dyssynergia. Autonomic hyperreflexia or dysreflexia is an important visceral alarm symptom usually due to a distended bladder or impacted rectum.

An acute episode is associated with throbbing headache, sweating, and bradycardia. There is a generalized sustained increase in sympathetic tone, usually below the level of the lesion, which leads to altered hemodynamics and a rise in arterial pressure by (1) elevating arteriolar resistance, (2) reducing the distensibility of postarteriolar capacity vessels, and (3) directly increasing myocardial contractility. Marked peripheral vasoconstriction below the level of lesion seems to be mediated by norepinephrine. Following an attack of autonomic dysreflexia there is marked increase of serum dopamine-β-hydroxylase (DBH), plasma catecholamine, and norepinephrine metabolites (such as normetanephrine) in urine.[25] Prompt drainage of the bladder usually relieves the acute episode. Local instillation of 0.25 per cent tetracaine HCl 25 to 50 ml in patients with a suprapubic tube or through an indwelling catheter may provide topical anesthesia of the vesical mucosa and reduce triggering impulses to the spinal cord. Gentle evacuation of fecal masses from the rectum and instillation of Nupercainal ointment (1 per cent dibucaine NF) may reduce impulses originating from the rectum.

The control of widespread sympathetic activity below the spinal lesion is the key factor in the management of autonomic dysreflexia. Therefore spinal anesthesia, ganglion blockers, adrenergic neuron blockers, adrenergic blockers, and drugs acting directly on the blood vessels are useful in controlling hypertension accompanying autonomic dysreflexia.[26] Figure 38–14 diagrammatically illustrates the principal site of action of hypotensive drugs useful in autonomic dysreflexia. Phenoxybenzamine

10 mg three or four times a day is usually sufficient to control acute dysreflexia.

Recurrent episodes of autonomic hyperreflexia are usually associated with detrusor-sphincter dyssynergia.[27, 28] Therefore, surgical management of detrusor-sphincter dyssynergia with adequate transurethral sphincterotomy will provide definitive management of the major primary problem provoking the stimulus for autonomic hyperreflexia. Long-term medical management with guanethidine (Ismelin) 10 to 20 mg/day does provide relief of hypertension but not adequate control of sweating. It also leads to side effects such as postural hypotension, nasal stuffiness, and diarrhea in some patients.

Those patients who show detrusor hyperreflexia as well as detrusor-sphincter dyssynergia could run the risk of developing vesicoureteral reflux and silent hydronephrosis.[29] Careful use of adequate dosage of anticholinergics, alpha blockers, and early transurethral resection of the sphincter may be very rewarding for an adequate and quick rehabilitation of the patient with complete lesions. Also an alpha

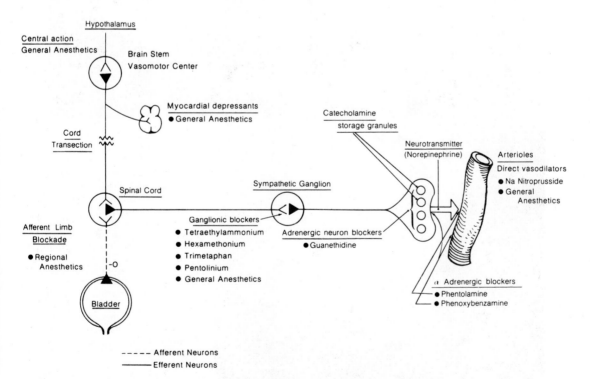

FIGURE 38–14. Principal site of action of hypotensive drugs useful in autonomic dysreflexia. (Reproduced by permission from Schonwald, G., Fish, A., and Perkash, I.: Anesthesiology, 55:550–558, 1981.)

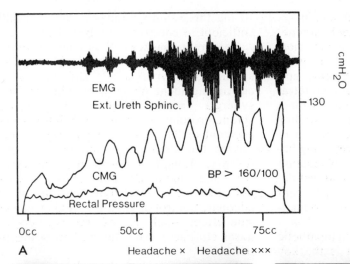

A

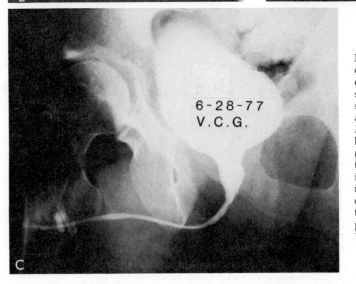

B

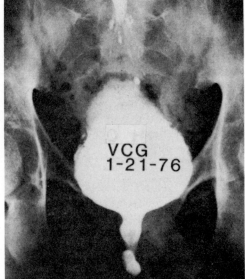

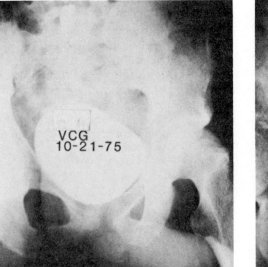

C

FIGURE 38–15. *A,* Simultaneous CMG and EMG recordings of external urethral sphincter show detrusor-sphincter dyssynergia in a C6 tetraplegic about four months after injury. *B,* Voiding cystourethrogram before (10–21–75) and after (1–21–76) transurethral sphincterotomy. *C,* Follow-up voiding cystourethrogram about 18 months later showed well-opened bladder neck and posterior urethra. (Reproduced by permission from Perkash, I.: J. Urol., 131:778, 1979.)

blocker such as phenoxybenzamine has been found very useful for long-term treatment of autonomic dysreflexia.[30] Simultaneous cystomanometry and periurethral striated E.M.G. are shown in Figure 38–15A, which illustrates detrusor-sphincter dyssynergia and detrusor hyperreflexia in a tetraplegic patient. Strong detrusor contractions are seen after filling the bladder with 50 ml of fluid; the blood pressure rose to 160/100, at which time he also complained of sweating and headache (autonomic dysreflexia). Following transurethral resection of the sphincter and the use of alpha blockers, marked relief from autonomic dysreflexia was noticed (Fig. 38–15B). During the follow-up for over four years, this patient has been voiding easily and has been uninfected. Voiding cystourethrogram two and one-half years after surgery shows well-opened bladder neck and posterior urethra (Fig. 38–15C).

Cauda Equina Lesions. Management of patients with cauda equina lesions needs special consideration. They usually have an areflexic (noncontractile) bladder and void with Credé/Valsalva manipulation. Their lesions are invariably incomplete or mixed and have a potential for recovery. Urodynamic evaluation may indicate an intact external urethral sphincter and therefore such patients may not be able to void unless they generate very high intravesical pressures. This could even lead to vesicoureteral reflux. Also in these patients with damage to the parasympathetic and an intact sympathetic innervation (which emerges above the cauda equina [Fig. 38–3]) the bladder neck may not open well on voiding. The excess sympathetic activity could be demonstrated on intravenous phentolamine testing. In such patients, voiding can be improved with the use of alpha blockers such as oral phenoxybenzamine 10 to 20 mg daily or by limited bladder neck incision.

Central Cord Syndrome. Neurogenic bladder due to incomplete lesions such as the central cord syndrome[31] may recover in over 50 per cent of patients. It is important to separate patients with central cord syndrome from other patients with incomplete tetraplegia. Despite severe neurologic dysfunction during the first few weeks, considerable bladder functional recovery can occur, particularly since the bladder fibers are the peripheral ones in the spinal cord. These patients are usually managed with intermittent catheterization and drug therapy. It is possible to cause incontinence by an early transurethral resection of sphincter and thus necessitate an external collecting device. Persisting detrusor-sphincter dyssynergia, severe spasticity, and hydronephrotic change may be indications for transurethral sphincterotomy after trial with alpha blockers, anticholinergics, and skeletal muscle relaxants such as dantrolene sodium.

Management of the neurogenic bladder in female patients with spinal cord lesions (upper motor neuron) is difficult; however, conal and cauda equina lesions (lower motor neuron) can be easily managed with the Credé/Valsalva maneuver. Intermittent catheterization is started every 4 or 6 hours, and with fluid restriction to about 1.5 liters a day, these patients may be managed with three catheterizations a day. To reduce stress incontinence between catheterizations, use of an anticholinergic such as oxybutynin 5 mg once or twice a day is helpful. Bladder irritability is increased with infection; therefore, treatment of infection is rather important to prevent leakage of urine. Long-term prophylaxis for urinary tract infection is strongly recommended. The patient is encouraged and trained to empty the bladder by the Credé/Valsalva maneuver periodically. Failure to manage with intermittent catheterization usually results in long-term placement of an indwelling catheter. Neurosurgical procedures such as selective sacral nerve root blocks and rhizotomies may be indicated to convert a reflex (contractile) into an areflexic bladder that, as mentioned above, can be managed easily by the Credé/Valsalva maneuver.

Management of Infection in Patients with Spinal Cord Injury

The use of antibacterial drugs in patients with a neurogenic bladder has been the subject of much debate. There is no disagreement as to the need for antibiotics when there are constitutional manifestions of an acute infection of the urinary tract.

At the start of intermittent catheterization, when the indwelling catheter is being removed, we start patients on a suitable antibiotic for the first five to seven days to prevent dissemination of urethral infection. Both

Pearman's study and our own[32, 33] indicate usefulness of bladder and urethal irrigation with antibiotics following each intermittent catheterization. There was significantly lower incidence of bacteriuria, and it also obviated the necessity for prophylaxis during intermittent catheterization. After each catheterization about 50 ml of polymyxin neomycin irrigant solution was instilled and removed and then 15 ml of this irrigant was left in the bladder and about 15 ml was used to irrigate the urethra while the catheter was being removed. All infections during intermittent catheterization were treated with an appropriate antibiotic.

Our patients on external condom drainage with a balanced bladder and off intermittent catheterization are prophylactically treated with methenamine or Macrodantin. Patients growing urea-splitting bacteria, such as *Proteus mirabilis*, are given trimethoprim-sulfamethoxazole.

Follow-up. All patients with spinal cord injury need periodic urologic follow-up for the rest of their lives. During the first year after discharge, blood urea nitrogen, urine culture (and sensitivities), and the patient's general well-being are reviewed. Unnecessary catheterizations for checking residual urine in someone who shows no clinical evidence of urine retention, infection, or lithiasis may not be warranted. In otherwise asyptomatic patients whose urodynamics had been previously studied, instead of routine annual intravenous pyelography, plain x-ray of the abdomen may be enough to rule out calculous disease. Most of the patients may need maintenance therapy with methenamine and ascorbic acid. All infections with urea-splitting organisms need to be treated to prevent urolithiasis.

THE BOWEL

Defecation, like the voiding of urine, is under volitional control. The reflex activity starts with the filling and distention of the sigmoid colon and rectum, when afferent impulses thus generated pass to the sacral spinal center in the conus. Efferent impulses emanate from the sacral center, leading to the evacuation process when the sigmoid and rectum contract along with a synergistic relaxation of the anal sphincter. Following emptying of the anal canal the anal sphincter and levator ani contract and there is relaxation of rectum and lower colon. This process repeats until all the lower bowel is empty. Under resting conditions, the external anal sphincter shows continuous electrical activity and tonic contraction.[34] However, this activity is absent during the spinal shock phase and following intrathecal injection of alcohol.[35]

Management During the Shock Phase

Complete spinal cord and cauda equina lesions or even severe incomplete transections result in the loss of reflex gastrointestinal function during the shock phase. This may last for two to three days. In some patients paralytic ileus may be present for several days and bowel sounds will be absent. There is abdominal distention (this is usually absent with lesions below T10), which may lead to regurgitation of food and could interfere with the diaphragmatic movements and thus produce respiratory distress in tetraplegic patients. Such patients need careful monitoring, along with gastric tube suction, parenteral alimentation, and fluid replacement. There is widespread venous paralysis during the shock phase, and unless careful fluid balance is maintained these patients could develop overhydration and pulmonary edema. Intramuscular injections of prostigmine 0.3 to 0.5 mg every 4 hours[36] or subcutaneous injections of bethanechol 2.5 mg every 6 hours may help restart intestinal activity. A further complication of gastric involvement is mucosal hemorrhages and stress ulceration in the stomach or duodenum. These usually develop within the first two weeks of injury. Patients with a previous history of gastric or duodenal ulceration are particularly susceptible and are therefore often given antacids to avoid this complication.

Bowel Retraining

Habit retraining for reflex bowel evacuation may be begun as soon as the patient is out of shock, capable of receiving instructions, and able to take food by mouth. The diet should be such as to produce a stool of normal consistency.

A specific time of day should be established for defecation, such as following breakfast or following the evening meal, to take advantage of the gastrocolic reflex. Until the time when the patient can tolerate sitting in a commode chair, the patient will have his bowel care in bed. The lower rectum is examined and, if it is full, the feces are removed. A suppository may then be inserted (glycerin or Dulcolax) to stimulate peristalsis reflexly and the movement of feces into the lower bowel or rectal vault. Some patients may need additional digital stimulation, which is accomplished by insertion of the gloved lubricated finger into the rectum and massage of the walls of the rectum in a wavelike motion. Digital stimulation may need to be repeated every 10 minutes for three or four times. Many patients can be managed with digital stimulation only and should be encouraged to experiment. Others may need a combination of suppository and digital stimulation and must use softeners such as dioctyl sodium sulfosuccinate (Colace) to keep their feces from becoming too hard.

Patients who have injuries to the cord at the conus or below often manage their bowel with manual removal on a daily or every-other-day schedule. These are the patients who may begin having accidental bowel movements as they begin to use a standing frame or to walk in parallel bars. Increasing the frequency of their bowel care from every other day to daily, accompanied by instructions on maintaining firm stool through diet management, may eliminate accidents.

When sitting tolerance permits, the patient should receive bowel care on a commode chair to allow gravity to assist in bowel evacuation. Massage of the abdomen from right to left may also facilitate movement of feces to the lower tract. On those occasions when no feces are evacuated with the standard methods, the patient may need to try a mild laxative and repeat the bowel program 8 to 10 hours later.

Muscular activity is enormously important. The patient who is up and exercising every day is seldom constipated. In this, as in many other respects, the quadriplegic is at some disadvantage because his activity is relatively limited. A good bowel habit can still be established, but there is a tendency to chronic moderate distention, more noticeable, perhaps, on the x-ray film than on physical examination. In the investigation of a patient suspected of intra-abdominal lesion, it is important not to interpret this as actual ileus. Once a good habit program has been established, involuntary defecation is unusual as long as the feces remain of normal consistency.

Diarrhea in a spinal cord–injured patient is a sorry experience for the patient and his attendants. It could be associated with impaction. Any such tendency must be promptly and vigorously investigated by a rectal examination. Scybala are prone to produce impactions that require manual extraction. High fecal impaction in the colon could present as an acute abdomen and may be associated with autonomic dysreflexia, which manifests as a rise in blood pressure and bradycardia and is accompanied with sweating and headache.

Intra-abdominal Gastrointestinal Problems

In spinal injury patients it is sometimes difficult to differentiate acute abdominal lesions from fecal impaction. Rectal examination and palpation of colon may reveal impaction. Patients using anticholinergics over a long period can develop megacolon. Barium enema examination shows a megacolon in a quadriplegic (Fig. 38–16) where transverse colostomy had to be done to provide adequate bowel evacuation. Accidental perforations of the rectum have also been reported following rectal manipulations with enema tips.[37] Also reported are silent perforations of the stomach and appendicitis. Diagnostic criteria for intra-abdominal catastrophe are (1) history of sudden illness "out of proportion" to the physical signs, (2) associated autonomic dysreflexia, (3) increased abdominal tone or increased generalized spasticity, (4) absent bowel sounds, and (5) shoulder pain due to diaphragmatic irritation with perforated viscus.[38, 39] Urgent intravenous pyelography and blood and urine examination provide additional help to seek out urinary tract pathology. Sometimes root pains may also be confusing. Chest x-ray, ultrasound B scan, abdominal tap, C.T. scanning, and even exploratory laparotomy may be necessary to diagnose or rule out intra-abdominal pathology.

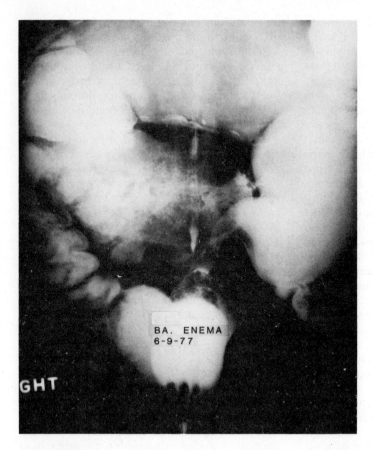

FIGURE 38–16. Barium enema shows megacolon in a quadriplegic patient.

REFERENCES

1. Winkler, G.: Contribucional estudeo de la innervation de la visceras pelvianas. Arch. Esp. Urol., 20:259, 1967.
2. Hutch, J. A.: Anatomy and Physiology of the Trigone, Bladder and Urethra. New York, Appleton-Century Croft, 1972.
3. Heiss, R.: Ueber der Sphincter vesicalis internus. Virchows Arch. Pathol. Anat., 220:367, 1915.
4. Hutch, J. A.: The internal urinary sphincters: A double-loop system. J. Urol., 105:375, 1971.
5. Gosling, J. A., and Dixon, J. S.: The structure and innervation of smooth muscle in the wall of the bladder neck and proximal urethra. Br. J. Urol., 47:549, 1975.
6. Nergardh, A., and Boreus, L. O.: The functional role of cholinergic receptors in the outlet region of the urinary bladder. An in vitro study in the cat. Acta Pharmacol., 32:467, 1973.
7. El-Badawi, A., and Schenk, E. A.: A new theory of the innervation of bladder musculature. J. Urol., 111:613, 1974.
8. Gil-Vernet, S.: L'innervation somatique et vegetative des organes genitourinaries. Acta Urol. Belg., 32:265, 1964.
9. Denny-Brown, D., and Robertson, E. G.: On the physiology of micturition. Brain, 56:149, 1933.
10. Ghoneim, M. A., Fretin, J. A., Gagnon, D. J., and Susset, J. G.: The influence of vesical distension

11. Tanagho, E. A., and Smith, D. R.: The anatomy and function of the bladder neck. Br. J. Urol., 38:54, 1966.
12. Weeks, J. R.: Prostaglandins. Ann. Rev. Pharmacol., 12:317, 1972.
13. Hedquist, P.: Autonomic transmission. In Ramwell, P. W. (Ed.): The Prostaglandins, Vol. 1. New York, Plenum Press, 1973, p. 101.
14. Ghoneim, M. A., Fretin, J. A., Gagnon, D. J., et al.: The influence of vesical distention on the urethra resistance to flow: A possible role for prostaglandins. J. Urol., 116:739, 1976.
15. Bradley, W. E., Rockswold, G. L., Timm, G. W., et al.: Neurology of micturition. J. Urol., 115:481, 1976.
16. Urmura, E., Fletcher, T. F., Dirks, V. A., et al.: Distribution of sacral afferent axons in cat urinary bladder. Am. J. Anat., 136:305, 1973.
17. Winter, D. L.: Receptor characteristics and conduction velocities in bladder afferents. J. Psychiat. Res., 8:225, 1971.
18. Bradley, W. E., and Teague, C. T.: Spinal cord organization of micturition reflex afferents. Exp. Neurol., 22:504, 1968.
19. Nyberg-Hansen, R.: Innervation and nervous control of the urinary bladder. Anatomical aspects. Acta Neurol. Scand., 42 (Suppl. 20):7, 1966.
20. Quesada, E. M., Scott, F. B., and Cardus, D.:

on urethral resistance to flow: the collecting phase, Br. J. Urol., 47:657, 1975.

entmarktrans.

Functional classification of neurogenic bladder dysfunction. Arch. Phys. Med. Rehabil., 49:17, 1968.

21. Awad, S. C., Downie, J. W., Lywood, D. W., Young, R. A., and Jarzylo, S. V.: Sympathetic activity in the proximal urethra in patients with urinary obstruction. J. Urol., 115:545, 1976.

22. Guttman, L., and Frankel, H.: Value of intermittent catheterization in early management of traumatic paraplegia and tetraplegia. Paraplegia, 4:63, 1966/67.

23. Perkash, A., Prakash, V., and Perkash, I.: Experience with the management of thromboembolism in patients with spinal cord injury: Part I. Incidence, diagnosis and role of some risk factors. Paraplegia, 16:322, 1978/79.

24. Perkash, I.: Intermittent catheterization failure and an approach to bladder rehabilitation in spinal cord injury patients. Arch. Phys. Med. Rehabil., 59:9, 1978.

25. Naftchi, N. E., Demeny, M., Lowman, E. W., and Tuckman, J.: Hypertensive crises in quadriplegic patients: Changes in cardiac output, blood volume, serum dopamine-β-hydroxylase activity, and arterial prostaglandin PGE$_2$. Circulation, 57:336, 1978.

26. Perkash, I.: Pharmacologic Management of Autonomic Dysreflexia. Pharmacology of the Urinary Tract and the Male Reproductive System. New York, Appleton-Century-Crofts, 1982, pp. 285–293.

27. Perkash, I.: Pressor response during cystomanometry in spinal injury patients complicated with detrusor-sphincter dyssynergia. J. Urol., 121:778–82, 1979.

28. Perkash, I.: Detrusor-sphincter dyssynergia and dyssynergia responses: Recognition and rationale for early modified transurethral sphincterotomy in complete spinal cord injury lesions. J. Urol., 120:469, 1978.

29. Perkash, I.: Detrusor-sphincter dyssynergia and detrusor hyperreflexia leading to hydronephrosis during intermittent catheterization. J. Urol., 120:620, 1978.

30. McGuire, E. J., Wagner, F. M., and Weiss, R. M.: Treatment of autonomic dysreflexia with phenoxybenzamine. J. Urol., 115:53, 1976.

31. Perkash, I.: Management of neurogenic bladder dysfunctions following acute traumatic cervical central cord syndrome (incomplete tetraplegia). Paraplegia, 15:21, 1977/78.

32. Rhame, F. S., and Perkash, I.: Urinary tract infections occurring in recent spinal cord injury patients on intermittent catheterization. J. Urol., 122:669–673, 1979.

33. Pearman, J. W.: Prevention of urinary tract infections following spinal cord injury. Paraplegia, 9:95, 1971.

34. Floyd, W. F., and Walls, E. W.: Electromyography of the sphincter ani externus in man. J. Physiol., 122:599, 1953.

35. Melzak, J., and Porter, N. B.: Studies on the reflex activity of the external sphincter ani in man. Paraplegia, 3:77, 1964.

36. Guttman, L.: Spinal Cord Injuries, Chapter 27. London, Blackwell Scientific Publications, 1973, p. 442.

37. Frankel, H. L.: Accidental perforation of the rectum. Paraplegia, 11:314, 1974.

38. Walsh, J. J., Nuseibeh, M. B., and El-Masri, W.: Perforated peptic ulcer in paraplegia. Paraplegia, 11:310, 1974.

39. Dollfus, P., Holderbach, G. L., Husser, J. M., and Jacob-Chia, D.: Must appendicitis be still considered as a rare complication in paraplegia? Paraplegia, 11:306, 1974.

39

REHABILITATION OF CHILDREN WITH BRAIN DAMAGE

DANIEL HALPERN

The results of brain injury in children are classified as prenatal, perinatal, or postnatal depending upon the age at injury.[1-3] Table 39–1 illustrates the most common etiologic factors in each of the important life periods of children.

In the prenatal period, athetosis, which 30 years ago was seen most commonly in the child of an Rh-negative mother, now occurs mainly as a result of prolonged moderate perinatal hypoxia in the mature neonate. As the anoxic process increases in severity, spasticity becomes more prominent. The election of cesarean section to avoid difficult vaginal extractions has reduced the incidence of perinatal anoxic spasticity and traumatic hemiplegia. Biologically active chemicals in the maternal environment are becoming recognized with increasing frequency as a cause of fetal brain injury. Drugs such as alcohol and tobacco, as well as narcotics, have been shown to contribute to fetal incompetence, underdevelopment, and respiratory distress as well as to structural abnormalities. To what extent other mood-altering compounds impair fetal metabolism remains to be defined. Prenatal factors causing prematurity are associated with

intracranial hemorrhage and play a significant role in the etiology of spastic diplegia.[4] Low birth weight and prematurity continue to represent significant risk factors for brain damage. Maternal malnutrition has been associated with mental subnormality, but no clear relationship has been established between this and brain damage giving rise to motor defects.

In the perinatal period,[5] accidents of the birth process — prolapsing cord, placenta previa, abruptio placentae — remain prominent as causes of acute brain damage. Changes in obstetrical practices have diminished the incidence of traumatic hemiplegia. Changes in the use of maternal sedation have reduced the anoxic damage resulting from respiratory obtundation. The development of sophisticated intensive care systems in newborn nurseries has increased the number of infants surviving prematurity, neonatal respiratory distress syndrome, and other congenital and perinatal abnormalities.[1-3]

Postnatally, bacterial or viral infections, trauma, asphyxia, drownings,[6] and gunshot wounds are causes of childhood brain damage. About one million children each year are injured in automobile accidents. A signif-

Supported in part by Grant No. 16-P-56810/5-17 from the Social and Rehabilitation Service, Department of Health and Human Services, Washington, D.C., for the University of Minnesota Medical Rehabilitation Research and Training Center.

TABLE 39–1. ETIOLOGY OF BRAIN DAMAGE IN CHILDREN

Prenatal	Perinatal	Postnatal
Hereditary Genetically transmitted and present at birth or soon after, e.g., hereditary athetosis, familial tremors, neurologic disorders, dermatologic syndromes	**Anoxia** Mechanical respiratory obstruction Respiratory distress syndrome Placenta previa Prolapsed cord Maternal anoxia or hypotension Breech delivery with delayed aftercoming head	**Trauma** Falls, motor vehicles, gunshot, abuse
Acquired in utero Gonadal irradiation Chromosomal defects Prenatal infections: toxoplasmosis, rubella, lues, or other maternal infections Developmental anomalies: meningomyelocele, hydrocephalus, CNS malformation Prenatal anoxia: maternal anoxia or trauma, anemia, hypertension, placental abnormalities (abruptio, infarcts) Chemical toxicity: alcohol, tobacco, prescribed psychoactive drugs and nonprescribed medications, dysmaturity in diabetic mothers	**Cerebral hemorrhage** Trauma: dystocia, obstetrical Following anoxia **Constitutional factors** Prematurity Hyperinsulinism Anemia of newborn Hypoprothrombinemia	**Infections** Acute: meningitis, encephalitis (viral or bacterial), thrombophlebitis Chronic: brain abscess, bacterial, granuloma, tuberculosis, mycoticfungal, lues **Vascular** Anomalies (with or without hemorrhage): arterial aneurysms, venous aneurysms, malformations, wall dysplasias Embolus Thrombosis Allergies: vascular occlusion
Prenatal cerebral hemorrhage Toxemia of pregnancy Vascular anomalies Maternal bleeding diathesis Trauma		**Anoxia** Carbon monoxide poisoning Drowning, food aspiration, croup, and other respiratory obstructions Ondine's curse (unexplained respiratory arrest)
Rh factor		**Inflammatory-immunologic** Lupus erythematosus Periarteritis nodosa Reye's syndrome
Metabolic disturbances		**Metabolic** Hyperinsulinism Electrolyte imbalance **Post-neoplastic**

icant number of these suffer head injury with permanent residual deficits.[7, 8] Many injuries would be totally preventable by use of appropriate seating restraints in motor vehicles and preventive measures against poisoning, falls, and other dangerous impulsive behaviors in children. A recently emphasized hazard is brain damage due to trauma at the hands of parents or other adults in whose care they are placed. In the rehabilitation of these children, the battered child needs to be identified in order to make appropriate decisions with regard to placement, parental support services, and education that will prevent further injury of the child and siblings.

The purpose of rehabilitation of children with central nervous system impairment is (1) to identify, develop, and train to the optimal level those abilities of which the child is capable and (2) to define the conditions of management under which the child is able to function optimally. This requires an assessment in the child, of abilities and dis-

abilities of motor function, behavior, receptive and expressive communication, and cognition; and in the community, of family and home resources and needs, schooling facilities, and residential or respite resources.

THE HANDICAPPED CHILD AS A SPECIAL PERSON

Intervention for the purpose of habilitation or rehabilitation implies the concept that it is possible to modify the responsiveness of a child with brain damage in a manner that is analogous to that in the normal child. There is much evidence that the developing central nervous system of the child with brain damage has potential for acquiring new responses to stimulation. Van Hof[9] has reviewed the hypothesis that recovery from brain damage in young individuals is better than that in adults. Although there has been wide acceptance as well as experimental support of this concept, he points out that it is still debatable. At the same time, Greenough et al.[10] and Yu[11] report that individuals with brain damage show recovery of some functions through environmental modification and experience.

Children have incomplete neuroanatomic structures and neurophysiologic processes. The growth of structures is still proceeding. The child is experiencing a broad variety of learning episodes. He/she still has not developed learned responses to a large number of experiences and therefore is open to new or different approaches to situations and problems provided that enough appropriate neural tissue is available. In addition, environmental management to augment learning is easier to provide for the child than it is for the adult.

NEUROPHYSIOLOGIC ORGANIZATION OF MOTOR FUNCTION

Motor activities are hierarchically organized in the central nervous system. The spinal cord, midbrain, cerebellum, basal ganglia, and cerebral cortex each possess characteristic motor functions. Each level contributes a specific quality of motor organization and responsiveness to the total motor activity. Dysfunction of each level contributes its own special qualities to the abnormality of function that is seen clinically. The clinical manifestations of dysfunction are the result of distortions of motor activities, sensory activities, or the effects of experience to modify functional performance. Damage to motor centers or pathways may cause impairment or loss of motor function on the one hand or loss of inhibition or modulation of activities of the residual central nervous system on the other. Sensory performance may be impaired by damage to pathways necessary for reception, perception, processing, or conceptualization. Deficiencies in these functions interfere with motor learning and guidance of coordination. The actual level of functional performance achieved depends on the opportunities for repetition of each motor activity under conscious perception. Each multimuscular activity in the repertory of coordination must be developed by this repetitive practicing. Finally the attitude and expectations resulting from past experiences determine the willingness of the patient to participate in the learning process, while the attitudes and behaviors of family members, peers, and professionals establish the rewarding or nonrewarding social environment in which the patient must work.

Spinal Activity

Independent activity of the spinal cord is characterized by reflex responses to somesthetic stimuli. These responses are based primarily upon the muscle spindle stretch-sensitive reflexes, modified by the gamma motor system.[12] A discussion of the spinal and supraspinal reflexes is presented in Chapter 11, page 218.

Clinically, these reflexes are manifested by increased muscle tone or hypertonia. The primary Ia annulospiral fibers respond to rapid stretch with a quick and brief contraction — the myotatic reflex. Animal models indicate that the secondary sensory endings show a prolonged discharge in response to elongation resulting in a persistent contraction, which increases in intensity with stretch. As a result, the muscle shortens progressively, giving rise to persistent contractures with functional shortening of the limb. The flexor musculature is involved preferentially. These two responses taken together constitute the typical patterns of behavior of dynamic and static *spasticity*.

The cutaneous stimuli of touch and pain may directly influence the activity of the anterior horn cells to increase the hypertonia independent of muscle spindles and also, by increasing the activity of the gamma motor system, to increase muscle spindle spasticity. The Golgi tendon organs inhibit alpha and gamma motor neuron activity and decrease muscular tension. The spinal reflex patterns produced by the long spinal, the crossed extensor-flexor, the extensor thrust, and the Marie-Foix reflexes possess the essential connections to enable the child to carry out effective reciprocation required for quadruped walking. However, the spinal cord does not possess the capacity to integrate these reflexes into an effective walking pattern because it lacks purposeful regulation to achieve balance, equilibrium, and progression. A center with the capacity to initiate reciprocation and support has been reported in the midbrain by Grillner.[13] Balance, adaptability, and purpose require control from a higher level.

The medulla and midbrain are sites of centers coordinating reflex activities at a higher level of organization. The symmetrical and asymmetrical neck, tongue, and mouth reflexes and the axio-derotational and labyrinthine reflexes are mediated in the midbrain, while those related to sucking and swallowing have centers at medullary levels. Therefore, these reflex activities may be elicited in response to somesthetic stimulation when there is no response to efforts at volitional movement. Thus, a patient with cerebral pyramidal and extrapyramidal impairment may show reflex tongue protrusion and retraction, biting, or a hyperactive gag reflex but not have the ability to chew, manipulate food, or swallow in a coordinated way. Speech may be dysarthric as well. He/she also may show tonic neck reflexes but be unable to carry out an appropriate reaching effort if the head is restrained. The child with brain damage who manifests hyperactive deep tendon reflexes and generalized persistent flexor posture of all four extremities with inability to extend the neck is demonstrating reflex motor activity originating predominantly from the level of the spinal cord. Some residual volitional supraspinal control may be evident in the form of bowel and bladder continence or restricted stereotyped voluntary motions that utilize the spinal reflex patterns for limited functional purposes.

Midbrain Activity — Decerebrate Motor Activity

The vestibular system contributes to extensor dystonia or rigidity due to uninhibited excitation of anterior horn cells from medial vestibular nuclear activity and exaggeration of spasticity by facilitation of muscle spindles through the lateral vestibular nucleus.[14] The patient showing extensor thrust, an opisthotonic posture, and all four limbs held in extension, internal rotation, and adduction shows exaggeration of spindle reflexes by vestibular reflex activity, because cerebral and cerebellar brain stem inhibition is deficient. In many patients, head position and acceleration are not significant contributing elements to the dystonia and spasticity. It is proposed that, in these patients, there is failure of inhibition of anterior horn cells to vestibular nuclear activity. In those patients who show changes of tone with changes in head orientation, there is loss of inhibition of the vestibular nuclei to postural changes. This response is mediated by activity of the cerebellar vermis. It is conceivable that electrical stimulation of the cerebellum, when it is effective, activates this inhibition.

In patients with lesions in which the functional control of motor activity is essentially at the level of the midbrain, the extensor dystonia is the characteristic decerebrate posture. Failure of cerebral inhibition of reflexes mediated through the brain stem gives rise to excessive responsiveness to tactile, auditory, visual, or vestibular stimuli. As a result of an uninhibited reticular activating system, startle responses are frequently exaggerated, with a generalized over-response to stimulation. On the other hand, patients with lesions in the reticular activating system show lethargy and impaired responsiveness.

CEREBELLAR REGULATION

The cerebellum[15] contributes elements of control and coordination in terms of force, direction, and distance. The number of motor units contracting in a unit period of time determines the force or speed. The muscles acting synergistically determine the direction; and the length of time they each contract determines the distance. Present concepts regard this control system to be effected by preprogrammed activity.[16] The program has been determined through prior experience and is engaged primarily in the execution of rapid, skilled, volitional, and automatic activities where feedback is not useful because of the speed of the motion.

Impairment of cerebellar function or interruption of cerebellar pathways to and from the rest of the central nervous system results in dysmetria, dyssynergia, and decomposition of movement. Intention tremor results during attempts to carry out purposeful motions. Taken together, these abnormalties constitute the symptom complex of ataxia. The patient is unable to carry out effective, rapid, accurate, smoothly coordinated or automatic movements or to maintain a stabilized posture.

BASAL GANGLIA

The function of the basal ganglia is to participate in the elaboration of volitional motor activities by organizing current and anticipated support for ongoing activity. Jung and Hassler[17] refer to the activities as ereismatic, referring to postural support for current activity and telekinesis for anticipated activity. Kornhuber[16] and DeLong[18] have shown that the basal ganglia participate in the generation of accurate ramplike motions where feedback is utilized for positional control. These activities are produced by integration, modulation, and inhibition of selected subordinate reflex motor patterns.

Impairment of function in the basal ganglia, therefore, results in failure of inhibition of reflex patterns of motor activity. The patient presents with varying degrees of increased motor tone and uncontrolled inaccurate movements. The increased motor tone is called dystonia. The excessive motion is described as chorea. Together the increased tone and motion may be regarded as dyskinesia. A progression in the clinical spectrum of dyskinesia may be viewed as either nonvoluntary or volition-related activity. *Ballism* is a grossly flailing movement in which the whole limb or side of the body is flung into violent activity. There is no persistent motor tone, and the movements appear to be spontaneous and nonvolitional. This type of movement is not seen in children with brain damage but is seen in adults with damage to the corpus Luysi. *Chorea* consists of flailing or jerky motions of segments of the extremities. There is considerable motion but very little persistent tone. The movements typically are nonvoluntary and are usually seen in Sydenham's or Huntington's chorea. *Choreiform movements* consist of flailing or jerky motions of the limbs, abnormal postures of the head, and facial grimaces that occur during attempts at voluntary movement, on generalized activity, or in response to emotional stimulation because of impaired capacity for inhibition. They are characterized by rapid movements of relatively small range but frequent occurrence and the absence of more than minimal levels of increased persistent tone. *Athetosis* consists of distortions of volition, producing motions that have often been described as writhing, twisting, or wormlike. There is moderate tension and the motions are limited in range. These motions are initiated by voluntary effort or by reflex stimulation. On examination, movement patterns can be recognized as partial or complete expressions of lower level reflexes that have occurred because of inadequate inhibition. *Dystonia* consists of spontaneous motion through a very limited range with a high degree of persistent tone during attempted voluntary activity. Dystonia is characterized by severe cocontraction of antagonistic muscles. The patients often go through severe contortions and gyrations exerting strong motor activity and frequently involving many muscles of the face, head, neck, trunk, and all four extremities. *Rigidity* is the result of constant cocontraction of antagonist muscles. Motion is absent or minimal. The tone is so great that the body part is fixed in position.

MOTOR AND PRE-MOTOR CORTEX

The motor and pre-motor cortex play an important part in the initiation and organization of complex skilled motor activities.[19] They contribute to the adaptability, deftness, complexity, and rapidity that is observed in well-learned motor behaviors in a normal individual. These characteristics of coordination may be encompassed in the general concept of praxis. An individual with a deficiency in the integrated functions of motor activity is regarded as dyspraxic or apraxic.

Dyspraxia is the impairment of ability to perform *learned*, complex voluntary movements. Dyspraxia may be expressed at different levels of complexity. Kinetic or motor dyspraxia represents impaired ability to execute appropriate motor patterns and sequences of muscular activity. Constructional dyspraxia refers to impaired ability to execute manipulative tasks guided by visual or spatial information. Ideomotor dyspraxia describes difficulty in applying motor activity in appropriate functional context. Ideational dyspraxia is an impaired ability to carry out purposeful motor activity in appropriate symbolic context.

Damage to the motor and pre-motor cortex is characterized, therefore, by loss of specific components of the repertory, related to the specific localization of the lesion and proportional to the amount of brain tissue involved. The quality described by Hughlings Jackson as "poverty of movement," or stereotypy, is a major characteristic of cerebral cortical damage.

The stereotyped motor patterns represent an inability to select appropriate muscle groups to carry out motor activity and also to modulate or inhibit synergic patterns generated by lower levels of the central nervous

TABLE 39–2. CLINICAL FEATURES OF MOTOR IMPAIRMENT IN BRAIN-DAMAGED CHILDREN

Spasticity	Athetosis
Monoplegia	Nontension
Hemiplegia	Tension
Paraplegia	Choreoathetosis
Diplegia	Dystonic
Quadriplegia	
Rigidity	Tremor
Ataxia	Mixed

TABLE 39–3. STATES INFLUENCING RESPONSIVENESS

State of Consciousness
  Obtunded consciousness
    Coma, stupor, confusion
    Seizure activity
  Hypoactive states
    Somnolence
    Lethargy
    Fatigue
    Febrile or metabolic illness
  Hyperactive states
    Mania
    Hyperkinesis
    Hyperirritability
  Seizure activity
Sensory and Perceptual Ability
  Blindness or impaired visual acuity
  Deafness or impaired auditory acuity
  Impaired pain perception
  Visual-perceptual defects
  Language-receptive deficit or auditory imperception
  Impaired kinesthesis — touch, proprioception
Cognitive Ability
  Situation comprehension
  Deficient symbolization
    Passive manipulation
    Gestures
    Verbal impairment
Attentiveness
  Ability to orient to significant stimuli
  Maintain focus on significant elements
  Distractibility
  Impulsivity
  Stimulus-bound behavior
Affective States
  Separation apathy or anxiety
  Dejection
  Hostility
  Rapport
  Psychiatric states
    Thought disturbance
    Autism
    Depression
  Rigidity to change — novelty rejection
  Paucity of rewards or reinforcers
Behavioral Background
  Inconsistent discipline
    Nonreinforcement of responding–habituation
    Reinforcement of nonresponding
  Promotion of dependency, passivity
  Promotion of inattention
  Suppression of initiative
Motivation
  Inner direction — rejection of external influence
  Cooperation
  Energy level
  Interest level in activities presented
    Previous background
    Rapport
    Value system
    Behavioral drives
    Available reinforcers
  Novelty effect
    Positive
    Negative
  Rapport — acceptance of nonfamiliar staff personnel
Motor Activity

system hierarchy. A familiar example is the flexion of the elbow that occurs during the attempt of a patient with hemiplegia to abduct the shoulder. Another example is the stiffly maintained angle of knee flexion during ambulation, representing inability to coordinate hip extension on the stance leg with knee extension on the swinging leg.

CLASSIFICATION OF MOTOR SYMPTOMATOLOGY

Understanding of the role of the hierarchical organization of the central nervous system and the integration of motor activity provides for the classification of individuals with brain damage on the basis of clinical features. The motor disability associated with continuing dysfunction occurring in the developmental phase of brain growth is called cerebral palsy. The current classification of motor disorders in cerebral palsy is generally accepted based on the clinical features of the motor impairment of children with brain damage (Table 39–2).

EVALUATION OF THE CHILD WITH BRAIN DYSFUNCTION

The physiatric evaluation of the child with brain dysfunction should include an assessment of the capabilities of the child to respond either to stimuli or to instruction. One also needs to differentiate between the ability to respond and the willingness to do so. It is also necessary to distinguish between the failure to respond because motor ability is impaired and because more general systemic or behavioral defects are present. Table 39–3 illustrates the elements to be considered in any evaluation of a child's abilities.

The evaluation of the motor activity of a child with brain injury should correspond to the basic concepts of motor organization that have been outlined above. *The movements and postures that the individual can achieve constitute the motor repertory, which provides a basis for the prescription of a training program.* The essential characteristic of the motor repertory is that it describes the motor activities of the child and of each of the component limbs in functional terms. The therapeutic program is based upon this analysis as it correlates with developmental expectations.

The normal sequence of motor development provides a general guide for the acquisition of new patterns of movement and posture for children with normal systems of motor control. A thorough knowledge of normal motor development is essential in order to make an accurate evaluation. Excellent reviews of this subject are provided by Gesell and Amatruda,[20] Illingworth,[21] and Lowrey.[22] Assessment of motor function in a child should include the history of the age at which key milestones of function were achieved. The motor developmental history also provides a screening technique to alert the examiner to the existence of a problem. However, it should not be considered to be a rigid track through which each child must pass regardless of the nature and location of the disturbance in the central nervous system. Evaluation of the motor repertory will identify the motor abilities and deficiencies in terms consistent with the neurophysiologic diagnosis.

Considerable confusion has been engendered by the manner in which the evaluation of development of function has been used in the assessment and planning of motor training. The motor capacity of a normal child is the result of the biologic changes that occur together with the experiential exposure. It is important to distinguish, therefore, between deficits in achievement of motor activities that are the consequence the injury or dysfunction of specific structures within the central nervous system that control specific types of motor activity, and the failure to develop these activities because of lack of the experiences necessary to establish the appropriate neuronal connections through a learning-developmental process. As an extreme example, it would be inappropriate to consider an adult hemiplegic patient developmentally delayed because his upper extremity is flexed at the elbow, wrist, and

fingers, and the thumb is adducted, even though this posture resembles that of a newborn infant. A child who has had an acquired brain injury and shows the same pattern should also be recognized as an individual whose central motor control system is creating these postures. Somewhat more confusing is the child who, as the result of an injury to the cerebellar pathway, has ataxia and does not stand. Lack of standing balance results from the ataxia rather than inability to develop the motor coordination for balance and walking because of "developmental delay."

The developmental sequence in a child with central nervous system damage and dysfunction may differ from that of the child with an intact central nervous system. As an example, it should not be expected that a child with a hemiparesis will learn to crawl on hands and knees before he learns to stand and walk. The creeping position is much too difficult to assume because of the paralyzed upper extremity, which cannot be extended to provide appropriate support and security. In fact, the child with hemiplegia may find that ambulation on his feet is easier after he achieves the coordination necessary for balancing, since the extensor spasticity of the lower extremity assists in providing support. It would be a mistake to restrain this child from walking or to attempt to train him first to creep on hands and knees because he has not followed the "normal" pattern of creeping before walking.

The motor repertory of a child is evaluated by observing the child's posture and movements as they occur spontaneously, in response to verbal or nonverbal instructions, in response to placement in various positions, and in response to the applications of somesthetic stimulation.

Voluntary Activity. In observing voluntary activity, the degree to which individuals demonstrate the freedom from or rigidity of association with undesired movements, i.e., stereotyping, must be evaluated. A child with a hemiplegia, for instance, may have difficulty in flexing the elbow without abducting the shoulder or vice versa. He may have difficulty in extending the hip without excessive adduction and internal rotation. The ability to carry out a specific and precise individual motion at will is an important indicator of the specificity of control and of the range of motor potential for that individual. The greater the stereotyping of function, the fewer are the possibilities for the acquisition of complex gross or fine motor coordination and speed. The normal child, of course, follows a developmental sequence in this regard, progressing from a reach with palmar grasp and the ulnar aspect of the hand down toward the working surface at six months to pronation of the hand with palmar grasp at eight months and eventual radial grasp with pinch and finger prehension at nine to ten months of age. The hemiplegic or quadriplegic child with pronator dystonia is exhibiting stereotypy with limited specific control, and not precocious maturation. Separate individual finger motions for the purpose of complex manipulations may not be acquired until three to four years of age. This specificity develops through practice by learning to inhibit the undesired components of the stereotyped patterns.

Conscious vs. Automatic Coordination. The degree to which each motion is carried out by conscious volitional planning or by automatic engrams should also be observed. Automatic engrams are the result of well-established learning and reflect the ability to execute motor activity at a skilled level which does not require the direct attention of the individual once the motion is set into progress. If the central nervous system has never developed the capacity to carry out skilled motor activity at an automatic level, as in many athetoid patients, then it can be carried out only under direct attention which, necessarily, is slower, and the number of activities that can be monitored at any time is limited. Prolonged correct practice is essential to develop automatic mechanisms. With continued training, the acquisition of automaticity can be achieved *if the structural substrate for those motions is available.* An assessment of the degree to which such automaticity has been achieved with similar motions or postures can, therefore, give the examiner an idea of the degree to which automaticity training is possible in a proposed skill sequence. As an example, the maintenance of head posture is normally achieved at an early age, and the lack of automaticity is generally a sign of serious impairment of this function. At the same time, it is possible, although unusual, to find individuals who have the ability to either stand or sit in the erect posture without being able to maintain head position, which indi-

cates that lack of head control is not a generalized impairment of balance but that there are specific elements relating to control of individual segments of the body.

Postural Adjustment vs. Prime Movers. The third aspect of voluntary motor control to be evaluated is whether the impairment is in the components of postural support or in the control of the prime movers. While individual motions occur utilizing specific or regional muscle groups, the effort may be ineffective because postural activity may be deficient. Similarly, postural coordination may be adequate but voluntary precise activity of those muscle may be impaired when the patient attempts to use them as prime movers. An example of this is the presence of a good extensor support reaction when a patient is placed upright in the standing position, but there is difficulty in getting good reciprocation for stair climbing because voluntary extension of the hip and knee is inadequate. This difference occurs because reflex mechanisms that are initiated in the support reaction cannot be appropriately inhibited to allow reciprocation or because specific volitional hip extensor activity, which is required for walking or climbing stairs, is not yet available to the child. The decisions for the training program offer the alternatives of exercises to improve the deficient aspects of function, substitution for deficiencies, or recognition that the disability is so great that improvement cannot occur.

Posture and maintenance of position require endurance. Active translational motions should be trained by repetitive motions involving action of the prime and synergic movers. Sensory reinforcement improves motor control. As the characteristic abilities of the voluntary motor activity are identified in each limb, the priorities for the therapeutic program are established.

Involuntary Activity. Involuntary activity is the result of uninhibited reflex activity of a simple or complex nature. The degree to which this reflex activity can be modulated is an essential element in determination of the therapeutic program. The specific reflexes to be observed are discussed in Chapter 11 (page 218). As a normal individual matures, the reflex activities of the spinal cord, medulla, and midbrain are integrated into the normal activity and appear as discrete reflex patterns as a rule only during severe exertion when the reflex acts as a facilitating mechanism. Under normal conditions, these reflexes are not apparent, although it is obvious that they are still present within the central nervous system as organized circuits, since they appear clinically when higher level central nervous system structures are damaged in later life. Reflexes are considered obligatory if they occur consistently when the appropriate stimulation is applied. They are considered facultative if they occur weakly, intermittently, or inconsistently in response to stimulation or if they can be inhibited by voluntary or automatic activity of the individual. In the rehabilitative program patients are trained to inhibit excessive tone or excessive reflex activity. Medications like diazepam, baclofen, or dantrolene may be helpful. When uninhibited motor activity is obligatory, intramuscular neurolysis may be useful as a temporary measure to assess the possibilities for learning of inhibition. Tendon lengthening and tendon transfers are effective procedures to decrease sensitivity of the muscle spindle stretch-sensitive endings to reduce obligatory spasticity.

Motor Control. The control of accuracy of use of each prime mover muscle needs to be evaluated. Defects in this function are referred to as dysmetria. Inaccuracy of force giving rise either to dystonia or to abnormal undesired velocity of movement is referred to as dyssynergia. Excessive motor activity gives rise to excessive velocity and force of movement. If the prime movers are opposed by cocontraction of antagonistic muscles, this produces dystonic movements. The force is controlled by the temporal organization of the contractions of individual motor units within a muscle. Impairment of the ability to synchronize or desynchronize motor unit contractions, therefore, gives rise to hypotonia, dyssynergia, or dystonia.

Impairment of coordination of synergic muscle groups and inhibition of antagonistic muscle groups with the desired motion constitute another aspect of dyssynergia. Another component of motor coordination is that of direction, which requires the coordinated contraction of a number of muscles at a specified velocity for a specific period of time to ultimately achieve the desired position. The ability to reach a desired position by the most efficient route requires the coordination of several muscles in an organized correlation of strength and time. A defect in this function produces the clinical picture of ataxia.

Evaluation of Motor Activity

The evaluation of a child's motor activity is carried out topographically. The response of head control in the supine, prone, and sitting positions is observed both in stable positions and during changes of posture. The responses to tilting and to traction on the upper extremities and the closeness of correlation between head raising and lower extremity and upper extremity positions are observed. The characteristics of head responses at the critical developmental ages are well-defined, and correlation between age and level of function will give an idea of the severity of involvement. It is helpful to quantify observations by specifying the angle of tilt of the body in each direction than can be applied while the head is held upright. If the head falls, it should be assisted to the erect position, and the length of time the head is held upright when assistance is removed should be observed. In the supine position when the arms are pulled, does the head come with the body, precede, or lag? If the head maintains a linear relationship with the trunk, is this a response to tilt or a function of overall rigidity?

In the recumbent position, the position of the head, the upper and lower extremities, the spine, and the pelvis are noted. The presence of the ability to roll over either from supine to prone or prone to supine spontaneously or with the facilitation of the body-on-body or head-on-body reflexes is observed. While the child is in the recumbent position, it is useful to look for tonic neck reflexes, either symmetrical or asymmetrical, in response to movement of the head. The symmetrical tonic neck reflexes are observed best in the lateral recumbent position, since the head can be flexed or extended without stimulating vestibular responses, which can overshadow the tonic neck reflexes. Changes in tone of the biceps and triceps may be the most sensitive indicators of persistent tonic reflexes.

Sitting posture is observed in the stable, supported short sitting position, tailor sitting position, and long sitting position. The degree to which sitting posture can be maintained independently by appropriately controlled trunk movements in the anterior, posterior, and lateral directions and the degree to which the upper and lower extremities carry out protective extension and compensatory equilibrium reactions are observed.

In the upright position, the posture of the lower extremities, back, and head is noted both in response to the suspended upright position and during standing. In the suspended upright position, the presence of excessive hip and knee extension and scissoring is indicative of abnormality, as is persistent hip or knee flexion after four months of age. In the weight-bearing position, the presence or absence of a support reaction adequate to maintain body weight is observed. Equinus of the feet or any deficiency in plantigrade foot posture is noted. Weakness of dorsiflexion also is significant. It is important to note whether the support reaction in the lower extremities is reflex or voluntary. When an adequate support reaction is present, are appropriate equilibrium responses available in the head, upper extremities, trunk, hips, and lower extremities? If equilibrium responses are not evident, can they be elicited either through facilitation or through verbal or nonverbal instruction. If adequate support and equilibrium responses are present, the performance of ambulation either with or without assistance is evaluated. While examining for reciprocation, assistance for balance may be given manually at the pelvis to aid a weak gluteus medius. Additional assistance may be given, if needed, for support of the trunk or chest. The requirements for ambulation are (1) support, (2) reciprocation, (3) dynamic equilibrium, (4) segmental coordination, and (5) gait sequence. Each of these components should be evaluated kinesiologically and the training program directed at improving deficiencies.

The function of the upper extremities can be subdivided into reach, grasp, manipulation, placement, and release. Palmar grasp may be ulnar or radial with or without shoulder rotation and forearm pronation or supination. Prehension requires finger and thumb coordination as three-finger pinch, two-finger opposed pinch, and two-finger lateral pinch.

A distinction must be made in the nature and degree of skill of reach and grasp, in impairments due to cerebral disconnection or injury, and in those of developmental delay. The developmentally delayed grasp is considered to be an ulnar type grasp, typical of the normal five- to six-month-old child. Between six and eight months of age, the radial grasp develops. However, the grasp of the child who has damage to the motor cortex is an excessively pronated grasp with weakness of supination.

The persistence of uninhibited reflexes is generally considered a prognostic sign indicating limited potential for motor learning.[23] Nevertheless, when voluntary movements are available or elicitable, they may be used as the basis for the establishment of a training program. Due regard without rigid adherence needs to be given to the level of motor achievement appropriate for age in order to establish appropriate goals.

Bracing and assistive devices may be used to provide support in the functional position if inadequate motor ability in a specific area interferes with functional performance. Thus, a child with equinus as a result of a weak anterior tibialis muscle will do well with a dorsiflexion brace if he has the ability to balance his trunk, support his weight at hips and knees, and reciprocate. Assistive devices like walkers, axillary or forearm crutches, or canes may also be used to assist balance as well as to provide support. Further assistance for support may be given by blocking the ankle joint of a short-leg brace at 80 degrees to prevent excessive dorsiflexion at the ankle and flexion of the knee. Occasionally a child may be helped by long-leg braces to learn to lock the knees in extension for support while practicing reciprocation and trunk balance. The knees can be unlocked for short periods of time to allow knee control to be practiced while providing the necessary assistance for balance. The basic principle here, as in any learning situation is to *present a specific task to each child in an isolated form and intensity at which the child can succeed.*

Some children with poor support reactions have general hypoactivity and show a flexed posture at hips, knees, shoulders, and elbows. They are sluggish in their responsiveness, slow in movement, and have high arousal thresholds. They can be aided by providing a strongly stimulating milieu. Commands should be clear, loud, and rhythmic. Fairly loud, rhythmic music is often useful to provide general reticular system activation. Extensor activity is improved in this way. At the same time, noise and motion that interfere with the child's perception of his training activities must be kept to a minimum. The fact that these children are hypoactive does not protect them against distractibility.

MOTOR TRAINING

Therapeutic management is based upon the determination of the level of functional ability represented in the motor repertory, in each of the topographical areas, together with an establishment of priorities for training the functional activities required to meet the patient's needs. As the more basic needs are met by learning improved skills, new goals may be added to the program. The modes of intervention are (1) training of improved motor function, (2) assistance of function by human or specialized devices, (3) substitution for function by specialized devices, (4) limitation of requirements by a modified environment, (5) training of substitute functions to compensate for a deficit, and (6) modification of anatomic or physiologic abnormalities by surgical procedures or medication.[24]

Motor training procedures[25] should be carried out in an attitude simulating relaxed play and emphasized by voice, manner, behavior, and approach that encourage participation in and enjoyment of the activity. At the same time, sufficient structure should be present to ensure that the activity to be performed is clearly discriminated from the background by the child. The milieu should not be overwhelmingly distracting by auditory or visual noise. The activity should be inherently pleasant, attractive, and rewarding to the child. Precise observation of the performance needs to be made by the therapist for recording progress and by the child to recognize the degree of success with which each motion to be trained is being performed. The experience of numerous studies of learning of motor skill in normal adults as well as handicapped individuals has shown that perception of motor response is important in the learning process.[26, 27] Proper structuring of the training situation will direct the child's attention to the details of each activity. When excessive motor tone is a significant element impairing motor control, volitional inhibition of dystonia — relaxation — should be taught. Techniques for inducing relaxation as advocated by Jacobson,[28]

Rood,[29] or Bobath[30] may be used to make the relaxation available for the learning process.

The movements to be trained are selected by evaluation of the motor repertory. Those activities that are inadequate for function are identified and priorities are set to develop to a more functional level the available but inadequate responses that can be elicited. The kinesiologic components of the motion to be trained are then identified. Desynthesis consists of simplifying motions to the level of components that the child can control during each training session (Fig. 39–1). These motions are practiced repeatedly until control is precise and dependable. As precise control of performance of each component is developed, the individual components are combined or resynthesized into progressively more complex activities that gradually approximate the complete motion.

It is important for the child to see that these components are, in fact, useful subordinate units in the final motion. It may be necessary, with some children, to demonstrate this by introducing during a portion of the training session the synthesized motion with sufficient assistance to perform it correctly. One method of isolating a functional component in an activity is to provide assistance by bracing or supporting other components so that the child is able to concentrate on the desired motor component (Fig. 39–2).

The motion to be trained should be isolated under conditions that guarantee optimal attention. Accessory motor activity is allowed only when the motion to be trained is easily performed, automatic, or well-learned. The isolation of an activity may be achieved by eliminating the need during training for any accessory motion by positioning the patient, providing assistance, manual manipulation, bracing, or requiring performance only of the single motions to be learned (Fig. 39–3). Progress is achieved by successively chaining components into a resynthesis of the primary pattern and gradually re-introducing the necessary accessory motor activity, so that the complex functional usefulness is approached.[31] See Chapter 19 (page 403).

Training of head control may be initiated by providing a wheelchair with adequate trunk support and stabilizing assistance for the head in the erect position (Figs. 39–4 to 39–6). The purpose of passive assistance is to accustom the child to the correct head posture during most of the time while sitting

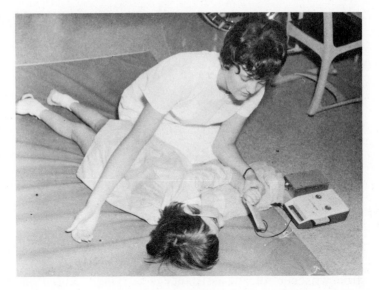

FIGURE 39–1. When the patient is positioned to remove all gravitational demands, she need not attend to body support or balance while concentrating on learning controlled pinch and grasp.

(Figs. 39–7 and 39–8). Short periods of active head control in response to a hinged head halter may then be introduced and carefully timed for endurance (Fig. 39–9).[32] Manual assistance is often necessary for cuing and guidance. As improvement occurs, rewarding auditory or visual feedback systems may be introduced[33] (Fig. 39–3). Stresses in the form of tilting and rocking may be utilized as head control develops to stimulate dynamic as well as static responses.

Upper extremity training may require stabilized posture in a wheelchair, splinting or manual assistance to isolate finger grasp

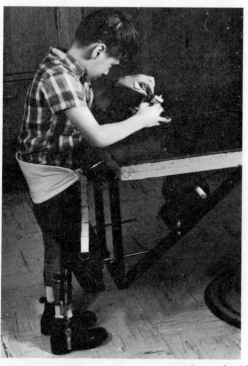

FIGURE 39–2. Minimizing extraneous demands aids in concentration on the assigned task. A short-leg brace, buttock sling, and blocking knee pad decrease demands for attention to support of the lower extremities while attending to a task that requires manual dexterity.

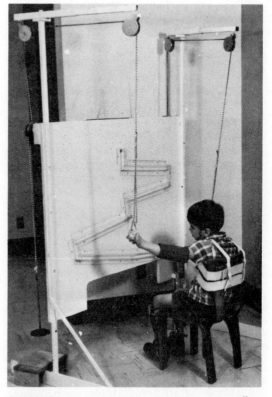

FIGURE 39–3. Assistance to maintain posture allows the patient to concentrate on exerting maximal effort for shoulder depressor activity.

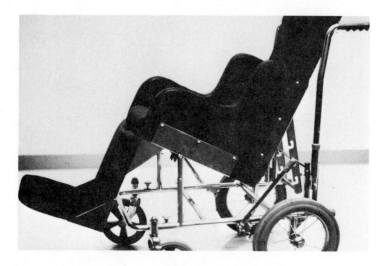

FIGURE 39–4. An adjustable tilting seat orthosis mounted on a Toronto wheel base provides corrected and comfortable support for a child with strong reflex flexion of the trunk and neck.

from wrist control, and assistance in carrying or reaching while grasping is being practiced (Fig. 39–11). Another useful technique for practice of hand control is to have the patient recumbent on a mat or table. All postural requirements for the trunk, head, and shoulder are eliminated by appropriate support. Adequate attention may then be focused on the activity of the hand (Fig. 39–1). Such isolated activity will of course have limited value in the child's understanding unless it is also clearly related to the training goal of a useful functional activity.

Identify the role of each motor component in the synthesized movement as postural or translational. For postural movements, the training goal will usually be to increase the duration and stability of the motor activity. For the translational or prime mover activity, the criterion would involve accuracy and timing, and to a lesser degree, strength or speed.

Elicit the activity repetitively by (a) Instruction. (b) Carrying out the motion repeatedly in the course of a purposeful act. For

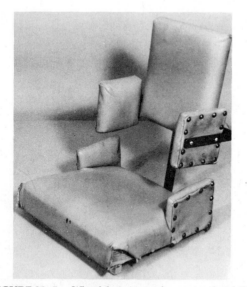

FIGURE 39–5. Wheelchair insert for postural stabilization. The anterior portion of the seat cushion is elevated 15 to 20 degrees to flex the hips. In this way, extensor thrust is reflexly inhibited and, with gravity assisting, the patient remains seated well back in the chair. The upper side pads are adjustable to fit against the lateral thorax at heights corresponding to lateral spinal curves. The lower side pads are thick enough, and set in to contact the trochanters, giving a three-point pressure system for support.

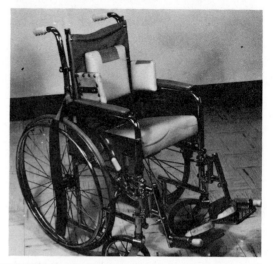

FIGURE 39–6. The wheelchair insert is relatively inexpensive and may be placed in the chair or removed as required for transportation.

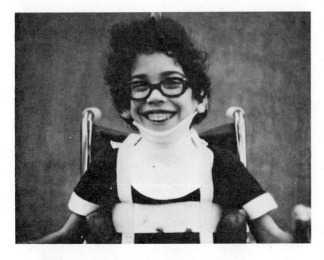
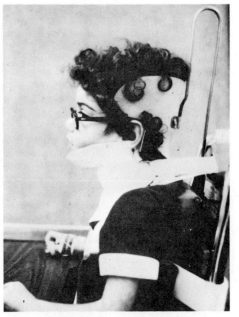

FIGURE 39–7.   When a child is unable to sit erect and maintain posture, a molded fitted neck collar may be attached to the chair. Its use should be coordinated with training of volitional head control and should be removed as head balance develops.

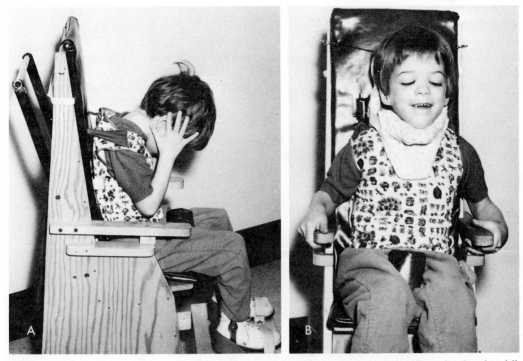

FIGURE 39–8.   Phases of training of head control. *A*, Without assistance the patient allows her head to fall and makes no effort to keep it vertical. *B*, With passive assistance she becomes accustomed to the vertical position as an acceptable one, and with appropriate reinforcement it becomes a desirable one.

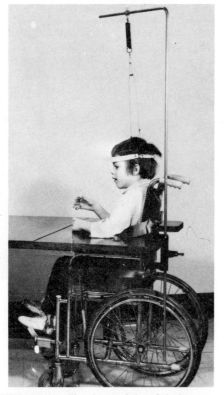

FIGURE 39–9. The hinged head halter provdes some active assistance but primarily provides tactile cues regarding correctness of head position.

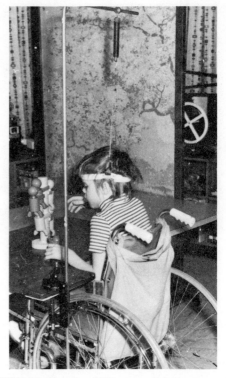

FIGURE 39–11. As ability to maintain an upright head is acquired, other tasks are introduced so that by practice automatic engrams of head control develop.

instance, in order to extend the neck, the command to look up or to turn the head, "Look at Mommy," may be used. (c) Providing assistance to the motion with instructions to "Move this way," or "I'll help you," or "You help me." For instance, during ambulation training when emphasizing reciprocation and support, assistance may be given for balancing by supporting the child at the trochanters to prevent lateral loss

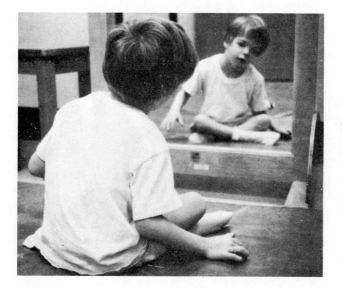

FIGURE 39–10. Visual information as a supplement to proprioception in a teaching format enables the child to progress to independent head posture.

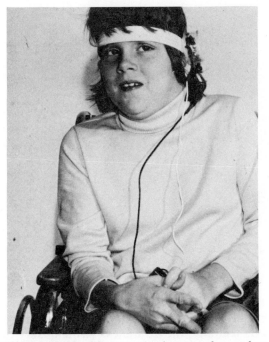

FIGURE 39–12. Mercury switches may be used to provide auditory cues, or music or television can be used as a reward to reinforce the maintenance of upright posture of the head.

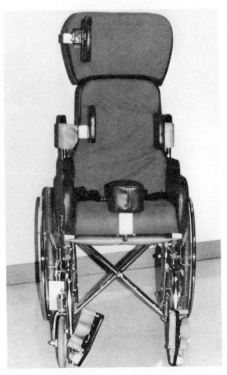

FIGURE 39–14. Difficult positioning problems occasioned by back deformities may be aided by a well-constructed fitted seating orthosis adapted to the needs of the individual child. The seat belt should always be attached at the level at which the seat meets the back of the chair.

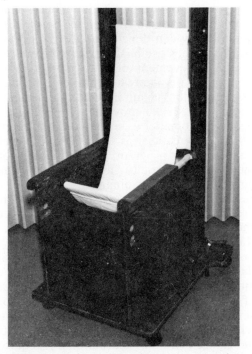

FIGURE 39–13. Special problems require adapted seating. A simple sling chair will prevent severe extensor thrust.

of equilibrium, or by placing one hand on the stance hip and the other under the axilla on the swing side to support against the drop of the pelvis and loss of balance. The child thus learns to carry out an effective compensated Trendelenburg gait. (d) Induce the activity by facilitation. Ankle dorsiflexion may be induced by exerting resistance against hip flexion (Bechterew reflex). Head extension may be elicited by tipping the patient forward or by elevating his head and asking him to hold it that way. Vestibular stimulation to elicit upper extremity protective extension may be introduced by rolling the child lying prone over a ball or rolling log. Functional electrical stimulation is a useful modality for such motions as wrist extension or elbow extension, or in the lower extremity for hip abduction, hip extension, or knee extension.[34] Elastic bands around the thighs have been used to stimulate abduction. Brushing, icing, or other cutaneous stimulation has been used to facilitate the responses of the underlying muscles.[29] It is important that

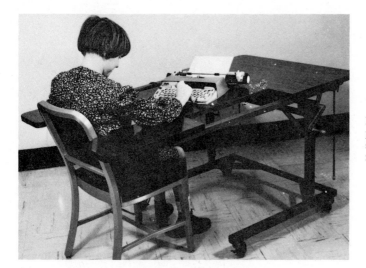

FIGURE 39–15. Even children with mild problems of balance during sitting need stability in order to learn upper extremity motor skills.

facilitation techniques elicit a clear and identifiable activity. When this occurs, the child can participate actively and simultaneously, in attempting to repeat the muscular activity voluntarily, and eventually can perform without the facilitation. If the desired response is not elicited, other more effective techniques should be sought.

Participation should be reinforced by a reward that is *observed* to be effective (Fig. 39–12). In the beginning, this should be done regularly and immediately as the performance meets the minimal criteria. Reinforcement for *cooperation* is a separate issue and should be carried out independently. In some children in whom cooperation is a major issue, especially in the beginning of the training program, reinforcement should be used for any attempt at cooperation, beginning with simply allowing the trainer to manipulate the child. Reinforcement for cooperation may be necessary to achieve and maintain cooperation. However, cooperation in itself does not enhance learning of motor activity. The fact that cooperation fosters repetition is helpful, but the quality of the repetition is governed by careful application of reinforcement or reward to elicit the correct performance of the specific motor activity. It is important, therefore, to set criteria within the ability of the child to succeed and gradually to increase the strictness of standards to be met as they become achievable.

Reinforcement serves also to direct attention to the specific motion and to the criteria for performance. By serving as a sensory feedback mechanism, it aids in developing the ability for self-monitoring. When carried out skillfully, the awareness of the quality of movement that develops becomes associated with the reward or reinforcement. A successful performance, therefore, begins to become rewarding in itself as the awareness of result of the motion becomes its own reinforcement.

With repetition and incorporation of the components of motion into functional, pleasurable, and inherently interesting activities, automaticity can develop as the praxic program becomes established as an engram.[31]

The achievement of criteria in a motor performance is the result of a learning process. Attention is an important element in learning of skilled movements. As learning occurs, automaticity develops through repetition. Automaticity is the result of a well-learned motor program.[27] With the development of automaticity, as the demands for conscious attention diminish, the ability to respond to multiple complex stimuli increases (Fig. 39–11). Automaticity requires the development of its own neural circuits. If this potential is not present, automaticity will not develop. Not all individuals with brain damage are able to achieve normal levels of automatic motor activity. The achievement of a voluntarily directed motion under conscious attention is not always associated with the later development of automaticity, indicating that the neurocircuitry required for voluntary and for automatic motor activity is different.

Facilitative techniques such as efflorage, tappotement, muscle percussion, vibration of a specific limb, body or head positioning, passive rocking, tilting, and elastic or nonflexible resistance may be used to assist training. Functional electrical stimulation is an extremely effective modality for facilitation.[34] Its application requires careful reinforcement. It is used by applying trains of brief direct or alternating current impulses and increasing the amplitude during successive voluntary efforts until successful contraction occurs. (See Chapter 16, page 372.) These techniques of facilitation generate cutaneous, muscle spindle, kinesiologic, or vestibular stimuli. They evoke reflex impulses that converge on anterior horn cells together with volitionally initiated impulses to exceed the excitatory threshold and produce a motor response. In addition, this type of sensory stimulation may also serve to direct attention to the limb being trained, thereby improving the ability of the child to monitor the activity and direct it.

Klein[26] and Keele[35] have shown that during the performance of a highly skilled task, learning and improvement of performance were better in those circumstances where repetition and attention were higher. According to Klein, knowledge of the criteria of performance was also shown to enhance attention, and, with it, to improve learning. See Chapter 19 (p. 403) for a more complete discussion of the training of coordination.

It has been a common observation that during the early teaching of a difficult task a greatly increased motor tone occurs in patients with motor disorders (Fig. 39–13). In fact, the same thing occurs in normal individuals learning a difficult task, especially when under stress. For the child with brain damage, this uncontrolled motor activity becomes a problem that interferes with learning the desired motor performance. It has been interpreted to be the result of "cortical" participation. Neurophysiologic studies, however, have shown that the motor cortex participates in the initiation of a learned motion, but once motion is initiated, activity in related neurons of the motor cortex disappears.[36] It does not follow, however, that learning is carried out best by nonparticipation of the cortex. To the contrary, the cortical neurons are essential to interact with the subcortical structures to produce the coordination pattern. The cortex is required for learning, and

the work of Evarts indicates that cortical participation occurs during the initiation of well-learned activities. Pyramidal neurons tend to be continuously active during a motion only when the motion is still being learned. The increased tone occurring during training of motor activities in brain-damaged children is due to increased excitation or insufficient inhibition (Fig. 39–15). Excessive excitation may result from persistence of preexisting response patterns, inappropriate training techniques, or a distracting milieu. It may also result from the child's efforts to please or the therapist's or parent's exhortation to "try harder." Ability to inhibit irradiation in the nervous system develops with practice and increased tone represents irradiation that exceeds the capacity for inhibition.

When structure is provided in the therapeutic session to specifically reinforce inhibition of excessive tone and encourage active motion from a state of relaxation, maximal learning of motor skill occurs. Because automatic activities can be carried out without paying attention to them some programs of training advocate repetition of activity without conscious attention. Studies on motor learning indicate that this is counterproductive. From a practical point of view, it has not been shown to be possible to "eliminate the cortex" from participation in motor learning to develop automatic coordination. More to the point, however, is the concept that learning of a motor skill is more rapid and effective when (1) there is knowledge of criteria for performance; (2) there is knowledge of results; (3) there is active participation of the learner in the motor process; (4) the greater the attention to the criterion-result relationship, the more effective is the learning process; (5) there is massive repetition; (6) the activity is sufficiently isolated from extraneous requirements to allow successful performance (Fig. 39–1).

Instruction does not have to be communicated verbally if the child has poor language ability or is immature. By positive reinforcement and passive structural modeling of the child's activity, communication can be established and the learning process fostered.

Maintenance of musculoskeletal posture and mobility of children with cerebral palsy is essential to the training of control and the development of coordination (Fig. 39–14). The prevention of deformity by regular careful range-of-motion exercises, stretching (see page 399), timely orthopedic surgery,[37] and regular observation and accurate measurement is important in management. Intramuscular neurolysis[24] is a useful procedure to achieve muscular relaxation for six months to a year or more while awaiting surgery, or to evaluate the functional benefits that might occur following a surgical procedure to relieve tone. Serial casting is useful to correct recent contractures. Scoliosis may be treated or its advance delayed by the use of an appropriate spinal supportive orthosis. Prompt surgical fusion is extremely useful in preventing serious structural and postural deformity. Special attention should be paid to the hip joints in the presence of simultaneous spasticity of the hip adductor and flexor muscles or adductor and hamstring muscles. This spasticity contributes to early dislocation that may be aggravated by vigorous stretching procedures. Early adductor releases with prolonged night splinting in abduction is often effective in preventing dislocation of the hip. Weight bearing in the quadruped position also is helpful if feasible.

Cognitive Function

Intellectual function requires synthesis into perception of the stimuli transmitted through the different sensory systems. This is then processed, analyzed, related to other information, and ultimately assigned a meaning to which some response is organized. In assessing cognitive function in children with brain damage, it is important, therefore, to attempt to define these cognitive processes in order to learn which intellectual systems are intact and which are disrupted. Certain tests of intellectual function place relatively strong requirements for performance on noncognitive functions such as behavior, attentiveness, inner drive of energy, and motor coordination. It is, therefore, desirable to identify those behavioral, attitudinal, attentional, and motor functions that are required for the comprehension of the task and for the execution of the response which is supposed to measure the cognitive function that is presumed to be tested.

The preferential processing of linguistic information in the left hemisphere and visual spatial information in the right hemisphere is well known, as is the important role of the corpus callosum for transmitting information between both hemispheres. Proprioceptive information is processed to a large extent in the posterolateral portion of the parietal lobes. As we learn more about the brain, subordinate functions are being localized to certain specific areas of the cortex.[38] It is helpful, when possible, to identify specific deficiencies, since a remedial program may be organized to take into account their influence on the functional capacity of child. It is of less value to be able simply to identify a child by an averaged I.Q. level. The intelligence quotient may be useful, for administrative purposes, to place a child with brain damage in a school program. To organize an individualized educational program for a brain damaged child, knowledge of the individual functional characteristics that affect learning ability in a specific educational area is necessary.

The major sensory areas in which cognitive functioning is mediated are auditory, visual, and somesthetic. Each has an expressive motor aspect as well as receptive aspects — verbal, visual-motor, and kinesthetic. Each may be considered to operate on three levels of abstractness versus concreteness. The most concrete level is that of sensory reception, e.g., hearing, seeing, and touch. A higher level of data processing is that of perception, in which characteristic patterns are identified or recognized: phonemes, sounds, or their combinations; forms, shapes, or designs; or specific body or limb movements. A still higher level of abstraction is reached when these perceptions take on meaning. They begin to be associated with patterns, perceptions, or concepts in other senses. A word becomes associated with a picture or an object; a movement signifies an emotional state or an instruction and becomes a gesture; or a series of standardized shapes on a piece of paper signifies a spoken word, an object or action, a quality, or an idea. Still higher levels of abstraction exist in the form of classification or symbolization.

Among the subordinate processes that have been recognized are those of visual perception — recognition and distinction of shapes and forms; identifying similarities and differences in orientation, shape, size, sequence, order, and spatial relationships; and discriminating a figure on a background. Each process individually contributes important modifications to meanings of visually presented material. A need for multiple tests arises from the fact that in practice, achievement on any of the test batteries and their subtests is influenced by a number of factors in addition to the one nominally being tested. In many cases these factors are not of primary interest in cognitive assessment, but they interfere with evaluation of significant functions. By a judicious selection of multiple test procedures, it is possible to deduce much information concerning the functional ability of the child in the school situation. It is then necessary to formulate these characteristics in terms that will be useful to the teachers in developing a remedial educational program. The clinical neuropsychologist can make essential contributions to understanding cognitive processing by the brain damaged child. The recognition of deficits in identifying or responding to these variables is important for establishing a remedial program.

PERSONALITY AND BEHAVIOR

The child who has suffered brain damage may have distortions of perception of incidents and interpersonal events that carry profound implications for future development of personality and behavior. Damage to specific structures of the brain has been associated with abnormalities of behavior. The frontal lobe, anterior to areas 6 and 8, receives contributions from the dorsal medial nucleus of the thalamus, which conveys impulses from the hypothalamus. These areas are connected by the cingulum and uncinate fasciculus to the anterior portion of the temporal lobe and to parietal and adjacent occipital and temporal association areas. These connections make possible the association of emotional values with sensory or affective input. From experimental evidence it is proposed that this mechanism allows the recognition of events that have an emotional meaning.[39, 40] Rewards or punishments are conceived to be monitored by the hypothalamus and recorded for memory in the frontal cortex. Attention and responses are organized and triggered in the limbic system. Thus, the mechanisms are available for focusing attention on relevant and significant material for the improvement of function and memory with training.

In his review of animal experiments, Isaacson[41] demonstrated that destruction of specific areas in the limbic system gives rise to disorders of concentration affecting the ability to respond appropriately to problem-solving situations. The limbic system is composed of the cingulum, cingulate gyrus, hippocampus, septal nucleus, amygdala, and hypothalamus. The locus ceruleus, midbrain reticular system, and midbrain tegmental nuclei are closely related structures. The forebrain structures, septal nucleus, hippocampus, and midbrain structures are connected by the median forebrain bundle. Deficits in function differ depending upon the specific localization of the lesion within the component structures of the limbic system. Laboratory studies[41] in animals have demonstrated that limbic system lesions result in the following abnormalities in behavior: (1) impairment of ability to withhold response to a stimulus, (2) increased activity level, (3) decreased attentive ability, (4) impaired ability to analyze problems systematically, (5) impulsivity, (6) perseveration, (7) rigidity or resistance to change. While evidence is still insufficient to correlate specific localization of lesions in humans with behavioral changes, these behavioral abnormalities are seen frequently in children with diffuse brain damage. Considerations of the behavioral alterations following limbic system lesions demonstrate that impairments of subordinate functions such as impulsivity or diminished attentive ability may manifest themselves by deficiency in higher cognitive functions.[42] Inability to withhold a response to a stimulus may manifest itself as a premature response to a question. Failure to observe that the response is incorrect because of impulsive behavior may lead to the conclusion that the child lacks the cognitive information required.

Similarly, inability to attend sufficiently will interfere with the solution of a problem if the problem is presented in a manner that exceeds the duration of attention of the child. The substance of the problem may be satisfactorily managed if the material is presented more succinctly. Attentive ability is limited not only in relation to its duration but in relation to background stimulation. Tests sensitive to figure-background discrimination, either visual or auditory, are useful, therefore, as indices of attentive ability.

Perseveration is another form of responding to previous experience. The child responds to certain criteria given previously without noticing that the conditions may have changed or even refusing to recognize that the conditions have changed. If there is difficulty in recognizing changing conditions this may provide a reason for responding incorrectly to a problem and may lead to incorrect conclusions concerning the child's ability to comprehend and solve problems. In a group of children with problems in school, the following behaviors were noted to relate closely to disorders of behavior seen in animals with limbic system lesions: tangential responses; distractibility; easy frustration; organizational deficits; visual, spatial, or temporal deficits; limitation of hypothesis formation; and impaired responses to internal cues.

There are conflicting views in the literature on whether deficits of attention represent organic brain damage, an affective disorder, or inadequate prior training. However, as in any other diagnostic exercise, the association of multiple behavioral manifestations of impaired ability to inhibit responses appropriately, a consistent demonstration of the impairment in different situations, and, in addition, signs of organic brain damage may be used as evidence to support an organic basis for the behavior. At the same time, it is necessary to eliminate the possibility of emotional or experiential bases. In practice, it is not unusual to find elements of all three etiologic factors operating in the child with brain damage. Management then becomes the problem of dealing with each of the contributory elements in proportion to its significance in the individual child.

PRINCIPLES OF MANAGEMENT IN ATTENTION-DEFICIT DISORDERS

A structured training situation that is consistent in all areas is probably the one essential management technique that applies to attentional deficits of any etiology. This structure requires careful establishment of criteria for tasks that provide challenge but are well within the capacity of the child. Distracting competitive stimuli — auditory, visual, social, and motivational — should be reduced to a level manageable by the child. The significant stimulus should be clearly discriminable from the background. There should be a guarantee of success in assigned tasks. This is made possible by a clear definition of the required response at a level at

which the child will succeed. This may be done by passively moving the child through the required response, providing a problem-solving protocol to follow with reinforcers of sensory-motor cues as necessary to assure success, e.g., using a series of verbal cues to solve a picture puzzle when verbal skills are better than visual. Assistance is provided at junctures where blocking occurs during a physical or problem-solving task and the assistance is diminished as progress is made. A consistent, meaningful reinforcement schedule is provided for correct or successful activity. Monitoring of the effectiveness of the reward is necessary, since not all children respond to the same rewards equally, and satiation may occur. There must be consistent structure, reinforcement techniques and schedules, behavioral management, and disciplinary techniques by all disciplines cooperating in the management of the child. This should include the school teacher, occupational therapist, physical therapist, speech pathologist, nurse, parent, physician, social worker, psychologist, and any other person working with the child. This requires that the therapeutic procedures in physical therapy, occupational therapy, speech therapy, and schoolroom be homogeneous and provide an appropriate milieu for learning.

Medications are useful for the child with deficits of attention of organic origin. Connors[43] has described a rating scale that is useful for some children with overt brain damage with hyperactivity. The criteria for observation of effects should be defined as precisely as possible. One or more target behaviors may be chosen and incidents counted in a unit period of time. Ad hoc rating scales constructed for individual children are preferable. Specific characteristic behaviors are identified and numerical as well as verbal values defined. Observations can be focused on one or two key items that are meaningful in the management plan for that child.

Useful medications have been dextroamphetamine, methylphenidate, amitriptyline, nortriptyline, and trifluperazine. To a lesser extent, the phenothiazines (chlorpromazine, promazine, thioridazine) and minor tranquilizers like hydroxizine are useful for limited periods of time. Since it is difficult to predict which medications will be effective in any one child, it is useful to proceed with the idea of carrying out a consistent and sequential series of therapeutic trials. A range of dosage levels should be tried to be certain that the best effect with minimal side effects has been achieved. A small percentage of children respond well to one medication for a few months and then proceed to adapt. If the child is followed closely, this may be detected early and a change to another medication may be helpful. Parents need to be educated regarding the rationale for the use of medications. The precise criteria for effectiveness should be defined behaviorally in measureable terms, e.g., number of minutes without reminders on a specific task, number of distractions of gaze per 5-minute period, number of impulsive or tangential responses per class hour, etc. Clear distinctions should be made between these measures and "social tolerance," or "tolerable" level of hyperactivity — which are highly subjective measures. The aim of therapy is not to make the child less active, but to permit him to focus his activity for better learning of cognitive as well as motor skills.

All behaviors exhibited by a child need to be recognized as a natural consequence of the interaction of the child with the adults who care for him, and, later, the peers who are part of his environment. The actions of parents, like those of the professionals, depend upon their own emotional, cognitive, and attitudinal backgrounds which they bring to the child. Most parents have had little training in child-rearing in general and no training in rearing a handicapped, brain-injured child. Their attempted support or protection often is inconvenient for professionals but does not deserve the epithets of "over-mothering" or "smothering." A realistic assessment of the origins of parental management styles should be included in the development of the program of management for the child.

MANAGEMENT OF EMOTIONAL AND
MOTIVATIONAL FACTORS

The most common emotional stress that the brain-injured child experiences during treatment is that of being surrounded by unfamiliar personnel. The immediate involvement of the parents or other familiar adults during the treatment of the child is frequently useful in assisting the transition to the professional. It may be sufficient for the parent to stand by and approve. Some children may do better if the parent handles the child under the direction of the professional in the beginning. Gradual transition to the professional may then be allowed.

However, successful rehabilitation of children cannot be considered to be achieved until the care and handling of the child has been returned to the parents or surrogates. The parents need to be skilled in techniques of management, and the child should behave as well with them as with the therapist, nurse, or teacher. The emotional lability often seen in children with diffuse brain damage of the pseudobulbar type may be managed by maintaining a nonstressful pleasant atmosphere in the educational or therapeutic program. Adequate opportunity for recreation is essential in a management program to provide diversional as well as functional activity in a highly motivating milieu so that there is opportunity to utilize newly learned skills. Emotional problems deriving from interpersonal relationships, familial interactions, disturbances of attitudes, and perspectives secondary to past experience need to be identified and programs of management for retraining of the undesired behavior included in the overall rehabilitation program. Alteration of disturbing behaviors of family members is essential and, although difficult, should be undertaken. Verbal counseling is usually less effective than behavioral management for children. Adolescents and older children may be amenable to verbal mediation, in which case it is a useful adjunct but rarely a mainstay of the program of management.

Programs of Therapeutic Intervention

Since the early 1950's, a number of different schools of thought have developed differing approaches to the therapeutic management of children with brain damage. Each has claimed to be based upon neurophysiologic concepts selected from the literature to support that particular point of view. Reference has been made to some of these authors in the preceding pages where the ideas developed coincide with the basic approach presented here. Primarily, this approach is based on current concepts of learning theory. The child can change his behavior only by a process of learning. The

Chapter 18, quantity and quality of learning is determined by the structural and physiologic integrity of the entire central nervous system. Therefore, an evaluation is required of the specific central nervous system functions that are available in the child for sensation, active participation, and repetitions of performance.[44, 45] If facilitation techniques make an activity available to a child by eliciting a motor response, then a learning process may take place, provided adequate cerebral volitional connections exist.

The reader is referred to discussions by Gillette,[46] Pearson and Williams,[47] and Harris[48] and to the proceedings of the NUSTEP Conference[49] for descriptions of these methods of therapy relating to training of motor activity. A more detailed presentation of the management of motor training based on principles of learning is presented elsewhere.[25, 31] Work by Ayres[50] was originally directed at children with learning disabilities but has been applied to children with mental and motor retardation and developmental disabilities as well. A number of attempts have been made to evaluate treatment techniques advocated by Doman and Delacato.[51] Brunnstrom has described the application of reflex activity for adult hemiplegic patients which has equal applicability to children with cerebral palsy.[52]

Evaluation of the efficacy of any of the methods proposed has been notoriously inadequate. Only a few studies have been published, and valid controls have been difficult to demonstrate.[53] Evidence for effect has been largely anecdotal. The ideas presented above have been subjected to several studies but suffer from similar deficiency in that these studies have not yet been published. Nevertheless, children need to be treated.

SUMMARY

In the present state of knowledge, the most prudent course, and one that is still rooted in a basic respect for each individual as possessing intrinsic human value, is to utilize established principles of learning and behavioral management together with careful neurophysiologic diagnosis, as a basis for teaching brain-damaged children new motor and behavioral skills. A judgment can be made of the effectiveness of a procedure if one defines the expected goal precisely in measurable terms and maintains accurate records of functional achievement. The strength of a motion, its voluntary range, the number of contractions or repetitions, the duration of activity, the resistance overcome, and the difficulty tolerated may all be used as criteria for measurement of progress. These should show evidence of positive change within a reasonable time. Significant improvement even though small should be demonstrable within two months of consistent application of treatment once appropriate rapport has been established. If this is not seen, it is incumbent upon the professional in charge to identify a reason for failure, change the conditions, change the treatment, or discontinue it as indicated. Even though improvement may be seen in this short time, training of coordination to the optimal level requires months or years. This long period of time essential for the formation of coordination engrams is the basis for the failure of short-term or intermittent therapies. Coordination must be trained until automatic engrams have developed and then been maintained by frequent practice.

When organizing a training program for a child with brain damage it is important to observe the child's ability to learn. Treatment methods, even if they are proven to be scientifically valid, need to be consistent in their effect upon the child's attentive ability, motivation, and retention, as well as have a demonstrable effect on motor activity. Choices will have to be made that depend on the motor, perceptual, and behavioral characteristics of the child as determined by the lesion in the central nervous system. This development of a plan of management is the responsibility of the physician concerned with the child's habilitation. The specific choices will also be influenced by the previous experience and attitude of the child in a learning situation. Where structure and discipline are required for scholastic work, the imposition of such structure in motor training is equally essential. Where training of attentive ability is required for cognitive learning, training and monitoring of attention also should be included in the program of motor training.

For children who do not have problems in attention, motivational energy, or initiative to undertake independent tasks, the "change of pace" provided by recreational periods is beneficial. However, this should not be confused with the therapeutic method selected for its intrinsic ability to develop identified cognitive or motor skills.

Since the children cannot be assigned responsibility for their own activities, the inclusion of parents or other responsible adults is necessary. Family attitudes, goals, and values must be considered. The physical, emotional, intellectual, and financial resources of the family all influence the degree and extent of participation of which the parents are capable. Their instruction in principles and techniques of management should be an ongoing process in which the parents work with the child, both under the observation of the professional staff and separately. Simple didactic instruction without hands-on application is insufficient to transfer the performance of the child while under the guidance of the therapist to a home program directed by the parents. It is not until the child is at his optimal level performing at home and at school that it can be said that rehabilitation has been successful.

REFERENCES

1. Nelson, K. B., and Ellenberg, J.: Epidemiology of cerebral palsy. *In* Schoenberg, B. S. (Ed.): Neurological Epidemiology: Principles and Clinical Applications. Vol. 19, Advances in Neurology. New York, Raven Press, 1978, pp. 421–435.
2. Kiely, J. L., Paneth, N., and Susser, M.: Low birthweight, neonatal care, and cerebral palsy. An epidemiological review. *In* Mittler, P. (Ed.): Frontiers of Knowledge in Mental Retardation. Baltimore, University Park Press, 1981.
3. Hagberg, B., Hagberg, G., and Olow, I.: The changing panorama of cerebral palsy in Sweden 1954–1977. Paediatr. Acta Scand., 64:187–192, 1975.
4. Bennett, F. C., Chandler, L. S., Robinson, N. M., and Sells, C. J.: Spastic diplegia in premature injuries. Etiologic and diagnostic considerations. Am. J. Dis. Child., 135:732–737, 1981.
5. Nelson, K., and Broman, S. H.: Perinatal risk factors in children with serious motor and mental handicaps. Ann. Neurol., 2:371–377, 1977.
6. Moyes, C. D.: Epidemiology of head injuries in children. Child Care Health Dev., 6:1–10, 1980.
7. Brink, J., Ganett, A. L., Hale, W. R., Woo-Sam, J., and Nickel, V. L.: Recovery of motor and intellectual functioning in children sustaining head injuries. Dev. Med. Child Neurol., 12:565–571, 1970.
8. Walker, A. E.: Head injury. *In* Caveness, W. F., and Walker, A. E. (Eds.): Conference Proceedings. Philadelphia, J. B. Lippincott, 1966, p. 15.
9. Van Hof, M. W.: Development and recovery from brain damage. *In* Connolly, K. J., and Prechtl, H.

F. R. (Eds.): Maturation and Development. London, Spastics International Medical Publishers, 1981.
10. Greenough, W. T., Foss, B., and Devoogd, T. L.: The influence of experience on recovery following brain damage in rodents — hypothesis based on developmental research. *In* Walsh, R. N., and Greenough, W. T. (Eds.): Environment as Therapy for Brain Dysfunction. New York, Plenum Press, 1976.
11. Yu, J.: Neuromuscular recovery with training after central nervous system lesions: An experimental approach. *In* Ince, L. P. (Ed.): Behavioral Psychology in Rehabilitation Medicine: Clinical Applications. Baltimore, Williams and Wilkins, 1980.
12. Kottke, F. J.: Reflex patterns initiated by secondary sensory fiber endings of muscle spindles, a proposal. Arch. Phys. Med. Rehabil., 56:1–7, 1975.
13. Grillner, S.: Descending control of spinal circuits. *In* Herman, R. M., Grillner, S., Stein, P. S. G., and Stuart, B. G. (Eds.): Neural Control of Locomotion. New York, Plenum Press, 1975, pp. 351–375.
14. Pompeiano, O.: Vestibulo-spinal relationships. *In* Naunton, R. F. (Ed.): The Vestibular System. New York, Academic Press, 1975.
15. Eccles, J. C., Ito, M., and Szentagothai, J.: The Cerebellum as a Neuronal Machine. Berlin Springer Verlag., 1967, p. 67.
16. Kornhuber, H. H.: Cerebral cortex, cerebellum, and basal ganglia: An introduction to their motor functions. *In* Schmitt, F. O., and Worden, F. G. (Eds.): The Neurosciences, Third Study Program. Cambridge, Mass., MIT Press, 1974.
17. Jung, R., and Hassler, R.: The extrapyramidal motor system. *In* Field, W., and Magoun, J. (Eds.): Handbook of Physiology, Neurophysiology. Sect. 1, Vol. II, Chapter 35, pp. 863–927, Washington, D. C., American Physiological Society, 1960.
18. DeLong, M.: Activity of basal ganglia neurons during movement. Brain Res., 40:127–135, 1972.
19. Evarts, E. V.: Sensorimotor cortex activity association with movements triggered by visual as compared with somesthetic inputs. *In* Schmitt, F. O., and Worden, F. G. (Eds.): The Neurosciences, Third Study Program. Cambridge, Mass., MIT Press, 1974, pp. 327–337.
20. Gesell, A., Amatruda, C. S., Knoblock, H., and Pasamanick, B.: Developmental Diagnosis, 3rd Ed. Hagerstown, Md., Harper and Row, 1974.
21. Illingworth, R. S.: The Development of the Infant and Young Child. Edinburgh, E. & S. Livingstone, 1967.
22. Lowery, G. H.: Growth and Development in Children. Chicago, Year Book Publishing Co., 1975.
23. Molnar, G., and Taft, E.: Pediatric Rehabilitation I. Cur. Probl. Pediatr. 7:3–155, 1977.
24. Easton, J. K. M., Ozel, A. T., and Halpern, D.: Intramuscular neurolysis for spasticity in children. Arch. Phys. Med. Rehabil., 60:155–158, 1979.
25. Halpern, D.: Therapeutic exercise for cerebral palsy. *In* Basmajian, J. V. (Ed.): Therapeutic Exercises, 3rd Ed. Baltimore, Williams and Wilkins, 1978, pp. 281–306.

26. Klein, R. M.: Attention and movement. *In* Stelmach, G. E. (Ed.): Motor Control, Issues and Trends. New York, Academic Press, 1976.

27. Keele, S. W., and Summers, J. J.: The structure of motor programs. *In* Stelmach, G. E. (Ed.): Motor Control, Issues and Trends. New York, Academic Press, 1976.

28. Jacobson, E.: Progressive Relaxation. Chicago, University of Chicago Press, 1938.

29. Stockmeyer, S. A.: An interpretation of the approach of Rood to the treatment of neuromuscular dysfunction. Am. J. Phys. Med., 46:900–956, 1967.

30. Bobath, K.: A Neurophysiological Basis for the Treatment of Cerebral Palsy. Clinics in Developmental Medicine. No. 75, pp. 1–98. Philadelphia, J. B. Lippincott, 1980.

31. Kottke, F. J., Halpern, D., Easton, J. K. M., Ozel, A. T., and Burrill, C.: The training of coordination. Arch. Phys. Med. Rehabil., 59:567–522, 1978.

32. Halpern, D., Kottke, F. J., Burrill, C., Fiterman, C., Popp, J., and Palmer, S.: Training of control of head posture in children with cerebral palsy. Dev. Med. Child Neurol., 12:290–305, 1970.

33. Harris, F. A.: Treatment with position feed-back controlled head stabilizer. Am. J. Phys. Med., 58:169–184, 1979.

34. Gracanin, F.: Use of Functional Stimulation in Rehabilitation of Hemiplegic Patients. Final Report Research Project No. 19-p. 58395-F-012-66. Dept. of Health, Education & Welfare. Ljubljana, The Institute of the S R Slovenia of Rehabilitation of the Disabled, 1972.

35. Keele, S. W.: Movement control in skilled motor performance. Psychol. Bull., 70:387–403, 1968.

36. Evarts, E. V.: Contrasts between activity of pre-central and post-central neurons during movement in the monkey. Brain Res. 40:25–31, 1972.

37. Samilson, R. (Ed.): Orthopedic Aspects of Cerebral Palsy. Clinics in Developmental Medicine, Nos. 52/53, pp. 1–301. Philadelphia, J. B. Lippincott, 1975.

38. Lutey, C.: Individual Intelligence Testing. Greeley, Col., Lutey Publishing Co., 1977.

39. Papez, J. W.: A proposed mechanism of emotion. Arch. Neurol. Psychiatry, 38:725–743, 1937.

40. MacLean, P. D.: The triune brain, emotion, and scientific bias. *In* Schmitt, F. O. (Ed.): The Neurosciences, Second Study Program. New York, The Rockefeller University Press, 1970, pp. 336–349.

41. Isaacson, R.: The Limbic System. New York, Plenum Press, 1974.

42. Kimble, D. P.: The effects of hippocampal lesion on extinction and "hypothesis behavior" in rats. Physiol. Behav., 5:735–738, 1970.

43. Connors, C. K.: Food Additives and Hyperactive Children. New York, Plenum Press, 1979, pp. 113–119.

44. Held, R., and Hein, A.: Movement produced stimulation in the development of visually guided behavior. J. Comp. Physiol. Psych., 56:872–876, 1963.

45. White, B. L: Experience and the development of motor mechanisms. *In* Connolly, K. (Ed.): Mechanisms of Motor Skill Development. New York, Academic Press, 1970.

46. Gillette, H.: Systems of Therapy in Cerebral Palsy. Am. Lecture Series No. 762. Springfield, Ill., Charles C Thomas, Publisher, 1969.

47. Pearson, P., and Williams, C. E.: Physical Therapy Services in the Developmental Disabilities. Springfield, Ill., Charles C Thomas, Publisher, 1972.

48. Harris, F. A.: Facilitation techniques. *In* Basmajian, J. V. (Ed.): Therapeutic Exercise, 3rd Ed. Baltimore, Williams and Wilkins, 1978, pp. 93–137.

49. Bouman, H. D.: Exploratory and analytical survey of therapeutic exercise. Northwestern University Special Therapeutic Exercise Project. Am. J. Phys. Med., 46:1–1108, 1967.

50. Ayres, A. J.: Sensory Integration and Learning Disorders. Los Angeles, Western Psychological Services, 1978.

51. Freeman, R. D.: Controversy over "patterning" as a treatment for brain damage in children. J.A.M.A., 202:385–388, 1967.

52. Brunnstrom, S.: Movement Therapy for Stroke Patients, A Neurophysiological Approach. New York, Harper and Row, Publishers, 1970.

53. Wright, T., and Nicholson, J.: Physiotherapy for the spastic child: An evaluation. Dev. Med. Child Neurol., 15:146–163, 1973.

40

REHABILITATION FOR RESPIRATORY DYSFUNCTION

H. FREDERIC HELMHOLZ, JR.
HENRY H. STONNINGTON

DISORDERS OF RESPIRATION

Respiration is transport. It is the process of moving oxygen from the air to the alveoli of the lungs by a mass movement of air, called ventilation, and in turn removing carbon dioxide from the alveoli by the same mass movement. Ventilation maintains a pressure (concentration) gradient between alveolar gas and venous blood so that gases exchange between blood and alveolar gas by diffusion. The circulatory system provides the transport between the lungs and the tissues.

The effort, or cost, of ventilation depends on the elastic properties of the lungs, thorax, diaphragm, abdomen complex, and accessory muscles and the resistance to flow through the multiple air passages between the outside and the alveoli.

Physiologic Basis of Disorders of Respiration

Respiratory disorders, then, are conditions that prevent adequate transport in and out of the lungs (exchange), thereby leading to retention of carbon dioxide and to oxygen lack. These disorders may be caused by (1) muscle weakness or inefficiency or increasing stiffness of elastic components or by (2) increased resistance to air flow through the tracheobronchial tree; hence they are classified as (1) *restrictive* or (2) *obstructive*. A third category, that of conditions due to an increase in thickness of, or a decrease in area of, the alveolar diffusing membrane, is usually associated with a restrictive disorder; it leads primarily to low oxygen tension in arterial blood without carbon dioxide retention because of the much greater diffusivity of carbon dioxide in body tissues.

In Figure 40–1 the lung volume relationships and definitions are shown, and the effect of position on the end-expiratory position relative to vital capacity is suggested. The end-expiratory position is that at which elastic recoil of the lung is exactly balanced by the tendency of the "chest" to expand (point O, for example, in Figure 40–2). This point of equilibrium differs with position: in the supine position, the weight of abdominal contents favors expiration; in the upright position, it favors inspiration. In the weak individual, this change can be used to produce adequate resting ventilation (for example, with the rocking bed).

Restrictive Disorders

Figure 40–2 illustrates the elastic properties of the lung and "chest" (by which is

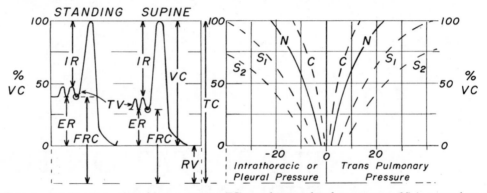

FIGURE 40–1. Subdivisions of total lung capacity (TC) are shown related to pressure (N) in normal respiratory maneuvers. Dotted lines indicate pressures required with different lung compliances. IR = inspiratory reserve volume; TV = tidal volume; ER = expiratory reserve volume; RV = residual volume; VC = vital capacity; FRC = functional residual capacity; C = more compliant than the normal; S_1 and S_2 = less compliant (stiffer) than the normal.

meant the entire complex of thoracic cage, diaphragm, abdomen, and relaxed abdominal muscles). Normally about 20 cm of water pressure would fill the isolated lung to vital capacity size (curve L, Fig. 40–2). Thus, full inspiration requires a transpulmonary pres-

sure of this magnitude, normally achieved by maintenance of the same pressure below atmospheric in the pleural space, i.e., the space around the lungs (curves N, Fig. 40–1). The dotted curves indicate the effect of varying the lung compliance (Fig. 40–1).

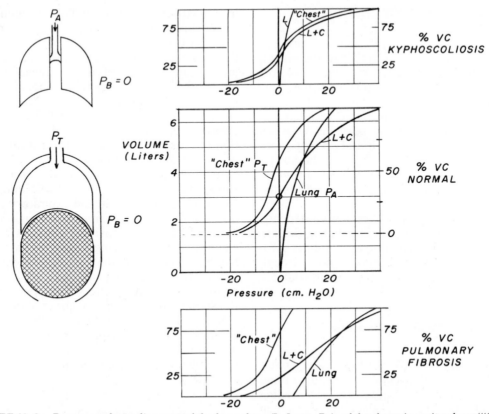

FIGURE 40–2. Pressure-volume diagrams of the lung alone (L; Lung; P_A), of the thoracic cavity alone ("Chest;" P_T), and of the combination (L + C) are constructed to indicate normal relationships and those found in two types of restrictive disorder. $P_B = O$ indicates that the atmospheric (barometric) pressure is the pressure to which the other pressures are referred.

Curves C are for increased compliance and curves S_1 and S_2, for lungs stiffer than normal.

If the lungs were removed and pressures above and below atmospheric were applied inside the remaining cavity, the characteristic curve marked "Chest" would be obtained (Fig. 40–2).

If, in the paralyzed individual, the combination of lungs and chest were similarly treated, one would obtain the combined curve relating volume to pressure indicated by "L + C" (Fig. 40–2). Such a curve describes the elastic properties of the system and the recoil that must be overcome in breathing. For any given tidal volume, the area between the line of zero pressure and the curve to this tidal volume represents work. If the time required is specified as well, one has an expression of power, or the rate at which work is done.

In Figure 40–2 the chart above the normal indicates the effect of chest deformity in changing the elastic properties of the chest and reducing the vital capacity. Note that the chest curve is the restricting element; thus, intrathoracic (pleural) pressure is never much below atmospheric, because the elastic lung is never stretched sufficiently to produce a large negative pressure.

The chart below the normal chart indicates the effect of increased stiffness of the lung (loss of compliance) in changing the elastic properties of the system and reducing the vital capacity. Note that this disorder leads to pressure well below atmospheric at all lung volumes, because of increased elastic recoil of the lung at all volumes.

Restrictive disorders are characterized by increased energy requirement to overcome elastic recoil of lung or chest structures at any given ventilation. Any disease that stiffens costovertebral or sternocostal connections or causes fibrosis of respiratory, abdominal, or shoulder girdle muscles or of the lungs themselves can lead to restrictive impairment of pulmonary function.

The same effect is produced by the loss of muscle or the loss of nerves that activate the muscles of respiration. The chart marked "normal" in Figure 40–2 shows the relationships that would occur if the vital capacity were reduced by a decrease in both the inspiratory and the expiratory reserve volumes. The restriction in such cases would be the inability to bring force to bear and do work against the recoil of the elastic system.

Obstructive Disorders

In any lung the air distribution system expands as the lung expands, and therefore there is a relationship between lung size and the resistance to gas flow (Fig. 40–3). One of the characteristics of asthma and emphysema is an increase in resistance to air flow as indicated in the curve marked "Emphysema." The dotted curve indicates the behavior in many cases of emphysema when expiration is forced. This is the phenomenon of air trapping, in which the airway develops such high resistance when transpulmonary pressure is high that air flow stops before emptying is complete. It has been shown that the obstructive phenomena in the emphysematous lung are characteristically nonuniform and are primarily brought out on expiration. Asthma tends to produce more uniform obstruction, which is evident to some extent during inspiration.

FIGURE 40–3. Resistance to air flow in a normal and emphysematous lung during expiration. Dotted line indicates effect of increased effort during a "forced expiration."

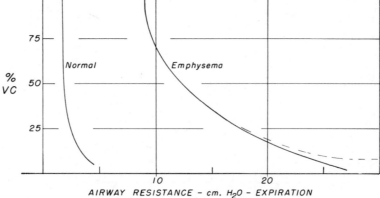

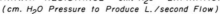

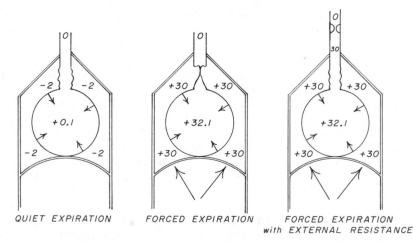

QUIET EXPIRATION   FORCED EXPIRATION   FORCED EXPIRATION
                                                with EXTERNAL RESISTANCE

FIGURE 40–4. Diagram to illustrate one possible mechanism of air-trapping and effect of resistance imposed by pursed-lip or grunting expiration. (This model requires rapid onset of positive intrapleural pressure to show the phenomenon. A resistance interposed between the "alveolus" and the compliant segment of airway converts this to a better demonstration model.)

A simple obstructing lesion of the trachea, when intrathoracic, can simulate emphysema if the involved trachea becomes collapsible. This kind of lesion serves here as a model in understanding air trapping (Fig. 40–4). When the lung empties because of its own elastic recoil, the pressure (intrathoracic) around the nonrigid trachea remains below atmospheric and the airway remains patent. If forced expiration is attempted and intrathoracic pressure rises above atmos-

pheric, the trachea collapses and prevents egress of the remaining air. It is theorized that multiple small air passages act the same way in emphysema. By obstruction of the airway *outside* the chest during exhalation, the pressure inside these passages is increased and the collapse is prevented. Hence, beathing out through pursed lips or grunting is often beneficial.

Obstructive disease can cause a decrease in arterial oxygen tension and retention of

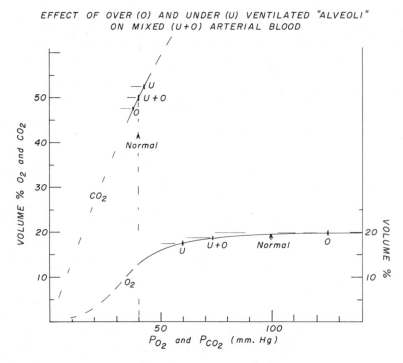

EFFECT OF OVER (O) AND UNDER (U) VENTILATED "ALVEOLI"
ON MIXED (U+O) ARTERIAL BLOOD

FIGURE 40–5. Plotting of oxygen and carbon dioxide dissociation curves together shows the effect of relative linearity of carbon dioxide solubility contrasted with alinearity of oxygen solubility on content of mixed (U + O) arterial blood content when it is made up of blood perfusing underventilated (U) and overventilated (O) areas of lung.

carbon dioxide when obstruction is relatively uniform, as in obstructing lesions of the trachea, for example.

Emphysema, however, and most cases of asthma characteristically cause a reduction in arterial oxygen tension without carbon dioxide retention because of the difference of the carbon dioxide and oxygen dissociation curves. Figure 40–5 illustrates how the retention of carbon dioxide in underventilated areas is compensated for in overventilated areas, whereas so little extra oxygen is taken up in the overventilated areas that the oxygen content and tension of arterial blood are below normal.

Diffusing Capacity Disorders

The amount of oxygen passing through the alveolar membrane of the lung depends directly on the difference between the alveolar oxygen pressure and the mean oxygen pressure of capillary blood, It depends also on the area of the membrane that separates air and blood; it is reduced by an increased distance between alveolar air and the hemoglobin of the blood (membrane thickness factor). Pulmonary fibrosis in its various forms causes thickening of the membrane and a decrease in alveolar surface, typically without obstructive disease.

Normally, increased oxygen uptake by the lung is caused by a decrease in the oxygen content of venous blood and an increase in pulmonary blood flow along with an increase in ventilation. A diffusion barrier can be compensated for to some extent by increasing ventilation, which reduces the carbon dioxide concentration in alveolar gas and thus raises the oxygen concentration (that is, pressure). In these cases the cost of maintaining a low alveolar carbon dioxide pressure is least when a rapid rate of breathing is used. Deep breathing would require excessive work because of decreased compliance.

Diagnostic Characteristics of Disorders

If the vital capacity, forced vital capacity (maximal expiratory effort following maximal inspiration), and the pattern and volume of ventilation with maximal breathing effort (so-called maximal breathing capacity) are measured with a suitable recording spirometer, the presence of obstructive disease can be detected. If no obstructive phenomena are found but dyspnea is present, the magnitude of the vital capacity may be used as an index of possible reduction in lung volume. Measurements of diffusing capacity of the lung can be made to detect abnormalities in such patients. The reader is referred to Comroe and associates[2] for details of testing procedures and, when dealing with children, to Polgar and Promadhat.[3]

Restrictive disorders are inferred when vital capacity and total capacity are reduced and no obstructive disorder is evident. Documentation of such disorders requires special tests that are beyond the scope of this presentation.

The table below gives findings in obstructive and restrictive disorders that can be obatined by a recording spirometer.

Estimates of lung size from physical examination and chest roentgenograms will indicate that total capacity is normal or increased in obstructive disorders and reduced in restrictive disorders.

Respiratory Muscles and Their Control

Normal ventilation at rest is accomplished by contraction of the diaphragm with enough activity of the external intercostal muscle to fix the chest cage. Initial shortening of the diaphragm muscle is associated with outward flare of the lower rib borders and rise of abdominal pressure, and there is concomitant relaxation of abdominal muscles. Expiration

	Vital Capacity	Forced Vital Capacity* (% in 1 second)	Maximal Breathing Capacity
Obstructive	Reduced	Less than 85%	Reduced
Restrictive	Reduced	85% or more	Normal or slightly reduced

*Many modifications of the method of estimating obstruction from a forced vital capacity are used. Any can be used when a recording is obtained.

is caused by gradual relaxation of the diaphragm with force being provided primarily by the elastic recoil of the lung.

Increased oxygen demand and carbon dioxide production during muscular activity are accompanied by an increase in ventilation immediately, owing to nervous impulses from active muscles and joints directly. (That due to fever is accompanied by increased ventilation as the result of increased activity of the respiratory center as the temperature rises.) Secondary mechanisms that also can increase ventilation are the effect of increased carbon dioxide tension (or fall of pH) in arterial blood on the respiratory center directly and the effect of a fall in arterial oxygen tension mediated through chemoreceptors (carotid and aortic bodies as well as specialized nerve endings on the surface of the medulla, sensitive to pH changes in the spinal fluid).

Increased activity of the respiratory center increases both the depth and the rate of breathing, and active expiration (lowering of the ribs by the internal intercostals and contraction of the abdominal muscles) begins. The stimulus to the respiratory center, if sufficiently intense, causes recruitment of accessory muscles of the neck, shoulder girdle, and abdomen to aid in inspiration and expiration.

Stimulation of the respiratory center also involves the circulatory centers nearby so that increases in ventilation are accompanied by increases in cardiac output. In addition, with deeper respiration the decrease in pressure inside the thorax increases the gradient of pressure between systemic veins and the right atrium, thereby tending to increase venous return, which increases the output of first the right side and then the left side of the heart.

In response to stimuli to the nose, pharynx, and tracheobronchial tree, coordinated reflexes are produced, i.e., the sneeze, the gag, and the cough. These involve all muscles of ventilation as well as the laryngeal mechanism for blocking the airway as the false vocal cords close the glottis. Effective cough or sneeze requires adequate abdominal muscle activity to raise pressure against the closed glottis so that the sudden release will cause velocity in the tracheobronchial tree adequate to provide turbulent flow. Laminar flow cannot move materials on the wall of the airway. Ciliary action is needed for this function.

When abdominal muscle power is lost or inadequate an effective cough can be produced by what is called exsufflation, originally introduced by Barach. The proper use of the cough machine is understood by few and the procedure is neglected in therapy today. Proper timing of inspiratory and expiratory periods is essential and can be provided by the COF-FLATOR produced to Dr. Barach's specifications.[4, 5]

Basis for Breathing Exercises and Chest Physical Therapy

Restrictive Disorders

When the nerves are intact or remnants of the neuromuscular system are underdeveloped, muscle weakness can be helped by suitable exercise. It should be emphasized that muscles of respiration cannot be put at rest and therefore they should be exercised voluntarily so that the increase in ventilation will make possible lessened activity of the muscles following therapeutic exercise. The margin between activity that will cause damage and activity that will cause hypertrophy can be narrow in patients with restrictive disorders and due caution should be observed when increased demands are put on respiratory muscles.

Chest deformities disturb the relations between the insertions and origins of respiratory muscles and may tend to flatten the diaphragm by increasing the anteroposterior dimension of the chest. Pulling in of the lower part of the rib cage with inspiration indicates inefficient use of the diaphragm. Often no increase in doming can be achieved in such patients, but the phenomenon should be noted and abdominal muscle exercises should be instituted when benefit is possible. Each case of deformity must be studied carefully before an exercise program is outlined. In many cases the only possible therapy is mechanical assistance to ventilation.

In treating any fibrosing or sclerosing disease of the chest cage and musculature the effect of loss of compliance should be kept in mind. Loosening of contractures and stiffened joints, when it is possible, decreases remarkably the work of breathing.

Loss of compliance of the lungs (fibrosis) is difficult to treat by physical means, but further development of respiratory muscles can be tried.

Obstructive Disorders

Obstructive disease is accompanied by fixation of the chest in a position larger than the normal end-expiratory level, with an increase in the functional residual capacity and residual volume. This condition tends to produce a flattening of the diaphragm and thus to lessen the usefulness of this muscle in inspiration. In some cases the abdominal muscles are contracted during inspiration and work against the inspiratory effort of the intercostal, neck, and shoulder muscles. In such cases help can be afforded by retraining to ensure relaxation of the abdominal muscles during inspiration. The best method is the use of exercises that contract the abdominal muscles during *expiration*.

Because the work of breathing increases rapidly when air velocity increases in obstructive disease, the following formulation is emphasized:

$$\dot{V}_A = (V_T - V_D)\, f$$

in which V_A = alveolar ventilation (liters per minute) BTPS, V_T = tidal volume (liters), V_D = dead space volume (liters), and f = frequency (breaths per minute). Since with each breath the dead space remains constant, the amount of dead space ventilation increases as frequency increases. With each breath the volume in excess of the dead space inhaled is the effective, or alveolar, ventilation; the greater the tidal volume, the smaller the fraction that is dead space ventilation.

Thus, the minimal total ventilation required for a given alveolar ventilation is attained by slow, deep breathing. Air velocities are also least when a given alveolar ventilation is attained by a *maximal tidal volume* and a *minimal frequency*. Since obstruction is primarily expiratory, fast inhalation ensures the lowest frequency. In addition, the phenomenon of air trapping should be kept in mind and rapid forced expiration should be avoided except through pursed lips or the partially closed glottis or vocal cords. With these principles in mind, a rational program of breathing exercises can be worked out that will help any patient who normally uses rapid, shallow breathing through an open mouth. The patient who already breathes slowly and deeply, and who exhales through pursed lips or grunts during expiration, will be helped less but can be reassured. Training can ensure deeper expiration when exercise produces stimulation of the expiratory muscles, if emphasis is put on deeper, faster inhalation and slower exhalation through pursed lips.

Underventilation

When restrictive disorders (including loss of muscle power) and obstructive disorders are of such severity that resting ventilation is insufficient to remove metabolic carbon dioxide, alveolar concentration of this gas rises as carbon dioxide is retained until increased alveolar concentration provides for removal of metabolic production again, according to the following formula:

$$\dot{V}_{CO_2} = \dot{V}_A \times F_{ACO_2}$$

in which $\dot{V}_{CO_2}$ = liters of CO_2 exhaled per minute BTP, V_A = alveolar ventilation (liters per minute) BTPS and F_{ACO_2} = fraction of CO_2 in alveolar gas.

Underventilation produces respiratory acidosis and, as carbon dioxide rises, oxygen falls to seriously low levels when air is breathed. However, cyanosis cannot be used as an index of adequacy of ventilation because of the variability in the amount of reduced hemoglobin in the superficial (visible) capillary beds. Severe oxygen deficiency in arterial blood is possible with cyanosis (for example, in peripheral vasoconstriction or anemia), and cyanosis occurs frequently in congestive failure when arterial blood is sufficiently saturated with oxygen.

Assistance to ventilation is the treatment of choice when the patient is capable of some respiratory effort. It can be accomplished by application of positive pressure to the airway during inspiration by an I.P.P.B.I. (intermittent positive pressure breathing, inspiration) machine. This device is so designed that a slight negative pressure starts a flow of gas, which continues until a preset positive pressure is reached; then the flow stops and the airway is vented to the outside. The pressure setting determines the tidal volume. The patient can slow the rate or speed it up, depending on the ventilation needed. The patient's own respiratory control mechanism thus becomes effective once more in regulating alveolar ventilation to metabolic needs.

When all respiratory activity has ceased, total control of ventilation must be undertaken by applying positive pressure to the airway, or negative pressure to the body, at regular intervals. It is impossible with the equipment currently available to adjust ventilation as precisely as does the respiratory control system of the body, but estimates made periodically of arterial blood levels of pH and carbon dioxide allow one to check adequacy by the following relationship (Henderson-Hasselbalch equation for the bicarbonate-carbon dioxide system):

$$pH = 6.1 + \log\frac{[HCO_3^-]}{0.03\ P_{CO_2}}$$

or

$$pH = 6.1 + \log\frac{[Total\ CO_2] - 0.03\ P_{CO_2}}{0.03\ P_{CO_2}}$$

Solution indicates that normal values approximate the following:

$$7.4 = 6.1 + \log\frac{20}{1} =$$

$$6.1 + \log\frac{24\ mEq/L}{0.03\ (40)\ mM/L} =$$

$$6.1 + \log\frac{25.2 - 1.2\ mM/L}{1.2\ mM/L}$$

25.2 = mM/L total CO_2 content of blood.
25.2 mM/L = 56.87 ml/dl or vol %.
0.03 mM/L/mm = solubility coefficient for CO_2 at body temperature.

In respiratory acidosis, P_{CO_2} goes up and pH goes down. Renal compensation will allow an increase in bicarbonate so that its ratio to P_{CO_2} increases again and pH returns toward normal.

Carbon dioxide retention can be tolerated for relatively long periods of time (although it causes narcosis when excessive), but lack of oxygen cannot; therefore, filling the lungs with high concentrations of oxygen will protect the individual from oxygen lack in emergency situations until definitive treatment can be instituted. Oxygen should always be administered first. When the lung contains only oxygen, carbon dioxide, and water vapor, cyanosis will never intervene if circulation is intact; thus, once oxygen has been administered, cyanosis cannot be an indication of ventilatory insufficiency in any sense at all.

When positive pressure is applied through the airway or negative pressure around the body to expand the lungs, the intrathoracic pressure relative to systemic venous pressure is inevitably raised and venous return is decreased. The normal circulatory system can compensate for this, but when it is hampered by blood loss or other abnormalities, serious decreases in cardiac output are produced. In those forms of restrictive disorder that are due to decreased compliance of the lungs, positive pressure applied to the airway causes much less circulatory disturbance than does negative pressure around the body. In other restrictive conditions, the two methods affect the circulatory system about equally. In obstructive disease, the application of positive pressure through the airway may be expected to affect the circulatory system more than would negative pressure around the body.

In those forms of restrictive disorder in which the primary abnormality is a barrier to diffusion of oxygen from alveolar gas to blood, a simple increase in the oxygen concentration of the inhaled gas will provide adequate compensation.

By studying the charts in Figure 40–1, with the additional information that lung compliance is usually within the normal range but the "chest" curve may be moved to the left in obstructive disease, one can work out the mechanical relationships that may be expected in various forms of pulmonary disorders. The circulatory disorders that affect lung function are those that cause pulmonary venous hypertension (such as mitral stenosis or left heart failure). They produce a decrease in lung compliance and, when pulmonary edema is present, a diffusion barrier.

Proper synchronization of muscular effort in producing ventilation is often lost in patients with obstructive lung disease so that accessory muscles, principally of the neck, are contracted to raise the chest while either the abdominal muscles are simultaneously contracted or there is little or no diaphragmatic contraction taking place. Sometimes this latter is due to excessive flattening of the diaphragm, i.e., loss of mechanical advantage. When flattening is severe one can note drawing in of the lower border of the chest on inspiration (see also discussion of chest deformity above).

Chest Injuries

The special case of chest injuries merits some consideration. Loss of integrity of the lung, which causes pneumothorax, is an emergency to be handled by a thoracic surgeon, but loss of integrity of the chest cage leads to a mechanical defect that tends to prevent inspiration. For example, negative pleural pressure developed by diaphragmatic contraction causes a nonrigid rib cage to collapse, thus preventing expansion of the lungs. Fixation of the ribs has been the treatment of choice. Positive pressure applied to the airway during inspiration has many advantages in that it ensures ventilation and splints the chest without operative measures. When the ribs are intact but muscle contraction causes pain, inspiration is limited. Therefore, intermittent positive pressure breathing is the treatment of choice in chest injuries that cause underventilation. It decreases pain as it increases ventilation. Apparatus delivering a set volume with each breath (volume preset) is usually preferred over pressure preset instruments in these cases. Decrease in venous return is the only complication; it should be considered whenever there has been loss of blood. Fall in blood pressure or increase in pulse rate, or both, indicate the need for blood replacement.

In the use of equipment for the support of or assistance to ventilation, certain principles are often forgotten. Any pneumatic system used is effective only if forces are applied to the elastic system including the lungs. Any leaks in the system prevent this application. A leak is the most frequent cause of failure and must not be permitted. Devices designed to compensate for leaks are unrealistic and lead to slipshod therapy.

Whenever the nasal passages are bypassed (by the use of tracheal tubes, pharyngeal catheters, mouth breathing, or tracheostomy), sufficient water must be added to the inhaled gas to ensure a relative humidity of 100 per cent at the body temperature of the patient. Gases below this temperature must contain particulate water. In practice, it is necessary to add heat to humidifiers in order to maintain this relative humidity.

The physical therapist will sometimes be called upon to assist in the retraining of individuals being weaned from ventilatory support after recovering from paralysis due to disease or produced to combat disease such as tetanus. Since the introduction of techniques of intermittent mandatory ventilation (IMV) the incidence of respiratory muscle incoordination following prolonged ventilatory support has decreased. IMV allows the patient to take breaths on his own while still supplying him with a determined number of mechanically produced breaths. Retraining involves emphasis on diaphragmatic contraction on inspiration with abdominal extra effort on expiration to increase the doming of the diaphragm.

Note: If ventilatory support has been prolonged or if the diaphragm is weakened by disease, one must remember that the diaphragm cannot be put at complete rest unless ventilatory support is resumed or provided. Any muscle will gain strength (hypertrophy) only if it is given rest periods or periods of minimal activity after being stressed. If a period of relative rest is not provided the muscle may be damaged. This can, of course, happen to the diaphragm as well as other muscles.

CHEST PHYSICAL THERAPY

It has been known since the days of Hippocrates that if a patient is left in one position for a prolonged period, particularly if depressed by disease (and in modern times by drugs), he will develop pneumonia. The actual steps leading to this pneumonia are atelectasis in dependent parts of the lung, retention of secretions, and growth of bacteria that ordinarily would be removed with the retained secretions.

Modern blood gas studies identify the first sign of atelectasis as a decrease in arterial oxygen partial pressure without a change in arterial carbon dioxide partial pressure.

All types of chest physical therapy and respiratory therapy techniques providing increased inspiratory effort by direction or incentive spirometry, or increased tidal volume by properly administered intermittent positive pressure breathing (IPPB), when combined with position changes and activity where possible, as well as coughing, will prevent atelectasis and hence the following pneumonia that so often is a complication postoperatively or in severely ill patients.

Chest physical therapy is the application

of physical methods to the respiratory care of patients with pulmonary disease. The range of treatment includes instruction in relaxation and breathing exercises; performance of postural drainage, percussion or clapping, and vibration; and splinting the chest or incision site to facilitate coughing. All these techniques assist in clearing pulmonary secretions. They are particularly indicated in patients with chronic obstructive lung disease manifested as asthma, bronchitis, emphysema, bronchiectasis, and cystic fibrosis; after major surgery of the upper abdomen, thorax, and cardiovascular system; and in all patients who are dependent on mechanical ventilation. A supportive program of chest physical therapy is necessary to assist patients with neuromuscular disease and a diminished cough reflex or effort who are unable to mobilize their pulmonary se-

cretions. All patients immobilized in bed can benefit from instructions in coughing and breathing exercises. Surgical patients are helped if they have developed confidence in the therapist before the operation. After the operation, it is difficult to gain the cooperation of a patient who is in pain and receiving analgesics. In the acutely ill, chest physical therapy is closely allied with inhalation therapy and intensive-care nursing. A working knowledge of oxygen and humidification equipment, mechanical ventilators, intermittent positive-pressure breathing devices, and endotracheal and tracheostomy tubes is essential.

Breathing Exercises. The therapist should instruct the patient in the techniques of breathing exercises (Fig. 40–6).

Postural Drainage. Optimal use of postural drainage requires a knowledge of the

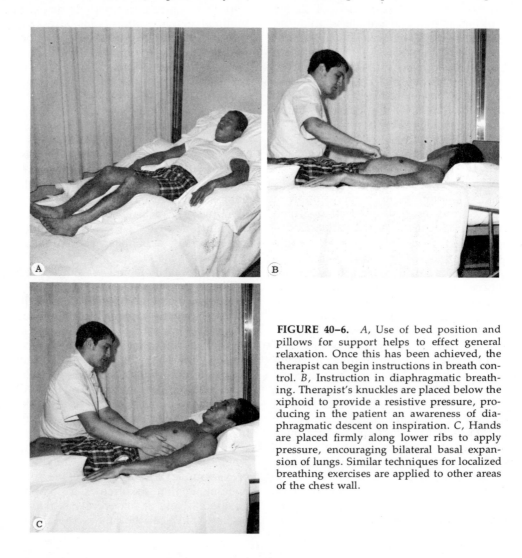

FIGURE 40–6. *A,* Use of bed position and pillows for support helps to effect general relaxation. Once this has been achieved, the therapist can begin instructions in breath control. *B,* Instruction in diaphragmatic breathing. Therapist's knuckles are placed below the xiphoid to provide a resistive pressure, producing in the patient an awareness of diaphragmatic descent on inspiration. *C,* Hands are placed firmly along lower ribs to apply pressure, encouraging bilateral basal expansion of lungs. Similar techniques for localized breathing exercises are applied to other areas of the chest wall.

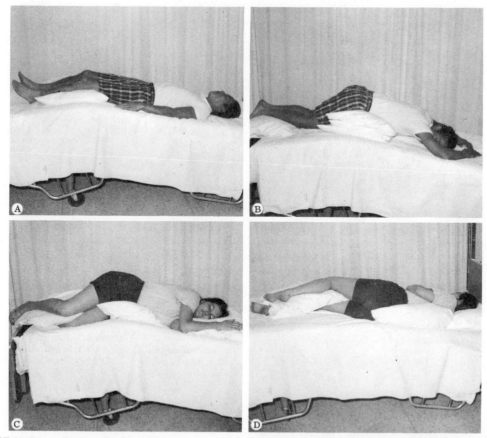

FIGURE 40–7. *A,* Patient should spend some time in the dependent position. Most patients will tolerate 10 to 15 degrees of head-down tilt for a brief period, several times a day. This position facilitates drainage by gravity of the anterior basal segments. *B,* Position used for draining the posterior basal segments. *C,* Position for drainage of right lower lobe and lateral basal bronchus. *D,* Position for drainage of the left upper lobe and for lower division of the superior and inferior bronchi.

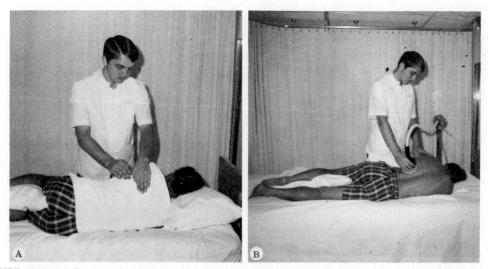

FIGURE 40–8. *A,* Position for chest percussion or clapping. *B,* Position for manual or mechanical vibration.

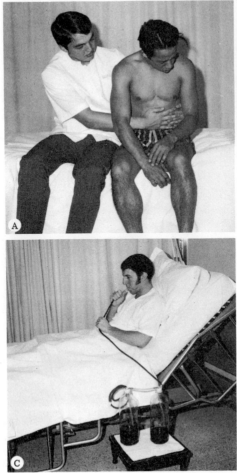
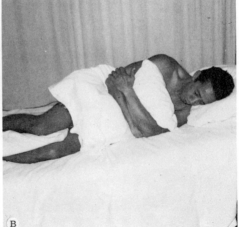

FIGURE 40–9. *A*, Manual splinting of chest or abdominal incision. *B*, While coughing, patient hugs pillow. *C*, Blow bottle helps lung expansion.

segmental anatomy of the lung.[6-8] References to more detailed manuals are listed at the end of this section. For the patient with a poor cough and widespread pulmonary secretions who is confined to bed, hourly turning from side to side may be inadequate to manage secretions. A modified program of postural drainage, practical even in many critically ill patients, can be developed (Fig. 40–7).

Other Maneuvers. In addition to the basic postural drainage maneuvers that the patient can be taught to do for himself, chest percussion or clapping (Fig. 40–8*A*) and vibration, either manually or mechanically (Fig. 40–8*B*), are necessary and useful adjuncts in clearing secretions.

Other techniques frequently used to help postoperative patients are manual splinting of the chest or abdominal incision by the therapist (Fig. 40–9*A*), patient coughing while hugging a pillow (Fig. 40–9*B*), and use of a blow bottle (Fig. 40–9*C*) for the patient to exhale against resistance in order to encourage increased tidal volume. Adaptations of the techniques can be useful in small children (Fig. 40–10).

Routine Chest Physical Therapy

In the acutely ill patient, chest physical therapy may be given as frequently as every two hours and should be closely coordinated within the overall respiratory program. For routine treatment given two to four times daily, the following sequence and procedures are ordered.

1. Mist Inhalation (20 Minutes). This will wet down the upper airways and help liquefy secretions. The mist may be cold for febrile patients but preferably is heated to deliver more water. Usually the carrier gas is oxygen-enriched air. Administration via a mask or into a tent may be by humidifier or nebulizer. Instruction for breathing exercises and

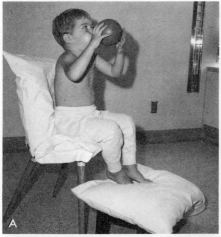

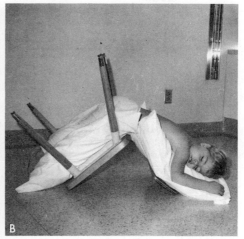

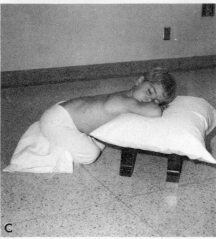

FIGURE 40–10. Techniques useful for small children.

cough control can be given at this time, if it is convenient for the physical therapist.

2. Intermittent Positive-Pressure Breathing (IPPB) (15 Minutes). These treatments are given by inhalation-therapy or nursing personnel and result in a period of mild hyperventilation and an increase in lung expansion. IPPB also provides an effective means of delivering bronchodilator, decongestant, and mucolytic agents to the airways and, in addition, continues to add moisture.

3. Chest Physical Therapy (20 Minutes). After the mist and IPPB are given, postural drainage, combined with vibration and percussion, usually produces good results in clearing secretions. Supplemental maneuvers performed at this time for patients on ventilators are stimulation of cough by direct tracheal suctioning, hyperinflation with oxygen by bag and mask, and instillation of saline through endotracheal and tracheostomy tubes prior to suctioning.

Within the range of respiratory care, chest physical therapy and inhalation therapy have complementary roles. Most patients who receive chest physical therapy also will use one or more pieces of oxygen equipment and likely will receive IPPB therapy as well. The physical therapist must be familiar with the operation of this equipment, just as the inhalation therapist must have experience in the technique of chest physical therapy.

MANAGEMENT OF RESPIRATORY COMPLICATIONS IN MUSCULOSKELETAL DISORDERS

Disorders seen by the physiatrist frequently have respiratory complications. Conditions such as arthritis, ankylosing spondylitis, muscular dystrophy, and debility, as well as stroke and spinal cord injuries, have the possibility of poor ventilation, secretion retention, and atelectasis. These complications are among the main causes of morbidity as well as death. It is, therefore, important to provide respiratory care for all of these conditions, but it is particularly important for the quadriplegic, and this is given in more detail a little later.

Inspiratory Incentive Spirometry

In recent years, the incentive spirometer has become an inexpensive and effective measure available to the physician and to the patient. Bartlett et al.[9] showed how important inspiratory exercises were in treating and preventing atelectasis. They showed that inspiratory incentive spirometers were even more effective than IPPB in conscious and alert patients and that older methods such as blow bottles that employed expiratory methods actually could aggravate atelectasis. The incentive spirometer can help all types of patients from those who are debilitated and bedbound to those with stroke and spinal cord injuries or muscular dystrophy. In all of these patients, collapse of individual alveoli can be a problem. As more alveoli collapse, significantly larger amounts of right-to-left shunting occur. There also will be a decrease of the functional residual capacity with a consequent decrease of lung compliance and an increase in the work of breathing. This may not be obvious on clinical observation because the tidal volume may remain constant despite restriction of functional residual volume. The normal individual prevents alveolar collapse with occasional deep breaths and yawns. This mechanism may not be present in some of the disabilities mentioned above. Thus, the regular use of these spirometers maintains the means of maximal lung inflation.

There are many such spirometers on the market. One example is "Voldyne" (Cheeseborough Pond's Incorporated, Greenwich, Connecticut) (Fig. 40–11), which is a hand-held compact spirometer that measures the volume of air inspired up to a maximum of about 4000 ml. Sustained maximal inspiration exercise can thus be combined with volume measurement, and it is the visualization of daily improvement in volume that provides incentive to the patient. Other varieties are "Spirocare" (Marion Laboratories Incorporated Pharmaceutical Division, Kansas City, Missouri) and Bartlett-Edwards "Incentive Spirometer" (McGaw

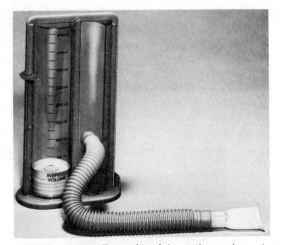

FIGURE 40–11. Example of incentive spirometer (Voldyne, made by Cheesebrough Ponds, Inc.) which allows up to 4000 ml of inspired air to be measured. This is a hand-held device that allows for visualization of daily improvement in volume, as well as giving a means of doing sustained maximal inspiration exercises.

Respiratory Therapy, Division of American Hospital Supply Corporation, Irvine, California).

The Quadriplegic Patient

Bellamy et al.[10] reported a fatality of 40 per cent within the first year after injury of the traumatic quadriplegic patient. They were able to show at autopsy that in the vast majority of cases, death was related to a pulmonary cause. There are various factors that play a part in this. Spontaneous ventilation is impossible if the lesion is above the fourth cervical segment. If the lesion is below the fourth cervical segment, spontaneous respiration is possible and the diaphragmatic function is unimpaired but, because of the lack of movement of intercostals and the initial flaccidity of the abdominal musculature, respiratory function is abnormal and respiratory complications occur frequently. As soon as the flaccidity is replaced by spasticity in both the abdominal and intercostal muscles, the patient's respiratory function improves and fewer complications occur. This is particularly so when in the sitting position. The flaccid abdominal muscles protrude and the diaphragm lowers, with the result that inspiration results in lesser movement of the diaphragm, and with expiration, no abdominal rebound occurs. In the supine position the patient has fewer problems. The main complications as a result of these problems are retention of secretions and atelectasis. McMichan et al.[11] describe a careful protocol that effectively prevents these complications from occurring. They stress the importance of turning the patient frequently, having the patient take four deep breathing exercises every four hours, the use of incentive spirometry, and chest percussion. With sputum retention, IPPB is used every four hours combined with aerosolization of the bronchodilator, isoetharine hydrochloride. Furthermore, once there is radiographic evidence of lobar atelectasis, fiberoptic bronchoscopy and bronchial lavage should be instituted immediately.

Electrophrenic Stimulation

Patients who sustain injuries high in the spinal cord fall into two categories: those who do not injure the anterior motor neurons of the phrenic nerve and those who do. Thus, if you have a cord lesion at C2, this leaves C3 and C4 intact, and you do not get denervation atrophy of the diaphragm. However, with an injury at C3 and C4 there is likely to be irreparable damage to the phrenic nerve. All of these patients initially need a respirator to stay alive. After a period of time, consideration can be given to the implanting of a phrenic nerve stimulator. Obviously, one cannot stimulate a damaged nerve and the only patients who are likely candidates are those with very high lesions or with incomplete lesions. Therefore, to see whether a patient is a candidate, an EMG of the diaphragm is a necessary preliminary study. A denervated diaphragm is a definite contraindication. Furthermore, one must wait at least six months before considering this. Before that, the flaccidity of the chest wall causes a flail chest syndrome with the movement of the diaphragm and the procedure fails. The chest wall needs to become noncompliant in order to give the diaphragm a chance to provide adequate respiration when stimulated.

The incomplete lesion is an interesting one and it is important to recognize it. For this to be understood, one needs to remember that voluntary respiration is controlled by the cerebral cortex and that automatic respiration arises from various areas of the brain stem. These various areas send tracts down to the spinal motor neurons. Thus, it is possible to damage only the automatic tract and leave the voluntary tract intact. If respiration entirely depends upon the voluntary system, sleep apnea occurs. A similar situation can occur in brain stem infarcts as well as in children with the syndrome known as Ondine's curse. This syndrome responds well to electrophrenic pacing.

The modern era of electrophrenic pacing was introduced by Glenn and associates.[12] They use an external battery-powered transmitter. This transmits trains of pulse-modulated radio frequency energy to a loop antenna. There are two receivers implanted subcutaneously in the right and left sides of the upper anterior chest wall. The receivers are connected to bipolar platinum electrodes that surround each phrenic nerve. The antenna is placed over one of the receivers and only one phrenic nerve is used at one time. For two weeks after installation, no pacing is done, and after that it is started for only short periods of time. Gradually, the system as well as the muscles are trained and can be used for the full 24 hours alternating right and left phrenic nerves. The pulse train for the transmitter is fixed to give 34 square impulses in 1.35 seconds. This is the inspiratory part of the cycle. There follows a period of 2.65 seconds without stimulation during which expiration is allowed to occur. The respiratory cycle lasts four seconds, making a rate of 15 breaths per minute. It is regulated in such a way that it starts the diaphragmatic contraction with a minimal current that gradually builds up over the inspiratory part of the cycle, giving the muscle a smooth contraction and not a sudden hiccup.

The advantage of this system over the constant use of a ventilator is that it allows that patient to move with much less difficulty; however, the patient still needs to have a tracheostomy for suction and proper suction equipment needs to be available at all times. In addition, the patient needs to have some other form of ventilation available in case the system breaks down. There now have been patients who have used this system for many years with few complications. The phrenic nerve does not appear to be damaged by the electrode.

CONCLUSION

This chapter has dealt with some basic concepts of respiration as well as with what happens during various respiratory disorders. It has touched on the management of some of these disorders. It will be clear that this management, particularly in the acute stages of the disorders, is complicated and really needs a physician who has specialized in this field. This may well be an anesthesiologist or chest physician. There are, however, prophylactic measures that any physician needs to know about when dealing with these patients.

REFERENCES

Disorders of Respiration

1. Campbell, E. J. M.: The Respiratory Muscles: And the Mechanics of Breathing. Chicago, Year Book Medical Publishers, Inc., 1958.
2. Comroe, J. H., Jr., Forster, R. E., II, Dubois, A. B., Briscoe, W. A., and Carlsen, E.: The Lung; Clinical Physiology and Pulmonary Function Tests, 2nd Ed. Chicago, Year Book Medical Publishers, Inc., 1962.
3. Polgar, G., and Promadhat V.: Pulmonary Function Testing in Children. Philadelphia, W. B. Saunders Company, 1971.
4. Barach, A. L., Beck, G. J., Bickerman, H. A., and Seanor, H. E.: Physical methods simulating cough mechanisms. Use in poliomyelitis, bronchial asthma, pulmonary emphysema and bronchiectasis. JAMA, 150:1380, 1952.
5. Barach, A. L., and Beck, G. J.: Exsufflation with negative pressure, physiologic and clinical studies in poliomyelitis, bronchial asthma, pulmonary emphysema and bronchiectasis. Arch. Int. Med., 93:825, 1954.

Chest Physical Therapy

6. Physiotherapy Department, Brompton Hospital, London: Physiotherapy for Medical and Surgical Thoracic Conditions, 1967.
7. Egan, D. F.: Fundamentals of Inhalation Therapy. St. Louis, The C. V. Mosby Co., 1969.
8. Halpern, D.: Techniques of Bronchial Drainage. Department of Physical Medicine and Rehabilitation, University of Minnesota Medical School, Minneapolis, 1967.
9. Bartlett, R. H., Brennon, M. L., Gazzaniga, A. B., and Hansen, E. L.: Studies on the pathogenesis and prevention of postoperative pulmonary complications. Surg. Gynecol. Obstet., 137:925, 1975.
10. Bellamy, R., Pitts, F. W., and Stauffer, E. S.: Respiratory complications of traumatic quadriplegia: Analysis of 20 years experience. J. Neurosurg., 39:596–600, 1973.
11. McMichan, J. C., Michel, L., and Westbrook, P. R.: Pulmonary dysfunction following traumatic quadriplegia. JAMA, 243:528–531, 1980.
12. Glenn, W. W. L., Holcomb, W. G., Shaw, R. K., Hogan, J. F., and Holschuh, K. R.: Long-term ventilatory support by diaphragm pacing in quadriplegia. Ann. Surg., 183:566, 1976.

41

COMMON CARDIOVASCULAR PROBLEMS IN REHABILITATION

FREDERIC J. KOTTKE

CARDIAC DISEASE

The heart diseases treated in rehabilitation programs may be divided into three general types.

Mechanical Derangements. Conditions in which the valves or chambers of the heart are faulty, resulting in interference with forward flow, regurgitation, or diversion of blood, fall into this category. The heart performs inefficiently like an obstructed or leaky pump. More work than normal must be performed by the myocardium to pump a given amount of blood into the arterial tree. As a consequence, there is increased myocardial strain and fatigue. If the myocardium cannot compensate by hypertrophy to meet the increased demand, cardiac failure ensues.

Increased Resistance to Blood Flow (Arterial Hypertension). In diseases of this type the heart must contract against a pressure that is greater than normal so that the myocardial work per liter of blood pumped is increased. Cardiac failure develops when the myocardium can no longer meet the increased demand for energy.

Decreased Energy Production. Pathologic changes in the myocardium or in coronary circulation reduce the energy output to below normal. Destruction or metabolic dysfunction of the myocardium or decreased circulation to the myocardium may limit its ability to do work. In each case the heart will be limited in its ability to respond to the demands of metabolic activities.

Work of the Heart

The function of the heart is to convert chemical energy from cellular metabolism into mechanical energy to pump the blood through the circulatory system composed of an expansible elastic-muscular network of vessels. The arteries by their elasticity and muscular tension maintain a positive pressure in the outflow system during the period between ventricular contractions and convert an intermittent, pulsatile flow into a steady flow at the capillary level. Such mechanical factors as abnormal resistance to flow through stenotic valves, regurgitation through leaky valves, and abnormal flow through shunts decrease the effectiveness of the pumping action.

The work performed by the heart depends upon the quantity of blood ejected, the pressure against which it is pumped, and the velocity imparted to the blood. If the valves are competent and if there are no intracardiac shunts, the work of the heart will appear as external work, represented by the formula:

$$W = QP + \frac{wV^2}{2g}$$

in which W = work of the ventricles, Q = volume of blood pumped, P = mean arterial blood pressure, w = weight of the blood pumped, and V = velocity of ejected blood.

For the patient who has valvular disease with insufficiency, all of the work of the heart does not appear as external work because of the repumping of a portion of the blood. Likewise, stenotic valvular disease produces an increased resistance to flow that is not apparent in the peripheral blood pressure. Consequently, the hearts of patients with valvular disease must do more work in proportion to the external work that is accomplished, and myocardial fatigue occurs more rapidly at any level of metabolic activity.

Cardiac output is determined by the volume of blood pumped per systolic contraction and the heart rate. Either or both of these may vary with the activity of the patient. For a normal healthy young adult, the maximal cardiac rate is approximately 180 to 210 beats per minute.[1] Although for each normal individual there is a linear correlation between pulse rate and metabolic work when that individual is in a constant posture, working at a nonfatiguing rate, in a steady state while working at a uniform type of work, variation of any of these factors will produce a nonlinear response.[2] Consequently, the pulse rate is not a reliable index of the demands on the heart for work during random activity. Moreover, patients with cardiac disease may differ markedly in their abilities to increase their heart rates and may be in cardiac distress at heart rates that are well within the safe working range for normal individuals.

The stroke volume of each ventricle at rest is approximately 60 to 70 ml of the 150 to 170 ml of blood contained in the ventricle. In trained athletes during maximal work stroke volumes of 120 to 190 ml have been reported.[1] The resting stroke volume is greater during recumbency than it is in the erect position. The increase in stroke volume during increased muscular activity may be due in part to increased diastolic volume and in part to increased systolic contraction. The cardiac patient with dilatation and hypertrophy of the heart may have a stroke volume that is considerably greater than normal.

The capacity of the normal heart to do work far exceeds the work requirement under basal conditions or during ordinary light activity (Fig. 41–1). The maximal cardiac output measured in young healthy men can be increased up to four times the resting cardiac output.[3] Under normal conditions of working and living, excluding recreation, metabolic demand rarely exceeds 6 METs. (1 MET is the metabolic oxygen requirement under basal conditions = 1 B.M.R. The energy requirements of activities are commonly expressed in METs.) Walking or cycling up to 6 METs increases cardiac output only 50 to 100 per cent above basal.[3, 4] Early methods for measuring human cardiac output based on gas or dye dilution in the blood had inherent methodologic errors that overestimated cardiac output.[1] All methods have significant error confounded further by continuous physiologic fluctuations in cardiovascular control. The method that currently produces the most reliable and reproducible index of relative change in cardiac output, if not the absolute volume of cardiac output, is impedance cardiography (ZCG).[5] The myocardial work may be increased up to eight times basal because blood pressure doubles and cardiac output increases fourfold at maximal work. Owing to extracardiac factors, the oxygen consumption can show a further increase to approximately 10 to 12 times the resting level. In persons who are not in good physical condition because of illness or age, the maximal working capacity of the heart is greatly reduced.

The difference between the capacity of the heart to do work and the demand for cardiac work is called the cardiac reserve. With age and heart disease the cardiac reserve is reduced. During prolonged muscular work above light levels the cardiac capacity to do work is reduced by fatigue in proportion to the intensity and the duration of the work. Therefore, the conditions of work and the intervals of rest as well as the condition of the myocardium influence the cardiac re-

RELATIONSHIP BETWEEN CARDIAC CAPACITY, CARDIAC WORK,

AND CARDIAC RESERVE OF THE NORMAL HEART.

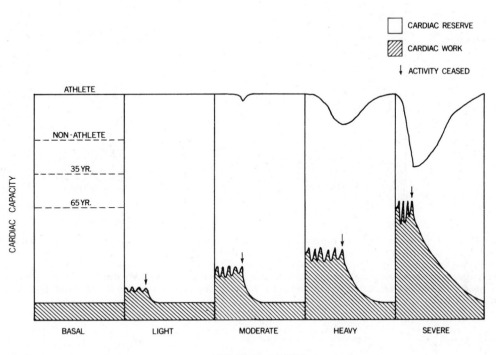

FIGURE 41–1. Relationship between the cardiac capacity, cardiac output, and cardiac reserve of the normal heart, showing the relative decrease of cardiac capacity with age. The cardiac work of the heart of a young athlete, at maximal capacity, is approximately eight times the basal requirement for the cardiac work. During heavy and severe muscular activity, the fatigue produced by the increased myocardial work causes a decrease of cardiac capacity, which recovers rapidly during the subsequent rest.

serve. When the work required of the heart reaches the capacity of the heart to do work, a cardiac reserve no longer exists and unless the work of the heart can be reduced below the capacity, the heart is decompensated and unable to continue to work at the level demanded of it.

Successful management of the patient with cardiac disease depends upon keeping he load imposed upon the heart below the cardiac capacity so that the patient maintains an adequate cardiac reserve. In myocardial disease, fatigue during muscular effort occurs more rapidly than it does in a heart in good condition. Consequently, the amount and duration of effort must be less and the period of rest during which recovery can occur must be longer (Fig. 41–2).

For the patient who has just experienced acute myocardial disease or infarction, a program must be planned that will eventually restore him to the greatest usefulness that is possible with his damaged heart. In view of the fact that 70 per cent of patients hospitalized for an acute episode of myocardial infarction survive, the initial care of the cardiac patient should include the beginning steps of the rehabilitation program, anticipating the return of the patient to his home and employment. This program of restoration is long and involved. The physician must make many decisions regarding activities that the patient may perform during the acute and convalescent stages of his illness as well as the limitations he must observe when he can return to work. It becomes imperative that the clinician know the relative cardiac stresses imposed by various activities so that he can intelligently prescribe activities that fall within the patient's cardiac capacity and advise the patient against activities that cause excessive cardiac stress.

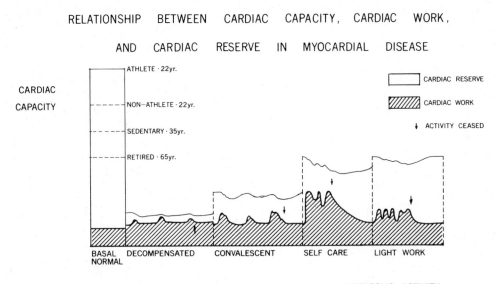

RELATIONSHIP BETWEEN CARDIAC CAPACITY, CARDIAC WORK, AND CARDIAC RESERVE IN MYOCARDIAL DISEASE

FIGURE 41–2. Relationship between cardiac capacity, cardiac output, and cardiac reserve in myocardial disease in relation to normal. In myocardial disease cardiac capacity is severely impaired. During decompensation, cardiac output approaches cardiac capacity. Cardiac capacity gradually increases during convalescence, but activity causes cardiac fatigue with decreasing cardiac capacity, and recovery occurs more slowly during rest than it does in the normal heart. The level of work that can be sustained for more than a few minutes is somewhat less than 50 per cent of cardiac capacity.[29]

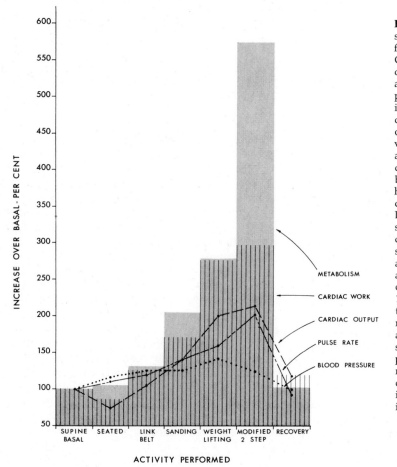

FIGURE 41–3. Variations of some parameters of cardiac performance during activities. Cardiac work parallels oxygen consumption more closely than any other single index of cardiac performance during upper extremity activity and deviates widely during the lower extremity work of stair climbing. Equicaloric activities of the upper extremities and lower extremities do not induce the same amount of work by the heart. The work of the heart is slightly less when sitting quietly than when lying supine. Light hand activities (link belt assembly) while sitting increase cardiac work to 125 per cent of the supine basal value. Bilateral arm activities (sanding) increase cardiac work to approximately 170 per cent of the supine value. Lifting a 10 pound weight through a distance of 15 inches 46 times per minute increases cardiac work to approximately 300 per cent of the supine value. The changes of the pulse rate and blood pressure do not correlate closely enough with changes of cardiac work to be good indices of cardiac work when used individually.

CARDIAC REQUIREMENT DURING ACTIVITY

Studies of the parameters of cardiac work show that changes in cardiac work are not indicated reliably by monitoring any single parameter. During upper extremity activity changes in cardiac work parallel changes in oxygen consumption more closely than any other single index, but there is a significant difference in these relationships during lower extremity activity[6-8] (Fig. 41–3). The pulse rate is an insensitive index of cardiac work in normal subjects carrying out a variety of activities and is probably less reliable for patients with cardiac disease. The blood pressure does not change linearly with cardiac work. Therefore, knowledge of the cardiac work or metabolic requirements of the activities performed by cardiac patients is necessary in order to establish reasonable regulation of those activities.

Although it has been customary to assume that when the patient is lying in bed he is maintained at the basal level of cardiac work, such is not the actual case. Any movement by the patient will increase oxygen consumption and cardiac output.[9] The patient who is confined to bed may move his extremities, shift his position, reach to his bedside stand, turn over, or even sit erect. All of these activities require lifting of the extremities or elevation of the body and increased oxygen consumption. Even under the best of circumstances the average oxygen consumption of the patient restricted to bed is above the basal level and during certain bed activities it increases greatly. Rising from the lying position to the sitting position in bed without assistance will temporarily double the oxygen consumption above the basal level.

There is also an increase in the blood pressure because of the contraction of the abdominal muscles as the patient sits up so that the work of the heart is increased to an even greater extent.

Posture affects the work of the heart through its influence on both the cardiac output and the blood pressure. Sitting in an easy chair, fully relaxed, with support for the head, back, arms, thighs, and feet is a position of minimal cardiac requirement in which the cardiac output is only approximately 85 per cent as great as when a person is lying in a supine position (Table 41–1). In that supported position a patient may relax while reading or listening to programmed music or may carry on light occupational therapeutic hand activities as he wishes with little increase of his metabolic demand or cardiac work (Fig. 41–4). The diversional activities decrease emotional tension and anxiety, which results in a decrease of blood pressure and with it a decrease of the pressure work of the myocardium. Sitting in a straight back chair or "dangling" the legs while sitting on the edge of the bed require less cardiac output than supine recumbency. Likewise, during quiet standing, cardiac output is only approximately 90 per cent of that during supine recumbency. On the other hand, when a patient is semireclining in a hospital bed (Fig. 41–5) with the backrest and the knee support elevated, as is customary for patients who are bedfast in the hospital, the cardiac output is greater (110 per cent) than the value when supine, although metabolism is not increased.[9]

In estimating the cardiac work required by an activity, it is necessary to take into consideration the peripheral distribution of the blood. Pooling of blood occurs when the feet

TABLE 41–1. THE EFFECTS OF POSTURE ON CARDIAC OUTPUT AND METABOLISM

Posture	Metabolism (METS)	Cardiac Output (COS)
Sitting in easy chair, full support	1.00 (0.90*)	0.85
Seated on straight-backed chair	1.10	0.95
Seated on edge of bed with feet supported	1.10	0.95
Standing, relaxed	1.20	0.90
Supine, basal	1.00	1.00
Lateral decubitus, up on elbow	1.10	1.00
Semireclining at 45° with knees up	1.00	1.10
Seated on high stool, forearms on table	1.25	–

COS—cardiac output, ratio to basal
METS—metabolism, ratio to basal
*Patients with old myocardial infarcts without orthopnea show a lower oxygen consumption during fully supported sitting than when lying supine.

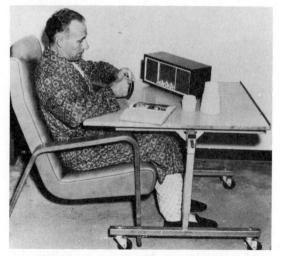

FIGURE 41–4. The fully supported sitting position in an arm chair with a high back for head support requires less cardiac output and cardiac work than that required when lying at supine rest in bed. A table, holding a water glass, a book, and light craft activities within easy reach, decreases physical exertion and encourages diversional activities to relieve anxieties.

and legs are dependent, decreasing the venous return and the drive on the heart. Under such conditions cardiac output is decreased (Fig. 41–6). If the patient is semireclining in bed with his knees elevated, the dependent vascular bed in which pooling may occur is decreased and the splanchnic area compressed, both of which augment venous return and increase the cardiac output. The patient with heart failure who insists on "dangling" his legs over the side of the bed rather than semireclining has found

that there is less cardiac effort involved even though unsupported sitting does slightly increase the demand for oxygen. The patient with myocardial insufficiency relaxes best with the least cardiac demand when he is sitting in a chair with support for his head, back, and arms but with his feet and legs dependent. Only if he has orthostatic hypotension does this become an adverse position. If, following myocardial infarction, a 30 per cent difference in the minimal requirement for cardiac work is of significance for survival, the patient should be in the fully supported easy-chair position rather than semireclining in bed with his knees elevated. Beyond this, the psychologically beneficial reassurance of being allowed to sit up rather than being confined to strict bed rest relieves anxiety and aids relaxation. It provides a subtle reassurance to the anxious patient. Minor nonstressful hand activities reinforce this sense that his condition is under control.

Studies of patients with myocardial disease indicate that cardiac patients respond to positional changes as do normal individuals except that their oxygen consumption as well as their cardiac output is slightly less in a sitting position than in a recumbent position (Table 41–1).

Minimal Cardiac Activity. Activities that require use of the hands and wrists while the patient is seated with the forearms supported increase metabolism and cardiac work less than 50 per cent above the supine resting level and increase the cardiac output no

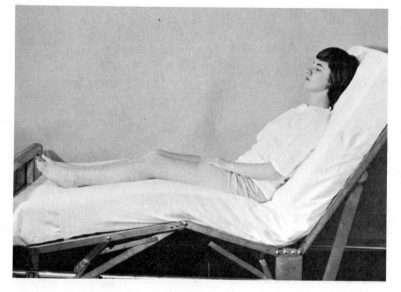

FIGURE 41–5. When a patient is semireclining in bed with the knee support elevated, the cardiac output is slightly greater than when the patient is lying supine.

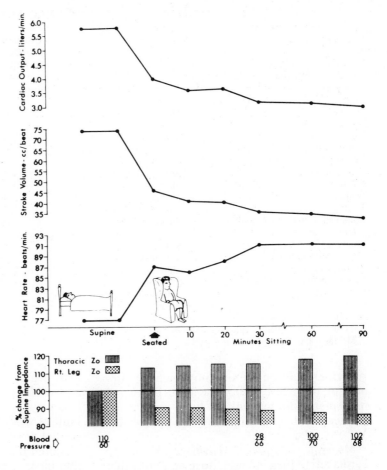

FIGURE 41–6. The parameters of cardiac work changed as a patient in the early stage of rehabilitation after myocardial infarction was transferred from supine to sitting. Pooling of blood in the lower extremities, indicated by the decreased ZCG impedance in lower extremities and increased impedance in thorax, resulted in decreased stroke volume and decreased cardiac output even though the heart rate increased. The combination of decreased cardiac output and slightly decreased blood pressure resulted in decreased work of the heart throughout the time the patient was sitting. (From Ramos, M. U.: Cardiovascular considerations in the rehabilitation of the elderly. Bull. Puerto Rico Med. Assoc. 20:67, 1978.)

more than 25 per cent (Table 41–2). Since the occasional moving in bed that any patient does will produce similar changes, activities at this level have been classified as minimal. Muscular tension or an increase of blood pressure due to anxiety may increase the cardiac work far above this level. Therefore, diversional activities that cause a patient to relax will decrease his cardiac work in the early stages following a myocardial infarction.

Light Cardiac Activity. Activity that increases cardiac work (or metabolism) from 1.5 to 2.5 times the basal value and cardiac output from 1.25 to 2.0 times the basal value has been classified as light cardiac activity.

TABLE 41–2. MINIMAL CARDIAC ACTIVITY

Activity	Position	Cardiac Work (CUBS) or Metabolism (METS)	Cardiac Output (COS)
Leather belt assembly	Sitting at table	1.25	1.10
Leather stamping	Sitting at table	1.35	1.10
Leather tooling	Sitting at table	1.30	1.20
Listening to radio	Sitting in easy chair	1.40	—
Bench assembly, light	Sitting at bench	1.40	1.10
Leather lacing	Sitting at table	1.45	—
Leather lacing	Lateral decubitus	1.55	1.20
Chip carving	Sitting at table	1.60	1.20

CUBS—cardiac work units, ratio to basal
COS—cardiac output, ratio to basal
METS—metabolism, ratio to basal

TABLE 41–3. LIGHT CARDIAC ACTIVITY

Activity	Position	Cardiac Work (CUBS) or Metabolism (METS)	Cardiac Output (COS)
Eating	Sitting	1.50	—
Sewing	Sitting	1.60	—
Clerical work	Sitting	1.60	—
Setting type	Standing	1.60	1.35
Getting out of and into bed	Bed to chair	1.65	1.45
Leather carving	Sitting on chair	1.70	—
Weaving, table loom	Sitting on stool	1.70	—
Clerical work	Standing	1.80	—
Writing	Sitting	2.00	—
Typing	Sitting on chair	2.00	1.35
Bimanual activity test sanding, 50 strokes/min.	Sitting on chair	2.00	1.40
Weaving, floor loom	Sitting on bench	2.10	1.75
Metal work, hammer	Standing	2.15	1.65
Printing, platen press	Standing	2.30	1.75
Bench assembly, moderate	Sitting	2.35	1.70
Hanging clothes on line	Standing — stooping	2.40	1.80

CUBS — cardiac work units, ratio to basal
COS — cardiac output, ratio to basal
METS — metabolism, ratio to basal

Activities that require full movement or support of the arms without a load, balancing movements of the trunk, or hand work while standing fall into this category (Table 41–3).[9, 10]

Moderate Cardiac Activities. Moderate cardiac activities include those activities that increase cardiac work (or metabolism) 2.5 to 3.5 times and cardiac output 2.0 to 2.5 times the supine resting value. Sedentary clerical or benchwork activities requiring periodic lifting of not more than 10 pounds, dressing, showering, preparing meals, driving a car, and walking at moderate speed fall into this category (Table 41–4).[11] This is the upper limit of work to which the patient with myocardial damage should be assigned. It should be noted that frequently vocational activities that have been prohibited require less cardiac work than self-care activities that the patient has been allowed to perform early in his convalescence.

Heavy, Severe, and Excessively Severe Cardiac Activities. Included in the category of

TABLE 41–4. MODERATE CARDIAC ACTIVITY

Activity	Position	Cardiac Work (CUBS) or Metabolism (METS)	Cardiac Output (COS)
Playing piano		2.50	—
Dressing, undressing		2.50–3.50	—
Sawing, jeweler's saw	Sitting	1.90	2.05
Sawing, hack saw	Standing	2.55	2.00
Driving car		2.80	—
Bicycling, slowly		2.90	2.45
Preparing meals		3.00	—
Weight lifting, 10 lb lifted 15″, 46/min	Sitting	2.80	2.00
Walking, 2.0 mph		3.20	—
Handsawing, wood	Standing	3.50	2.35
Warm shower		3.50	—

CUBS — cardiac work units, ratio to basal
COS — cardiac output, ratio to basal
METS — metabolism, ratio to basal

TABLE 41–5. HEAVY AND SEVERE CARDIAC ACTIVITY

Activity	Position	Metabolism (METS)	Cardiac Output (COS)
Bowel movement	Toilet	3.60	
Bowel movement	Bedpan	4.70	
Making beds	Standing	3.90	
Hot shower	Standing	4.20	
Walking fast (3.5 mph)		5.00	
Descending stairs		5.20	
Scrubbing floor	Kneeling	5.30	3.00
Master two-step climbing test		5.70	3.00
Weight lifting, 10–20 lb lifted 36", 15/min		6.50	3.50
Bicycling, fast		6.90	3.30
Running		7.40	4.0
Mowing lawn		7.70	
Climbing stairs		9.00	

METS—metabolism, ratio to basal
COS—cardiac output, ratio to basal

heavy cardiac activity are those activities that increase cardiac work 3.5 to 5.0 times or cardiac output 2.5 to 3.0 times basal values (Table 41–5). Such activities should be avoided by the patient with myocardial disease, or they should be restricted to short intervals of activity followed by prolonged periods of rest. The upper limit of this level of activity is the greatest that a normal person can maintain during daily work without evidence of metabolic deterioration and has been classified by Müller as the "endurance limit" of work.[12] Activities that require lifting, pushing, pulling, and carrying may exceed this category and should be avoided by persons who have suffered a myocardial infarction. Activities that increase cardiac work (or metabolism) 5.0 to 7.0 times the basal value and cardiac output 3.0 to 4.0 times the basal value are classified as severe, and activities that exceed these ranges are classified as excessively severe. Climbing slopes or stairs rapidly or running increase the cardiac work to such an extent that they are excessively severe cardiac work.[7, 10] Rapid work or strong emotion may transform a lighter activity to one of heavy cardiac work. Activity in a hot environment that interferes with the dissipation of the heat of the body also increases the cardiac work that must be performed. Heavy manual labor, climbing with heavy loads, and many athletic activities are excessively severe and can be carried on only for short periods of time by healthy individuals (Fig. 41–7).

On the basis of studies of the physiologic parameters of cardiac function, muscular activities have been classified in Table 41–6

according to the stress imposed on the myocardium. With the knowledge of the relative cardiac demands of various activities, the physician is able to protect the patient

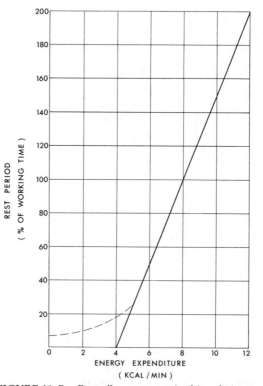

FIGURE 41–7. Rest allowance required in relation to the energy expended for normal work up to 2000 kilocalories per eight hour shift. Based upon a maximal work capacity of 4.0 kilocalories per minute plus basal metabolism of 1.0 kilocalorie per minute. (From Müller, E. A.: The physiological basis of rest pauses in heavy work. Q.J. Exp. Physiol., 38:205–215, 1953.)

TABLE 41–6. CLASSIFICATION OF NORMAL ACTIVITIES BASED ON CARDIAC OUTPUT DURING THE ACTIVITY

Activity	Metabolism (METs)	Cardiac Output (COs)
Minimal	<1.5	<1.25
Light	1.5–2.5	1.25–1.5
Moderate	2.5–3.5	1.5–2.0
Heavy	3.5–5.0	2.0–2.5
Severe	5.0–7.0	2.5–3.0
Excessively severe	>7.0	3.0–4.0

COs — cardiac output, ratio to basal
METs — metabolism, ratio to basal

against excessive myocardial effort in the acute and subacute stages of his disease.

CARDIAC REHABILITATION

Cardiac rehabilitation programs following myocardial infarction are of two general types: acute and delayed. There are fundamental differences in the philosophies, pathophysiologic concepts, and psychosocial values in the two approaches. Both programs aspire to protect the patient through the period of maximal risk and then safely restore him to a near-normal home life and appropriate vocational activity. Both programs assume that physical activity and emotional stress increase the work of the heart and with it increase the likelihood of ventricular fibrillation. The amount of protection and the return to activity are programmed to minimize the risk and maximize the recovery.

Acute Cardiac Rehabilitation. At the time of the acute myocardial infarction the patient is at greatest risk of sudden death (Fig. 41–8). More than 90 per cent of these deaths are due to ventricular fibrillation. Immediate transfer to an intensive coronary care unit is indicated so that the patient may be monitored continuously and appropriate antiarrhythmic and supportive therapy maintained. During the time that the patient is in the ICCU, a cardiologist assumes responsibility for his program. Even at this stage protective posture may be used to minimize the work of the heart (Fig. 41–9). The medical, nursing, and therapist staff members begin to introduce the concepts of the rehabilitation program both to prepare the patient and also as a means of reassurance. Activity is maintained at or below 1.5 METs. When, after two to

four days, it is determined that the myocardium is adequately stabilized the patient is transferred to cardiac rehabilitation, where, under continuing monitoring, a program of activity is instituted.[13] Twice daily a therapist supervises calisthenic exercises requiring 1.2 METs of energy for 20 seconds followed by a two-minute rest and repeated twice. The duration of the exercises is gradually increased at each succeeding exercise period until two-minute exercises are in-

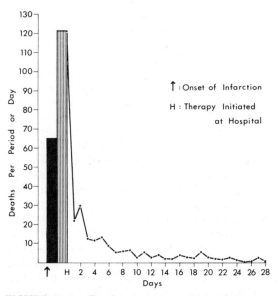

FIGURE 41–8. Deaths per time period or per day from onset of myocardial infarction through 28 days of hospitalization. The black bar indicates deaths with patient unattended. Vertical lined bar indicates deaths from time patient received first assistance until he reached the ICCU. Points on line indicate deaths per day over the next 28 days. (From Gazes, P.C., et al.: Mortality by days and weeks up to one year after myocardial infarction. Comparative study. JAMA, 197:906–908, 1966.)

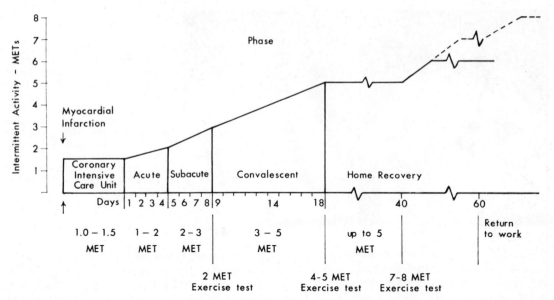

FIGURE 41-9. Schematic diagram of the intensity of activity in METs allowed to patients each day of an acute cardiac rehabilitation program. The patients were tested on an upper extremity 2 MET test for 6 minutes on day 8, and on a 3 MET, 4 MET, or 5 MET lower extremity ergometer test before being discharged home at the end of the convalescent period.

terspersed with one-minute rest periods during which pulse rates are recorded and any arrhythmia noted. Initially activities are controlled to keep pulse rates below 60 per cent of the maximal rate for age (Fig. 41-10). In the later convalescent period at the discretion of the physician and in the home recov-

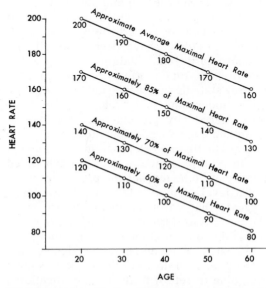

FIGURE 41-10. Decline of maximal heart rate with age and proportional heart rates used as limiting rates during activities for rehabilitation after myocardial infarction. (Courtesy of H.W. Blackburn.)

ery period, the limiting heart rate is 70 per cent of the maximal rate for age. During this same time occupational therapy activities are begun at low intensity and increased in time and intensity proportional to the increase of the calisthenic exercises.

Each day the intensity, number, and duration of the calisthenic exercises[14] are increased in orderly progression if the patient shows no untoward symptoms as indicated below for representative days:

Day 2 1 to 2 METs calisthenics and O.T. = 21 minutes

Day 5 2 METs calisthenics and O.T. = 39 minutes

Day 9 3 METs calisthenics and O.T. = 84 minutes + 7.5 min. walking

Day 12 4 METs calisthenics and 3 METs O.T. = 105 min. + 15 min. walking

Day 15 4.6 METs calisthenics and 3 METs O.T. 3 METs bicycling; stair climbing = Total activity 115 min. + 15 min. walking.

Periodically throughout the rehabilitation program the patient is tested for endurance on progressively more vigorous activities. On Day 8 he performs a standardized 2 MET bilateral upper extremity alternating activity for six minutes using a sanding block

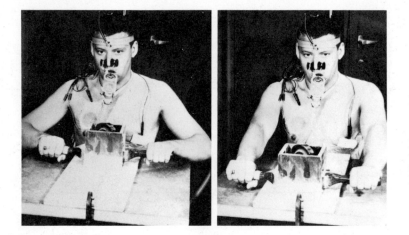

FIGURE 41–11. Patient performing an upper extremity exercise test at a 2 MET level consisting of sanding a pine board using a double-handled sanding block loaded with 2 kilograms. (From Kottke, F.J., Kubicek, W.G., Olson, M.E., Hastings, R.H., and Quast, K.: Five stage test of cardiac performance during occupational activity. Arch. Phys. Med. Rehabil., 43:228–234, 1962.)

(Fig. 41–11) as a test for endurance.[7] If he passes this text he continues on into the convalescent program and adds periods of walking to his schedule. Before the patient is discharged home he is tested for six minutes on a bicycle ergometer progressively at 3 METs, 4 METs, and 5 METs as tolerated to ascertain his level of endurance. A patient who can maintain 5 METs activity for six minutes can safely perform all of the usual sedentary activities at home, whereas a patient who cannot complete six minutes of a 3 MET activity must be cautioned regarding physical and emotional stresses at home and has a much more guarded prognosis.

At home the patient continues his calisthenic and occupational therapy activity for two hours each day plus walking which is increased to 30 to 40 minutes at a speed of 3, 3.5, or 4 miles per hour, as determined by his doctor based on his rate of recovery. At six weeks he returns for a bicycle or treadmill endurance test at 6 to 8 METs for six minutes. Any patient who completes this program on schedule is ready to return to moderate work at 60 days.

It was reported by Schoening in 1972 that of 540 patients who were treated following myocardial infarction, 64 per cent completed the program on schedule, completed the 3 MET endurance test for six minutes, and returned to their premorbid work or activity at the end of two months.[15] More than 90 per cent of patients who had been working prior to the infarction were working at the end of one year. There were no deaths during the rehabilitation program and no morbidity resulting from the rehabilitation activities. Four programs have been set up on this prototype with essentially similar results.[16]

Furthermore it has been reported that failure to successfully complete the 2 MET test at 8 days or the 3 MET test at 15 days is predictive of a high risk for further coronary accidents.[17]

The major advantage of initiating an acute cardiac rehabilitation program at the time when the patient is admitted to the coronary care unit is that it shortens morbidity time. Ninety per cent of these patients will survive to need a rehabilitation program. Early institution of an optimal plan of reactivation prevents both muscular and neurovascular deconditioning, whereas a delayed program is not introduced until the patient has experienced considerable deconditioning. As this program of controlled activities is teaching the patient what he can and should do, it is also teaching him what not to do and how to observe when he is performing safely. Although no studies have been reported that compare early rehabilitation with late rehabilitation or with no formal rehabilitation, the general statistics available indicate that patients undergoing early rehabilitation have not suffered any greater risk of injury or death and even suggest that survival may be better. The three-week program of training in the hospital plus the six weeks of scheduled activity at home teaches the patient to maintain a level of moderate activity. Evidence suggests that coronary incidents are more likely to occur during or following excessive physical and/or emotional stress. Training to avoid such incidents may be significantly protective. Two thirds of these patients have been able to return to their prior vocational activity at two months after the infarction and 85 per cent have returned to work at six months. This is a significant psychosocial improvement over situations in which cardiac rehabilitation is not instituted. Harpur et al.[18] reported on a study of 199 patients either maintained at bed rest for eight days and then mobilized and discharged home on the fifteenth day, or kept at minimal activity for 21 days and then mobilized and discharged on the twenty-eighth day. Of those discharged home on the fifteenth day, 41 per cent had returned to work at the end of two months, but of those discharged home on the twenty-eighth day, only 17 per cent had returned to work after two months. There are extensive data, similar in nature, indicating that emphasis on prolonged rest implies that any activity, and especially return to work, is dangerous. Such management conditions the patient psychologically to a life of inactivity.

Delayed Cardiac Rehabilitation. The majority of cardiac rehabilitation programs are of the delayed type. The patient is maintained on minimal activity in the ICCU and in his hospital room for about a week. Gradually he is allowed to increase his activity in his room and later to begin walking in the hospital corridor.[19, 20] When he is discharged home he is advised to restrict his activities. More recently hospitalizations of three to four weeks have been reduced to approximately two weeks for uncomplicated myocardial infarction, and specified activity is being introduced earlier in the hospital stay.[21] The major emphasis, however, remains on the rehabilitation exercise program, which is initiated two to three months after discharge from the hospital if the patient has had no further complication. With minor variations the patient goes through a program of reevaluation, exercise stress testing to establish his exercise tolerance, and a prescribed program of reconditioning exercises.[22] Three or more sessions of group exercises are carried on each week under the guidance of a physician or exercise physiologist. Exercises consist of calisthenics, walking-jogging, and group games. Each participant is tested for treadmill or bicycle ergometer performance at regular intervals to determine the adjustment of his activity level. The basic assumption in these reactivation programs is that the greater the capacity for endurance activity, the less likely it is that the person will suffer further coronary disease. However, this assumption still remains to be documented in a convincing study. It does appear, nevertheless, that persons who follow a reasonable activity program, maintain a good diet, and abstain from smoking do better than persons who ignore these coronary risk factors.

SEXUAL ACTIVITY

Conventional wisdom recognizes that sexual intercourse with its attendant excitement and muscular activity increases cardiac work. For many years the increased stress of sexual excitement has been listed as one of the common causes of sudden death of patients with coronary disease. However, carefully documented studies in recent years indicate that this is a relatively rare cause of sudden cardiac death.[23] Bartlett, measuring pulse rate, respiratory rate, and volume, found that during coitus between young (22 to 30 years) married couples heart rates might increase to 60 to 70 per cent of maximal over a period of 3 to 10 minutes and peak near 80 per cent of maximal at orgasm (Fig. 41–12). Respiration followed a similar course.[24] The study appears to confirm the conventional wisdom that vigorous and emotional sexual intercourse, although usually of only a few minutes duration, represents intense physical activity. This evaluation receives further support from Ueno,[23] who reported that the majority of deaths related to coitus occurred outside of wedlock under conditions indicating intense excitement. To date there have been no studies reported during intense intercourse by unmarried couples nor outside of the inhibiting atmosphere and paraphernalia of the laboratory. A best guess based on the available data is that younger couples during active intercourse show responses equivalent to 5 to 6 METs activity, while intense and emotional intercourse may peak at an intensity equivalent to 7 to 8 METs activity.

However, Hellerstein and Friedman[25] equipped men who had had myocardial infarctions with portable electrocardiographic recorders, which they wore continuously through the working day and through the night. They found that conjugal sexual intercourse increased the pulse rate equivalent to the exertion associated with climbing two flights of stairs or walking briskly on the street. The mean maximal heart rate at orgasm was 117 beats per minute (range, 90 to

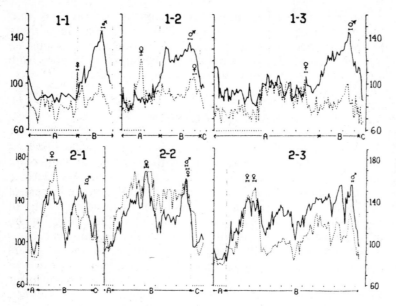

FIGURE 41–12. Physiological arousal during sexual activity as indicated by increase of heart rate in men and women. *A*, Foreplay. *B*, Coitus. *C*, Relaxation. Time in minutes. Solid line represents male response; dotted line, female response. (From Bartlett, R.G., Jr.: Physiologic responses during coitus. J. Appl. Physiol., 9:469–472, 1956.)

144 beats per minute). Tests of physical activity to produce a similar increase in heart rate in these patients showed that during physical activity producing an equivalent increase in pulse rate the blood pressure was 162/89 mm Hg and the maximal oxygen consumption was less than that required for the Master two-step test. Nemec, Mansfield, and Kennedy reported similar findings with no difference between male-on-top and male-on-bottom positions and a decline of both pulse and blood presure to normal within two minutes after orgasm.[26] There have been fewer studies on the physiologic responses of women to sexual stimulation. This presumably correlates with experience that there are fewer sex-related deaths among women.

In counseling a patient regarding rehabilitation, the physician plays a key role in advising the patient regarding his sexual activity, as well as other activities. The patient's happiness and successful re-entry into the family dynamics depends upon his sexual adjustment. If the patient can exercise at the level of 6 to 8 calories per minute, such as the Master two-step test, without symptoms, abnormal pulse rate or blood pressure, or ECG changes, it is generally safe to recommend the resumption of sexual activity. Even when abnormal responses indicate caution, he may still be able to perform these activities which are comparable to the requirements for climbing two flights of stairs.

CARDIAC WORK EVALUATION

Graded exercise tests may use treadmills, bicycle ergometers, or step tests, applying the principles and methods developed by work physiologists as an appraisal of the cardiac status of the patient. Maximal oxygen intake during treadmill exercise has been used as an index of maximal cardiac performance.[27, 28] The maximal oxygen intake for normal healthy young men was nearly 11 times the basal requirement (11 METS). The maximum oxygen intake rate ($\dot{V}O_{2\,max}$) is the accepted index of cardiac capacity for work per kilogram of body weight per minute (ml/kg-min). $\dot{V}O_{2\,max}$ will vary from 60+ ml in adolescent boys and trained young men, to 35 ± 7 ml in sedentary men over age 45, to 25 ± 4 ml in sedentary women over age 45. Deconditioning and heart disease decrease the $\dot{V}O_{2\,max}$. Astrand has proposed that the capacity for sustained work is somewhat less than 50 per cent of the rate of O_2 consumption during acute maximal exercise.[29] This would convert to the need for a patient to perform 3 MET activities to have a $\dot{V}O_{2\,max}$ = 21 or more. To perform 5 MET activities for a sustained period would require a $\dot{V}O_{2\,max}$ = 35. Cardiac work evaluation, therefore, provides useful information for counseling patients regarding both short-term and sustained activities.

In a multistage progressive test of cardiac capacity, the individual begins the exercise

TABLE 41–7. AVERAGE ENERGY COSTS OF TWO MILE PER HOUR TREADMILL TEST*

METs	Kcal/min	O₂ ml/kg-min	Pulse Rate	Per Cent Grade
2	2.5	7.0	97	0
3	3.7	10.5	105	3.5
4	5.0	14.0	114	7.0
5	6.25	17.5	126	10.5
6	7.5	21.0	135	14.0
7	8.7	24.5	144	17.5

*The energy costs of treadmill walking at 2.0 mph at various slopes are tabulated in terms of the oxygen intake, Kcal per minute, and METs. The pulse rate figures represent average values measured in healthy, middle-aged sedentary men. (From Naughton, J.: J. S. Carolina Med. Assoc., 65 [Suppl.]: 96, 1969.)

with a brief period of warm-up at about 2 METS. Following a short rest the individual begins exercising at a relatively low effort of energy expenditure, which is increased either intermittently or continuously until the patient approaches a predetermined endpoint such as heart rate, respiration, symptoms, or maximum oxygen uptake.

In the Naughton modification of the maximal aerobic work capacity the patient begins walking on a treadmill at a speed of two miles per hour on a level grade.[30] The speed is held constant while the slope of the treadmill bed is elevated 3.5 per cent every three minutes. Blood pressure and pulse rate are recorded by auscultation during the last half of each minute. A single ECG continuously monitors heart rate and regularity. Minute ventilation and metabolism are measured by collecting and analyzing expired gases. The increments of energy expenditure are in multiples of the resting metabolic states, or METs, as shown in Table 41–7. This test is adequate for most clinical appraisals, since the averge man has an aerobic working capacity of 9 to 10 METs.

A bicycle ergometer may be used to evaluate working capacity on either a continuous or an intermittent basis.[31] In the intermittent work capacity test, the patient begins pedaling at an energy requirement of 300 kpm*/min (oxygen intake approximately 500 ml per minute) for six minutes followed by a four-minute rest. Each subsequent step is increased 150 kpm (170 ml O₂ per min), with six minutes of exercise and four minutes of rest. The patient continues the exercise until the heart rate reaches 150 beats per minute. In this test the data that should be recorded include blood pressure, pulse rate, and electrocardiogram (Table 41–8).

Another method for estimating the safe working level for the damaged heart has utilized upper extremity activities of standardized intensity and recorded the cardiovascular responses of the patient as he works through the stages from light to heavy work.[6]

---

*Kpm = kilopondmeter. A kilopondmeter is the work of moving one kilogram against the gravitational force of the earth through a distance of one meter = 10 Newtons.

TABLE 41–8. AVERAGE ENERGY COSTS OF UPRIGHT BICYCLE ERGOMETER TESTS*

METs	Kcal/min	O₂ ml/kg-min	Kpm/min	Watts
2.6	3.2	10.4	305	50
4.0	4.9	15.8	458	75
5.2	6.4	20.9	610	100
6.5	8.1	26.2	763	125
7.8	9.6	31.4	915	150
9.2	11.3	36.6	1068	175
10.5	12.9	41.9	1220	200

*The energy costs of pedaling a bicycle ergometer at various loads are compared for a 70 kg man in terms of METs. Kcal/min, and oxygen intake.

This table is constructed on the basis that each watt of resistance is equivalent to 6.1 Kpm of work and that each Kpm requires approximately 2.4 ml O₂. (From Naughton, J.: J. S. Carolina Med. Assoc., 65 [Suppl]: 96, 1969.)

TABLE 41–9. PARAMETERS OF CARDIAC PERFORMANCE OF NORMAL SUBJECTS AT SIX LEVELS OF PROGRESSIVE ACTIVITY

Level of Activity	Response — Ratio to Basal				
	Cardiac Work	Cardiac Output	Metabolism	Heart Rate	Blood Pressure
I Supine, basal	1.00	1.00	1.00	1.00	1.00
II Sitting at table with forearm support	0.85	0.75	1.05	1.10	1.15
III Light hand activity with forearm support	1.25	1.05	1.30	1.20	1.25
IV Bilateral arm motion, sanding pine board	1.70	1.40	2.10	1.40	1.25
V Bimanual lifting, 10 lb lifted 15″, 46/min	2.80	2.00	2.80	1.60	1.40
VI Master double two-step test	3.00	2.14	5.75	2.03	1.26

The demonstrated ability to carry on sustained activity at any stage without adverse effect indicates the capability of the patient to carry on the same intensity of activity at home or at work. Five levels of activity have been studied and related to the supine basal resting condition as the reference level of metabolism (METs) or cardiac output (COs). There activities in increasing order of effort are shown in Table 41–9, together with the requirements of the Master two-step test as reported by Dawson.[7] As shown in Figure 41–3, none of the parameters of cardiac performance remain proportional to the cardiac work throughout these activities. Therefore it is highly desirable to measure cardiac output and blood pressure during an activity in order to have a more precise estimate of the work of the heart.

A radio-frequency impedance cardiograph has been developed, which is, in essence, a thoracic impedance plethysmograph responding to the increased column of blood in the aorta with each systole[32] (Fig. 41–13). The change of impedance provides a measure of the left ventricular systolic stroke volume. The stroke volume times heart rate gives minute cardiac output and, multiplied by blood pressure, gives potential work performed per minute by the left ventricle. During systole the impedance, ΔZ, through the chest, from neck to lower thorax, decreases (Fig. 41–14). The rate of change of impedance, dz/dt, is proportional to the stroke volume. From the record in Figure 41–14 it is clearly evident that dz/dt begins at the closure of the mitral valve and ends at the closure of the aortic valve. The magnitude of $(dz/dt)_{min}$ is directly proportional to the stroke volume. The time of maximal deviation of dz/dt is the moment of maximum energy release by the myocardium. The im-

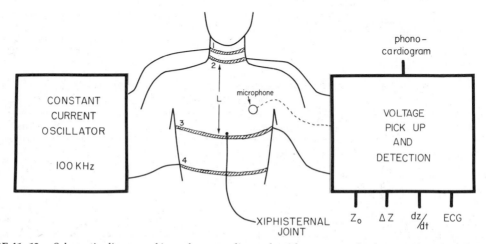

FIGURE 41–13. Schematic diagram of impedance cardiograph with cutaneous leads around neck and chest Z_0, impedance through chest. ΔZ, change of impedance during systole. dz/dt, rate of change of impedance which represents rate of energy release by ventricle. (From Kubicek, W.G., From, A.H.L., Patterson, R.P., Witsoe, D.A., Castaneda, A., Lillehei, R.C., and Ersek, R.: Impedance cardiography as a noninvasive means to monitor cardiac function. J. Assoc. Advancement Med. Instrum., 4:79–84, 1970.)

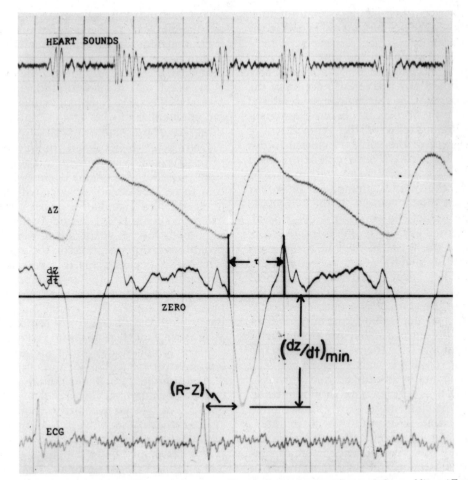

FIGURE 41–14. Record from impedance cardiometer. Top tracing, phonocardiogram. Second line, ΔZ, change in impedance through thorax with systole. Third line, dz/dt, rate of change of impedance with systole. Fourth line, electrocardiogram. (From Kubicek, W.G., From, A.H.L., Patterson, R.P., Witsoe, D.A., Castaneda, A., Lillehei, R.C., and Ersek, R.: Impedance cardiography as a noninvasive means to monitor cardiac function. J. Assoc. Advancement Med. Instrum., 4:79–84, 1970.)

pedance cardiograph provides a precise noninvasive method for comparing changes of stroke volume from which cardiac output can be calculated during exercise testing or rehabilitation activities.[33-35]

PERIPHERAL VASCULAR DISORDERS

See Chapter 42, Management of Peripheral Vascular Disease.

LYMPHEDEMA

Lymphedema of the extremities may be primary or it may be secondary to the surgical removal of lymphatic vessels or obstruction by infection. In any case the water and protein balance across the capillary membrane is disturbed, resulting in the accumulation of extravascular, extracellular fluid. The endothelium of the lymph vessels is more permeable than is that of the blood capillaries. Protein molecules and particles of microscopic dimensions are able to enter the lymph capillaries and by passing through the lymph vessels are removed from the tissue spaces. The main function of the lymph vessels is to remove plasma proteins that filter through the capillaries into the tissue spaces. When the lymphatic vessels are absent or obstructed, the proteins are retained in the tissue spaces, where they increase the colloid osmotic pressure, upset the water balance across the capillary endothelium, and stimulate the production of fibrosis in the tissue spaces.

The flow of lymph in the limbs of several mammals,[36] including man,[37] is normally produced primarily by active vasomotion of the lymphatics. If this mechanism is rendered inoperative by fibrosis or chemical inactivation of the muscles of the lymphatics or incompetence of the valves, external forces assume a larger role. These include the force of gravity, skeletal muscle action,[38] motion of the joints, the thoracic pump, and pulsation of adjacent blood vessels. If the lymphatic valves are intact, this motion is centripetal. During normal activity lymph is moved from the feet to the thoracic duct in a few minutes.[39] During inactivity the pressure in the extravascular spaces and the lymphatics rises to a level slightly below that of the pressure in the veins.[40] The venous pressure in the inactive dependent extremity rises to equal the pressure exerted by a column of water extending from the dependent extremity to the level of the heart.[41]

Lymph contains fibrinogen and thrombin but, owing to a deficiency of thromboplastic substance, it clots more slowly than blood, usually clotting in from 10 to 20 minutes. However, if traumatized cells or bacteria are present they will provide the deficient thromboplastic substance and then thrombosis in the lymph vessels will occur readily. When a lymph vessel thromboses, the thrombi contract and shrink away from the wall of the vessel, leaving adequate space for circulation of lymph. Recurrent thrombi may completely fill the vessel, however.[42]

At a site of severe inflammation, particles of colloidal size or larger will pass through the capillary endothelium into the tissue spaces but will not be removed because fibrin thrombi in the lymphatic vessels obstruct the flow of lymph away from the inflammatory process.[43] When the protein content of lymph increases, collagen is laid down more rapidly. This fibrosis contributes to further stasis. As a result of the increased quantity of lymph and protein in the tissues, there is increased susceptibility to infection. Recurrent inflammation produces progressive thrombosis of the lymph vessels, more stasis of lymph, more fibrosis, and a progressively increasing edema.

Lymphatic vessels have remarkable powers of regeneration. When a large lymphatic vessel is cut, a new channel develops across the scar of the incision and physiologic regeneration may be complete by the eighth day.[44] Collateral vessels also develop extensively. However, if the flow of lymph is so great that it markedly dilates the collateral vessels, the lymphatic valves become incompetent and the lymph flows in the direction of pressure or gravity.

Olszewski[45] has studied the development of postsurgical lymphedema in dogs. A transient postoperative edema occurs which lasts four to six weeks and subsides with regeneration of fine lymphatics across the gap. There ensues a latent period lasting several months to several years during which time a progressive deterioration of the obstructed lymphatics occurs. This is followed by the appearance of chronic lymphedema.

Lymphedema most frequently occurs secondary to surgery in which the regional lymph nodes are extensively removed, such as in radical mastectomy with removal of the axillary lymph nodes or in surgery of the lower extremity with resection of the inguinal lymph nodes. Edema in the arm and hand causes considerable distress due to the increased weight, sensory disturbance in the skin, stiffness of the fingers, and interference with the fit of clothing. In the lower extremity, lymphedema causes stiffness and discomfort and increases fatigability. In both cases resistance to infection in the edematous extremity is decreased, and recurrent attacks of cellulitis occurring spontaneously or following minor trauma are common results.

Treatment of lymphedema by physiatric means involves reduction in the volume of the extremity, support of the affected area to prevent recurrence of the edema, and measures to prevent recurrent infection.

The rationale for management of edema is based on knowledge of the Starling cycle of exchange of water across the capillary membrane. Movement of water across the capillary membrane into the tissue spaces is promoted by the hydrostatic pressure of the blood in the capillary and the osmotic pressure of protein in the tissue fluid. The movement of water from the tissue spaces into the capillary is promoted by the hydrostatic pressure in the tissue fluids and the osmotic pressure of proteins in the plasma. Any excess fluid and protein filtering into the tissue spaces is normally removed through the lymphatic channels. Disturbance of the normal balance by increased capillary pressure, whether it is due to venous congestion or arterial dilatation, or by increased colloidal osmotic pressure in the extravascular space must be offset by increased lymph flow or increasing edema until the increasing tissue pressure restores a balance of exchange of water across the capillary membrane. When the extremity is dependent, the flow of venous blood and lymph will be opposed by the force of gravity.

Management of lymphedema involves attempts to increase venous and lymphatic drainage and tissue hydrostatic pressure. The movement of fluid out of the limb is aided by elevation, mechanical and manual massage, and increased tissue pressure by the application of elastic support.[46] In addition, it is necessary to use measures to prevent the recurrence of cellulitis and lymphangitis. The reduction of lymphedema may require several weeks of intensive therapy to be effective.

Reduction of Edema. For the treatment of lymphedema, the extremity is elevated on a bolster at an angle of 30 to 45 degrees to take advantage of gravity flow. Intermittent mechanical compression is applied by a pneumatic sleeve which is inflated to a pressure of 60 to 100 mm Hg. Tinkham and Stillwell report that they rarely use pressures above 80 mm Hg for 2.5 minutes on and 0.5 minutes off (the longest time cycle of the Jobst hospital model intermittent compressor).[47] Other compressors cycle faster. The combination

of "on" and "off" time can be adjusted as desired, but usually compression time is more than three times as long as decompression time. If pressures are higher than 80 mm Hg a long compression time may not be tolerated; neither has it been demonstrated that a higher pressure is more effective. This mechanical pressure may be applied for periods of 30 minutes to two hours. It appears that the major effect is obtained in the first 60 minutes. Following this mechanical massage, deep stroking and kneading manual massage is applied in a centripetal direction for 10 minutes in an attempt to strip more fluid from the lymphatics. The volume of the arm may be determined by measuring the amount of water displaced from a large cylinder before and after treatment (Fig. 41–15). In addition, the circumferences along the extremity may be recorded as further indices of the effect of the treatment.

Following this therapy the extremity is snugly wrapped with a double-length elastic bandage 3 inches wide. On occasion a 4-inch bandage is used for a mammoth arm. The patient is also instructed to hold the extremity elevated 45 degrees and perform isometric contractions of all the muscles in the extremity four times daily. These isometric contractions are held to the count of 10 and repeated four times a minute for five minutes. Following the isometric exercises the extremity should be unwrapped and wrapped again with the elastic bandage so that a firm compression is obtained. Progressive reduction

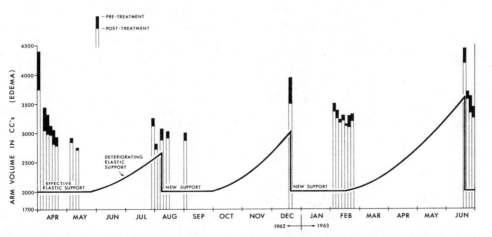

FIGURE 41–15. Changes in volume of an upper extremity with massive lymphedema following radical mastectomy. The volume of the contralateral normal extremity was 1700 cc. Black sections of columns indicate changes in limb volume during one to three hours of intermittent compression treatment using a pneumatic sleeve. The line graph indicates the effectiveness of elastic support of the arm from an Ace bandage or an elastic sleeve. Deterioration of the elastic support without therapy resulted in increase of the lymphedema.

in the size of the arm with decreased turgor of the tissues and decreased arm volume usually occurs over the period from about the second to the tenth day of treatment. At the end of four to six weeks, when limb volume has been reduced as much as possible, the patient is fitted with an elastic sleeve that provides a tissue pressure of 40 mm Hg. The amount of compression required probably is greater with a larger limb in accordance with the law of Laplace, $P = \dfrac{T}{R}$.[48] The patient is instructed to wear the sleeve throughout the day at home. She is also instructed to continue her isometric exercises four times each day at home and to sleep with the arm elevated 30 degrees on a bolster. On this regimen, patients report a continuing slow decrease in the size of the arm after they return home.

The decrease of the volume of edema during a six-day period of therapy has been reported to be greater than 20 per cent in 82 per cent or more of cases, greater than 30 per cent in 64 per cent of cases, and 40 per cent in 41 per cent of cases.[49]

Prevention of Infection. Frequently the patient with lymphedema has a history of recurrent cellulitis and lymphangitis. Minor trauma such as insect bites, cat scratches, needle or thorn pricks, small burns, infected hangnails, and epidermophytosis are commonly associated with the history of recurrent cellulitis in the edematous extremity. Such conditions should be treated appropriately. Clinical findings of induration and increased temperature in the forearm and medial surface of the arm or in the calf, with or without pain or fever, may be taken as evidence of chronic subclinical infection. Frank cellulitis or lymphangitis obviously represents an acute infection that should be treated by penicillin or a broad-spectrum antibiotic.[50] Antibiotics have also been given prophylactically to prevent recurrent lymphangitis and excellent results have been reported. Benzathine penicillin G injections of 1,200,000 units monthly; penicillin V monthly; phenethicillin potassium, 250 milligrams twice daily for five days each month; or oxytetracycline, 250 milligrams four times daily for five days each month if the patient is allergic to penicillin have been reported effective in preventing recurrent lymphangitis in cases of lymphedema.[51]

In addition to the avoidance of infection

(which may with inflammation increase lymph production and the concentration of macromolecular debris, as well as occluding more lymphatics), it is important to avoid other things that increase the lymph load and may precipitate or aggravate the edema. These include:

1. Prolonged use of the muscles of the limb, even for relatively light tasks. Usually 30 to 45 minutes is the maximum at any one time, followed by activity (or inactivity) that does not use the limb for an hour.

2. Local application of heat.

3. Hot environment.

REFERENCES

1. Asmussen, E., and Nielsen, M.: Cardiac output during muscular work and its regulation. Physiol. Rev., 35:778–800, 1955.
2. Berggren, G., and Christensen, E. H.: Heart rate and body temperature as indices of metabolic rate during work. Arbeitsphysiol., 14:255–260, 1950.
3. Tracy, R. A.: Case Studies of the Effect of Systematic Training on Maximal Oxygen Consumption, Myocardial and Circulatory Function and Running Performance Among Selected Middle Distance Runners. Thesis, University of Minnesota, Minneapolis, 1971.
4. Mancini, R., Kottke, F. J., Patterson, R. P., Kubicek, W. G., and Olson, M. E.: Cardiac output and contractility indices: Establishing a standard in response to low-to-moderate level exercise in healthy men. Arch. Phys. Med. Rehabil., 60:567–573, 1979.
5. Kubicek, W. G., Kottke, F. J., Ramos, M. U., Patterson, R. P., Witsoe, D. A., LaBree, J. W., Remole, W., Layman, T. E., Schoening, H. A., and Garamella, J. T.: The Minnesota impedence cardiography—theory and applications. Biomed. Engin., 9:410–416, 1974.
6. Kottke, F. J., Kubicek, W. G., Olson, M. E., Hastings, R. H., and Quast, K.: Five stage test of cardiac performance during occupational activity. Arch. Phys. Med. Rehabil., 43:228–234, 1962.
7. Dawson, W. J., Jr., Kottke, F. J., Kubicek, W. G., Olson, M. E., Harstad, K., Bearman, J. E., Canner, P. L., and Canterbury, J. B.: Evaluation of cardiac output, cardiac work and metabolic rate during hydrotherapy and exercise in normal subjects. Arch. Phys. Med. Rehabil., 46:605–614, 1965.
8. Hershfield, S., Kottke, F. J., Kubicek, W. G., Olson, M. E., Boen, J., Lilquist, C., and Stradal, L.: Relative effects on the heart by muscular work in the upper and lower extremities. Arch. Phys. Med. Rehabil., 49:249–257, 1968.
9. Kottke, F. J., Kubicek, W. G., Danz, J. N., and Olson, M. E.: Studies of cardiac output during the early phase of rehabilitation. Postgrad. Med., 23:533–544, 1958.
10. Passmore, R., and Durnin, J. V. G. A.: Human energy expenditure. Physiol. Rev., 35:801–840, 1955.

11. Gordon, E. E.: Energy costs of various physical activities in relation to pulmonary tuberculosis. Arch. Phys. Med. Rehabil., 33:201–209, 1952.

12. Müller, E. A.: The physiological basis of rest pauses in heavy work. Q. J. Exp. Physiol., 38:205–215, 1953.

13. Schoening, H. A., Remole, W., and LaBree, J. W.: Cardiac rehabilitation program of St. Mary's hospital, Minneapolis. (Mimeo, 1968; revised 4-25-1972.)

14. Weiss, R. A., and Karpovich, P. V.: Energy cost of exercises for convalescents. Arch. Phys. Med. Rehabil., 28:447–454, 1947.

15. Schoening, H. A. (Panelist): Evaluation and Treatment of Cardiopulmonary Disease and Physical Activity Impairment in Patient with Pre-existing Physical Disability. American Congress of Rehabilitation Medicine 49th Annual Session, Denver, Aug. 23, 1972.

16. Monzon de Briceño, Y., Carrasco, H., Fuenmayor, A. M., Parra, A., and Sanchez, C.: Seguimento de Pacientes con Infarta Agudo del Miocardio no Complicado Sometidos a un Programa Precoz de Rehabilitacion Cardiaca. Hospital Universitario de Los Andes, Merida, Venezuela, 1981.

17. Rimer de Casanova, M., and Carrasco, H.: Valor Prognostico de las Pruebas de 2 y 3 Mets, en Pacientes con Infarto de Miocardio no Complicado Sometidos a un Programa de Rehabilitacion Cardiaca Precoz. Hospital Universitario de Los Andes, Merida, Venezuela, 1981.

18. Harpur, J. E., Conner, W. T., Hamilton, M., Kellett, R. J., Galbraith, H.-J. B., Murray, J. J., Swallow, J. H., and Rose, G. A.: Controlled trial of early mobilization and discharge from hospital in uncomplicated myocardial infarction. Lancet, 2:1331–1334, 1971.

19. Wenger, N. K., Hellerstein, H. K., Blackburn, H., et al.: Uncomplicated myocardial infarction. Current physician practice in patient management. J.A.M.A., 224:511–514, 1973.

20. Rose, G.: Early mobilization and discharge after myocardial infarction. Mod. Concepts Cardiovasc. Dis., 41:59–63, 1972.

21. Fletcher, G. F., and Cantwell, J. D.: Exercise and Coronary Heart Disease. Springfield, Ill., Charles C Thomas, Publisher, 1973.

22. Boyer, J. L.: Adult fitness starter program for individuals considered to be at high risk for coronary heart disease. J. S. C. Med. Assoc., 65 (Suppl. 1):99, 1969.

23. Ueno, T.: The so-called coition death. Jap. J. Legal Med., 17:333–340, 1963.

24. Bartlett, R. G., Jr.: Physiologic responses during coitus. J. Appl. Physiol., 9:469–472, 1956.

25. Hellerstein, H. K., and Friedman, E. H.: Sexual activity and the postcoronary patient. Arch. Intern. Med., 125:987–999, 1970.

26. Nemec, E. D., Mansfield, L., and Kennedy, J. W.: Heart rate and blood pressure responses during sexual activity in normal males. Am. Heart J., 92:274–277, 1964.

27. Taylor, H. L., Buskirk, E., and Henschel, A.: Maximal oxygen intake as an objective measure of cardio-respiratory performance. J. Appl. Physiol., 8:73–80, 1955.

28. Bruce, R. A., Kusumi, F., and Hosmer, D.: Maximal oxygen intake and normographic assessment of functional aerobic impairment in cardiovascular disease. Am. Heart J., 85:546–562, 1973.

29. Åstrand, P. O.: Experimental Studies of Physiologic Working Capacity in Relation to Age and Sex. Copenhagen, Ejnar Munksgaard, 1952.

30. Naughton, J., Sevelius, G., and Balke, B.: Physiological responses of normal and pathological subjects to a modified work capacity test. J. Sports Med., 3:201–207, 1963.

31. Hellerstein, H. K., and Hornsten, T. R.: Assessing and preparing the patient for return to a meaningful and productive life. J. Rehab., 32:48–52, 1966.

32. Kubicek, W. G., From, A. H. L., Patterson, R. P., Witsoe, D. A., Castaneda, A., Lillehei, R. C., and Ersek, R.: Impedance cardiography as a noninvasive means to monitor cardiac function. J. Assoc. Advancement Med. Instrum., 4:79–84, 1970.

33. Ramos, M. U.: An abnormal early diastolic impedance waveform: A predictor of poor prognosis in the cardiac patient? Am. Heart J., 94:274–281, 1977.

34. Mancini, R., Kottke, F. J., Patterson, R., Kubicek, W. G., and Olson, M.: Cardiac output and contractility indices: Establishing a standard in response to low-to-moderate level exercise in healthy men. Arch. Phys. Med. Rehabil., 60:567–573, 1979.

35. Wilde, S. W., Miles, D. S., Durbin, R. J., Sawka, M. N., Suryaprasod, A. G., Gotshall, R. W., and Glaser, R. M.: Evaluation of myocardial performance during wheelchair ergometer exercise. Am. J. Phys. Med. Rehabil., 60:277–291, 1981.

36. Hall, J. G., Morris, B., and Woolley, G.: Intrinsic rhythmic propulsion of lymph in the unanaesthetized sheep. J. Physiol. (Lond.), 180:336, 1965.

37. Olszewski, W. L., and Engeset, A.: Intrinsic contractility of leg lymphatics in man. Lymphology, 12:81–84, 1979.

38. Ladd, M. P., Kottke, F. J., and Blanchard, R. S.: Studies of the effect of massage on the flow of lymph from the foreleg of the dog. Arch. Phys. Med. Rehabil., 33:604–612, 1952.

39. Elkins, E. C., Herrick, J. F., Grindlay, J. H., Mann, F. C., and DeForest, R. E.: Effect of various procedures on the flow of lymph. Arch. Phys. Med. Rehabil., 34:31–39, 1953.

40. Irisawa, A., and Rushmer, R. F.: Relationship between lymphatic and venous pressure in leg of dog. Am. J. Physiol., 196:495–498, 1959.

41. Pollack, A. H., and Wood, E. H.: Venous pressure in the saphenous vein at the ankle in man during exercise and changes in posture. J. Appl. Physiol., 1:649–662, 1949.

42. Opie, E. L.: Thrombosis and occlusion of lymphatics. J. Med. Res., 29:131–146, 1913.

43. Menkin, V.: Biochemical Mechanisms in Inflammation, 2nd Ed. Springfield, Ill., Charles C Thomas, Publisher, 1956.

44. Middleton, D. S.: Congenital lymphangiectatic fibrous hypertrophy (elephantiasis congenita fibrosa lymphangiectatica). Br. J. Surg., 19:356–361, 1932.

45. Olsezwski, W.: Pathophysiological and clinical observations of obstructive lymphedema of the

limbs. Chap. 6, pp. 79–102. *In* Clodius, L.: Lymphedema. Stuttgart, Georg Thieme Verlag. (Supplement to Lymphology, 1977.)

46. Stillwell, G. K., and Redford, J. W. B.: Physical treatment of postmastectomy lymphedema. Proc. Mayo Clin., 33:1–8, 1958.

47. Tinkham, R. G., and Stillwell, G. K.: The role of pneumatic pumping devices in the treatment of postmastectomy lymphedema. Arch. Phys. Med. Rehabil., 46:193–197, 1965.

48. Stillwell, G. K.: The law of Laplace: Some clinical applications. Mayo Clin. Proc., 48:863–869, 1973.

49. Stillwell, G. K.: Physical medicine in the management of patients with postmastectomy lymphedema. JAMA, 171:2285–2291, 1959.

50. Britton, R. C., and Nelson, P. A.: Causes and treatment of postmastectomy lymphedema of the arm. JAMA, 180:95–102, 1962.

51. Babb, R. R., Spittell, J. A., Jr., Martin, W. J., and Schirger, A.: Prophylaxis of recurrent lymphangitis complicating lymphedema: Preliminary observations. Proc. Mayo Clin., 37:485–491, 1962.

52. Gazes, P. C., et al.: Mortality by days and weeks up to one year after myocardial infarction. Comparative study. JAMA, 197:906–908, 1966.

42

MANAGEMENT OF VASCULAR DISEASE

GARY FELL

D. E. STRANDNESS, JR.

The clinical management of patients presenting with peripheral vascular disease is dependent upon an understanding of the natural history of the disease process combined with an accurate diagnosis of the degree of severity of the patient's disease. Recently, advances have been made in the noninvasive assessment of the pathophysiologic state of the limb circulation which are of assistance in the clinical assessment of the patient with regard to both the diagnosis and the therapy.

ARTERIAL DISEASE

Acute Arterial Occlusion

Acute arterial occlusion secondary to either embolus, acute thrombosis, or trauma may result in severe ischemia and gangrene of the limb. The major factors that affect the outcome in acute arterial occlusion are the location of the obstruction, the available collateral circulation, and the extent to which thrombus propagation occurs. Emboli most commonly lodge at sites of branches or bifurcations of major vessels, which is also the most common area for the development of atherosclerotic plaques. Propagation of thrombus proximal and distal to the obstruction may occur, resulting in further reduction in flow to the distal limb.

The heart is the most common source of emboli to both the upper and the lower limbs. Less common sources of emboli include ulcerated atherosclerotic plaques and aneurysms of proximal major arteries. In the lower limb, emboli most commonly lodge in the superficial femoral and popliteal arteries, although occlusion of the abdominal aorta is seen in about one sixth of all cases.

If the distal perfusion is inadequate to sustain viability, cutaneous sensation is usually lost within one hour, and after six hours the calf muscles become edematous and tender and begin to undergo ischemic contracture. Shortly thereafter fixed staining of the skin occurs, which is a certain sign of inevitable tissue loss.

The symptoms and signs that develop in response to acute occlusion are in large part related to the site and extent of the occlusion. The five major features of acute arterial occlusion are pain, paresthesia, paralysis, pallor, and pulselessness. If the collateral

This work supported by NIH grant # HL20898.

circulation is adequate, numbness is the most prominent early symptom and may rapidly disappear. Pain in the foot or hand clearly indicates that the collateral circulation is inadequate and should prompt immediate action. Physical examination with this degree of ischemia reveals a cool, pale distal limb with absent palpable pulses distal to the site of occlusion.

The proximal extent of the obstruction can usually be localized by tracing out the major vessels with a Doppler ultrasonic velocity detector. In addition, the measured ankle pressure can help in deciding the most appropriate course of action. It is rare for a patient with an acute arterial occlusion and an ankle pressure of 40 mm Hg or greater to proceed to loss of tissue with nonoperative therapy.

The diagnosis of acute arterial occlusion with evidence of an inadequate collateral circulation demands urgent operation to restore an adequate circulation. Failure to operate will lead to the onset of tissue death in as little as six hours after the onset of symptoms.[1] If viability of the limb is not in question, then the indications for operative intervention will depend upon the location of the occlusion. If the occlusion is proximal to or in the popliteal artery, claudication will result. Thus, for obstructions in these locations, operation is generally indicated because removal of emboli is most easily accomplished in the first 48 to 72 hours after the event.

Embolectomy is usually easily accomplished with an inflatable balloon-tipped catheter under local anesthesia. The operative mortality is in the 15 to 30 per cent range, with cardiac disease being the most common cause of death. In survivors, limb salvage occurs in 80 to 90 per cent in most reported series.[2, 3]

Full systemic anticoagulation with heparin initially and oral anticoagulants later may reduce the extent of propagation of secondary thrombosis and is not a problem should the patient require operation. Pain relief usually is required along with the correction by intravenous fluids of metabolic acidosis and hypovolemia. Protection of the extremity is very important, since the ischemic limb is very susceptible to even minor trauma, both mechanical and thermal. The application of direct heat is inappropriate and may produce significant thermal damage to the skin. In addition, the raised temperature increases the metabolic requirement of a limb unable to maintain even the basic metabolic requirements. The head of the bed should be raised six to eight inches, thereby increasing tissue perfusion with the aid of gravity. Vasodilator drugs have not been found to be useful.

Acute thrombosis may occur in patients with marked arteriosclerosis obliterans, as a complication of peripheral aneurysms (popliteal, femoral), or as a result of compression associated with thoracic outlet or popliteal artery entrapment syndromes. The degree of ischemia is variable, and therapy is more difficult than with acute embolism. In addition to noninvasive studies to measure the perfusion pressure to the limb, arteriography should be performed, since direct arterial surgery is often required.

Arteriosclerosis Obliterans (ASO)

Atherosclerosis involves primarily the large and medium sized arteries, where progressive stenosis may lead to occlusion of the most severely involved vessels. Limb survival is possible because of the extensive network of pre-existing collateral vessels that increase in size in response to disease. These collateral pathways are high resistance conduits that produce an abnormal pressure drop across the diseased segment. Multisegmental stenoses and occlusions are common and in ASO result in an even greater decrease in the perfusion pressure to the distal limb. The most common sites of disease are the superficial femoral artery at the level of the adductor canal, followed by involvement of the aortoiliac segment.

Patients with arteriosclerosis obliterans typically present with a slow progression of symptoms unless the disease process is complicated by acute thrombosis on a preexisting plaque. Intermittent claudication, the ischemic pain related to exercise, is the most common symptom of arteriosclerosis obliterans. The amount of exercise required to induce the pain remains relatively constant on a day-to-day basis, and pain usually subsides rapidly upon cessation of walking. As the disease progresses to involve more than one segment, exercise tolerance is progressively reduced. The terminal stage of the disease is manifested by the appearance of ischemic rest pain of the foot and digits, which may be partially or completely relieved by dependency. Ulceration and gangrene are common when the perfusion pressure falls below 40 mm Hg at the level of the ankle and/or digit.[4]

It should be noted that claudication always involves a more distal limb segment than the actual level of occlusion. Therefore, superficial femoral artery occlusion is associated with calf claudication, while aortoiliac disease may produce thigh and buttock pain in addition to that which occurs in the muscles of the calf.

The physical examination usually supports the clinical diagnosis made from the patient's history. The appearance of the limb in single segment disease is normal, but absent or diminished pulses may be noted. In more advanced stages of disease, dependent rubor and delayed capillary filling may be noted together with evidence of poor skin nutrition with the absence of hair, skin ulceration, and perhaps gangrene of the digits or foot. Careful auscultation for the detection of bruits in the abdomen and over the common femoral and popliteal arteries may confirm suspected arteriosclerotic arterial disease.

NONINVASIVE ASSESSMENT

Noninvasive evaluation and confirmation of the presence, severity, and rate of progression of ASO and of the results of reconstructive vascular surgery are now possible with simple, relatively inexpensive bedside equipment. A number of techniques have been developed, including strain gauge plethysmography, pulse volume recording, and Doppler ultrasonic velocity detection. The sensor is usually placed over the digits, foot (plethysmography), or the dorsalis pedis or posterior tibial artery (ultrasonic velocity detector). The systolic blood pressure can be estimated at the level of the ankle and then compared with the brachial systolic pressure.[5] The ankle systolic pressure is normally equal to or above the brachial systolic pressure. Arterial occlusions at one or more sites result in a pressure drop that can be expressed as a ratio of arm/ankle pressure which is less than 1.0. This arm/ankle index is used to adjust for changes in systemic blood pressure. The absolute level of the ankle or digit pressure is of importance in alerting the physician to the development of rest pain. Pressures at or below 40 mm Hg are marginal in terms of tissue perfusion.

The recordings and measurements can be used to confirm the clinical suspicion of occlusive vascular disease, to assist in differentiating vascular from neurogenic pain, to follow patients on medical regimens, and to evaluate the patency and effectiveness of reconstructive vascular surgery.

THERAPY

The patient and the patient's family must be fully acquainted with the natural history of the disease, in particular the expected chance of loss of a limb or the indications for and outcome of reconstructive vascular surgery. The expected rate of a major amputation after the onset of intermittent claudication is 1.4 per cent per year, while the prospect of dying inside five years is about 15 per cent.[6] Diabetics, however, have a much increased rate of amputation, 34 per cent in 10 years in one study.[7]

Medical management, which is always required whether surgery is performed or not, is palliative, supportive, and preventive, but not curative. Surgical intervention is not indicated for those patients with intermittent claudication that does not limit employment or the ability to maintain usual daily activities. Of course, after surgery, the basic atherosclerotic disease process is still present, and continuing care is necessary to prevent progression and the potential threat of limb loss.

Clearly, for the patient with symptoms, the elimination or reduction of risk factors is mandatory. The cessation of smoking and recognition and control of diabetes, hypertension, and hyperlipidemias may, if properly managed, contribute to the reduced progression of the disease. Vasodilating drugs and long-term anticoagulation have not been found to be efficacious in the treatment of chronic arteriosclerosis obliterans.

Exercise on a daily basis to the limit imposed by claudication may result in an increased walking distance. If there are no contraindications, it is advisable to ask patients with intermittent claudication to walk up to their limit twice to three times daily. Fungal infections, minor wounds, contusion, scratches, blisters, rubbing from shoes, and minor surgical operations around the toes frequently precipitate episodes of local skin necrosis, ulceration, and sepsis and must be avoided or recognized and treated promptly.

Patients with severe lower limb ischemia, as evidenced by rest pain, cyanosis, rubor, ulceration, or gangrene, in whom surgical reconstruction is not feasible require bed rest in a warm environment with the head of the bed elevated six to eight inches. Analgesia is often required, although the necessity for using narcotics may be an indication for amputation. Protection of the feet from trauma — mechanical, thermal, or chemical —is mandatory or healing of damaged tissue will have even less of a chance of occurring.

Daily physical therapy is used to prevent disuse atrophy and joint contractures, particularly of the hip and knee joints. Patients who remain in bed because of severe ischemia are at considerable risk of developing ulceration secondary to the effects of pressure on the heels.

Reconstructive vascular surgery is indicated for rest pain, nonhealing ulcers, and severe progressive disabling intermittent claudication. Moderate or mild intermittent claudication that is incompatible with the patient's work is only a relative indication for operation. All patients must be fully acquainted with the risks of surgery, particularly the 1 to 5 per cent mortality rate associated with aortoiliac reconstruction and the prospect of graft occlusion of 15 per cent at five years.[8, 9] For femoropopliteal revascularization, the mortality rate is considerably less, although the rate of graft failure is higher, approximately 40 to 50 per cent at five years.[10, 11]

Operation is contraindicated in the absence of threatened tissue loss if the patient is sedentary or unable to walk for other reasons such as paralysis or general debility. Significant extracranial cerebrovascular and ischemic coronary artery disease should be fully evaluated and treated prior to revascularization of the lower extremities.

Amputation is considered when there is no alternative procedure available and it is certain that the patient will benefit from the proposed operation. Indications include gangrene of the limb with sepsis, nonhealing ulceration, and intractable rest pain. Dry gangrene of individual digits or ulceration on non–weight-bearing areas can be managed expectantly and amputation withheld.

Further consideration prior to amputation should be given to the expected quality and length of life. One third of vascular amputees will be dead within two years and two thirds within five years; loss of a limb poses a further threat to the enjoyment of remaining life. The early mortality associated with below-the-knee amputation is approximately 5 per cent, although with advancing age and increasing numbers of associated illnesses, the figure may be higher.

Thromboangiitis Obliterans (Buerger's Disease)

In contrast to arteriosclerosis obliterans, which is multisegmental and involves the large and medium sized arteries, Buerger's disease has a different distribution. Thromboangiitis obliterans commences in the smaller arteries of the feet and hands and progresses proximally to involve the medium sized vessels. It is primarily an inflammatory process involving the entire neurovascular bundle.

The typical patient with thromboangiitis obliterans is a male cigarette smoker in the 20 to 40 year age range. The first symptom is usually intermittent claudication, often of the instep initially and of the calf with further progression of the disease. Recurrent episodes of superficial thrombophlebitis in short nonvaricose segments of veins are seen in about 40 per cent of patients. Upper extremity involvement and cold sensitivity are seen frequently. Ischemic rest pain in the digits is often associated with ulceration and then frank gangrene.

The clinical course of the disease is greatly influenced by whether or not the patient stops smoking. Unfortunately, many patients with Buerger's disease continue to smoke in the face of progressive disease, and first minor and then major amputations are required to remove the gangrenous tissue.

VENOUS DISORDERS

The development of acute venous thrombosis, when it involves the deep venous system,[12] is potentially complicated by pulmonary embolism. In contrast, involvement of the superficial venous system usually resolves without significant complications or long-term sequelae.

Numerous factors are associated with an increased risk of deep venous thrombosis: (1) age, (2) immobility and prolonged bed rest, (3) obesity, (4) malignancy, (5) oral contraception, (6) polycythemia rubra vera, (7) pregnancy and the postpartum state, (8) orthopedic injuries, (9) congestive heart failure, and (10) the postoperative state. Although all these factors are associated risk factors, the specific etiologic agent or hemodynamic factor involved in the development of venous thrombosis remains unknown.

Approximately 50 per cent of patients with deep venous thrombosis will present with commonly recognized features, which include calf pain, swelling, deep calf tenderness, and discoloration of the leg. The remaining 50 per cent of patients with deep venous thromboses will go undetected unless noninvasive techniques or phlebography are utilized in patient evaluation.[13, 14] Occlusions involving the iliofemoral venous segments are reliably detected using the ultrasonic velocity detector. Isolated involvement of the calf veins can be detected by ^{125}I-labeled fibrinogen, although this technique has too many limitations for widespread clinical usage. Phlebography, although an invasive technique, remains the most reliable and accurate method of making the diagnosis, but it too has a number of limitations that must be recognized: (1) complete filling of involved veins is required; (2) it is difficult to visualize the entire leg and major pelvic veins; (3) repeat examination is difficult; and (4) exacerbation or initiation of deep venous thrombosis occurs in about 7 per cent of cases.

THERAPY

The treatment of acute superficial thrombophlebitis includes rest, elevation of the limb, and local heat in the early inflammatory period. Ambulation may be begun as soon as the pain subsides.

Established deep venous thrombosis is treated by full systemic heparinization. The heparin is administered by continuous intravenous infusion after an initial loading dose is administered.[15] The partial thromboplastin time is checked prior to the commencement of therapy and then on a daily basis to maintain a value of at least two times that of the control. Intravenous heparin is continued for 10 days, at which point oral anticoagulants commenced prior to the cessation of heparin should be in the therapeutic range.

The duration of oral anticoagulant therapy is unsettled, although recent evidence suggests a six-week course for uncomplicated isolated calf vein thrombosis.[16] Following major iliofemoral vein thrombosis or pulmonary embolism, a 3- to 6-month course of anticoagulants is required.

In the acute phase of the deep venous thrombosis, the patient should remain in bed with the foot of the bed elevated. No other local measures are required. Ambulation should be encouraged early, and no patient should be allowed to remain sitting or standing still; he should either be actively walking or resting with the legs elevated. During ambulation, support stockings should be used if edema develops.

Post-thrombotic Syndrome

Following single or multiple episodes of deep venous thrombosis, the deep and perforating veins are often subject to both obstruction and destruction of the venous valves. Blood in the deep veins is thereby forced by the calf muscle pump via abnormal pathways into the superficial venous system during exercise, when in the normal situation the reverse occurs. Over a prolonged period, chronic interstitial edema and rupture of small subcutaneous vessels occurs; hemosiderin (stasis pigmentation) deposition occurs along with fibrosis, cutaneous atrophy, and lymphatic obstruction. These chronic changes in the skin of the leg may lead to the development of stasis ulceration.

The first clinical manifestation of chronic venous insufficiency is the development of dependent edema of the limb, which is worse at the end of the day and tends to clear after a period of recumbency and elevation. Secondly, stasis pigmentation is noted followed by induration and less resolution of the edema with elevation of the limbs. Ulceration is common and usually develops following minor episodes of trauma. The ulcers commonly occur in the region of the medial malleolus but may extend all the way around the ankle. Multiple organisms can often be cultured from the base of the ulcer and secondary infection may occur, leading to episodes of cellulitis, further fibrosis, induration, and the prevention of healing of the ulcer.

THERAPY

The major goal in all patients with the post-thrombotic syndrome is to reduce the ambulatory venous pressure. This may usually be accomplished by the wearing of tailored, graduated pressure support stockings, bandages, or both, combined with elevation of the legs whenever possible.

In cases with ulceration, healing can always be achieved by persistent, prolonged bed rest and elevation. For most patients this is not feasible and the ulcer must be healed while the patient remains active and ambulatory. Healing can usually be achieved by the use of the Una boot applied from the base of the toes to below the knee. The dressing is applied directly to the ulcer and changed weekly or sooner if drainage is excessive. The patients remain ambulatory and when complete healing has occurred a tailored pressure gradient stocking is used. For large ulcers that do not respond to this form of therapy, skin grafting may became necessary.

LYMPHATIC DISORDERS

Lymphedema occurs secondary to congenital or acquired lymphatic obstruction. It always involves the dorsum of the digits, foot, or hand, which is rare with edema secondary to venous obstruction. It is often brawny in nature and does not respond as rapidly to elevation. Ulceration is rare, but cellulitis secondary to streptococcal infection is not uncommon. For this reason, prophylactic penicillin is commonly used, since repeated episodes of cellulitis lead to edema that is worse after each episode.

Since the edema is difficult to manage once it gets out of control, it is essential that daily care include the following: (1) limb measurements recorded in a diary; (2) graded, heavy elastic support; (3) prophylactic penicillin; and (4) the use of intermittent pneumatic compression devices at night to assist in the control of the edema.

Lymphangiography has been recommended to confirm the diagnosis, but this is rarely required. Further, if lymphangitis occurs secondary to the procedure, the edema is always worse. The lifetime nature of the problem must be emphasized to the patient, and frequent medical follow-up is mandatory to insure compliance with recommended therapy. Surgical removal of the involved tissue is only rarely required if proper conservative therapy has been used and followed.

REFERENCES

1. Tibbs, P. J.: Acute ischemia of the limbs. Proc. R. Soc. Med., 55:593, 1962.
2. Levy, J. F., and Butcher, H. R.: Arterial emboli: An analysis of 125 patients. Surgery, 68:968, 1970.
3. Blaisdell, F. W., Steele, M., and Allen, R. E.: Management of acute lower extremity arterial ischemia due to embolism and thrombosis. Surgery, 84:822, 1978.
4. Strandness, D. E., Jr.: Diagnostic considerations in occlusive arterial disease. Vasc. Surg., 11:271, 1977.
5. Carter, S. A.: Role of pressure measurements in vascular disease. In Bernstein, E. F. (ed.): Noninvasive Diagnostic Techniques in Vascular Disease. St. Louis, The C. V. Mosby Co., 1978.
6. Boyd, A. M.: The natural course of arteriosclerosis of the lower extremities. Proc. R. Soc. Med., 53:591, 1962.
7. Silbert, S., and Zazeela, H.: Prognosis in arteriosclerotic peripheral vascular disease. J.A.M.A., 166:1816, 1958.
8. Mozersky, D. J., Sumner, D. S., and Strandness, D. E., Jr.: Long term results of reconstructive aortoiliac surgery. Am. J. Surg., 123:503, 1972.
9. Hill, D. A., McGrath, M. A., Lord, R. S. A., and Tracy, G. D.: The effect of superficial femoral artery occlusion on the outcome of aortofemoral bypass for intermittent claudication. Surgery, 87:133, 1980.
10. Reichle, F. A., Rankin, K. P., Tyson, R. R., Finestone, A. S., and Shuman, C.: Long term results of 474 arterial reconstructions for severely ischemic limbs: A fourteen year followup. Surgery, 85:93, 1979.
11. Szilagyi, D. E., Hageman, J. H., Smith, F. R., Elliott, J. P., Brown, F., and Dietz, P.: Autogenous vein grafting in femoro-popliteal atherosclerosis: The limits of its effectiveness. Surgery, 86:836, 1979.
12. Strandness, D. E., Jr., Ward, K., and Krugmire, R., Jr.: The present status of acute deep venous thrombosis. Surg. Obstet. Gynecol., 145:433, 1977.
13. Sumner, D. S., and Lambeth, A.: Reliability of Doppler ultrasound in the diagnosis of acute deep venous thrombosis both above and below the knee. Am. J. Surg., 138:205, 1979.
14. Strandness, D. E., Jr.: Invasive and noninvasive techniques in the detection and evaluation of acute venous thrombosis. Vasc. Surg., 11:205, 1977.
15. Salzman, E. W., Deykin, D., Shapiro, R. M., and Rosenberg, R.: Management of heparin therapy: Controlled prospective trial. N. Engl. J. Med., 292:1046, 1975.
16. Hull, R., Delmore, T., Genton, E., Hirsh, J., Gent, M., Sackett, D., McLoughlin, D., and Armstrong, P.: Sodium versus low-dose heparin in the long-term treatment of venous thrombosis. N. Engl. J. Med., 301:855, 1979.

Suggested Reading

Bergan, J. J., and Yao, J. S. T. (Eds.): Venous Problems. Chicago, Year Book Medical Publisher, Inc., 1978.
Haimovici, H. (Ed.): Vascular Surgery, Principles and Techniques. New York, McGraw-Hill Book Company, 1976.
Rutherford, R. B. (Ed.): Vascular Surgery. Philadelphia, W. B. Saunders Co., 1977.

43

RECONSTRUCTIVE SURGERY OF THE EXTREMITIES

JOACHIM L. OPITZ

With the advent of total joint replacement during the last 15 years, reconstructive surgery of the extremities has entered a new and promising era. Substantial advances also are being made in tendon transfers and other areas. The following chapter outlines the principles related to common reconstructive procedures in the extremities and to the subsequent postoperative management.

TOTAL JOINT REPLACEMENT

General Considerations

Purposes. The purposes of total joint replacement are to relieve pain, to correct deformities, to re-establish function, and to prevent or ameliorate painful secondary effects on adjacent joints. The combination of high-density polyethylene and highly polished resilient metal alloys (nickel, chrome, molybdenum), as first described by Charnley[2] in his total hip prosthesis, has led progressively to replacement of all major joints in both lower and upper extremities. Many different prostheses of various degrees of constraint are being used, most of which have the combination of high-density polyethylene and metal in their components or are joint spacers made of special Silastic rubber elastomers. Clinical experience of more than 10 years has indicated very little wear of the polyethylene-on-metal prostheses, less than 0.15 mm per year in total hip arthroplasty, with maintenance of the low-friction features and no foreign body reactions. The optically polished metal components have usually satisfactory resilience, excellent tissue acceptance, and no appreciable wear.

Limitations. The greatest, initially unanticipated, source of late failures relates to loosening of prosthetic devices in bone. Methylmethacrylate, a cementing compound, provides major advantages over the press fitting of components. The methacrylate is well tolerated by tissues, although it is less than ideal as a grouting agent. The higher the degree of constraint built into a total joint replacement and the rougher its use in the absence of pain in the young and in the overweight person, the higher the incidence of late loosening tends to be.

Infection in total joint replacements, even though of low incidence, is also a worrisome cause of failure. Hematogenous spread of organisms is the usual cause of late infection and often necessitates the temporary removal of the prosthetic components. Therefore, the prophylactic use of antibiotics is justified in total joint replacements when transient bacteremia is to be expected, such as with tooth extractions, thorough professional dental cleansing, urinary tract infection, systemic infections, etc.

Total replacement of hip and knee have given reliable and satisfactory long-term results.[22] The replacement of wrists, metacarpophalangeal joints, and shoulders is in a developmental stage but is showing promising results.[21] The total replacement of elbows and ankles is in the early state of evolution.

Indications. The main indications for total joint arthroplasties exist in patients afflicted with degenerative joint disease, destructive rheumatoid arthritis, and to some extent, post-traumatic arthritis. Total joint replacement for post-traumatic arthritis is at present limited to the hip, knee, thumb, shoulder, and perhaps elbow.

In general, requirements for total joint replacements of the lower extremity have precedence over those of the upper extremities, except on occasion when a patient otherwise would be totally dependent in feeding and self-care. Oftentimes, joints of the upper extremity improve remarkably once they are relieved of the severe stress of assisting the lower extremities in weight-bearing after total hip or knee replacement.

Contraindications. Absolute contraindications for total joint arthroplasties exist in patients with recent septic arthritis, paralysis about the joint to be replaced, and neuropathic joint disease. Relative contraindications exist in patients with severe osteoporosis, severe and incorrectable ligamentous defects about the joint, and other physiologic or psychologic deficiencies of proportion.

Goals. The goals of postoperative physiatric management need to be in line with the purposes of total joint replacement. They are relief of pain, redevelopment of comfortable musculoskeletal functions, and development of living habits that avoid excessively stressing the joint replacement.

1. RELIEF OF PAIN. For practical purposes, pain can be defined for patient and therapist as the degree of discomfort that causes motor incoordination, such as unreasonable cocontraction of the antagonistic muscle groups (splinting). This definition allows for a gradual increase in strain of therapeutic exercises as the patient maintains smooth neuromuscular function about the replaced joint. The patient who undergoes total joint replacement usually has had years of progressive pain about the joint in question. Long-term expectation and experience of joint pain, progressive limitation of

range of motion, and the decrease of strength due to diminished use of the extremity have led to deep-seated changes in coordination and motor behavior. Muscle misuse, that is, unreasonable cocontraction of antagonistic muscles, usually has become firmly established before total joint replacement. The effects of muscle misuse tend to perpetuate vicious circles of pain. As a result of muscle misuse, which is the natural response to pain, a number of undesirable effects evolve. Range of motion becomes unnecessarily limited by heavy cocontraction of antagonistic muscle groups. Joints are exposed to high compression forces because such cocontractions occur during attempted motion, causing increased wear and synovial irritation. Lastly, the involved muscles themselves become overused. With chronic joint pain, muscle contractions often last much longer than needed. Continued low-grade to moderate muscle contraction, therefore, may result in chronic muscle overuse with associated tension myalgia, muscle attachment pain, and tenosynovitis. Such pernicious interrelationships contribute substantially to the increase in pain and the limitation of functions. Because pain is also a very effective inhibitor of muscle contraction, it causes progressive decrease of strength as a result of muscle misuse.

When the patient is seen postoperatively in the Department of Physical Medicine and Rehabilitation, the motor behavior of muscle misuse usually has been further reinforced by the substantial bone and soft-tissue trauma during the joint replacement procedure and by the apprehension of the patient, who often expects the postoperative program to be a painful experience. The examination tends to be less threatening to the patient if the evaluator first takes inventory of the uninvolved extremities and then inspects the involved extremity. Slow, passive motion of the involved limb follows. Avoidance of pain is important. Testing for clinically apparent deep venous thrombosis, peripheral nerve injury, deep infection, and substantial hematoma usually can be done without considerable and potentially threatening movements of the involved extremity. The assessment of the total passive range of motion is of questionable value at this point, because it is usually limited by muscle guarding, which should be avoided. Thus, during the evaluation process, the patient can be relieved of some anxiety and can become better pre-

TABLE 43–1. PRIORITIES OF SUCCESSIVE EXERCISES AND ACTIVITIES AFTER TOTAL JOINT REPLACEMENT

Passive relaxed motion and neuromuscular re-education

Active (assisted) range-of-motion exercises

Light functional activities of daily living, hobby, and self-care

Redevelopment of maximal desirable range of motion (with gentle, prolonged stretching)

Formal strengthening (if indicated)

Modified from Opitz, J. L.: Total joint arthroplasty: Principles and guidelines for postoperative physiatric management. Mayo Clin. Proc., 54:602–612, 1979. By permission.

pared to work for improvement of normal function. The negative effects of muscle misuse on the joint, periarticular structures, range of motion, strength, and normal joint function make it logical that the first and perhaps the most important therapeutic goal after operation is to eliminate abnormal motor behavior resulting from expected or actual pain.

Pain usually can be eliminated because the total joint replacement has rendered the joint itself free of pain. The patient should know that the therapeutic exercises and subsequent therapeutic functional activities can be practiced smoothly and without pain.

Priorities of successive exercises in activities should be carefully considered (Table 43–1). These priorities need to be adhered to in order to eliminate pain, avoid muscle misuse and substitution patterns, and ensure the efficient attainment of the overall goals of total joint replacement. Generally, it is advisable first to re-establish a satisfactory range of motion — with gentle, prolonged stretching, if necessary — before advancing to formal strengthening (if indicated).

2. RE-ESTABLISHMENT OF NORMAL FUNCTION. Neuromuscular re-education is the initial therapeutic exercise system that is designed to assist the patient in the re-establishment of pain-free, well-coordinated motor activities. In neuromuscular re-education, the patient's undesirable old pattern of muscle misuse is consciously dismissed by allowing the therapist to move the extremity passively through the pain-free range of motion. The patient should permit passive movement without interference through many repetitions. As the patterns of muscle misuse are eliminated in this fashion, the therapist then, through various tech-

niques, coaches the patient to contract the prime mover of a specific motion, free of associated, undesirable cocontraction of antagonistic muscles. Motion through the pain-free arc is then accomplished by gentle contraction of the prime mover while assistance is given by the therapist. In this way, normal motor behavior is re-established and incorporated in range-of-motion exercises and light functional activities of daily living. Dysfunctional motor behaviors, if they reappear, are recognized at their inception by experienced therapists. These behaviors are promptly and gently discouraged. Usually, motor tasks that cause motor incoordination should temporarily be made simpler for the patient. If this measure is unsuccessful, techniques of neuromuscular re-education need to be reapplied. Often, simply a temporary reduction in speed, force, and perhaps arc of motion permits the return of an acceptable motor pattern. In such fashion, the patient progresses most efficiently to more difficult tasks, with clear, acceptable, and comfortable motor performance.

Because the potentially available range of motion can be developed at mild-to-moderate, usually pain-free muscle contractions, and because strengthening exercises usually require potentially painful, strong muscle contraction, strengthening exercises are best postponed until the full range of motion has been redeveloped. For strengthening exercises, muscle contractions about the joint should be free of pain and have become nonthreatening to periarticular structures.

Some uncertainty exists concerning when stretching exercises can be applied safely to increase the range of motion more efficiently than by the active-assisted or active range-of-motion exercises alone. The reasons for such uncertainty relate to the difficulty in estimating the tensile strength of periarticular structures as healing progresses and to the degree of stretching force applied by the individual therapist during stretching exercises.

If exposed to pain-free, mild-to-moderate stretching forces for 15 to 30 minutes several times a day, maturing scar tissue should elongate without injury. Such stretching forces can be applied 4 to 6 weeks after operation without threatening essential periarticular structures. In fact, such gentle, prolonged stretching forces are probably important for the proper alignment of collagen

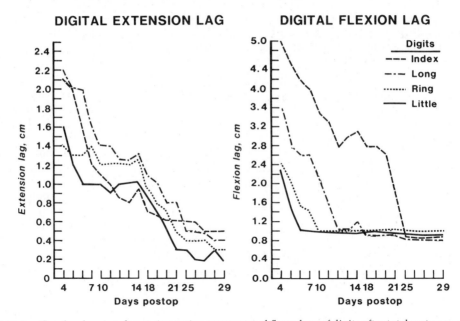

FIGURE 43–1. Graphs showing decreasing active extensor and flexor lags of digits after total metacarpophalangeal joint replacement in a patient with rheumatoid arthritis. (From Opitz, J. L.: Total joint arthroplasty: Principles and guidelines for postoperative physiatric management. Mayo Clin Proc., 54:602–612, 1979. By permission.)

bundles and, thus, lead to better connective tissue structures about the joint as healing progresses. Forceful stretching should be avoided because it is likely to result in pain, splinting of the muscles being stretched, and irritation of the joint. Such stretching also threatens the integrity of periarticular structures and causes protective motor behavior (muscle misuse) with its negative consequences.

When rapid increases in range of motion are not forthcoming, the daily measurement of active range of motion (goniometry) with the patient in a gravity-eliminated position of the joint at the end of the last exercise period of the day is helpful in assessing progress (Fig. 43–1). Results of goniometry are likely to be reproducible only if the motion is done actively by the patient without assistance. The results of daily goniometry are particularly helpful in motivating the patient for range-of-motion exercises, because the patient is then exercising in competition with himself. If the daily results are recorded on a graph, the patient, the therapist, and the physician can easily follow and appreciate advances in range of motion. Slowing of progress, lack of progress, or actual regression of performance is recognized early.

After increases in range of motion have stopped, further increases often may be achieved by heating the connective tissue to be stretched with ultrasound at the time of gentle, prolonged stretching. This technique has been described by Lehmann and associates.[11] For practical purposes, ultrasound may be applied safely in the presence of metallic or plastic implants.

Restrengthening of the involved extremity, as mentioned earlier, is last in the list of priorities because of the associated strong muscle contractions, which are potentially painful and possibly injurious to periarticular structures recently operated on. Often, formal strengthening exercises are not necessary because the extremities with total joint replacements, when kept free of pain, strengthen spontaneously to substantial levels as they are made to perform the daily functional activities during the first three to six months after operation. Because of the relatively high incidence of loosening of components in total joint replacement when the extremities are exposed to heavy mechanical stresses, formal restrengthening to a maximal degree may be unnecessary or even contraindicated. If strengthening is needed, it should be postponed until it can be done comfortably. Pain is a very potent inhibitor of muscle contraction and usually prohibits strengthening.

3. ADEQUATE RELIEF OF WEIGHT-BEARING. Reliable reduction of weight-bearing after hip, knee, and ankle replacements con-

tinues to be of concern. Examinations of reproducibility of reduction in weight-bearing in biomechanic laboratories have shown that the only consistently reproducible method for relief of weight-bearing identified is to "touch only" with the involved lower extremity during gait. This reduces weight-bearing to 20 lb (9 kg) or less. "Touch-only" weight-bearing can be checked simply by the physician and therapist during gait training of the patient. In order to check "touch only," one assesses the friction between the shoe and the floor resulting from the superimposed body weight of the patient by means of a few gentle, rapid knocks against the heel of the patient's shoe by the examiner's foot during the stance phase. Weight-bearing is minimal ("touch only") if the patient's foot is easily (and minimally) displaced by gentle knocking during stance. The foot cannot be displaced by this method if weight-bearing is substantial.

Often, however, weight-bearing can be reduced enough postoperatively for the patient to be free from discomfort. Such an order might read: "Weight-bearing on the left (or right) lower extremity as tolerated comfortably." It permits progressive increase in weight-bearing without overly stressing recently operated soft tissues, provided that, in the patient with total hip replacement, the greater trochanter has not been osteotomized and reattached. If substantial muscle or bone had to be divided and reapproximated, the formal method of "touch only" is the only reliable method of preventing overexposure to weight-bearing.

Evaluation before starting physical therapy and occupational therapy (when indicated) requires review of the written referral, of the operative report, and of the appropriate preoperative and postoperative roentgenograms in order to determine whether unusual circumstances exist that necessitate modification of the postoperative program. Any personal input from the surgeon by word or (preferably) in writing helps serve the same purpose. Nevertheless, the operative report and roentgenograms still should be reviewed carefully. If any question remains, clarification by the surgeons is imperative before a treatment program is started.

Lower Extremities

Total Hip Arthroplasty. Total hip replacements are done routinely in patients with painfully decompensating primary or secondary degenerative joint disease, rheumatoid arthritis, or congenital hip disease. Total hip replacement also may be done to salvage other arthroplasties of the hip if the hip has become painful or to salvage arthrodeses of the hip, provided that the hip musculature is adequate (Fig. 43–2). Since 1961, when Charnley[2] reported on total hip arthroplasty, low-friction arthroplasty with a high-density acetabular polyethylene component, and the corresponding optically polished Vitallium femoral head prosthesis, progress in total joint replacement has been phenomenal. The advantages of metalloplastic prostheses have been confirmed for several of the major joints in terms of no pain, no wear, good mobility, adequate stability, and durability if not overly stressed. The components of total hip replacement are cemented into bone with methylmethacrylate. Relief of pain is most gratifying in 90 per cent of patients. Reoperations occur at approximately 1 per cent per year, mostly for late infection, dislocation, and loosening of the femoral component. Stress fractures of the femoral components have been prevented by the use of stronger stems. Loosening and dislocation of the femoral component are greatly reduced by removing all cancellous soft bone, by injecting the cement under pressure, and by proper seating with proper alignment of the components in kinesiologically sound positions.

Several modifications of the Charnley prosthesis are being used for special conditions that require greater stability by virtue of a larger prosthetic head (Mueller, Aufranc-Turner). Resurfacing arthroplasty of the femoral head, such as the total hip articular internal eccentric shell (THARIES), in association with a polyethylene acetabulum, is an interesting new development that has had promising initial success. Special long-stemmed femoral components as part of a total hip arthroplasty may replace en bloc resection of tumors involving the proximal femur where amputation of the lower extremity by hip disarticulation was previously necessary.

The patient is referred to Physical Medicine and Rehabilitation during the third to the fifth day after total hip arthroplasty. The exercise program consists of individual brief periods of neuromuscular re-education for active-assisted range of motion of ankle, knee, and hip. Gait training should be started on a tilt table to ascertain whether the patient

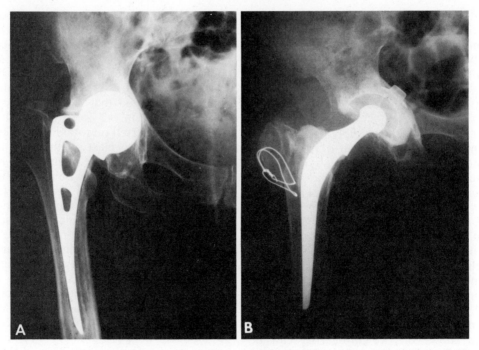

FIGURE 43–2. *A*, Anteroposteriør view of loose femoral head prosthesis with arthrocathadesis. *B*, Anteroposterior view of the same hip salvaged by Charnley total hip arthroplasty.

is free from orthostatic hypotension; such hypotension should be treated. The therapist should check the patient's pulse and blood pressure during the tilting and at intervals up to 5 to 7 minutes of standing. The patient is advanced to standing, in parallel bars, once major orthostatic responses in blood pressure and pulse have been controlled. After standing balance has been achieved with the help of parallel bars, neuromuscular re-education re-establishes proper motion of the involved extemity during the swing phase in the parallel bars. Also, the stance phase of the involved lower extremity is practiced ("touch only" or "weight-bearing as tolerated comfortably") initially while standing with the help of parallel bars. If several repetitions of the isolated swing phase and stance phase are performed satisfactorily, the patient is asked to take a single step. If the single step is performed well, the patient should attempt to take two consecutive steps. The number of consecutive steps is increased progressively as acceptable performance permits. A decrease in speed and accuracy of performance indicates fatigue and signals the need for a short pause or a longer rest period. Once an uninterrupted gait with the help of parallel bars has become smooth and acceptable (three-point gait for

unilateral and four-point gait for bilateral hip involvement), the patient is advanced to the use of crutches. Again, one should start and advance with the same sequence as was done with the use of parallel bars before beginning gait training on curbs and stairs.

Isometric contraction of the quadriceps muscle of the involved extremity against gravity through 10 repetitions is usually tolerated well. Formal isometric strengthening of the quadriceps muscle of the uninvolved side, however, also may be very beneficial for rapid development of a safe gait, especially in relation to curbs and stairs.

Restriction of hip flexion initially to 90 degrees requires the patient to learn to use assistive devices for dressing below the waist (socks, undergarments, and shoes) (Fig. 43–3).

Written home instructions concern the restrictions of weight-bearing and a maximum of 90 degrees of hip flexion (usually during the first three months), as related to the usual activities of daily living and of self-care. A program of range-of-motion exercises is generally not necessary, since pre-existing hip flexion contractures are usually released surgically and hip flexion increases with sitting. Written home instructions and isometric strengthening of quadriceps may be indicat-

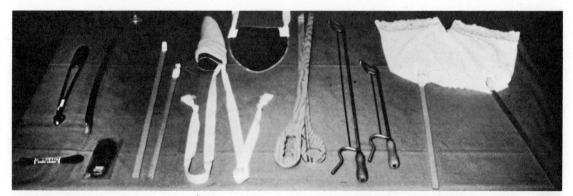

FIGURE 43–3. Assistive devices initially used by patients after total hip replacement. (From Opitz, J. L.: Total joint arthroplasty: Principles and guidelines for postoperative physiatric management. Mayo Clin. Proc., 54:602–612, 1979. By permission.)

ed. The patient is usually ready for dismissal within two weeks after surgery.

During recheck visits, deficits of function are identified and are treated on an individual basis with physical therapy. Transition from crutches to canes occurs usually at 4 to 12 weeks after operation. In order to have adequate support during stance phase on the involved side with the use of a cane, the quadriceps muscle of the involved side should have an isometric 10 RM of at least 8 kg (approximately 18 lb).

Total Knee Arthroplasty. Severe progressive gonalgia with increasing instability and increasing deformity in primary or secondary degenerative joint disease and in destructive rheumatoid arthritis are the usual indications for total knee arthroplasty. En bloc resections of low-grade neoplasms of the distal femur or proximal tibia may be replaced with fully constrained prostheses when previously above-the-knee amputations had to be done. Total knee prostheses are available with minimal constraint (polycentric and similar modular designs), partial constraint (geometric, anametric, total condylar, UCI, and many others), and full constraint (the Guepar, Tavernetti, spherocentric, and others) (Figs. 43–4 to 43–6). With the present designs of minimal or moderate constraint, one can expect freedom from pain, normal stability, and satisfaction in 85 per

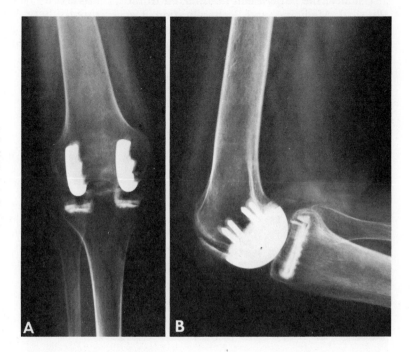

FIGURE 43–4. Polycentric knee arthroplasty. *A,* Anteroposterior view showing four-component nature of prosthesis. *B,* Lateral view. (From Peterson, L. F. A., Fitzgerald, R. H., Jr., and Johnson, E. W., Jr.: Total joint arthroplasty: The knee. Mayo Clin. Proc., 54:564–569, 1979. By permission.)

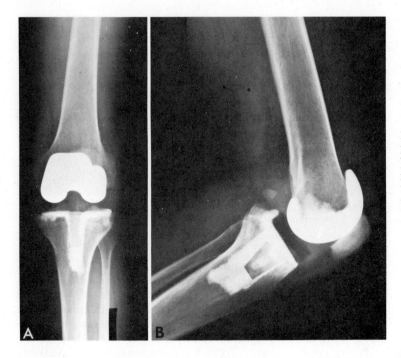

FIGURE 43–5. Total condylar prosthesis. A, Anteroposterior view. B, Lateral view. (From Peterson, L. F. A., Fitzgerald, R. H., Jr., and Johnson, E. W., Jr.: Total joint arthroplasty: The knee. Mayo Clin. Proc., 54:564–569, 1979. By permission.)

cent of patients. The five-year rate of loosening is approximately 6 per cent with a prosthesis of minimal constraint,[22] and the two-year rate is 11 per cent with a prosthesis of moderate constraint. With designs of full constraint, satisfactory results were achieved in 80 per cent of patients, with a higher revision rate of 20 per cent, mostly because of loosening and fracture of the prosthesis.

Usually, the patient can be referred to the Physical Medicine and Rehabilitation Department between the third and the fifth postoperative day. Initial therapeutic exer-

cises consist of neuromuscular re-education to gentle, active-assisted range-of-motion exercises. There is a substantial advantage if range-of-motion exercises can be begun from a fully extended knee position if the knee has been immobilized postoperatively in full extension. Difficulties in achieving full active extension of the knee are common in patients in whom the knee was immobilized postoperatively in flexion. Adhesions, which form rapidly between the quadriceps mechanism and the surrounding tissues, are likely the cause of the difficulties. These adhesions can

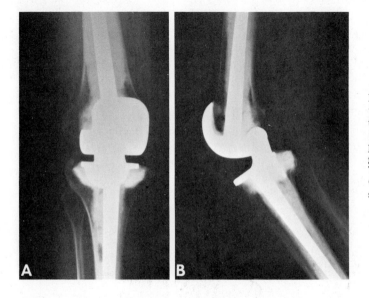

FIGURE 43–6. Guepar total knee prosthesis of hinge variety. A, Anteroposterior view. B, Lateral view showing patella resting on anterior flange of prosthesis. (From Peterson, L. F. A., Fitzgerald, R. H., Jr., and Johnson, E. W., Jr.: Total joint arthroplasty: The knee. Mayo Clin. Proc., 54:564–569, 1979. By permission.)

be stretched, reduced, and eliminated much more easily by the weight of the leg during assisted flexion from full extension than by the proximal pull of the quadriceps muscle alone in a proximal direction if the knee had been kept previously in flexion. Under such circumstances, adhesions of the quadriceps mechanism, which formed with the knee in flexion, often effectively block the transmission of quadriceps power for full knee extension to the patellar tendon and tibia. For this reason, postoperative immobilization of the knee in extension is strongly advised.

Gentle, pain-free, prolonged stretching (10 to 20 minutes four times per day) to increase knee flexion or extension usually may be started after the second postoperative week if progress is inadequate with range-of-motion exercises. The force of stretching must, of necessity, be very mild. For increase of knee flexion, in an antigravity position, part of the weight of the leg is borne by the therapist. For increase of knee extension, part of the weight of the lower extremity is supported by the plinth, bed, or chair with the patient in a semi-sitting position.

The principles for gait training are the same as those outlined for total hip arthroplasty. Usually, they involve the "touch only" category. Redevelopment of adequate knee flexion and ankle dorsiflexion during the swing phase, along with adequate knee extension during the stance phase, is emphasized.

At times, mild isometric quadriceps strengthening can be started toward the end of the second postoperative week, when satisfactory range of motion has been developed and gait training on the level is essentially complete. Isometric strengthening should not be painful and should not increase joint stiffness or swelling or cause joint effusion. Also, the opposite quadriceps muscle is strengthened if desirable.

Patients are usually ready for dismissal within three weeks after operation. The written home program consists of active assisted range-of-motion exercises and mild isometric quadriceps strengthening (10 repetitions per day), with weekly increases in resistance that are comfortably tolerated without producing evidence of joint irritation.

During recheck visits, transition from crutches to a cane is done when adequate healing of bone and soft tissues has progressed and antigravity quadriceps strength

has progressed to at least 8 kg (approximately 18 lb).

Total Ankle Arthroplasty. Total ankle arthroplasty is currently available as a totally constrained metalloplastic prosthesis.[22] The procedure is indicated in patients with destructive rheumatoid arthritis and post-traumatic degenerative joint disease who are more than 60 years old and is contraindicated in patients less than 60 years of age who have post-traumatic degenerative joint disease or failed arthrodeses. Satisfactory results currently can be anticipated in approximately 70 per cent of patients.

Therapeutic exercises are started when swelling and postoperative discomfort have sufficiently subsided. At that time, active, gentle, assisted range-of-motion exercise for flexion and extension and for pronation and supination of the foot can be given twice daily.

Gait training is also started in essentially the same fashion as described for total hip arthroplasty ("touch only"), with special emphasis on adequate dorsiflexion of the ankle during the swing phase.

Because the patient favors the involved lower extremity for a while, isometric quadriceps strengthening (10 repetitions only) is regularly done on the involved side and is continued at home, as are the active, gentle, assisted range-of-motion exercises. Progression from crutches to a single cane is usually achieved after three months, when the bony and periarticular structures of the ankle have healed adequately, the gait pattern is acceptable, and quadriceps strength is satisfactory.

Upper Extremities

Total Shoulder Arthroplasty. Because total shoulder arthroplasty is still in the developmental stage, it should be used only when a fusion of the glenohumeral joint is indicated for pain and lack of function in primary or secondary degenerative joint disease, rheumatoid arthritis, avascular necrosis, and similar conditions of the shoulder. Special long-stem prostheses are available to replace large humeral bone defects after en bloc tumor resection.[21] Generally, pain relief, shoulder function, and cosmesis are better with total shoulder arthroplasty than with shoulder arthrodesis. The incidences of loosening of the glenoid component and of limited range of motion are higher with fully constrained and semiconstrained total shoulder prostheses than with nonconstrained, resurfacing prostheses. Because the latter procedure relies on the stability of the repaired rotator cuff, particular care should be taken during the postoperative management. Heavy use of the upper extremity should be permanently avoided. With the resurfacing total shoulder arthroplasty (Fig. 43–7), satisfactory relief of pain can be anticipated in approximately 90 per cent of patients. Also, in 90 per cent of patients, active range of motion can be anticipated to degrees that permit the usual activities of daily living and light work.[21] Contraindications to total shoulder arthroplasty are related to paralysis, recent septic arthritis, poor bone or soft-tissue structures, and other substantial physiologic or psychologic inadequacies.

Referrals for gentle mobilization occur at about the fourth postoperative day. During the initial two weeks after the arthroplasty, the upper extremity is held in a neutral position in a shoulder immobilizer along the thorax, with the elbow in flexion, except during the therapeutic exercises, which are done twice daily. The therapeutic exercise program consists of gentle, passive, relaxed range-of-motion exercises in the supine position with the avoidance of pain as well as of neuromuscular re-education of the shoulder groups for active, gentle, assisted range-of-motion exercises. Combinations of external rotation, abduction, and extension are carefully avoided because of the anterior surgical approach to the joint.

During the first two weeks, all shoulder exercises are done in the supine position for better relaxation of the shoulder girdle musculature during exercises. Active range-of-motion exercises are also done for the elbow, wrist, and hand.

During the second week, sitting posture is practiced in order to achieve a balanced position of the head in relation to the upper part of the back. Once the head no longer represents overhanging weight, the nuchal muscles and the trapezius muscles are likely to relax spontaneously. As the trapezius muscles relax, the pectoral muscles also tend to relax spontaneously. Postural relaxation

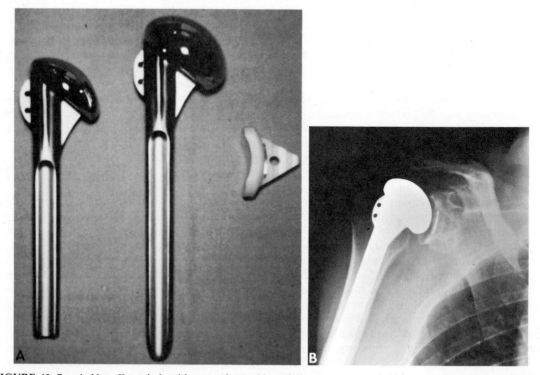

FIGURE 43–7. *A,* Neer II total shoulder prosthesis. Note different sizes available of humeral head, also polyethylene glenoid component viewed from its side. Triangular "keel" is placed within neck of scapula. *B,* Total shoulder arthroplasty with a Neer II prosthesis. (From Cofield, R. H.: Total joint arthroplasty: The shoulder. Mayo Clin. Proc., 54:500–506, 1979. By permission.)

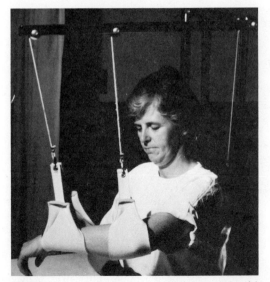

FIGURE 43–8. Deltoid aid as used after total shoulder replacement. (From Opitz, J. L.: Total joint arthroplasty: Principles and guidelines for postoperative physiatric management. Mayo Clin. Proc., 54:602–612, 1979. By permission.)

of the shoulder girdle musculature is desirable during the postoperative phase, especially when, during the third postoperative week, the supine shoulder exercises are also done in the sitting position (with assistance given by the therapist). During the third postoperative week, light functional hand activities (such as light assembly work, knotting, mosaic work, puzzles, and the like) are started in occupational therapy, with the upper extremity supported in a deltoid aid (Fig. 43–8). Throughout the postoperative period, passive, relaxed ranging, however, is continued; ranging is done twice daily with the elbow flexed and the patient in the supine position.

The patient is usually dismissed toward the end of the third week. The home exercise program consists of the aforementioned passive, relaxed (supine), active-assisted (supine and sitting) range-of-motion exercises. The patient continues to practice a balanced sitting posture and light functional activities of the upper extremity. Frequent rest periods are advisable (semi-sitting or supine).

During recheck visits, the exercise program is updated in terms of emphasizing advancement of certain ranges that are particularly needed and shoulder girdle relaxation. Gentle, comfortable, prolonged stretching in gravity-eliminated positions (supine and side-lying) is added to range-of-motion exercises, if necessary. If tolerated without discomfort, pain-free isometric contractions (10 repetitions) of the shoulder abductors, adductors, external rotators, and internal rotators, with the shoulder in neutral position, may be started. In occupational therapy, the patient advances to light self-care, dressing, and household activities when these activities can be performed free of substitution patterns (free of discomfort) without the use of much force.

During additional recheck visits, the exercises may be further modified for needed increases of range of motion and for some further increase in strength. Careful emphasis is placed on relaxation, freedom from substitution patterns, freedom from pain, and increase in range of motion. Initial strengthening can be done isometrically against absolute resistance with the shoulder in an adducted and otherwise neutral position.

Patients with substantial repairs of the rotator cuffs, especially when fascial grafts are needed, may require that the upper extremity be kept in an airplane splint for four to six weeks. During this period, only passive, relaxed (supine) range-of-motion exercises are done "above the splint level." The mobility of the distal joints is also maintained while the extremity is resting on the splint. Sitting posture for enhancement of nuchal and shoulder girdle release is especially important in these patients. Gradual mobilization of the shoulder after removal of the splint follows the guidelines previously described.

Total Elbow Arthroplasty. The usual indications for total elbow arthroplasty are severe pain and permanent limitation of essential function that are not amenable to synovectomy and resection of the radial head in rheumatoid arthritis or to nonresection arthroplasty in degenerative arthritis. Constrained and semiconstrained prostheses, usually interfacing polyethylene with stainless steel, are available. Because these prostheses are associated with a relatively high incidence of loosening, newer prostheses have lesser constraint and are essentially resurfacing arthroplasties. The minimal or nonconstrained prostheses are preferred when periarticular structures can be adequately repaired. When a nonconstrained prosthesis fails, usually there is the option of

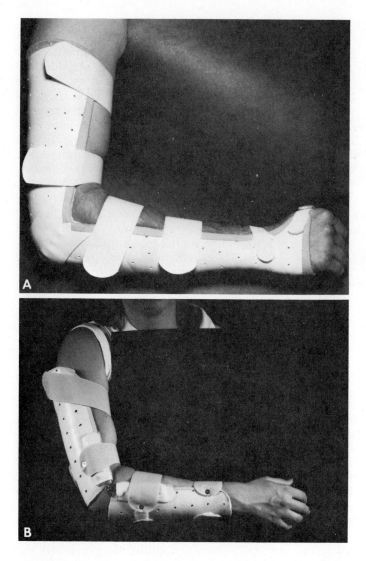

FIGURE 43–9. Static (*A*) and dynamic (*B*) splints used after total elbow replacement. (From Opitz, J. L.: Total joint arthroplasty: Principles and guidelines for postoperative physiatric management. Mayo Clin. Proc., 54:602–612, 1979. By permission.)

changeover to a resectional arthroplasty, which allows the elbow to remain fairly stable and with fairly satisfactory, pain-free flexion-extension ranges.

Postoperatively, once the swelling has definitely begun to subside, static and dynamic elbow splints are made in occupational therapy, usually between the fourth and the sixth postoperative days (Fig. 43–9). The dynamic splint has plastic hinge joints, which allow flexion and extension to occur in a fixed neutral plane. Usually during the next day, neuromuscular re-education for active, gentle, assisted elbow flexion and extension (pronation and supination if the prosthesis allows) is started. Range-of-motion exercises are done with gravity eliminated by means of a raised powder-board. Active, gentle, assisted range-of-motion exercises are done to maintain shoulder mobility in the supine po-

sition. Active ranging is done also for wrist and hand at the same time.

Initially, active-assisted ranging of the elbow allows flexion only to about 60 degrees. The range of flexion thereafter is only slowly allowed to advance to 100 degrees in order to preserve the reattachment of the triceps muscle. No forcing, no stretching, no pain, and no resistance to the triceps muscles are permitted during the first two weeks (or longer).

During the third postoperative week, light activities of daily living and light diversional activities are practiced in occupational therapy free of substitution patterns.

If indicated, gentle, prolonged stretching utilizing only the weight of the upper extremity distal to the elbow and free of any pain may be started after the third week and may be included in the home exercise program, if tolerated without evidence of joint irritation.

The home exercise program consists of active, gentle, assisted range-of-motion exercises and gentle, prolonged stretching (15 to 20 minutes two to four times daily), if indicated. Formal strengthening usually is not emphasized at this point, but it may become part of the home program during later recheck visits.

Total Wrist Arthroplasty. Arthritic and post-traumatic conditions of both wrists may be amenable to total joint replacement to relieve pain, to salvage function, and to improve cosmesis. Total wrist arthroplasty can be done when other surgical procedures, such as synovectomy, soft-tissue repair, and other arthroplasties, are inadequate. Periarticular structures should be sufficiently strong or adequately repairable to assure stability and a balanced transmission of power across the replaced joint. Total wrist arthroplasty has come of age, mostly in its semiconstrained version (Volz) and in its nonconstrained version (Meuli), both of which interface polyethylene with metal components (Fig. 43–10). Relief of pain and improvement of range of motion usually are satisfactory.[1] Potential loosening of the components requires permanent restriction of forceful engagement of the upper extremity.

Postoperatively, the wrist is kept immobilized in slight extension and in neutral abduction for approximately 10 days. During this period, the extremity distal to the elbow is usually elevated.

Because re-establishment of tensile strength of periarticular connective tissue in a proper position is of utmost importance for proper functioning of the semiconstrained and the nonconstrained total wrist prostheses (Meuli, Volz), particular care and proper balancing of powers during surgery continue postoperatively during mobilization and functional training.

At approximately the tenth postoperative day, an isoprene (Orthoplast) resting splint with 20 to 40 degrees of wrist extension and with the thumb positioned in abduction is made. In addition, a dynamic Orthoplast wrist splint (Fig. 43–11) is made with a plastic hinge on each side. This splint permits only wrist flexion and extension to occur in a neutral abduction-adduction stance, so that the second and third metacarpals are aligned in the direction of the long axis of the radius.

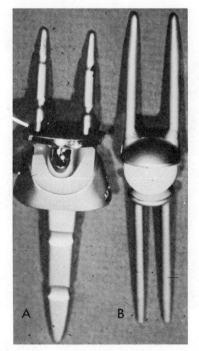

FIGURE 43–10. Total wrist prostheses. *A*, Volz (semiconstrained). *B*, Meuli (nonconstrained).

On the same day, active control of edema is started, with wrapping and rewrapping of the digits, the hand, and the wrist with soft rubber wrappings. Decongestive massage to the same area may be added (except for the incisional area) and continued until the postoperative edema has subsided. The hand, wrist, and forearm can be maintained in an elevated position during rest.

Therapeutic exercises are started on the same or the following day. They consist of neuromuscular re-education to redevelop active, gentle, assisted flexion and extension of the wrist with a dynamic splint in place. Active, gentle, assisted digital flexion, extension, intrinsic-minus and intrinsic-plus positions of the digits, and opposition of the thumb are also practiced free of substitution patterns. Active range-of-motion exercises are done for the elbow and the shoulder.

As soon as patterns of isolated hand movements and of isolated wrist flexion and extension are acceptable, the dynamic splint may be left off during some of the exercises. Neuromuscular re-education is then started in order to redevelop a balanced wrist function, including radial and ulnar abduction.

The next goal of therapeutic exercises is the redevelopment of properly coordinated digital flexion with wrist extension and of

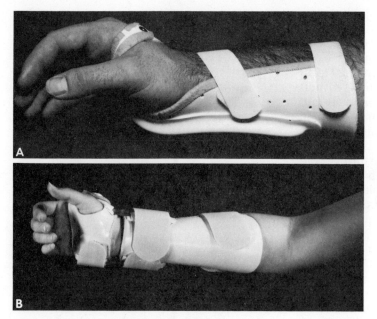

FIGURE 43–11. Static (*A*) and dynamic (*B*) splints used after total wrist replacement. (From Opitz, J. L.: Total joint arthroplasty: Principles and guidelines for postoperative physiatric management. Mayo Clin. Proc., 54:602–612, 1979. By permission.)

digital extension with wrist flexion in a proper wrist abduction-adduction stance. Lastly, isolated digital and thumb movements are practiced with the wrist in various positions of extension (and flexion) and ulnar (and radial) abduction.

Light functional hand activities are started (at first in the dynamic splint) as soon as synergistic hand-wrist movements, as well as the basic hand functions, are smooth in various wrist positions. The patient usually accomplishes this within the third postoperative week. The light functional hand and wrist activities consist of simple placement of objects, to light assembling (leather work, mosaics, puzzles), to simple painting, feeding, and simple knotting. Great care is taken to ensure that the light functional hand activities are free of substitutional patterns, such as undesirable associated elbow and shoulder motions, inappropriate wrist flexion with digital flexion, and inappropriate radial abduction instead of slight ulnar abduction stance of the wrist. When the patient is not in therapy, the dynamic wrist splint continues to be worn most of the time. The patient is dismissed when, under supervision, the exercises can be done securely and smoothly, without evidence of stress and increasing joint irritation. Written instructions are provided for the above-described coordinated wrist-hand exercises, range-of-motion exercises, and light functional hand activities.

At six weeks (if necessary), gentle, prolonged (15 to 20 minutes four times a day) stretching is taught during several sessions for increase of missing ranges, especially wrist extension and ulnar deviation. Rarely is it necessary to add an elastic extension assist to the dynamic wrist splint. If necessary, mild isometric strengthening of wrist extensors also can be added. Exercises for further advancement of proper combined wrist and hand motions, as well as of light-to-moderate activities of daily living (complete dressing, self-care, and kitchen, household, and diversional activities), are added progressively.

Total Metacarpophalangeal Joint Replacement. Total arthroplasty of metacarpophalangeal joints is useful in patients with destructive rheumatoid arthritis who have metacarpophalangeal subluxation, usually associated with ulnar drift. Total metacarpophalangeal arthroplasties can be done if the tendons can be repaired satisfactorily, skin and bone are adequate, the neurovascular status is satisfactory, and the patient is physiologically and psychologically stable. Usually, one can expect to obtain relief of pain, improvement of function,[18] and improvement of cosmesis. At the present time, pinch force and power grip are not improved over preoperative levels.[18] For metacarpophalangeal joint replacement, the most common prostheses are those made of silicone rubber (Swanson or Niebauer types) (Fig.

43–12). These prostheses act as joint spacers. Careful reconstruction of capsular and ligament structures about the metacarpophalangeal joint is very important. Like the Steffee prosthesis, other prostheses (Mayo, Shultz, Walker), using snap-fitted, semiconstrained metal-on-plastic components, are cemented with methylmethacrylate within the marrow cavities (Fig. 43–12).

After the acute postoperative tissue responses have subsided adequately with the hand kept elevated, static and dynamic Orthoplast splints are made (Fig. 43–13). The splints should fit comfortably and should be checked daily for proper fit. Adjustments are made as swelling decreases and range of motion increases. The resting splint needs to support the metacarpophalangeal joints in extension and in proper radioulnar alignment. Swan-neck deformity of the proximal interphalangeal joints is prevented by providing support for the proximal interphalangeal joints in moderate flexion or simply by supporting the proximal phalanx. Ulnar deviation is prevented, if necessary, by incorporating dividers at the proximal phalangeal level. The dynamic splint assists metacar-

pophalangeal extension by supporting function of the extensor digitorum communis with elastic slings across the proximal phalanges, and it allows the digits to track properly in a radioulnar alignment. The dynamic splint is worn for 6 to 12 weeks. The patient may remove the splint only for exercises, bathing activities, and during dressing, when the splint would be in the way. If needed for increase of the metacarpophalangeal range of flexion, an elastic flexion assist may be added during the third week or later (Fig. 43–13).

Antiedema measures are started promptly on referral as needed. These have already been described in the section on total wrist arthroplasty.

The initial therapeutic exercise program consists of neuromuscular re-education for active, gentle, assisted exercises, especially digital extension and flexion, of which digital extension has definite priority so that as much grasp opening as possible can be achieved. Grasp opening in the rheumatoid hand is usually substantially decreased because of the dislodgment of the metacarpophalangeal extensor hood mechanism and

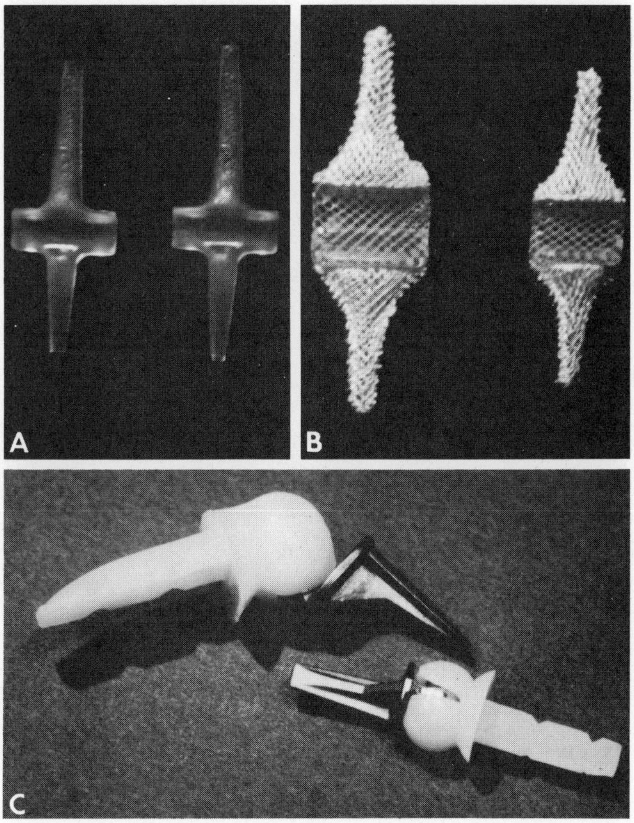

FIGURE 43–12. Total metacarpophalangeal joint prostheses. A, Swanson (silicon elastomer). B, Niebauer (silicon elastomer with Dacron). C, Steffee (metalloplastic). (A and B from Linscheid, R. L., and Dobyns, J. H.: Total joint arthroplasty: The hand. Mayo Clin. Proc., 54:516–526, 1979. By permission.)

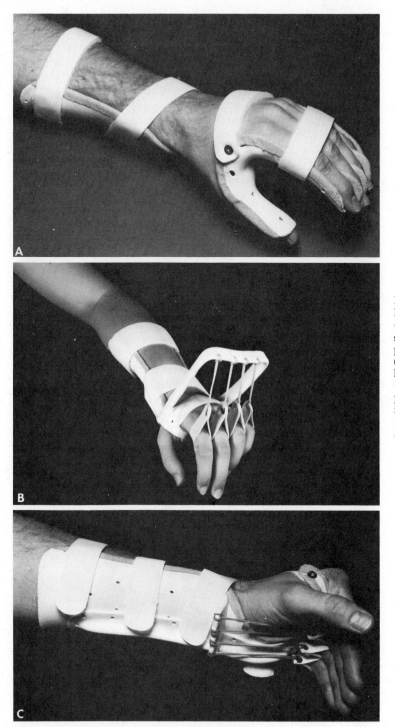

FIGURE 43–13. Static wrist and hand splint (*A*), dynamic metacarpophalangeal extension-assist splint (*B*), and dynamic metacarpophalangeal flexion-assist splint (*C*) used after total metacarpophalangeal joint replacement. (From Opitz, J. L.: Total joint arthroplasty: Principles and guidelines for postoperative physiatric management. Mayo Clin. Proc., 54:602–612, 1979. By permission.)

the adduction contracture of the thumb. Neuromuscular re-education is also concerned with the redevelopment of smooth execution of the intrinsic-plus and intrinsic-minus digital positions, of digital radial abduction, and of thumb opposition. All of these movements constitute the six classic digital exercises practiced routinely and are included in the home program for the subsequent 6 to 12 months.

A number of common substitution patterns are encountered by patients after meta-

TABLE 43–2. COMMON HAND AND FOREARM SUBSTITUTION PATTERNS AFTER TOTAL JOINT REPLACEMENT OF WRIST AND HAND

Task	Substitution by Use of
Digital flexion	Intrinsic muscles at metacarpophalangeal joint with interphalangeal joint in extension
Digital extension	Intrinsic muscles at interphalangeal joint with metacarpophalangeal joint in flexion
Thumb abduction	Ulnar digital intrinsic muscles for associated digital ulnar abduction
Thumb opposition	Thenar muscles for thumb adduction and flexion
Grasp opening	Wrist flexors for associated wrist flexion
Forearm supination	Associated shoulder external rotation and adduction
Forearm pronation	Associated shoulder internal rotation and abduction

From Opitz, J. L.: Total joint arthroplasty: Principles and guidelines for postoperative physiatric management. Mayo Clin. Proc., 54:602–612, 1979. By permission.

carpophalangeal replacement (Table 43–2). Substitution patterns indicate motor incoordination and should be avoided carefully in their early beginnings. Retraining uses the basic techniques of neuromuscular re-education. Once the exercises are progressing, basic grasp functions of the hand (tip or power prehension, lateral prehension or key grip, cylindrical grasp, and spherical grasp) are also practiced.

Active, gentle, assisted range-of-motion exercises are also given for the more proximal joints of the upper extremities, as indicated. Light functional hand activities are started as soon as the basic grasp functions of the hand are performed smoothly in slow but correct motion. The light functional hand activities have been described in the section on total wrist arthroplasty. Forceful use of the hand is carefully avoided in order to maintain the repaired periarticular structures in their optimal positions. Special instructions are given and practiced to protect the hands from unnecessary strain during common activities of dressing, self-care, kitchen and other housework, and avocational activities, in part by using different techniques and in part by using assistive devices. Printed home instructions for work simplification may be helpful.

Very gentle, prolonged stretching (20 minutes four times per day) may be added after three to six weeks if the redevelopment of range of motion is lacking. Pain should be carefully avoided. As mentioned, a digital flexion assist may be added to the dynamic hand splint and applied intermittently as long as they can be worn comfortably. Such a digital flexion assist either has rubber bands attached to little hooks that are glued to the

distal regions of the nails (if the interphalangeal, as well as the metacarpophalangeal, joints need stretching) or makes use of leather loops across the proximal phalanges to stretch the metacarpophalangeal joints gently toward increased flexion. Daily graphic representation of the still-missing active digital flexion and extension is useful. Thus, the developing ranges are easily followed on the graph by the patient, the therapist, and the physician. Any lack of progress or regression is quickly noticed, and appropriate corrective measures can be taken (see Fig. 43–1). The patient can be started on a home program of exercises, usually after the third postoperative week. The home program consists of active, gentle, assisted range-of-motion exercises, light functional hand activities, and work simplification to avoid overuse of the hand.

Rarely is it necessary in rheumatoid patients to increase the strength of the extensor digitorum communis and of the flexor digitorum profundus and superficialis with the use of progressive resistive exercises during later recheck visits.

TENDON TRANSFERS

General Considerations

Purposes. Tendon transfers can be most helpful for re-establishment of power in patients with isolated, nonprogressive deficits of the lower motor neuron (such as peripheral nerve injuries), tetraplegia in spinal cord injury, and post-traumatic reconstruction of the upper extremities. Especially in post-traumatic reconstruction, the use of tendon transfers has increased substantially during the past decade. However, the usefulness of tendon transfers in stable upper motor neuron deficits such as hemiplegia or cerebral palsy is not so common, is not easy to predict, and needs to be highly individualized.

Surgical Considerations. Since tendon transfers are usually the final step in reconstructive surgical efforts, other applicable procedures for correction of deformities (capsulotomies, osteotomies, tendon lengthening), for stabilization (arthrodeses, tenodeses, insertion of bone blocks), or for reconstruction of peripheral nerves (neurolysis, nerve reanastomosis, nerve transfer, nerve graft) usually should be done before or at least at the time of tendon transfer. Likewise, prior to tendon transfer, sufficient range of motion and maximal strength of muscles involved in tendon transfers, as well as maximal redevelopment of sensation to touch, pain, and kinesthesis, need to have been developed by appropriate nonsurgical and possibly surgical methods.

Transfer of spastic muscles is often contraindicated. If selected for transfer, they should function fully in phase with that of the lost voluntary motor power because of otherwise insurmountable difficulties later with neuromuscular re-education in the presence of spasticity.

Poor results in tendon transfers also can be expected if the patient is still bedridden, does not really want surgery, is mentally inactive, or has not yet adequately accepted his major physical disability for a lifetime.

As Moberg[16] has pointed out, sensory function in the area of the tendon transfer is very important. In the absence of other than ocular afference, only a single, simple transfer can be expected to develop satisfactory function. Further, no tendon transfer should impair any existing function. Moberg believes that a tendon transfer should be fully reversible if the result is unsatisfactory. Having received a tendon transfer, the patient should retain the option of returning to his preoperative condition.

Optimal team intercommunication before and after tendon transfers is important among the specialties involved, such as the primary service, Orthopedics, Physical Medicine and Rehabilitation, Neurology, and Neurosurgery. Such interrelationships usually take time to develop, but they are of utmost importance for optimal decision making, patient motivation, postoperative management, follow-up care, and the management of possible complications.

Decisions regarding tendon transfers in traumatic tetraplegia should be delayed at least for one year in order to have full return of function present, all spasticity apparent, and maximal strength developed in all muscles to be used in transfer. Patients should be sufficiently far along educationally, emotionally, sociovocationally, and physically in their readaptation to spinal cord injury. In peripheral trauma, similar considerations are often true, depending on extent and severity of injury and the resulting impairment.

Orientation of the patient prior to tendon transfers involves a realistic description of the limited goals of the procedure itself, time and cost involved, the necessary preoperative and postoperative efforts of the patient, and the number and duration of needed follow-up visits.

Preoperative Program. Ideally, the preoperative program concentrates on three basic issues: re-establishment of a full passive range of motion for the expected function of the transfer; maximal strengthening of the presumptive new muscle power; and initial training of conscious perception of kinesthetic sensations relating to neuromuscular re-education of the transfer.

Preoperative mobilization re-establishes the passive motion of the expected function. Shortened connective tissue about the joint capsule, intra-articular connective tissue, and adhesions about tendons and muscle bellies usually can resist even strong stretching forces of short duration. Therefore, stretching needs to be done gently over prolonged periods (20 to 30 minutes four times per day). Within limits, connective tissue usually can elongate without trauma during gentle prolonged stretching. If needed, serial, static splinting or casting or prolonged, gentle pull of rubber bands may, in time, assist in providing adequate passive range of motion. If not, combined ultrasound heating with stretching of the area[11] is likely to give further increase in range of motion.

Graphic recording of daily measurements of range of motion is helpful in motivating patients to continue their stretching exercises for weeks as well for one's quick orientation regarding progress of range of motion (see Fig. 43–1).

With early and persistent use of such range-of-motion exercises, surgical release procedures often can be limited substantially, or even avoided, thus lessening trauma and increasing chances of successful tendon transfers.

Before transfer, the muscle to be transferred should be as strong as possible. Once the muscle is transferred, its effective strength usually decreases by one grade owing to the change in routing of its tendon. During the postoperative period of complete immobilization (usually three weeks), the strength of the transferred muscle decreases exponentially to approximately half of its preoperative strength. Adhesions form between the tendon at the site of its anastomosis and wherever vascular injury to tendon or muscle occurred, causing segmental necrosis. While assistive power can mobilize such adhesions of the tendon in a distal direction, the proximal mobilization of the tendon can be done only by the power of the transferred muscle itself. For such reasons, maximal preoperative strengthening is highly desirable. Maximal restrengthening of muscles to be used in second-stage transfers is also essential.

Kinesthetic sensory training can be started preoperatively in preparation for neuromuscular re-education of the transferred muscle. Conscious perception of related joint movement, joint position, related muscle contraction and relaxation (with augmented sensory feedback through the palpating free hand of the patient), force of muscle contraction, and conscious perception of tendon tapping and stroking of the skin overlying the muscle to be transferred can be practiced preoperatively in order to increase kinesthetic awareness of the patient.

In the selection of a suitable muscle for transfer, if at all possible, a synergistic muscle should be chosen, especially in patients with upper motor neuron deficit and with transfers in the lower extremity. During transfer, the routing of the tendon should be done with the least possible disturbance of its mesotenons, as noted, in order to avoid segmental tendon necrosis with the associated formation of adhesions and possible stretching of the necrotic tendon segment during mobilization.

Routing of the transferred tendon should be as straight and as superficial as possible, since adhesions tend to be more extensive and firmer at tendon angulations and in deeper tissues.

Tendon anastomosis should be done with nonconstrictive suturing and with the least irritating suture possible in order to lessen adhesions at that site.[8]

Strength and amplitude of the muscle to be transferred should be equal to or, if possible, larger than that of the original muscle.

Immobilization after tendon transfer should be kept at a safe minimum so that the adhesions that form regularly about the transferred tendon are capable of elongation with gentle range-of-motion exercises. Thus, they can, in a nontraumatic fashion, mature to become mesotenons of adequate length and provide adequate blood supply to the transferred tendon.[8]

Early prolonged tension of the transferred tendon should be avoided in order to prevent gap formation at the site of tendon anastomosis, which predisposes the anastomosis to rupture during remobilization. Gap formation also increases the formation of adhesions.[9] During postoperative immobilization, the extremity should be positioned in such a way that the transferred muscle is at its shortest resting length. In this way, adhesions about the transferred tendon can be mobilized with controlled external pull, moving the tendon distally, rather than by the uncontrolled pull of the weakened transferred muscle in a proximal direction.

Postoperative Management. This usually consists of the following components: antiedema measures; gentle, prolonged passive ranging; neuromuscular re-education of basic movements; gentle, active (assistive) ranging; redevelopment of proper use of the transferred muscle in light functional activities; and redevelopment of accuracy and speed (coordination).

The postoperative antiedema measures are the same as those used after total wrist or metacarpophalangeal joint replacement. If hydrotherapy is being used for cleansing and relaxation purposes, one should carefully avoid increases in edema during immersion by keeping the duration of hydrotherapy relatively short (10 to 15 minutes) and the water temperature relatively low initially (35° C or less).

As mentioned previously, gentle, well-controlled, small, passive movements can be used to cause progressive elongation of adhesions around the tendon without rupturing. In this fashion, new mesotenons of adequate length are being formed at a time when the new fibrovascular tissue is still immature, without embarrassing the tendon anastomosis. This may be started as early as three or four days to one week after operation.[13] Such gentle passive motions may be done four times a day, without pain, through a very small range that is being increased in very small increments during the subsequent two weeks. As mentioned previously, gentle, early passive motion has the most advantage, if the limb is immobilized postoperatively in a position with the transferred muscle at its shortest resting length.

Three weeks after operation, neuromuscular re-education of the transferred muscle is started. Passive range of motion of approximately 30 degrees (as needed for neuromuscular re-education) has been developed by then. During neuromuscular re-education of the transferred muscle, one should never ask the patient primarily for the performance of the motion for which the tendon transfer has been done. Rather, the patient should be asked to produce that motion for which the transferred muscle was originally responsible. The original motion then is being blocked manually by the therapist, so that the transferred tendon can now execute the new motion. In this fashion, the patient will be able to perceive the new set of kinesthetic sensations: the feeling of muscle contraction, the tendon tension of the transferred muscle, and the sensation of the new motion affected. This new set of combined kinesthetic input, when consciously perceived, recalled, and reproduced by the patient through many correct repetitions, forms the new engram and the intended new motor skill. The old engram then is being progressively forgotten and left with the function of previously synergistic muscles of the transfer.

As soon as the new, basic movements can be executed deliberately in clear and acceptable patterns actively (usually in physical therapy), functional training with light functional activities is started (usually in occupational therapy). Six weeks after operation, the resistance demanded during functional activities can be increased to moderate levels, if they can be performed without pain or fatigue. Performance should always be kept fully acceptable and at its peak, because negative training with deterioration of the new engrams or motor patterns is likely to

occur if functional training is done until the patient is fatigued (with decreasing accuracy and speed).

After successful neuromuscular re-education, increases in range of motion may be accomplished by active, gentle, assistive range-of-motion exercises between three and six weeks after operation. After six weeks, gentle prolonged (10 to 20 minutes four times per day) stretching exercises may be added to the daily program. As mentioned before, daily graphing of active ranges is particularly helpful for the maintenance of motivation of the patient and for the quick orientation regarding success (see Fig. 43–1). Ultrasound heating in combination with stretching may be used when increases in range of motion have leveled off.[11] If needed, operative tenolysis rarely is indicated before completion of tendon healing, at approximately six months.

Strengthening of the transferred muscle best occurs with its use in functional activities after two weeks. Single transfers may be strengthened formally with progressive resistive exercises. However, the associated overflow of motor activities, which is likely to occur with maximal or near-maximal efforts, may weaken or destroy the engrams, especially when done with multiple tendon transfers or single transfers that either are spastic or are transferred out of phase. Usually, formal strengthening exercises are neither needed nor advisable.

Upper Extremities

In patients with deltoid paralysis, numerous attempts at transfer of biceps, triceps, trapezius, and other muscles have been made, yet when such transfers are accomplished, not the desired substitution of deltoid function but rather effects of tenodesis may be noted around the glenohumeral joint.

Arthrodesis of the shoulder in painful, flail shoulders with presence of major portions of the scapular rotators still is likely to be the best reconstructive choice. In medial winging of the scapula due to serratus anterior paralysis, the pectoralis minor muscle, lengthened by a fascial graft, may decrease winging and stabilize the scapula when transferred to its inferior angle. When lateral winging of the scapula is caused by trapezius paralysis, levator scapulae may be transferred to a more lateral position on the scapula in association with fascial fixation of the vertebral border of the scapula to the thorax.

Biceps Paralysis. Missing biceps function often can be replaced in part by proximal advancement (by 3 to 4 cm) of the common origin of flexor carpi radialis, flexor carpi ulnaris, and palmaris longus (Steindler), if these muscles are strong. Since these muscles normally cross the elbow, proximal transfer of the origin further lengthens the lever arm for elbow flexion. The muscles, however, should be opposed by strong wrist and digital extensors at the wrist.

Commonly used tendon transfers in peripheral nerve injuries have been well described.[14]

Radial Nerve Paralysis. Radial nerve paralysis results in the absence of extension of the wrist, thumb, and proximal finger joints and the loss of brachioradialis and thumb abductor muscles. Suggested transfers are pronator teres to extensor carpi radialis longus and brevis; flexor carpi ulnaris or flexor digitorum superficialis to extensor digitorum communis; and palmaris longus to translocated extensor pollicis longus.

Ulnar Nerve Paralysis. Such paralysis may result in absent or inadequate lateral stability of the index finger (first dorsal interosseus muscle). Lateral stability of the index finger is essential for tip and lateral prehension between the thumb and the index finger. To substitute for a paralyzed first dorsal interosseus muscle, the tendon of the extensor indices proprius or the tendon of the extensor pollicis brevis may be transferred to the tendon of the first dorsal interosseus. Paralysis of the fourth and fifth digits may not require any transfer of tendons.

Median Nerve Paralysis. Such paralysis results in loss of sensation of the medial surface of the palm. Every attempt should be made to restore sensation. In low median nerve paralysis, the motor loss of consequence may be opposition of the thumb. The pronator teres or adductor pollicis muscle may be used in transfer for opposition of the thumb. High median nerve paralysis results in loss of finger flexion of the first, second, and third digits (flexor pollicis longus, flexor digitorum superficialis, and the radial half of flexor digitorum profundus) and loss in opposition of the thumb (opponens pollicis, flexor

pollicis brevis, abductor pollicis brevis, and flexor pollicis longus). Possible tendon transfers in high median nerve paralysis may be as follows: the ulnar half of the flexor digitorum profundus muscle or the brachioradialis to the flexor tendons of the second and third digits, the extensor carpi radialis longus to the flexor pollicis longus and to the opponens pollicis. Arthrodesis of the metacarpophalangeal joint of the thumb may be necessary. Other combinations of tendon transfers are possible.

Forearm and Hand Trauma. Repair of a deep cut or replacement of a crushed tendon in the forearm and hand is a challenging problem. There is a rapidly increasing understanding of the anatomy of vascular supply to tendons, pulley systems, maintenance and replacement of peritendinous structures, tendon grafting, and principles of early mobilization.[13] The postoperative management follows principles similar to those described under tendon transfers in the upper extremity.

Spinal Cord Injury

In spinal cord injury that spares C5 and C6, active elbow extension can be restored to moderate antigravity levels using the mobilized posterior deltoid muscle in transfer to the olecranon, with interposition of a tendon graft from toe extensors.[15] Elbow extension is essential for independence in reaching above the level of the shoulder, driving, and when further power is needed in transfers. During the postoperative mobilization of elbow flexion and re-education of the posterior deltoid for triceps muscle function, one needs to progress extremely slowly to avoid stretching of the tendon graft. If the graft elongates, it compromises the limited contractile amplitude of the deltoid muscle for elbow extension. Various static and dynamic elbow splints are used to allow increments of only 10 degrees of elbow flexion per week from a fully extended position after initial immobilization of six weeks, until tendon healing is complete after six months.

In spinal cord injury that spares C5 in which only a fairly strong brachioradialis muscle is available in the forearm, wrist extension and key grip (lateral prehension) can be restored through transfer of brachioradialis to extensor carpi radialis brevis, tenodesis of flexor pollicis longus at the distal radius with resection of the annular ligament, allowing the tenodesed tendon to bowstring, and through arthrodesis of the interphalangeal joint of the thumb.[15] Sensory function at this level of deficit is often preserved in the thumb. This procedure allows for moderate grip opening of lateral prehension during passive wrist flexion and fairly adequate key grip prehension during active wrist extension in persons that otherwise would have no hand or wrist function. The postoperative re-education of the brachioradialis to wrist extension is not difficult. Fine tuning of tension of the thumb flexor tenodesis may require a simple reoperation.

In spinal cord injuries that spare C6, strong extensor carpi radialis longus and brevis, pronator teres, and brachioradialis functions may be preserved. It may be possible to restore digital extension, digital flexion, and lateral prehension of the thumb through transfer of extensor carpi radialis longus to extensor digitorum communis and extensor pollicis longus (first stage) and through transfer of pronator teres to flexor digitorum profundus and of brachioradialis to flexor pollicis longus (second stage).[12] Sufficient time should elapse between the two stages in order to allow for neuromuscular re-education of extensor carpi radialis longus to extensor digitorum communis and extensor pollicis longus function, restrengthening of pronator teres and brachioradialis, and remobilization of the wrist and hand with careful preservation of flexion contracture at the metacarpophalangeal joints of the digits.

Other tendon transfers in the tetraplegic patient are possible and have been proposed.[3, 10, 23] All tendon transfers into the tetraplegic hand may be doomed to failure unless, by some means, clawing of the hand as a result of intrinsic muscle paralysis is prevented. The prevention of the claw-hand deformity should be started at the onset of tetraplegia through deliberate development of a metacarpophalangeal joint flexion contracture. Such a flexion contracture may develop with the use of static forearm- and hand-based splints. Later, the hands should be used as fists during mat activities and transfers. It may be necessary to wear a hand-based splint during such activities in order to elevate the rest of the hand 2 to 3 cm from the supporting surface so that the metacarpophalangeal and interphalangeal joints

may remain in flexion. In patients with an inadequate metacarpophalangeal flexion stance in the tetraplegic hand, metacarpophalangeal flexor tightness can be regained by long flexor tenodesis or by volar metacarpophalangeal capsulorrhaphy (Zancolli) or by both. However, both procedures will stretch out again, provided the hand is not protected from overstretching the achieved metacarpophalangeal flexion contractures, especially during independent transfer activities.

Lower Extremities

Hip Group Paralysis. In hip abductor paralysis, two tendon transfer procedures are available. Tensor fasciae latae may be freed up, together with a strip of fascia lata. The strip of fascia lata is then attached to the greater trochanter, is continued posteriorly, and is anastomosed to the lateral two thirds of the mobilized erector spinae muscles. The erector spinae muscles can be placed in such a position as to act more as an extensor or more as an abductor of the hip. Usually the effect of this transfer is predominantly that of a tenodesis, providing increased stability during stance phase. Only in partial paralysis of gluteus medius can one expect to abolish the typical abductor lurch by transfer of tensor fasciae latae.

In 1952, Mustard[17] described the transfer of the iliopsoas muscle through a large window in the iliac wing to the greater trochanter for the same purpose. Adequate function of the sartorius and rectus femoris, however, is essential to provide adequate hip flexion.

Quadriceps Paralysis. In isolated quadriceps paralysis, the transfer of the biceps femoris and of one of the medial hamstring muscles into the quadriceps tendon gives power for climbing stairs, getting in and out of chairs, and walking up and down hills. Care should be taken to avoid this transfer in patients with weakness of the posterior thigh and leg muscles because further weakening of these groups by the described transfer will result in genu recurvatum and its associated gait disturbance.

Cerebral Palsy

Tendon transfers in cerebral palsy[6] and hemiplegia are often unpredictable in their final outcome because movement patterns rather than individual muscle functions are represented in the brain and are changed. Oftentimes the immediate results appear to be satisfactory, only to change progressively back to a similar abnormal postural stance. Severe spasticity, athetosis, mental retardation, and ataxia are usually regarded as contraindications for tendon transfers.

The pronation deformity of the upper extremity in hemiplegia may be improved by transfer of the flexor carpi ulnaris across the dorsal aspect of the forearm to the extensor carpi radialis longus with release of the pronator teres.[20] Knee flexion deformity may be improved by transferring the hamstring insertions proximally to the femoral condyles.[5] In rotational deformities of the thigh in patients with cerebral palsy, derotational femoral osteotomy again brings the long axis of the foot parallel to the line of progression. A similar procedure can be done at the tibia, if indicated. Both procedures can be very helpful adjuncts in the corrective treatment of cerebral palsy. Rebalancing of the spastic ankle and foot deformities by transferring tendons needs to be considered individually. Oftentimes, it requires combinations with bone stabilization procedures, tendon lengthening, tenotomy, or neurectomy.[19] Spastic equinovarus deformity due to overactive gastrocnemius-soleus muscles often can be improved by sectioning of the gastrocnemius origin, with subsequent reattachment of the gastrocnemius in a shortened length distally. Often, it is advisable to weaken the gastrocnemius muscle at the same time, with selective sectioning of parts of its motor nerves in the popliteal fossa. If a contracture of the soleus or both the soleus and gastrocnemius muscles is present, the preferred operation is the Z-plasty of the Achilles tendon. Judicious, regular stretching of the posterior calf muscles remains essential for maintenance of the achieved dorsiflexion range at the ankle.

OTHER RECONSTRUCTIVE PROCEDURES

Shoulder

Arthrodesis of the shoulder may be done unilaterally in severe degenerative joint disease provided that scapular rotator muscles of the shoulder are normal and the other shoulder is essentially unimpaired. Arthrodesis of the shoulder is not advisable in women because of its anticosmetic effects and should not be done in persons whose occupation requires humeral rotation of that side. Total shoulder replacement is becoming a viable alternative.

Recurring dislocation of the shoulder oftentimes happens in a downward and anterior direction. The Bankart operation is repairing the anteroinferior portion of the capsule, especially when it is often torn away from the glenoid rim. The Putti-Platt operation, in addition, reinforces the tendon of the subscapularis muscle in order to prevent the forward and downward dislocation of the humeral head. Postoperatively, until tendon healing is complete, shoulder mobilization should avoid stretching of the repaired structures in abduction or external rotation (or both). General principles of mobilization are the same as those in total shoulder arthroplasty.

Wrist and Hand

In unilateral, severe, painful, posttraumatic degenerative arthritis of the wrist, arthrodesis may still be a good choice, since it provides pain-free stability, especially when forceful use of the upper extremity is required.

Boutonnière, swan-neck, and other rheumatoid hand deformities of digits and thumb may be amenable to highly skillful tissue reconstruction procedures (especially when done early), in addition to total joint replacement or arthrodesis (or both) of digital joints or thumb joints.[4]

Dupuytren's contracture of the palmar fascia, oftentimes involving the flexor tendon sheaths, may be excised. Early postoperative mobilization, including gentle prolonged stretching for digital extension, is essential for optimal outcomes of the procedure. The digital extension ranges, however, need to be maintained indefinitely, if possible, by a reasonable stretching routine.[7]

Hip and Thigh

Spasticity of the hip adductor muscles may result in impairment of gait due to scissoring of the lower extremities. When scissoring is excessive, it may impair the accessibility of the perineum. Adductor tenotomy or obturator neurectomy (or both) may relieve the hip adductor contractures. Postoperative stretching is essential for the maintenance of gains made in range of motion.

Decreased leg length may occur, with predominantly unilateral impairment of a lower extremity in the growing child. The most commonly used corrective measure is designed to slow down the growth of the uninvolved lower extremity. The procedure should be done some years before the growth centers are closed, usually between the ages of 10 and 12 years. Steel staples are placed in the epiphysis of the lower portion of the femur or upper part of the tibia. They may be removed at any time as required. The operation is usually considered if the leg length discrepancy is in excess of 2.5 cm. If growth is complete, excision of a segment of the femur may be done to accomplish equal leg length.

Knee

Ligaments, menisci, and articular surfaces of the knee are often subject to injury. Repair of these structures is done frequently in common surgical procedures of the knee, such as removal of a torn medial or lateral meniscus, internal fixation of fractured bone segments involving the joint surfaces, or repair of torn cruciate or collateral ligaments. Torn major ligaments of the knee may be successfully repaired if operated on soon after the injury occurred. Later repairs often are not successful in restoring good stability of the knee. Remobilization after adequate healing of repaired tendons should be done initially strictly in planes of motion that do not injure the repaired structures yet provide slowly increasing flexion range of the knee that had been immobilized in an extended position. Mobilization of a knee that had been immobilized in a semi-flexed or flexed position may be difficult because of adhesions of the quadriceps mechanism, which a deconditioned, weak quadriceps muscle cannot mobilize proximally. In such a case, passive extension of the knee may be regained relatively easily, yet active extension is not forthcoming adequately. Eventually, tenolysis of the quadriceps mechanism may be required.

Operations to restore reasonable function in knees damaged by degenerative joint disease or rheumatoid arthritis, yet not requiring total joint replacement, include debridement of hypertrophic joint ridges, synovectomy, and osteotomy. The principles of postoperative remobilization and of quadriceps and hamstring strengthening are, in general, the same as those described for total knee arthroplasties.

Ankle and Foot

Several arthrodeses are available to prevent footdrop or to prevent and correct deformities of the foot (or both). Usually, the arthrodeses are delayed until the growth centers are closed. Among the most common procedures is the triple arthrodesis. It is a classic operation in which the three major joints of the posterior part of the foot (the talocalcaneal, the calcaneocuboid, and the talonavicular joints) are fused. The procedure may be used for any condition in which the posterior part of the foot is unstable or in a varus or valgus position. It may be combined with tendon transfers. An arthrodesis of the tibiotalar joint will prevent the dropping of the foot into an equinus position. However, a fused ankle causes a definite limp and requires pain-free mobility of the foot in order to allow a reasonably good gait.

Resection of part of the proximal phalanx of the first toe (Keller) may be done for the usual hallux valgus deformity with or without bunionectomy. Resectional arthroplasties of other metatarsophalangeal joints also may be helpful in treating painful, destructive arthritis or metatarsalgia (usually affecting the digital nerves in the third and fourth metatarsal spaces).

The deformity of hammer toe consists of dorsiflexion of the proximal phalanx, plantar flexion of the middle phalanx, and flexion or extension of the distal phalanx. Usually, the deformity affects most severely the second toe and to lesser degrees the third to fifth toes. Treatment is either by partial resection or by arthrodesis of the proximal interphalangeal joints.

REFERENCES

1. Beckenbaugh, R. D.: Total wrist arthroplasty: The wrist. Mayo Clin. Proc., 54:513–515, 1979.
2. Charnley, J.: Arthroplasty of the hip: A new operation. Lancet, 1:1129–1132, 1961.
3. Curtis, R. M.: Tendon transfers in the patient with

spinal cord injury. Orthop. Clin. North Am., 5:415–423, 1974.

4. Dobyns, J. H., and Linscheid, R. L.: Rheumatoid hand repairs. Orthop. Clin. North Am., 2:629–647, 1971.

5. Eggers, G. W. N.: Transplantation of hamstring tendons to femoral condyles in order to improve hip extension and to decrease knee flexion in cerebral spastic paralysis. J. Bone Joint Surg., 34A:827–830, 1952.

6. Eggers, G. W. N., and Evans, E. B.: Surgery in cerebral palsy. J. Bone Joint Surg., 45A:1275–1305, 1963.

7. Fietti, V. G., Jr., and Mackin, E. J.: Dupuytren's disease. *In* Hunter, J. M., Schneider, L. H., Mackin, E. J., and Bell, J. A. (Eds.): Rehabilitation of the Hand. St. Louis, The C. V. Mosby Co., 1978, pp. 147–153.

8. Ketchum, L. D.: Primary tendon healing: A review. J. Hand Surg., 2:428–435, 1977.

9. Ketchum, L. D., Martin, N. L., and Kappel, D. A.: Experimental evaluation of factors affecting the strength of tendon repairs. Plast. Reconstr. Surg., 59:708–719, 1977.

10. Lamb, D. W., and Landry, R.: The hand in quadriplegia. Hand, 3:31–37, 1971.

11. Lehmann, J. F., Masock, A. J., Warren, C. G., and Koblanski, J. N.: Effect of therapeutic temperatures on tendon extensibility. Arch. Phys. Med. Rehabil., 51:481–487, 1970.

12. Lipscomb, P. R., Elkins, E. C., and Henderson, E. D.: Tendon transfers to restore function of hands in tetraplegia, especially after a fracture-dislocation of the sixth cervical vertebra on the seventh. J. Bone Joint Surg., 40A:1071–1080, 1958.

13. Mackin, E. J., and Maiorano, L.: Postoperative therapy following staged flexor tendon reconstruction. *In* Hunter, J. M., Schneider, L. H., Mackin, E. J., and Bell, J. A. (Eds.): Rehabilitation of the Hand. St. Louis, The C. V. Mosby Co., 1978, pp. 247–261.

14. Magness, J. L., and Elkins, E. C.: Tendon transfer: A review of patient selection and commonly used procedures. Arch. Phys. Med. Rehabil., 48:1–11, 1967.

15. Moberg, E.: Surgical treatment for absent single-hand grip and elbow extension in quadriplegia: Principles and preliminary experience. J. Bone Joint Surg., 57A:196–206, 1975.

16. Moberg, E.: Helpful upper limb surgery in tetraplegia. *In* Hunter, J. M., Schneider, L. H., Mackin, E. J., and Bell, J. A. (Eds.): Rehabilitation of the Hand. St. Louis, The C. V. Mosby Co., 1978, pp. 304–311.

17. Mustard, W. T.: Iliopsoas transfer for weakness of the hip abductors: A preliminary report. J. Bone Joint Surg., 34A:647–649, 1952.

18. Opitz, J. L., and Linscheid, R. L.: Hand function after metacarpophalangeal joint replacement in rheumatoid arthritis. Arch. Phys. Med. Rehabil., 59:160–165, 1978.

19. Phelps, W. M.: Long-term results of orthopaedic surgery in cerebral palsy. J. Bone Joint Surg., 39A:53–59, 1957.

20. Steindler, A.: Postgraduate Lectures on Orthopedic Diagnosis and Indications, Vol. 2. Springfield, Ill., Charles C Thomas, Publisher, 1951, pp. 32–51.

21. Total Joint Arthroplasty Symposium: Part I. Mayo Clin. Proc., 54:489–526, 1979.

22. Total Joint Arthroplasty Symposium: Part II. Mayo Clin. Proc., 54:557–612, 1979.

23. Zancolli, E.: Surgery for the quadriplegic hand with active strong wrist extension preserved: A study of 97 cases. Clin. Orthop., 112:101–113, 1975.

44

REHABILITATION AND MANAGEMENT OF AUDITORY DISORDERS

JEROME D. SCHEIN
MAURICE H. MILLER

Nearly 14 million persons in the United States suffer a significant hearing impairment.[59] Of these, nearly two million have profound losses preventing the discrimination of speech: they are *deaf*. Despite its substantial prevalence and harsh consequences, hearing impairment does not receive the attention it merits from rehabilitation personnel, government agencies, and the general public.

In the sections that follow, we first consider the numerical and social significance of impaired hearing. Then we discuss the auditory system from a functional-anatomical viewpoint. The various causes of hearing loss come after a review of techniques for diagnosis of hearing impairment. The remaining sections turn from diagnosis and evaluation to remediation of hearing problems, considering, in turn, aural rehabilitation, hearing aids, education, and related matters.

NATURE AND EXTENT OF HEARING IMPAIRMENT

Impairment of hearing is the most prevalent chronic physical disability in the United States. There are more common acute conditions (e.g., the common cold), and mental illness reportedly occurs more frequently than any physical disability. But arthritis, heart conditions, blindness, and other chronic physical disabilities do not individually strike as many of our citizens as does hearing impairment.

Table 44–1 summarizes some recent data on this condition. *Hearing impairment* in the table refers to any deviation in the ability to hear which is sufficient to be reported by a person when asked about it. A *significant, bilateral hearing impairment* is such a deviation affecting both ears. The final entry in the table, *deafness*, refers to the inability to understand speech solely by audition. Of the nearly 14 million hearing-impaired persons, almost half have bilateral impairments, and about one fourth of the latter group (the deaf persons) cannot depend upon their hearing for communication.

These figures clearly establish the great prevalence of this disorder in the population. They are, however, applicable only to the United States in 1971. Rates reported for hearing impairment differ widely from country to country.[54] Some differences are due to lack of uniformity of definitions. But differ-

TABLE 44–1. PREVALENCE AND PREVALENCE RATES FOR HEARING IMPAIRMENTS IN THE CIVILIAN, NONINSTITUTIONALIZED POPULATION: UNITED STATES, 1971

Degree of Impairment	Age at Onset	Number*	Rates per 100,000
All degrees	All ages	13,362,842	6,603
Significant bilateral	All ages	6,548,842	3,236
Deafness	All ages	1,767,046	873
	Before 19 years	410,522	203
	Before 3 years	201,626	100

*Entries are not to be added. For example, deafness is subsumed under Significant bilateral.

From Schein, J. D., and Delk, M. T.: The Deaf Population of the United States. Silver Spring, MD., National Association of the Deaf, 1974.

ences in rates may also reflect disparate conditions. Within the United States the prevalence rates for hearing impairment also vary substantially by locale, as shown in Table 44–2. The figures come from one study; hence, the definitions are the same across the regions. The Northeast has the smallest proportion of hearing-impaired and deaf persons, while the West has the highest proportion of hearing-impaired and the North Central the highest proportion of deaf persons. The differences in these rates are both statistically and practically significant. Thus, planning of services for deaf persons based on the national average of 870 per 100,000 would overprovide substantially in the Northeast (700 per 100,000) and underprovide in the North Central area (960 per 100,000).

Similar findings apply to prevalence rates for deafness by age. As will be discussed below, the cause of hearing impairment is partly exogenous. Hence, sizable differences in incidence rates are expected from year to year. Table 44–3 displays the age and sex distribution of estimated prevalence, not incidence, rates for significant bilateral hearing impairments in the United States in 1971. The age-relatedness of the data suggests that the incidence rates are likewise associated with specific periods in the life cycle. Other studies support both inferences. Older persons tend to become hearing impaired, especially after the fifth decade of life; and cases of deafness are noted to increase following epidemics. By the year 2030, demographers project 20 million hearing-impaired persons at and over 65 years of age alone. Widespread incidence of noise, infectious disease, ototoxic drugs, and other causal agents

TABLE 44–2. DISTRIBUTION OF HEARING-IMPAIRED POPULATION: UNITED STATES, 1971

Geographical Region	Classification of Loss		
	Hearing Impaired	*Deaf*	*Prevocationally Deaf*
United States	13,362,842	1,767,046	410,522
Northeast	2,891,380	337,022	83,909
North Central	3,683,226	541,465	135,653
South	4,280,177	562,756	123,260
West	2,508,059	325,803	67,700
	Rates per 100,000		
United States	6,603	873	203
Northeast	5,977	697	173
North Central	6,563	965	242
South	6,807	895	196
West	7,170	931	194

*Do not add entries horizontally. Of the 13.36 million hearing-impaired persons, 1.77 million are deaf, and of the 1.77 million deaf persons, 0.41 million are prevocationally deaf.

From Schein, J. D., and Delk, M. T.: The Deaf Population of the United States. Silver Spring, MD., National Association of the Deaf, 1974.

TABLE 44–3. PREVALENCE AND PREVALENCE RATES FOR SIGNIFICANT, BILATERAL HEARING IMPAIRMENT: UNITED STATES, 1971

Sex and Age (in years)	Number	Rate per 100,000
Both Sexes	6,549,643	3,237
Under 6	56,038	262
6 to 16	384,557	852
17 to 24	235,121	862
25 to 44	642,988	1,356
45 to 64	1,870,356	4,478
65 and over	3,360,583	17,368
Females	2,706,124	2,583
Under 6	23,771	227
6 to 16	155,738	701
17 to 24	81,923	568
25 to 44	243,403	990
45 to 64	610,741	2,783
65 and over	1,590,818	14,257
Males	3,843,519	3,938
Under 6	32,267	295
6 to 16	228,819	997
17 to 24	153,198	1,191
25 to 44	399,585	1,749
45 to 64	1,259,885	6,535
65 and over	1,769,765	21,606

doubtless will contribute to the increased future occurrence of hearing impairment at all ages. Thus, prevalence rates for hearing impairment will likely fluctuate over time.

Note in Table 44–3 the sex differences in proportions affected. The male preponderance is usually found in ascertainments of hearing impairment in unselected populations. Between 17 and 24 years of age, males appear to experience severe bilateral hearing impairment almost *twice* as frequently as females. By 65 years of age and beyond, the reported discrepancy declines to a still-large difference in rate of about 50 per cent. Some genetic and some environmental explanations for the sex discrepancy have been advanced.[21] Of importance to the rehabilitator, regardless of explanation, are the contributions of this fact to provisions for service delivery and to appreciation of the economic impact on families in which male heads of household predominate.

Hearing impairment ranks high in severity of consequences. When it occurs early in life, a hearing impairment, even a relatively mild one, tends to interfere with education, especially speech and language development.[9, 17, 51] A conductive impairment that raises the threshold in the better ear by as little as 20 dB above the normal threshold can markedly interfere with acquisition of both verbal and nonverbal learning, particularly if sustained during the first two years of life when the child is biologically programmed for rapid language development.

Profound hearing losses occurring during or before speech development are associated with failure to acquire intelligible speech — a frequent, although not a necessary, correlate.[11, 34] Delay in language acquisition, too, is a usual concomitant of early hearing losses. Later onsets of hearing impairment, while less likely to affect speech and language, may result in social isolation, loss of principal occupation, and major emotional upheavals — all consequences that are dependent, to some degree, upon the extent of impairment and the remedial steps taken to counteract it.[1, 50, 66]

Hearing loss poses barriers to human communication. The result of impaired hearing, then, is frequently a social handicap. Because it attacks the base of interpersonal relations, disruption of communications is no trivial matter. Without vigorous, effective rehabilitation, the hearing-impaired person suffers as much as does one afflicted by any other physical disability — typically more. This chapter focuses on what are now considered sound rehabilitation practices. To understand them, however, the reader must address the prior considerations that are discussed below.

FUNCTIONAL ANATOMY OF THE EAR

The auditory system is composed of the peripheral mechanism (the outer, middle, and inner ear) activating a series of intricate connections within the central nervous system via the eighth nerve and terminating in the auditory receptive areas of the temporal cortex. The anatomy and physiology of this complex system will be briefly reviewed here as a basis for understanding the different types of hearing loss. The reader desiring more detailed information should consult the relevant references.[3, 15, 16, 69-73, 77]

Figure 44–1 schematizes the human ear. The *outer ear* consists of the *pinna* or *auricle* and the *external auditory canal*. The pinna adds slightly to sensitivity for high frequen-

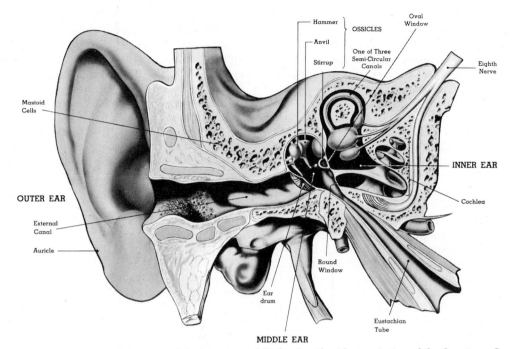

FIGURE 44–1. Sectional diagram of the human ear. (Reproduced with permission of the Sonotone Corp.)

cies and helps to direct sound waves into the external auditory canal.

The *tympanic membrane* or *eardrum* divides the outer ear from the middle ear. The *middle-ear cavity* contains a chain of three tiny bones, the *ossicles,* whose names are *malleus, incus,* and *stapes.* Suspended in the cavity by a system of ligaments, the ossicles increase the effective pressure of sounds conveyed to the inner ear, because of the large difference between the area of the tympanic membrane and the footplate of the stapes which is attached to the oval window (*condensation effect*). The ossicles function as a lever, because the length of the manubrium and neck of the malleus is greater than that of the long process of the incus, so that the force at the tympanic membrane is increased by a factor of 1.3 at the stapes. Thus the pressure increase by a factor of 17 resulting from the area difference of the tympanic membrane and stapes footplate is further amplified by 1.3, resulting in a theoretical maximum total pressure increase of 17×1.3, or 22, which corresponds to 27 dB.[76]

Dividing the middle ear from the inner ear are two membranes: the *oval window,* to which the stapes is attached, and the *round window.* The latter acts to compensate for the changes in pressure caused by impres-sion and expression of the oval window. Encased in the temporal bone is the *inner-ear cavity,* which houses a series of canals in the bony foundation called the *osseous labyrinth.* It is filled with *perilymph,* a liquid similar in chemical composition to cerebro-spinal fluid. The perilymph circulates through the three principal subdivisions of the labyrinth: the *semicircular canals,* the *vestibule,* and the *cochlea.* The semicircular canals are so arranged as to provide the stimuli an individual uses to orient himself in space. The conch-shaped cochlea contains the *organ of Corti.* The conversion of mechanical to electrical (neural) energy takes place at this point. The organ of Corti has over 30,000 hair cells on its inner and outer portions. The auditory nerve interacts with the hair cells by synaptic junctions. Vibrations of the inner ear fluids bend the cilia of the hair cells, initiating a change of neural potential. The resulting impulses are transmitted along the auditory pathways to the temporal cortex.

THEORIES OF HEARING

The exact manner in which the cochlea functions as an analyzer of sound is the subject of vast research and continuing discussion. Four theories predominate as explanations of how hearing takes place.

Place theory states that pitch perception is related to the point of maximum stimulation along the basilar membrane of the organ of Corti. This theory proposes that the hair cells function as a series of tuned resonators. It is generally accepted for stimuli with a frequency at or above 5000 Hz.

Frequency theory relates pitch perception to the frequency of a current of impulses in the auditory nerve. For example, a sound with a frequency of 500 Hz would cause the fibers within the auditory nerve to fire at a rate of 500 times per second. Since no auditory nerve fiber is capable of firing faster than 1000 times per second, this theory could account for pitch perception only at frequencies around 1000 Hz or less.

A compromise between the place and frequency theories is the *volley theory*. It holds that pitch perception for frequencies up to 1000 Hz can be explained primarily on the basis of the frequency theory and that the place theory accounts for pitch perception at the higher frequencies.

Traveling wave theory postulates, on the basis of meticulously performed experiments with cochlear models, that sound is propagated in the form of a wave traveling from the base to the apex of the cochlea. The maximum amplitude of the wave occurs at a point on the basilar membrane corresponding to the frequency of the stimulus.

These four theories of hearing cover present-day views. They appear here for two purposes. First, the fact that four different explanations persist indicates the complexity of the process. The rehabilitator can use this perspective in approaching hearing impairment. Second, these theories serve to introduce the next topic, the measurement of hearing and diagnosis of hearing impairment.

INTRODUCTION TO AUDIOMETRY

Two common-sense aspects of sound have sophisticated analogs in the measurement of hearing: pitch and loudness. Objectively, *sound* is a form of wave motion resulting from a change in pressure or particle displacement in an elastic medium, such as air. The wave form is characterized by alternate pressure peaks and valleys called *compres-*

sions and *rarefactions*. One successive compression and rarefaction constitute one cycle of a sound wave. The more rapidly these vibrations occur the higher the *frequency* symbolized by the abbreviations Hz (for *hertz*) or cps (for *cycles per second*). A sound wave whose cycles occur 500 times per second would be designated as 500 Hz; one vibrating twice as fast would be written 1000 Hz. The psychological equivalent of frequency is *pitch;* the more rapidly the wave oscillates, the higher the pitch is perceived by the listener, although pitch is affected by other factors. Middle "C" on the piano, for example, has a frequency near 256 Hz, while the next higher octave is 512 Hz. The human ear is theoretically capable of hearing sounds as low as 20 Hz and as high as 20,000 Hz. For purposes of hearing and understanding connected discourse in quiet surroundings by persons whose hearing was normal early in life, however, the critical frequencies range from 500 to 3000 Hz. This point has considerable importance to testing hearing and to rehabilitation, as will be discussed below.

The *intensity* (loudness) of sound is measured by the amount of its pressure. *Sound-pressure level* (SPL) is the difference between a given pressure and 0.0002 dynes/cm^2, the standard reference. The amount of the difference is expressed in decibels (dB), a log unit in which 0 dB = 0.0002 dynes/cm^2, the standard value. The reader unfamiliar with logarithms should note that to increase from 1 dB to 100 dB requires 100,000 times more energy, not a mere 100 times. This relative measure can also be confusing, because the same unit, dB, is used in measuring hearing sensitivity. However, in the latter case, the standard reference is not 0.0002 dynes/cm^2 but is a statistically determined amount of energy needed by a "normal" person to hear that particular sound (the *hearing-threshold level,* HTL). To avoid confusing the two concepts, decibel values should carry the reference level as part of the notation, e.g., 40 dB SPL or 40 dB HTL. The amount of energy expressed by the former differs significantly from that expressed by the latter.

The weakest amount of sound pressure that the human ear experiences as sound is a very small quantity, but the range of sound pressure that the ear can perceive is extremely large. Subjectively, a listener may describe some sounds as causing a tickling or painful sensation. The sound pressure that corresponds to very loud sounds is 1,000,000,000,000 (10^{12}) times greater than the sound pressure of barely audible sounds. That is why a log scale is used to express this tremendous range of pressures that the human ear can experience as sound. The range on the decibel scale would be expressed as 0 to 120 dB HTL, a more manageable set of numbers.

Another term of importance to measuring hearing is *threshold,* the point at which correct responses are elicited 50 per cent of the time. Hearing sensitivity is defined by the amount of energy (in decibels) required by a listener to respond appropriately to the stimulus half the time. It follows, then, that the higher the threshold, the poorer the hearing. A person whose threshold is 0 dB HTL has no deviation from normal and, therefore, has more sensitive hearing than someone whose threshold for the same stimulus is, say, 20 dB HTL. That a larger number signifies poorer hearing sensitivity must be borne in mind as audiograms are read.

The Audiometer and the Audiogram

Audiometry is the measurement of hearing. Basic testing to determine the degree and type of hearing loss is performed with a *pure-tone audiometer,* an instrument for measuring hearing sensitivity which provides pure tones of selected frequencies at calibrated sound-pressure levels. The results of such testing are recorded on an *audiogram,* which is a graph showing hearing sensitivity as a function of frequency.

In the audiogram shown in Figure 44–2, "Zero dB Hearing Level" represents the zero reference level. The range between –10 dB and 25 dB in the audiogram is considered to be "within normal limits." This definition has been appropriately questioned in relation to the hearing of children going through major periods of speech and language development, when a threshold increase even to 20 or 25 dB may significantly impede language acquisition and development of academic skills.

At thresholds above this "normal-hearing range," differing degrees of hearing impairment are indicated by higher numbers. The audiogram in Figure 44–3 shows normal hearing throughout the tested range in the left ear. However, at 4000 Hz in the right ear, the hearing threshold is 35 dB greater than that of the normally hearing person — a deviation indicative of a problem in the auditory system, albeit a small one in this example.

The test results shown in Figure 44–3 represent thresholds for *air conduction,* i.e.,

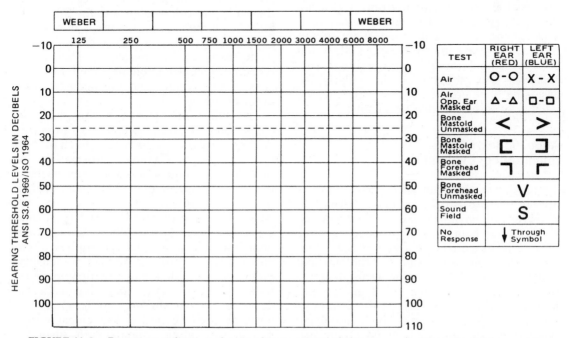

FIGURE 44–2. Pure tone audiogram showing hearing threshold levels as a function of tonal frequency.

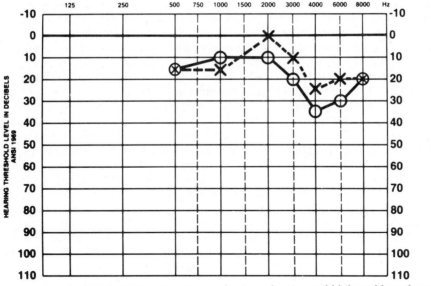

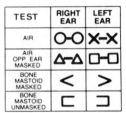

FIGURE 44–3. Pure tone audiogram showing mild bilateral loss above 3000 Hz.

for stimuli transmitted to the external ear through earphones. Another way of presenting stimuli to the ear is *bone conduction,* in which a vibrator is placed on portions of the skull, usually the mastoid process.

The general anatomic area of the ear which is involved in the patient's hearing impairment can be determined by comparing air-conduction to bone-conduction thresholds. Bone-conduction measurements must be performed with the judicious use of *masking,* i.e., presenting a complex signal to the contralateral ear to prevent it from picking up the sound presented to the ear under test. Through the bone-conduction test an attempt is made to bypass the middle-ear system and conduct sound directly to the inner ear. Judicious use of masking, particularly for assessing bone conduction, is critical to the validity of this important procedure.

Acoustic Impedance (Immittance) Evaluation

Impedance or immittance measurements are not hearing tests in the usual sense, and the term *audiometry* should not be employed to describe them. These procedures have become an essential component of the evaluation of persons with auditory problems and constitute one of the most powerful diagnostic tools available. Some clinicians use impedance measurements at the beginning of the evaluation to determine which audiologic procedures are indicated, while others use them to obtain site-of-lesion data and to provide additional diagnostic information.[29, 42]

Impedance measurements are an objective method for assessing the integrity and performance of the peripheral auditory system. The electroacoustic impedance meter contains a probe tip that is sealed in the external auditory meatus. The probe tip has three holes: (1) one for a probe tone of about 220 Hz, (2) one for a cavity air-pressure control, and (3) one for a pick-up microphone to compare the sound-pressure level (SPL) in the ear canal with reference to the SPL in the impedance meter. A test tone is introduced, and the sound that is reflected by the tympanic membrane is measured. The amount reflected depends upon the mass and stiffness of the system and the acoustic resistance of the air.

The basic immittance battery includes *tympanometry, static compliance,* and measurement of the *acoustic reflex.* Each of these tests provides valuable information, although static compliance is the least useful of the three measurements. The index of diagnostic accuracy is significantly improved when the entire immittance battery is used, especially in relation to other audiologic and nonaudiologic site-of-lesion studies. Tympanometry is probably the most sensitive indicator of middle-ear function available today. Acoustic-reflex and stapedial-reflex decay tests are useful in the differential diagnosis of cochlear and retrocochlear lesions and in evaluating patients with suspected functional hearing problems. Reflex levels can be used in selection and adjustment of hearing aids for difficult-to-test children. Some abnormality in the acoustic reflex (i.e., elevated or absent reflex or the presence of significant reflex decay) is related to an acoustic tumor in as many as 85 per cent of cases.

Speech Audiometry

Speech audiometry is a measure of overall hearing performance for functional speech stimuli. It is also used to estimate the degree of actual handicap imposed by the auditory deficit. Calibrated speech materials are used to assess two aspects of auditory performance: speech-reception thresholds (or spondee thresholds) and speech discrimination.

Speech-reception thresholds (SRT) are obtained by asking the patient to repeat a series of spondee words (those that have roughly equal stress on the two syllables, e.g., "cowboy," "mushroom," "airplane"). The materials are presented at successively louder levels via monitored live voice or a recording into earphones worn by the patient. Threshold is the level at which the patient is able to repeat just 50 per cent of the words correctly.

Speech discrimination (SD) is a test of the patient's ability to understand speech when the level of presentation is not a factor in determining the number of words repeated correctly. Lists consisting of 50 words are presented that theoretically reflect the frequency of occurrence of the various phonetic elements in everyday conversational speech (i.e., are phonetically balanced). The level of presentation is usually 30 to 40 dB above the patient's SRT, although in some cases it is important to obtain a complete articulation function reflecting the patient's ability to understand speech as the intensity of the signal is gradually increased. SD is widely used in differential diagnosis and hearing-aid evaluation. Jerger and his associates developed lists of synthetic sentence material consisting of seven-word sentences that are grammatically correct but meaningless ("Small boat with a picture has become").[68] They can be presented with a competing speech message introduced into the contralateral or ipsilateral ear. The procedure has been suggested for diagnosis of brain stem and cortical lesions as well as for hearing-aid evaluation.

Pure-tone air- and bone-conduction audiometry, speech audiometry, and the impedance (immittance) battery compose the basic audiologic evaluation should be performed on all persons with known or suspected auditory problems. On the basis of the results of these tests and the case history, some or all of the procedures described next may be indicated.

The Audiologic Site-of-Lesion Battery

An impressive array of audiologic procedures is now available to elucidate the nature of the auditory problem and to determine, in conjunction with nonaudiologic procedures, the site of lesion within the auditory system. While each test has a different index of accuracy in predicting the locus of pathology, the accuracy increases significantly when each test is viewed as part of a comprehensive battery and carefully evaluated with a recognition of the advantages and weaknesses of each procedure for different groups of hypacusic patients. A number of audiologic procedures have been "sensitized" to provide additional diagnostic information, particularly in difficult-to-diagnose early and mild lesions. These modifications will not be discussed in the following brief review of some of the audiologic site-of-lesion studies now in use.

Loudness Balance Tests.   A tone of a given frequency is presented alternately to the two ears of the patient, who is asked to match its relative loudness. This procedure, called the *Alternate Binaural Loudness Balance* (ABLB) test, allows the demonstration of recruitment in certain pathologic ears. *Recruitment* is an abnormal growth in the loudness of sound when its intensity is increased above the impaired threshold. It is characteristically present in persons with cochlear lesions (e.g., Ménière's disease, ototoxic deafness, noise-induced hearing loss) and frequently, but not invariably, absent in persons with eighth-nerve tumors and other lesions affecting the auditory nerve. The test is optimally suited for cases of unilateral sensorineural losses but can be used in persons with asymmetric losses in whom the difference in hearing sensitivity between ears exceeds 30 to 40 dB at some frequencies and when the better, reference ear is known to be nonrecruiting.[12]

A loudness balance test that can be used

when there is no difference in sensitivity between ears and both have a symmetrical loss of approximately equal degree is called the *Monaural Loudness Balance* test or the *Alternate Monaural Loudness Balance* (AMLB) test. It involves a comparison of the relative loudness of two frequencies, one at an impaired and one at an unimpaired frequency, presented alternately to the same ear of the patient. The test is more difficult for the patient than ABLB because a comparison of two sounds of disparate frequencies is involved and results can be affected by the musical sophistication of the subject and, to a greater extent than with some other audiologic tests, by a practice effect. Persons with eighth-nerve lesions, a major concern of the diagnostician, are more likely to show a unilateral or asymmetrical loss in which the ABLB is the procedure of choice rather than bilateral, symmetrical losses in which the AMLB would be employed.

Short Increment Sensitivity Index. The short increment sensitivity index (SISI) measures the patient's ability to detect small changes in intensity. A pure tone is presented to the patient at 20 dB above his threshold. Twenty one-dB increments are superimposed upon the constant tone at periodic intervals. Persons with pathologic cochleas are able to detect these small increments while those with lesions elsewhere usually cannot.[30]

Békésy Audiometry. Békésy audiometry uses a self-recording technique to determine pure-tone thresholds. The patient is told to push a button and keep it depressed as long as he hears the signal and to release it when the tone is no longer audible. The audiometer is connected to an X-Y recorder which traces the patient's audiogram as a series of vertical excursions of the marking pen. In a version widely used today, thresholds are established first for periodically interrupted and then for continuous pure tones. The relationship of thresholds for the two types of stimuli is compared to differentiate various pathologies, including pseudohypacusis.[28] ABLB, SISI, and Békésy testing have fallen into some disrepute of late because of their failure to detect many cases of acoustic neurinomas and to an increasing degree are being replaced by newer techniques, e.g., stapedial reflex measurements and brain stem evoked-response audiometry.

Abnormal tone decay or auditory adaptation is a loss of sensitivity which occurs during exposure to an auditory stimulus. It is a symptom that in its most bizarre forms is characteristic of eighth-nerve lesions, although various degrees and patterns of abnormal tone decay can occur in cochlear and brain stem lesions. Tone decay of 30 dB or more is generally considered to reflect retrocochlear pathology. However, the likelihood of a retrocochlear lesion increases when tone decay of only 30 dB is found in association with normal or near-normal thresholds at the frequency at which the test is performed. Any conventional audiometer can be used to perform this test, which is a powerful screening and diagnostic tool in differential diagnosis.[23]

Electrophysiologic (Neuroelectric) Tests of Auditory Function

For many patients, tests that do not involve active cooperation in the form of voluntary, conditioned responses are essential. Among the patients in whom objective procedures are most useful are children who are too young or too involved to respond to standard pediatric audiologic measures (e.g., children under 18 months of age and those who are retarded, neurologically impaired, or severely disturbed psychologically) and persons with suspected functional auditory problems. For the latter, such tests may play an important but still controversial role in medicolegal proceedings. Finally, some forms of electrophysiologic measures are extremely sensitive detectors of eighth-nerve, brain stem, and cortical lesions and thus compose an important part of the site-of-lesion battery.

Electroencephalic audiometry (EEA) quantifies changes in the electroencephalogram which result from auditory stimulation. *Evoked response audiometry* (ERA) is a general term used for the different forms of audiometry which tap a number of electric responses that can be evoked from different parts of the auditory system by auditory stimulation. All of these responses are very small and require repetitive stimulation and the summation of many responses by use of a response-averaging computer. The responses, which are time-locked to the acoustic stimuli, add in the memory of the computer, and the random background activity of the brain and muscles is cancelled out.

The most widely used of the electric auditory responses today is *brain stem evoked-response audiometry* (BERA).[36]

With BERA, a measurement is made of auditory-evoked potentials believed to originate between the eighth nerve and the inferior colliculus. The responses appear quite reliable and not difficult to identify. BERA has become the most accurate noninvasive procedure in the diagnosis of acoustic neurinomas and has the lowest false-positive rate.[8] For purposes of determining hearing thresholds, BERA can measure within 10 dB of the individual's psychophysical threshold for the stimulus used, when appropriate signal characteristics and recording techniques are used.

Electrocochleography (ECoG) measures the electrophysiologic activity that originates within the cochlea or the auditory nerve. The compound action potential (AP) of the auditory nerve is the basis for most ECoG studies. Recording sites are the transtympanic membrane, where needle electrodes make contact with the promontory of the cochlea, the intrameatal surface, and the surface of the external auditory canal. For the uncooperative patient, an anesthesiologist is necessary to monitor and control levels of anesthesia, and life-support equipment must be available should complications of general anesthesia occur. An otolaryngologist inserts the electrodes and is responsible for pre- and postrecording medical care of the patient. The test procedure is carried out by an audiologist. The AP response appears to be a sensitive indicator of cochlear and auditory nerve activity. *Cochleograms* can be obtained which reflect recruitment, sensorineural losses of various degrees and configurations, and total hearing impairment. Recordings obtained from sites other than the promontory of the cochlea appear to be of limited value.[13] This invasive technique has been largely replaced by BERA in most laboratories, although ECoG provides data on certain aspects of cochlear function not yielded by BERA.

CLASSIFICATION OF TYPES OF HEARING IMPAIRMENT

Peripheral, organic hearing impairments can be usefully divided into three categories for rehabilitation purposes. These three categories are based on the locus of the lesion responsible for the impairment. *Conductive impairments* prevent or interfere with transmission of sound to the cochlea. Such lesions occur in the outer or middle ear. Hearing loss resulting from damage to the cochlea and/or the auditory nerve is called *sensorineural impairment*. When these structures are defective, interpretation of the auditory stimulus may be difficult or impossible. When both conductive and sensorineural impairments are present, the loss is referred to as *mixed* or *combined*.

The value of this three-part classification of peripheral hearing impairment is that some rehabilitative strategies are directly associated with them. These strategies will be discussed later. Here we concentrate on the procedures for determining the site of the lesion.

Pure-tone air-conduction audiometry provides quantitative information about hearing sensitivity only. To determine the type of hearing impairment present, other tests are required. Table 44–4 relates the degree of hearing loss on the pure-tone audiogram to the degree of difficulty in understanding conversational speech. This relationship is far from an exact one, because the ability to understand speech cannot be directly predicted from responses to pure-tone stimuli. Difficulty in understanding speech is also related, in part, to the configuration of the audiogram and to the amount and type of distortion present. Persons with significantly greater losses in the high frequencies (above 1000 Hz) usually have noticeable problems in speech discrimination, although low-frequency sensorineural losses can also be related to poor speech discrimination, e.g., Ménière's disease. The degree of difficulty in understanding speech with or without amplification is also dependent upon the type of hearing loss present, the age at onset, and other factors. Nonetheless, the table relates the approximate degree of difficulty that most persons in each category will experience.

Figure 44–4 shows the air-conduction thresholds of an individual with an average pure-tone loss of 60 dB. Bone-conduction measurements fall entirely within normal limits. This individual has a *conductive* hearing impairment. A conductive hearing impairment reflects damage or disease to the outer or middle ear. Conductive hearing im-

TABLE 44–4. RELATION OF DEGREE OF HEARING LOSS TO ABILITY TO UNDERSTAND SPEECH

Class	Classification Category of Hearing Loss	Average Hearing Threshold Level for 500, 1000, and 2000 Hz in the Better Ear* More Than	Not More Than	Ability to Understand Speech
A	Within normal limits		25 dB	No significant difficulty with faint speech
B	Slight or mild	26	40 dB	Difficulty only with faint speech
C	Moderate	41	55 dB	Frequent difficulty with normal speech
D	Moderately severe	56	70 dB	Frequent difficulty with loud speech
E	Severe	71	90 dB	Can understand only shouted or amplified speech
F	Profound	91		Usually cannot understand even amplified speech

*Re: 1969 ANSI reference threshold. Adapted from Davis, H.: Guide for the classification and evaluation of hearing handicapped. Trans. Am. Acad. Ophthalmol. Otolaryngol., 1965, 69:740–751.

pairments are potentially correctable by a variety of medical and surgical means.

Hearing-conservation programs in schools often do not detect many auditory problems, especially those associated with secretory otitis media (vide infra). The schools set screening levels for air conduction at 20 or 25 db HTL, levels too high for early detection. The hearing tests are given too infrequently to uncover many fluctuating losses. Most critically, a better test than air conduction for such problems would be tympanometry,

a measure of the change in eardrum compliance that has been described above.

Figure 44–5 shows a bilateral *sensorineural* hearing impairment in a noise-susceptible individual who has worked in a very noisy environment without using personal hearing-protective devices. Note that there is no air-bone gap; i.e., bone-conduction values closely parallel the air-conduction thresholds.

Figure 44–6 shows a *mixed* hearing impairment. In this case the loss of hearing below

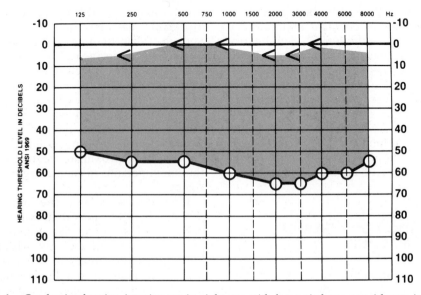

FIGURE 44–4. Conductive hearing impairment in right ear with large air-bone gap (shown in shaded area) associated with otosclerosis.

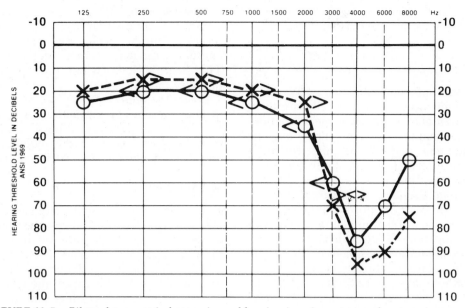

FIGURE 44–5. Bilateral symmetrical sensorineural hearing impairment secondary to noise exposure.

1000 Hz is primarily conductive and secondary to otitis media, while the loss above 1000 Hz is primarily sensorineural and secondary to presbycusis. Specifying the cause of the impairment, of course, requires more than an audiogram. An inferential diagnosis involves careful history and additional non-audiologic tests, as well as thorough physical examination.

MAJOR CAUSES OF HEARING IMPAIRMENT BY LOCUS OF LESION

Principal causes of hearing impairment are arranged below in the order of anatomical structures involved. The first group describes impairments associated with the outer ear. Note, however, that a given patient may simultaneously suffer more than

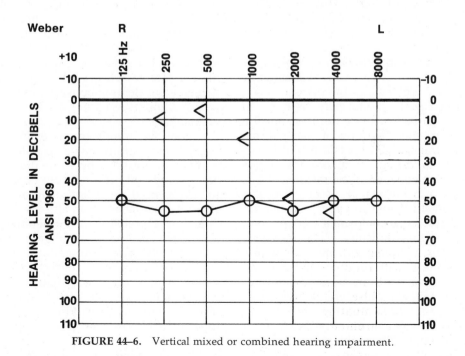

FIGURE 44–6. Vertical mixed or combined hearing impairment.

one disorder, although this presentation treats each disorder separately.

Outer Ear

Disorders of the outer ear may affect sound conduction. They generally are amenable to treatment restoring normal functioning of the auditory system. They may be associated with middle- and inner-ear problems whose management is considered in subsequent sections.

Congenital Atresia of the External Auditory Canal. Failure to develop an opening in the external meatus affecting sound conduction to the tympanum is often associated with microtia and multiple rudimentary or auricular tags of accessory auricles. These obvious malformations may be accompanied by deformities of the middle ear or inner ear as well as of other organs, e.g., the kidneys. These conditions may be unilateral or bilateral and may present both auditory and cosmetic problems.

Foreign Bodies. Tumors involving skin, cartilage, and bone are found in the external auditory canal and may require surgical removal. By far the most common problem is impacted cerumen (ear wax), which can cause up to a 40-dB conductive loss. As long as a pinhead opening of the tympanic membrane remains visible, cerumen is unlikely to affect hearing significantly. However, when the eardrum is completely obstructed by cerumen, removal by an otologist is indicated. Osteomas, hyperostoses, and exostoses require surgical management only when they completely obstruct the external meatus or present other problems to the patient.

Collapsed Canal. Some persons have an anatomical variant of the outermost portion of the cartilaginous portion of the external canal and tragus. The pressure of the earphone used to test air-conduction thresholds can produce a collapse of the meatus. While this is not a lesion per se, it may cause a pseudoconductive loss to appear on the audiometric test, unaccompanied by any complaint of auditory difficulty. Such problems do not occur in tuning-fork measurements. These patients will require "propping" of the ear canal with an earmold or other plug to prevent this false conductive hearing loss from contaminating the results of audiologic measurements performed under earphones. The problem occurs quite frequently in elderly persons.

External otitis. This is usually the result of a bacterial infection in the skin of the external auditory canal. Redness, swelling, and discharge may accompany the infection. The hearing loss, when present, is conductive.

Treacher-Collins Syndrome. This syndrome combines abnormalities of the mandible with hearing loss resulting from the first-branchial-arch origin of the mandible, malleus, and incus. The loss is conductive.

Middle Ear

A variety of congenital lesions of the middle ear may occur, including absent or fused ossicles, congenital fixation of the stapedial footplate, and occasionally a complete immobilization of the ossicular chain. Again, hearing losses resulting from these disorders are conductive, unless other auditory structures are involved. These conditions often respond well to surgical management.

Otitis Media. Acute infections of the middle ear are accompanied by pain, fever, and malaise. Widespread use of antibiotics has dramatically reduced the incidence of acute mastoiditis arising from otitis media, but their use may mask the classic symptoms of infection and lead to a latent form *(silent or occult otitis media)* accompanied by varying degrees of conductive hearing loss.

Serous or *secretory otitis media* is by far the most prevalent cause of conductive hearing loss in preschool and school-age children. The child suffering from this condition is typically not constitutionally ill and is attending school but experiencing a fluctuating conductive hearing loss that is often not detected by hearing-conservation programs in the school (see earlier discussion of tympanometry).

Among the complications of inadequately treated serous otitis media is *cholesteatoma,* a squamous cyst that begins in the middle ear and extends into the mastoid antrum, often to the mastoid tip. Cholesteatomas can destroy the ossicular chain and are potentially fatal. Irreversible sensorineural hearing losses may also occur in children with silent, inadequately treated serous otitis.[22] In long-standing cases of serous otitis media, conservative management is usually ineffective, and surgery, consisting of adenoidectomy, myringotomy, and insertion of ventilation tubes into the eardrum to replace a malfunctioning eustachian tube, is the treatment of choice. Treatment of an underlying allergy, often to food rather than inhalants, may be required for some intractable cases.

Otosclerosis. Otosclerosis is a common cause of hearing loss in adults. The disease affects the otic capsule and in its early stage often involves a softening of the oval window anterior to the stapes footplate. It is twice as common in women as in men and is relatively rare among blacks. The condition can also involve cochlear structures and may even have its primary effect on the inner ear, a form of the condition known as *labyrinthine otosclerosis.*

Persons with otosclerosis whose lesions involve primarily the oval window and who audiometrically show large air-bone gaps and good speech discrimination are typically excellent candidates for stapedectomy, a surgical procedure in which the involved portion of the stapes is removed and the ossicular chain is reconstructed in a variety of ways. Stapedectomy can restore hearing to within 10 dB of the preoperative bone-conduction curve in over 90 per cent of carefully selected patients. Some far-advanced otosclerotics who may have unmeasurable air-bone gaps may be helped through stapes surgery to regain sufficient hearing to allow them to use amplification or to allow the use of ear-level rather than body-mounted instruments. The specific objectives of surgery in such cases must be carefully explained to these patients, so that they are not led to believe that the surgery can eliminate the need for hearing aids.

Discontinuities of the Ossicular Chain. Mechanical damage to the ear from blows to the head (as in vehicular or bicycle accidents) can cause a dislocation of the ossicular chain and varying degrees of conductive hearing loss. Surgical procedures are available to reconstruct the ossicular chain and restore hearing, often to normal or near-normal levels. Impedance evaluation (vide supra) is extremely helpful in distinguishing ossicular-chain discontinuities from otosclerosis, an important consideration in cases involving medicolegal litigation.

Inner Ear

By far the largest number of hearing-impaired persons in the general population have disease or damage to the cochlea. A smaller number have lesions affecting the eighth nerve, while some have combinations of cochlear and eighth-nerve involvement.

Conditions such as acoustic tumors have serious life-threatening implications, and early diagnosis and management are essential. Lesions affecting the cochlea, in general, are not correctable by medical or surgical techniques, and patients with such lesions represent the largest population of candidates for hearing aids and various forms of audiologic rehabilitation. They are suffering from sensorineural hearing impairments.

Noise-induced Hearing Loss. Noise, in and out of the work place, is believed to account for more cases of hearing impairment than all other causes combined. It is certainly the major cause of new cases of hearing loss. Over five million individual work areas have been identified as having potentially hazardous noise levels. More than 40 million workers are exposed each work day to a noise level of over 90 dBA, and 16.5 million persons have already sustained some permanent sensorineural hearing loss from noise exposure. The federal government, through the Occupational Safety and Health Administration of the Department of Labor, passed a final regulation on occupational noise exposure which became effective 22 August 1981. It requires a hearing-conservation program for all workers exposed to noise level equal to or greater than 85 dBA for a time-weighted equivalent of 8 hours.[37] Exposures greater than 90 dBA are permitted for various periods of time (e.g., 100 dBA for two hours and 105 dBA for one hour), but the cumulative noise exposure in any eight-hour period must not exceed an average of 90 dBA. The hearing-conservation program must include noise monitoring, audiometric testing, worker education, and use of personal hearing-protective devices.[39]

Noise measurements are made on a *sound-level meter,* an instrument that measures noise at the source. It consists of a microphone, an amplifier, a calibrated attenuator, an indicating meter, and a series of circuits (networks) which adjust the overall frequency characteristics of the input. The "A" network (signified in the symbol dBA) simulates the response of the normal ear to low-frequency sounds; it is the most commonly used setting for studies of work place and environmental noise.

Noise exposure first damages the outer hair cells of the organ of Corti and later involves its inner hair cells, the sensory and vascular epithelium of the cochlea, and the

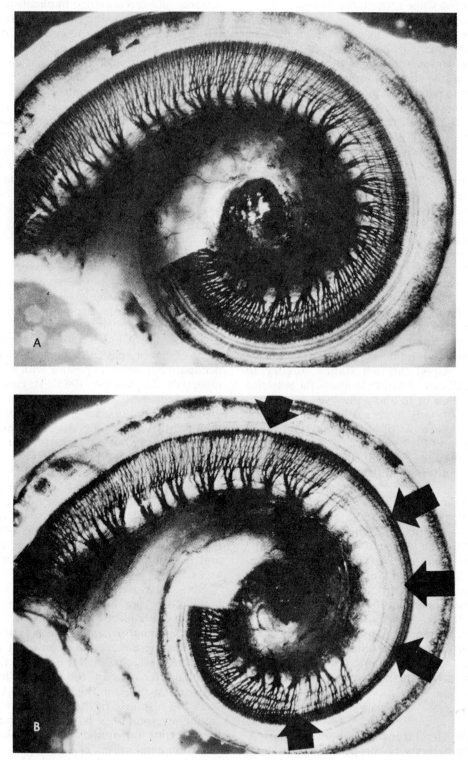

FIGURE 44–7. *A,* The cochlea of a normal, healthy ear seen under an electron microscope. *B,* Noise-damaged cochlea. Further deterioration from noise exposure may be prevented by use of hearing protection.

capillary vessels. Eventually the organ of Corti disappears and is replaced by a layer of simple epithelial cells. Audiometrically, a threshold elevation is first noted at 4000 Hz and less often at 3000 and 6000 Hz. As exposure increases in susceptible individuals, particularly those not using any personal hearing-protective devices, the noise-induced loss increases and spreads to lower and higher frequencies. In addition to the hearing loss, *tinnitus* (noises heard without external stimulation) becomes a major symptom (vide infra).

While occupational noise exposure accounts for the greatest incidence of noise-induced hearing loss, excessive noise exposure affects people in virtually every area where they live or play. Rock-music concerts and discotheques, trap and skeet shooting, power lawn mowers, chain saws, snowmobiles, motor-driven bicycles, garbage disposals, blenders and ice-jets, personal earphones attached to stereo cassettes and radio devices, and home stereo units are a few of the avocational sources of significant noise exposure. An example of auditory damage from gunfire exposure is shown in Figure 44–7. The illustration on the bottom shows damage to the sensory elements of the cochlea responsible for reception of high-frequency stimuli. The figure on the top shows an intact sensory mechanism on the contralateral nonexposed side.

Presbycusis is the term applied to the various ways in which the auditory system degenerates with age. All portions of the system are subject to such changes from atropic alterations in the skin of the external auditory canal and a flaccidity of the tympanic membrane to a nonspecific osteitis and sclerosis of the auditory ossicles. However, auditory changes with age involve primarily the sensorineural and central mechanisms and not the conductive system.

Audiologically, age changes associated with presbycusis are usually characterized by a gradual loss of pure-tone sensitivity in the high frequencies. Figure 44–8 displays data based on eight different studies from four countries, with hearing level for 25-year-old adults used as a reference. Note that males lose hearing for high frequencies more rapidly than females, but the general trend applies to both sexes.

More significant than the decrease in high-frequency sensitivity among the elderly is the disproportionate drop in speech discrimination which is frequently encountered in this population, particularly in the presence of noise. Such an abnormal breakdown in the understanding of speech has been termed *phonemic regression* and has important rehabilitative implications. Persons having this condition benefit less from hearing aids and require more intense audiologic rehabilitation than those with good discrimination.

A neural form of presbycusis involves a loss of neurons in the central nervous system and is often seen in persons with severe arteriosclerosis. This variety of the condition does not lend itself to simple correction by existing forms of electroacoustic amplification. Specifically designed geriatric audiologic-rehabilitation programs using a team approach and involving both individual and group sessions are required to achieve success with such cases. However, the neural form of presbycusis is only one of at least four forms of the condition that have been identified, and each group shows a different potential for audiologic rehabilitation. A *sensory form* involves degeneration of the sensory and supportive cells of the basal turns of the cochlea. Atrophy of the stria vascularis, which is believed to be the site of endolymph production, produces a *metabolic type* of presbycusis. *Mechanical presbycusis* results from a disorder of the motion mechanics of the cochlear duct caused by stiffening of the basilar membrane.[62, 63] Each of these forms of presbycusis is accompanied by a different constellation of audiologic findings and by varied histories. The patient with metabolic presbycusis has an excellent prognosis for successful use of amplification, often with relatively short periods of audiologic rehabilitation. In contrast to this group, the neural form requires massive rehabilitation, and amplification alone will play a less decisive role in achieving any success. The presbycusic population, which represents the largest number of new patients seen by audiologists, has not been adequately served by many hearing professionals, who have tended to view presbycusis as a single entity, usually unresponsive to hearing aids and audiologic rehabilitation. Since over 20 million hearing-impaired persons over the age of 65 are expected by the year 2030, it is critical that the most creative and resourceful professional talent available be mobilized to provide services to

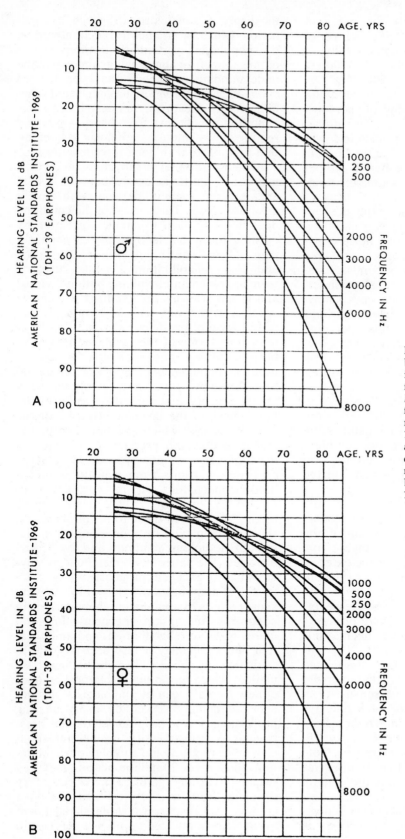

Figure 44–8. *A*, Composite presbycusic curves for males, according to Spoor, modified to conform to ANSI-1969 standard. *B*, Composite presbycusic curves from females, according to Spoor, modified to conform to ANSI-1969 standard. (From Lebo, C. P., and Reddell, R. C.: The presbycusis component in occupational noise-induced hearing loss. Laryngoscope, 82:1399–1409, 1972.)

this challenging population. Fortunately, signs of such efforts are beginning to emerge.

Ototoxic Drugs. Inner-ear structures are susceptible to damage by a wide variety of pharmaceutical agents. Some drugs, such as aspirin and quinine, exert transient effects on the auditory system, while others, such as the aminoglycoside antibiotics (neomycin, kanamycin, etc.) can cause irreversible changes. Even those drugs whose ototoxic effects are reversible may produce permanent hearing loss through interactions with other factors, e.g., noise exposure. A factor that complicates the relationship between drugs and hearing damage is the delayed effect that some medications have on the auditory system. Dihydrostreptomycin, for example, may produce damage to the auditory system up to six months after cessation of therapy.

Virtually all ototoxic effects are signaled by tinnitus, which characteristically precedes audiometric changes. Patients taking any known or suspected ototoxic drug should be told to inform their physician at once if tinnitus occurs so that adjustments in medication can be made when feasible. Serial audiometric monitoring and vestibular studies using electronystagmography are essential in such instances. Since ototoxic drugs affect primarily the cochlear hair cells, the potential for severe irreversible sensorineural hearing loss from these agents should be considered whenever they are prescribed, particularly to patients with any of the noted risk factors.

Ménière's Disease. Ménière's disease, while not nearly as frequent as any of the causes of sensorineural hearing loss previously described, probably causes more suffering and anguish than all other auditory disorders combined. The typical patient complains of a true *rotary vertigo* (illusion of movement); a fluctuating, low-frequency sensorineural hearing loss; tinnitus; nausea and vomiting; and a sensation of "fullness" in the ear. Attacks come in clusters, with periods when the patient is free from symptoms. The hearing loss is unilateral in about 80 per cent of cases, but some of these patients will show bilateral involvement if studied over a period of many years. Audiologically, patients show evidence of a cochlear site of lesion, and speech discrimination is markedly affected during the Ménière's

attack. Ménière's disease is believed to involve a dilatation of the endolymphatic spaces (endolymphatic hydrops) resulting from an increase of endolymph, and a specific etiologic agent can be established in 55 per cent of affected patients.[48] Patients should be evaluated for food allergy with one of the newer diagnostic procedures (RAST, cytotoxic test) as well as for possible endocrine disturbances, including impaired glucose metabolism.[32, 47, 64]

Ménière's disease has been called the number one unsolved problem in clinical otology. It has been treated with an extraordinary array of medical and surgical approaches, few subject to controlled investigation of any kind. Some patients with intractable forms of the disease require surgical intervention. The long-term benefits of surgery, particularly those procedures designed to preserve hearing, are controversial. There is a persistent danger that a patient who has had a total ablation of cochlear and vestibular function may at some time in the future develop symptoms in the opposite ear. In addition to ongoing care by the otolaryngologist, patients with Ménière's disease should be evaluated and managed by audiologists who can select specially designed hearing aids for use during periods when hearing sensitivity and speech discrimination are sufficiently depressed to warrant assistance. Special modifications of existing hearing-aid circuits may be required by these patients to compensate for various forms of nonlinear distortion and for severely reduced tolerance. Auditory training and speechreading are strongly indicated for many of these patients.

Viral and Bacterial Disease. The most common viral cause of unilateral sensorineural hearing loss is *mumps,* which typically produces a total unilateral loss without involvement of the vestibular system. *Measles* and *chicken pox* can cause bilateral hearing impairment. *Bacterial meningitis* may damage both the cochlear and vestibular systems. Other bacterial diseases implicated in sensorineural hearing loss are *typhoid fever, diphtheria,* and *scarlet fever.* Scarlet fever can cause a purulent otitis media in addition to inner-ear damage, resulting in a mixed hearing loss. The importance of immunization against diseases such as measles and mumps cannot be overemphasized. Prenatal rubella is discussed below.

Sudden Deafness. While most sensori-neural hearing loss is typically characterized by insidious onset, some persons lose their hearing suddenly, often reporting the condition upon awakening. The etiology is obscure but is believed to result from either a viral labyrinthitis causing inner-ear changes, similar to those occurring in mumps deafness, or a vascular occlusion (spasm, embolism) affecting the blood supply to the inner ear. Some persons report sudden loss of hearing after exposure to cold. Since approximately 50 per cent of affected persons show spontaneous hearing recovery, often to within normal limits, it is difficult to evaluate the efficacy of any therapeutic regimen. Audiologists, by the performance and interpretation of sophisticated site-of-lesion studies, can usually determine whether the cochlea or the eighth nerve is involved, and treatment can be based in part upon such diagnostic data. Since sudden deafness is a dramatic, frightening condition, most otologists advocate vigorous treatment including vasodilation, anticoagulation, and corticosteroids, the latter particularly when audiologic tests localize the lesion in the auditory nerve.

Familial and Congenital Hearing Loss. There are over 60 types of hereditary hearing loss which can be separated from one another by type of impairment, age at onset, severity, mode of genetic transmission (dominant, recessive, and sex-linked), and associated abnormalities in other systems caused by the same genetic agent. Forty per cent of profound childhood deafness is autosomal recessive in origin, 10 per cent is by dominant transmission, and 3 per cent is by sex-linked gene. A large proportion of affected persons have profound, bilateral sensorineural hearing loss and require special educational facilities. In many cases, the auditory problem is progressive. Genetic counseling represents the major approach to prevention of these conditions.[21]

Congenital hearing losses arise from conditions affecting the birth process, such as birth trauma, or those appearing in the first few days of life, such as icterus neonatorum and kernicterus. Congenital hearing loss also applies to impairments secondary to viruses and other agents that affect the mother during pregnancy. *Maternal* or *prenatal rubella* is the best example. In the 1963-64 rubella epidemic, at least 45 per cent of the children born of mothers with confirmed prenatal rubella showed significant hearing loss, either as the primary deficit or in association with heart and eye defects. Almost any infection, particularly if contracted during the first trimester of pregnancy, can damage the fetus's auditory system.

The Joint Committee on Newborn Hearing has recommended complete otologic and audiologic evaluations on infants with the following conditions:

1. Familial deafness (congenital sensorineural hearing loss in first cousin or closer).
2. Hyperbilirubinemia: 20 mg/100 ml of serum or over.
3. Rubella (or other nonbacterial intra-uterine infection such as cytomegalovirus) during pregnancy.
4. Congenital malformations of ear, nose, or throat (cleft lip and/or palate, multiple anomalies, any first-arch syndrome).
5. Birthweight 1500 grams or less.
6. Apnea and cyanosis (Apgar score 1-4).
7. Severe infection (neonatal).

Lesions of the Eighth Nerve. Acoustic neurinoma accounts for over half of all tumors involving the cerebellopontine angle.[19] The tumor is believed to produce signs and symptoms typically between 30 and 40 years of age and older. However, with modern diagnostic techniques, the identification of these tumors can be made at an early age, and it is not unusual for these conditions to be diagnosed in the second decade of life.

The usual site of origin of an acoustic tumor is the vestibular portion of the eighth cranial nerve in the region of Scarpa's ganglion. These tumors are believed to originate frequently in the internal auditory canal. They enlarge slowly within the canal and can produce bony erosion extending toward the cerebellopontine angle. The initial symptoms of these tumors are hearing impairment, unsteadiness of gait, and tinnitus. Tinnitus typically develops in association with hearing impairment but can be the only presenting symptom. Patients may report only a distortion or alteration of the quality of sound in the affected side, with no significant impairment in hearing sensitivity. Abnormal tone decay and abnormalities of the stapedial reflex are often present. Dizziness in the form of an unsteadiness occurs as an early symptom in about 80 per cent of patients. True vertigo is less common, occurring in about a third of patients, but may become a significant symptom as the tumor enlarges. Other early complaints are a prickling sensation, an itching sensation, and pain in the affected ear.

Diagnostic evaluation of these conditions includes an audiologic battery with tests for abnormal auditory adaptation and BERA, vestibular evaluation using electronystagmography, neuroradiologic studies using polytomography, and posterior fossa myelography with contrast media when the suspicion of a tumor is high. Abnormalities in the stapedial reflex are found in 83 to 85 per cent of acoustic tumors. However, BERA is believed to be the most accurate audiologic method of identifying tumors, with a reported success rate of 95 to 98 per cent correct identification. It is important to note that audiologic site-of-lesion studies cannot at this stage determine the *nature* of the lesion, although the *site* of the lesion is correctly identified in an impressive percentage of patients. Degenerative, inflammatory, and vascular lesions of the eighth nerve often show a constellation of audiologic responses identical to those found in space-occupying lesions of the eighth nerve.

Persons with Exaggerated Hearing Levels. "Emotionally based" hearing problems are of two types: psychogenic and malingering. *Psychogenic deafness* is a form of conversion hysteria in which a serious emotional problem is converted into an apparent inability to hear. *Volitional hearing impairment* or *malingering* is a conscious simulation of hearing loss on the part of an individual who wishes to convince the examiner that his hearing problem is greater than is actually the case. The wide variety of tests for the detection of these conditions (also referred to as *nonorganic* or *functional* hearing impairments or *pseudohypacusis)* include various forms of electrophysiologic audiometry, such as BERA, that do not involve any voluntary response on the part of the patient under evaluation.

Central Auditory Impairments. Central auditory impairments result from lesions affecting the brain stem pathway in the lateral lemniscus and the primary auditory project area on the superior temporal gyri of the temporal cortex (Heschl's gyrus). In general, tests of auditory function that are used in the evaluation of peripheral auditory disorders will be useless in the demonstration of a central auditory lesion. Patients with unilateral temporal-lobe disease typically show a deficit in understanding distorted speech on the ear contralateral to the affected temporal lobe. Tests for central auditory lesions involve a variety of frequency-distorted word tests, speech in the presence of a competing message presented either ipsilaterally or contralaterally, periodically interrupted speech stimuli, and other methods of reducing the external redundancy of the speech message.[6, 32]

Tinnitus

Tinnitus is a subjective sensation of sound in the head which may be localized in one or both ears or perceived in the cranial area. It may be described as a throbbing, hissing, whistling, booming, clicking, buzzing, roaring, or high-pitched tone or as noise. Tinnitus may result from an auditory impairment in any location within the auditory pathway. It may have a vascular, muscular, or hormonal origin. Any disease or injury capable of affecting the auditory system may be accompanied by tinnitus.

Tinnitus is believed to affect over 37 million Americans. For some individuals, tinnitus may be as disabling as a hearing loss or more so. Desperate sufferers have submitted to a variety of surgical procedures that sometimes involve sacrificing the hearing of the affected ear, and some patients have not obtained relief of tinnitus even after such destructive procedures have been performed, suggesting a central rather than a peripheral basis for the symptom. Suicide attempts have been reported in some tinnitus sufferers unable to obtain relief from the condition.

Occasionally, tinnitus is objective and can be heard by the examiner. Among the reported causes of objective tinnitus are palatal myoclonus, tensor-tympani or stapedial myoclonus, and an abnormally patent eustachian tube. Vascular abnormalities can also cause objective tinnitus and include arteriovenous fistulas and hemangiomas of the external ear. A plaque in the internal carotid artery may also cause this condition. It is *subjective tinnitus,* also called static, nonvibratory, or intrinsic tinnitus, which accounts by far for the largest number of patients suffering from the condition.

Tinnitus is a symptom that may reflect a wide array of otic and auditory problems, many of which are treatable by medical, surgical, and rehabilitative measures. All patients complaining of this condition should receive a complete diagnostic evaluation, including careful case history, physical examination, audiologic site-of-lesion studies, and, when indicated, neuroradiography and vestibular studies.

A large number of patients have disabling tinnitus related to noise exposure, head injury, or ototoxic medication. Some patients obtain relief by medical management. Vasodilators, histamine, large doses of vitamin A, xylocaine, and Tegretol are among the substances that are used. Patients who are "borderline" hearing-aid candidates may obtain relief from a hearing aid that masks the tinnitus when the instrument is in use. The hearing aid should be used in the ear in which the tinnitus is more severe, and binaural aids should be considered for patients with bilateral tinnitus.

Biofeedback and tinnitus maskers are now employed for some patients with intractable tinnitus unresponsive to other therapies. Biofeedback seeks to achieve muscle relaxation and increased circulation.[27] An electromyographic device allows the patient to experience the electrical output of the frontalis muscle by viewing a voltmeter and listening to clicks relayed to him by earphones. The peripheral vasculature is dilated by raising the temperature of the finger. Some patients can learn muscle relaxation in 12 one-hour visits. Biofeedback appears to be most useful in patients who are extremely anxious about the condition. Tension appears to exacerbate the patient's perception of his tinnitus, causing it to become subjectively louder. When the patient learns to relax physically, it is hoped, he is able to reduce his apprehension and tension and achieve greater control of his response to the problem.

Tinnitus maskers are usually built into a postauricular hearing-aid chassis, although they can also be mounted in an all-in-the-ear housing. The object is to mask the patient's tinnitus with a band of white noise.[46] A volume control allows the patient to adjust the gain of the instrument to a level that just masks his tinnitus. The majority of tinnitus sufferers match their tinnitus with a frequency of 2000 Hz or higher. The tinnitus masker is a relatively innocuous, noninvasive method of providing relief from this condition and should be considered for patients whose auditory problems have been comprehensively evaluated by competent specialists who have ruled out significant organic and psychological pathology. Double-blind studies are necessary to determine whether the masker provides significant improvement rather than a distraction or a placebo effect. Long-term follow-up of patients using the maskers is essential to determine persistence of the benefits and any as-yet-unknown side effects.

Additional Disabilities

The patient's presenting complaint, hearing impairment, or deformity of the ears may so occupy the rehabilitator's attention that secondary disabilities are overlooked. Yet these additional problems are often critical factors in the patient's rehabilitation. Another disability tends to multiply, rather than add to, the problems of hearing loss. As a rule, the presence of a hearing impairment raises the probability of another disability. Among deaf school children, for example, about one in three has an additional educationally handicapping condition.[53] Similar findings emerge in studies of hearing-impaired adults. Of critical importance is the intactness of visual functioning. The more impaired the individual's hearing, the more dependent he or she becomes on vision.[57] Planning for auditory rehabilitation must take into account all of a patient's limitations and assets, not hearing ability as an isolated factor.

TREATMENT OF HEARING IMPAIRMENT

Treatment of hearing impairment depends generally on three factors: type of loss (conductive, sensorineural, or mixed), degree, and age at onset. Available treatments, in turn, fall into three large categories: surgical-medical intervention, corrective amplification, and education. These treatments often overlap, of course, with patients receiving two or more procedures from among these broad categories. The management of hearing impairment should also include counseling at every stage in treatment. Because of the ubiquitous need for it, counseling is alluded to in each section.

Surgical-Medical Intervention

Conductive losses are generally amenable to medical and/or surgical management of impairment. The degree of conductive impairment and the status of the patient's bone conduction and speech discrimination influence the decision to operate. However, the age at onset does not. Regardless of how long or short the duration of the loss, its reversal is considered worthwhile. Procedures range from repair and reconstruction of the tympanic membrane (myringoplasty) to replacement of the ossicles. In some instances, plastic surgery on the outer ear may be indicated to construct an absent pinna or otologic surgery to open the external canal. The vastly increased ability to surgically correct conductive hearing problems reinforces the value of prompt, accurate diagnosis. Mixed losses do not provide the same degree of hearing recovery that conductive losses do. Nonetheless, consideration should be given to removing the conductive component of the loss, thus restoring a portion of the hearing ability.

Many eighth-nerve tumors are surgically removed and, depending on the surgical route employed, hearing may be preserved. However, hearing preservation is not the primary objective of such procedures. Various surgical procedures are employed by some otologists for patients with Ménière's disease, but the primary objective in these cases is relief from intractable vertigo. The extent to which surgery improves hearing is controversial. Prevention is critical in the case of noise-induced hearing loss, ototoxicity, and prenatal rubella, but medical-surgical treatment is of little avail for such conditions as presbycusis. (Inner-ear surgery to improve hearing is not yet deemed appropriate by most otologists; however, see the section below on cochlear implants, a procedure now being investigated.)

In addition to surgery, medication, and related tactics, complete management should include counseling directed at adjusting to the emotional impact accompanying sensory impairment and preparing the patient to accept limitations and overcome handicaps that remain after treatment (vide infra). In particular, patients should be given an opportunity to realistically appraise their condition and any therapeutic limitations.

The Cochlear Implant

The object of the cochlear implant is to provide hearing in a deaf ear by electrical stimulation of the auditory nerve. Efforts have been directed at implanting one or more electrodes permanently in the cochlea of patients with no residual hearing. The indwelling prosthesis is designed to deliver electrical stimuli to remaining nerve fibers and to provide selective stimulation, related to acoustic frequency, for different nerve fibers through multiple electrodes — a goal that has not yet been successfully achieved. Implants in use in the United States employ, for the most part, a single intracochlear electrode. One or more fine-wired electrodes are introduced through the round window or through holes drilled into the scala tympani. Such implants have not rendered speech intelligible, but implanted subjects report the ability to recognize familiar environmental sounds and an improved ability to maintain some auditory contact with the world around them. Intensity discrimination in implants subjects is reportedly good, but frequency discrimination is poor.[44]

At this time, the use of cochlear implants must be considered experimental. Some implant subjects are initially pleased by their ability to detect certain sounds but later become frustrated by their inability to discriminate speech. Candidates for implants should be adults with adventitious hearing loss and no residual hearing in the ear to be implanted. Only patients with sensory, rather than neural, deficits should be considered. Candidates should be told to expect some improvements in auditory awareness and gross discrimination but not in speech discrimination. The human cochlea contains 25,000 to 30,000 nerve fibers working together to allow the auditory discriminations necessary for normal function. We are not yet near the point at which this system can be reproduced with a cochlear prosthesis. Special, intensive audiologic rehabilitation is indicated for implanted patients.

Hearing Aids

The hearing aid is the major tool of audiologic rehabilitation and should be considered for all persons with medically irreversible forms of hearing impairment. A hearing aid is any device which brings sound more effectively to the ear of the listener and, by this broad definition, includes the ear trumpet, the hand cupped behind the ear, and the acoustic fan.

With rapid development of various forms of electroacoustic amplification, few persons with hearing impairments seriously consider the nonelectronic forms. Microminiaturized transistor circuits allow us to present speech at a comfortable and tolerable level to virtually all hearing-impaired persons, except those with profoundly impaired speech discrimination and no measurable hearing responses. Persons whose hearing impairment is too severe to enable them to comprehend speech may still benefit from amplification sufficient for detection of low-frequency components of some of the vowels as well as nonspeech sounds, thus improving contact with their auditory environment and providing clues that can aid speechreading.

Many persons with "borderline" auditory problems who would not have accepted a body-mounted hearing aid (Fig. 44–9) now derive significant benefit from small, easily carried hearing aids mounted entirely in or near the ear and used for selected listening situations. Because of improvements in hearing-aid design during the last 20 years, virtually all individuals with any degree of significant difficulty in social or professional listening situations can derive sub-

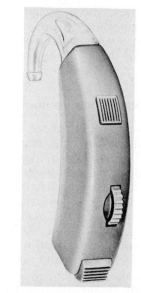

FIGURE 44–10. A postauricular (behind-the-ear) hearing aid.

stantial benefit from ear-level amplification. Increasingly, audiologists question the classic indications for hearing-aid candidacy (a pure-tone average of 40 dB or more in the better ear) and evaluate suitable forms of wearable amplification for *all* persons reporting difficulty in listening situations important to their daily lives.[38]

All hearing aids have the following basic components: a microphone that converts sound into electrical energy, an amplifier that increases the strength of the electrical signal, and a receiver or an earphone that converts the amplified signal back into acoustic energy. The system is energized by a battery. The output may be fed into either an air-conduction receiver or a bone-conduction vibrator.

The basic types of electroacoustic hearing aids are:

Behind-the-Ear or Postauricular Hearing Aid. This type of instrument accounts for 60 to 65 per cent of hearing aids purchased today and is shown in Figure 44–10. Postauricular hearing aids do not interfere with the wearing of eyeglasses, so the hearing aid can be used with or without spectacles, an advantage for persons whose use of hearing aids and eyeglasses does not coincide. Figure 44–11 pictures an *eyeglass* hearing aid in which the amplifier, microphone, and receiver are built into the temple of the spectacles.

All-in-the-Ear Hearing Aids. These have

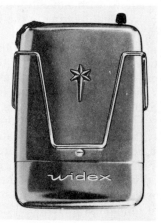

FIGURE 44–9. A body-mounted hearing aid.

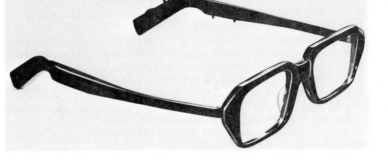

FIGURE 44–11. An eyeglass hearing aid.

grown in popularity enormously in recent years and now account for 20 to 25 per cent of new hearing aids purchased (see Fig. 44–12). Improvements in design significantly reduce the problems of acoustic feedback, expand the frequency response, reduce distortion, and allow the incorporation of features formerly available only with larger instruments, e.g., compression circuits to limit the saturation SPL of the instrument.

Body-Worn Hearing Aids. These were the predominant method of mounting hearing aids in the pretransistorized era, but they have shown a sharp decrease in popularity and now account for only 3 to 5 per cent of hearing aids purchased (see Fig. 44–9). The decline in these instruments has paralleled the improved performance of ear-level aids. True binaural hearing is not possible with body-mounting hearing aids, one of a number of advantages of mounting the entire instrument in or near the ear. Other disadvantages of the body-type aid are the noise that results from layers of clothing rubbing against the microphone and the awkward position required for use of the telephone with this type of instrument.

In terms of its functions, the hearing aid must also have the following characteristics:

Gain. A hearing aid must provide sufficient amplification to compensate for the degree of hearing loss present. The gain of an amplifying system refers to the difference between the input (microphone) and output (receiver) of the system.

Output. Output is the level of the input signal plus the gain of the hearing aid. *Maximum output* or *saturation sound-pressure level* refers to the maximum-power-handling capacity of the aid. Every amplifying system must impose a restriction on the strength of the signal delivered by the hearing aid so that the user's tolerance level for loud sounds is not exceeded. Maximum output must be achieved without excessively distorting the speech signal. *Peak clipping* (eliminating the crests of sound waves) has traditionally been used to achieve output control, but this is often accomplished at a sacrifice of speech intelligibility, particularly when only the positive portion of the sound waves is clipped. Various forms of compression amplification are now available in which the gain of the hearing aid is automatically reduced when the intensity of the input signal reaches a predetermined level. Time constants must be carefully specified to prevent degradation of the speech signal and a "flutter" or "thump" sound in the system. Careful selection of the appropriate maximum-output levels represents a critical factor in determining successful adjustment to a hearing aid, especially in hearing-impaired persons with *recruitment* (an abnormal increase of the loudness of the sound as its

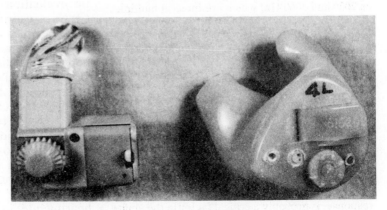

FIGURE 44–12. Two types of in-the-ear hearing aids.

intensity is raised above the impaired threshold) and a restricted range of comfortable loudness. Patients who are "overfit" will find the hearing aid an unpleasant and uncomfortable experience. The recognition of the significance of this factor in affecting hearing-aid performance and the conduct of tests of tolerance as part of the hearing-aid evaluation has led to successful use of hearing aids by many previously "unfittable" patients.

Frequency Response. This refers to the range of frequencies that a particular hearing aid amplifies. The microphone generally limits the low-frequency response of the system, while the receiver limits the high-frequency response. There is a strong relationship between the high-frequency response of the hearing aid and the user's ability to discriminate speech in quiet and in noise. Since frequencies over 1000 Hz contribute 60 per cent of the intelligibility of speech (but account for only 5 per cent of total power), excessive amplification in the low frequencies can mask the weak consonant sounds and adversely affect the understanding of speech. Furthermore, many hearing-aid users have relatively good unaided hearing for low frequencies and require less amplification in this portion of the range. Appropriate modification of the frequency response so that greater amplification is provided in the high-frequency range (through 6000 to 7000 Hz, when indicated) is, second only to proper control of maximum output, the most important determinant of successful hearing-aid use.

Distortion. Distortion occurs when the output of an amplifying system is not a faithful reproduction of the input signal. All amplifying systems distort to some extent and the relatively low fidelity of portable hearing aids tends to produce significant distortion. To add to the problem, current hearing-aid users are invariably persons with some form of sensorineural hearing loss for whom even low levels of distortion may be unacceptable.

Most audiologic attention has been directed to *harmonic distortion*. This occurs when signals other than the input are produced at the output. When a tone of 1000 Hz is introduced into a hearing-aid microphone, other frequencies, such as 2000 and 3000 Hz, which are integral multiples of the basic frequency, may occur at the output. *Intermodulation distortion* occurs when the output contains a greater number of components than the input. These frequencies are arithmetic sums and differences of two or more frequencies. *Transient distortion* is present whenever the hearing aid is unable to duplicate accurately the initial onset or sudden decay of a sound. The result is a "lingering" of the wave form, causing a ringing sound. Many speech sounds such as /p/ and /k/ are transient in nature, and the ringing referred to can seriously hamper speech discrimination. Transient distortion, which appears related to the presence of sharp resonant peaks in the frequency response, is probably a critical factor in the ability of persons with sensorineural hearing loss to discriminate speech in noise. Unfortunately, current hearing-aid standards do not specify the conditions for measurement of this form of distortion, and manufacturers generally do not include transient distortion data in their specifications.

New Developments in Hearing Aids. A detailed discussion of the various developments in hearing aids is beyond the scope of this chapter, and the reader is urged to consult one or more of the excellent references on the subject.[5, 10, 46] Among these advances are directional microphones, the electret condensor microphone, various sophisticated output-limiting circuits, and open earmolds. Hearing aids that pick up a signal from the side of a poorly or nonfunctioning ear and route to the side of the better-hearing ear (Contralateral Routing of Signals, or CROS, aids) have been developed in an almost endless number of variations providing great assistance for persons with audiograms characterized by precipitous high-frequency dropoffs as well as those with other "hard-to-fit" configurations. Wearable, ear-level, binaural hearing aids are available and are in widespread use by many hearing-impaired persons, including prelingually hearing-impaired children and blind-deaf persons. Their use should be evaluated by audiologists who can make appropriate selections in relation to specific audiologic manifestations and in carefully controlled sound-field evaluations with different systems. Hearing aids should always be evaluated both in quiet and in noise; the signal-to-noise ratios should simulate those the patient will be likely to encounter in everyday listening.

Management of the Sensorineural Hearing-Impaired Patient. After a complete diagnostic evaluation has been done and the patient's sensorineural hearing impairment is established as medically irreversible, the audiologist is a key professional in meeting the patient's audiologic rehabilitative needs. Under controlled conditions, he determines first whether the use of a hearing aid is justified. If such indication is established, he will, through tests of aided performance in properly sound-isolated environments, seek the answers to a series of important clinical questions. On which ear should the hearing aid be used, or should the aid be alternated from one ear to the other? Is a binaural hearing aid indicated? Air conduction or bone conduction? Earmold type? Special circuit modifications? In one widely used system of hearing-aid evaluation, he will then select from representative samples of current hearing aids several that are appropriate for the type and degree of hearing loss present. On the basis of the patient's performance with these instruments in the *hearing-aid evaluation,* he will recommend an amplifying system that meets the needs of the patient. He will either sell the hearing aid himself or refer the patient to a reliable hearing-aid dealer in the patient's community. Follow-up services after the hearing aid is obtained are critical to the overall success of the rehabilitation and should be arranged when the aid is acquired.[24, 52]

Emotional Impact

The rehabilitator who ignores the emotional impact of hearing loss cannot hope to be optimally effective. Wright[75] has illuminated the natural history of any acquired physical disability: from initial shock to mourning to revised values and eventual positive adjustment. At each phase, the rehabilitator has an important role to play. Most importantly, the rehabilitator must be aware of any tendencies to pass over or move too quickly through any phase. Wright's thesis, supported by subsequent research, is that the phases are *natural*; newly disabled persons need to go through them and resolve the powerful emotions aroused at each step. An important task of rehabilitators, in addition to implementing the technical knowledge at their command, is to assist the patient to gain emotional acceptance of the new status imposed by the impairment. Without that acceptance, rehabilitation will be impeded.[50, 65]

Dealing with the emotional concomitants of acquired physical disability may require skills beyond those the rehabilitator has acquired. In such instances, competent psychiatric and psychological assistance should be sought. Counseling or psychotherapy may be conducted in one-to-one, group, or a combination of individual and group sessions.[7, 57] It may precede other therapeutic intervention, follow it, or be coincident with it. Even if the rehabilitator manages the counseling personally, consultation with mental health experts may prove to be a valuable therapeutic adjunct.

What about congenital hearing impairments? The gradual awareness that typically occurs tends to cushion the emotional shock for the born-deaf and prelingually deafened child. That is not true, however, for parents who are told that their young child is deaf.[41] For them, it is a shock. Parental counseling should be routinely offered to parents who receive such information. They will tend to pass through the same phases mentioned above, even though their child, not they, has suffered the loss. Attempting to undertake education and rehabilitation of young children without first attending to the parents' emotional adjustment will prove partially, if not wholly, ineffective.[61] Parents frequently report that they heard nothing the professional said after giving them the child's diagnosis, despite vigorous efforts on the practitioner's part to inform them about critical next steps in treatment.

Most unfortunate are parents who have been told of their child's deafness by a diagnostician whose entire demeanor suggests a death sentence rather than a diagnosis. Equally incongruous is being cheerful when confronting parents with what they regard as very bad news. The appropriate attitude might best be characterized as *understanding* and *hopeful* — understanding of the parent's bitter feelings and hopeful about the child's future.[41] Above all, the practitioner must recognize the function of time. Parental adjustment will not be instantaneous even in the most competent practitioner's hands. Some time is essential for recovery from depression, working through of anger, and resolving the value hierarchy they have acquired over years. How much is needed will vary from person to person. The practitioner must monitor the reactions, set aside or provide time for counseling, and in these ways assist the clients and parents to acquire facilitating attitudes toward their own or their child's rehabilitation. If an emotional disorder coexists with a hearing impairment, it will require the special skills of psychologists and psychiatrists in its management. Hearing impairment and psychosis may be present in such disorders as prenatal rubella.

Auditory Training

After the aid has been selected, the audiologist will schedule a series of visits to work with the patient on initial adjustment to the hearing aid. Trial or rental periods are often arranged so that the hearing aid can be returned with a minimum of expense to the patient, if a satisfactory level of performance cannot be achieved. An extended period of audiologic rehabilitation will be necessary for some individuals. Patients with very poor discrimination, excessive recruitment, and a narrow dynamic range should not be issued a hearing aid unless first enrolled in an extensive audiologic rehabilitative program in which adjustment to various amplifying systems is carefully monitored (see discussion of phonemic regression above). Systematic training in speech discrimination in various listening situations will be necessary for many persons with sensorineural hearing impairments. For others, acceptance of and adjustment to hearing aids are realized early.

The hearing-aid user should be counseled about the limitations of amplification in relation to his particular auditory problems and needs. His concerns and fears about his hearing loss and its interaction with the hearing aid must be managed with consummate professional skill. The initial fear that many persons feel about using an electronic apparatus must be confronted. The loss of manual dexterity, particularly among elderly persons, affects their ability to manipulate the small controls of the hearing aid, to change the battery, and to insert the earmold into the ear. These seemingly simple mechanical operations must be demonstrated to them over and over again, with support and assistance offered until success is finally achieved. Audiologists' role in the acceptance of and adjustment to amplification and their ability to improve receptive listening skills through special training are potent determinants of the successful use of hearing aids. In a very real sense, their responsibility to the hearing-impaired patient *begins* on the day when the patient obtains the recommended hearing aid.

Other Adaptive Devices

Hearing impairments diminish or eliminate the ability to use telecommunications. Also, hearing losses affect many everyday activities that involve devices that emit auditory signals. Recently, means have been developed to surmount auditory barriers to using the telephone and to enjoying television,[60] as well as to compensate for hearing loss in other mundane activities.

Telephone Adaptation Devices. Telephone adaptation devices (TADs) send audible signals over the telephone lines to machines at the receiving end, which convert the signals to visible form. At present, there are a half dozen versions. Each has a keyboard, a coupler which attaches to the telephone mouthpiece, and a message display. The machines differ in size, portability, type of keyboard, and display. They are important to deaf people, because they provide easy access to facilities not otherwise possible. Deaf people, of course, can make telephone calls through interpreters, friends, and relatives. TADs give the deaf person some added independence and increased employability. As more and more TADs come into place, the social and economic disadvantages the telephone imposes on deaf people will be lifted.

Captioned Television. Since early 1980, many television programs have carried *captions* — printed versions of the spoken transmission. The captions are "hidden"; i.e., they are broadcast over the vertical blanking interval (line 21 on U.S. television sets), so they are seen only on sets equipped with a special decoder. Organizations interested in hearing-impaired people, particularly the National Association of the Deaf, have fought vigorously to win this concession from the television industry. Captioned television promises to greatly alleviate the social isolation caused by severe hearing impairment.[55]

Home Appliances. Appliances can usually be fitted with light-signaling adaptations to replace the auditory signal. The doorbell can be wired so that when it is rung it flashes the lights in any or all rooms in the house. Alarm clocks can turn on lights or activate a vibrator placed under the deaf persons's pillow. The National Association of the Deaf (814 Thayer Avenue, Silver Spring, Md., 20910) issues a catalogue describing a variety of these and other pieces of equipment for the deaf householder. Merely knowing such devices are available can give the newly hearing-impaired person a psychological boost, for their abundance and ready availability indicate that many people share the same problem.

Education and Training

Loss of hearing confers on the afflicted individual no compensatory gains. What must be done to overcome the disability must be learned. The task of the rehabilitator is to teach the adaptive means for coping with the problems hearing loss engenders and for using devices, especially hearing aids, designed to compensate for the loss. Hearing aids and other adaptive devices have been discussed above, along with auditory training. What follows are educational strategies for living with a hearing loss.

Since hearing loss principally interferes with interpersonal communication, these strategies are directed toward the communication barriers and their emotional accompaniments. The age of the individual at the time hearing is impaired heavily affects educational and rehabilitation planning. This fact will be indicated with respect to each of the ensuing discussions of educational intervention.

Speech. Speech, once established, is usually not lost because of a hearing impairment, but articulation and voice quality may deteriorate in cases of progressive or sudden hearing loss.[66] Early, severe hearing loss does, however, affect speech development. Prelingually deaf children can learn to speak well, but few currently do.[11, 34] These frequent failures, in view of the occasional successes, are more likely due to lack of adequate education than to inherent inability to acquire speech (see section on language which follows). Readers may wrongly infer that the preceding statement unfairly condemns the valiant teachers who struggle so hard to develop deaf children's speaking abilities. Readers might alternatively assume the statement merely urges that more of the educational day be devoted specifically to developing speech. Neither position reflects our view. We recognize the awesome task of teaching speech via proprioceptive, tactual, and visual clues, in the absence of auditory feedback. To us, the solution to prelingually deaf children's present lack of success in developing more intelligible speech lies not in the amount of time expended but in the methods selected to teach speech. When success is not attained, the procedures, not the child, should be suspected, and new approaches should be sought to attain the educational objectives.[11, 34, 40] Admittedly, excellent speech development for every born-deaf child may be an overly idealistic goal for educators. However, even a little speech can be useful in our highly oral culture. Socioeconomic success has been, and

probably can continue to be, attained without it.[59] The development of language, however, is another matter, for we distinguish between speech (a motor ability) and language (a symbol system).[14]

For the person deafened after speech has been established, the problem becomes one of maintaining its good quality. Postlingually deafened children must not only be encouraged to continue using their speech, but they must also be given feedback to assist them with melody, rhythm, articulation, and loudness. While less critical as age at onset increases, speech conservation retains an important place in rehabilitation of children and adults.[66] They need instruction on how to adjust the volume of their speech in response to extra-auditory cues, to avoid misarticulations, and to retain normal voice quality. Retention of good speech after hearing impairment is far less difficult than developing speech without auditory feedback; however, the value of retaining this ability makes critical the provisions for speech conservation in the rehabilitation process for hearing-impaired adults.

Speechreading refers to determining what a speaker is saying by observation rather than hearing per se. An alternative term, *lipreading,* suggests that the observations are of the lips alone. However, other cues, especially situational and contextual ones, are usually critical in deciphering a particular message. For that reason, we prefer the term *speechreading,* because it implies that a broader range of stimuli are involved. That information other than lip movements is essential to speechreading is established by the disparity between the 40 or more phonemes in spoken language and the 16 discriminable shapes of the lips.[4] By observing one's own lips in a mirror while successively saying "time" and "dime" or "bare," "pair," and "mare," one quickly can grasp the speechreader's major difficulty — *homophenes,* words that look exactly or almost alike on the lips.

To what extent can speechreading be taught? Some people seem to acquire the skill readily, others not.[4, 43, 45] Since less than half the visual differentiation of speech can be determined from the principal source, the lips, the good speechreader must make use of other information. Knowledge of the language appears critical, as does familiarity with the culture. If a well-dressed stranger stops you on the street and asks, "Do you have (a dime)/(the time)?'' the latter choice is the likely one. At a party, you would have little difficulty choosing the correct choice from among "Do you want a (bear)/(mare)/(pair)/(beer)?'' Of the four homophenes, the last has the highest probability in the circumstances. Making use of cultural-linguistic cues is easier for the person who loses hearing later in life than for the born-deaf person. The former has more exposure to language and generally more acquaintance with the culture. That is why, contrary to popular belief, normally hearing adults, as a group, are better speechreaders than the average prelingually deaf person.

Prospective speechreaders can be taught to make use of their residual hearing. They need to be alerted to variations in speech rhythms and to ways of combining visual with whatever auditory information they can perceive. In addition, they can learn to imitate what they see, in order to make use of proprioception. Such instruction can bolster the speechreader's confidence, another major factor. Good speechreaders appear to be good linguistic gamblers; they bet on the most likely outcome. When subsequent reactions indicate it, they must also be willing to drop an apparently poor guess and make another.

Sharpening visual perception and sensitizing the speechreader to language nuances can be achieved in the instructional setting. The personality qualities contributing to speechreading may not be developed in the classroom. Some rehabilitation programs use group strategies to help speechreaders overcome their reluctance to approach a conversational situation flexibly and with minimal embarrassment. Sharing frustrations and emotional upset with similarly affected persons seems to increase many speechreaders' confidence in their eventual ability to succeed.

There are a number of methods of teaching speechreading. Each offers its own emphases, sequence of lessons, and drills.[4, 43, 45] No one method will be optimal for all persons. The speechreading instructor should have a variety of methods and materials to meet the varying needs of hearing-impaired students. Counseling must help avoid the disastrous consequences of overly high expectations. Speechreading cannot fully compensate for a hearing loss. The hearing-impaired person who continually finds he is not getting precise information may feel depressed by his own inadequacy. He must understand that the process itself is not wholly adequate; it is a good supplement but a limited one. Understanding the limitations of speechreading will add to, not subtract from, its usefulness.

Language. Language deficits are common among prelingually deaf persons. On standardized tests of English, the average deaf 18-year-old student scores at about a fourth-grade level — a score indicating virtual illiteracy.[51] The extent of the language deficit correlates with age at onset, as well as degree, of hearing impairment. As noted above, even relatively mild losses of hearing may give rise to academic retardation.

Linguists now recognize that American Sign Language (Ameslan), used by most early deafened adults, meets all the criteria for a language.[2, 25, 33, 74] As will be discussed next, the language deficit found among early deafened persons is an English-language deficit. The same individuals may be fluent in Ameslan. Thus, their language deficiency, as with their speech defects, may be due more to inadequate educational strategies than to any inherent weakness in learning potential. Indeed, considerable ancillary evidence supports that conclusion.[40] Most instruction in public schools is auditory; instruction by visual means has not received the same attention from educators.

The language deficits associated with early hearing impairments call for special education. Where to provide this education — in residential schools, day schools, special classes, or regular classes — depends upon many factors: the child, his family, and available community resources.[9] Regardless of where it is given, special attention to language is critical to the academic development of deaf children.

Manual Communication. A great deal of emotion has clouded the consideration of manual communication in rehabilitation. "Talking with one's hands" has negative connotations in our culture. Manual communication, however, has undeniable advantages for hearing-impaired persons. It requires no special equipment. It is entirely visual. Anything that can be expressed through speech can be expressed manually.

Manual communication basically takes two forms in the United States: Manual English (ME) and Ameslan. ME has a

NATIONAL ASSOCIATION OF THE DEAF

The Manual Alphabet
(as seen by the receiver)

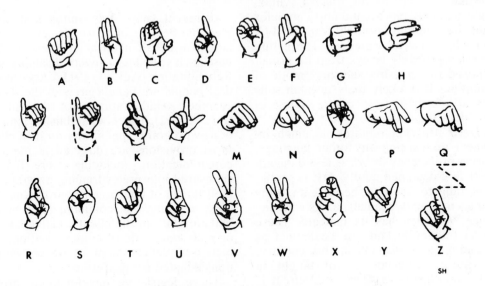

The Manual Alphabet
(as seen by the sender)

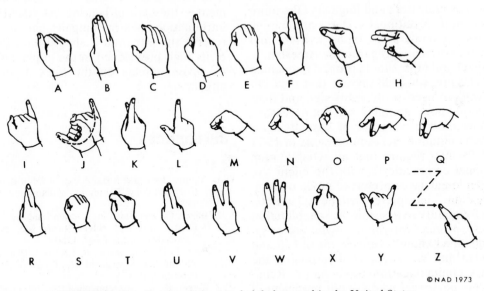

© NAD 1973

FIGURE 44–13. One-handed manual alphabet used in the United States.

number of variations, but they all present English on the hands. *Fingerspelling* (see Fig. 44–13) is a special case of ME: it represents each letter of the alphabet with a distinct hand configuration. To communicate by fingerspelling, one spells each word, letter by letter. Almost all manual communicators make some use of fingerspelling, whether or not they also use signs; it is useful at least to indicate proper names.

Signs are hand-motion configurations that represent concepts. In ME, signs generally stand for words. Signs in ME follow English syntax. In the most elaborate forms of ME, the appropriate linguistic forms are differentiated by adding signs for the suffixes.[25]

Ameslan does not follow English syntax. A single sign may represent a fairly complex thought, i.e., be appropriately translated by an English phrase or sentence.[2] The nature of Ameslan probably grows from its visual, as opposed to English's auditory, mode of presentation. It is likely that Ameslan suits the visual information-processing system as English does the auditory.

To learn Ameslan requires as much involvement as learning any other language. Acquiring proficiency in ME is less demanding. For late deafened adults, ME is probably preferable to Ameslan, because it closely resembles their native language. As with any language, Ameslan has its dialects. These occur as frequently and are as distinct as American English dialects in this country. Furthermore, Ameslan is not taught in schools and classes for deaf children. It is passed from person to person with all the possibilities for variation which attend an unwritten language that is not formally taught. This situation, however, is about to change, as educators and linguists take more interest in it. Notational systems are coming into use, grammars are being written, and curricula are being prepared for Ameslan.

The rehabilitator should properly conclude from the preceding discussion that deaf clients will not necessarily know sign and that, if they do know sign, they will not necessarily understand all varieties of sign. Because the Rehabilitation Act Amendments of 1978 (P.L. 95–602) require that all rehabilitation personnel communicate with the client "in his own language or preferred mode of communication," interpreters will be called upon more frequently to assist in the rehabilitation process. *Manual interpreters* who are properly qualified know several forms of ME and Ameslan and are adept at determining the client's communication preferences. Rehabilitation personnel who are not proficient in manual communication and who have deaf clients will need to learn how to use interpreters effectively. A good beginning will be made with the realization that employing an interpreter introduces a new element in rehabilitation and that teamwork will be enhanced by consultation with the interpreter before the client is seen. In that way, many problems can be avoided and the client-interpreter-rehabilitator interaction smoothed.[58]

Legislation

In recent years, the United States Congress has become increasingly active in legislating on behalf of disabled persons. Deafness is classified as a severe disability in the Rehabilitation Act of 1973. Accordingly, deaf people are beneficiaries of the recently enacted Rehabilitation Act Amendments (P.L. 95–602). This law establishes a number of new programs specifically for deaf clients. Most provisions are directed at improving communication, including more federally sponsored interpreter-training programs, establishment of interpreter-coordinating facilities, requiring that communication in rehabilitation be "in the client's native language or preferred mode of communication," and increased development of telecommunications adapted for deaf users.[58, 60]

These legislative developments promise greatly increased success in rehabilitation of deaf clients. However, similar attention needs to be directed toward those persons who have lesser degrees of hearing impairment — the hard of hearing. As stated in the introduction, hearing impairment does not receive the attention it should have in view of its high prevalence in the population and its severe effects on the lives of those it afflicts.

REFERENCES

1. Alpiner, J. G. (Ed.): Handbook of Adult Rehabilitative Audiology. Baltimore, Williams and Wilkins, 1978.
2. Baker, C., and Battison, R.: Sign Language and the Deaf Community. Silver Spring, Md., National Association of the Deaf, 1980.
3. Bast, T. H., and Anson, B. J.: The Temporal Bone and the Ear. Springfield, Ill., Charles C Thomas, Publisher, 1949.
4. Berger, K. W.: Speechreading Principles and Methods. Baltimore, National Educational Press, 1972.
5. Berger, K. W., and Millin, J. R.: Hearing aids. *In* Rose, D. E. (Ed.): Audiological Assessment, 2nd Ed. Englewood Cliffs, N.J., Prentice-Hall, Inc., 1978.
6. Bolla, E., and Calearo, C.: Central hearing processes. *In* Jerger, J. (Ed.): Modern Developments in Audiology. New York, Academic Press, Inc., 1963.

7. Bowe, F. G., and Schein, J. D.: Group strategies with deaf and hearing-impaired patients. *In* Seligman, M. (Ed.): Group Counseling and Group Psychotherapy with Rehabilitation Clients. Springfield, Ill., Charles C Thomas, Publishers, 1977.

8. Brackman, D. E., Selters, W. A., and Don, M.: Electric response audiometry. *In* Paparella, M., and Shumrich, D. A. (Eds.): Otolaryngology. Philadelphia, W. B. Saunders Company, 1980.

9. Brill, R. G.: The Education of the Deaf. Washington, D.C., Gallaudet College Press, 1974.

10. Briskey, R. J.: Binaural hearing aids and new innovations. *In* Katz, J. (Ed.): Handbook of Clinical Audiology, 2nd Ed. Baltimore, Williams and Wilkins, 1978.

11. Calvert, D. R., and Silverman, S. R.: Speech and Deafness. Washington, D.C., A. G. Bell Association for the Deaf, 1975.

12. Carver, W. F.: Loudness balance procedures. *In* Katz, J. (Ed.): Handbook of Clinical Audiology, 2nd Ed. Baltimore, Williams and Wilkins, 1978.

13. Crowley, D. E., Davis, H., and Beagley, H.: Clinical use of electrocochleology: A preliminary report. *In* Ruben, R. J., Elberling, C., and Salomon, G. (Eds.): Electrocochleology. Baltimore, University Park Press, 1976.

14. Cutting, J. E., and Kavanagh, J. F.: On the relationship speech to language. Asha, 17:500–506, 1975.

15. Dallos, P.: The Auditory Periphery: Biophysics and Physiology. New York, Academic Press, Inc., 1973.

16. Davis, H.: Anatomy and physiology of the auditory system. *In* Davis, H., Silverman, S. R. (Eds.): Hearing and Deafness, 4th Ed. New York, Holt, Rinehart and Winston, 1978.

17. Downs, M. P.: The handicap of deafness. *In* Northern, J. L. (Ed.): Hearing Disorders. Boston, Little, Brown and Company, 1976.

18. Durrant, J. D.: Anatomic and physiologic correlates of the effects of noise on hearing. *In* Lipscomb, D. M. (Ed.): Noise and Audiology. Baltimore, University Park Press, 1978.

19. Evans, V., and Courville, C. B.: The nervous acousticus. Pathologic conditions involving the eighth nerve and cerebello-pontine angle. Laryngoscope, 42:432–455, 1932.

20. Feldman, A. S.: Acoustic impedance admittance battery. *In* Katz, J. (Ed.): Handbook of Clinical Audiology, 2nd Ed. Baltimore, Williams and Wilkins, 1978.

21. Fraser, G. R.: The Causes of Profound Deafness in Childhood. Baltimore, Johns Hopkins University Press, 1976.

22. Ganzer, A. W., and Kleimann, H.: Sensory neural hearing loss in mucous otitis. Arch. Otolargyngol., 215:91–93, 1977.

23. Green, D. S.: Tone decay. *In* Katz, J. (Ed.): Handbook of Clinical Audiology, 2nd Ed. Baltimore, Williams and Wilkins, 1978.

24. Hodgson, W. R.: Hearing aid counseling and orientation. *In* Katz, J. (Ed.): Handbook of Clinical Audiology. Baltimore, Williams and Wilkins, 1978.

25. Hoemann, H. H.: Communicating with Deaf People. Baltimore, University Park Press, 1978.

26. Hopkinson, N. T.: Speech reception threshold; and Goetzinger, C. P.: Word discrimination testing. *In* Katz, J. (Ed.): Handbook of Clinical Audiology, 2nd Ed. Baltimore, Williams and Wilkins, 1978.

27. House, J. W., Miller, L., and House, P. R.: Severe tinnitus: Treatment with biofeedback training. (Results in 41 cases.) Trans. Am. Acad. Ophthal. mol. Otolaryngol., 84:697–703, 1977.

28. Hughes, R. L., and Johnson, E. W.: Békésy audiometry. *In* Katz, J. (Ed.): Handbook of Clinical Audiology, 2nd Ed. Baltimore, Williams and Wilkins Co., 1978.

29. Jerger, J. F., and Northern, J. L. (Eds.): Clinical Impedance Audiometry, 2nd Ed. Hudson, New Hampshire, American Electromedics Corp., 1980.

30. Jerger, J., Shedd, J., and Harford, E.: On the detection of extremely small changes in sound intensity. Arch. Otolaryngol., 69:200–211, 1959.

31. Keith, R.: Central Auditory Dysfunction. New York, Grune and Stratton, 1977.

32. Kinney, S. E.: The metabolic evaluation in Ménière's disease. Otolaryngol. Head Neck Surg., 88:594–598, 1980.

33. Klima, E., and Bellugi, U.: The Signs of Language. Cambridge, Mass., Harvard University Press, 1979.

34. Ling, D.: Speech and the Hearing-impaired Child: Theory and Practice. Washington, D.C., A. G. Bell Association for the Deaf, 1976.

35. Lybarger, S. F.: Earmolds. *In* Katz, J. (Ed.): Handbook of Clinical Audiology, 2nd Ed. Baltimore, Williams and Wilkins, 1978.

36. McCandless, G. A.: Neuroelectric measures of auditory function. *In* Rose, D. E. (Ed.): Audiological Assessment, 2nd Ed. Englewood Cliffs, N.J., Prentice-Hall, Inc., 1978.

37. Miller, M. H.: OSHA Hearing Conservation Amendment: 1910. 95, Occupational noise exposure. *In* Miller, M. H. (Ed.): Occupational Hearing Conservation: State of the Art. Upper Darby, Pa., Instrumentation Associates, Inc., 1981.

38. Miller, M. H.: Hearing Aids. Indianapolis, Bobbs Merrill, 1972.

39. Miller, M. H., and Harris, J. D.: Hearing testing in industry and hearing conservation in industry. *In* Harris, C. M. (Ed.): Handbook of Noise Control, 2nd Ed. New York, McGraw-Hill Book Company, 1979.

40. Moores, D. F.: Educating the Deaf. Boston, Houghton Mifflin, 1978.

41. Naiman, D., and Schein, J. D.: For Parents of Deaf Children. Silver Spring, Md., National Association of the Deaf, 1978.

42. Northern, J. L., and Grimes, A. M.: Introduction to acoustic impedance. *In* Katz, J. (Ed.): Handbook of Clinical Audiology, 2nd Ed. Baltimore, Williams and Wilkins, 1978.

43. O'Neill, J. J., and Oyer, H. J.: Visual Communication for the Hard of Hearing. Englewood Cliffs, N.J., Prentice-Hall, Inc., 1961.

44. Paparella, M. M., and Davis, H.: Medical and surgical treatment of hearing loss. *In* Davis, H., and Silverman, S. R. (Ed.): Hearing and deafness, 4th Ed. New York, Holt, Rinehart and Winston, 1978.

45. Perry, A. L., and Silverman, S. R.: Speechreading. *In* Davis, H., and Silverman, S. R. (Eds.): Hearing and Deafness. New York, Holt, Rinehart and Winston, 1978.

46. Pollack, M. C.: Special application of amplification. *In* Pollack, M. C. (Ed.): Amplification for the Hearing Impaired, 2nd Ed. New York, Grune and Stratton, 1980.

47. Proctor, C. A.: Abnormal insulin levels and vertigo. Laryngoscope, 91:1657–1662, 1981.

48. Pulec, J. L.: Ménière's disease. *In* Northern, J. L. (Ed.): Hearing Disorders. Boston, Little, Brown and Co., 1976.

49. Pulec, J. L., House, W. F., and Hughes, R. L.: Vestibular involvement and testing in acoustic neuromas. Arch. Otolaryngol., 80:677–681, 1964.

50. Ramsdell, D. A.: The psychology of the hard-of-hearing and deafened adult. *In* Davis, H., and Silverman, S. R. (Eds.): Hearing and Deafness, 4th Ed. New York, Holt, Rinehart and Winston, 1978.

51. Ries, P.: Further studies in achievement testing, hearing impaired students. United States: Spring 1971 Series D, No. 13. Washington, D.C., Office of Demographic Studies, Gallaudet College, 1973.

52. Sanders, D. A.: Hearing aid orientation and counseling. *In* Pollack, M. C. (Ed.): Amplification for the Hearing Impaired, 2nd Ed. New York, Grune and Stratton, 1980.

53. Schein, J. D.: Multiply handicapped hearing-impaired children. *In* Bradford, L. J., and Hardy, W. G. (Eds.): Hearing and hearing impairment. New York, Grune and Stratton, 1979.

54. Schein, J. D.: Hearing Disorders. *In* Kurland, L. T., Kurtke, J. F., and Goldberg, I. D. (Eds.): Epidemiology of Neurologic and Sense Organ Disorders. Cambridge, Mass., Harvard University Press, 1973.

55. Schein, J. D.: From zero to line 21: Closing the TV gap for deaf viewers. J. Educ. Technol. Systems, 9 (3):241–245, 1980.

56. Schein, J. D.: How well can you see me? Teaching Exceptional Children, 12:55–58, 1980.

57. Schein, J. D.: Group techniques applied to deaf and hearing-impaired persons. *In* Seligman, M. (Ed.): Group psychotherapy and counseling with special populations. Baltimore, University Park Press, 1982.

58. Schein, J. D.: Model State Plan for Rehabilitation of Deaf Clients. Silver Spring, MD., National Association of the Deaf, 1980.

59. Schein, J. D., and Delk, M. T.: The Deaf Population of the United States. Silver Spring, MD., National Association of the Deaf, 1974.

60. Schein, J. D., and Hamilton, R.: Impact 1980. Telecommunications and Deafness. Silver Spring, MD., National Association of the Deaf, 1980.

61. Schlesinger, H. S., and Meadow, F. P.: Sound and Sign. Berkeley, CA., University of California Press, 1972.

62. Schuknecht, H.: Presbycusis. Laryngology, 65:402–419, 1955.

63. Schuknecht, H.: Further observations on presbycusis. Arch. Otolaryngol., 80:369–382, 1964.

64. Shambaugh, G. E., and Wiet, R. V.: The diagnosis and evaluation of allergic disorders with food intolerance in Ménière's disease. Otolaryngol. Clin. North Am., 13(4):671–679, 1980.

65. Shontz, F. C.: Physical disability and personality. *In* Neff, W. S. (Ed.): Rehabilitation Psychology. Washington, D.C., American Psychological Association, 1971.

66. Silverman, S. R.: Conservation and development of speech. *In* Davis, H., and Silverman, S. R. (Eds.): Hearing and Deafness, 4th Ed. New York, Holt, Rinehart and Winston, 1978.

67. Sims, D. G.: Visual and auditory training for adults. *In* Katz, J. (Ed.): Handbook of Clinical Audiology. Baltimore, MD., Williams and Wilkins, 1978.

68. Speaks, C., and Jerger, J.: Method for measurement of speech identification. J. Speech Hear. Res., 8:185–194, 1965.

69. Stevens, S. S. (Ed.): Handbook of Experimental Psychology. New York, John Wiley and Sons, 1951.

70. Tobias, J. V. (Ed.): Foundations of Modern Auditory Theory, Vol. 1. New York, Academic Press, Inc., 1970.

71. Von Békésy, G.: Experiments in Hearing. New York, McGraw-Hill, 1960.

72. Wever, E. G.: Theory of Hearing. New York, John Wiley and Sons, 1949.

73. Wever, E. G., and Lawrence, M.: Physiological Acoustics. Princeton, N.J., Princeton University Press, 1954.

74. Wilbur, R. B.: American Sign Language and Sign Systems. Baltimore, University Park Press, 1979.

75. Wright, B. A.: Physical Disability — A Psychological Approach. New York, Harper and Row, 1960.

76. Yost, W. A., and Nielsen, D. W.: Fundamentals of Hearing. An Introduction. New York, Holt, Rinehart and Winston, 1977.

77. Zemlin, W. R.: Speech and Hearing Science. Englewood Cliffs, N.J., Prentice-Hall, 1966.

45

FOOTWEAR AND FOOTWEAR MODIFICATIONS

RITA BISTEVINS

GENERAL CONSIDERATIONS

Shoes consist of the upper, the sole, and, in most cases, an added heel. The material and style of each of these components contribute to the overall appearance and utility of the shoe. The commonly worn footwear styles include the oxford, pump, sandal, moccasin, tennis shoe, clog, and various types of boots (Fig. 45–1). The heel height varies from a negative heel that is lower than the forefoot position (Fig. 45–1*b*) to 2 or 3 inches high (Fig. 45–1*c*). The shoe upper is made of a flexible material — leather, woven fabrics, or synthetic materials such as urethane or vinyl. Leather is the most suitable of all available materials, as it has the ability to "breathe," is moisture absorbent, and tends to mold to the shape of the foot with wear.[14] This is not the case with most synthetic materials. Because of their poor ability to handle moisture, the man-made materials may be more useful for open style shoes such as sandals. In the oxford style shoe, the upper consists of at least three pieces that are cut from a pattern. The anterior part, covering the instep and toes, is known as the vamp. The pieces that make up the posterior

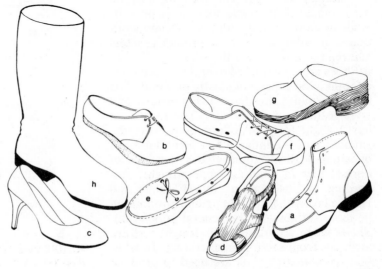

FIGURE 45–1. Commonly worn footwear styles. *a*, Laced work shoe; *b*, oxford — shown here with a negative heel; *c*, pump; *d*, sandal; *e*, moccasin; *f*, tennis shoe; *g*, clog; *h*, boot.

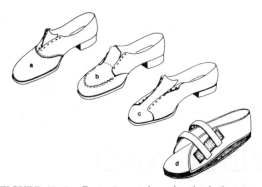

FIGURE 45-2. Fastening styles of oxford shoes. *a,* balmoral; *b,* blucher; *c,* open to the toe; *d,* convalescent.

part of the shoe are known as the quarters. Prior to lasting, these pieces are sewn together and fitted with a lining made of leather or canvas. The cut of the upper determines the fastening style of the shoe, which may be open to the toe, balmoral, blucher, or convalescent type (Fig. 45-2). The sole consists of three layers — the insole, the outsole, and the filler between them. The insole may be made of thin leather or man-made material. The filler usually consists of cork dust and latex. The outsole may be made of leather, rubber, crepe, plastic, wood, or other materials. The same variety of materials is available for the heels. The structural stability of the shoe is enhanced by the heel counter, the shank, and the toe box (Fig. 45-3). The heel counter, which is made of firm leather or other stiff material, supports the posterior part of the shoe. The shank, usually made of steel, is used to provide additional support for the shoe in the region corresponding to the arch of the foot. The toe box may be hard, made of synthetic materials, or soft, made of cloth coated with latex. Some work boots, in addition, have a protective steel cap reinforcement over the toes.

Shoes are constructed over a last, which is a footlike form made of plastic or wood. The last determines the desired dimensions and style features of the shoe.[14] The usual last has a slight forefoot inflare. However, the suitability of the inflared last form has been questioned. Bleck[3] found that 85 per cent of normal feet in children were straight. According to observations by Holscher and Hu,[12] a last with a straight medial border may be more suitable for the general population. Shoes made according to a straight last are available from some manufacturers. In addition, combination lasts are used to produce

footwear of combined dimensions such as a medium width forefoot and a narrow fitting heel. During the lasting process, the insole is temporarily tacked to the bottom of the last. After positioning of the heel counter and the toe box, the upper is applied snugly over the last so that the shoe upper adapts to the form of the last in every detail. It is then secured to the insole. Some steps of the lasting process include handling of the materials in a high-humidity environment. This softens the leather for shaping. The lasting process is followed by attachment of the outsole and the heel. In most footwear manufactured today, the upper is secured to the sole by rubber-based adhesives. The heel is attached by either gluing or nailing. For some outdoor footwear, heavy duty workshoes, and tennis shoes, a rubber or plastic sole is applied with vulcanizing or injection molding utilizing plastic materials.[14] In the so-called welt construction shoe, first a strip of leather known as the welt is sewn to the upper, the lining, and the insole. After the shank is attached, the outsole is stitched to the welt followed by heel attachment and trimming of the heel and edges of the sole to the required contour. The welt construction shoes are quality shoes. They provide comfort because of a seam-free insole. They hold their shape well

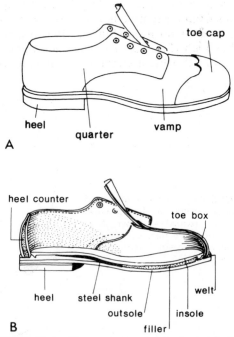

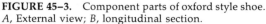

FIGURE 45-3. Component parts of oxford style shoe. *A,* External view; *B,* longitudinal section.

and have good structural stability, but they may be somewhat heavier and less flexible.

Shoes are worn for protection of the feet from rough terrain, cold, moisture, and dirt. Shoes are also important fashion items and are usually selected according to the current fashion trends. Our footwear needs change from infancy to old age. The infant needs shoes for protection from cold only. At other times, the shoes may be left off. When the child is just beginning to stand, his or her shoes should have a firm heel counter, a soft leather top, and soft flexible sole approximately ⅛ inch thick.[7] The soft flexible sole is also of advantage for the crawling child, as shoes with stiff soles tend to roll into a toe-in or toe-out attitude, thus aggravating any toe-in or toe-out tendencies.[15] As the child begins to walk, he or she should have a shoe with a firm heel counter and a firm sole approximately ¼ inch thick.[7] The heel height may be ¼ inch or ⅜ inch. During the first two years of life, a high top shoe will fit more securely. After this age, the foot and the heel have developed sufficiently to stay in a low shoe, although the heel width in many children's shoes is too great. For ages 3 years to 9 years, a round toe shoe is recommended to accommodate the growing foot. The heel height may be ¼ to ⅜ inch. The shoe should have a steel shank, but flexibility should be allowed for the forefoot. The shoe of the active adolescent also should have a steel shank and a firm heel counter to prevent rapid shoe breakdown. Shoes for the growing foot should be fitted to allow ½ to ¾ inch distance between the longest toe and the end of the toe box during weight bearing. In all cases, the counter should fit the heel snugly. Frequent evaluation of footwear fit is needed, as children may outgrow their footwear in three to four months. The shoes should be replaced when the foot size has increased so that the toes approach the end of the toe box or when there is other evidence of tightness or loss of shape of the shoes. A shoe with a firm heel counter and a snug fit at the heel is recommended for adults of all ages. In weight bearing, there should be ½ inch distance between the toes and the end of the toe box to ensure adequate length. In a shoe of proper width, there should be no bulging at the welt. Tested over the widest portion of the foot, the upper should be loose enough to permit grasping a small fold of the material between the forefinger and thumb. With increasing age, the foot tends to become wider

and less flexible. A wider shoe with a soft flexible sole and a soft upper is recommended for the elderly person. A cushioned insole and a low heel may provide a more comfortable fit. However, shoes with soft soles are not suitable for elderly persons who tend to shuffle their feet when walking. The soft soles, especially those made of crepe, may cause tripping. To ensure maximum stability and safety in walking, special care must be taken to have the elderly person's footwear always securely fastened.

Shoe sizes are indicated by numbers referring to the length and by letters referring to the width. In the United States, children's shoe sizes range from 1 (infant size) to 13, starting again at size 1 on the adult scale. Although this is variable, men's shoes up to size 14 or 15 and women's shoes up to size 12 or possibly size 13 are available in shoe stores. Larger sizes may need to be ordered from the manufacturer or specialty houses. The width ranges from A (narrow) to E (wide). Some manufacturers record the width as N (narrow), M (medium), or W (wide). With each increase in the length or the width of the shoe there will be an increase in both the length and the width. The shoe retailer may not stock all sizes in width so extra narrow or extra wide shoes may need to be ordered specially. Lasts and sizes change with the manufacturer and with changing fashions, so correct fit can be determined only by trying the shoe on the foot. Functionally, the shoe should be comfortable for several hours of uninterrupted wear. The shoe should bend easily where the foot normally bends and remain rigid where the foot is normally rigid.[15] The shoe should not interfere with the normal lateral stability of the foot and should not cause loss of balance due to insecure fit. These important functional considerations have been disregarded in the design of some fashion footwear. The thick inflexible platform sole limits the normal motion of the foot during walking. The normal lateral stability of the foot is reduced if the shoe is constructed with a convexity in the sole permitting the foot to rock from side to side. The narrow base of a high heel also contributes to instability. Backless shoes tend to slide off the feet and cause loss of balance. In addition, the shank curve and a forward slanting heel seat permit the foot to slide forward in the shoe, crowding the toes in the toe box and causing skin irritation and foot deformities. The negative heel may cause discomfort due to tension on the triceps surae. These undesirable consequences of fashion footwear are by no means limited to women's shoes. Some problems related to footwear result from the materials utilized for modern shoe construction or the processing of these materials. Common allergens in footwear are rubber-based adhesives, coloring agents, and, in leather shoes, chrome and formaldehyde present in most leathers as tanning agents.[8] Moisture from perspiration may leech chemicals out of one area and transfer them to distant sites, thus causing apparent spread of the dermatitis. White buck or other undyed leather or tennis shoes may need to be substituted. When the tanning agents are at fault, vegetable-tanned or glutaraldehyde-tanned leather shoes may be needed. Excessive moisture is a particular problem with synthetic materials and some specially treated leathers. Ventilation holes similar to those in some tennis shoes may need to be made in the upper using a leather punch. Wearing of two pairs of cotton socks is also helpful. Prospective allergy testing of shoe components may be appropriate in some cases.[8] In general, the adult has a wide choice of footwear materials and styles. Time spent in selection of a well-fitting shoe is time well invested, as the result will be comfort and walking ease during many months.

FOOTWEAR MODIFICATIONS

Welt process shoes are best suited for modifications because the sole and the upper can be separated and reattached without disturbing the structural stability of the shoe. This type of shoe can support orthotic devices, including metal braces. The so-called "orthopedic" shoe is a welt shoe. In addition, it has an extended heel on the medial side known as the Thomas heel, an extended medial heel counter, and a rigid steel shank. Shoes that have soles attached by adhesives do not lend themselves to modifications that require separation of the sole and the upper because of difficulty of reattaching the soles. However, some shoes of this type may be suitable for simple external modifications such as heel elevations or metatarsal bars. Various internal shoe modifications can be fabricated from a heat-moldable polyethylene foam (Plastazote).[11] A full-molded insole requires an extra-depth shoe. In the manufacture of these shoes extra depth has been provided to accommodate a removable insole of 1/4 to 5/8 inch thickness in the different shoes. The insole can be removed to provide extra space in the shoe to accommodate deformities, or it can be replaced by an insole individually molded for each patient. Sandal kits* consist of a heat-moldable soft insole material, microcellular rubber, soling, and the appropriate materials for the upper. The inventive physician or orthotist will adapt them to a variety of conditions.

Footwear modifications should be detailed in a written prescription that defines the type of footwear to be modified and the desired modifications. A simple diagram attached to the prescription may convey added information and clarify the request. If the shoes are to be supplied by the orthotist, the prescription should indicate the freedom the patient may be permitted in shoe selection, for example, selection of color, lacing, or style. When the situation warrants it and regularly in some clinics the physiatrist and the orthotist may examine the patient together. It is the physician's responsibility to evaluate the modified shoe to confirm that the desired effect has been achieved.

The style and appearance of the shoe are of great importance to the patient and should never be disregarded in the prescription of shoes and shoe modifications. It is common sense to use the simplest and most cosmetically acceptable modification that will achieve its purpose. The patient should clearly understand the purpose of the modification and have an opportunity to communicate his or her preferences to the physiatrist and the orthotist. The following paragraphs contain some practical guidelines for footwear selection and modification in the conditions commonly seen in the physiatrist's practice.

Elevations. Heel and sole elevations, also known as heel and sole lifts, are prescribed when there is a need for length adjustment of the lower limb. A lift of 3/8 inch or less can be worn under the heel inside a suitable shoe. This type of lift may be made of felt, firm rubber, or other materials and lightly glued into its position. Higher elevations will require external modification. For adjustment of up to 1 inch, heel elevation alone will be sufficient. When the length adjustment exceeds 1 inch, both heel and sole elevations

*Quickie Sandal Kit, available from AliMed, 138 Prince Street, Boston, Massachusetts 02113.

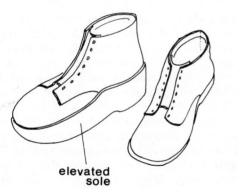

FIGURE 45–4. Sole and heel elevations. Note the upward tapered distal portion of the elevated sole.

are used. Care should be taken to maintain the heel height greater than the sole height in order to avoid a negative heel effect. Tapering of the distal portion of the sole upward will aid in walking by allowing easier weight transfer over the forefoot, as the elevated sole is usually not flexible (Fig. 45–4). Although the usual soling materials can be used for heel and sole elevations, lightweight materials such as cork are recommended if the lift is relatively high. When covered with leather matching the shoe upper, the elevated portion is less conspicuous.

Forefoot Deformities. Deformities of the forefoot such as a bunion require a wide shoe with a soft upper. Extra room for the deformity may be provided by slitting the upper close to the sole or along seams or excising a portion of the upper. A patch of material similar to the upper material is then sewn into place over the excised portion, making sure that the needed width adjustment has been achieved. This simple modification can be done in most shoe repair shops. It will provide comfortable walking in a shoe of acceptable appearance.

Painful Heel Spurs and Plantar Fasciitis. In most cases, heel pain will subside with decreased amount of weight bearing and an insert of soft rubber or soft grade polyethylene foam (Plastazote) cut to fit under the heel inside the shoe. This provides a cushion under the heel and relieves tension on the plantar fascia slightly. Campbell and Inman[6] report good success in resistant cases using the UC-BL (University of California Biomechanics Laboratory) shoe insert that provides an alternate method to elevate the arch. The theory of the UC-BL shoe insert is to hold the foot in a position that relieves tension on the plantar fascia. By holding the heel in inversion with forces against the

navicular and the outer border of the forefoot, this is accomplished without direct pressure on the soft tissues under the longitudinal arch. The insert is a plastic shell made by laminating layers of nylon and fiberglass, constructed according to a plaster cast. The cast is made from a negative that is taken with the leg externally rotated while the forefoot is held in pronation and slight adduction.

Flat Feet. Adults with mildly pronated feet that are asymptomatic require no special shoes or shoe modifications. If there is evidence of longitudinal arch strain, a Thomas heel shoe that also has a long medial heel counter will provide some support despite the fact that the Thomas heel extends only part way under the arch. Supports of the longitudinal arch can be added. Although some commercially available supports may fit, individually molded arch supports made of polyethylene foam may be better tolerated. Only the flexible flat foot will adjust to these modifications. The rigid flat foot needs to be fitted for comfort only. In the usual case, this means selection of a wide shoe with a comfortable fit. A molded polyethylene foam insole backed by microcellular rubber may increase the patient's comfort. If the molded insole is used, an extra depth shoe is also needed. The insole should be molded to the foot as is without incorporating an arch support, as the arch support may produce undesirable pressure and cause pain under the inflexible arch.

Footwear modifications using a Thomas heel and a medial heel wedge are recommended for children with flexible flat feet who have leg pain in the evening following a long day of activity. Pain may be expected to subside as early as within two to three days. Cowell[7] believes that the Thomas heel and medical heel are most appropriately used for the flexible flat foot. This type of correction should not be used for flexible flat feet that do not form an arch in either sitting or standing position, as pressure in the arch region will aggravate the discomfort.[7] The need of footwear corrections for children with asymptomatic flat feet is questionable.

For the medial heel wedge and the Thomas heel to be effective, the shoe fit should be satisfactory and the heel counter should fit snugly and resist distortion.[1] If the heel of the shoe is too wide, a fitted heel counter will be needed. The medial heel counter should be extended, but not as far forward as the

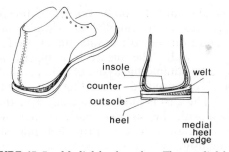

FIGURE 45–5. Medial heel wedge. The medial heel wedge is positioned between the insole and the outsole. The wedge tapers to 0 laterally.

navicular if spot pressure on this bone is to be avoided. The medial heel wedge should be placed between the outsole and the insole (Fig. 45–5). The wedge should be highest on the medial side, tapering to 0 laterally. For children up to age 2 years, the wedge should measure $^1/_{16}$ inch; from age 2 to 5 years, $^1/_8$ inch; after age 5 years, $^3/_{16}$ inch.[7] In some cases, a small pad just anterior to the os calcis weight-bearing area may be needed to maintain the heel in its proper position.

The Insensitive Foot. Impaired lower extremity sensation may result from peripheral nerve or spinal cord injury, myelodysplasia, stroke, neuropathies, and other conditions seen in the physiatrist's practice. The foot with impaired sensation requires a careful evaluation prior to footwear selection. The evaluation should include assessment of skin condition and the distribution of plantar pressure in standing and walking. Attention must be paid to the thickness of fat pads, calluses, and scarring on the plantar surface of the foot. With the use of the Harris mat, the plantar pressure evaluation can be carried out in the physiatrist's office. The footprint made by the patient bearing weight on the inked mat indicates areas of high pressure that may need to be protected by special shoe modifications. A thin form of the Harris mat can be used inside the shoe for additional evaluation.[5, 16] The Microcapsule Sock Test developed at the U.S. Public Health Service Hospital at Carville, Louisiana, also may be used for evaluation of pressures inside the shoe.[5, 9]

If the evaluation reveals that the sensory-impaired foot has no soft tissue or skeletal deformity, carefully fitted regular shoes are acceptable.[9] In cases in which an area of concentrated pressure has been demonstrated by plantar pressure evaluation, a microcellular rubber insole will distribute the

stress over a larger area. An extra-depth shoe may or may not be needed. If the foot is scarred on the plantar surface from previous trauma, the risk of further injury is increased. In this case, a combination insole of molded polyethylene foam backed by microcellular rubber is recommended for the active patient. Molded polyethylene foam with latex cork backing is another useful combination of materials. Soft grade and medium grade Plastazote may be used for the same insole (Fig. 45–6). The insoles are fitted inside extra-depth shoes. If bony deformity on the plantar aspect of the foot is also present, a soft molded insole of polyethylene foam is recommended, with areas of relief under the prominences to prevent plantar ulceration.[9] A metatarsal bar attached to the flexible sole in its correct position with the high point of the bar located just proximal to the metatarsal heads will relieve stress off the metatarsal heads. When the sole is rigid, a rocker bar can be fitted by the orthotist.[5] This allows the substitution of a rocking motion for direct pressure on the metatarsal region (Fig. 45–7). A sandal with a soft molded insole can be made from a kit or from assembled materials in a relatively short time and may be of value for patients who need temporary footwear during healing of foot lesions (Fig. 45–8). Individually made rigid-soled rocker shoes are used in special cases for patients with Hansen's disease.[5] Unfortunately, the expert craftsmanship and experience required to make these shoes, as well as the appropriate facilities, may not be available in all locations.

Regardless of whether the sensory impairment is considered permanent or transient,

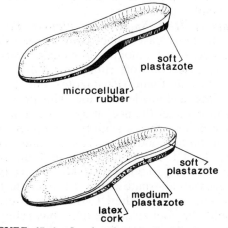

FIGURE 45–6. Insoles for use inside extra-depth shoes. Note combinations of materials.

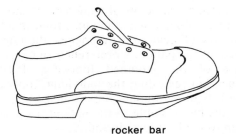

FIGURE 45–7. Oxford shoe with a rocker bar.

the patient must be taught techniques of preventive foot care. Because of decreased or absent sensory feedback, the patient may not be aware that his footwear is too tight or that skin breakdown is imminent from trauma due to other causes. For the same reason, he or she is not able to adjust the gait to lessen the repetitive pressure of walking on the skin areas that may be already inflamed.[4] The preventive program includes daily foot examination to detect areas of tissue trauma and examination of shoes and socks.[16] In the hospital setting, diagnostic aids such as thermography and volumetric studies may be available to detect signs of inflammation. At home, however, the patient will need to monitor for these signs visually and by touch. Particular attention must be paid to the areas that receive the greatest pressure, especially the region of the metatarsal heads. This region is particularly vulnerable, as the forefoot carries the greatest load in walking by sustaining the weight for a longer period of time than the heel.[2] The multiply handicapped patient may not be able to carry out the examination independently and may require assistance from a member of the family. In some cases, gait training may be needed to minimize the effects of repetitive stress. Usually, this involves teaching the patient to walk slowly and to take shorter steps. Shoes should be changed at midday and again in the evening.[4] At first, new shoes should not be worn longer than two hours without examining the feet. If spasticity complicates .the clinical picture, additional trauma to the foot may result as the spastic muscles force the foot against the shoe. When the patient exerts effort in ambulation, the level of spasticity may increase; therefore, the fit of the shoe may be different in ambulation than during non–weight-bearing or while standing. Repeated evaluation of the footwear and of orthotic and assistive devices, combined with judicious use of medication or intramuscular neurolysis for control of spasticity, may be necessary in the management of the difficult case. Inquiry into the patient's daily activities often reveals the need for work simplification techniques in order to reduce the total distance walked each day. The skin of the insensitive foot may lack the normal perspiration moisture, leading to scaling and fissuring. Daily foot soaks followed by application of an emollient to retain skin moisture may be needed.[16] We have found Albolene, with its main ingredients of mineral oil, petrolatum, and paraffin, useful for this purpose. It also seems to be well accepted by the patients.

The Arthritic Foot. The foot is involved in 90 per cent of all patients who have had rheumatoid arthritis for any period of time.[13] The metatarsophalangeal joints are affected early in the disease, and tenosynovitis, rheumatoid nodules, and inflamed bursae are common. Atrophy of fat pads also occurs. A wide shoe with a soft upper is recommended to avoid painful mediolateral compression of the metatarsophalangeal joints. It should have a flexible sole. A soft heel counter is useful for those patients who have heel pain due to rheumatoid nodules and inflamed bursae. The common abnormalities of the foot in advanced arthritis include hallux valgus, clawing of the toes, spread of the forefoot, and a rigid flat foot. When there is clawing of the toes an extra-depth shoe should be prescribed to avoid pressure on the dorsum of the toes. The shoe should be wide and have a soft toecap that can adjust to the deformities. Spot stretching may be needed to further enlarge the upper. A commonly prescribed modification for relief of pressure on the painful metatarsal heads is a metatarsal pad attached inside the shoe. This localized modification has disadvantages. As the shoe loosens with wear, the pad may no longer be in

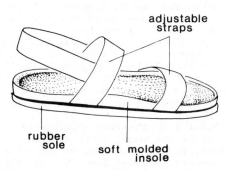

FIGURE 45–8. Sandal with soft molded insole and adjustable straps. It is similar to sandals made from a kit.

its correct location and can cause undesirable pressure in other areas of the weight-bearing surface of the foot. For this reason, a full-molded insole is preferable to distribute weight over the entire weight-bearing surface. As for the insole used for the insensitive foot, heat-moldable or a combination of moldable and nonmoldable materials may be used. External modification in the form of a metatarsal bar applied to a flexible sole may serve to reduce pressure over the painful metatarsophalangeal region. The severely deformed foot requires a custom-made shoe. The shoe is made according to a plaster cast of the foot. Whenever possible, leather should be used for the upper. Also of value for indoor use and in warm climate outdoors are sandals with soft soles and the straps adjusted or altered so that they avoid pressure on sensitive areas. High heel shoes are not suitable for the arthritic foot, as in the high heel shoe extra weight is placed on the already painful metatarsal heads.[10] Also, in general, the arthritic foot is not flexible enough to fit well into a high heel shoe. The use of physical therapy measures to maintain foot flexibility is of advantage to the patient, as the flexible foot will have a greater choice of footwear styles and in some instances may even tolerate a moderate heel. The choice of suitable footwear and footwear styles for the foot with severe deformities such as hallux valgus and fixed deformities of the toes may be increased by corrective surgical procedures that restore the foot to near normal shape.[17] The patient with severe rheumatoid arthritis and decreased function of the hands often requires assistive devices for dressing his or her feet and adaptations for closure of the shoes.

CONCLUSION

The changing styles and materials of fashion footwear make the selection of suitable shoes an ongoing challenge for everyone, including persons whose feet are considered normal. This challenge is considerably greater for persons whose feet require special consideration because of deformity, disease, or nonconformity to the usual last. The amount of experimental data relating to the usefulness and long-term effects of various types of footwear and footwear modifications is limited. For the most part, the clinician will need to rely on his or her own evaluation and clinical judgment regarding footwear selection and modification. In addition, the clinician must recognize the importance of the patient's preference and acceptance of the modified footwear. Patient education regarding the individual footwear needs is of paramount importance. It should always be available to the patient, as it may help to avoid future disability.

Acknowledgment

The author wishes to express thanks to Winkley Orthopedic Laboratories of Golden Valley, Minnesota, for information regarding currently available adaptations for shoes and to Jean Magney for preparing the illustrations for this chapter.

REFERENCES

1. Allison, J. D.: Change in heel width following support of pronated foot. Arch. Phys. Med. Rehabil., 48:195–200, 1967.
2. Blackburn, P. A., et al.: An investigation of the centres of pressure under the foot while walking. J. Bone Joint Surg., 57B:98–103, 1975.
3. Bleck, E. E.: The shoeing of children: Sham or science? Dev. Med. Child. Neurol., 13:188–195, 1971.
4. Brand, P. W.: Management of the insensitive limb. Phys. Ther., 59:8–12, 1979.
5. Brand, P. W.: Repetitive Stress on Insensitive Feet: The Pathology and Management of Plantar Ulceration in Neuropathic Feet. U. S. Public Health Service Hospital, Carville, Louisiana, 1975.
6. Campbell, J. W., and Inman, V. T.: Treatment of plantar fasciitis and calcaneal spurs with the UC-BL shoe insert. Clin. Orthop., 103:57–62, 1974.
7. Cowell, H. R.: Shoes and shoe corrections. Pediatr. Clin. North Am., 24:791–797, 1977.
8. Dahl, M. V.: Allergic contact dermatitis from footwear. Minn. Med., 58:871–874, 1975.
9. Hampton, G. H.: Therapeutic footwear for the insensitive foot. Phys. Ther., 59:23–29, 1979.
10. Haslock, D. I., and Wright, V.: Footwear for arthritic patients. Ann. Phys. Med., 10:236–240, 1970.
11. Hertzman, C. A.: Use of Plastazote in foot disabilities. Am. J. Phys. Med., 52:289–303, 1973.
12. Holscher, E. C., and Hu, K. K.: Detrimental results with the common inflared shoe. Orthop. Clin. North Am., 7:1011–1018, 1976.
13. Potter, T. A.: Correction of arthritic deformities. In Hollander, J. E., and McCarty, D. J.: Arthritis and Allied Conditions. Philadelphia, Lea & Febiger, 1972, pp. 629–672.
14. Rossi, W. A.: Shoes and the shoe industry—reality versus illusion. J. Am. Podiatry Assoc., 68:215–229, 1978.
15. Schuster, R. O.: The effects of modern footgear. J. Am. Podiatry Assoc., 68:235–241, 1978.
16. Shipley, D. E.: Clinical evaluation and care of the insensitive foot. Phys. Ther., 59:13–18, 1979.
17. Thomas, W. H.: Surgery of the foot in rheumatoid arthritis. Orthop. Clin. North Am., 6:831–835, 1975.

46

PREVENTION AND REHABILITATION OF ISCHEMIC ULCERS

MICHAEL KOSIAK

Ischemic ulcers are localized areas of cellular necrosis of the skin and subcutaneous tissues that have been subjected to supracapillary pressure for prolonged periods. Ulcerations occur with special frequency over weight-bearing bony prominences covered only by skin and small amounts of muscle and subcutaneous tissue. The areas over the sacrum, trochanters, and ischial tuberosities are most frequently involved. Obviously, the distribution depends to a great extent on the patient's functional status. That is, trochanteric and sacral ulcers are more prevalent in the bedridden patient, and ischial ulcers are found almost exclusively in patients who are able to sit for long periods of time. Among the severely debilitated, ulcers also occur over the knees, heels, malleoli, scapulae, and spine.

INCIDENCE

The exact incidence of ischemic ulcers is unknown. Studies in the past would indicate that up to 28 per cent of the hospital population might be afflicted.[1] In patients with spinal cord injuries an incidence of 24 to 85 per cent has been reported, with 7 to 8 per cent of the deaths in these patients being attributed to complications arising from the presence of ischemic ulcers.[2-4] Most read-

missions to spinal cord injury centers are for treatment of ischemic ulcers.[5]

ETIOLOGY

Primary Factors

Pressure

Ischemic ulcers arise from prolonged tissue ischemia caused by pressure exceeding the tissue capillary pressure. Recent studies of the changes in capillary blood flow using several experimental methods have established important facts regarding vascular hemodynamics. Remarkable instability in capillaries at low perfusion pressures with cessation or temporary reversal of flow at a low positive pressure has been demonstrated.[6, 7]

Because the hydrostatic pressures in capillaries are relatively low (from 13 to 32 mm Hg) and because cessation of flow occurs even in the presence of positive arterial pressure, it would seem that complete tissue ischemia does occur when pressures of the order of capillary blood pressure are applied to the body.[8]

Pathologic changes following ischemia have been shown to be due to disturbances in capillary circulation. The presence of edema and cellular infiltration 24 hours after the

881

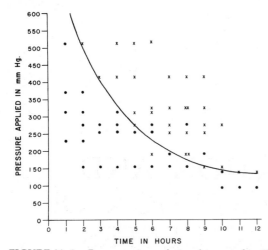

FIGURE 46–1. Pressure-time relationship noted in 62 separate experiments in 16 dogs: X = ulceration; • = no ulceration.

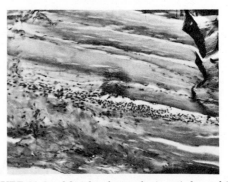

FIGURE 46–3. Muscle of paraplegic rat's leg subjected to 70 mm Hg constant pressure for four hours. The section shows an isolated fiber undergoing necrosis associated with extensive phagocytosis by neutrophils and macrophages. Stained with hematoxylin and eosin. Magnified 170 ×.

application of moderate pressure would indicate changes in capillary permeability due to capillary membrane ischemia. Increasing the degree or duration of ischemia not only increases the changes in capillary membrane permeability but also interferes with cellular metabolism to a degree sufficient to produce cellular necrosis and inflammatory reaction in muscle tissue.[9]

The application of 60 mm Hg pressure for one hour has been shown to produce edema, cellular infiltration, and extravasation in the tissue of dogs. An inverse relationship, resembling a parabolic curve, was found to exist between the amount and duration of pressure that normal tissue could tolerate before pathologic changes would occur (Fig. 46–1).[10]

Microscopic examination of rat muscle 24 hours after being subjected to 70 mm Hg pressure for one hour demonstrated a decrease or loss of cross striations and myofibrils, hyalinization of fibers, and neutrophilic infiltrations.

When complete relief of pressure was provided at regular five-minute intervals, such as in an alternating pressure support system, the tissue showed consistently less evidence of ischemic change or no change at all when compared with tissue subjected to an equivalent amount of constant pressure. This was true even at pressures as high as 240 mm Hg for three hours (Table 46–1).[11]

In the sitting position resting pressures can assume alarming magnitudes, while the pressures encountered by the patient in the prone and supine positions may also exceed capillary pressure.[12-16]

Friction and Shearing

The importance of shearing force as a factor in the production of ischemic ulcers was first reported by Reichel.[17] Although his work was primarily a clinical study, it clearly showed that shearing and stretching of blood vessels tended to compound the ischemic changes produced by external pressure, therefore increasing the rate of tissue breakdown.

Dinsdale,[18] working with animals, demonstrated a significant increase in the rate and frequency of skin breakdown when the tissue of swine was subjected to both pressure and friction, as opposed to changes produced by pressure alone.

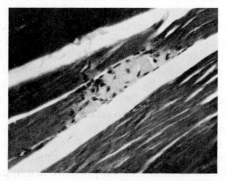

FIGURE 46–2. Muscle of normal rat's leg after application of 115 mm Hg constant pressure for two hours. The section shows early involvement of an isolated fiber consisting of hyaline degeneration and phagocytosis. Stained with hematoxylin and eosin. Magnified 380 ×.

TABLE 46–1. MICROSCOPIC CHANGES NOTED IN MUSCLE OF ANIMALS 24 HOURS AFTER APPLICATION OF PRESSURE*

Pressure Transmitted to Muscle	Time in Hours	Normal		Paraplegic	
		Constant Pressure	Alternating Pressure (5 min intervals)	Constant Pressure	Alternating Pressure (5 min intervals)
35 mm Hg	1	None	None	None	None
	2	None	None	None	None
	3	None	None	None	None
	4	None	None	None	None
70 mm Hg	1	None	None	None	None
	2	Moderate	None	Moderate	Minimal
	3	Moderate	Minimal	Moderate	Minimal
	4	Moderate	Minimal	Marked	Minimal
115 mm Hg	1	None		None	
	2	Minimal		Moderate	
	3	Marked		Marked	
	4	Moderate		Moderate	
155 mm Hg	1	None	None	None	None
	2	Moderate	None	Minimal	None
	3	Marked	Minimal	Minimal	None
	4	Moderate	Moderate	Moderate	Minimal
190 mm Hg	1	None		Minimal	
	2	Minimal		Moderate	
	3	Marked		Marked	
	4	Marked		Marked	
240 mm Hg	1	Minimal	None	Moderate	None
	2	Moderate	Minimal	Moderate	None
	3	Moderate	None	Moderate	Minimal
	4	Moderate	Moderate	Marked	Minimal

*None = No microscopic change.
Minimal = Involvement of isolated fibers.
Moderate = Involvement of up to 10 per cent of muscle examined.
Marked = Involvement of more than 10 per cent of muscle examined.

Temperature

Very little research has been done regarding the combined effects of temperature and pressure in the production of ulcerations. However, a skin temperature rise of 3° C beneath the sitting surface was reported in subjects resting on foam-rubber cushions.[19]

Since the metabolic rate increases 10 per cent with every one degree Centigrade rise in body temperature, any increase in tissue temperature in conjunction with tissue ischemia may further compromise the metabolism of the ischemic cells.

Aging

The incidence of ischemic ulcers appears to increase with age. After the third decade, a progressive decrease in skin pliability and elasticity has been reported, while after the fifth decade a rapid decrease in skin blood flow occurs.[20, 21]

Other reasons for the increased incidence of ischemic ulcers in the elderly could be attributed to a greater lack of mobility, poorer state of nutrition, higher incidence of complicating medical problems, and longer periods of confinement.[22]

Contributing Factors

Nutrition

Recently, increased emphasis has been placed on the role of nutrition during the acute and convalescent phases of illness, especially on the negative nitrogen and calcium balance that inevitably appears after an acute insult. After almost any illness or injury, such as a fracture, tooth extraction, or even a mild infection, a negative nitrogen, phosphorus, sulfur, and calcium balance with evidence of osteoporosis, wasting of tissue, and loss of weight generally results. The reaction is much more pronounced, of course, in a severe insult than in a mild one. This negative balance reaches its peak in about two to eight days and does not return to normal for several months. No dietary product can completely reverse the negative balance, although the degree of negativity of the nitrogen balance can be reduced.[23]

Because of the severe alteration of body metabolism produced by almost any illness and the additional changes produced by the bed rest that usually follow injury or illness, it would seem that rather drastic changes in the dietary intake would be indicated, if only to counterbalance the metabolic losses.

Edema

Edema of varying degrees is undoubtedly a contributing factor in the production of ischemic ulcers. An increased amount of interstitial fluid increases the distance from the capillary to the cell. Since the rate of diffusion of oxygen and food from the capillary to the cell decreases in proportion to this distance, it is clear that edema has a profound influence on the supply of nutrients to the cell.

Anemia

Anemia is also a contributing factor of great significance in determining whether cellular hypoxia and necrosis will occur. It is obvious that the possibility for ischemic tissue to survive is greatly enhanced when the hemoglobin content and the supply of oxygen within the blood are normal, even though blood flow is reduced. If in ischemia there is also a decreased oxygen content in the blood, cellular metabolism is further restricted.

PREVENTION

Ischemic ulcers are preventable. They need not occur. However, prevention requires knowledge of the correct techniques of management of patients at risk and then the conscientious and continuous application of those techniques. Since ischemia lasting only 30 to 60 minutes causes metabolic impairment that may lead to necrosis of cells, the program of preventive maintenance must be continuous. Patients who have multiple etiologic factors that impair cellular metabolism are at greater risk than those with a healthy metabolism, but all are threatened by cellular necrosis if the tissues are exposed to complete ischemia for a period of somewhat less than one hour. Moreover, the effects of exposure to repeated ischemia are cumulative. The results of allowing ischemic ulcers to develop are devastating. Ulcers are always disabling; if prolonged they are debilitating and occasionally lead to the patient's death. Treatment of ischemic ulcers after they have developed is difficult, time-consuming, and very expensive.

General Preventive Measures

Education

Education is the basis of any comprehensive preventive program. Intensive, informative educational efforts for hospital personnel as well as the patient and the family are absolutely essential. All involved persons must be kept continuously aware and informed regarding the primary cause of pressure sores, the serious consequences that can develop, and the patient morbidity that invariably results.

New equipment and adaptations must be thoroughly evaluated by the medical and nursing personnel and information regarding new materials, and improved methods must be provided to all the hospital staff. Above all, the patient and the medical staff must be made to realize that ischemic ulcers can be prevented but that no device or treatment measure, regardless of its cost or design, can effectively substitute for informed, conscientious skin care.

Identification of High-Risk Patient

Because of the critical time-pressure relationship, it is essential that efforts be made to identify every patient whose mobility is limited or restricted at the time of admission to the hospital or nursing facility. Those persons with impaired mobility, especially in combination with decreased sensation or alteration in the level of mental awareness, are obvious candidates for skin breakdown if neglected. Identification of these persons at the time of admission to the hospital and institution of appropriate, preventive skin-care programs will effectively preclude ischemic ulcers.

Special consideration must be given patients who require sedation or mood-altering drugs. In the process of providing relief of pain and limiting mental anguish and anxiety, the patient's mobility and response to the discomfort of pressure are depressed, with the result that the patient does not move enough to relieve the pressure areas.

The comatose, decerebrate, or spinal cord–injured patient is a prime candidate for skin breakdown because of the above-mentioned factors. These people, at the time they are admitted to the medical-care facility, must be identified and intensive, preventive skin-care measures must be instituted immediately.

The postsurgical or multiply traumatized patient also falls into this category because extensive surgical procedures, casting, and postoperative sedation all tend to interfere with mobility, thereby promoting skin breakdown.

Recognition of Impending Skin Breakdown

All personnel working with these patients must be taught the early recognition of those skin changes that are an indication of an impending skin breakdown. The earliest clinical evidence of skin damage is indicated by inflammation of the skin, which blanches on the application of digital pressure. This process originally presents as a hyperemic response except that the inflammation, unlike the hyperemic response, persists for a longer period of time. Whereas hyperemia lasts up to one half to three fourths as long as the occlusion, this preulcer inflammatory reaction may persist for several hours after the pressure has been relieved. At this stage, the condition is usually a completely and readily reversible process. Prevention of progression to more serious damage can be effected by the immediate complete elimination of pressure to the involved area. The time needed for complete resolution of the inflammation depends on the length of time the tissue has been subjected to pressure in excess of capillary pressure. Without prompt attention, this condition progresses to increasing inflammation and erythema that persists for more than 24 hours and does not blanch on digital pressure. The skin and underlying tissue become indurated, and there may actually be some vesicle formation. However, even at this stage, prompt preventive measures are generally effective.

Failure to recognize the skin changes noted above and to immediately relieve the involved area of all pressure will result in rapid progression to frank ulceration. The ability to recognize clinically the pre-existing skin changes involving only the dermis with its associated inflammatory response is infinitely more important than any classification of the deep, undermined, and infected ulceration. Recognizing the impending skin changes and instituting immediate preventive measures can lead to prevention of frank breakdown.

Specific Preventive Measures — Elimination or Reduction of Pressure

If we accept the proposition that pressure in excess of capillary pressure is the chief cause of ischemic ulcers, then our primary preventive efforts must be directed toward reducing or eliminating pressure over susceptible areas.

Intermittent pressure relief must be provided all patients, but especially those who have been identified as highly susceptible to skin breakdown. Position changes must be made not less frequently than every two hours around the clock. Patients with multiple risk factors must be turned or shifted more frequently. The skin must be carefully assessed each time the position is changed and areas showing evidence of inflammation must then be completely relieved of support pressure.

Since pressure relief, within the range of capillary pressure, is not possible on a static supporting surface, complete relief of pressure for each resting surface must be provided at regular intervals. The intermittent pressure support system appears to offer the greatest advantage because relief from pressure is provided to each resting surface at regular predictable intervals.[24]

Pressure extremes on alternating pressure relief surfaces frequently exceed those resting pressures of static surfaces. Although short periods of high pressure are not desirable, these pressures do not have the destructive effect of low pressures (above capillary pressure) when applied for prolonged periods of time.[25]

MANAGEMENT

General Measures

Since any major infectious or traumatic process requiring enforced bed rest results in dramatic changes in the body metabolism, appropriate dietary measures must be initiated if only to counteract the effects of infections and bed rest. Wound repair is influenced by the nutritional disorders stemming from the altered metabolic processes associated with severe injury, as well as by the patient's previous nutritional status.

Superimposed on these disturbances are other problems posed by contaminating microorganisms and compromised blood supply to the injured tissues. Obviously, maintenance of the patient in a good state of nutrition should be of high priority both to sustain healing and to avoid infection.

Specific Measures

Conservative

Conservative treatment methods share three common objectives: pressure relief, wound debridement, and infection control.

Pressure Relief. Since pressure is the primary cause of ischemic ulcers, complete relief of pressure of the involved area is essential if healing is to take place. The ulcerated area should never be subjected to any pressure unless absolutely necessary for resting support.

When multiple support areas are involved, these areas must be provided complete relief of pressure at regular intervals. This can be accomplished physically by frequent turning of the patient or mechanically by means of an alternating pressure support system. The alternating-pressure air mattress is the best mechanical method of providing pressure relief for the supine patient. However, over areas of maximum support, the pressures often may exceed capillary pressure so that even the patient, so confined, must be turned.

Debridement. Because all ischemic ulcers exhibit some degree of tissue necrosis, cleansing of the ulcer and the surrounding area is important.

MECHANICAL DEBRIDEMENT. Various forms of mechanical debridement are accepted in the treatment of ischemic ulcers. Cleansing of the ulcer and the surrounding tissue is best accomplished through the use of a bland antiseptic soap and warm water. The area can then be rinsed well with warm water and normal saline.

Hydrotherapy in the form of whirlpool or Hubbard tank baths is beneficial in assisting in the cleansing of large necrotic ischial or sacral ulcers. Minor surgical debridement is frequently necessary in small necrotic lesions while major surgical debridement, requiring the facilities of the operating room, may be needed in the treatment of the larger lesions.

CHEMICAL DEBRIDEMENT. Enzymes, in the form of ointments, solutions, powders, and sprays, have been used in the treatment of pressure sores with varying degrees of reported success. Enzymes physiologically debride eschar and necrotic tissue, thus tending to reduce infection.

Enzymatic substances are either fibrinolytic (capable of dissolving fibrin), proteolytic (capable of splitting protein by hydrolysis), or collagenolytic (capable of dissolving collagen). Although these enzymes assist in wound debridement, they have no healing effect per se.

Enzymatic measures are indicated especially when simple mechanical debridement is ineffective and surgical debridement is not indicated. Repeated, prolonged use of enzymatic compounds causes lysis of normal protein as well as necrotic material and actually delays wound healing. Enzymatic solutions are usually equally effective with fewer undesirable side effects.

OTHER DEBRIDING AGENTS. Numerous other agents, usually in the form of packs, poultices, and baths, have been used in the treatment of ischemic ulcers. The physiologic actions of some of these substances have been debated and the end results have at times been of questionable value. Almost without exception, the primary action of these methods of treatment is simple mechanical debridement combined with relief of pressure.

Infection Control. Wound cultures should be obtained at the time of admission of the patient to the hospital. While the results of the culture are being awaited, conservative debridement may be initiated. Because of the reported high incidence of anaerobic organisms cultured from ischemic ulcers, specific efforts must be made to isolate these organisms.

Once the organisms have been identified, specific antibiotic measures should be instituted. The mode of administration depends on the degree of involvement: generally topical antibiotic ointments are least effective in combating infection, while oral antibiotics may be the treatment of choice for the outpatient with a superficial, infected lesion. For the inpatient, especially the debilitated patient with extensive infection, intravenous antibiotic administration is indicated.

Surgical

Although conservative treatment measures are obviously the treatment of choice whenever indicated, surgical intervention plays a very important part in the treatment of ischemic ulcers.

No attempt will be made to review or discuss the technical nature of surgical intervention. Since this subject has been thoroughly discussed and reviewed in the surgical literature, the reader is referred to the surgical journals for a more complete and comprehensive assessment of the problem.

SUMMARY

Ischemic ulcers continue to constitute a major medical problem that interferes with the care of elderly and debilitated patients and patients with paralysis and anesthesia, such as spinal cord–injured patients. In spite of the great advances made in modern medical care, too little attention has been paid to the prevention of pressure ulcers. As a result, even though pressure ulcers are completely preventable, a great number still develop in patients in hospitals and nursing homes as well as those at home.

Preventive measures must be based on education of the patient, his family, and all involved professional personnel. Patients and personnel must be constantly reminded of the etiology, pathology, and cost of ischemic ulcers. They must also be convinced that ischemic ulcers can be prevented through diligent and enlightened nursing and self-care. The importance of providing pressure relief to the support areas must continue to be stressed, and materials and methods must never be substituted for sound nursing care.

REFERENCES

1. Munro, D.: Care of the back following spinal-cord injuries. N. Engl. J. Med., 223:391–398, 1940.
2. Dietrick, R. B., and Russi, S.: Tabulation and review of autopsy findings in fifty-five paraplegics. JAMA, 166:41–44, 1958.
3. Kuhn, W. G., Jr.: Care and rehabilitation of patients with injuries of spinal cord and cauda equina. J. Neurosurg., 4:40–68, 1947.
4. Freed, M. M., Bakst, H. J., and Barrie, D. L.: Life expectancy, survival rates and causes of death in civilian patients with spinal cord trauma. Arch. Phys. Med. Rehabil., 47:457–463, 1966.
5. Conference on care of patients with spinal cord injury. Palo Alto, Ca., Veterans Administration Hospital, 1975.
6. Nichol, J., Girling, F., Jerrard, W., Claxton, E. B., and Burton, A. C.: Fundamental instability of small blood vessels and critical closing pressures in vascular beds. Am. J. Physiol., 4:330–344, 1951.
7. Burton, A. C., and Yamada, S.: Relation between blood pressure and flow in human forearm. J. Appl. Physiol., 4:329–339, 1951.
8. Landis, E. M.: Micro-injection studies of capillary blood pressure in human skin. Heart, 15:209–228, 1930.
9. Harman, J. W.: A histological study of skeletal muscle in acute ischemia. Am. J. Pathol., 23:551–565, 1947.
10. Kosiak, M.: Etiology and pathology of ischemic ulcers. Arch. Phys. Med. Rehabil., 40:61–69, 1959.
11. Kosiak, M.: Etiology of decubitus ulcers. Arch. Phys. Med. Rehabil., 42:19–29, 1961.
12. Bush, C. A.: Study of pressure in skin under ischial tuberosity and thighs during sitting. Arch. Phys. Med. Rehabil., 50:207–212, 1967.
13. Houle, R. J.: Evaluation of seat devices designed to prevent ischemic ulcers in paraplegic patients. Arch. Phys. Med. Rehabil., 50:587–594, 1969.
14. Souther, S. G., Carr, S. D., and Vistnes, L. M.: Wheel chair cushions to reduce pressure under bony prominences. Arch. Phys. Med. Rehabil., 55:460–464, 1974.
15. Mooney, V., Eisbund, M. J., Rogers, J. E., and Stauffer, E. S.: Comparison of pressure distribution qualities in seat cushions. Bull. Prosthet. Res., (Spring), 129–143, 1971.
16. Lindan, O., Greenway, R. M., and Piazza, J. N.: Pressure distribution on the surface of the human body: 1. Evaluation in lying and sitting position

using a "bed of springs and nails." Arch. Phys. Med. Rehabil., 46:378–385, 1965.

17. Reichel, S. M.: Shearing force as a factor in decubitus ulcers in paraplegics. JAMA, 166:762–763, 1958.

18. Dinsdale, S. M.: Decubitus ulcers in swine, light and microscopy study of pathogenesis. Arch. Phys. Med. Rehabil., 54:51–56, 1973.

19. Fisher, S. V., Szymke, T. E., Apte, S. Y., and Kosiak, M.: Wheelchair cushion effect on skin temperature. Arch. Phys. Med. Rehabil., 59:68–72, 1978.

20. Alexander, H., and Cook, T.: Variations with age in the mechanical properties of human skin in vivo. *In* Kenedi, R. M., Cowden, J. M., and Scales, J. T. (Eds.): Bedsore Biomechanics. Baltimore, University Park Press 1975, pp. 109–117.

21. Tsuchida, Y., and Tsuya, A.: Measurement of skin blood flow in delayed deltopectoral flaps using local clearance of ^{133}Xenon. Plast. Reconstr. Surg., 62:763–770, 1978.

22. Exton Smith, A. N.: *In* Kenedi, R. M., Cowden, J. M., and Scales J. T. (Eds.): Bedsore Biomechanics. Baltimore, University Park Press, 1975, pp. 133–139.

23. Deitrick, J. E.: Effects of immobilization on metabolic and physiological functions of normal men. Bull. N.Y. Acad. Med., 24:364–375, 1948.

24. Kosiak, M.: A mechanical resting surface: Its effect on pressure distribution. Arch. Phys. Med. Rehabil., 57:481–484, 1976.

25. Hussain, T.: Experimental study of some pressure effects on tissues with reference to the bed sore problem. J. Pathol. Bacteriol., 66:347–358, 1953.

47

REHABILITATION OF PROBLEMS OF SEXUALITY IN PHYSICAL DISABILITY

THEODORE M. COLE
SANDRA S. COLE

If one reflects on the images that may come to mind when the word "sex" is spoken, many people would think pleasant thoughts such as lovemaking, fun, warmth, and pleasure — both giving and taking. On the other hand, if one considers the imagery evoked by the word "disability," it would not be surprising for many people to think in such concepts as alone, ugly, incapable, and painful. A significant realization may occur when these two sets of concepts are put into juxtaposition. The emotional reaction to the concepts of sex and disability together might include such thoughts as impossibility, frustration, withdrawal, disinterest, or vulnerability. It is clear that a conscious effort will be needed by health professionals and disabled people alike to alter the attitudes that lead to such thoughts.

Although physicians are generally informed about the pathophysiology of genitourinary and reproductive function, they may not be informed about contemporary sexual behavior. The information they do possess may be colored by personal preferences, aversions, and taboos that may further foster ignorance. The uneasiness and anxiety that result from misinformation may make it difficult for the physician to hear or treat the patient's complaints. Patients and their families can also be ill informed or uncomfortable with sexuality, thereby impeding the physician's ability to obtain a cogent sexual history or initiate a referral for sexual intervention. The presence of a physical disability does not erase the years of socialization that may make it difficult for patients and families to discuss sexuality with the physician. That same discomfort or anxiety may lead to sexual dysfunction and marital strife, and the foundation for sexual dysfunction may be passed on to children. However, a patient's unwillingness to talk about sexuality does not necessarily mean disinterest. Unwillingness may mean that the patient is anxious or fearful about the sexual implications of the physical disability. The physician may be able to reduce the anxiety by taking positive actions to facilitate comfort and set the expectation with the patient that sexuality, like any other important aspect of living, is an appropriate area of concern for physicians and the patients who seek their services.

While studying human sexuality curricula in American medical schools, Ebert and Lief[1] pointed out that although reproductive physiology and pathology were commonly taught, sexuality training programs for medical students were almost nonexistent before 1954. In the early 1960's there were only three programs. However, by 1968 there were 30 medical schools offering sexuality curriculum and by 1975 nearly all medical schools reported substantial sex education programs for their students. Interest in sexuality and physical disability has followed a similar course of recent expansion.

A physical disability is a condition of impairment that can usually be described by a physician. A handicap is a collective result of all the hinderances that a disability places between an individual and optimum functional potential. It is more accurate to refer to *an individual with a disability* rather than *a disabled person* because the term "disabled" subordinates all areas of function to the disabling aspect. These are not irrelevant attitudinal distinctions. The degree to which a physical disability is handicapping is relative to each situation and social role. Not all people perceive the same disability as particularly handicapping, especially with respect to sexuality. A physical condition that is not necessarily disabling or handicapping may become so owing to social stigmatization. Roberts and Roberts[2] conclude that a physical attribute becomes a handicap only when it is seen as a significant obstacle to the accomplishment of a particular goal and that a physical attribute may become handicapping not because it imposes actual limitations but because it interferes with social relations or is in conflict with the individual's value systems.

SEXUALITY: ITS MEANING FOR REHABILITATION

Some physical disabilities affect sexuality directly by disablement of genital function. However, most do not. Blindness does not affect genital function, but it certainly affects communication. Myocardial infarction is frequently followed by impotence in a high percentage of males and may also affect the libido and activities of the patient's partner because of fear of sudden death precipitated by sexual activity. The individual with a disfiguring burn may want acceptance and contact but instead withdraws and covers up. In these examples sexuality is defined by and expressed in how people present themselves — their bodies, activities, relationship preferences, and aversions. Understood in broad terms, it becomes clear that sexuality may influence and be influenced by physical disability. Sexuality is an avenue toward intimacy.[3] The imposition of a life devoid of intimacy may have a devastating effect upon the person with a physical disability and may compound the health care problems with which the physician must deal.

Medical rehabilitation has been defined in many ways. For the purposes of this chapter it is defined as a process that promotes a stabilization of the disabling condition, maximizes restoration of lost functions, and institues adaptive mechanisms that allow resumption of responsibility for part or all of one's own life. If a physical disability is complex and moderately severe, pursuit of these goals will require the efforts of an integrated team of practitioners who can provide an array of health care services in medical, psychosocial, vocational, and educational areas. Such a team will discover that fruitful work with a person with a physical disability mandates a rapport of trust and openness that must be maintained over the duration of the handicap and its treatment. Trust is not easily achieved and may be hampered by aloofness, impaired communication, or distance between the physician and the patient. Sensitive attention given to sexuality, however, can play a facilitating role in building rapport by emphasizing caring, comprehensiveness, and openness, while minimizing aloofness and barriers to communication.

FOUNDATIONS OF SEXUAL HEALTH

When one accepts a broad definition of human sexuality one can better see and understand the sexuality of people with handicapping conditions. One may then understand when and in what ways the handicapped person may have concerns about expressing sexuality.

As for any other aspect of health care, the practitioner should be trained in how to initiate questions and interventions relative to sexuality. Consideration of the physician's own sexuality may help him or her become more effective in dealing with the sexuality of others. Lief[1] points out that a physician learns about sexuality differently than he or she learns about other scientific topics. One can effectively employ a body of knowledge about chemistry without emotionally understanding one's own chemistry. However, one cannot effectively employ a body of knowledge about sexuality and apply it to a patient without thinking about one's own sexuality. The absence of self-understanding about sexuality may lead the physician to do harm to the patient and disservice to the medical profession.

Sexuality is a health issue. Rehabilitation, perhaps more than most other medical specialties, concerns itself with the whole patient. Sexuality is part of the whole and is a natural function. However, naturalness may be impeded by many things, including previous experiences or physical conditions. The physician can be helpful as diagnostitian, educator, or therapist by employing the medical model. The medical model should not be abandoned when dealing with the area of sexuality. It is not sufficient for a physician to ask "How is your sex life?" A similar abandonment of the medical model would cause the physician to ask a patient with ulcerative colitis "How is your defecation life?" Specific questions and answers can lead to diagnoses and therapy.

Sexual health is different for different people. However, there are several components of sexuality that are common to a state of sexual health. These include a positive self-esteem, freedom from prohibiting attitudes and ignorance, and a willingness to risk intimacy with another person. For some people sexual health also involves a measure of physical competence. Like other physical activities sex requires a certain amount of practice and skill. Unfortunately, our culture does not provide physically disabled people with a sufficient array of sex education materials to allow them to become educated about themselves and the world in which they live. Thus, many people with physical disabilities either learn little about themselves or possess spotty if not erroneous information about their physical capabilities. Remediation of this misinformation is clearly within the province of the physician.

PSYCHOSEXUAL DEVELOPMENT OF CHILDREN

During infancy and the first decade, boys experience penile erections at regular intervals. These may be reflexogenic during infancy but later on result from deliberate self-stimulation. Females also engage in self-stimulation. Their early sexual character is described as being more diffuse than that of the male. The early sexual experiences of girls may result from a wider assortment of stimuli than direct genital stimulation. During these years, both boys and girls are having their attention drawn to sex with such tasks as toilet training, learning sex differences between parents, siblings, and friends, and learning or adopting sexual modesty codes. During these same years, the child is developing a language base that will include "acceptable" and "dirty" words for conveying sexual information. Facility with sexual language becomes exceedingly important if the youth is to understand the world, communicate with peers, and avoid problems that arise from ignorance.

Learning differences between right and wrong is a major task during these growing years. It is hoped that the child will build wholesome attitudes toward self while at the same time learning how to get along with peers. The development of a conscience becomes evident at a time when the child is learning appropriate sex roles, acquiring moral and ethical standards, and beginning to project attitudes toward social groups and institutions which have direct sexual associations.

The child grows within the framework of a society that adopts, projects, and enforces a set of attitudes which impact back on the child's sexuality. The able-bodied and the physically disabled child must both contend with society's attitudes towards menstruation, wet dreams, masturbation, and sexual fantasies. Society's admiration of the "perfect body" may convey the message that physical disability desexualizes the child. The family's efforts to protect the child from rejection or exploitation may lead to avoidance of the topic of sex and normal family interactions. The child may thus be insulated from exposure to sexual situations and may be thought of by peers as "less than" other children. The gaps in the sex education of a child may lead to problems that can become insurmountable in later years. Parents, in turn, may be isolated by the child's fear of admitting ignorance or of revealing fantasies and concerns. Like able-bodied children, the disabled child worries about being normal, over- or under-sexed, attractive or unattractive. It is clear that the physician can help to provide the child with an adult role model that recognizes sexuality in the formative years and helps the child and the family develop a growing sense of sexual health.

SEXUAL PHYSIOLOGY AND RESPONSIVITY

It is not the purpose of this chapter to provide a comprehensive discussion of the physiologic and behavioral aspects of sexuality. For such information the reader is referred to appropriate texts.[5-10] However, a brief review is appropriate to establish a common basis of understanding between the authors and readers.

The sexual response cycle has been described by many workers. The work of Masters and Johnson may be the best known and identifies four phases of the cycle.

The excitement phase can be psychological or physical. It begins when the person is first aware of being sexually stimulated. Both men and women show increases in muscle tension, heart rate, blood pressure, and breathing rate. If stimulation continues in the male, erection of the penis occurs. In the female, vaginal lubrication begins with continued stimulation. If stimuli cease to be effective, the next phase will not occur and the body will return to the unaroused state. If sexual stimulation continues, however, the second phase begins.

The plateau phase is the second phase and extends from the end of excitement until the beginning of orgasm. Owing to neurovascular influences, congestion of the primary sexual organs occurs. If stimulation is ineffective or ceases, the body will show a gradual reduction of the physiologic phenomena that are part of this phase. With continued effective stimulation, the third phase will commence.

Orgasm is the third phase. If no psychologic or physical discomfort occurs, the person will progress through one or more orgasms. Orgasms customarily last from 30 to 60 seconds but have been described as lasting from as little as a few seconds to as long as several minutes. Most often, the male ejaculates during orgasm and is aware of a rhythmic contraction of his perineal muscles. Women also experience rhythmic contractions of the pubococcygeal muscles, and in both sexes anal sphincter contraction occurs synchronously with contractions of the pelvic floor. Immediately after orgasm, a refractory period commences during which time more stimulation will not produce further sexual arousal. The refractory phase may last from minutes to days, depending upon such factors as age and intensity of sexual arousal. Women have brief refractory periods and may be multiorgasmic.

The fourth phase is called resolution. During this phase the body returns to its prearoused and relaxed state.

Inability to achieve orgasm is often equated with sexual dysfunction. However, as can be seen from the description of the sexual response cycle, dysfunction can occur at any phase in the cycle. Educating patients about their natural responsiveness and physiology, while encouraging them to become comfortable with themselves and their sexuality, can be very therapeutic for people with or without physical disabilities.

Although sexuality, intimacy, and genital function can be separated, they are usually interconnected. It is helpful, therefore, to define the more common genital dysfunctions so that one can understand how they can cause or be caused by personal or interpersonal problems. It should be kept in mind that genital aspects of sexual function have an impact upon the entire personality. Changes in genital function will almost always create reverberations throughout the personality structure of the individual.

Female Sexual Dysfunctions

Preorgasmia. Women who have never experienced an orgasm by any means are considered preorgasmic. In the absence of physical disability, the roots of preorgasmia are usually found in the religious upbringing, the family environment, or childhood sexual trauma.

Secondary Nonorgasmia. Secondary nonorgasmia is often situational. Women who experience orgasm with masturbation or with a partner's stimulation but not with sexual intercourse are included in this group.

Also included are women who experience physical orgasm but do not experience a psychological component and women who experienced orgasm during an earlier part of their life but not currently.

Dyspareunia. Women who experience disabling pain during intercourse are considered to have dyspareunia. Prior to counseling, a woman should receive a thorough medical examination to exclude organic causes of vaginal pain.

Sexual Aversion. Women who are repulsed or terrified by sex are described as being sexually aversive. Etiologic factors may include one or more of the following: doubts about her own sexual adequacy; over-reaction to body odors, penis size, or semen; early traumatic sexual experience; or extremely prohibiting religious views leading to feelings of guilt and shame regarding sex.

Vaginismus. Vaginismus occurs during attempted penetration of the vulva by the erect penis and is characterized by involuntary spasms of the muscles of the pelvic floor which surround the outer third of the vagina. This dysfunction is also frequently associated with sexual fears and anxieties about intercourse. Its roots can frequently be found in the woman's lack of self-acceptance, an underdeveloped ability to form sexual relationships, inability to trust a partner, religious prohibitions, or previous sexual trauma.

Male Sexual Dysfunctions

Premature Ejaculation. A man is said to prematurely ejaculate if he ejaculates before he wishes. This is one of the most common sexual dysfunctions of men, and, fortunately, one of the easiest to treat.

Primary Erectile Dysfunction. A condition of primary erectile dysfunction exists when a man states that he has never been able to maintain an erect penis for the purpose of sexual penetration. He may, however, be capable of having erections during masturbation and may report erections during sleep. Physical examinations should be carried out to eliminate organic etiologies, which will be described later. Anxieties, which may be rooted in sexual trauma in early life, male sex role stress, feelings of inadequacy, or prohibiting religious or moral views may also be etiologically significant.

Secondary Erectile Dysfunction. Men who have been able to achieve erections on some occasions but not on others are said to have secondary erectile dysfunction. Erection may be possible during foreplay but may disappear as coitus is attempted. Some men report achievement of erections with some partners but not with others. Common causative factors include excessive use of alcohol, relationship stresses, and secondary effects of some therapeutic medicines to be described later.

Retarded Ejaculation. Men whose ejaculatory reflexes are inhibited while erection remains are experiencing retarded ejaculation. Such men sometimes experience ejaculation through manual or oral stimulation but are unable to ejaculate while the penis is contained in the vagina. Etiologic factors often include guilt feelings surrounding sex in general or guilt feelings with specific sexual partners. Sexual identity conflicts, fear of pregnancy in a partner, and moral and ethical considerations also may play a part.

As this brief description of the more common sexual dysfunctions shows, the etiology is often related to dysfunctional sexual attitudes, behavioral problems, relationship problems, or early traumatic sexual experiences. However, none of them presuppose the presence of a physical disability as a causative factor or an initiating event leading to sexual dysfunction. Any of the above sexual dysfunctions can be seen in a physically disabled adult. In addition, a sexual dysfunction may have its onset after the occurrence of a physical disability. The physician should therefore be acquainted with the ways in which sexual function may be altered by a physical disability.

SEXUAL EVALUATION OF THE DISABLED PATIENT

Why Ask?

The physician asks questions of the patient in order to make diagnoses, develop a plan of management, assess effectiveness of therapy, and make modifications in relation to progress. Restoration to optimal function as an individual in his community is the goal. Specific diagnoses of sexual dysfunctions that are amenable to correction can be made by an alert clinician who asks the right questions in a sensitive way.

Masters and Johnson have asserted that sexual dysfunction occurs at one time or another in at least 50 per cent of the general population. There is a probability that problems of sexuality are even more frequent in persons with disabilities. Many sexual dysfunctions are treatable if identified. The problems associated with sexual dysfunction often are substantive and concrete. Although many sexual dysfunctions become intertwined with the personality structure, there are often functional problems that can be remedied by brief therapy.

How to Ask

The rehabilitation model serves us well in the area of sexuality. Just as with rehabilitation, issues such as mobility, self-care, and weakness are treated within the context of the disabilities. Questions about intimacy may be integrated into genitourinary inquiries and into questions dealing with pain, alterations in bodily sensations, disfigurements, etc. Segregating questions about sexuality from the medical and rehabilitation history conveys the message that sex is not really a health issue or is less acceptable to the physician than other aspects of the patient's health.

Since in our culture discussion of sex usually carries an emotional loading that is stressful to the patient, questions should be discretely and privately asked and an understanding of confidentiality should be established early in the interview. Difficult questions can often be made easier if the physician will frankly ask the patient for permission to delve into personal and even sensitive areas. When the patient understands that if the physician is informed in these areas he is able to treat the problems that stem from the physical disability, then willingness is usually freely expressed. Identifying personal areas as sensitive is a useful technique for eliciting the patient's permission. The patient may be more prepared to answer questions if there is a clear relationship between the question and the disability under consideration. Thus, questions to an arthritic patient about pain on movement, especially freedom of movement of the hips, can easily be seen to be a sex-related topic. Similarly, the medical ramifications of diabetic peripheral neuropathy should properly include questions relative to erections in the male, vaginal lubrication in the female, and orgasmic function in both.

The physician can make the socially stressful situation of the medical interview more comfortable by indicating to the patient that it may seem awkward when a person is asked to reveal personal areas of self to a relative stranger. Simply saying so may do much to allay anxiety and allow for a sensitive exploration of sexual issues.

Some physicians are reluctant to commence a sexual interview because they fear that once begun a comprehensive review of material with which they are not familiar must be carried out. However, most physicians do not need to conduct a comprehensive sexual interview in order to go over information useful for the rehabilitation team. Specific questions may be all that are needed to identify the sexual problems and concerns of some patients. Lief[4] points out that perhaps 25 per cent of patients with sexual dysfunctions can be benefited solely by providing information within an atmosphere of friendliness and permission to talk. The sexual partner of the patient is an important person to be interviewed, either separately or with the patient. Not only may the physician gain new and important insights about the patient's sexuality, but bringing the partner along at the same rate as the patient may avoid future pitfalls created by unevenness of information and expectations between the patient and the sexual partner.

Reactions from the patient and/or partner may indicate areas of need. Thus, the patient who displays apparent indifference after questions about sexuality may really be displaying anxiety or fear of discovery. Very few people are genuinely disinterested in their own sexuality. A skilled clinician can return in the future with further questions if the indifference persists throughout the initial interview. Denial of sexual concerns may genuinely reflect a lack of concern on the part of the patient. However, the lack of concern may stem from lack of information rather than an informed reason to be unconcerned. For example, a patient in the early stages of severe stroke may believe that he or she will return to the premorbid vocation, and it may not be until weeks later that he or she recognizes the vocational disability that has resulted. So too, a return to questions of sexuality and intimacy at a later date may reveal that the denial has been replaced by a genuine interest, and even by fear of dysfunction. The use of comfort-producing techniques such as brief anecdotes about similar situations can do much to forge a basis for subsequent productive discussions on intimate issues.

Some patients may react with frank hostility. Often hostility is strong evidence of a serious problem that deserves further exploration if not consultation by professionals skilled in human sexuality and physical disability. All the while, the physician must remember to avoid becoming defensive or feeling a need for lengthy explanations of sexually related questions.

The language of sex may be as personal as the activities themselves. The physician should make an effort to understand the patient and provide a language that is comfortable and communicative. Resorting to strictly medical terms is often as undesirable in the area of sexuality as it is in any medical area where accurate communication is essential. However, the physician may learn that the patient's sex-related words and language are different from his or her own. The physician should be prepared to use the patient's preferred language in order to communicate. Thus, for some people ''come'' may be a more effective word than orgasm and ''hard-on'' may be more communicative than erection.

What to Ask

The patient should be encouraged to express his or her needs, concerns, and fears about the disability and expressions of intimacy. The type and duration of the disability are important, since a disability having its onset during childhood usually has a different effect upon sexuality than a disability that has its onset after psychosexual development has been completed. Information having to do with sexual techniques, frequency, sexual fantasy, and personal values and ethics is important to gather in order to be helpful. The physician should remember not to put a person into conflict with his God, his morals, or his ethics in the area of sexuality. Specific questions should be asked in order to gain an understanding of a couple's sexual patterns. Information about sexual practices, either solitary or with the sexual partner, should be gathered. Masturbation, anal sex, oral genital stimulation, manual genital manipulation, and use of sexual devices are frequently practiced among adults in western culture. The patterns of sexual expression are important for a physician to know, just as he would find it important to know about a patient's daily living activities or vocational interests in setting goals for a rehabilitation plan. The physician must not overlook the fact that some people engage in homosexual activities either exclusively or in addition to heterosexual activities. Thus, the sexual orientation of the patient should be determined. Questions about sexual partners other than the primary partner also should be asked, especially in cases of erectile dysfunction or loss of libido.

In interviewing a physically disabled person, as with a person without an apparent disability, sex should be considered in a broad sense, not only as genital function. Sex is a major avenue of communication between people and involves not only coitus and self-pleasuring but any other physical activity that is mutually acceptable and pleasurable. The physician's inquiries about sexual history should be made in a way that is acceptable and/or satisfying to both the patient and the physician. An interview can be not only diagnostic but sometimes therapeutic as well.

The physician's examination should also assess the patient's general knowledge about sexuality. The physician can help patients by having available, for educational purposes, printed material and examples of equipment or devices used by disabled persons. This may include not only items that a disabled person may use to accomplish activities of daily living, such as catheters, fecal drainage bags, etc., but also equipment related to sexual function, such as an electrical vibrator.

PHYSICAL EXAMINATION

As with any other aspect of the physical examination, the physician's examination of the patient with respect to sexual function should be organized and systematic.

Sensory testing should include testing of the genitals and the perineal area. In addition, other erogenous zones, whether identified by the patient or believed to be important by the physician, should also be examined for sexual function. In many cases of spinal cord injury, erogenous zones change dramatically with the onset of sensory paralysis. Frequently, the dermatomal levels just above the anesthetic area of the body become erogenous, whereas they may not have been so prior to the disability. Sensory examination should also include the urinary and rectal sphincters, and special attention should be paid to the S_1, S_2, and S_3 dermatomes on the buttocks and legs.

Motor testing should include the S_1 to S_3 motor segments of the lower extremities as well as sphincter tone strength of the pelvic floor and the rectum. The bulbocavernosus reflex should be tested in both the male and the female. Its absence may indicate a lesion of the reflex arc between the pelvic floor and the spinal cord. The force of the urinary stream, either audibly or visibly monitored, may help to provide information about detrusor S_1 to S_3 function, which can be influenced in a parallel way with organic sexual function.

Vascular lesions in the large vessels of the legs and pelvis may explain the lack of pelvic congestion following sexual stimulation. They may also be responsible for erectile dysfunctions in both men and women. The shaft of the penis should be examined for the plaques of Peronie's disease and the vagina should be examined for mechanical obstructions and inflammation.

Examination of the urinary tract should include not only a thorough examination of the external genitals but also electrical studies of the bladder and the pelvic floor. A cystometrogram can provide the physician with important information about the function of the bladder, which is served by many of the same nerve roots that serve sexual function. EMG studies of the external urinary or rectal sphincter may also help to diagnose upper or lower motor neuron disease, which in turn may affect not only erectile function but ejaculation in the male and lubrication in the female as well. Investigation of nocturnal penile tumescence is a technique that has become popular in recent years and may be useful to the physician in diagnosing erectile dysfunction in the male. Erections varying in length from 15 to 30 minutes occur several times a night during periods of rapid eye movement (REM) sleep in the neurologically intact male. The absence of such a phenomenon may indicate an organic basis for the erectile dysfunction.

The physician should also examine the patient for target organ disease elsewhere, as in patients with diabetes mellitus. A history of changes in bowel function, loss of esophageal motility, or gastric atony may help confirm the autonomic neuropathy of diabetes. Ten to 25 per cent of diabetics have disturbances of pupillary function. Decreased sudomotor function is also seen in the peripheral neuropathy of diabetes mellitus. Orthostatic hypertension, changes in peripheral pulse rate with positional changes of the body, alterations in the R-R interval on the ECG during and after the Valsalva maneuver, and cardiovascular responses to forceful gripping are all measures of autonomic nervous system function.

CLASSIFICATION OF PHYSICAL DISABILITIES

Physical disabilities can be grouped into four categories, depending upon age of onset and the progressive or stable nature of the disability.

Type I Disabilities — Preadolescent Nonprogressive

Type I disabilities are those that begin before puberty and are not progressive. Congenital brain injury, limb amputation in early life, and congenital loss of organs of special sensation are examples. People with these disabilities experience a lifetime of being different from their peers. Protective or guilt-laden attitudes by society or parents may have an inhibiting effect on their sexual maturation. They may be deliberately or inadvertently deprived of important adolescent experiences. Such individuals emerge from adolescence with maturational deficits and lack of social skills. They find themselves in an adult world, wanting to be sexually sophisticated but lacking the requisite education.

Developmental Disabilities. Public Law 94–103 states that a developmental disability is a physical or mental impairment resulting in limitations of major life activities. It is manifested before the age of 22 and is likely to continue. It often produces a lifelong need for special or extended care. Public Law 94–142 specifically provides for public education for all school age children who are physically disabled. The education is mandated to occur in the least restrictive manner.

Easton[11] points out that addressing the sexuality of such a person may require considerable and continuing effort. The individual who has been disabled from birth or early childhood has been different for a lifetime. Together with the usual self-consciousness of adolescence, the developmental disability may prevent the child from mixing with other children. The child may focus much energy into academic achievement. Many children are delayed in reaching independence due to physical, mental, or emotional barriers occurring within themselves, within others, or within the environment. Added to this is the fact that growing up takes place in a society that is uneasy about sex, where sexual activity begins at earlier and earlier ages, and where there is not enough communication between the child and the adult world. Robinault[12] states that the physician can take the role of healer, educator, and counselor. However, the role of healer may be conflicted by the chronicity of the disease, the role of educator by the diversity in which the child lives, and the role of counselor by the many options for sexual education and expression that are available and practical in our society.

Easton[11] states that the handicapped child may not learn because of limited physical and social experience, low demands or expectations from the family and school, and limited teaching in the skills of adolescence and adulthood. Learning may also suffer from a lack of honest feedback about inappropriate behavior, problems attendant to separation from the family, and informational deficits in street language and innuendo. The child may lack an orientation to peer values and many manifest egocentricity and preoccupation with physical or academic activities that are encouraged by the family and society. Added to these may be learning or perceptual problems, deficits in special sensation, and expressive or receptive communication problems. The mosaic may be complicated by a limited supply of energy that is drained by demands placed upon the child for independence and mobility. The result is often a child who does not know how to take responsibility for his or her own social and sexual success.

The physician must understand the very real limitations imposed by the child's disability and at the same time make use of the child's environment and strengths. The child whose family provides healthy, warm, and loving support will generally do better in psychosexual development. Most important is the need to consider the child as a sexual person from the very beginning. School personnel may also play a role as the child progresses to a larger world. The goals of education may need to be different for the child with a physical handicap, and more emphasis may have to be placed on social abilities than on pure academics. In providing services to such a child and family, the physician should respect the family's value system. Sensitive issues or different standards of ethics, religion, and sex will require sensitivity from the physician.

Deafness. Deafness is the most common chronic disability in the United States today (see Chapter 44). In approaching the deaf child and the family, the physician should recognize that 90 per cent of deaf children have parents with normal hearing abilities. Usually children with congenital deafness receive their education and much of life's experiences in residential schools where they may stay until age 21.

Since the average deaf child achieves a reading level between the fourth and fifth grade, they are handicapped by a dearth of sex education material available at that level. The deaf child or young adult may have had difficulties in learning about sexuality due to limited auditory observational opportunities. Added to this is the fact that sex-related sign language is very regional in the United States and very private and personal. It is often not readily available to the developing child. In those few schools for the deaf where sex education is provided, it is necessary that the signing interpreter be comfortable with sexuality. Graphics have been found to be helpful, especially when prepared specifically for deaf children.

The physician's approach to a deaf child and family must be directed toward helping the child achieve social skills and a positive self-image while encouraging the caretakers in the family and schools to facilitate the sexualization of the child as a normal and healthy development.

Type II Disabilities — Preadolescent Progressive

Type II disabilities also begin before puberty and may produce effects similar to those of Type I. However, these disabilities are progressive and the child becomes more dysfunctional with time. Examples include juvenile rheumatoid arthritis, childhood-onset diabetes mellitus, muscular dystrophy, and cystic fibrosis. Because of the nature of the disability, these patients are involved in regular treatment programs that require much of their energy. This produces an inadequate body image, a feeling of being sick, and an unwillingness to regard their bodies as able to provide sensual pleasure.

Neuromuscular diseases are typical examples of Type II physical disabilities. A child who is growing up with muscular dystrophy may experience many of the physical difficulties described in Type I above and, in addition, is handicapped by progressive deterioration of physical abilities.[13, 14] The child may face loss of mobility, reduced endurance, and difficulties with muscular coordination. Contractures may necessitate special and conspicuous external equipment such as a wheelchair and orthotic devices. The physician should recognize that the child's orientation may be toward a continually declining base of health and physical and emotional expectations.

Type III Disabilities — Adolescent and Adult Nonprogressive

Type III disabilities are those that occur in adolescent or adult life and are nonprogressive. Examples include traumatic spinal cord injury, amputation, and disfiguring burns. Individuals with these disabilities have already experienced a "normal" adolescence and have probably been sexually socialized. This reference point may be helpful in their efforts to reestablish their psychosexual identity. Further, they may already have learned the interpersonal skills necessary for the development of healthy adult sexual relationships. These skills may serve them after they become disabled.

Spinal Cord Injury. Injury to the spinal cord usually has its onset after puberty and is nonprogressive. The concept of self is severely stressed by spinal cord injury.[17]

Soon after the injury, depression frequently becomes a dominant personality pattern as the patient begins a relative acceptance of an unpleasant reality.[18] Teal and Athelstan[18] state that depression is primarily due to the perception of a diminished self-worth. They point out that the paralyzed person's sexuality can have a powerful effect upon a sense of self-worth. Similarly, self-worth can have a significant effect upon sexuality. They followed 256 patients for 2 to 20 years after spinal cord injury and learned that sexual satisfaction is often lacking. In comparison to other aspects of postdisability adjustment, their subjects showed less satisfaction with their sexual lives than they did with their employment situations, living arrangements, social lives, and general health.

Bregman and Hadley[15] report that only 50 per cent of spinal cord–injured women whom they studied had received even the basic information about sexuality during their initial hospitalization and rehabilitation. Cole and his co-workers[16] compared able-bodied single and married medical students to a group of single and married men and women with spinal cord injury living in the community. They found that spinal cord–injured people were more ready than the medical students to talk about sex and displayed less defensiveness and more openness. They also found that the role of fantasy was stronger in the spinal cord–injured population than in the medical students.

Cole[20] and his co-workers studied sexual attitudes and experiences of spinal cord–injured people at the time of discharge from their initial hospitalization, one year later, and again two years after injury. Approximately one fourth to one third of their patients reported that the importance of sex declined within the first year after injury, but at the end of the second year interest had returned to the pre-injury level or had become heightened. Approximately one third of the patients reported that the spinal cord injury did not produce a change in the sexual activity they enjoyed the most, but many expressed a wish for more sexual counseling while in the hospital. Fifty per cent considered their sexual adjustment to be good two years after their injury, but more than half of the patients reported that they were not as sexually active as they would have liked. The most common reason offered one year after injury was lack of partners. Two years after injury, lack of activity was attributed not only to lack of partners but also to fear of rejection, health concerns, and problems with erections. Three years after injury, males listed problems with erections as being the major reason for lack of activity.

Berkman[21] worked with veterans in the United States military and tested the hypothesis that improved sexual adjustment would be accompanied by proportionate increases in psychological, social, physiologic, and vocational adjustment. She applied an Index of Sexual Adjustment to 104 sexually active spinal-injured adults living in the community and found that sexual adjustment was more favorable among the young and among those whose financial resources were greater. She also found that the Index of Sexual Adjustment varied directly with companion indices measuring physical function and community participation. Lastly, the ability of the person to function in the worker role also varied directly with scores obtained on her Index of Sexual Adjustment.

McCluer[22] studied contraceptive practices of spinal cord–injured women through questionnaires to the women and to rehabilitation physicians. Although most physicians she sampled had not seen complications from contraceptives, those who had seen them described phlebitis or complications secondary to the use of intrauterine contraceptive devices. She also questioned 227 spinal cord–injured women, 25 per cent of whom were sexually active paraplegic women and 57 per cent of whom were sexually active quadriplegic women, and found that 21 per cent of the paraplegic women had become pregnant, as had 7 per cent of the quadriplegic women. The most frequent methods of contraception were oral contraceptives and intrauterine devices.

Brain Injury. Injury to the brain by trauma or vascular disease falls in the category of Type III disabilities. The sexual correlates of damage to the frontal lobe are related to learning and behavioral problems. Loss of fantasy and loss of moral and ethical restraints are often seen. However, increases in libido have not been described. Temporal lobe dysfunction is associated with a change in the sexual activation system. Usually this is associated with a decreased libido and decreased genital and sexual arousal. Rarely, excessive libido may be seen.

Other correlates of brain dysfunction are associated with hemianesthesia, which may accompany left or right hemispheric damage. Patients may be unaware of touch, or touch may be perceived as painful or uncomfortable. If the language centers are damaged the ability of the patient to participate in the verbal communication of sex may be impaired. Urinary and bowel continence may not be reliable. Autonomic nervous system abnormalities may lead to alterations in tumescence of the sex organs or lubrication of the vagina. Added to these are the kinesiosexual dysfunctions that can result from weakness, spasticity, incoordination, limitation of motion, or pain associated with the physical activities and postures associated with sexual expression.

Patients may manifest several sexual concomitants during the stages of recovery from brain damage. During the coma phase no recognizable sex focus is seen. However, during progression from the vegetative to the community reintegration stages, a progression of sexual foci can be seen. Early in the awakening stage patients may manifest sexual interest through auto-stimulation of the genitals. This has been said to resemble the prepubescent phase of normal development. Coital interest and masturbatory activity begin to appear as the patient becomes more alert. Efforts by the staff to appropriately channel these interests can be useful.

Family education is extremely important at this point. As the patient is reintegrated into the community, the main sexual focus is to increase the psychosexual skills of the patient. A fuller understanding of pleasuring and an appreciation of the consequences of actions can also be taught to many patients. As with all other aspects of sexuality, it is important to establish awareness of the self as worthwhile and deserving of physical and intimate experiences. Most patients can be taught to express their desires and to focus them on appropriate people.

Type IV Disabilities — Postadolescent Progressive

Type IV disabilities include the degenerative diseases that affect most adults who live to be old. Examples include degenerative heart disease, stroke, cancer, and chronic renal disease. Their onsets are often gradual and their courses progressive, thus allowing for slow adjustment to the disabling process. However, like Type II disabilities, the Type IV disabilities produce an unstable base from which one can plan a lifetime. People with these disabilities may find it necessary to invest considerable energy in maintaining their health and thus have great difficulty in looking upon themselves as "well," even though physically disabled.

Heart Disease. Hellerstein and Freidman[23] have found that the postcoronary sexual activity will depend upon such factors as precoronary sexual drive and performance, the customary effects of aging, pre-illness personality, emotional reaction to heart disease, current socioeconomic status, and the health attitudes and decisions of the sexual partner. The physician should investigate these factors in addition to focusing upon the contractile functions of the heart. Furthermore, pharmacologic management of heart disease, edema, and hypertension may require use of medications that also can affect sexual function. Hellerstein and Freidman have proposed a social class hypothesis that describes individuals who may be at lower risk for coronary heart disease. These people are not only more sexually active but are better educated, more affluent and verbally fluent, less obese, and less hypertensive.

With proper sexual counseling and taking into account age and other medical conditions, the development of fears in both the patient and the mate can be averted. Depression, reduced self-esteem, and preoccupation with life or death are obvious deterrents to sexual health. Patient and family education should point out that postcoronary sexual activity is feasible in 80 per cent of patients. The nature of the physical activity can be altered if resumption of precoronary patterns of sexual activity produces angina or respiratory symptoms. Episodes of sexual contact can be shorter and less physically strenuous so as not to place excessive demands upon the heart. The cardiac demand of sexual activity can be held down to that experienced by other customary activities of everyday living and work.

Arthritis. Arthritis may be associated with chronic pain, depression, and disfigurement, and these characteristics may produce sexual dysfunctions as part of the clinical picture. Chronic pain may produce or be produced by depression, and the libido may be affected. Some patients may experience enough pain on joint motion that physical activities of sexual expression may sometimes be precluded. It should be noted, however, that some patients describe a dramatic reduction in pain following genital stimulation and orgasm. The possible role of endorphins has been implicated, as has been the psychological role of caring and being cared for by another person.

Ehrlich[24] reports that specific locations of arthritis may be more commonly associated with sexual dysfunctions. A prime example is arthritis of the hips in a woman, causing inability to abduct and externally rotate them for intercourse in the traditional male-on-top position. Arthritis of the spine may cause pain on motion and arthritis of the knees may limit leg flexion or kneeling for men and women during sexual intercourse. Deforming arthritis of the hands may not only be unattractive but may also limit manual dexterity for purposes of stroking, caressing, and genital manipulation. Interferences in hygiene may result from arthritic involvement of hips and hands, preventing adequate toileting of the perineum and genitals.

Some arthritides are associated with rashes or ulcers of the skin or mucocutaneous areas, for example psoriatic arthritis, Sjögren's syndrome, or Behçet's disease. Dryness of the vagina may also occur in Sjögren's syndrome.

Lung Disease. Chronic progressive lung disease generally includes chronic bronchitis, emphysema, chronic obstructive pulmonary disease (COPD), and chronic obstructive lung disease (COLD). The distinguishing factor of all four is the progressive destruction of the lungs' ability to adequately exchange gases and clear excess mucus. The result is increasing shortness of breath in association with anxiety and chronic cough.

Chronic progressive lung disease is a dramatic example of a physical condition that may produce sexual disabilities. With the progression of lung disease the patient's ability to perform even the simple daily activities of bathing, dressing, and household chores may be affected. Patients can often benefit from a medical regimen that also includes instruction in relaxation, diaphragmatic breath control with pursed lip breathing, and postural drainage techniques. Specific kinesiologic instruction in sexual expression is also helpful. Positions that have been found effective for postural drainage of the lungs can be adapted for methods of sexual expression. Patients and partners can be counseled in options to traditional positions so that sexual intercourse can be accomplished in the sitting, standing, side-lying, and kneeling positions. Simultaneous use of oxygen in association with deliberate relaxation is also helpful. Sometimes a period of preparation with nebulization of bronchodilators and bronchial drainage may be helpful immediately preceding sexual activity.

Diabetes Mellitus. Diabetes mellitus usually has its onset in adult life and is progressive. It has been reported that half of all male diabetics have erectile dysfunction and about one third of diabetic women experience orgasmic dysfunction. Although diabetic neuropathy appears to be the primary etiologic factor in a majority of cases, some sexual problems in diabetics are due to correctable causes such as vascular occlusions.

In the diabetic male erectile dysfunction may have an abrupt onset but, more commonly, the onset is gradual. In 85 per cent of cases, the erectile dysfunction is due to organic causes and is the most common sexual disturbance.[25] Usually libido is unaffected, as is ejaculation in the diabetic male.

The physician may be able to separate the psychologic from the physiologic causes for erectile dysfunction by the use of nocturnal penile tumescence testing, although this method is not entirely accurate. The diabetic patient is no less susceptible to psychogenic reasons for erectile dysfunction than the nondiabetic male and, thus, it is important to consider nervous, vascular, and psychic functions simultaneously. In many men the organic dysfunction is accompanied by a psychological one, and the clinician should think of both etiologies rather than simply one or the other. In the male, retrograde ejaculation may also occur owing to diabetic neuropathy and is, of course, associated with the impaired fertility. Sensation of orgasm is usually retained, however, as is the sense of light touch and pinprick on the genitals.

It has been reported[25] that 35 per cent of diabetic women have orgasmic dysfunction, whereas only 6 per cent of nondiabetic women report this problem. Usually the onset in women is five to seven years later than sexual dysfunction in the man and its occurrence is often associated with the decrease in vaginal lubrication, chronic vaginitis, and dyspareunia. Libido is usually unimpaired.

The treatment of sexual dysfunction in diabetes includes metabolic regulation of the diabetes, correction of localized vascular disturbances, sexual counseling, and, in the male, consideration of implantation of a penile prosthesis.

End-stage Renal Disease. Sexual rehabilitation of the hemodialysis patient has been described by Levy.[31] There are over 30,000 new cases of end-stage renal disease occurring each year in the United States, most of which are a result of chronic pyelonephritis and glomerulonephritis. Although 15 years ago most of these patients would have died, most are now able to live on the artificial kidney and, thus, are coming to the attention of clinicians who are concerned about sexual function. A number of metabolic disturbances accompany this syndrome, including bone pain, chronic anemia, peripheral neuropathies, anorexia, and fatigue. Most patients receive treatment six hours a day, three times a week, and many have to go to a medical care facility to receive it. Only 30 per cent of men on chronic hemodialysis return to full vocational productivity.

The sexual dysfunction that was first recognized in this patient population was erectile dysfunction among men. However, lubrication problems and anorgasmia have recently been described in women on chronic hemodialysis. The prevalence of impotence in men on hemodialysis is probably 70 per cent, and the lack of improvement on hemodialysis is all the more remarkable because the same patients usually sustain improvements in all other physical functions during the same period of time. Although endocrinologic abnormalities have been described, there is no evidence that they correlate directly with sexual dysfunctions. Another factor that may play a role is the frequent necessary use of antihypertensive medications which, by themselves, may adversely influence sexual function by decreasing tumescence in males and libido in both sexes.

As for the other disabilities, psychological factors also play an important role. A man's sense of his masculinity and a woman's sense of her femininity may be severely stressed by inability to function in traditional or previous roles, inability to assume previous employment, or dependency upon outside support mechanisms. For men, role reversal is often experienced as the wives go back to work to help support their families. Role reversal may affect the man's sense of his masculinity. As with other progressive disabilities, depression, anxiety, and chronic fatigue may play important roles in sexual activity and satisfaction.

Treatment must take into consideration the medical and the psychological components. Recent research has shown that depletion of trace amounts of zinc may be linked to reduced testosterone production in patients on hemodialysis.[32] Probably the most important treatment is prevention of future difficulties and counseling with the patient and the sexual partner.

EFFECTS OF MEDICATIONS ON SEXUALITY

Increasingly, physicians are becoming aware of the host of effects that some drugs may have on the body. Some drugs have a potentiating effect on one another, while others have an inhibiting effect.

If one regards sexuality in a broad sense, not limited to genital function, one can see that many medications are capable of affecting sexual function. Any drug that produces or reduces pruritis or a skin rash will have a sexual effect through affecting appearance and distractability. Drugs that treat bone pain caused by neoplasms or osteoporosis or that reduce inflammation of joints and permit greater range of motion will have a sexual effect. Medications that control spasticity, increase strength, or reduce muscle pain will have a salutary effect upon kinesiosexual function. Medications that control seizures, diminish the rigidity of Parkinson's disease, or alter a mood may affect sexual function in obvious ways. Heart and lung disease treated by pharmacologic agents that reduce circulatory symptoms, heart pain, and shortness of breath may affect sexuality. Medications used to treat peptic ulcer may produce dryness of the mouth and thus affect oral activities associated with sex. Medications that are used to treat diarrhea or that influence rectal sphincter function may play a role in sexual activities. Contraceptives or antibiotics that weaken resistance to the development of vaginitis may produce dyspareunia and thus affect sexual function. Drugs thought to be sexually innocuous may in fact have significant side effects. When a patient believes that he or she is experiencing an iatrogenic, drug-induced sexual difficulty, the drug may simply be stopped without informing the physician and the patient will become a silent noncomplier.

Antihypertensive diuretic drugs may produce an effect on sexual function by depleting potassium stores and producing fatigue. Thiazide diuretics may also produce diabetes. If taken for a long period of time they may contribute to the diabetic syndrome described earlier. Spironolactone, on the other hand, has a potassium-conserving effect but produces other sexual side effects such as breast tenderness, galactorrhea, and gynecomastia, which is not always reversible in the male. In high doses spironolactone may reduce circulating testosterone and increase circulating progesterone.[33] In 25 to 40 per cent of men, spironolactone is known to produce erectile dysfunction and decrease sperm production. Spironolactone also may influence the hormonal events of the menstrual cycle.

Reserpine produces depression in 5 to 15 per cent of patients and in this group may adversely affect the libido. Guanethidine is a ganglionic blocker that in two thirds of male patients may lead to a reduction of ejaculatory ability. Propranolol, a beta blocker, has been known to produce erectile dysfunction in some men.

Hydralazine is considered to be innocuous as measured by its effect upon sexual function. Although it produces an increase in heart rate when used with propranolol, heart rate changes alone may not be deleterious. Sexual side effects often associated with other antihypertensive medications may be reduced in up to 85 per cent of patients thus treated. Alpha-methyldopa is one of the most widely used antihypertensives. In doses of less than 1 gm per day, erectile function, libido, and ejaculatory ability are seldom affected. However, as daily dosages approach 1.5 to 2 gm per day, up to half of men questioned report erectile dysfunction and decrease in libido. The physician must be sensitive to the direct as well as to the peripheral side effects of medications upon sexual function. Therapy can include adjustments in medication schedules and dosages as well as counseling to minimize or prevent the effects of anxiety or depression that may follow alterations of sexual function.

Almost all men with traumatic spinal cord injury are interested in regaining their potency and fertility. Ninety per cent of spinal-injured men are unable to ejaculate using physical stimulation of the penis. Early work by Guttman et al.[34] described the intrathecal injection of prostigmine, which produced ejaculation in some spinal-injured males. However, side effects, including autonomic hyperreflexia and hypertension, have been severe in some cases, making physicians and patients reluctant to employ this method. Recently the European literature has reported successful electroejaculation in the human male.[35-37] Although the methods used have not yet found widespread application, there is now the possibility that electrostimulation may be effective in paraplegic and quadriplegic men, even those injured many years ago. Successful impregnations have been accomplished in able-bodied women from sperm obtained from spinal cord–injured husbands. In a number of cases the pregnancies have progressed to term and the infants have been normal.

EFFECTS OF SURGICAL PROCEDURES ON SEXUALITY

Penile Prostheses. The urologic surgeon can implant a penile stiffener or penile prosthesis when there is organic erectile dysfunction, and some urologic surgeons are willing to install the device in selected cases of psychogenic erectile dysfunction. Confirmation of the presence of erectile dysfunction requires an adequate history and physical examination, a search for localized vascular insufficiency, and examination of the abdomen, penis, and scrotum. Manual dexterity also is important if the surgeon is installing a hydraulic stiffener as described by Bradley et al.[26] If the surgeon is considering a semirigid prosthesis, such as developed by Small and Carrion,[27] Finney,[28] or Jonas,[29] then the absence of prostatic obstruction must be assured. Bladder instrumentation may be difficult or impossible after the semi-rigid prosthesis is installed. In the hands of some surgeons the surgical success rate is greater than 90 per cent, and mechanical complications are negligible with a semi-rigid device. Although the surgical success rate may also be greater than 90 per cent with the inflatable prosthesis, mechanical complications may be as high as 15 per cent.

However, the penile prosthesis should not be adopted without adequate assessment and evaluation of each individual case. Maddock[30] has emphasized the importance of preoperative evaluation even though the patient himself may adamantly request implantation of the device. Maddock points out that there is no such thing as a totally organic erectile dysfunction. A psychological component is always present in the form of a discrepancy between male performance standards and the reality of any physical limitation. He also points out that in some men in whom sexual dysfunction coexists with diabetes, the dysfunction may be a psychological defense mechanism against anxiety or threat.

Maddock found that problems of self-esteem and overall psychological disturbances of patients treated surgically were generally greater than for patients treated with psychotherapy. There was also a greater incidence of excess alcohol consumption among the VA population who were treated surgically. Although surgery did not appreciably increase the frequency of sexual intercourse after adequate time for healing, most patients were satisfied with the result. Surgery did not significantly affect self-esteem levels or personal adjustments of patients with their wives, even though motivation for surgery appeared to be largely interpersonal, i.e., probably related to feelings of self-worth or "manliness" and/or relational rather than "sexual" per se. Maddock concluded that the outcome of surgery and possibly even the motivation to have the surgery were strongly linked to the attitudes and behavior of the female partner. Whether or not the surgery was deemed to be successful by the patients, particularly the married patients, was a function of how the female partner responded sexually after the procedure.

Gynecologic Problems. Surgical procedures frequently performed by the gynecologist include vulvectomy, hysterectomy, tubal ligation, abortion, vaginal repair, cystocele repair, hymenectomies, and clitoral hood resections. In each of these cases a mechanical alteration of the women's genitals may bring about changes in libido as well as in sexual activity. When the ovaries are removed circulating testosterone is reduced and the woman may experience a decrease in libido. A loss of the uterus may result in a change of pelvic sensation for women who have been accustomed to feeling the penis touch the uterine cervix during sexual intercourse. Vaginal repair must be carried out by a surgeon who is sensitive to reconstruction of the vagina without making it either too tight or too short for sexual intercourse.

Vulvectomy can have a severe psychological effect on the inadequately prepared woman and her sexual partner. Grief, depression, fear, and mood swings have been described by vulvectomized women, many of whom have expressed fear of establishing new sexual relationships. Those who are married state that they are glad that they are married so that they do not have to risk rejection in the establishment of a new sexual relationship. Some women have described a dramatic decrease in libido, self-image, and sexual activity following vulvectomy. Most women have asked for better preoperative counseling and education, especially of their husbands.

PHYSICIAN INVOLVEMENT IN PROBLEMS OF SEXUALITY

Depending upon skills, interest, and job responsibilities, each physician can find a level of involvement appropriate to himself or herself. Annon[38] has suggested a four-tiered scheme of involvement. The first tier is that level at which the physician generates an attitude wherein the disabled person senses permission to express and discuss sexual concerns. This can be done by asking leading questions, initiating talk about sensitive subjects, or simply by listening to the spoken or body language of the patient. All physicians should be able to function at level 1. Not to do so may deny patients permission to discuss the very real problems and concerns that they may be facing.

The second tier is a level at which the physician provides limited information for general problem solving. Typically, the limited information is educational and nonpersonal and deals with the disability and its implications on sexual health in a general sense.

The third tier of involvement is the level at which the physician provides specific suggestions about sexual concerns and dysfunctions. This implies that the physician has taken a sexual history and is knowledgeable about sexuality and the particular physical disability under consideration.

The fourth tier is the level of intensive therapy. This is provided by professionals who have been thoroughly trained in sex counseling and who also understand physical disabilities. Intensive therapy often involves intrapersonal and psychological issues and frequently requires relationship counseling. It goes well beyond providing permission, limited information, or even specific suggestions. It implies a thorough understanding and training in psychodynamics, especially as they relate to sexuality. It also implies a thorough understanding of physical disabilities, medical rehabilitation, and personal and family reactions to disability in the rehabilitation environment.

Guidelines for Working with People with Physical Disabilities

The following are a few guidelines that may help the physician and the patient in the area of sexuality and physical disability.

1. Genital function alone does not make a functional relationship.

2. Urinary incontinence does not mean genital incontinence.

3. Absence of sensation does not mean absence of feelings.

4. Inability to move does not mean inability to please or be pleased.

5. The presence of deformities does not mean the absence of desire.

6. Inability to perform does not mean inability to enjoy.

7. Loss of genitals does not mean loss of sexuality.

8. Sexual dysfunction is not synonymous with personal inadequacy.

REFERENCES

1. Ebert, R. K., and Lief, H. I.: Why sex education for medical students? *In* Green, R. (Ed.): Human Sexuality, A Health Practitioner's Text. Baltimore, Williams and Wilkins, 1975, pp. 1–6.
2. Roberts, M., and Roberts, A.: Psychosocial Rehabilitation of the Handicapped. Proc. 1st International Conference on Lifestyle and Health. A. S. Leon and G. T. Amundson (Eds.). Minneapolis Dept. of Conferences, University of Minnesota, 1979.
3. Cole, T. M., and Glass, D. D.: Sexuality and physical disabilities. Arch. Phys. Med. Rehabil., 58:585–586, 1977.
4. Lief, H. I.: New developments in the sex education of the physician. JAMA, 212:1864–1867, 1970.
5. Kolodny, R. C., Masters, W. H., and Johnson, V. E.: Textbook of Sexual Medicine. Boston, Little, Brown & Company, 1979.
6. Sandler, J., Myerson, M., and Kinder, B. N.: Human Sexuality: Current Perspectives. Tampa, Mariner Publishing Company, 1980.
7. McCary, J. L.: McCary's Human Sexuality, 3rd Ed. New York, D. Van Nostrand and Company, 1978.

8. Katchadourian, H. A., and Lunde, D. T.: Fundamentals of Human Sexuality, 2nd Ed. New York, Holt, Rinehart and Winston, 1972.

9. Kaplan, H. S.: The New Sex Therapy. New York, Brunner Mazel Publication, 1974.

10. Kelly, G. F.: Sexuality: The Human Perspective. Woodbury, Barron's, 1980.

11. Easton, J.: Children, Parents, and Schools. Paper presented at Sexuality and Physical Disabilities: Medical Aspects and Clinical Care Seminar University of Michigan Medical Center, November, 1980.

12. Robinault, I.: Sex, Society and the Disabled — A Developmental Inquiry into Roles, Relationships, and Responsibility. Hagerstown, Md., Harper and Row, 1978.

13. Anderson, F., Bardach, J., and Goodgold, J.: Sexuality in Neuromuscular Diseases. Monograph 56, New York Institute of Rehabilitation Medicine, 1979.

14. Goodgold, J., Bardach, J., and Anderson, F.: A Study of Sexuality in Muscular Dystrophy and Related Diseases. Muscular Dystrophy Assoc.

15. Bregman, S., and Hadley, R. G.: Sexual adjustment and feminine attractiveness among spinal cord injured women. Arch. Phys. Med. Rehabil., 57:448–450, 1976.

16. Cole, T. M., Chilgren, R. A., and Rosenberg, P.: A new programme of sex education and counseling for spinal cord injured adults and health care professionals. Int. J. Para., 11:111–124, 1973.

17. Nagler, B.: Psychiatric aspects of cord injury. Am. J. Psychiatry, 107:49–56, 1950.

18. Teal, J. C., and Athelstan, G. T.: Sexuality and spinal cord injury: Some psychosocial considerations. Arch. Phys. Med. Rehabil., 56:264–268, 1975.

19. There is no reference 19.

20. Cole, T. M.: Unpublished data for Regional Spinal Cord Injury Center of Minnesota, Theodore M. Cole, M.D., Director, 1977.

21. Berkman, A. H., Weissman, R., and Freilich, M. H.: Sexual adjustment of spinal cord injured veterans living in the community. Arch. Phys. Med. Rehabil., 59:29–33, 1978.

22. McClure, S.: Contraception and the Spinal Injured Woman, Paper presented at Sexuality and Physical Disabilities: Medical Aspects and Clinical Care Seminar, University of Michigan Medical Center, November, 1980.

23. Hellerstein, H. K., and Freidman, E. H.: Sexual activity and the post coronary patient. Arch. Intern. Med., 125:987–999, 1970.

24. Ehrlich, G. E.: Sexual problems of the arthritic patient. In Ehrlich, G. E. (Ed.): Total Management of the Arthritic Patient. Philadelphia, J. B. Lippincott Company, 1973, pp. 193–208.

25. Kolodny, R. C., Masters, W. H., and Johnson, V. E.: Textbook of Sexual Medicine. Boston, Little, Brown & Company, 1979.

26. Scott, F. B., Bradley, W. E., and Timm, G. W.: Management of erectile impotence. Use of implantable, inflatable prosthesis. Urology, 2:80, 1973.

27. Small, M. P., Carrion, H. M., and Gordon, J. A.: Small-Carrion penile prosthesis. Urology, 5:479, 1975.

28. Finney, R. P.: New hinged silicone penile implant. J. Urol., 118:585, 1977.

29. Jonas, U., and Jacobi, G. H.: Silicone-silver penile prosthesis: Description, operative approach, and results. J. Urol., 123:865, 1980.

30. Maddock, J. W.: Assessment and evaluation protocol for surgical treatment of impotence. Sexual. Disabil., 3:39–49, 1980.

31. Levy, N. B.: The sexual rehabilitation of the hemodialysis patient. Sexual. Disabil., 2:76–81, 1979.

32. Antoniou, L. D., Sudhakar, T., and Shalhoub, R. J., et al.: Reversal of uremic impotence by zinc. Lancet, 2:895–898, 1977.

33. Caminos-Torres, R., Ma, L., and Snyder, P. J.: Gynecomastia and semen abnormalities induced by spironolactone in normal men. J. Clin. Endocrinol. Metab., 45:255–260, 1977.

34. Guttman, L., and Walsh, J. J.: Prostigmin assessment test of fertility in spinal-injured man. Paraplegia, 9:38–51, 1971.

35. Francois, N., Maury, M., Jouannet, D., David, G., and Vacant, J.: Electroejaculation of a complete paraplegic followed by pregnancy. Paraplegia, 16:248–251, 1978.

36. Brindley, G. S.: Electroejaculation and the fertility of paraplegic men. Sexual. Disabil., 3:223–229, 1980.

37. Hachen, H. J.: Bilan endocrinien et spermatogenese chex le traumatise medullaire. Ann. Med. Phys., 21:403–417, 1978.

38. Annon, J.: The Behavioral Treatment of Sexual Problems: Brief Therapy. New York, Harper and Row, 1976.

48

UPPER EXTREMITY PROSTHETICS

LEONARD F. BENDER

The absence of all or part of the limb comes about either from congenital skeletal deficiency or from amputation by trauma or surgery. The word *amputation* should be reserved for surgical, traumatic, and disease-created limb losses. Avoidance of the confusing term *congenital amputation* would help to clarify the distinction between congenital skeletal deficiencies and amputations.

CONGENITAL SKELETAL DEFICIENCY

Of cases of skeletal deficiency involving the upper extremity, in all age groups, the deficiency is congenital in 22 per cent.[1] Analysis of the age group from birth to 10 years shows that 75 per cent of limb losses are congenital and only 25 per cent traumatic or surgical. Then, as children grow to adulthood, traumatic amputation and tumors account for an increased percentage of upper limb deficiencies, and, when all age groups are considered together, trauma is the etiologic agent in 70 per cent.

The reasons for congenital malformations are largely unknown. Hereditary abnormalities identified as leading to limb deficiency are extremely rare.[2] Teratogenic agents have received considerable attention as a result of the thalidomide catastrophe in Europe between 1960 and 1963. Excessive radiation is

often implicated;[3] cortisone and tolbutamide are highly suspect. Positive proof of the teratogenic effect of many chemical agents and environmental pollutants remains to be demonstrated.

The most common congenital skeletal deficiency in the upper limb is absence of the distal two thirds of the forearm, the wrist, and the hand. According to the Dundee classification promulgated in 1974, this would be a transverse deficiency, forearm, upper one-third. Previous classifications used the term *hemimelia,* and later, *meromelia,* combined with the type and level of deficiency. The latest classification was developed at an international conference held in Dundee, Scotland.[4] It simplifies the terminology and divides all congenital skeletal deficiencies into transverse or longitudinal. Transverse is defined as absence of all skeletal elements distal to the deficiency along a designated transverse axis; the axis is described by a two-letter abbreviation of the area of the limb (SH = shoulder, AR = arm, FO = forearm, CA = carpals, MC = metacarpals, PH = phalanges) plus the level in that area (total, upper one-third, middle one-third, distal one-third). Longitudinal deficiency is an absence extending parallel to the long axis of the limb; all bones missing are named in two-letter abbreviations plus the term *partial* or *total.* Arranged in order of decreasing frequency, congenital upper limb skeletal deficiencies in the United States are forearm, upper one-third; wrist, total; arm, lower one-third; forearm, total; arm, total; and metacarpal, middle one-third.[1]

CAUSES OF ACQUIRED LIMB LOSS

Amputation of upper limb segments in children below 10 years of age is rare; motor vehicle accidents, tumors, and trauma from natural disasters such as earthquakes and high winds are among the etiologic agents. Children 10 to 20 years old subject themselves to more hazardous situations than younger children do, and malignancy is also more likely to develop in this age group.

Trauma is the cause of upper limb amputation in 70 per cent of patients over age 18. In Michigan, the preponderance of amputations in adults is caused by stamping presses, conveyor mechanisms, and farm machinery such as corn pickers, threshers, and balers. Diseases account for only 6 per cent of all arm amputations, which is in sharp contrast to lower limb amputations, 40 per cent of which are necessitated by peripheral vascular syndromes. Malignancies constitute one half of the disease-related causes of arm amputation and appear predominantly in the 10 to 20 year age group.

AMPUTATION

Levels of Amputation

Upper extremity amputation stumps are classified by level of amputation, using ter-

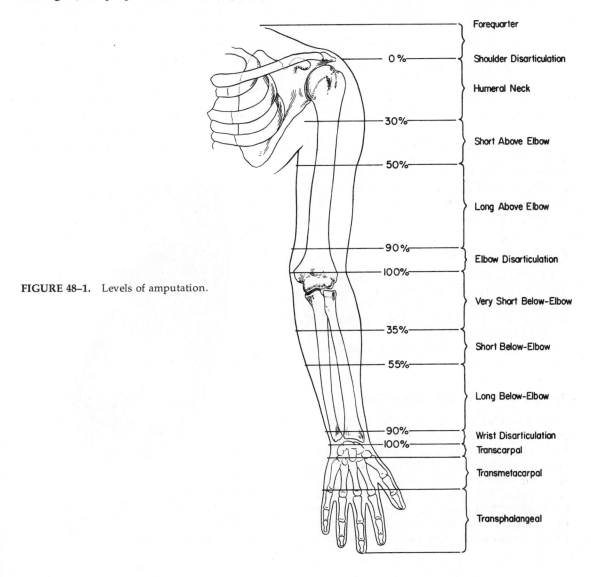

FIGURE 48–1. Levels of amputation.

minology different from that used for congenital skeletal deficiency. First, the length of the stump must be measured. Above-elbow stumps are measured from the tip of the acromion to the bone end; this measurement is compared to the sound side distance from acromion to the lateral epicondyle and is expressed as a percentage of normal side length. Below-elbow measurement is made from the medial epicondyle to the end of the ulna or radius, whichever is longer in the stump, and to the ulnar styloid tip on the sound side. Levels of amputation are as follows (see also Fig. 48–1):

Per Cent of Normal	Classification
Above Elbow	
0	Shoulder disarticulation
0–30	Humeral neck
30–50	Short above-elbow
50–90	Long above-elbow
90–100	Elbow disarticulation
Below Elbow	
0–35	Very short below-elbow
35–55	Short below-elbow
55–90	Long below-elbow
90–100	Wrist disarticulation

In bilateral amputations, where no normal segment remains for comparative measurement, the normal upper arm length is estimated by multiplying the patient's height by 0.19, and normal forearm length is estimated by multiplying by 0.21.[5, 6]

Elective Amputation

Elective amputations may be performed when the hand or the entire limb is sensationless and functionless. The hand may also be swollen, painful, and limited in range of motion. The most frequent cause is brachial plexus injuries or multiple cervical root avulsions.

Preoperative Rehabilitative Care

Only on rare occasions do the physiatrist and therapists knowledgeable in prosthetics have an opportunity to examine and to advise a patient prior to amputation. When such an occasion does arise — in elective amputation, for instance — the patient can be instructed in postoperative range of motion exercises and shown some of the prosthetic components available to amputees.

One-handed techniques for some basic activities of daily living can be demonstrated and a degree of psychologic support can be developed through this early contact.

Postoperative Rehabilitative Care

The immediate postoperative period offers a few days during which the physician, physical and occupational therapist, and nurses may provide specialized care and give instructions to the patient, which will shorten the period of stump conditioning and help to reduce psychologic depression. Range-of-motion exercises for the remaining joints of the arm, one-handed ways of performing activities of daily living, and proper skin care techniques can be taught early.

A variety of methods are utilized by surgeons to care for the stump. Some begin application of elastic stump shrinkers or elastic bandages the day after amputation; others wait until the stitches are out. Rigid plaster dressings may be used instead of elastic bandages. When applied properly, elastic bandages are effective in shaping the stump and reducing edema. Six to eight weeks of wrapping usually will bring the stump to satisfactory condition for fitting with a pros-

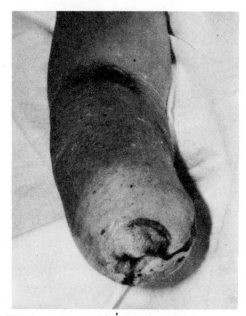

FIGURE 48–2. Early postoperative below-elbow stump following electrical burn and amputation. (From Bender, Leonard F.: Prostheses and Rehabilitation after Arm Amputation, 1974. Courtesy of Charles C Thomas, Publisher, Springfield, Illinois.)

thesis, but wrapping must be continued until the prosthesis is received.

Immediate Postoperative Fitting

The advantages of immediate postoperative fitting were first described for lower extremity amputations.[7] A similar procedure has been tried during elective amputation in the forearm or arm when it is possible for the physician and prosthetist to make arrangements in advance. When prior arrangements cannot be made, it is possible to make an early postoperative prosthesis a day or two after surgery. The application of a prosthesis immediately after amputation minimizes pain and edema in the stump, facilitates healing, and reduces waiting time for the standard prosthesis.

Persons with simultaneous bilateral upper extremity amputations are ideal candidates for immediate or early postoperative fitting with a plaster prosthesis. The frustration of being totally dependent on others can largely be avoided by use of a temporary prosthesis on one or both sides.

The construction of an immediate postoperative plaster prosthesis is usually done in the operating room or an adjoining cast

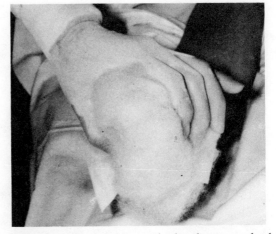

FIGURE 48–4. Lamb's wool placed over end of stump to provide padding. (From Bender, Leonard F.: Prostheses and Rehabilitation after Arm Amputation, 1974. Courtesy of Charles C Thomas, Publisher, Springfield, Illinois.)

room. Sterile technique is maintained until the inner wall of the plaster socket is completed. The surgical incision is first covered with one layer of non-adhering gauze and one or two 4 × 4 inch gauze pads. Sterilized lamb's wool is then applied over the end of the stump and a knitted Orlon stump sock, which has been previously sterilized, is unrolled up the stump. Since this portion of the process may be painful, analgesia may be necessary. An elastic plaster bandage is then applied to the stump sock, creating a plaster socket. Cotton webbing straps for suspen-

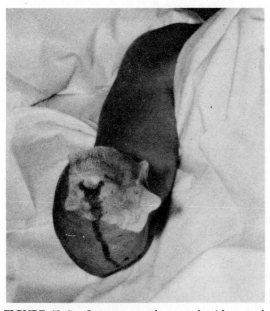

FIGURE 48–3. Stump wound covered with nonadherent dressing after cleansing. (From Bender, Leonard F.: Prostheses and Rehabilitation after Arm Amputation, 1974. Courtesy of Charles C Thomas, Publisher, Springfield, Illinois.)

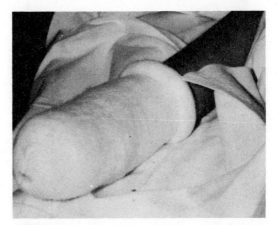

FIGURE 48–5. Knitted orlon sock rolled up stump. (From Bender, Leonard F.: Prostheses and Rehabilitation after Arm Amputation, 1974. Courtesy of Charles C Thomas, Publisher, Springfield, Illinois.)

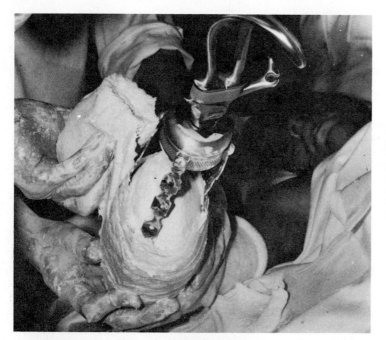

FIGURE 48–6. Friction wrist unit attached to long metal straps, which are incorporated into plaster socket. (From Bender, Leonard F.: Prostheses and Rehabilitation after Arm Amputation, 1974. Courtesy of Charles C Thomas, Publisher, Springfield, Illinois.)

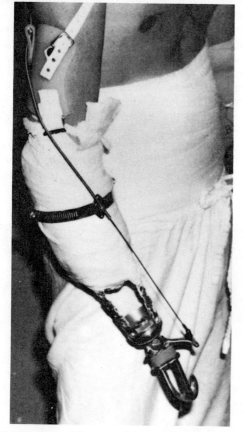

FIGURE 48–7. The completed early postoperative plaster prosthesis. (From Bender, Leonard F.: Prostheses and Rehabilitation after Arm Amputation, 1974. Courtesy of Charles C Thomas, Publisher, Springfield, Illinois.)

sion of the prosthesis and steel straps attached to either a wrist unit or an elbow unit are placed in the proper positions relative to the socket and are secured to the thin plaster socket with a roll of regular plaster bandage. The prosthetist can then incorporate a base plate laterally on the plaster socket and proceed to construct and fit a harness and control cable. In a week to 10 days, the socket should be removed by slipping it off. The wound can be examined and either the first socket replaced on the stump if it is still a good fit or a new plaster socket constructed in a process similar to that just described. When the stump is well healed and appropriately contoured, the standard prosthesis can be constructed.

PROSTHETIC SOCKETS

The most important component of the prosthesis is the inner wall of the socket. If it does not fit satisfactorily, the prosthesis may not function effectively and may be uncomfortable. Almost all sockets are made with two walls: an inner wall that fits the amputation stump comfortably and an outer wall that has the general contour of the normal arm or forearm. In special cases, such as elbow disarticulation, there may be no space between the inner and outer walls, and the socket is considered to have a single wall.

With infants, it is customary in our clinic to use a three-walled socket. The inner wall fits the stump. A middle wall is constructed over a thin wax build-up and is designed to fit the stump a year or two after the prosthesis is first fitted to the patient. The outer wall again corresponds to the normal contour of that segment of the arm. The inner wall of such a socket can be removed by the prosthetist as the child grows and needs more room inside the socket. This extends the useful life of the prosthesis considerably and reduces cost.

The upper rim of the usual below-elbow socket should be located 1.5 cm below the epicondyles of the humerus as the elbow is held at a right angle. The trimline should come straight volarly from the ulnar side and then curve distally on the volar surface to allow adequate room for the tendon of the biceps brachii muscle. Long stumps may have a longer volar relief area.

Very short below-elbow stumps will often be fitted with a modified Munster type of socket. In this socket, the trimline comes proximal to the epicondyles and the socket is fitted while the elbow is held slightly flexed. The posterior portion of the socket presses above the olecranon on the triceps tendon as the elbow is extended. The anterior portion of the socket is contoured snugly around the biceps tendon. When fitted properly, a suspension harness may not be necessary for this design of socket; this makes it well suited for electric hands with myoelectric control systems.

Very short below-elbow stumps with limited range of motion at the elbow may benefit from a split socket with a step-up hinge; the forearm outer shell moves 2 degrees for each degree the stump moves at the elbow. The gain in motion in this type of prosthesis is accompanied by reduction in power, whereas the Munster socket retains power through a limited range of motion. Very short below-elbow stumps with marked reduction in strength may also be fitted with a split socket, but the motion of the stump is utilized to operate an elbow-locking mechanism instead of utilizing it for elbow flexion and extension.

For short and long above-elbow stumps, the standard socket is trimmed approximately 1 cm lateral to the acromion on a line that runs around to the axilla anteriorly and posteriorly. If the above-elbow stump is less than 35 per cent of humeral length (humeral neck), the socket will have to be constructed so that it extends 2.5 cm medial to the acromion.

Sockets for shoulder disarticulation level of amputation require extensions over a portion of the scapula posteriorly and over a small portion of the rib cage anteriorly. Sockets for forequarter amputations require a large area of contact over the rib cage anteriorly and posteriorly.

TERMINAL DEVICES

Terminal devices are made in the shape of a hand or a variety of hooks. Some are functional, and others are not. Special terminal devices are also available in the form of adapted standard or special tools.

Voluntary opening terminal devices are opened by tension placed on the control cable and are closed by rubber bands or springs. They have a two-cycle action: pulling the control cable opens the device and releasing the control cable permits the device to be closed by its rubber bands or springs. Voluntary opening devices operate quickly with a minimum of control motions and are preferred by most persons with amputations. All Dorrance hooks and hands are voluntary opening devices.

Voluntary closing terminal devices provide a degree of graded prehension that is generally not possible with voluntary opening devices. They usually have a four-cycle action: pulling the control cable closes the

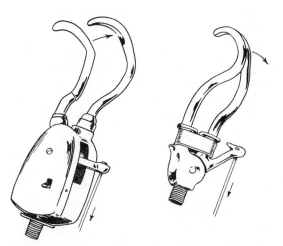

FIGURE 48–8. Voluntary closing (left) and voluntary opening (right) terminal devices. Tension applied to the control cable closes VC devices and opens VO devices.

hook partially or fully; releasing the control cable tension causes the hook to lock in the attained position; a slightly stronger pull unlocks the hook; and release of the pulling force allows the hook to spring open.

Motor driven terminal devices are manufactured primarily in Europe and are operated by a small electric motor. Both opening and closing of the hands and hooks are provided by the reversible electric motors.

Cosmetic hands are nonfunctional hands constructed of rigid or semi-rigid material and covered by a cosmetic glove. They may also be molded out of a semi-rigid material in the size and shape of a normal hand. They may have the standard stud that screws into a friction wrist unit or they may be secured to the stump by a zipper on the volar surface of the glove. They are available in many color shades to match the appearance of the skin.

Which Terminal Device to Use

In the United States it is convenient to select a Dorrance voluntary opening hook and hand. The Dorrance hand is frequently used because the thumb moves away from the palm simultaneously with finger extension as tension is exerted through the control cable. No passive prepositioning of the thumb by the other hand is necessary, as is done with the APRL hand. Dorrance hands are available in four sizes from glove size 6 through 8.

The selection of appropriate terminal devices for a patient is part of writing the prescription for a prosthesis. The team needs detailed information about the patient in order to perform this function; this information includes the patient's size, level of amputation, previous occupation and future vocation, avocational interests, and the willingness to accept a functional terminal device.

An infant needs a small hook, such as a Dorrance 12P, which is the smallest available. There is no functional hand small enough for an infant. As the child grows, a slightly larger hook will be needed, the Dorrance 10X or 10P. P indicates plastisol coating and X indicates neoprene lining of the hook. Depending on the child's size, a larger hook may be needed at about six years of age. A Dorrance No. 99X is 1.3 cm longer

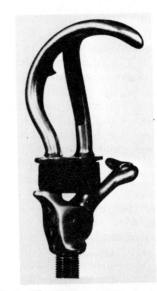

FIGURE 48–9. The Dorrance 5XA hook is light in weight, neoprene lined, and popular with adults for desk work. (From Bender, Leonard F.: Prostheses and Rehabilitation after Arm Amputation, 1974. Courtesy of Charles C Thomas, Publisher, Springfield, Illinois.)

than a 10X; a Dorrance 88X is 2.5 cm longer than a 10X. Either the 99X or 88X may be used up to age 12 or 13. The two most popular hooks for adults are the Dorrance Model 5XA and 7. Model 5XA is used for

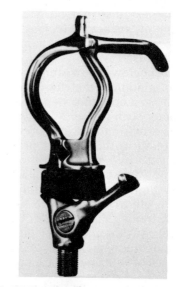

FIGURE 48–10. The Dorrance 7 hook is used by many male adults because it is durable and can hold a number of tools or a knife or a nail. (From Bender, Leonard F.: Prostheses and Rehabilitation after Arm Amputation, 1974. Courtesy of Charles C Thomas, Publisher, Springfield, Illinois.)

light activities, since it is made of aluminum, and Model 7, made of steel, is used for heavy work. If it is important to have the terminal device lock firmly around a handle or other cylindrical objects, the Dorrance Model 6 superlock hook may be preferred. For wrist disarticulation and long below-elbow length stumps, it may be necessary to use a shorter hook, such as Dorrance Models 88X or 8, to avoid having the hook-fingers lower than the tip of the thumb on the normal side.

Electric hands, manufactured by Otto Bock and Viennatone, are available in several sizes; however, none of these is small enough for a child. The electric hand is customarily controlled myoelectrically and is applied to short or long below-elbow stumps when the patient wants a functional hand but does not desire a functional hook. No conventional harness is needed because a modified Munster style socket is used. This eliminates harness straps across the chest and the back and shoulders.

All hooks and hands made in the United States have the same one-half inch, 20-thread stud for attachment to wrist units and all are interchangeable. Most foreign manufactured terminal devices also use the same stud and, therefore, are also interchangeable. A patient who wishes a cosmetic or functional hand need only select the proper size of hand and color of cosmetic glove. It can then easily and quickly be interchanged with a functional hook-type terminal device.

In addition to commercially available hands and hooks, devices to meet special requirements are sometimes needed. A locking tool chuck screws into standard wrist units or can be adapted to quick-disconnect wrist units. Many different tools can be held in this chuck. Many specially adapted standard and special tools are also available for direct insertion into terminal devices or into the wrist unit. Detailed descriptions of these terminal devices are available in catalogues provided by various prosthetic component manufacturers and in text books.[8]

Wrist Components

Terminal devices must be attached to a below-elbow socket or to a forearm shell in the case of above-elbow amputations. Wrist units provide a mechanism for the attachment of terminal devices in either case. A wrist unit is laminated into and becomes an integral part of a below-elbow socket or a forearm shell. There are two basic designs of wrist units. Most are threaded sockets that limit rotation of the terminal device through a friction ring but do not lock in any position. Other units provide both a locking feature and a mechanism for quickly changing from one terminal device to another. These quick-change wrist units require a metal adapter that is screwed onto the stud of each terminal device and fits snugly into the wrist unit. Quick-change wrist units are preferred by persons who need to lock the terminal device

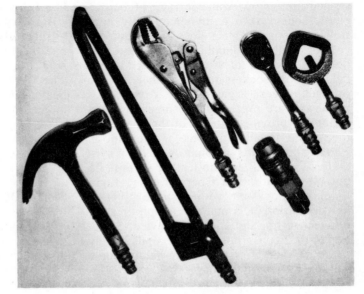

FIGURE 48–11. A tool chuck with a rotating locking ring accepts a hexagonal shaft that can be attached to many different tools. (From Bender, Leonard F.: Prostheses and Rehabilitation after Arm Amputation, 1974. Courtesy of Charles C Thomas, Publisher, Springfield, Illinois.)

to prevent rotation of it as they lift and manipulate heavy objects and by those who frequently change from one terminal device to another.

Friction wrist units are available in various sizes, from infant through adult, and in two shapes, circular and oval. Quick-change wrist units are all circular. A thin friction wrist unit is available for use with wrist-disarticulation stumps; it reduces the length of the socket by nearly 1 cm.

A unit that provides flexion at the wrist may be added to a standard wrist unit or may be an integral part of a special wrist unit. This unit permits the terminal device to be positioned close to the body and is appropriate for persons with bilateral short above-elbow amputations because some dressing, grooming, and toileting activities require it. Most other amputees find that they do not need it.

A few wrist units have been developed which enhance pronation and supination of the terminal device through either mechanical linkage or electric power. These have generally not found acceptance and they are not readily available.

ELBOW COMPONENTS

Most persons with below-elbow amputations require a harness for suspension of the prosthesis and for control of the terminal device. The straps that fasten the below-elbow socket to the harness are generally termed *hinges*. A Munster type of below-elbow socket with a myoelectrically controlled terminal device does not require a control cable and should not need the suspension portion of a harness. All other below-elbow sockets require either flexible or rigid hinges. Rigid hinges are made of metal and are preferred by some for short stumps to provide stability of the socket on the stump in all positions of the elbow. Flexible hinges are customarily made of synthetic fabrics rather than leather so they do not stretch or absorb perspiration. Rigid hinges are available with a single pivot, a polycentric pivot, a multiple action or step-up mechanism, and a locking device. Selection of the appropriate hinge depends largely upon the characteristics of the below-elbow stump and the type of harness used.

Above-elbow prostheses for all levels of

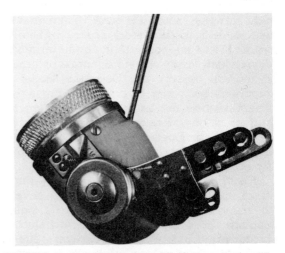

FIGURE 48–12. Hosmer positive locking elbow with forearm lift assist. (From Bender, Leonard F.: Prostheses and Rehabilitation after Arm Amputation, 1974. Courtesy of Charles C Thomas, Publisher, Springfield, Illinois.)

above-elbow amputation except elbow disarticulation utilize an elbow unit that locks in different positions between 5 and 135 degrees of elbow flexion. It also has a friction plate turntable above the elbow that permits the forearm shell to be positioned through a limited range of rotation which simulates internal and external rotation of the arm. An adjustable spring mechanism mounted on the medial aspect of the unit assists elbow flexion by partially counterbalancing the weight of the prosthesis distal to the elbow.

Elbow disarticulation stumps require rigid hinges on the outside of the socket, since the customary elbow unit, when installed distal to the socket, would place the axis of elbow motion at least 5 cm lower than on the sound side. Electric elbow units that are myoelectrically controlled are available, but they are heavy and expensive. Specific criteria and indications for their use remain to be developed; they appear to be most helpful to persons with short above-elbow stumps and limited range of motion or strength.

SHOULDER COMPONENTS

Shoulder units are needed for forequarter levels of amputation as well as for shoulder disarticulations and some amputations at the level of the humeral neck. Shoulder units may be either a ball joint or two friction hinges or plates that create a universal joint. In the completed prosthesis, their position is not changed by control cables or electric motors; they must be prepositioned with the sound arm or by pressing the prosthesis against a solid object.

A cosmetic shoulder pad may be all some patients desire rather than a functional upper extremity prosthesis. Such a pad can be constructed from a block of polyfoam and held on with a chest strap. It will provide a normal shoulder contour.

PROSTHETIC SUSPENSION AND CONTROL

The prosthesis must ordinarily be held on the stump through some arrangement of straps called a harness. In addition to suspension of the prosthesis, the harness provides an attachment for the control cable, which operates the terminal device and, in above-elbow amputations, the elbow unit. The harness most commonly used is shaped like the figure eight. The straps should cross in back just to the sound side of the lowest cervical vertebra, and they are sewn to each other at that point. If a ring is inserted at the point where the straps cross, the length of each strap can be adjusted through a buckle and the harness is called an O-ring harness. The anterior strap, which lies in the delto-pectoral groove on the amputated side, attaches directly to the socket of an above-elbow prosthesis or to the Y-strap and triceps pad of a below-elbow prosthesis. The posterior strap on the amputated side pro-

vides the attachment for the proximal end of the control cable. In some persons, the loop that runs through the sound axilla creates compression of the neurovascular components on that side when the prosthesis is used for heavy lifting; this occurs because the harness transfers the pull on the suspension strap of the prosthesis across to the axillary loop.

Persons who do heavy work may prefer a modified shoulder saddle harness. It suspends the prosthesis through a Bowden cable (a braided steel cable inside a tubular housing) which runs over the top of the shoulder on the amputated side, attaching anteriorly and posteriorly to the socket of an above-elbow prosthesis with the cable housing anchored through baseplates and retainers on the anterior and posterior aspects of the saddle. In a below-elbow prosthesis, the suspension cable attaches to the Y-strap anteriorly and to the triceps pad posteriorly. The shoulder saddle, Y-strap, and triceps pad may all be constructed of clear polyethylene, and a chest strap must be used to hold it in the correct position over the top of the shoulder. The shoulder saddle provides a large weight-bearing area and permits the lifting of heavy axial loads with comfort and without pull being transferred to the sound axilla.

In forequarter amputations, shoulder disarticulations, and humeral neck amputations, a chest strap alone will usually provide adequate suspension and a proper attachment for the control cable. This chest strap attaches both anteriorly and posteriorly to the socket of the prosthesis.

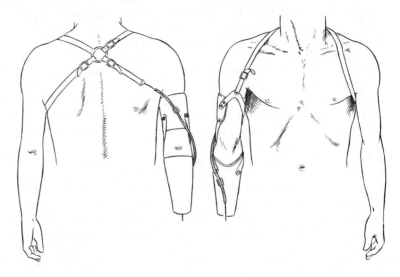

FIGURE 48–13. O-ring harness.

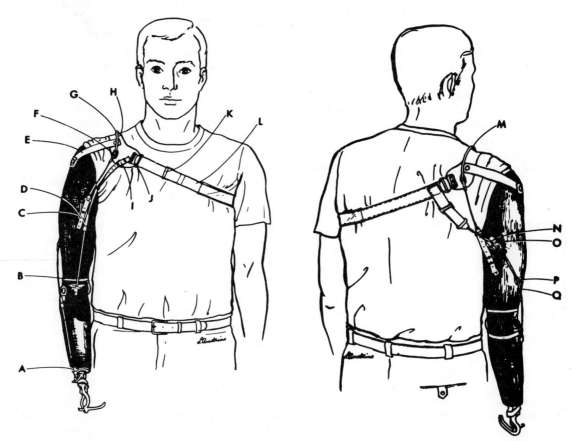

FIGURE 48–14. Modified shoulder saddle harness for above-elbow prosthesis. *A,* Button placed midline to dorsum of socket. *B,* Turntable aligned perpendicular to parasagittal line, and as close to the body as possible. *C,* Strap and buckle for adjustment. *D,* Retainer for elbow lock cable. *E,* Elastic "V" strap to eliminate excessive internal rotation and to hold top of socket snugly against shoulder. *F,* Point in cable where sharp angle must be avoided. *G,* Suspension cable. *H,* Polyethylene saddle 1½ inches wide. *I,* Strap and buckle for adjustment. *J,* Snap buckle. *K,* Three-prong safety buckle. *L,* Nylon webbing 1⅜ inches wide and 1/16 inch thick. *M,* Suspension cable housing should not touch saddle. *N,* Slit, do not cut out piece of cross-bar hanger strap. *O,* Use two rivets on cross-bar hanger strap. *P,* Attach base plate here. *Q,* Dual control cable. (From Bender, Leonard F.: Prostheses and Rehabilitation after Arm Amputation, 1974. Courtesy of Charles C Thomas, Publisher, Springfield, Illinois.)

Mechanical control of functional terminal devices and elbow units is achieved by metal cables running through a housing that guides the cable from its point of origin to the point of attachment on the device. The cable is composed of braided stainless steel wire with a smooth surface; the housing is stainless steel wire tightly wound to form a small tube. The housing is attached to the socket and to the forearm shell of an above-elbow prosthesis through retainers and baseplates. In a below-elbow prosthesis, the control cable housing is attached to the triceps pad through a crossbar hanger assembly and to the socket through a baseplate and retainer. A Bowden control system utilizes a single control cable inside a single piece of housing attached at two or more points to the prosthesis or the harness.

The fair-lead control system is similar to a Bowden control except that the single control cable slides through two separate pieces of cable housing. This system provides two actions: (1) a force transmitted to the terminal device to operate it, and (2) a force applied to move the two pieces of housing toward each other. The second force can be used to flex the elbow, as long as it requires less force to flex the elbow than it does to operate the terminal device. A single control cable thereby becomes a dual control system for above-elbow prostheses.

Myoelectric control has recently been utilized with proportional type switches to operate electric motor driven hands, hooks, and elbows. Surface electrodes are placed inside the inner wall of the socket and press against the skin over analogous or appro-

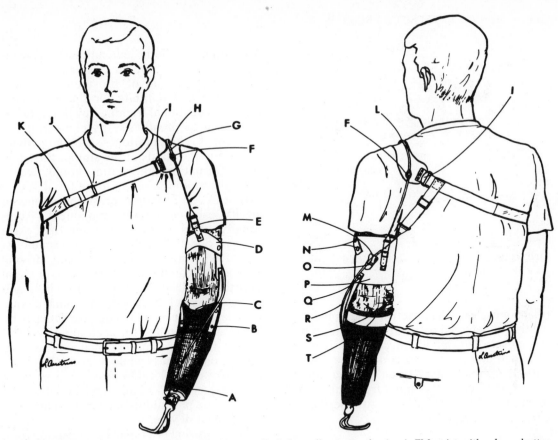

FIGURE 48–15. Modified shoulder saddle harness for below-elbow prosthesis. *A*, FM wrist with release button placed in midline. *B*, Rivets fastening the flexible elbow hinges. *C*, Cut-out for biceps tendon. *D*, Polyethylene Y-strap, 1/8 inch thick. *E*, Strap and buckle for adjustment of suspension cable. *F*, Point in cable where sharp angle must be avoided. *G*, Bowden suspension cable and housing. *H*, Polyethylene saddle 1½ inches wide. *I*, Snap-buckle for chest strap fastener. *J*, Three-prong safety buckle for chest strap adjustment. *K*, Nylon chest strap. *L*, Suspension cable housing should not touch saddle. *M*, Slit, do not cut out a piece of cross-bar hanger strap. *N*, Use two rivets. *O*, Use two rivets on cross-bar hanger strap. *P*, Polyethylene triceps pad. *Q*, Use one rivet to attach flexible elbow hinge to triceps pad. *R*, Single control cable. *S*, Flare socket to avoid pressure on olecranon. *T*, Place hinge cross strap (proximally) within ¼ inch of edge of socket. (From Bender, Leonard F.: Prostheses and Rehabilitation after Arm Amputation, 1974. Courtesy of Charles C Thomas, Publisher, Springfield, Illinois.)

FIGURE 48–16. *A*, Bowden control. *B*, Fair-lead control. (From Bender, Leonard F.: Prostheses and Rehabilitation after Arm Amputation, 1974. Courtesy of Charles C Thomas, Publisher, Springfield, Illinois.)

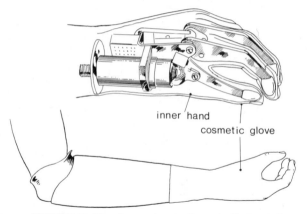

inner hand

cosmetic glove

FIGURE 48–17. A myoelectrically controlled prosthesis with electric hand.

priate muscles. The electromyographic signal that is detected by these electrodes when the muscle beneath them contracts can be amplified and utilized to control the flow of current from a battery to an electric motor. This type of control is most frequently used in below-elbow prostheses to operate an electric hand or hook.

PROSTHETIC PRESCRIPTION

Both the amputee and the prosthetist are served best by having an amputee clinic or team compose the elements of a prescription. The team may consist of a social worker, a prosthetist, an occupational therapist, a rehabilitation nurse, a physical therapist, an orthotist, a vocational counselor, and a physician. Their roles are consistent with their background and training. To write an appropriate prosthetic prescription, the team must have adequate information about the patient; this should include educational achievements, previous jobs, age, distance from his home to the clinic or prosthetist's office, motivation and aptitude for further educational or vocational training, level of interest in wearing a prosthesis, psychological adjustment to amputation, secondary diagnoses, and the status of the stump. Based on this information, the team should decide when the stump is ready to be fitted with a prosthesis. The written prescription should specify each structural component. Additionally, it is helpful to order one extra harness, one extra control cable assembly, a pair of band appliers, and as many driving rings as indicated. A driving ring is a metal loop that attaches to a steering wheel and accepts the hook fingers of a terminal device in its center; these are needed particularly by the left arm amputee for each motor vehicle driven. The extra harness makes it possible to wash one harness while wearing the other. The extra control cable provides a spare in case one breaks. Band appliers allow the amputee to put additional rubber bands on his terminal device.

The following is a typical prescription for a short below-elbow stump in a person who has good to normal range of motion and strength at the elbow and shoulder, who wishes to use the prosthesis in farming, and who also desires a cosmetic hand for social events:

Socket — Double wall, below-elbow with trimline just below epicondyles

Terminal Device — Dorrance Model 7 hook and Dorrance Model 4 hand plus cosmetic glove

Wrist — Hosmer FM (quick-disconnect)

Elbow — Flexible Dacron elbow hinges

Harness — Polyethylene shoulder saddle,

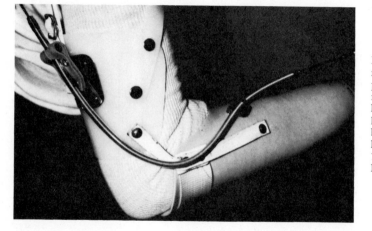

FIGURE 48–18. A standard prosthesis for a short below-elbow stump using a polyethylene triceps pad with attachments of flexible Dacron below-elbow hinges, polyethylene Y-strap, and leather cross-bar hanger strap. (From Bender, Leonard F.: Prostheses and Rehabilitation after Arm Amputation, 1974. Courtesy of Charles C Thomas, Publisher, Springfield, Illinois.)

triceps pad and Y-strap; Bowden control system

If this same amputee performed desk work instead of farming, it would be possible to use a Munster socket with electric hand and myoelectric control.

Similar specific prescriptions can be written for each level of amputation and for each set of constraints.[8]

PROSTHETIC CHECK-OUT AND TRAINING

After the prosthesis has been fabricated, it should be delivered to the amputee team for initial check-out on the amputee. The initial check-out takes only a few minutes and involves primarily an inspection of the components and their function. Conformance with the prescription should be checked along with the efficiency and workmanship of the prosthesis. After the patient dons the prosthesis, the fit of the socket and the position of the harness on the amputee should be observed.

Training proceeds during the completion of the check-out process. The amputee is taught to don the prosthesis by slipping it on like a jacket or a pull-over sweater. Control of each of the mechanisms of the prosthesis is then taught. When isolated movements have been mastered, the amputee moves on to performing specific integrated activities of daily living. Finally, skills useful in vocations and avocations are taught.

When a satisfactory level of control and use dexterity has been achieved, the training process is terminated and the amputee is asked to come back for periodic rechecks at lengthening intervals. These rechecks help provide preventive maintenance when the wearer does not recognize declining efficiency of the prosthesis and also provides continuing contact with the amputee during his readjustment.

PARTIAL HAND AMPUTATIONS

Amputation of part of a hand creates significant functional limitations and special prosthetic and/or orthotic problems. A variety of patterns of partial hand amputation can be observed, and the needs for devices vary considerably. Some persons are in-

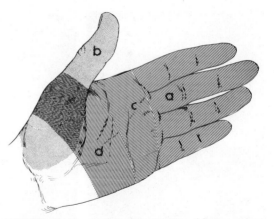

FIGURE 48–19. Levels of partial hand loss: *a*, transphalangeal; *b*, thenar; *c*, transmetacarpal, distal; *d*, transmetacarpal, proximal.

terested primarily in appearance while others desire function.

The causes of partial hand amputation are primarily traumatic and may involve such devices as punch presses, metal shears, conveyor belts, grinders, threshers, power saws, shredders, and corn pickers. They may also be caused by bullet wounds, explosions, freezing, and burning. Congenital skeletal deficiencies of the hand occur in many forms and add to the confusing variety of partial hand losses.

Analysis of these losses permits development of a classification of losses that will help guide the amputee clinic team toward the most appropriate prosthetic or orthotic solution. Levels of loss can conveniently be classified as follows:

1. Transphalangeal with involvement or sparing of the thumb
2. Thenar
3. Transmetacarpal distal with involvement or sparing of the thumb
4. Transmetacarpal proximal with involvement or sparing of the thumb

Transphalangeal levels of amputation usually require no device. The amputee may desire cosmetic fingers or even a portion of a cosmetic glove. These are available in a variety of skin tones, but they will provide little or no increased function. If the need can be defined, an orthosis may be specially designed to permit a needed function.

Thenar amputations are infrequent. Loss of only the distal phalanx usually necessitates nothing other than possibly a cosmetic thumb tip. Loss of part or the entire proximal phalanx usually is best handled by construct-

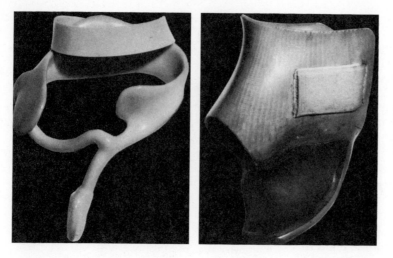

FIGURE 48–20. Open steel prosthesis (*left*) and mitt-shaped prosthesis (*right*) used in transmetacarpal amputations.

ing a prosthetic thumb of epoxy resins with a neoprene volar surface and a strap around the wrist to hold it in place.

Transmetacarpal distal and proximal levels of amputation can be fitted with three different devices: a cosmetic glove, a mitt-shaped prosthesis, or an open steel prosthesis shaped like an opposition semicircle. The mitt-shaped prosthesis is constructed like other double-walled sockets, but the exterior contour is that of slightly flexed fingers with no separation between the digits. It may be constructed with no strap to hold it on so that the amputee can merely slide his partial hand stump into the prosthesis and easily remove it when he has no need for it. The open steel prosthesis has a foundation shaped like a hand orthosis but has a steel rod attached to the foundation which extends out approximately in the contour of the previous fingertip positions; the intact thumb can then use it as an opposition device. The more proximal the level of amputation, the more difficult it is to construct the device.

In proximal transmetacarpal amputations, it may be possible and desirable to utilize functional fingers that can be attached to a short double-wall socket and controlled by a Bowden cable coming from a standard O-ring harness.

REFERENCES

1. Davies, E. J., Friz, B. R., and Clippinger, F. W.: Amputees and their prostheses. Artif. Limbs, 14:19, 1970.
2. Lamy, M., and Marteaux, P.: The genetic study of limb malformations. *In* Swinyard, C. A. (Ed.): Limb Development and Deformity: Problems of Evaluation and Rehabilitation. Springfield, Ill., Charles C Thomas, Publisher, 1969, pp. 170–175.
3. Cohlan, S. Q.: A review of teratogenic agents and human congenital malformations. *In* Swinyard, C. A. (Ed.): Limb Development and Deformity: Problems of Evaluation and Rehabilitation. Springfield, Ill., Charles C Thomas, Publisher, 1969, pp. 161–170.
4. Kay, H. W.: Clinical applications of the new international terminology for the classification of congenital limb deficiencies. Inter-Clinic Information Bull., Vol. XIV, No. 3, 1975.
5. Carlyle, L.: Using body measurements to determine proper lengths of artificial arms. Artificial Limbs Research Project, UCLA, Pamphlet Series No. 2, 1951.
6. Carlyle, L.: Fitting the artificial arm. *In* Klopsteg, P. E., and Wilson, P. D.: Human Limbs and Their Substitutes. New York, McGraw-Hill, 1954, pp. 637–652.
7. Weiss, M.: Neurological implications of fitting artificial limbs immediately after amputation surgery. Report of Fifth Workshop Panel on Lower-Extremity Prosthetics Fitting, Committee on Prosthetics Research and Development, National Academy of Sciences, February, 1966.
8. Bender, L. F.: Prostheses and Rehabilitation after Arm Amputation. Springfield, Ill., Charles C Thomas, Publisher, 1974.

49

MANAGEMENT OF THE LOWER EXTREMITY AMPUTEE

EMERY K. STONER

The "modern" approach to the rehabilitation of the amputee uses the combined efforts of the patient, the physician, the prosthetist, and the therapist as a team. No single individual is expected to have expert knowledge in all these areas. Success is achieved by the "team approach" in which each member sees clearly his own function and that of each of the other members. The principal duties of the group are to consider each individual case and to follow through with appropriate measures at the proper times. The steps are prescription, fitting, training, evaluating, and follow-up. It has been clearly demonstrated that amputees under the care of a clinical team become far better adapted to return to their place in society than those not fortunate enough to receive such guidance and support. In order for the patient to return to as full a life as possible he must be trained to use his remaining abilities to the best effect and assisted back to employment.

It is obvious that all these goals cannot be attained by one individual and that a number of workers, each an expert in his own field, must work together in the care of each amputee. The concept of the team approach has evolved and been put into practice. Amputee clinics, consisting of the association of physicians, therapists, prosthetists, social service workers, and vocational counselors, have been set up in many parts of our country.

Clinic procedures usually involve the following steps: preclinic examination; detailed prescription including surgical, physical, and prosthetics factors; preprosthetic therapy; prosthetic fabrication; initial checkout to determine whether the fit, alignment, and mechanical functions are such that training can be instituted; prosthetic training; final checkout to assure that the fit, alignment, and appearance of the prosthesis are acceptable and that the amputee's use of the limb is satisfactory; and follow-up examination. Prescription, initial check-out, and final check-out are the steps that require full clinic team participation.

PREPARATION FOR AMPUTATION

When the decision for amputation has been made, it is the physician's duty to explain to the patient the necessity for operation, the extent of surgery, and the deficit that will remain postoperatively. It is well to

921

describe the plan for postoperative care, preprosthetic conditioning, fitting with a prosthesis, and training in its use. In addition, the phenomenon of phantom sensation should be discussed.

SITES OF AMPUTATION

The trend has been toward more conservative surgery in amputations. Improved surgical techniques, use of antibiotics, and the development of new prosthetic materials and devices have made this possible. Maintenance of the knee joint preserves proprioception, which is important for balance and decreases the energy required for walking. The stump should be long enough to provide an adequate level to exert sufficient torque to move the prosthesis without excessive muscular effort. The aim of the surgeon is to produce a firm uniformly tapered or cylindrical stump, free of sensitive scarring, with the bone well padded along its length and covered at its tip by nonadherent fascia and skin.

POSTOPERATIVE CARE

Prevention of joint contracture is of prime importance. The stump should be positioned in good posture and mobilized as soon as possible. Compression bandaging, which is started early to prevent hemorrhage or edema and to promote shrinkage, is continued until the prosthesis is fitted. All joints proximal to the amputation should be moved through their full ranges of motion at least

three times a day as soon after amputation as possible. After the stump has healed, the patient is instructed and encouraged to exercise the residual muscles of the stump. As soon as possible the exercise should be of the progressive resistive type.

The stump should be washed daily with soap and water and dried thoroughly. For normal stumps the application of alcohol or any other agent to "toughen" the skin is not recommended.

COMPONENTS OF THE LOWER EXTREMITY PROSTHESIS[1]

Foot and Ankle. The prosthetic foot has generally been a solid block to which the ankle joint and toe section are attached. Conventional models of ankle joints provide flexion and dorsal flexion only, with rubber bumpers to restrain and restore these motions. The axis consists of a horizontal shaft, the outer ends of which rotate on plain bushings. Many variations have been tried. Lateral and transverse rotations are provided by rubber blocks or coil springs.

The SACH (Solid Ankle, Cushion Heel) foot is widely used at present. Rubber is molded or laminated over a "keel" of wood or metal. The foot permits inversion-eversion and plantar-dorsiflexion by compression of part of the foot. No ankle joint is used with it. The heel is made of layers of rubber of varying degrees of hardness. When the heel strikes, the rubber compresses and gives the appearance of ankle motion. The SACH foot is excellent cosmetically and it is the foot of choice for the wearing of high

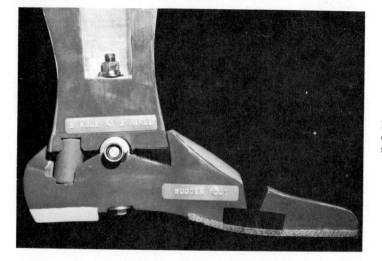

FIGURE 49–1. Conventional prosthetic foot. (Courtesy Dr. M. H. Anderson.)

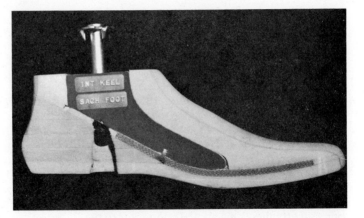

FIGURE 49–2. The solid ankle, cushion heel (SACH) foot. (Courtesy Dr. M. H. Anderson.)

heels. The main disadvantage is the gradual loss of elasticity in the material used (Figs. 49–1 and 49–2).

Knee Joints. Many prosthetic knees are available that partially satisfy the basic requirements of stability, gait, durability, comfort, and cosmesis.

Stability for weight bearing is provided by the backward force the stump exerts within the socket. The prosthesis may be aligned so that the knee is placed in slight hyperextension during weight bearing, or auxiliary mechanical aids, manual or automatic, may be added to stabilize the knee by locking it.

The types of prosthetic knees commercially available may be classified as constant friction, constant friction with friction lock, hydraulic, and polycentric. The "conventional single axis" knee is low in initial cost, and maintenance is simple. The friction or braking action does not vary during the swing phase of locomotion. The amount of friction may be increased or decreased by a simple adjustment.

If the amputee has impaired stump musculature, poor balance, or generalized weakness, a knee joint that provides constant friction with a friction lock may be used. In this type the ends of the knee bolt are not fixed but are allowed to slide in a short slot. When the leg bears weight the shank comes closer to the socket and a braking surface of each segment makes contact and a "friction lock" has been formed. During the swing phase a spring holds the two braking surfaces apart. The primary advantage of this type of knee is its stability. It is commonly used by elderly amputees.

The other types of knees are not often used. The hydraulic knee, of which there are several models, permits an excellent gait, but it is highly complex and very expensive.

Knee Extension Stops and Extension Aids. Limitation of extension of the prosthetic knee is usually accomplished by a radial arm or projection fitted around the knee bolt and to the shank, which stops the extension movements when the knee strikes it. The impact is usually lessened by a compressible bumper or cushion placed between the two parts. If the arm is made of spring steel it may also provide assistance in initiating knee flexion. When this principle is used the device is commonly referred to as a "hickory stick" kicker. It may also be designed to provide assistance in bringing the leg into full extension. An elastic strap in the back of the knee will assist in initiating knee flexion. An elastic strap in front of the knee will aid in extension, prevent excessive heel rise, and aid slightly in maintaining knee stability during weight bearing.

Above-knee Sockets. Sockets for above-knee prostheses are generally made of willow wood. Until recently the socket was shaped to the contour of the stump and called a "plug-fit" socket, and the body weight was borne on the tissues of the upper thigh over its entire circumference. With the development of the so-called "suction socket," the shape of the socket was changed to that of a "pressure" contour of the upper thigh and became roughly quadrilateral in shape.[1] The weight is borne more on the ischial tuberosity and gluteal muscle group. Most prescriptions now call for a quadrilateral-shaped wooden socket.

A more recent development has been the "total contact socket" for above-knee amputees. In this type the stump is in complete contact with the socket even though the bulk of the weight is carried on the ischial tuberosity and the gluteal tissues. The socket is suspended by suction and the valve is flush with the inner wall of the socket. Claims are made that the amputee has better control of this socket, that he gets more "feedback" from it so that he knows more confidently the position of his artificial limb, and that edema of the stump tends to disappear in a short time. Experience has proved the value of these sockets and they are used routinely today.

Suspension for Above-knee Prosthesis. Suspension may be provided by suction, the Silesian bandage, the pelvic belt, shoulder suspenders, or a combination of methods. A Silesian bandage is a light webbing band with one end attached by a swivel connector to the lateral aspect of the socket in the region of the greater trochanter. The other end is attached to the socket anteriorly in the midline at a point level with the ischial seat. The belt rests between the crest of the ilium and the trochanter on the sound side. This device is a valuable aid in stabilizing the prosthesis against rotation and lateral instability. The Silesian bandage is sometimes used concurrently with suction.

The pelvic belt may be used with a rigid or flexible pelvic band. It has the advantage of being easy to put on and it gives the new amputee a greater feeling of security and allows him to use one or more stump socks, which in turn permits longer tolerable socket fit.

PROSTHETIC PRESCRIPTION

Hip Disarticulation. This classification includes the true hip disarticulation and amputations as far as about 2 inches below the level of the perineum. In a hip disarticulation prosthesis, socket stability must be obtained at the pelvic level, energy for use of the limb must come from pelvic movement, and weight must be borne by the pelvic area. This requires a prosthesis that can be suspended from the pelvis and that possesses hip and knee joints that are reasonably stable during standing and capable of permitting the amputee to walk, sit, or stand with minimal discomfort, minimal energy cost, and maximal cosmesis. The Canadian type hip disarticulation prosthesis (Fig. 49–3) comes nearest to meeting these requirements.

Short Above-knee Stump. This division includes stumps from 2 inches below the perineum to the upper border of the middle third

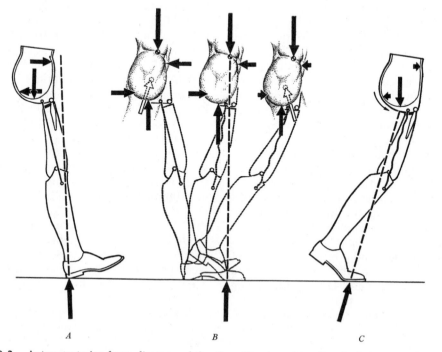

A   *B*   *C*

FIGURE 49–3. Anteroposterior force diagram of the Canadian type hip disarticulation prosthesis. *A*, Forces acting on prosthesis at heel contact. *B*, Forces acting on stump at heel contact, mid-stance, and push-off. *C*, Force acting on prosthesis at push-off. (From Radcliffe, C. W.: The Biomechanics of the Canadian Type Hip Disarticulation Prosthesis. Artif. Limbs, 1957.)

of the thigh. Socket stability and energy must come mainly from the pelvic area and the optimal weight-bearing area is the ischial tuberosity and the gluteal fold. Some stumps may permit suction suspension. The prosthesis used is an ischial weight-bearing socket, auxiliary suspension plus suction, if possible, with adequate knee stability.

Mid-thigh Stump. A mid-thigh stump results from amputation at any point within the middle third of the thigh. Socket stability is usually obtained from the femoral area, with the use of suction suspension. Power comes from flexion-extension of the hip. Weight is borne on the ischial tuberosity and the gluteal fold. Prescription calls for an ischial weight-bearing socket with suspension by suction or auxiliary suspension. Moderate knee stability is needed.[4]

Long Above-knee Stump. This stump ends below the middle of the thigh but it is not capable of end bearing. Socket stability is obtained in the femoral area with suction suspension, and power comes from flexion-extension of the hip and has the advantage of the longer lever arm and longer muscles. Weight is borne on the ischial tuberosity and the gluteal fold (Fig. 49–4). An ischial weight-bearing socket with suspension by suction (or auxiliary) suspension is prescribed. Minimal knee stability is necessary.

End Bearing Above-knee Stump. This group includes the various amputations at and above the knee which yield an end bearing stump: the Gritti, Krik, Callander, epicondylar, supracondylar, and others. Socket stability is supplied by both the femoral area and the end bearing stump. Weight is divided between the stump end and the ischial-gluteal area. This stump yields the maximum of power for use of an above-knee prosthesis. Prescription of this prosthesis includes an ischial weight-bearing socket with provision for partial end bearing, suction (or auxiliary) suspension, and minimal knee stability.

Short Below-knee Stump. This includes stumps with not more than 2 inches of the tibia remaining. Stability of the socket is dependent on accurate fitting of the stump plus side hinges and a thigh corset if necessary. Weight-bearing surfaces are the patellar ligament, the flares of the tibial condyles, and the anteromedial wall of the tibia. If necessary a thigh corset can support part of the weight load and, if needed, ischial weight

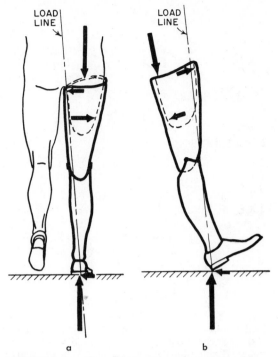

FIGURE 49–4.   Forces acting upon typical above-knee prosthesis during the stance phase. (From Klopsteg, P. E., and Wilson, P. L.: Human Limbs and Their Substitutes. New York, McGraw-Hill Book Co., Inc., 1954. Used by permission of McGraw-Hill Book Company.)

bearing can be provided. Power is provided by the quadriceps and hamstring muscles.

Standard Below-knee Stump. These stumps end at any point from 2 inches below the top of the tibia to the muscle-tendinous juncture of the gastrocnemius. Stability, power, and weight bearing are derived from the knee area. The patellar-tendon–bearing (PTB) prosthesis appears to be the best below-knee prosthesis at this time[2] (Figs. 49–5 and 49–6).

Below-knee Sockets. The conventional below-knee prosthesis, in which the socket was a plug fit and weight bearing and suspension were provided by side joints and a thigh lacer, was used almost universally for over 200 years. The development of the patellar-tendon–bearing (PTB) prosthesis was the result of a conference of leading prosthetists at the University of California at Berkeley in 1957. The original description of the PTB prosthesis was for a plastic laminate socket formed over a modified plaster-of-paris model of the stump. It contained a soft inner

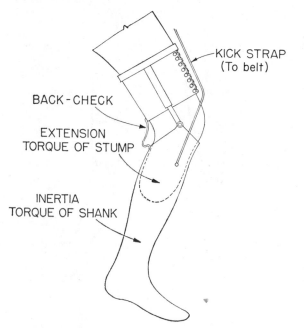

KICK STRAP
(To belt)

BACK-CHECK

EXTENSION
TORQUE OF STUMP

INERTIA
TORQUE OF SHANK

FIGURE 49–5. Conventional below-knee prosthesis with back check and kick strap, side joint and thigh corset. (From Klopsteg, P. E., and Wilson, P. D.: Human Limbs and Their Substitutes. New York, McGraw-Hill Book Co., Inc., 1954. Used by permission of McGraw-Hill Book Company.)

lining that contacted the entire surface of the stump. The weight was borne mainly by the medial flare of the tibia and the patellar tendon. Suspension was provided by a fabric strap around the thigh just above the femoral condyles.

The PTB concept has gained widespread acceptance and today the PTB socket is considered standard for below-knee amputations. Recently, modifications have been introduced as improvements to the basic concept.[7]

The Hard Socket. The original PTB socket had a liner of leather or plastic backed by sponge rubber. The plastic did not allow the moisture to escape and the leather quickly rotted from perspiration. A trial of elimination of the liner proved to be successful and now the hard PTB socket is widely used.

THE PATELLAR-TENDON–SUSPENDING SOCKET. The suspension strap was satisfactory in most cases but improved suspension was desired. The proximal border of the socket was extended above the femoral condyles and the patella and this was found to suspend the limb adequately. This is known as the PTS socket. It may be used with or without a liner.

WEDGE SUSPENSION SOCKET. A small wedge inserted between the proximal area of the socket and the area of the stump along the medial condyle of the femur proved to suspend the limb satisfactorily. It is known as the supracondylar-wedge suspension and is normally used with a hard socket.

AIR CUSHION SOCKET. The air cushion PTB consists of an elastic inner sleeve suspended from the level of the tibial tubercle in a rigid outer sheet that is closed distally. Tension of the sleeve and compression of the air in the chamber between the inner and outer layers produce stump support. This socket has been found to be particularly helpful in patients with very tender stumps. More time is required to make this socket and little modification can be made after fabrication.

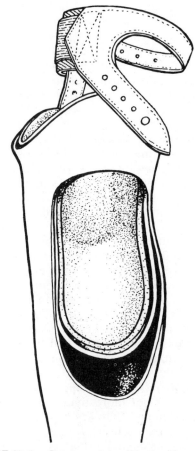

FIGURE 49–6. Cutaway view of the patellar-tendon–bearing socket incorporated in a thin-walled plastic shank. Note especially the cuff-suspension strap, the high lateral and medial wall, and the total contact features. (From Murphy, E. F., and Wilson, A. B., Jr.: Anatomical and Physiological Considerations in Below-knee Prosthetics. Artif. Limbs, 6:4-15, 1962.)

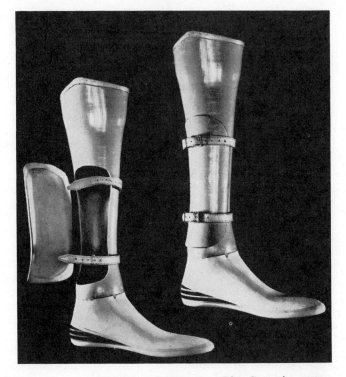

FIGURE 49–7. Syme prosthesis developed by the Veterans Administration Prosthetics Center, New York. The nylon-Dacron-polyester socket is provided with an opening in the medial wall. Weight bearing may be divided in any proportion between the proximal rim and the distal portions of the socket. (From Wilson, A. B., Jr.: Prosthetics for Syme's Amputation. Artif. Limbs, 6:52-75, 1961.)

POROUS SOCKET. Problems of perspiration have led to much effort to develop a satisfactory porous plastic laminate. Early porous laminates were too weak for lower extremity application. However, with the use of epoxy resins, a porous laminate socket can be made suitable for below-knee sockets. Problems with perspiration are minimized and the socket is lighter in weight.

CASTING METHODS. For fabricating the PTB socket the stump is wrapped with plaster and shaped by hand. The male mold is further modified and the socket is cast over the mold. A number of attempts have been made to simplify this procedure.

In the suspension-casting technique, the stump is wrapped while it is held in a vertical position that simulates weight bearing during standing. Felt pads to provide relief for sensitive area of the stump are applied directly to the stump. A synthetic rubber, Polysar X414,* has been found to have properties that make it suitable for forming a socket directly over the stump. Temporary or provisional below-knee prostheses made of this material are proving to be useful. Polysar X414 becomes pliable at temperatures tolerated by the skin and can be applied directly over the stump.

*Registered trademark of Polysar Corp. Ltd.

Ankle Disarticulation. The Syme's amputee has lost the foot and ankle but retains essentially the full length of the shank and weight-bearing characteristics that approach those of the normal heel. The problem is to restore the equivalent of foot and ankle function, to extend the stump to accommodate the loss of the tarsus and of the calcaneus, to furnish adequate body support during walking and standing, to provide suitable suspension for the prosthesis during the swing phase, and to do all these things so that the final result is acceptable to the wearer.

The Canadian type Syme prosthesis ("Plastic Syme") is a vast improvement over the older type because it is lighter in weight, is stronger, requires less maintenance, is less expensive, and is much improved in appearance (Fig. 49–7). The socket is made from laminated fiber glass or plastic-impregnated nylon stockinet; there is no ankle joint and the foot is of the SACH type. This prosthesis permits full or partial end bearing, depending upon the tolerance of the stump.

It must be emphasized here that Syme's amputation is indicated for all destructive, infective, or other disabling lesions of the foot that cannot be dealt with by a transmetatarsal amputation. Lisfranc's and Chopart's amputations are apt to be unsatisfactory.

Transtarsal Amputation. Transtarsal amputations are to be avoided.

Transmetatarsal Amputation. No prosthesis is necessary for transmetatarsal amputees. There is an excellent surface for weight bearing and a regular shoe can be worn. The front of the shoe may be stuffed with lamb's wool or some other material and covered with leather. To aid in toe-off a plate of spring metal is placed between the inner and outer sole.

Toe Amputation. Loss of the small toes leads to no particular gait difficulty. Absence of the great toe, however, prevents a good gait in rapid walking because of loss of toe-off. Here again the front of the shoe can be stuffed and a spring metal plate placed between the soles of the shoe.

TREATMENT

Preoperative Care of the Leg Amputee. Before surgery the patient should be prepared psychologically as well as physically for the procedure to guard against needless anxieties and to help him withstand the psychologic trauma of amputation. The patient wants to know the level of amputation, how he will look, and how disabled he will be. Before or soon after surgery he should be told about phantom limb sensation. The steps in his rehabilitation program should be outlined to him and he should be given an estimate of the time it will require.

Early Postoperative Care. The first three postoperative days are often uncomfortable ones for the amputee. By the fourth day steps should be taken to prevent contractures. The aim is to prevent abduction, flexion, and external rotation at the hip and flexion deformity at the knee. The amputee is taught to lie flat with no pillow under the stump, to lie face down part of the day, and to keep his pelvis level. Prolonged sitting in a wheelchair, especially during the first 10 days after surgery, should be avoided. The same care must be taken even though the amputee is not considered to be a candidate for a prosthesis.

Preprosthetic Training. General conditioning exercises may be started three to five days after surgery. Crutch walking is begun as soon as feasible. After the sutures are removed the patient is taught stump bandaging, a program of specific exercises for the stump, and stump hygiene.

Fitting of the Prosthesis. The clinic team — physician, prosthetist, therapist, and vocational counselor — decide on the limb for the amputee. Each in his own field can point out factors that should be considered in prosthesis selection. The patient's readiness for fitting is determined by many factors, such as the rapidity of healing, the presence of complications, his general condition, and his ability to use crutches.

Experience has shown that the amputee who can swing through in crutch walking and can negotiate stairs on crutches will use an artificial limb satisfactorily. If the economic factors were eliminated these patients could be fitted and trained very early. However, in three to six months a new socket would be needed. The amputee is usually measured by the prosthetist 8 to 10 weeks after surgery. By this time most of the stump shrinkage will have taken place and only minor changes will be necessary to keep the socket well fitted.

At the Hospital of the University of Pennsylvania we have found a number of patients who, although they never learned to use crutches, learned to use an artificial leg in a satisfactory fashion. The energy cost of using a prosthesis, with or without the assistance of crutches or canes, is less than that required for using crutches alone.

Prosthetic Training. Training in the use of his prosthetic limb is an important aspect of the rehabilitation of an amputee. Occasionally an individual is able to learn on his own but certainly this is not to be recommended. A set of parallel bars and a full length mirror are needed for training. Stairs and ramps can usually be found nearby although it is handy to have them in the gymnasium. An exercise mat is helpful for exercising and for practicing falling and getting up.

Training begins with instruction in how to put on the limb. Because an elderly person may have difficulty in putting on a limb with a socket suspended by suction, we rarely prescribe suction suspension for individuals over 50 years of age with recent amputations but prefer to use a pelvic band and belt.

Standing is started in the parallel bars and weight shifting is done forward, backward, and sideways. The patient learns to balance on one leg and steps are begun by putting the "best foot" forward and letting the momentum of the body help swing the prosthesis forward. Emphasis is placed upon keeping the steps even in length and keeping the trunk moving forward steadily. Side stepping is practiced, as is the act of getting up and down from chairs — wheelchairs, armchairs, and straight back chairs. Negotiation of steps, ramps, curbs, and finally rough ground is taught. Falling and getting up are practiced in suitable cases, as are running, pivoting, and overcoming obstacles.

Ordinarily training requires about 12 sessions for a below-knee amputee and 18 periods for an above-knee amputee. Training can be done on an outpatient basis, and it is my opinion that training three times a week is sufficient for the elderly amputee. The bilateral above-knee amputee requires prolonged inpatient training (six to eight weeks).

From various reports it seems that walking with a unilateral above-knee prosthesis requires an expenditure of 20 to 25 per cent more energy than walking on two normal legs.[3, 6] Although many geriatric amputees are successfully fitted and trained, the metabolic cost of using their prosthesis may be 10 to 15 per cent more than for the younger amputee and 25 to 35 per cent higher than the energy cost to a younger unimpaired person. Studies by Peizer[6] indicate that a general increase in efficiency of performing standard exercises can be expected with time and practice.

Many amputees can walk with a good gait but fail to do so in daily practice, adopting a more comfortable, less costly in energy, but less esthetic, gait. Walking very slowly is uneconomical because of the partial loss of momentum and the resulting necessity of overcoming inertia at each step. Fast walking is uneconomical because of increased internal friction within the body tissues as well as increased movement of the arms, shoulders, and trunk. The tension in postural muscles is increased. All of these adjustments require extra energy. It appears that each person has an optimal rate of walking for which the least energy is required. Normally this rate is the one that feels comfortable or "natural" to the individual.

Stump Bandaging. After the sutures are removed, elastic compression bandages are used to shrink and shape the stump. This is continued until the patient receives his prosthetic limb. If for any reason he is unable to wear his prosthesis, bandaging should be reinstituted until he again wears the limb.

The elastic bandages may be plain woven cotton or the elastic reinforced type. The above-knee stump usually requires a 6-inch bandage, the below-knee stump, a 4-inch bandage, and other stumps, appropriate widths. Wrapping should be done at least twice daily and continued all day.

Bandages should be applied so that the pressure is greatest at the tip of the stump and decreases from the distal to the proximal end. The bandage turns should be diagonal rather than horizontal. The above-knee bandage should be carried high into the groin and the below-knee bandage should reach to the lower pole of the patella.

Swelling. During healing after amputation there is usually some swelling in the stump. This may be minimized by elevating the stump and by wrapping it with elastic bandages. A poorly fitting socket can also cause edema of the stump.

Stump Hygiene. By following a simple routine of stump care consistently, the amputee can avoid many problems. Stump hygiene includes skin cleansing and care of the socket, socks, and bandages.

The stump should be cleansed with soap and water daily, preferably at night. A liquid antiseptic solution or cake soap containing hexachlorophene (e.g., pHisoHex, Dial, Gamophen) may be used. The skin must be rinsed and dried thoroughly.

The stump sock should be changed daily. It should be washed in warm water with a mild soap, rinsed thoroughly, and allowed to dry completely. Elastic bandages should be washed in the same way and allowed to dry on a flat surface.

The socket is washed with warm water and mild soap, wiped with a cloth, and permitted to dry thoroughly before the limb is worn. This is to be done at night and should be done on a daily basis in hot weather.

Phantom Pain. After loss of an arm or leg the missing part may leave its phantom to cause much mental and physical suffering. Phantoms usually include only distal portions of the missing members. An amputation of the lower extremity is most likely to be represented by a phantom foot; an upper extremity by a phantom hand. If the phantom is painless it is known as "phantom sensation" but if there is any unpleasant feeling or pain it is known as "phantom pain."

When phantom pain develops it is usually immediately after surgery and it characteristically persists. It has been described as cramping, squeezing, burning, sharp, shooting, or lancinating. Some patients describe the phenomenon in terms of numbness, pins and needles sensations, and variations in temperature, position, and pressure.

Various theories have attributed the cause of phantom pain to the peripheral and central nervous systems and to psychogenic factors. According to the peripheral theory, painful sensation originates from excitation of nerve endings in the scar, neuroma, or infected stump. Impulses from cut nerves set up a reverberating circuit that forms a self-perpetuating vicious circle between the thalamus and the cerebral cortex. Removal of the neuroma or further local surgery usually fails to relieve phantom pain, however. Occasional success with sympathetic block or anterolateral chordotomy has provided a strong argument against the psychogenic theory.

The central nervous system (body image) theory holds that during growth from childhood to adulthood multiple sensory impressions traveling to the cerebral cortex and its association center make us increasingly aware of parts of our body. Subsequently this image shows resistance to change and provides the basis for phantom pain. In favor of this theory is the complete absence of phantom sensation in children with agenesis of limbs and in those who have had amputations before the age of five years.

Treatment of phantom pain is as controversial as the theories of etiology. Positive findings such as a neuroma, painful scar, and tender spur call for treatment, but it is often unsuccessful in relieving the phantom pain.

Phantom pain and sensation have not been explained satisfactorily in terms upon which appropriate treatment may be founded. Methods such as firm bandaging day and night, ultraviolet radiation, diathermy, galvanism, ultrasound, paraffin baths, and repeated percussion of palpable tender neuromas have satisfactory transient effects that can be prolonged indefinitely by providing and maintaining function with a prosthesis. An artificial limb that functions like the missing part greatly lessens the pain. Restoration of function as soon as possible after amputation, together with psychotherapy and removal of local irritants, has been used as an efficient means of relieving phantom pain. A psychologic approach has been to "exercise the phantom" through carrying out motions which were formerly done by the missing extremity.

EMPLOYMENT OF AMPUTEES

After the amputee has completed training in the use of his prosthesis, the next step is reemployment. The handicapped have much less difficulty in finding employment now than they did a few years ago. If the amputee is unable to return to the same type of work he did formerly, provision is made for retraining for some other job.

The unilateral below-knee amputee has minimal disability. If he has a well-fitted prosthesis and has been properly trained in its use he can do almost everything he did before amputation, except for running. This type of amputee usually returns to his former employment.

The unilateral above-knee amputee cannot perform a job that will require carrying heavy objects and it must be understood that he will walk more slowly than the normal person.

The bilateral above-knee amputee has an extreme disability. He cannot be expected to stand for long periods or do much walking although he can stand for short periods and ambulate for short distances. He should be employed where he can sit down for most of the day or, if it is necessary to move, he can use a wheelchair.

The bilateral below-knee amputee can walk and stand well but he should be employed where he can be seated much of the day.

IMMEDIATE POSTSURGICAL FITTING OF PROSTHESES

Excellent results are being obtained worldwide with the use of immediate postsurgical fitting of prostheses. Sufficient experience has been gained so that it is now safe to form and train new teams in its use. The concept of fitting patients with prostheses immediately after surgery and initiating ambulation training the next day was first carried out by Berlemont in 1958, and reported on in 1961 at the Congress of Physical Medicine at Nancy. Weiss, in Warsaw, is given credit for the worldwide acceptance of this method. Burgess perfected the technique of the immediate prosthesis.[2]

A number of benefits result from the use of immediate fitting: less pain for the patient, more rapid healing of the wound, psychological benefits, early weight bearing with maintenance of postural reflexes, quicker maturation of the stump, and earlier fitting with the definitive prosthesis.

Every effort should be made to preserve the knee joint, even if it means a very short stump. As the surgeon gains experience he will be operating more frequently at the limits of viability and the chances of primary wound healing will correspondingly decrease. Techniques of amputation that provide for secure fixation of the muscle at the end of the stump at physiologic tension result in a firm well-shaped stump.

Wound hematoma is the main complication in amputation surgery and usually it is advantageous to use a drain.

The plaster cast using elastic plaster is applied at the completion of the operation and it prevents swelling of the stump. Because of change in the shape of the stump, such as that induced by changing position from bed rest to weight bearing, some resilient material needs to be placed between the plaster and the soft tissue. Zettl et al. studied various types of "interface" materials and found that reticulated polyurethane foam, 20 pores per inch, is ideal for use. It is available in preformed pads of suitable sizes.[9]

The general principles of management have been spelled out by Burgess et al.[2] They are:

1. A "team" approach which includes all relevant disciplines.
2. Definitive surgery is carried out at the lowest suitable level. The amputation is essentially a plastic-surgery procedure with conservation of dynamic stump function.
3. The immediate postsurgical prosthesis is applied as a rigid supportive pressure dressing designed to accept a temporary prosthesis.
4. Early ambulation is permitted consistent with the patient's condition.
5. A progressive program from amputation to definitive prosthesis involves continuous wound support and progressive ambulation with controlled weight bearing. Serial socket changes are made as needed.

Postoperative Management. The goals of immediate postsurgical fitting of a prosthesis are prompt primary wound healing, early ambulation, and rapid maximum rehabilitation of the patient. A patient who is unable to ambulate still benefits from the rigid dressing.

The initial period of standing on the prosthesis is limited to minimal, involving no more than 10 pounds of measured weight. The prosthesis unit must be aligned accurately with the patient standing. Usually the patient stands on the first or second postoperative day from 1 to 5 minutes. When endurance has increased to allow standing for several 5 minute periods twice daily, then ambulation is begun in the parallel bars. Weight on the amputation side should not exceed 20 pounds until primary wound healing is assured.

The patient begins and ends each training session by standing on paired scales to get the "feel" of the permitted weight bearing.

On the first postoperative day the therapist goes to the patient's room with a Walkerette and assists him to stand with minimal weight bearing on the prosthesis for 5 minutes or less. The pylon and foot are removed after the patient is returned to bed. On the second postoperative day the patient usually starts going to the physical medicine department in a wheelchair twice daily for periods of standing and exercises for the arms. From then until two weeks postoperatively, the patient gradually begins ambulation in the parallel bars. Approximately 20 to 30 pounds is the maximum weight permitted on the amputation side.

In the second two weeks after surgery the patient can usually progress to crutch walking. Forearm crutches are used if appropriate. They permit a more normal gait. Continue to limit weight bearing to 30 pounds.

Measurement for the definite prosthesis can be taken about one week following the second cast change if the sutures are removed and the wound is well healed. It is well to avoid any interruption that would leave the stump without support. Elastic bandaging is commonly used for several weeks after the definite prosthesis is delivered. At times a night cast may be necessary if the patient is not skillful in bandaging.

THE GERIATRIC AMPUTEE

Amputees in the older age group are beset with additional problems. Whereas in the child amputee factors such as growth, development, coordination, and muscular strength present problems, in the elderly amputee there are a multitude of medical complications and degenerative changes. Although the geriatric amputee is by far the most common patient seen in the amputee clinic of a general hospital, most efforts in the field of prosthetics have been for the young adult amputee.

Aged people walk with a significantly slower cadence. There is a decrease in the average speed of walking as age increases. In addition, aged people walk in a less vigorous fashion. There is a less dynamic transfer of the body weight onto and off the stance leg.

In the adult population peak aft shear stresses occur before double support begins, while in the elderly maximum aft shear stresses are generated after double support begins.[6] Apparently older people attempt to improve stability by increasing the period of double support.

Some biologic aging becomes symptomatic between 50 and 55 years of age. Biologic and chronologic aging are frequently not identical. It seems logical to use age 55 as a guide for classifying an amputee as a "new amputee" or an "old amputee" — it is clear that a patient whose limb was amputated earlier in life and attains age 55 presents different problems from the individual who loses a limb after the age of 55 years.

In the geriatric amputee about one third of the amputations are done because of the factor of atherosclerosis. About 39 per cent are secondary to atherosclerosis associated with diabetes mellitus. Thus, over 70 per cent of geriatric amputees have loss of limb directly attributable to vascular disease.

Care of the Amputation Stump

Stump care of the geriatric patient is similar to that for other amputees. Generally the sutures remain in place longer (10 to 14 days), since wound dehiscence is more frequent in this group. Prevention of contractures is of primary importance in the geriatric patient. Supervised active resistive exercise is the best means of preventing contractures.

Criteria for Prosthetic Fitting

Most geriatric amputees should be fitted with limbs. Many will not function at a very high level, but this is not to be considered reason for denying the patient an artificial limb and training in its use. This is not true for the elderly bilateral above-knee amputee.

It is difficult to set up clearly defined criteria for fitting, but certainly if the amputee can use crutches satisfactorily he will make good progress with a prosthesis.

Somewhat easier to list are factors which absolutely contraindicate limb fitting. These include (1) lack of motivation, (2) threatened gangrene of the remaining leg, (3) class IV heart disease, (4) severe neurologic problems, (5) unyielding stump problems, and (6) multiple major physical impairments.

Except in the case of absolute contraindications there is seldom justification for failing to recommend prosthetic fitting for the elderly amputee.

Prosthetic Factors

Comfort, fit, alignment, and appearance are criteria for an acceptable prosthesis for all amputees. Additional factors are important in fitting the elderly amputee. These include (1) minimum weight of prosthesis, (2) a stable knee joint, and (3) easily applied and effective suspension.

All means should be used to minimize the weight of the prosthesis while still retaining sufficient structural strength. Lightweight woods, reinforced duralumin ankle, knee, and hip joints with Teflon washers in areas of metal-to-metal contact, and rawhide finishing help in keeping the total weight very low. The socket thickness need not be as great as that for a young vigorous amputee. Lightweight knee units are available. A new type of molded SACH foot is now made which is about half the weight of the laminated type.

There is a definite need for a knee unit which has a positive lock during the stance phase and which permits motion during the swing phase. The Otto Bock safety knee is used frequently for the elderly amputee. A manual knee lock may be used for severely unstable knee conditions. It is true that a knee lock is associated with a circumducted gait with or without vaulting on the remaining foot. It is preferable to have a poor gait than not to walk at all. At times softening of the SACH foot will aid in stability.

Initial flexion for the above-knee amputee should be built into the socket so that the amputee can stand erect without unlocking the knee. Hip flexion contractures in the elderly are prevalent and very resistive to correction.

Suspension of the prosthesis can present a

difficult problem. The amputee must be comfortable while sitting for long periods, and the prosthesis must also be easy to put on and give effective suspension. Suction would be ideal except that it is difficult for an elderly person to put the limb on. It is seldom indicated in an older amputee. A pelvic band and belt with hip joint is easier to put on and adjust and gives effective suspension but is not comfortable on prolonged sitting. A good compromise is a pelvic belt (without the pelvic band) and a single-axis metal hip joint. A Silesian bandage is quite comfortable and easy to apply, but many amputees feel that the suspension is ineffective.

Because of weakness of hip musculature the elderly above-knee amputee may have difficulty in clearing the floor with his prosthesis. During the training period the artificial limb may be about one half inch shorter than his remaining leg. As training progresses the limb is lengthened until leg lengths are equal and the iliac crests level.

Energy Costs

Walking speed is greatly limited in the above-knee amputee. Even at low speeds a high metabolic effort is needed. This amounts to about 700 ml of oxygen per minute — roughly the same as maximum effort in older people. The energy costs for the elderly bilateral above-knee amputee are overwhelming. Wheelchair locomotion has been shown to require the least effort and energy expenditure.

Psychosocial Aspects

The process of aging has a detrimental effect on physical and psychological function. The trauma of amputation is added disaster. Thus, the older amputee must struggle with two negative forces which make it difficult for him to adjust — amputation and aging.

Self-image is constantly being adjusted. Slow changes permit gradual modification in self-image. A person losing a limb must drastically revise his body image. This reorganization of self-image is a major and at times an overwhelming task.

Prosthetic restoration plus the activity necessary to learn to use the limb should help with this adaptation or modification in self-image. For this reason alone, to institute

training in the use of a prosthetic device might be considered a proper decision even though the chance of ultimate success is very slim.

THE JUVENILE AMPUTEE

Amputation in children is usually traumatic, congenital, or secondary to the treatment of malignancy. The prosthetic management of the child amputee is essentially the same as that of adults. For the most part nearly all the prosthetic components are scaled-down versions of adult models.[8] This is not an ideal approach, but this is the way it has evolved.

The flexibility of the child, with his greater reserve of all tissues, permits him to adapt quickly to prostheses. The young amputee grows up with his appliance and accepts it as a necessary item for his daily life.

Amputation done on an individual in whom bone growth is not complete leads to certain alterations in form and internal structure of the long bones and the axial skeleton. Below-knee amputation occurring before the age of 10 years will show bowing and kyphosis of the stump after some time. Above-knee amputation is accompanied by hemiatrophy of the pelvis on the same side as the amputation. Complications of amputation seen in adults, such as painful spurs, symptomatic neuromata, bursitis, and phantom pain, are relatively rare in children. However, stump overgrowth is a complication seen only in the child amputee.

Between the ages of six and ten there is a disproportionate growth between the skin and bone, as shown by a long thin spindle of bone growing from the end of the amputation stump. Clinically the stump becomes red, swollen, and tender, and unless surgery is done the bony end protrudes from the stump. This occurs most commonly with the fibula and less frequently with the tibia and humerus. Surgical revision relieves this complication promptly. This phenomenon has not been observed in the true congenital amputee unless the periosteum has been altered by surgery.

Age for Prosthetic Fitting

Children with lower extremity defects should be fitted with their first prosthesis when they start making efforts to stand. The average age for children to stand and attempt walking is between 10 and 18 months. When this stage of development is reached, a prosthesis should be fitted even if it is quite simple. As balance is developed a conventional type of limb is indicated.

A variety of components are available for prescription by the clinic team for the child amputee. In uncomplicated cases satisfactory functional results are obtained, but many problems remain for the more complicated, severely disabled children. Special devices may need to be designed and fabricated for a particular case. Constant efforts are being made to improve the prostheses available for children.

Lower Extremity Components

Most lower extremity components are copied from adult models. The SACH (solid ankle/cushioned heel) foot is used routinely for children and is quite satisfactory. The Syme type of prosthesis is like that of the adult. The PTB (patellar-tendon–bearing) socket is used routinely in many clinics for the below-knee child amputee. There are still unanswered questions as to the effects of wearing a PTB socket on the knee joint in a growing child. When the PTB socket is not used, the conventional open-end socket and laced leather thigh corset are applied. A single-axis knee with constant-friction is used for the above-knee patient. Additional stigmata are seen in these children — saddle nose, coloboma or other eye defects, microtia, nevi of the forehead and face, and sometimes atresia of the external meatus. When there is upper extremity amelia or functionless phocomelia, the feet must be trained as prehensile organs. When the legs are involved and the child is unable to sit, a sitting socket must be furnished at the age the child would normally sit. When the child is able to sit independently, functionless upper extremities should be fitted. Further functional components can be added as the child develops more skill. The child with severe upper and lower extremity deformities will probably not walk and a motorized chair will be needed.

Lower Extremity Congenital Defects. Absence of the forefoot is seen at times. A modified shoe can be used, but the tendency for the development of equinovarus position may require a Syme amputation. Absence of the fibula is relatively common. This is associated with a valgus ankle and frequently with absence of the lateral two digital rays and bowing of the lower tibia. A strong shoe constructed to correct the valgus ankle is often all that is needed. A modified Syme amputation gives better cosmetic results and may be preferable if a plantigrade foot cannot be attained. Amputation for cosmetic reasons should not be done until the child is old enough to share in the decision.[2] However, when amputation is necessary to improve or promote function it should be done promptly. Absence of the tibia is manifested by total instability at the knee and ankle. The legs are unsatisfactory in an extension prosthesis and surgery is necessary. Disarticulation at the knee may be the most functional procedure. Femoral defects may range from simple coxa-vara to complete absence of the femur. Numerous surgical procedures have been tried for these cases but often the only gain has been in cosmesis, with some decrease of function. These patients usually learn to use an extension prosthesis quite satisfactorily.

Complete bilateral lower limb amelia (with normal upper extremities) has been managed by the use of stubbies of increasing height. Finally a pair of Canadian-type hip-disarticulation prostheses is fitted and the patient walks with a four-point gait.

Conversions

In the case of a severely deformed extremity, amputation, or ablation, correcting it to a more functional and cosmetically acceptable stump is termed *conversion*. This is used basically for congenital deformities. Conversion may simply be amputation at the required level or may be associated with proximal joint fusions to increase the remaining skeletal stability and length. Disarticulation in the lower extremity usually results in full weight bearing.

Training

The training of a child amputee is done with the playing of games. The child is shown how the prosthesis can help him accomplish something that he wants to do. Then he becomes willing to learn. When a child first receives an active device he is given inpatient training sessions for a time, with further training as an outpatient if feasible. Active participation by the parents is of great benefit in the child's learning to make use of a prosthesis.

Since children are generally very active and have periods of rapid growth, frequent adjustments and replacement of the prosthesis are required.

Psychosocial Problems[5]

Parental reaction to a deformed child may vary from complete rejection to overprotection. When possible the mother should be involved in the prosthetic "team." The feeling of guilt and inadequacy of the parents may lead to emotional problems in the congenital amputee.

The adolescent period is particularly painful for the congenital amputee. Appearance becomes important — for the first time the amputee realizes the various reactions that his disability brings forth in other people. He questions whether he is accepted as a person or because of his deformity. Reaction of the amputee may vary from withdrawal to denial of his difference. In either extreme there is the tendency to make neurotic use of the disability. However, child amputees as a group do not appear to show more emotional disturbances than those seen in other severely handicapped children.

REFERENCES

1. Anderson, M. H., and Sollars, R. E.: Manual of Above-Knee Prosthetics for Physicians and Therapists. University of California (Los Angeles), 1959.
2. Burgess, E. M., Romano, R. L., and Zettl, J. H.: The management of lower extremity amputation. TR 10–6, August, 1969.
3. Erdman, W. J., II, Hettinger, T., and Saez, F.: Comparative work stress for above-knee amputee using artificial legs or crutches. Am. J. Phys. Med., 39:225–232, 1960.
4. Klopsteg, P. E., and Wilson, P. D.: Human Limbs and Their Substitutes. New York, McGraw-Hill Book Co., Inc., 1964.
5. McKenzie, D. S.: Children — Medical and psychosocial consideration. Prosthet. Int., 2(1):7, 1964.
6. Peizer, E.: On the Energy Requirements for Prosthesis Use by Geriatric Amputees. The Geriatric Amputee. Washington, National Academy of Sciences, National Research Council Bulletin 919, 1961.
7. Wilson, A. B., Jr.: Recent advances in below-knee prosthetics. Artif. Limbs, 13(2):1–12, 1969.
8. Wilson, A. B., Jr.: Limb prosthesis for children. Prosthet. Int., 2(1):2, 1964.
9. Zettl, J. H., Burgess, E. M., and Romano, R. L.: The interface in the immediate postsurgical prosthesis. Orthot. Prosthet., 24(1):1–7, 1970.

50

MANAGEMENT AND REHABILITATION OF BURNS

EDWARD J. O'SHAUGHNESSY
DAVID HEIMBACH

Between 200,000 and 300,000 Americans are hospitalized each year because of trauma from burns.[12] Forty-one per cent of burn patients are between 17 and 40 years of age. This age group comprises the majority of those engaged in competitive occupation and with growing social and economic responsibilities. Sixty-six per cent of the burns, however, occur in home-related accidents and thus deprive patient and family of the economic aid of work-related insurance.

A greater percentage of patients survive after extensive burns today. The survival rate in the decade from 1965 to 1975 rose from 81 per cent to 90 per cent. The most dramatic improvement has been in survival rate from burns covering 20 to 70 per cent of body surface area. Now young adults with a burn over 65 per cent of the body surface are expected to survive. As patients survive following more severe burns, the sequelae of initial intensive treatment and of the healing process increase in importance. Over the past three decades nutritional maintenance, effective cardiopulmonary support, early debridement, skin replacement with readily available temporary biological covering, and

adequate and definitive autografting have improved. This also has increased the complexity of care of the burn patient.

The fact that the severely burned patient may now survive with disabilities from limb loss, contractures, and restricting and disfiguring scars makes rehabilitation a necessary and integral part of the management of the burned patient. The team concept of patient care is a *sine qua non* of good burn care. The immediate integration of positioning, splinting, and exercises; crisis management of patient, family, and staff; and reduction of disability and return to a vocation call for the constant collaboration of the surgeon, nurse, occupational therapist, physical therapist, physiatrist, medical social worker, psychologist, dietitian, and recreational therapist.

CLASSIFICATION OF BURNS

Depth of Burn

Modern classification of burns differentiates the depth of the burn in relation to the loss of the integument: epidermal (first degree), superficial partial thickness or deep partial thickness (second degree), and full thickness burns (third degree).

Epidermal burns involve only the epidermis. Such burns are red from dermal vasodilation and never blister. They heal without treatment, never scar, and in about a week the epithelium sloughs, as characterized by the peeling following sunburn.

Partial thickness burns are those that have destroyed the epidermis and a portion of the dermis. They may be divided into those that are superficial and those that are deep. The dermis, although a highly metabolically active and important framework, cannot regenerate epidermis. Once the epidermis has been destroyed, burns into the dermis must heal by wound contraction and proliferation of the epithelial cells within surviving pilosebaceous units and eccrine sweat glands. These appendages originate at two differing depths within the dermis; superficial burns have many appendages from which to regenerate, while deep burns have only a few. It is extremely difficult, but very important, to distinguish clinically between superficial and deep partial thickness burns.

Superficial burns are defined as those that heal in less than three weeks and deep partial thickness burns as those that require more than three weeks. The distinction is important because superficial burns rarely scar or cause functional impairment, while deeper burns usually scar and may limit function.

Superficial partial thickness burns blister and are extremely painful. When the blisters are debrided the dermis is homogeneous, pink, and wet. The base is exquisitely sensitive when cleansed, is usually raised above the surrounding skin, and blanches with pressure. Unfortunately, the transition from a superficial to a deep burn is difficult to detect clinically. Furthermore, the burn wound is dynamic and changes occur within days or even hours. The etiology of the burn may be helpful in determining the depth.

Areas of thin skin (eyelids, ears, genitalia, inner arms, the backs of hands, and the entire skin surface of infants) rarely sustain superficial burns. The most common superficial partial thickness burns are caused by scalds with a brief exposure to liquids of less than 71°C (160°F). Hot air explosions of less than 204°C (400°F) and propane or natural gas explosions are generally superficial.

Deep partial thickness burns also blister and may be relatively painful. The patient usually complains of discomfort rather than pain when the wound is debrided, the base is usually dry, and sensation to pinprick is perceived as pressure. A cherry-red wound that does not blanch with pressure is always a deep partial thickness or full thickness burn. After debridement a reticulated pattern with a white background interspersed with multiple red dots (representing the deep dermal vascular plexus) is indicative of a very deep dermal burn. Again, the etiologic agent is frequently of help. Scalds caused by liquids hotter than 71°C, even with brief exposure, usually cause deep burns. Gasoline explosions or high concentrations of propane at close range also fall in this category. Most grease burns and almost all flame burns are deep.

Full thickness burns destroy the entire thickness of the dermis and, since there are no epithelial remnants left, they must heal by contraction from the periphery or must be closed with skin grafting. In the extreme, these wounds have the dry inelastic appearance of tanned leather, but they may also be an extension of the white insensitive deep partial thickness burn. They are usually dry, depressed, and painless.

Area of Total Body Surface Burned

In addition to the depth of the burn, the area of the body surface involved must also be taken into account. The size of burn is calculated by the "rule of nines." The surface area of the body can be divided into multiples of nine. In adults each lower extremity and the anterior and posterior trunk amount to 18 per cent each, while the upper extremities and head are each 9 per cent. A reasonably close estimate of the size of the burn can be made from these simple calculations. In children the head accounts for nearly 18 per cent of the body surface area, while each lower extremity is closer to 13 per cent.

In addition to burn depth and area of body surface burned, other factors that characterize the severity of a burn are location, age, pre-existing illness, associated injuries, smoke inhalation, psychological orientation, and etiologic agent. The American Burn Association and the American College of Surgeons Committee on Trauma recommend hospitalization for any individual with superficial burns amounting to more than 15 per cent of the total body surface in adults and 10 per cent in children. Deep burns of more than 3 per cent of the total body surface should be admitted. Our own experience dictates that while a 10 per cent burn can sometimes be successfully managed on an outpatient basis, the difficulty in cleansing and exercise and the continuous pain make only a few highly intelligent and cooperative patients candidates for this treatment. Based on our experience, we admit most patients with burns greater than 5 per cent for at least 24 to 48 hours in order to instruct family members in the proper care of the burn wound.

The location of the burn is highly significant when considering the patient for admission. Unless the burn is very superficial and the patient very reliable, burns of the feet, face, hands, and perineum indicate that the patient should be admitted to the hospital. Of all the burns we attempt to handle on an outpatient basis, the most difficult are burns of the feet. The relatively poor blood supply, the inability of most patients to maintain elevation and refrain from weight bearing, and the pain associated with daily cleansing frequently lead to infection and need for hospitalization. Outpatients find it difficult to avoid pressure on burned ears and frequently develop chondritis that will require hospitalization and can lead to disastrous cosmetic results. The inability to maintain elevation and mobilization exercises of burned hands at home and the exquisite pain associated with the necessary cleansing leads to a high incidence of infection, and, without appropriate physical therapy, can lead to delayed recovery of normal function. A perineal burn is uncommon as a small isolated burn, but when it occurs the patient or the family may find it difficult to prevent contamination and subsequent infection.

Age

The age of the patient is also important. Children under two have very thin skin and probably an incompetent immune system. Not only are they prone to infection with conversion to full thickness injuries, but their discomfort frequently prevents them from eating adequately and their pain and suffering can lead to serious disruption of the family. Patients physiologically older than 65

years frequently have associated diseases or poor psychosocial support. Patients at both extremes of age should be admitted to the hospital unless the physician can be assured that the burn is trivial and that the family support system is strong.

Pre-existing Illness and Associated Injuries

Pre-existing illness and associated injuries usually necessitate admission. Diabetics, patients on steroids, and immunosuppressed patients would be in this category. All burn patients should be examined for associated injuries to the viscera and extremities. Their presence dictates inpatient care.

Smoke inhalation likewise mandates admission. It may be indicated by injury in an enclosed space, facial burns, debris in the pharynx, stridor, or respiratory distress.

Psychological Orientation

Consideration must be given to the psychosocial circumstances surrounding the burn. Heavy users of ethanol or other drugs, especially if the burn was related to drug abuse, are unlikely to fare well as outpatients. In the case of a child, the question of abuse or neglect versus accident should be investigated with the responsible caretaker. A detailed discussion of child abuse is beyond the scope of this chapter, but burns are among the commonest forms of child abuse seen by physicians; therefore, the treating physician must ascertain whether the circumstances and the pattern of burn are consistent with the history. Approximately 10 per cent of our pediatric burn center admissions are subsequently proven to be a direct result of abuse or gross neglect. Abused children should never be treated as outpatients, and any patient without adequate social support or facilities at home requires admission.

Etiologic Agent

Flame, hot liquids, chemicals, and electricity are the major etiologic agents causing burns. Hot liquids and flame are the most common agents and their effects have been discussed above. Electrical burns are unique in their presentation and complications.

Electricity from a 100-volt line may cause

immediate cardiac arrhythmia or, if bitten by a child, may cause oral burns. However, this low voltage rarely causes large cutaneous burns or deep injury. A high-voltage current with significant amperage, on the other hand, may cause severe cutaneous burns as well as severe thermal damage to structures beneath the skin. There may be cardiac arrhythmias, muscle necrosis, fractures, nerve damage, and myelopathy, resulting in long-term sequelae. For this reason all patients with electrical burns from lines greater than 110 volts are admitted and monitored for at least 24 hours.

TREATMENT

Resuscitation

Burns, like other trauma, require evaluation of the airway, respiration, and circulation immediately, and then a complete history and physical examination. As described above, the treatment is influenced by associated diseases and injuries that must be diagnosed at the outset. A history of immunization against tetanus must be obtained. If the previous immunization was more remote than five years, a booster should be administered. In the absence of previous immunization, an immunization program should be started on day one. If the wound can be kept clean the emergency use of hyperimmune human globulin probably is not required except for extensive deep burns.

Immediate resuscitation has greatly improved initial survival and markedly decreased the incidence of renal failure, an almost always lethal complication. Many formulas for administering fluids and electrolytes to burned patients have been developed in the past few years. Some of these are quite complex and some are potentially hazardous. All of them successfully resuscitate the patient, so the prudent physician should choose the simplest formula, one which uses a single solution and requires minimal electrolyte monitoring. The most commonly used formula is the so-called "Baxter" or "Parkland" formula.[6, 19] This formula recommends Ringer's lactate solution in a quantity of a 4 ml/kg/per cent burned area in the first 24 hours. One half of the total is given in the first eight hours and one fourth in each of the next two eight-hour segments. A quick calculation reveals that a 70-kilogram patient with a 50 per cent total body surface area (TBSA) burn will require 14 liters in 24 hours, or nearly one liter per hour for the first eight hours. The prodigious amount of fluid required sometimes leaves the inexperienced physician incredulous.

The formula is only a guideline; signs of adequate resuscitation include normal mentation, urine output of 30 to 50 ml/hour in adults (1.5 to 2.5 ml/kg/hr in a child), a normal central venous pressure, and relatively normal vital signs. With very large burns, careful monitoring of pulmonary artery wedge pressures, cardiac outputs, and blood gases have enabled almost all burned patients to undergo successful initial resuscitation. When resuscitation has been initiated, unless the patient is to remain at the local hospital, contact should be made with a specialized burn treatment facility and planning should proceed jointly.

Nutrition

A burn provides the greatest sustained stress and highest metabolic response of any known physiologic insult. The degree of hypermetabolism is to some extent related to the area of the burn, and metabolic rates can be at least double by the time the burn reaches 40 per cent of the total body surface area. The appreciation of this fact, and the ability to provide increased nutrition, both enterally and parenterally, have had a major impact on survival following extensive burns. Few patients with major burns can voluntarily eat enough to provide for their metabolic requirements. The provision of continuous enteral tube feeding has enabled many burn centers to maintain patients at 90 to 95 per cent of their original weights. A specially trained dietitian is an integral member of the staff of a burn center. Careful records of nitrogen balance studies and weight and accurate assessment of intake are provided daily on every patient by the dietitian. Nutrition is continued, even during episodes of sepsis, with provision of additional insulin, alteration of nutritional formulas, and adjustment of the route of administration. Most burn surgeons agree that adequate nutritional support has been directly responsible for increasing the survival rate of 50 per cent (lethal burn size 50 or LBS/50) for burns covering 50 per cent of body surface area to the current LBS/50 for burns covering 70 to 75 per cent of body surface area.

Immunity Response and Infection Control

Virtually every aspect of cellular and humoral immunity is disrupted following a severe burn. The cellular impairment extends to both macrophages and lymphocytes. T suppressor cells are actually increased, perhaps owing to the large amount of denatured protein and other inflammatory products from the burn, with the result that most defenses are even further compromised. Patients may develop humoral antibodies to antigens such as tetanus toxoid, but anergy to cellular antigens is very common and can be decreased but not eliminated by adequate nutrition.

Infection continues to be the commonest killer of burn patients. Surprisingly, the bacteriology has changed on a nationwide basis. In our own unit, burn wound sepsis has markedly decreased, while pneumonia and pulmonary failure remain relatively constant in patients who have suffered smoke inhalation. The advent of several effective topical antibacterial agents in the 1960's brought the LBS/50 from 30 to about 50 per cent of body surface area. All of these agents have a very broad spectrum, but none of them has uniform success against all bacteria. Prior to World War II, gram-positive cocci killed 30 per cent of burn patients during the first week after the burn. The use of penicillin diminished this, but patients still died during the second and third week from gram-negative infection. Topical agents kept overall bacterial growth under control in moderate size burns, but in larger burns gram-negative organisms prevailed and caused invasive burn wound sepsis. By the later 1960's and early 1970's infections with Klebsiella and Pseudomonas were the commonest causes of death. For reasons that are not entirely clear Pseudomonas has once again become a relatively unimportant pathogen. At the present time *Pseudomonas aeruginosa* accounts for fewer than 8 per cent of the cases of bacteremia seen in our burn center. Gram-positive organisms, particularly coagulase-positive staphylococci, have again become prevalent.

In the presence of adequate topical chemotherapy, the use of prophylactic penicillin has been shown to be ineffective in preventing cellulitis in the burn wound. The appreciation that antibiotics are not delivered to the avascular burn wound has convinced most burn surgeons to use systemic antibiotics infrequently and then only for specific infections when blood cultures are positive or for severe gram-negative sepsis.

Wound Closure

The ultimate goal of burn treatment is to replace the lost integument either through regrowth from wound edges or by autografting. To prepare the site for grafting, either debridement or excision of the burned area must be accomplished.

Hydrotherapy

If early excision and grafting are not utilized, then debridement of necrotic tissue is an important and daily requirement in the care of the hospitalized burn patient. The removal of the dressing as well as necrotic tissue is facilitated by the use of a water jet or a tub.

The Hubbard tank has traditionally been used, and in many areas it is still used for this purpose. While submerging a denuded part in water at 37°C (95 to 98°F) may increase the comfort of removal of the dressing, it is frequently a frightening experience to patients. Hartford et al. have recently compared tubbed to non-tubbed patients and have found no significant difference in the two methods in mortality, incidence of patients with positive blood cultures, or length of hospital stay.[9] Concern has been expressed that the use of the Hubbard tank may promote the leaching of electrolytes through the denuded areas. A physiologic Hubbard bath can be prepared by adding approximately 9.6 kg (21 lb) of salt (0.85 gm NaCl per liter) and 34 gm (1.25 oz) of KCl (0.03 gm/liter) to 300 gallons of H_2O.[13] The water jet used in association with a wash table allows for a rapid debridement with minimal use of water and staff and reduces the need for extensive "down-time" for cleansing and refilling of the larger tank.

Early aggressive wound excision and grafting have reduced the average hospital stay by 50 per cent. This concept, while not new, is now technically more feasible due to careful patient monitoring, improved anesthesia, availability of blood, and increased surgical skills. Patients with deep burns can not only be spared weeks of painful daily debridement and exercises, but can look forward to essentially normal function, improved cosmetic results, and less time away from home, work, or school. There are two basic surgical techniques involved. For deep dermal burns (those that require more than three weeks to heal) and small full thickness burns, the burn wound is sequentially shaved until a bed is formed of viable dermis or healthy fat. Immediate autografts can be applied to this bed, using sheet graft on cosmetically important areas and grafts run through a special meshing machine for all other areas. If done correctly, graft take approaches 100 per cent, and by the time the donor sites are healed (10 days to 2 weeks) the patient is well. Technical judgment regarding the depth of excision is important, and blood loss can be impressive. An excision of 20 per cent of the body surface may require transfusion of patient's entire blood volume. This technique is also useful for small burns usually treated on an outpatient basis. These small areas can be excised and grafted as a "day surgery" procedure with the same good results. The key to excisional therapy is the immediate coverage of the wound with an autograft or in some cases a homograft.

Since graft "take" on a subcutaneous bed is uncertain, large full thickness burns are best excised with removal of the burn and subcutaneous tissue down to the investing muscle fascia. Excision to fascia can be performed with a scalpel or electrocautery; recently, new tools such as the laser-assisted quartz scalpel have been introduced. Blood loss is less and graft take is more certain, but the cosmetic results are not much better than the older method of allowing separation of the burn eschar with placement of the graft on granulation tissue. Although it is difficult to prove, we believe that these techniques have decreased our mortality in large burns, and they clearly have diminished the length of hospitalization for surviving patients with major burns.

The very advances that now allow patients to survive what was previously a lethal burn put these patients at risk of surviving with disfiguring or disabling complications. Immediate and continued attention must be given to both the psychological and the physical consequences of the burn wound and its treatment.

Psychological Aspects of Burn

The period of hospitalization associated with a burn injury is an extremely stressful one to patient, family, and staff. The problems of adjustment that the patient must face during hospitalization are isolation, dependency, prolonged pain, monotony, and threats to his identity. The family is threatened with the possible death of a family member or with a painful period of survival; thus they perceive the family member perhaps in delirium and pain and certainly in a threatening and unfamiliar environment. They also perceive the staff to be engaging the patient in activities that are obviously painful and distressing.

The staff members caring for burn patients are subjected to failure in the resuscitation of some patients who are placed under their care, and for those resuscitated, they must engage in treatment activities that are obviously painful to the patient. The staff is frequently subjected to abuse and hostility by patients or families to whom they are giving a considerable amount of time and energy. The stress that the staff undergoes results in job dissatisfaction and frequent staff turnover, so that symposia are now often directed at the alleviation of the "burn-out" of the staff members on acute burn wards.

Steiner has attempted to chart the course of the burn patient throughout the period of initial hospitalization. The first stage is one of denial, which encompasses the patient's period of resuscitation, when the prime concern is whether he will survive the burn or not. The second stage occurs when the threat to life has passed and qualitative questions are asked. This is a transition from denial to the recognition of the severity of the burns and of the sequelae that may ensue. This is generally at the time of debridement and grafting. Poor adjustment at this particular stage may result in regressive behavior, temper tantrums, withdrawal, failure to comply with treatment, and rejection of staff or family. The third stage is one from discharge through the first burn year, and it is during this stage that the patient must undergo a stepwise desensitization in many cases so that he may cope with the curiosity and even hostility of those around him. The complications in this stage may include depression and traumatic neurosis.[22] Andreasen et al.[2] attempted to enumerate the factors influencing the poor adjustment of burn patients during hospitalization. They noted that 50 per cent of the patients adjusted quite well to the various stressful problems with which they were faced. Those who did poorly had pre-existing problems. Those who suffered from a severe depression had a history of a disturbed family situation that existed prior to the burn injury. Those undergoing severe regression had premorbid psychopathology or physical disability or decreased normal intelligence. Those who become hostile or presented management problems also had a history of premorbid psychopathology such as alcoholism, thought disorder, or impulsive behavior as a premorbid life-style. Delirium was associated with increased age and severity of burns. However, the long-time sequelae of burn injuries were fewer psychiatric or psychological problems than might have been anticipated. Feller reports that 85 per cent of patients had made an adjustment to life as good as or better than they had prior to the accident.[7] Andreasen reports that only 10 per cent of patients had a mild psychiatric problem, which he defines as traumatic neurosis and mild depression.[3]

Management of the psychological crises that occur during the acute hospitalization in the patient, family, and staff requires a psychologist and a social worker who are attuned to the management of these crises as members of the burn team.

CONTRACTURES

Contractures of the limbs resulting in the loss of range of motion of joints should not be confused with the contracture of skin, autografts, or hypertrophic scar. Contractures are the result of shortening of connective tissues of supporting structures over or around joints, such as muscles, tendons, and joint capsules. This shortening will result over time if the joint is allowed to remain in a constant position.[21] Contractures in burn patients fall into one of four etiologic categories: (1) contractures of convenience and/or neglect, (2) contractures secondary to contraction of the wound or graft, (3) contrac-

tures secondary to hypertrophic scarring, and (4) contractures of comfort.

Contractures of Convenience and/or Neglect

Positioning or malpositioning of the non-burned part to accommodate for equipment or therapeutic endeavors or neglect of positioning against gravity occurs easily in a busy intensive care unit where attention is directed to maintaining life. However, the results of such adaptation to equipment or neglect to observe the ill effects of gravity may result in permanent contractures, which then cause either permanent disability or a prolonged reconstructive period after the burn has healed. Gatching of the bed to elevate the extremities in order to reduce edema is an example of malpositioning. This maneuver results in hip flexion contractures. The placing of the arms close to the body in a posture of adduction to accommodate to narrow beds or to allow ease and maintenance of intravenous lines results in adduction contractures of the shoulders. Neglecting to maintain feet

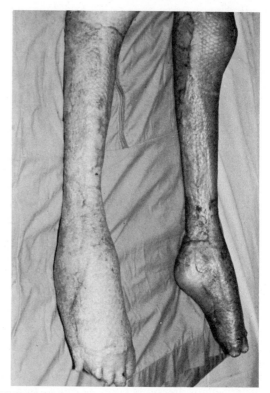

FIGURE 50–1. Plantar flexion contracture. Neglect to maintain feet in neutral dorsiflexed position resulted in a non–burn-related contracture.

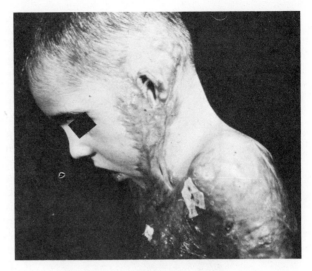

FIGURE 50–2. Flexion contracture of neck. This contracture resulted from a non-splinted burn scar.

in a neutral anatomical position, particularly for patients lying in a supine position, results in plantar contractures of the ankles (Fig. 50–1).

Contractures Secondary to Contraction of Wounds and Grafts

Contractions of grafts and skin will result in permanent contractures. The most frequent example of this is the contracture of the burn scar or graft of the anterior neck, which if inadequately managed will result in a flexion contracture of the neck (Fig. 50–2). Burns of the dorsum of the hand and fingers are notorious for resulting in a hyperextension contracture of the wrist and proximal phalanges and flexion contractures of the middle and distal phalanges (Fig. 50–3).

Contractures Secondary to Hypertrophic Scarring

The occurrence of hypertrophic scarring is a major cause of loss of range of motion of major joints and cosmetic distortions of the mouth and neck (Fig. 50–4). This is particularly true in the period after hospitalization.

Contractures of Comfort

The healing burn is painful and is least uncomfortable if held in a position that avoids tension on the healing wound or newly applied graft. The result of such a posture is the development of contractures of the joints in the position of maximum comfort (Fig. 50–5). This situation gives the rise to the useful motto that "the most com-

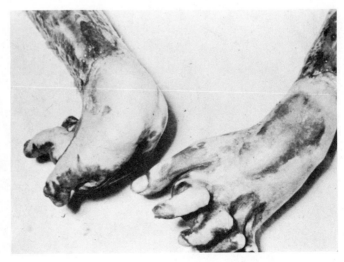

FIGURE 50–3. Classic contractures of dorsal hand burns. This complex of contractures of wrist and proximal phalanges in extension and distal phalanges in flexion is the classic result of allowing the wound to heal without splinting.

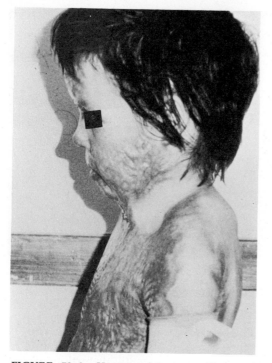

FIGURE 50–4. Hypertrophic scars. Hypertrophic scarring results in both loss of range of motion and disfigurement.

fortable position of the burn area is the wrong position." Prevention of contractures requires the immediate and continued institution of positioning, splinting, and range-of-motion exercise.

Range of Motion

Early and continued range-of-motion exercise of all joints, both those involved in the burn area and those not involved, is the basic maneuver to prevent contractures (Fig. 50–6). Active range of motion is preferred in the nonconfused patient. Assisted range of motion or passive range of motion may be more appropriate in the confused or combative patient. Gentle passive range of motion may be indicated in joints recently grafted. As a general rule, a graft should not be stressed by moving the joint through the range of motion until five days after grafting. The therapist must be empathetic with the patient's discomfort but at the same time persistent in maintaining the normal range of motion of all joints. Range-of-motion exercises should begin on the day of injury and should be continued throughout the convalescent period.

Positioning

Proper positioning will help to prevent contractures and should be maintained throughout the period during which the patient is bed-bound and is being grafted.

The patient should be positioned to counteract the lines of contraction of the burn. In the case of a burn involving the axilla, the arm should be positioned in abduction, which may require an abduction trough attached to the bed (Fig. 50–7). If the patient has a burn of the anterior neck, the neck can be positioned in extension by placing foam pads on the mattress from feet to shoulders, allowing the head to rest on the mattress with neck in extension (Fig. 50–8).

Skeletal traction may be required to maintain position during autografting of circum-

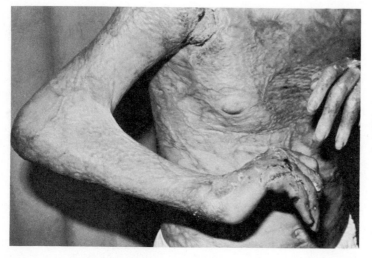

FIGURE 50–5. Contractures of malpositioning. These disabling contractures resulted from the patient's rejection of splinting and opting for a "position of comfort."

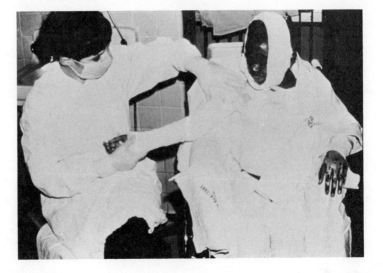

FIGURE 50–6. Early range of motion exercises must be instituted and maintained even in the acute stage of treatment.

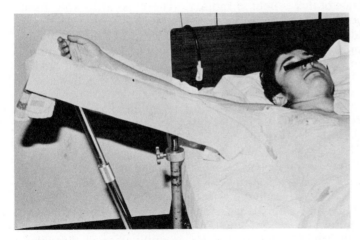

FIGURE 50–7. Abduction trough. Abduction aids attached to narrow beds are necessary to maintain proper positioning.

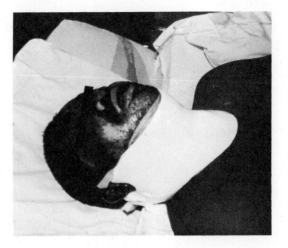

FIGURE 50–8. Extension positioning. Neck extension positioning can be achieved by multiple layered foam cushions.

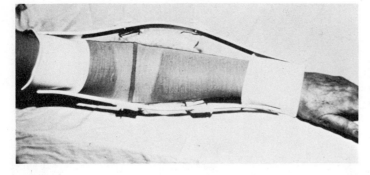

FIGURE 50–9. Static splinting. A three-point orthoplast brace can be used to maintain position and can be applied over pressure dressings.

ferential burns of the limbs or in the case of burns of the hands when the interphalangeal joints may be held in the desired position with Steinmann pins or Kirschner wires.

Splinting

While range-of-motion exercises and positioning are important, the maintenance of the burned part in a predetermined position to offset the contracting of the wound or in an appropriate position for the sleeping, confused, or painful patient will depend on appropriate splinting. Splints should be adapted to each patient and must be constantly modified as the wounds heal or are grafted or as various degrees of contractures evolve. Splints may be of the resting type, which maintain the part in a static position (Fig. 50–9), or the dynamic type, which allow exercise along a predetermined axis and resistance (Fig. 50–10).

Each splint should be made to maximize the position of the burn against the pattern of contracture anticipated. Thus the therapist must be cognizant of the pattern of contracture of burns. A burn of the dorsum of the

hand, for example, should be splinted in slight extension of the wrist with the proximal metatarsal joints at 65 degrees of flexion and the MP's and DP's in full extension (Fig. 50–11).

The hand is one of the most frequently burned parts of the body and if allowed to heal with a contracture there may be permanent disability. There is little soft tissue between the skin, tendons, and joint capsules. Burns of the fingers are frequently circumferential. Thus early grafting, proper positioning, and early movement all are needed simultaneously. Especially adapted skeletal traction that allows for open dressing, positioning, and guided movement have evolved as hay rakes and halos (Fig. 50–12). In the halo with the use of Kirschner wires through the distal phalanges, the fingers can be held in extension. The hay rake, while requiring additional skeletal pinning to position the wrist, the metacarpal heads, and the phalanges, permits open dressing, observation, and movement. The position of the fingers can be carefully moved throughout the entire arc of range of motion in increments that can be changed every two hours (Fig. 50–13).

Exercise

Active exercise should be initiated as soon as the patient is physiologically stable and need not wait until healing and grafting have been completed (Fig. 50–14). Early ambulation within the burn unit and progressive strengthening exercises will prevent debilitation and allow the patient to take an active role in his or her own treatment.

Allowing the patient to exercise in the general physical therapy gym institutes an early desensitization of the patient with major cosmetic complications. This reduces pain and sick behavior as the burned patient

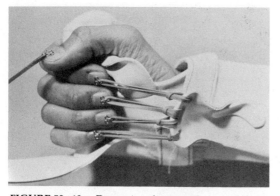

FIGURE 50–10. Dynamic splinting. The use of elastic bands attached to hook glued to fingernails allows for dynamic constant stretch.

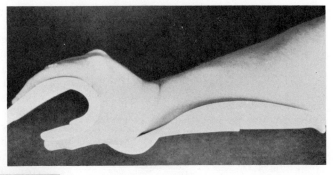

FIGURE 50–11. Wrist and hand splint. This traditional hand splint for dorsal hand burns prevents "claw" contracture deformity.

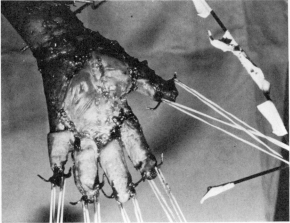

FIGURE 50–12. Halo traction. Fingers are held in extension connected to coat hanger wire bent in a halo configuration.

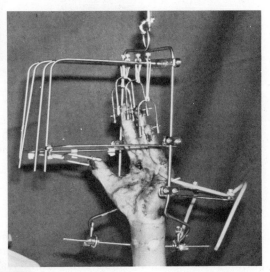

FIGURE 50–13. Hay rake traction. This configuration allows the fingers to be moved throughout entire arc of range of motion.

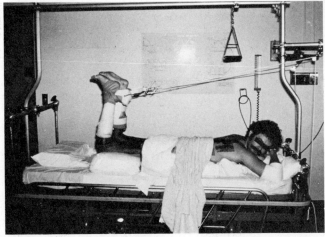

FIGURE 50–14. Active exercise. The patient should engage in active progressive strengthening exercises while still confined to bed.

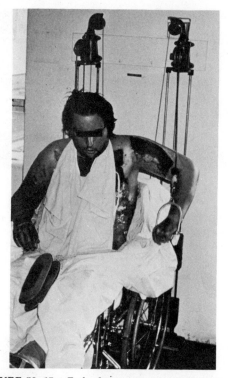

FIGURE 50–15. Early desensitization. Early exercise in a general physical therapy gym is a positive reenforcement of the healing process.

formation of granulation tissue with the appearance of fibroblasts, the production of collagen oriented parallel to stress lines, and the subsequent overgrowth of epithelium. The normal wound will be healed within about eight weeks and the scar evolved will be stabilized in about six to eight months.

The healing of a burn wound that penetrates the dermis, on the other hand, leads to a voluminous unesthetic scar with marked contractile properties that may remain active for a period of 8 to 15 months.[16] The healing of the burn wound is characterized by a marked cellular activity in the dermis, with increased capillary production and edema of the granulation tissue.[18] In addition to this, however, there is a marked increase of fibroblasts called myofibroblasts that have characteristics of smooth muscle cells with contractile actomyosin filaments.[5] Collagen is invaded by the fibroblasts, and the bundles are coated with a matrix rich in proteoglycans. The proteoglycan reduces the ability of the collagen to be denatured and hence prolongs the activity of the scar formation.[15]

The myofibroblasts that are attached by their filaments to the collagen bundles appear to have an influence on the disarray that

mixes with other patients in the general gym. This rotation off the burn unit provides to the patient a positive indication that healing and recovery are occurring (Fig. 50–15).

HYPERTROPHIC SCARS

Burns that involve the integument to the depth of the dermis heal with the formation of a voluminous heaped-up contracting scar that remains within the confines of the original area of the burn. These hypertrophic scars are differentiated from a keloid by the fact that a keloid is a tumor-like growth that spreads beyond the initial boundary of the injury. The hypertrophic scar that accompanies a burn has both cosmetically and functionally disabling characteristics. Its tendency to contract causes the loss of range of motion when it pulls across a joint and disfiguring bizarre contortions of the face, chin, and mouth when it occurs on the face and neck (Fig. 50–16).

Normal healing of a wound, which includes the loss of surface epithelium and penetration into the dermis, involves the

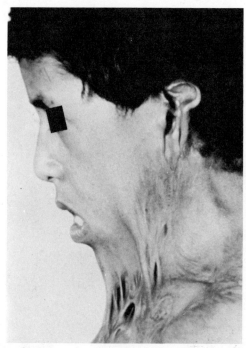

FIGURE 50–16. End-stage hypertrophic scar. The natural course of hypertrophic scarring results in major physical and cosmetic disability.

occurs in their orientation. The collagen within the burn wound forms whorls and nodules, which cause the gross heaped-up appearance of the hypertrophic scar.[1] The combination of the prolonged presence of myofibroblasts in an inordinate number and the disoriented configuration of the collagen results in a marked contraction of the dermis that is laid down in the healing process. This results in shrinking of the area of the graft or wound, which produces the deformities associated with hypertrophic scarring.

The coalescence of these adverse reactions results in unsightly scars and contractures of the joints, skinfolds, and orifices, which may persist for years.

PRESSURE GARMENTS

Fujimori in 1968 noted that excessive scars followed burns, trauma, and surgical intervention. It was his opinion that continuous pressure might prevent the hypertrophy and contraction of the scar. He treated his patients using an adhesive sponge pressure dressing. This device in his hands reduced the time for scar maturation from twelve months to six months.[8]

Larson and his associates noted that when the burned limb was subject to pressure by the firm application of isoprine splints held in position with elastic bandage, the expected hypertrophic scar did not develop. When the pressure was released, early signs of hypertrophy began with subepithelial nodules and rigidity of tissue. One patient was then used as her own control. The distal portion of the burned limb was kept in pressure dressings and the proximal portion was not. After five

months the patient returned with hypertrophic scarring confined to that portion of the burned limb that had not been subjected to pressure. Biopsy of the scar on the proximal part of the limb revealed a characteristic nodular pattern of the collagen, whereas in the distal portion, there was no such nodular formation.[14]

Baur and his associates in 1976 undertook a study of the ultrastructure of hypertrophied scars treated both with and without pressure.[5] While there was no change in the cellular type present in either group, there was a more rapid maturation of those wounds that were subject to continuous pressure than of those that were not. Their observations indicated that the cellular elements from which hypertrophic scarring evolved remained active even with pressure for a period of six to eight months.

All burn wounds extending into the dermis, including those treated with split thickness grafts, are at risk for formation of hypertrophied scar.[4] Since the scar formation begins to evolve within three weeks, all wounds should be treated with pressure dressings as soon as epithelialization begins or the graft has taken.[17] Considerable experience in the treatment of burns using pressure dressings has evolved. The pressure dressing consists initially of the use of an elastic bandage of appropriate width wrapped in a figure-eight dressing over the limbs (Fig. 50–17). This also can be used on the torso. It is frequently advisable to incorporate splints within the pressure dressing.

When the wound is healed an elastic cloth garment tailored specifically for the patient is a more efficient method of applying pressure (Fig. 50–18). The major supplier for pressure

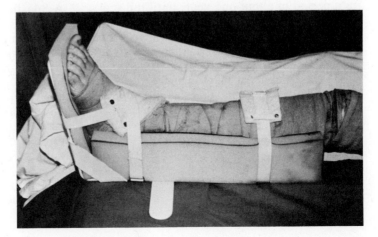

FIGURE 50–17. Early pressure dressing. Ace bandage in a figure-eight dressing is a satisfactory early pressure dressing.

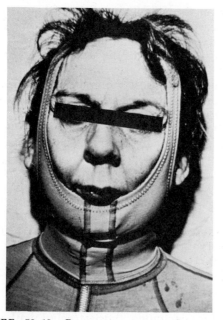

FIGURE 50–18. Pressure garments. Appropriate pressure can be maintained by tailored pressure garments.

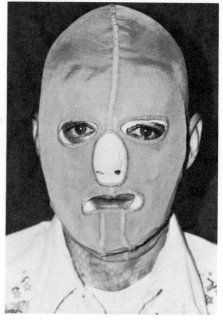

FIGURE 50–19. Elastic cloth face mask maintains pressure but may present a sinister appearance.

garments in this country is the Jobst Institute, Inc.* This company will provide measuring kits and a catalogue of their garments, which range from gloves to face masks to total body garments. It takes approximately two to three weeks to obtain delivery, although the company does maintain a "hotline" that speeds the process. Garments should be ordered in pairs, since they must be worn 24 hours per day, and the principle of "one garment on, the other in the wash" is a "must" for efficacious treatment. Garments will have to be remeasured and reordered as elasticity is lost or the patient's girth changes. Pressure garments must be worn for a period of about one year, until the scar matures. It is frequently necessary to reinforce garments or elastic bandages with foam or Silastic conformers to accommodate to the body's contours such as the axilla or face.

The elastic cloth garment is uncomfortable in the hot weather, must be laundered frequently, is frequently difficult to don, and is not cosmetic in the areas that are exposed to the public. Because of this, patient compliance may vary. It is important, therefore,

that both patients and parents understand the need for the continuous and long-term use of the pressure garments and the high risk of the formation of hypertrophic scars and contractures if the garments are not used.

The elastic cloth face mask has several disadvantages, one being that it does not fit the contours of the face snugly because it tents over the nose. In addition, the mask with apertures for eyes and mouth gives the patient a sinister appearance (Fig. 50–19). Because of this, an elastic face mask may either be a true barrier to school or employment or be perceived as such by the wearer.

A Silastic mask molded to conform to the concavities and convexities of the face exerts a more uniform pressure under an elastic mask (Fig. 50–20).

A clear plastic mask made of a material similar to plexiglass will provide uniform pressure on the face while eliminating the need to wear an opaque mask in public (Fig. 50–21). Moreover, the amount of pressure exerted over any area can be observed by the degree of blanching. The mask is not porous and hence must be removed every two hours for cleansing. Rigid masks must be monitored frequently and changed to conform to

_____

*Jobst Institute, Inc., P.O. Box 653, Toledo, Ohio 43694.

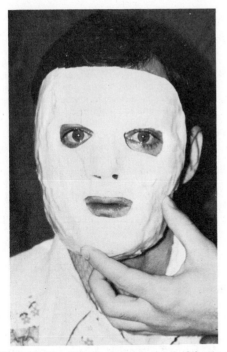

FIGURE 50–20. Silastic face mask. A Silastic face mask will conform to the surface of the face and can be worn under an elastic cloth mask.

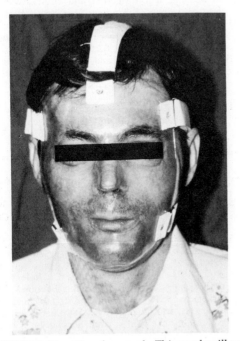

FIGURE 50–21. Clear face mask. This mask will provide pressure and is less threatening than the opaque elastic cloth mask.

the changes in the wound or the scar. These masks are made from a positive mold that can be made either in the operating room or at the bedside and are within the competence of the occupational therapist to fabricate.

NEUROPATHY

Damage to both the central nervous system and the peripheral nervous system is frequently observed in the burn patient. Damage to the central nervous system is frequently a result of an electric burn and may cause seizure disorders, quadriplegia, paraplegia, or spasticity.[20] Injury to the spinal cord may not be appreciated immediately because it may take several days for paralysis or spasticity to develop. It is difficult to make an accurate prognosis for such injuries, since some patients have a complete return of neural function over a period of weeks to months, while for other patients the damage is permanent. Henderson et al. called attention in 1971 to the prevalence of peripheral polyneuropathy in burn patients. The nerve deficits were unrelated to the areas of injury from the burns.[11] Our experience has been that focal neuropathy is associated with the area burned or results from positioning of the limb or pressure from assistive devices used. A brachial plexus injury may result from an excessive position of abduction; a peroneal injury, especially in the elderly, from unguarded bed positioning; and median or ulnar nerve injuries from splinting or skeletal traction. Helm recently reported a similar experience in which 43 per cent of patients with a peripheral neuropathy had preventable damage if proper care had been used in positioning, exercise techniques, and rotation of injections.[10]

TEAM CONCEPTS

A burn induces one of the most complex physiologic responses known to modern medicine. An understanding of both the physiologic and psychologic responses, as well as the realization that optimum care can return these patients to a nearly normal condition, has led to the development of specialized burn care facilities.

These facilities are usually self-contained

units devoted specifically to the care of the burned patient. While the proper physical environment is important, the development of a multidisciplinary team, all of whom understand the problems unique to the burned patient, is the crucial factor.

These facilities are usually self-contained units devoted specifically to the care of the burned patient. While the proper physical environment is important, the development of a multidisciplinary team, all of whom understand the problems unique to the burned patient, is the crucial factor.

The team is led by a surgeon with a special interest and training in burn care and includes nurses, physical therapists, and occupational therapists who also have the interest and specialized training in the care of the burned patient. The complete team includes a physiatrist, clinical psychologist, recreational therapist, medical social workers, and dietitian. The skin bank technician is also a valuable member of the burn team if the center has developed a skin bank with techniques for harvesting and storage of cadaver allografts.

The multiple personnel required and the specialized equipment used make burn care expensive. Although cost per day is high, cost accounters can show a saving in "cost per disease" because the hospital stays of these patients have been markedly shortened.

The re-integration into the community of individuals capable of resumption of a normal productive work life is cost-effective to society as a whole by any parameter of measurement.

REFERENCES

1. Alexander, S. A., and Donoff, R. B.: The histochemistry of glycoaminoglycans within hypertrophic scars. J. Surg. Res., 28:171–181, 1980.
2. Andreasen, N. J. C., Noyes, R., and Hartford, C. E.: Factors influencing adjustment to burn patients during hospitalization. Psychosom. Med., 34:517–524, 1972.
3. Andreasen, N. J. C., Norris, A. S., and Hartford, C. E.: Incidence of long-term psychiatric complications in severely burned adults. Ann. Surg., 174:785–793, 1971.
4. Baur, P. S., Larson, D. L., Stacey, T. R., Barratt, G. F., and Dobrovsky, M.: Ultrastructural analysis of pressure-treated human hypertrophic scars. J. Trauma, 16:958–967, 1976.
5. Baur, P. S., Larson, D. L., and Stacey, T. R.: The observation of myofibroblasts in hypertrophic scars. Surg. Gynecol. Obstet., 141:22–26, 1975.
6. Baxter, C. R., Curreri, W. P., and Marvin, J. A.: The control of burn wound sepsis by the use of quantitative bacteriologic studies and subeschar clysis with antibiotics. Surg. Clin. North Am., 53:1509–1517, 1973.
7. Feller, I., Koepke, G., Richards, K. E., and Withy, L.: Symposium on Treatment of Burns, Vol. 5. St. Louis, The C. V. Mosby Co., 1973.
8. Fujimori, R., Hiramoto, and Ofuji, S.: Sponge fixation method for treatment of early scars. Plast. Reconstr. Surg., 42:322–327, 1968.
9. Hartford, C. E., Panoc, C. L., and Swennson, A.: To tub or not to tub. (Abstract) Am. Burn Assoc. 12th Annual Meeting, 1980.
10. Helm, P. A.: Muscle weakness in the burn patient: Electrodiagnostic and clinical correlation. (Abstract) Am. Burn Assoc. 12th Annual Meeting, 1980.
11. Henderson, B., Koepke, G. H., and Feller, I.: Peripheral polyneuropathy among patients with burns. Arch. Phys. Med. Rehabil., 52:149–151, 1971.
12. Jay, K. M., Bartlett, R. N., Danet, R., and Allyn, P. A.: Burn epidemiology: A basis for burn prevention. J. Trauma, 17:943–947, 1977.
13. Koepke, G.: The role of physical medicine in the treatment of burns. Surg. Clin. North Am., 50:1385–1399, 1970.
14. Larson, D. L., Abston, S., Evans, E. B., Dobrovsky, M., and Linares, H. A.: Techniques for decreasing scar formation and contractures in burned patients. J. Trauma, 11:807–823, 1971.
15. Linares, H. A., and Larson, D. L.: Proteoglycans and collagenase in hypertrophic scar formation. Plast. Reconstr. Surg., 62:589–593, 1978.
16. Nicoletis, C., Bazin, S., and LeLous, M.: Clinical and biochemical features of normal, defective, and pathologic scars. Plast. Surg., 4:347–358, 1977.
17. Peacock, E. E., Madden, J. W., and Trier, W. C.: Biologic basis for the treatment of keloids and hypertrophic scars. South. Med. J., 63:755–760, 1970.
18. Robitaille, A., Halpern, D., Kottke, F. J., Burrill, C., and Payne, L.: Correction of keloids and finger contractures in burn patients. Arch. Phys. Med. Rehabil., 54:515–520, 1973.
19. Shires, T., Carrico, J., Baxter, C. R., et al.: Advances in Surgery. Ed. Claude E. Welch. Chicago, Year Book Medical Publishers, 1970.
20. Solem, L., Fischer, R. P., and Strate, R. G.: The natural history of electrical injury. J. Trauma, 17:487–492, 1977.
21. Stolov, W. C., and Thompson, S. C.: Soleus immobilization contracture in the baboon. (Abstract) Arch. Phys. Med. Rehabil., 60:556, 1979.
22. Steiner, H., and Clark, W. R.: Psychiatric complications of burn adults. Ann. Surg., 174:785–793, 1971.

51

REHABILITATION OF PATIENTS WITH CANCER

MYRON M. LaBAN

There are many complex problems that arise in the management of the cancer patient as the disease progresses from one stage to another. The specialist in physical medicine and rehabilitation, joining with his medical and surgical colleagues, can contribute his special skills to both the diagnosis and the management of complications related to neoplastic diseases and their treatment. The multifaceted team approach — blending the skills of the physiatrist and physical, occupational, and speech therapists, as successfully employed in the rehabilitation of chronic neuromuscular disability — can with equal facility be utilized in the management of the cancer patient. Although the rehabilitative goals of caring for patients with syndromes of hemiplegia, paraplegia, quadriplegia, amputation, neuropathy, and myopathy may remain essentially the same, treatment time is often telescoped by progressive disease requiring frequent alterations in the "staging" of functional levels of locomotion and self-care. The direct or remote effects of the cancer itself, the residua of radical surgery, and the toxic side effects of chemoprophylaxis and radiotherapy, combined with a sympathetic understanding of the "dying process," individually or collectively are the challenges the physiatrist must master to be a successful member of the "oncology treatment team."

DIRECT INVOLVEMENT OF ORGAN

Brain

Cerebral metastasis is the most frequent neurologic complication of systemic neoplasia.[1] The number of patients with brain metastasis is increasing as systemic cancers are more effectively controlled and as longevity is increased. Lung and breast carcinoma are the most frequent primary tumors metastasizing to the brain, with large bowel, pancreas, and renal carcinoma also important primaries. Approximately 20 to 40 per cent of all tumors eventually metastasize to the brain, with 10 per cent of these cases having multiple sites of brain metastasis. In more than half the cases, patients with carcinoma of the lung and malignant melanoma also develop brain metastasis.

Primary tumors of the central nervous system as a group account for 2 to 5 per cent of all tumors, with 80 per cent of those involving the brain. Gliomas account for 50 per cent of all primary brain tumors, with the majority being glioblastomas. Meningiomata are the most prevalent of the nongliomatous tumors. Pituitary adenomas, primarily chromophobic in origin, represent 12 to 18 per cent of intracranial neoplasms.

Most primary brain tumors of children are located in the posterior cranial fossa. Medul-

953

loblastomas and astrocytomas are each present in 30 per cent of cases, with ependymomas found in only 12 per cent.[2]

Approximately 40 per cent of patients presenting with hemiplegia secondary to brain metastasis can be restored to greater independence and improved quality of life during their period of survival. An additional 30 per cent gain some degree of palliation with early identification followed by surgical decompression, corticosteroids, and external irradiation.[3] The symptoms of hemiparesis and aphasia may clear dramatically when compared to the often slower resolution of symptoms following a vascular occlusive episode.

Rehabilitation treatment should be initiated as soon as medically feasible, with a prescription addressed to reasonable goals. When an intracranial metastasis is rapidly progressive and associated with symptoms of headache, intractable focal seizures, mentation changes, or debilitating vomiting, palliative treatment goals to prevent the development of contractures, decubiti, and bladder or bowel complications are most appropriate. Restorative and/or supportive rehabilitation goals utilizing proven techniques successfully employed in the noncancer patient are appropriate in those patients whose level of mentation and cardiopulmonary reserve are sufficient to tolerate the physical stress of activity.

Spinal Cord

Four thousand new cases of primary spinal cord tumor are detected annually. Meningiomas and neurofibromas account for 50 per cent of all cord tumors and occur most frequently at thoracic cord levels. Gliomas, primarily of the ependymoma type, represent another 23 per cent, with half arising in the filum terminale or conus medullaris. Less common are those of a miscellaneous group, which include the epidermoid and dermoid cysts as well as hemangioblastomas and chordomas.[4]

Epidural metastases with spinal cord compression are all too frequent complications of systemic cancer. Autopsy studies have demonstrated epidural metastases in over 5 per cent of all cancer patients. The most common primary sources are breast, lung, Hodgkin's disease, and prostatic carcinoma. Ninety per cent of these patients initially present with pain localized to the site of spinous

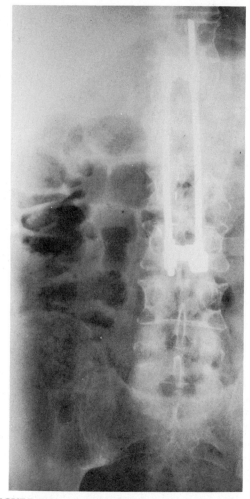

FIGURE 51–1. Surgical decompression and stabilization by Harrington rods of vertebra invaded by metastatic renal cell carcinoma.

metastasis. Too often, weeks to months pass before a radicular pattern of pain and weakness develops sufficient to demand intensive diagnostic study. In 50 per cent of patients with metastatic disease, initial "negative" x-rays and nuclear scan examinations can delay appropriate treatment.[5, 6] In these early stages electromyographic examination can be useful in suggesting the presence of paraspinous muscle metastasis when the neurologic, nuclear scan, and x-ray examinations are otherwise normal.[7] Earlier identification and aggressive surgical or radiotherapeutic treatment of spinal metastasis are more promising to maintain independent, ambulant patients than is expectant delay.

Paraplegia secondary to the pressure of an epidural metastasis responds poorly to decompressive laminectomy alone except at the level of the cauda equina, where prolonged pressure is tolerated better. Wright reported on 38 patients who were paraplegic or severely paraparetic prior to treatment. Of the 17 treated with combined radiotherapy and surgery, 50 per cent were ambulant following therapy. Twenty-one were treated by surgery alone, and only three (14 per cent) were ambulant postoperatively.[8]

A pathologic fracture-dislocation compromising the spinal cord or associated with painful vertebral instability secondary to an infiltrative carcinoma should be stabilized. Wiring of adjacent cervical vertebral processes combined with a bony fusion is used to produce stability, whereas at thoracic and lumbar levels Harrington compression rods are similarly employed (Fig. 51–1).[9] It was reported that external supports, including corsets, braces, and molded plastic jackets, were often poorly tolerated, particularly when metastases were generalized.

The prognosis for functional recovery is much better for primary spinal canal tumors such as meningiomas and neurofibromas than for metastatic tumors even after treatment with additional high-voltage irradia-

tion. Similarly, metastatic tumor types demonstrate a marked variability of response to treatment. Prostatic carcinoma and myeloma both are often responsive to combined surgery, chemotherapy, and irradiation, while breast and lung carcinomas are less so. Both these tumors have an additional propensity for early and widespread metastasis. Radiosensitive tumors within the spinal canal, such as Ewing's sarcoma, lymphomas, neuroblastomas, and leukemias, may be effectively treated with irradiation therapy without laminectomy.[10, 11]

The paraparetic patient with cancer requires the same immediate attention to bladder, bowel, and skin care that all patients with spinal cord dysfunction demand.[12] A rehabilitation program should be initiated immediately, adjusted to the postoperative limitations of a decompressive laminectomy and the associated debilitating effects of irradiation and chemotherapy. In this regard, therapeutic decisions related to mobilization, sitting, and lower extremity weight-bearing must be made with full knowledge of the primary malignancy and evaluation of any metastases that might cause a pathologic

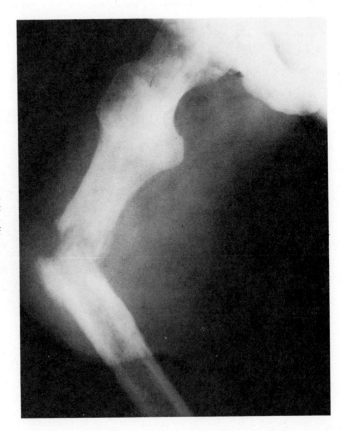

FIGURE 51–2. Flexibility exercises with stretching in chronic multiple sclerosis patient produced a pathological fracture in a femur invaded by metastases from occult carcinoma of the breast.

fracture if therapy is too vigorous (Fig. 51–2).

Although the mechanics of rehabilitation treatment are similar to those utilized for spinal cord–injured patients, the cancer patient often has more pain and less endurance for physical treatment. An initial rapid improvement in functional self-sufficiency may be followed by a steady decline. In this regard, all ADL equipment should be ordered with the potential of managing a patient who is likely to become functionally more impaired than when initially evaluated.

PAIN

To the layman, cancer is synonymous with prolonged intractable pain. Segmental neuromuscular or musculoskeletal pain is a concomitant of bony metastases, and pain may be the harbinger of an occult metastasis. Successful management of this debilitating and demoralizing symptom depends upon the identification of the anatomic site of neoplastic involvement. This task can be expedited by an understanding of the natural history of the type of tumor (Fig. 51–3).

Spinal metastases with or without involvement of the paraspinal muscles have associated local pain in 96 per cent of patients. Radicular or regional pain is present in 80 to 90 per cent of cervical and lumbar lesions and in 55 per cent of thoracic tumors. Pain usually precedes and may mask other neurologic signs and symptoms by several weeks. There may be rapid progression from minor motor deficits to total paralysis. Bony metastases can cause pain, but development of this and other neurologic symptoms and signs should not be attributed to the bony metastases without at least considering an associated epidural metastasis. An expanding epidural metastases can cause a rapid and often permanent loss of motor function if not identified early and the cord decompressed. Well-intended but misguided treatment, including cervical traction therapy, also has the potential for accelerating paresis when an occult extradural metastasis is masked by cervical osteoarthritis (Fig. 51–4).[13]

Spinal metastasis may be vertebral, epidural, or paraspinal. Metastases that cause instability of bone produce excruciating pain by distortion of the rich supply of pain endings in the periosteum or the more meager supply of pain endings in the endosteum.

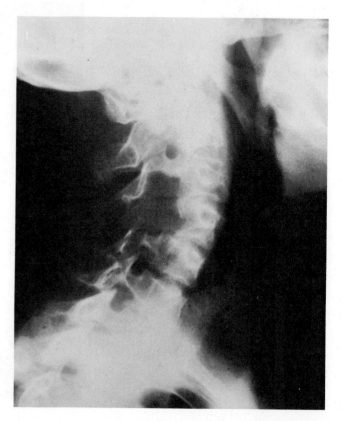

FIGURE 51–3. Invasion of cervical vertebrae by metastases from carcinoma of the esophagus one month after normal x-ray studies.

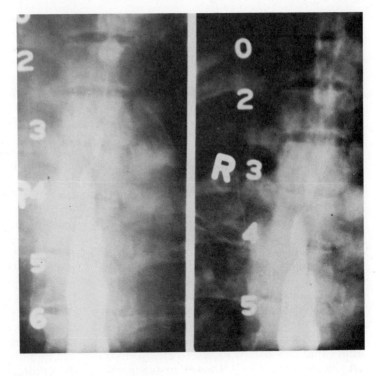

FIGURE 51–4. Epidural metastases from an occult prostatic carcinoma in a patient who developed quadriparesis while being treated with traction therapy for cervical radiculopathy.

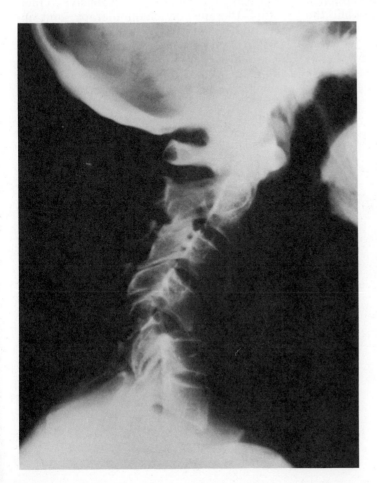

FIGURE 51–5. Vertebral collapse from metastases from primary carcinoma of the lung presenting as "neck stiffness" without pain in a neurologically normal patient.

Metastases to vertebrae or other bones, with or without fractures or dislocations, may be identified radiographically and confirmed both by radioisotope scanning and by bone biopsy (Fig. 51–5). Epidural metastases may cause distortion of pain endings or may be silent until symptoms of myelopathic loss due to compression become evident; once suspected, confirmation can be made by myelography.

Paraspinal muscle metastasis may be identified electromyographically even when unassociated with neurologic dysfunction or x-ray evidence of metastasis.[14] A pattern of segmental paraspinal muscle denervation confined to the distribution of the posterior primary rami with sparing of the anterior rami may be the earliest objective evidence of paraspinal muscle metastasis (Fig. 51–6).

Locally invasive carcinomas of the bladder, cervix, lung, and prostate can produce lumbosacral or brachial plexus dysfunction as well as extremity-compressive mononeuropathies that can also be localized electromyographically (Fig. 51–7). In each instance, the electrodiagnostic abnormalities are confined to the anterior rami distribution, while the posterior rami are spared.

Whenever metastases invade a vertebra and make it unstable enough to allow distortion of the periosteum, excruciating pain is produced. There may or may not be fracture lines evident on x-ray. Appropriate spinal bracing to prevent this distortion gives prompt relief of pain, allowing relaxation of the associated muscle spasm and resumption of sitting and ambulation by the patient (see Chapter 27, Spinal Orthoses). Heat and massage have been used effectively since the time of Hippocrates for analgesia and the relief of muscle spasm and are followed by mobilizing exercises leading to a level of ambulation and resumption of more than sedentary activity. As long as the patient is adequately braced so that there is no periosteal distortion, he or she is relatively free from pain. Transcutaneous electrical stimulation plays a role in physiologic blockade of pain perception in a significant proportion of patients. Beyond this, narcotic analgesics, when necessary, have recently been supplemented by various tricyclic drugs. As pain is ameliorated, the patient is able to relax, to sleep at night, and to participate in his own rehabilitation program while concurrent high-voltage radiation or chemotherapy is used for a direct attack on the tumor.

When pain is no longer responsive to radiation therapy or chemotherapy and increased narcotics are required for comfort, ablative surgical procedures are useful.[15, 16] These procedures should always be directed initially at the peripheral rather than the central nervous system. Preferred surgical

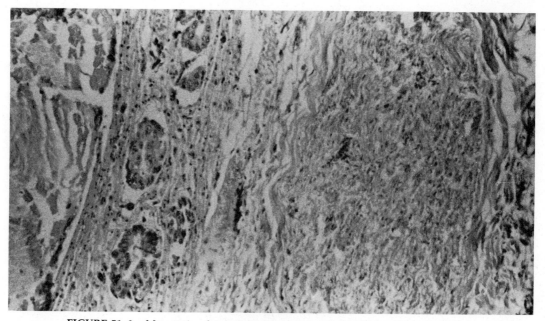

FIGURE 51–6. Metastatic adenocarcinoma in paraspinal muscle adjacent to nerve.

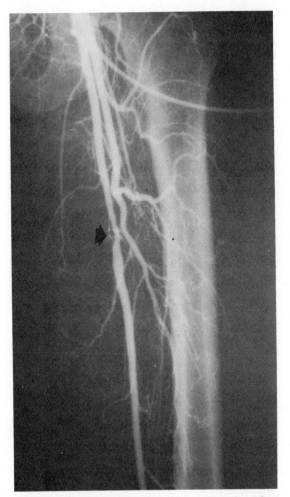

FIGURE 51–7. Adenocarcinoma associated with a partial vascular occlusion of the deep femoral vessels was identified initially by electromyographic compromise of branch of femoral nerve to vastus medialis.

procedures include chemical rhizotomy, or celiac block with alcohol, or surgical thoracic chordotomy may be required.

Percutaneous cervical chordotomy and dorsal column electroanalgesia are both relatively new procedures. Percutaneous cervical chordotomy, unlike the open thoracic procedure, can be performed under local anesthesia. Both procedures have the potential of compromising sphincter and lower extremity control, especially when done bilaterally. Chordotomy, percutaneous or open, is generally reserved for patients with a life expectancy of less than one year. The resultant anesthetic block fails in 40 per cent of open thoracic chordotomy procedures in less than one year and in 100 per cent of all percutaneous cervical procedures.

Direct dorsal column electrostimulation of the low threshold touch and proprioceptive fibers of the spinal cord theoretically should inhibit pain transmitted over C fibers. Electrodes are placed on the thoracic spinal cord four to eight segments above the level of entrance of pain impulses into the cord and stimulated with one milliamp pulse at 0.3 millisecond duration at a frequency of 50 to 200 hertz with a subcutaneously implanted stimulator. Although direct dorsal column-stimulation can raise the pain threshold 60 to 100 per cent, there are serious risks associated with subdural implantation, and this technique has been superseded largely by transcutaneous electrical stimulation.[17]

SECONDARY EFFECTS OF CARCINOMA

Neuropathy, polymyositis, and myasthenic syndrome are frequently associated with neoplasia and may be present preceding its clinical identification. Each syndrome can be identified by electrodiagnostic studies.[18]

Carcinomatous neuromyopathy, the combined clinical presentation of proximal extremity weakness and atrophy with a distal reduction of deep tendon reflexes, has been found associated with many types of neoplasms. It is, however, more likely to occur with ovarian or lung carcinoma. Evidence of neuromyopathy has been identified in 16 per cent of patients with these two neoplasms. Electrodiagnostic studies demonstrating slowing of nerve conduction velocities with proximal myopathic and distal neuropathic motor units is typical of carcinomatous neuromyopathy.[19]

Twelve per cent of all patients with dermatomyositis have an associated malignancy. However, over the age of 50, half or more will have an associated neoplasm. In the vast majority of cases the combined symptoms of periorbital rash and proximal extremity weakness precede those of an underlying tumor. An electromyographic pattern of muscle membrane hyperirritability associated with myopathic motor units, histologic evidence of muscle necrosis, and elevated serum enzymes are typical of this syndrome. Although there has not been a specific tumor type associated with dermatomyositis, carcinomas of the breast, lung, stomach, ovary, and uterus have been frequently reported.[20, 21]

The myasthenic syndrome most often associated with oat cell carcinoma of the lung, although similar in its curare sensitivity and initial symptomatic complaint of weakness, differs from typical myasthenia gravis in several important features. These include sparing of the cranial muscles, decreased or absent deep tendon reflexes, and no diagnostic response to neostigmine. Tetanic nerve stimulation tests at or in excess of 20 stimuli per second produce an increment of evoked action potentials rather than a decrement typical of myasthenia gravis at slower rates of stimulation.[22] Guanidine hydrochloride has been more effective than anticholinesterases in the management of this syndrome.

COMPLICATIONS OF TREATMENT

Radiotherapy

Progressive radiation myelopathy or plexopathy following radiotherapy of malignant disease near the vertebral column is a well-recognized complication of treatment (Fig. 51–8). An irreversible transverse myelitis

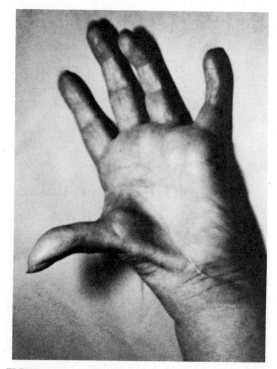

FIGURE 51–8. Postirradiation brachial plexopathy with impairment of hand function.

usually begins 9 to 12 months after irradiation. Two per cent of patients receiving over 4000 rads to the cord will develop paresis at the level of treatment.[23]

Less disabling but occurring with greater frequency are complaints of pain and stiffness in previous fields of irradiation treatment, especially in and around the pelvis. Arthralgias from the sacroiliac joints and the pubic symphysis are not uncommon following irradiation for endometrial carcinoma. Radiographic evidence of osteoarthritic degeneration of the underlying joints may be accompanied by electromyographic evidence of prolonged insertional potentials, and increased resistance to electrode insertion suggests fibrosis of the irradiated muscles. This particular group of patients often responds well to a combination of interarticular steroids, diathermy, and flexibility exercise.

Chemotherapy

Chemotherapy of systemic cancer utilizing a multi-drug approach assumes that drug effectiveness will be additive, whereas their individual toxicity will be diminished as well as diversified.[24] Among the host of side effects of common chemotherapeutic agents are drug-specific neurologic disorders such as sensorimotor peripheral neuropathy, cranial nerve dysfunction, meningoencephalopathy, cerebellar ataxia, paraplegia, and cerebral dysfunction. The use of some myelosuppressive drugs results in hemorrhages, especially when the platelet count falls below 10,000 per cubic millimeter. Disseminated intravascular coagulation and direct tumor invasion also have this potential for hemorrhage. Each can produce secondary neurologic dysfunction, especially when bleeding occurs in a closed area such as the retroperitoneal space.[25] Although usually dose related, complications of drug therapy are highly unpredictable, with some patients demonstrating severe toxic side effects with only modest treatment dosages. When an early neuropathy is suspected, electromyography and nerve conduction velocity studies are appropriate. These studies can be both diagnostic and prognostic, permitting a more judicious administration of drug and rehabilitation therapy. Patients with a clinically symptomatic neuropathy are managed with flexibility, coordination, and strengthening exercises and the use of ambulatory aids and light-weight bracing when indicated.

Surgical Therapy

Surgical resection of a primary or metastatic neoplasm, whether performed as a cure or as a palliative measure, is associated with the inherent risk of complications. Cervical nerve lesions associated with facial and neck surgery and intractable cervical pain as a result of loss of supporting shoulder girdle muscle following a radical neck dissection remain continuing challenges to reconstructive and rehabilitation treatment. Peripheral nerve and nerve plexus palsies are occasionally products of the risk associated with meticulous dissection. Although occurring less frequently than in the past, they still occur even with the more recent surgical procedures. Lymphedema following radical mastectomy may require management, but its incidence has been greatly reduced by the recent acceptance of the modified mastectomy procedure. Even in this group, however, trauma to the shoulder or postoperative infection can produce lymphedema requiring intermittent pneumatic pumping supplemented by a retention sleeve and hand gauntlet.[26]

Amputation surgery may vary from localized extirpation to radical and massive amputation. Hemicorpectomy with its attendant ostomy management problems and plastic jacket supports is among the most radical of these procedures.[27] The long-established doctrine for amputation for a neoplasm in an extremity was transection above the joint proximal to the lesion. Today some surgeons are suggesting amputation only 5 to 8 cm proximal to bone reactive on x-ray or bone scan.[28] In other instances bone resection rather than amputation has been used, with the bony segment replaced by an intramedullary rod or bone grafts in an effort to preserve the length of the extremity. These approaches have been made acceptable by effective combination drug therapies.

The technique of immediate postoperative prosthetic fitting of the cancer patient has resulted in a faster physical and psychological recovery for both patient and family.[29] An additional benefit is the ease with which the temporary and permanent sockets can be modified to accommodate for stump shrinkage attendant to early ambulation and ongoing chemotherapy. Although expensive, the prosthetic fitting of the young above-knee cancer amputee is no more costly than providing a prosthesis for the elderly vascular amputee. Prosthetic wearing time in both is roughly equivalent at 2.2 years.[30]

COPING

Complete restoration of function should always be the objective of rehabilitation. When not obtainable the maintenance of functional capacity to its fullest extent remains the goal. The efforts of the rehabilitation team often can return the cancer patient to an active and productive life. Frequent evaluations are necessary to adapt to increasing disability. The initial efforts may be directed to ambulation and self-care. Later it may be necessary to reorient to wheelchair and assisted self-care activity. Finally, supportive care of the nonmobile patient may be the objective. Early in the evaluation every effort should be made to mobilize family and community resources to provide assistive and supportive care at home if discharge planning is to be expedited. Family involvement, necessary at all levels of function, is imperative during final states of supportive care. Equipment including hospital beds, wheelchairs, lifts, and other nursing items can be obtained on loan through the "cancer closet" of the local unit of the American Cancer Society. Nursing assistance provided by the Visiting Nurse Association (VNA) is an invaluable adjunct to management of the patient at home. Although instruction in patient bed care, including ostomy and catheter management, should be provided to the family prior to hospital discharge, continuing supervision by the visiting nurse is essential.

The awareness of the status of the cancer patient depends upon close and attentive follow-up. Pain during assistive joint range-of-motion exercise may be the first indicator of a new metastasis or pathologic fracture. Increased weakness may be a sign of an increasing pressure myelopathy or neuro-myopathy.

Through its positive, supportive approach to therapy, the rehabilitation team can help to overcome the sense of despair and helplessness that accompanies the diagnosis of disseminated cancer. The patient may be less fearful of death itself than overwhelmed by the ''process of dying'' with its attendant anxieties, increasing dependency, and fear of abandonment. Patients who do not receive adequate support may withdraw completely and refuse all therapeutic overtures. However, most patients never lose hope and welcome all emotional and physical support. A continuing major effort must be made by the rehabilitation team to bridge the gulf between those who treat and cannot cure and those who will otherwise die abandoned to grief and loneliness.[31, 32] At the terminal stage of cancer all medical and rehabilitation team members need to continue the efforts to maintain contact with and support of the patient so that he or she will not feel abandoned and alone.[31, 32]

REFERENCES

1. Markesberg, W. R., Brooks, W. H., Gupta, G. D., and Young, A. B.: Treatment for patients with cerebral metastasis. Arch. Neurol., 35:754–756, 1978.
2. Simionescu, M. D.: Metastatic tumors of the brain. J. Neurosurg., 17:361–373, 1960.
3. Posner, J. B., and Shapiro, W. R.: The management of intracranial metastasis. In Morley, T. P. (Ed.): Current Controversies in Neurosurgery. Philadelphia, W. B. Saunders Co., 1976, pp. 356–366.
4. Epstein, B. S.: Spinal canal mass lesions. Radiol. Clin. North Am., 4:185–202, 1966.
5. Gilbert, H., Apuzzo, M., Marshall, L., Kogan, A. R., Crue, B., Wagner, J., Fuchs, K., Rush, J., Rao, A., Nussbaum, H., and Chan, P.: Neoplastic epidural spinal cord compression — A current prospective. JAMA, 240:2771–2773, 1978.
6. Moersch, F. P., Winchell, McK. C., and Christoferson, L. A.: Spinal cord tumors with minimal neurologic findings. Neurology, 1:39–47, 1951.
7. LaBan, M. M., and Grant, A. E.: Occult spinal metastasis — early electromyographic manifestation. Arch. Phys. Med. Rehabil., 52:223–225, 1971.
8. Wright, R. L.: Malignant tumors of the spinal extradural space — results of surgical treatment. Ann. Surg., 157:227–231, 1963.
9. Raycroft, J. F., Hockman, R. P., and Southwick, W. O.: Metastatic tumors involving the cervical vertebrae: Surgical palliation. J. Bone Joint Surg., 60A:763–768, 1978.
10. Barron, K. D., Hirano, A., Araki, S., and Terry, R. D.: Experiences with metastatic neoplasms involving the spinal cord. Neurology, 9:91–106, 1959.
11. Millburn, L., Hibbs, G. G., and Hendrickson, F. R.: Treatment of spinal cord compression from metastatic carcinoma. Cancer, 21:447–452, 1968.
12. Dietz, J. H.: The physician's viewpoint. In Symposium on Rehabilitation and Cancer Proceedings. New York, American Cancer Society, 1969, pp. 16–22.
13. LaBan, M. M., and Meerschaert, J. R.: Quadriplegia following cervical traction in patients with occult epidural prostatic metastasis. Arch. Phys. Med. Rehabil., 56:455–458, 1975.
14. LaBan, M. M., Meerschaert, J. R., Perez, L., and Goodman, P. A.: Metastatic disease of the paraspinal muscles: Electromyographic and histopathologic correlation in early detection. Arch. Phys. Med. Rehabil., 59:34–36, 1978.
15. Miller, R. N.: The control of pain in the cancer patient. In Rehabilitation of the Cancer Patient. Chicago, Year Book Medical Publishers, Inc., 1972, pp. 129–138.
16. Leavens, M.-E.: The neurosurgeon's role in rehabilitation of the cancer patient. In Rehabilitation of the Cancer Patient. Chicago, Year Book Medical Publishers, Inc., 1972, pp. 139–156.
17. Hardy, R. W.: Current techniques in the management of pain. Cleve. Clin. Q., 41:177–183, 1974.
18. Brain, L., and Norris, R., Jr.: The Remote Effects of Cancer on the Nervous System. New York, Grune & Stratton, 1970.
19. Norris, F. H., Rudolph, J. H., and Barney, M. O.: Carcinomatous neuropathy. Rare complication of cancer of the cervix uteri. Neurology, 14:202–205, 1964.
20. Bohan, A., and Peter, J. B.: Polymyositis and dermatomyositis. N. Engl. J. Med., 292:344–347, 1975.
21. Bohan, A., and Peter, J. B.: Polymyositis and dermatomyositis. N. Engl. J. Med., 292:403–407, 1975.
22. Lambert, E. H.: Defects of neuromuscular transmission in syndromes other than myasthenia gravis. Ann. N.Y. Acad. Sci., 135:367–384, 1966.
23. Coy, P., Baker, S., and Dolman, C. L.: Progressive myelopathy due to radiation. Can. Med. Assoc. J., 100:1129–1133, 1969.
24. Krakoff, I. H.: Cancer chemotherapeutic agents. CA, 27:130–143, 1977.
25. Belt, R. J., Leite, C., Haas, C. D., and Stephens, R. L.: Incidence of hemorrhagic complications in patients with cancer. JAMA, 239:2571–2574, 1978.
26. Stillwell, G. K., and Redford, J. W. B.: Physical treatment of postmastectomy lymphedema. Proc. Mayo. Clin., 33:1–8, 1958.
27. Easton, J. K. M., Aust, J. B., Dawson, W. J., and Kottke, F. J.: Fitting of a prosthesis on a patient after hemicorporectomy. Arch. Phys. Med. Rehabil., 44:335–337, 1963.
28. Sim, F. H., Ivins, J. C., and Pritchard, D. J.: Surgical treatment of osteogenic sarcoma at the Mayo Clinic. Cancer Treat. Rep., 62:205–211, 1978.
29. Sarmiento, A., May, B. J., Sinclair, W. F., McCullough, N. C., and Williams, E. M.: Lower-extremity amputation. The impact of immediate postsurgical prosthetic fitting. Clin. Orthop., 68:22–31, 1970.
30. Aitken, G. T.: Prosthetic fitting following amputation for bone tumor: A preliminary report. Inter-Clinic Information Bull., 3:1–2, 1964.
31. Kubler-Ross, E.: On Death and Dying. New York, MacMillan Publishing Co., 1969.
32. Vanderpool, H. Y.: The ethics of terminal care. JAMA, 239:850–852, 1978.

52

BODILY RESPONSES TO IMMOBILIZATION

CARLOS VALLBONA

One of the most prevalent syndromes encountered by rehabilitation specialists is that resulting from prolonged bed rest and immobilization. This is not surprising, since the syndrome occurs whenever illness or injury causes loss of mobility, or whenever a patient is on prolonged bed rest.

The basis of the immobilization syndrome is an imbalance of the normal relationship between rest and physical activity, two biologic processes that are essential to preserve man's optimal physical condition. The prescription of bed rest is a time-honored, common-sense therapeutic measure widely used by physicians in the presence of a serious illness. The value of physical exercise as an equally important treatment modality had been recognized by the Spanish physician Cristóbal Mendez, who in 1533 wrote a treatise on the physiologic responses to exercise and its therapeutic indications.[1] Yet physicians have often neglected exercise prescriptions in spite of the fact that cardiologists, physiatrists, and sports physicians have long documented the excellent results derived from exercise in a variety of clinical conditions.

The literature on the effects of immobilization clearly reflects the interest of numerous investigators in elucidating the pathophysiologic responses to various forms of immobilization. The first experimental study recorded in modern literature was that of Cuthbertson in 1929,[2] followed by the classic investigations conducted in the 1940's by Taylor et al.,[3] Deitrick et al.,[4] and Widdowson.[5] As a result of the interest in human space explorations, there was a new flurry of research in the early 1960's with the goal of measuring the adaptation of the human body to simulated weightlessness.[6, 7] From the moment that men started making brief orbital flights until their recent prolonged stays in space laboratories, several investigators have systematically collected data on the performance of astronauts and cosmonauts in the zero-gravity (0-G) environment.[8-11] Simultaneously, rehabilitation researchers started documenting the pathophysiologic changes exhibited by patients with extensive paralysis[12-15] and found some striking similarities between the clinical manifestations of prolonged immobilization in paralyzed patients and in healthy subjects after bed rest or sustained weightlessness.

Modalities of Immobilization

There are four types of inactivity which by themselves may cause the syndrome of immobilization:

1. Prolonged bed rest prescribed for the treatment of an acute illness or injury

2. Restricted neuromuscular activity due to paralysis

3. Continuous stay in a given position (e.g., sitting or recumbent), which effectively reduces the influence of gravity forces

4. State of weightlessness experienced

during space travel (especially if the traveler does not perform isometric or isotonic exercises while in flight) or simulated through prolonged immersion in water

Each one of these modalities of inactivity may produce subtle physiologic changes within a short period of time. Obvious clinical manifestations (e.g., orthostatism) occur within five to seven days, while others (e.g., ankylosis, renal lithiasis) do not become apparent until the individual has remained inactive for weeks or months. The first two modalities are of greatest interest in rehabilitation medicine because they prevail in the majority of physically disabled persons.

Basic Physiologic Concepts

As a prerequisite to a discussion of the pathophysiology of immobilization, it is appropriate to define and discuss the concepts of functional capacity, physiologic maximal potential, and functional reserve.

1. **Functional Capacity** is the maximum metabolic rate achieved by a subject during exertion.

2. **Physiologic Maximal Potential** is the maximum metabolic rate that the same individual is capable of achieving after a systematic program of physical training.

3. **Functional Reserve** is the difference between the functional capacity and the physiologic maximal potential.

Kottke discussed these concepts in an article in which he reviewed the impact that bed rest, exercise, and illness may have on an individual's functional capacity, physiologic maximal potential, and functional reserve.[14] As shown in Figure 52–1, the average sedentary person has a certain functional capacity that is considerably lower than his/her physiologic maximal potential. If the individual undertakes a program of physical training, the functional capacity will gradually increase to a point where it almost equals the physiologic maximal potential. On the

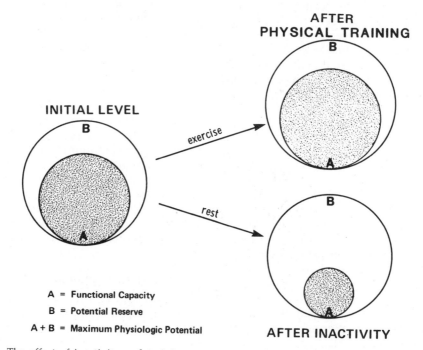

A = Functional Capacity

B = Potential Reserve

A + B = Maximum Physiologic Potential

FIGURE 52–1. The effect of inactivity and training on a person's functional capacity, potential reserve, and maximum physiologic potential. Area A inside of the left circle shows the functional capacity of an average sedentary person. Area B in the same circle represents that person's potential reserve. Area A + B represents the person's maximum physiologic potential. After physical training, the individual's functional capacity, as shown by area A on the top circle on the right side, will increase considerably. Similarly, there will be a slight increase in the potential reserve as shown by area B. On the contrary, after prolonged inactivity, there will be a marked decrease in functional capacity, as shown by the smaller size of area A in the bottom circle on the right side. The potential reserve will be high, but the maximum physiologic potential will, at best, remain the same as before the period of inactivity. (Modified from Kottke, F. J.: The effects of limitation of activity on the human body. JAMA, 196:117–122, 1966.)

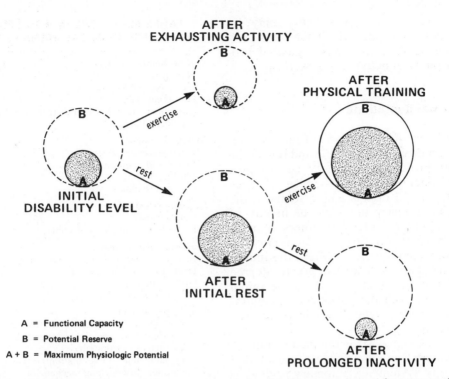

AFTER
EXHAUSTING ACTIVITY

AFTER
PHYSICAL TRAINING

INITIAL
DISABILITY LEVEL

AFTER
INITIAL REST

A = Functional Capacity

B = Potential Reserve

A + B = Maximum Physiologic Potential

AFTER
PROLONGED INACTIVITY

FIGURE 52–2. The impact of illness or injury on a person's functional capacity, potential reserve, and maximal physiologic potential. As a result of disability, both functional capacity and potential reserve (as shown by areas A and B in the circle on the left side) are much smaller than in the healthy state. The maximum physiologic potential (area A + B) is also smaller. A period of initial rest is necessary to achieve partial recovery. This leads to an increase in areas A and B, as shown in the bottom circle of the middle section. Exhausting activity rather than rest during convalescence would cause further losses, as shown by the smaller sizes of areas A and B in the top circle of the middle section. Judicious physical training is necessary beyond the period of convalescence in order to facilitate recovery, as shown by the larger areas A and B in the top circle on the right side of the graph. Prolonged inactivity would result in a serious decrease in functional capacity, as shown by the smaller area A in the bottom circle on the right. (Modified from Kottke, F. J.: The effects of limitation of activity upon the human body. JAMA, 196:117–122, 1966.)

other hand, continuing lack of exercise or prolonged inactivity will lead to a decline in functional capacity. Figure 52–2 depicts the sudden drop in functional capacity, as well as in functional reserve, which was experienced by the disabled person at the onset of a severe acute illness or injury. The prescription of exhaustive physical activity to an acutely ill or injured person would cause a further drop in functional capacity. At that stage, it is necessary to institute a program of bed rest in order to allow for a gradual recovery of the functional capacity and functional reserve. However, prolongation of bed rest beyond the initial convalescence would cause a new drop in functional capacity and functional reserve. It is for this reason that the patient must start a gradual program of physical activity with the goal of regaining the predisease levels of functional capacity and functional reserve (assuming, of course,

that the initial illness or injury has not caused permanent damage).

The magnitude of these changes in functional capacity, functional reserve, and maximal potential depends on the severity of the disease or injury, the duration of bed rest, and the intensity of exercise. They are also dependent on the individual's age, since children recover at faster rates than young adults,[16, 17] and these, in turn, at faster rates than the elderly.[18]

Individuals who participate in a regular program of physical exercise reach levels of functional capacity that are close to physiologic maximal potential. By contrast, deconditioned individuals have a marked reduction of functional capacity and eventually may lose the major part of their functional reserve. The process of aging also results in a gradual and irreversible decrease of an individual's functional capacity and functional reserve. However, the process may be slowed down considerably if the aged individual participates in a well-regulated program of physical activity and exercise.

Clinical Manifestations

The clinical manifestations of the immobilization syndrome are multiple and reflect the fact that prolonged inactivity causes profound physiologic and biochemical changes in practically all organs and systems of the body. The primary involvement in any of them may, in turn, affect the others, thereby setting up a pathophysiologic vicious circle of deleterious consequences. Often, the immobilization syndrome leads to a greater degree of disability than that caused by the initial illness or injury, jeopardizes the rehabilitation process, and significantly increases the cost of care.[19]

Table 52–1 summarizes the manifestations of the immobilization syndrome in each one of the body systems. A summary review of the pathophysiology of these manifestations is provided in the following paragraphs. The interested reader can find a detailed description of the functional pathology of immobilization in a recent monograph by Steinberg.[20]

Central Nervous System

Prolonged immobilization causes disturbances in the central nervous system. Their number and intensity depend, of course, on the primary illness that caused the inactivity. The major manifestations include the following:

Altered Sensation. This occurs because of a general decrease in sensory input. The problem is readily apparent in the paralyzed individual with involvement of the sensory afferent pathways and resulting anesthesia or hypesthesia below the level of the lesion. In some patients, prolonged inactivity in accompanied by paresthesias and a low threshold for pain.

Decreased Motor Activity. Unless the individual carries out frequent isometric or isotonic exercises while in bed (or in a weightless state), the overall motor output of the immobilized person will be consistently lower than that of a sedentary person performing activities of daily living. This prob-

TABLE 52–1. THE IMMOBILIZATION SYNDROME: CLINICAL MANIFESTATIONS

Central Nervous System
 Altered sensation
 Decreased motor activity
 Autonomic lability
 Emotional and behavioral disturbances
 Intellectual deficit

Muscular System
 Decreased muscle strength
 Decreased endurance
 Muscle atrophy
 Poor coordination

Skeletal System
 Osteoporosis
 Fibrosis and ankylosis of joints

Cardiovascular System
 Increased heart rate (adrenergic state)
 Decreased cardiac reserve
 Orthostatic hypotension
 Phlebothrombosis

Respiratory System
 Decreased vital capacity (restrictive impairment)
 Decreased maximal voluntary ventilation (restrictive impairment)
 Regional changes in ventilation/perfusion
 Impairment of coughing mechanism

Digestive System
 Anorexia
 Constipation

Endocrine and Renal Systems
 Increased diuresis and extracellular fluid shifts
 Increased natriuresis
 Hypercalciuria
 Renal lithiasis

Integumentary System
 Atrophy of the skin
 Bed sores

lem is especially serious in patients whose restricted physical activity is the result of flaccid paralysis. Patients with spastic paralysis maintain a significant level of muscle activity, thereby preventing atrophy (see below).

Autonomic Lability. The autonomic nervous system of immobilized persons becomes either hyperactive or hypoactive and, as a result, it is difficult to maintain a stable level of autonomic activity and the individual cannot adapt readily to daily stresses (e.g., changes in posture). The effect of autonomic lability on the cardiovascular system is described below.

Emotional Disturbances. Limited sensory input combined with a personal awareness of unproductivity is the major contributor to the anxiety-depression syndrome that occurs so frequently in the immobilized person.[21, 22] The underlying pathology may be the major factor leading to depression. Contrariwise, a prolonged stay in bed may be a manifestation of depression, since oftentimes a depressed person feels that by staying in bed and sleeping through a chronic illness all the worries will go away and the depression will disappear.

Intellectual Deficit. The capability of an individual to perform intellectual activities may decrease significantly as a result of prolonged inactivity and confinement.[23] Indeed, immobilized persons often experience difficulty in performing arithmetic or other complex tasks. The resulting frustrations contribute to the state of anxiety-depression previously mentioned.

Muscular System

The most obvious signs of prolonged immobilization occur in the muscular system. This is particularly true in patients who have suffered a paralytic condition. The most common manifestations are the following:

Decreased Muscle Strength. It is a well-known fact that whenever an individual does not carry out a program of moderate physical activity, his/her muscle strength decreases significantly. Studies conducted by Hettinger and Mueller[24] showed that after one week of bed rest there may be up to 20 per cent loss of the initial strength level and another 20 per cent decline in residual strength for each week of bed rest. For example, in the absence of any motor neuron lesion, a man whose grip strength on the dominant side is 50 kg will have a strength of 40 kg after one week of immobilization, 32 kg after two weeks, 25 kg after three weeks, etc. This has major implications in rehabilitation, because the rate of recovery is much slower; i.e., there is only a 10 per cent increase of initial strength per week if the individual participates in a program of daily exercise at 100 per cent of maximal muscle strength.

Decreased Endurance. The loss of endurance after prolonged immobilization is a consequence of the decrease in muscle strength and occurs at a similar rate. Physical exercise, on the contrary, improves muscular endurance in proportion to the overall increase in functional capacity.

Muscle Atrophy. Undoubtedly, the loss of muscle mass is one of the most visible manifestations of prolonged immobilization and it, in turn, accounts for the decrease in muscle strength and endurance. The degree of atrophy varies according to the modality of immobilization. It is quite evident in cases of flaccid paralysis, where for each involved lower motor unit there is abolition of its neuron's action potentials and loss of contraction of all the muscle fibers (tens or hundreds) innervated by that neuron. A totally denervated muscle may lose its normal bulk by as much as 90 to 95 per cent.[25] If denervation is not reversible, the muscle fibers undergo permanent degeneration and are replaced by fat and connective tissue. In patients with spastic paralysis as a result of an upper motor neuron lesion, or in patients immobilized by splinting, the degree of muscle atrophy is only 30 to 35 per cent of normal.

Poor Coordination. The combination of atrophy, decreased strength, and limited endurance leads to poor coordination of movements. It is manifest in both upper and lower extremities, and it seriously jeopardizes the individual's capacity to perform activities of daily living and causes severe frustration. In patients with CNS lesions the major factor leading to incoordination is the pathologic process affecting the motor units or higher centers, but the immobilization per se will also be a contributory factor.

Skeleton System

There are several changes in the bones that result mainly from the muscular disturbances described above. The integrity of man's bone metabolism and the equilibrium between accretion and resorption of skeletal mass depend in great part on the daily stresses and strains imposed by the pulling action of the tendons and by the force of gravity during the standing position. Paralysis and a prolonged stay in the horizontal position will cause profound changes in the skeletal system. The most common manifestations are the following:

Osteoporosis. It results not only from decreased muscular activity but from complex endocrine and metabolic reactions that take place as a result of bed rest (see below). Both organic and inorganic constituents of bone suffer the consequences of immobilization. The well-documented increased excretion of hydroxyproline and calcium after immobili-

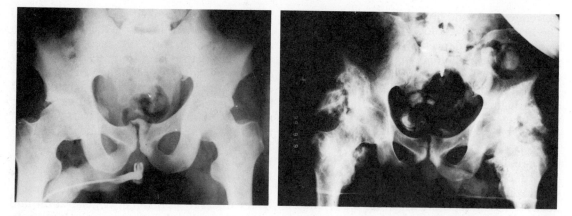

FIGURE 52–3. Radiographs of the pelvis of a 30-year-old paraplegic man. The x-ray on the left was taken within a few days after the onset of a spinal cord injury. It shows an indwelling catheter in place, but the bony structures are intact. The radiograph on the right was obtained at the time of admission to a rehabilitation center, 10 months after the injury. The patient had remained in bed during all this time. The radiograph shows abundant soft tissue calcification around the head of both femurs.

zation clearly shows that there is a depletion of organic and inorganic compounds.[12, 26, 27] The net result is a substantial decrease in total bone mass. The profound metabolic changes that occur in the skeletal system have repercussions in other systems mainly because of the mobilization of bone calcium that causes transient slight hypercalcemia, protracted hypercalciuria, and frequent deposition of calcium in injured soft tissues (ectopic calcification). The x-ray films of Figure 52–3 show clearly the development of ectopic calcification in a paraplegic patient subjected to prolonged immobilization.

Fibrosis and Ankylosis of the Joints. These two impairments are also a major manifestation of the syndrome of immobilization. They occur in varying degrees whenever a joint is not subjected to active or passive motion. Eventually, the overlying muscles are replaced by connective tissue. The joint then becomes stiff, unable to go through a full range of motion, and may become irreversibly deformed. As an example, oftentimes the patient who has suffered a stroke cannot walk well, not only because of paresis and spasticity but also because of ankyloses of the hip and ankle which occur if the patient remains in a recumbent position with the hip slightly flexed and the ankle in plantar flexion.[14] Ectopic calcification of the soft tissues around a joint may cause permanent ankylosis of that joint.

Cardiovascular System

As a result of prolonged immobilization, the cardiovascular system suffers major im-

pairments and cannot respond adequately to metabolic demands above the basal state. The clinical manifestations are as follows:

Increased Heart Rate. Several clinical investigators have pointed out that physical deconditioning leads to a preponderance of the sympathetic or adrenergic system over the cholinergic or vagal system. This accounts for an increase in the basal heart rate. Raab,[28] using two hypothetical examples, contrasted the process of chronic adjustment of the heart rate to daily exercise and to prolonged inactivity:

Professor A. D., an eminent scientist and noted Alpinist, former head of the Department of Physiology at the University of Vienna (eighty seven years old) has lived alone for the past twenty years with his paralyzed wife and a library of several thousand volumes in a 15th century isolated log cabin above Schruns, Vorarlberg, at an altitude of 5,000 feet. He cuts trees for firewood, raises his own vegetables, does all household chores, digs a path through deep snow on a precipitous slope, fetches mail and groceries twice weekly from a village in the valley and carries them up one and one-half hours to his abode. He makes extensive climbing excursions alone to high peaks (up to eighteen hours in a stretch) nearly every weekend, he does daily calisthenics at home. He still follows the scientific literature, writes articles and lectures occasionally. In recent years he had a few episodes of auricular fibrillation, but no signs of cardiac failure. His heart rate at rest is 48 to 60, at arrival on mountain peaks, about 90.

Miss B. C., a sixty-nine year old spinster, former piano teacher, decided at the age of thirty-seven, when her father died, to spend her life in bed. She stayed in bed for thirty years without interruption (except for one walk around the house after two years), wrote a large book about the courtship of her father, numerous poems and musical compositions. At the age of sixty-seven, when her older sister and house keeper died, she learned again slowly to walk and now spends a few hours out of bed every day. She does not do any housework. She has a small pliable thyroid nodule, but there are no signs of thyrotoxicosis. Her protein-bound iodine is low. Her heart rate, which has been over 100 for many years, is now up to 140 despite digitalization.

It is not clear why inactivity leads to a preponderance of the sympathetic (adrenergic) over the parasympathetic (cholinergic) system, but it is clear that a constellation of metabolic, endocrine, and mechanical factors interact to produce an adrenergic state with an increased cardiac rate as one of its manifestations. Increased basal heart rates (e.g., greater than 80 per minute) are indeed very common in sedentary persons and in those who remain in bed for long periods of time (several weeks). They are also common in paralyzed patients except in cases of high spinal cord injury, which causes complete denervation below the C4 level and which interrupts the transmission of sympathetic impulses to the sinoauricular pacemaker.

Decreased Cardiac Reserve. Under predominantly adrenergic influences there is an increased heart rate, which accounts for less diastolic filling time than at slow heart rates, a smaller systolic ejection, and a greatly diminished capacity of the heart to respond to metabolic demands above the basal level. The importance of maintaining low basal heart rates is evident if we take into consideration that at low rates the diastolic phase of the cardiac cycle is longer than the systolic phase, whereas at high rates the systolic phase is longer than the diastolic phase (e.g., at a heart rate of 60/min the electromechanical systole lasts 0.40 second and diastole 0.60 second, whereas at a rate of 150/min the systole time is 0.25 second and diastole 0.15 second. Since coronary blood flow occurs mainly during diastole, it is clear that at low rates there is greater blood flow through the coronary arteries per minute than at high cardiac rates. A greatly diminished cardiac reserve accounts for the patient's inability to carry out limited physical efforts. Such efforts may cause marked tachycardia and anginal pain, which often is masked in the quadriplegic individual.

Orthostatic Hypotension. This is one of the most common manifestations of cardio-vascular deconditioning following bed rest. Whenever a deconditioned individual attempts to sit up or stand up there is marked pooling of blood in the lower extremities, thereby decreasing the circulating blood volume and the venous return, preventing adequate ventricular filling during diastole, and causing the ventricle to eject a stroke volume that may be too small to achieve effective cerebral perfusion. In some instances, the blood pressure reaches levels as low as 60/30 mm Hg within 10 to 20 seconds of sitting with the legs hanging unsupported at the side of the bed. The pooling of blood in the lower extremities occurs because, in spite of an increased adrenergic state with concomitant stimulation of the vascular alpha-receptors, the arterioles and venules of the legs do not constrict sufficiently well to offset the effect of gravity on the column of blood that falls from the heart to the feet. As a result, there is increased hydrostatic pressure in the capillary bed, extravasation of fluid in the interstitial tissue, and marked dependent edema. The orthostatism that is so evident after prolonged immobilization contributes to the endocrine and metabolic disturbances that are also part of the immobilization syndrome[29] (see below).

Phlebothrombosis. One would expect that during prolonged bed rest there would be considerable venous stasis in the legs if we consider that in the horizontal position there is infrequent intermittent constriction of the arterioles and venules as well as a reduced or absent pumping action by the skeletal muscle. Yet prolonged bed rest in healthy subjects does not slow down significantly the ankle-to-groin venous flow time.[30] In spite of this, it is well known that paralyzed patients have a greater tendency to develop phlebothrombosis than the general population. The incidence of phlebothrombosis in patients with spinal cord injuries is considerably higher than in the normal population.[31, 32] In hemiplegic patients, phlebothrombosis is more frequent in the paralyzed than in the nonparalyzed side. It is evident that some hemodynamic changes in the venous return do occur in all paralyzed persons. These changes, coupled with a disturbance in the clotting mechanism, constitute a major determinant factor in the pathogenesis of phlebothrombosis. Possible changes in the production of prostaglandins or other disturbances of the platelet-aggregating mechanisms may play a role in the phlebothrombosis of immobilized persons, but this has not been clearly elucidated. The presence of sepsis or of infection in the wall of a major vein may precipitate the clotting process.

Respiratory System

The changes in respiratory function that occur in immobilized persons may also contribute to the severe disability that occurs as a result of immobilization, especially in patients with CNS lesions. The typical picture is that of a restrictive respiratory impairment which is manifested by the following:

Decreased Vital Capacity. Although healthy subjects subjected to prolonged bed rest do not show any significant reduction in the total lung capacity and its subdivisions (vital capacity, inspiratory capacity, expiratory reserve volume, functional residual capacity, and residual volume),[33] most immobilized patients, especially those with quadriplegia, show a greater reduction in vital capacity than one would expect from their underlying musculoskeletal pathology. Indeed, the inactive patient while in the supine position will seldom contract the intercostals, diaphragms, and abdominal muscles in order to accomplish a maximum inspiration or a forceful expiration. The overall decrease in muscle strength that was mentioned previously (see above) may eventually affect the respiratory muscles. If, in addition, the costovertebral and costochondral joints are not submitted to a full range of motion, they may become fixed in an expiratory position, thereby decreasing even further the capacity of the chest to achieve maximum inspiration. Thus, in the immobilized paralytic patients there can be a 25 to 50 per cent decrease in vital capacity and in functional respiratory capacity.

Decreased Maximal Voluntary Ventilation. The same mechanisms that account for a decrease in vital capacity lead to inability to sustain a maximal ventilatory effort and to decreased respiratory endurance. The observed values of maximal voluntary ventilation in the inactive person are significantly lower than predicted (by as much as 25 to 50 per cent below that of a nonparalyzed person).

Regional Changes in the Ventilation/Perfusion Ratio. As a result of the restrictive impairment described above and of the effect of the horizontal posture on the pulmonary circulation, there are marked regional differences in the ventilation/perfusion ratio.[20] Normally, these differences are not significant because the individual consciously or unconsciously mobilizes the thorax sufficiently to prevent underventilation and overperfusion of major parts of the lung. This does not happen in the immobilized person and, consequently, the dependent areas become poorly ventilated and overperfused. As a result, there is a significant arteriovenous shunt that lowers the arterial oxygen tension (Pao_2). Although this may not be significant while at rest, if the patient has an increased metabolic demand (because of an infection or exercise), hypoxia becomes apparent.

Impairment of the Coughing Mechanism. As a result of immobilization, even in healthy subjects, there is a significant decrease in the normal ciliary efficiency.[12] Because of this, the respiratory mucus secretions tend to accumulate in the dependent bronchioles, become more viscous than usual, interfere with the normal ciliary motion, and adhere to the airway epithelium. Coughing may fail to clear the bronchial tree, the problem being compounded if there is abdominal muscle weakness due to a motor lesion. Under these conditions, a mild upper respiratory infection may cause severe secondary infection of the lower airway and of the lung tissue.

Digestive Apparatus

An often overlooked aspect of the immobilization syndrome is an overall decrease in gastrointestinal activity, which affects not only the motility but also the secretory functions of the digestive glands (salivary, pancreas). The major manifestations are the following:

Anorexia. It is not surprising that the decreased caloric demands of the inactive individual result in significant loss of appetite. Often the anorexia is also a manifestation of the anxiety-depression that accompanies the immobilized state. The profound endocrine changes that occur in this state may further decrease the person's appetite.

Constipation. The adrenergic preponderance that occurs in the immobilized state inhibits peristalsis and constricts the sphincters. The overall result is a decrease in gastrointestinal motility. Contributing factors may be an increased intestinal absorption of water and a low dietary intake of liquids and/or fiber. In some instances, the protracted constipation causes severe fecal impactions.

Endocrine and Renal Systems

The profound metabolic and renal changes that occur in the immobilization syndrome result from the interaction of the endocrine system with others. There is an abundant literature on the nature of the endocrine and metabolic alterations that occur after bed rest[12] and in paralyzed persons.[34] Claus-Walker and Halstead have done a thorough review of the literature and have compiled the results of the most significant studies in a series of articles.[35] The most important endocrine and metabolic manifestations of the immobilization syndrome are the following:

Increased Diuresis. It occurs predominantly in the early phase of bed rest because the placement of the body in a horizontal position causes a temporary increase in circulating blood volume. This is due to a shift of some extracellular fluid to the venous side of the capillary bed with the subsequent increase in venous return. As a result, there is a stimulation of the volume receptors of the right atrium and a reflex inhibition of the antidiuretic hormone (ADH). The initial diuresis of bed rest does not pose a problem in the patient who receives intravenous fluid therapy.

Increased Natriuresis. This is also a temporary occurrence concomitant with the initial diuresis and it represents an attempt to maintain the plasma osmolality at a normal level.

Hypercalciuria. As mentioned previously (see above) osteoporosis is one of the major complications of prolonged inactivity. From a clinical standpoint, an important consequence is the constant mobilization of calcium from the bone matrix into the blood and eventual urinary excretion of the excess calcium. In addition to the previously mentioned mechanical factors that intervene in the development of osteoporosis, one has to consider the contributory role of the adrenal corticosteroids that may be released in excessive amounts because of the stress that accompanies the immobilizing disease or injury as well as the transient stress that occurs when the immobilized person starts sitting up or standing and develops orthostatic hypotension.[29] Under these conditions, and in an attempt to compensate for the decrease in circulating blood volume, there is a reflex release of fluid-retaining hormones (ADH, aldosterone, cortisol). Although the compensatory effect of these substances is not too efficacious in preventing orthostatism, it nevertheless has a lasting metabolic influence and eventually facilitates gradual adaptation to the upright posture.

Renal Lithiasis. The triad of hypercalciuria, urinary stasis, and urinary tract infection, when present, is dangerous because it leads to the production of calculi in the renal pelvis or in the lower urinary tract. The problem is of greater magnitude in paralyzed persons because of their marked hypercalciuria, their impaired bladder function, and the inevitable urinary tract infection that occurs in catheterized patients. Staghorn calculi develop in the renal pelvis (Fig. 52–4), and stones of various sizes may settle in the urinary bladder. Urinary obstruction poses serious problems, especially in the anesthetized spinal cord injury patient who does not feel the usual pain of renal colic. Repeated episodes of urinary tract infection and calculi may cause gradual impairment of renal function and eventually lead to a clear-cut picture of renal insufficiency.

Integumentary System

The skin and adnexa are not immune to the pathophysiologic changes that result from prolonged immobilization. The most common manifestations are the following:

Atrophy of the Skin. The subtle changes in extracellular fluid volume that occur in the dependent parts of the body affect the consistency of the subcutaneous tissues and dermis and lead to a gradual loss of skin turgor. Insufficient appetite and inadequate nutrition result in loss of subcutaneous fat and contribute to changes in skin turgor. Inadequate hygiene may worsen the problem and lead to skin breakdowns as well as to paronychia and ingrown toenails.

Bed Sores. They are common manifestations of prolonged immobilization and account for a great part of the cost of the rehabilitation of inadequately treated paralyzed individuals.[19] Chapter 46 discusses the problem of decubitus ulcers in detail.[36] It is important to state here that extensive bed sores produce considerable loss of protein, especially albumin. At the capillary level, the

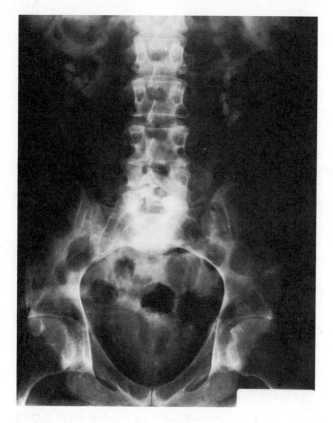

FIGURE 52–4. Radiograph of the abdomen of a quadriplegic person eight months after a cervical spinal cord injury. The patient had been inactive most of the time. Notice the kidney stones in the right and left kidney areas. There is extensive osteoporosis of the spine and pelvis.

decrease in serum protein results in a drop in oncotic pressure. This facilitates extravasation of fluid to the extracellular space when the individual sits up or gets up from bed. The extravasation aggravates the decreased circulating blood volume that occurs under the influence of gravity and contributes to the orthostatic hypotension that is so common in immobilized individuals (see above).

Prevention and Treatment

In order to prevent or to minimize the physiologic changes that occur as a result of immobilization, it is necessary to institute the following measures:

Sensory Stimulation. The institution of a program of sensory stimulation is the most effective means of preventing or treating the CNS manifestations of immobilization. A good comprehensive rehabilitation program must provide for environmental stimuli in order to ensure adequate sensory input to high cerebral areas and to compensate for whatever losses of sensation have occurred because of a CNS lesion. Participation in occupational and recreational therapy while in the hospital and stimulation by the patient's family to participate in discussions, watching of television, etc., may provide an antidote to sensory deprivation and may help overcome the emotional disturbances that occur frequently in the immobilized patient. Similarly, it is necessary to provide intellectual challenges to these patients and make them perform specific tasks (e.g., arithmetic, comment on news) in order to preserve intellectual function at a level similar to that before immobilization.

Active Muscle Exercise. A nonparalyzed person who must remain in bed should keep all muscle groups active to prevent muscular deconditioning. If there are no cardiovascular contraindications, the patient should be able to perform a variety of isotonic exercises such as the leg movements necessary to activate bicycle pedals mounted on a board that can lie on the patient's bed.[37] The exercise should take place at least once daily for 5 to 10 minutes.

Another useful way to preserve the integrity of the musculoskeletal and circulatory systems while in bed is the performance of simple isometric exercises. A particularly good one consists in making the supine patient apply pressure with the feet against a board placed perpendicular to the surface of the bed. This requires active isometric contraction of practically all muscle groups, especially those of the back and legs. Initially, the patient should do this once or twice a day by applying sustained pressure against the board for 5 seconds, relaxing for 10 seconds, and repeating the isometric contraction-relaxation three or four times. This type of exercise is obviously contraindicated in patients with spinal problems. In order to achieve effective isometric contractions of the arm muscles the patient should make a bilateral strong grip action for a few seconds with the arms extended. This exercise should take place at the same rate and frequency as the trunk and leg isometric exercises.

Adequate Positioning and Range-of-Motion Exercises. Both are necessary to prevent the skeletal changes that occur in immobilized, heavily sedated, or debilitated patients. The extremities should be properly positioned by maintaining each joint in its functional position to avoid ankylosis and deformities. Furthermore, the physician should prescribe range-of-motion exercises to be performed by a physical therapist, a nurse, or a member of the patient's family after proper training. A judicious program of range-of-motion exercises consists of making three to five consecutive full-range movements of each joint at least once (preferably twice) daily. The bathing of the patient offers an excellent opportunity for the nursing staff (or the family) to achieve passive range-of-motion exercise of practically all the joints.

Cardiovascular Reconditioning, Passive Tilt. The programs of muscular exercise previously described are helpful in preventing severe cardiovascular deconditioning. It is important, however, to avoid the patient's exhaustion by imposing excessive metabolic demands. During bed rest it is also prudent to maintain a heart rate at less than 120/min while performing isotonic or isometric exercises.

Individuals who are not paralyzed should assume the sitting and the standing postures as soon as feasible. This should take place

gradually, and as stated previously, the first attempts to sit up should consist in propping up the head of the bed at gradually increasing angles while keeping the legs horizontal. As the patient begins to sit at the edge of the bed and to stand up it is useful to prevent orthostatic hypotension by covering the legs with elastic stockings.

If the patient is unable to sit up because of paralysis or other disabling condition, it is highly advisable to impose the effect of gravity upon the body through passive assumption of the upright posture on a passive tilt table. Initially, the patient should reach a slight degree of tilt (e.g., 30 degrees), remain there for one minute, and gradually increase the duration of tilt to 30 minutes twice a day. As the patient's tolerance improves, the degree of tilt is increased by 5 to 10 degrees every week until the patient tolerates the 70 degree position (equivalent to 1G force) for about half an hour twice a day.

Elastic stockings help to minimize the effects of gravity because they prevent stasis of blood and edema in the lower extremities. The patient should wear the stockings most of the time while lying in bed, but especially in the periods of sitting or standing. In instances of severe orthostatic hypotension, the stockings should be extra firm in order to counteract the hydrostatic pressure exerted by the blood which pools in the lower extremities. Spinal cord–injury patients who cannot tolerate a gradual program of passive tilt in spite of wearing extra firm stockings may benefit from an especially tailored garment fashioned after a lower body G-suit.[38]

Respiratory and Coughing Exercises. The prescription of respiratory exercises is an essential component of the management of immobilized patients. While in bed, the inactive person must take three to five slow, deep breaths at least every hour while awake. A forced expiration should accompany each maximum inspiratory effort to maintain all lung compartments at a normal level. In order to reach a full inspiration, the person must learn to use equally the intercostals and the diaphragms. A useful approach is to concentrate on expanding the abdomen during inspiration. As the individual contracts both diaphragms, he lowers their position and pushes the viscera against the abdominal wall. If the abdominal muscles are weak a good contraction of the diaphragms results in marked expansion of the abdomen because of the limited resistance offered by the flabby abdominal wall. If the patient has respiratory muscle paralysis with a decrease in vital capacity below 60 per cent of normal, it is useful to carry out three to five passive lung inflations twice daily with a positive pressure apparatus at high settings of pressure, flow, and volume.

The nonparalyzed immobilized person should make a conscious effort to cough forcefully several times a day to prevent accumulation of tracheobronchial secretions and to facilitate periodic ventilation of all alveolar areas. Paralyzed persons can achieve effective coughing with weak expiratory abdominal muscles by applying pressure in the abdominal cavity at the end of a deep active inspiration or a passive inflation with a positive pressure apparatus.

Appropriate Nutrition and Fluid Intake. They are the mainstays of the prophylaxis of severe digestive and metabolic complications of immobilization. The caloric intake should be commensurate to the metabolic needs of the patient while at bed rest (these needs are greater if the patient is on an exercise program or has fever). Under most circumstances, there seldom is a problem of excessive caloric intake because the patient's inactive state leads to loss of appetite. The diet, of course, must be adequately balanced and should have a high fiber content to facilitate bowel movements. If the diet is nutritious, there is no need for vitamin supplements.

A stool softener (e.g., dioctyl sodium sulfosuccinate) may be useful in preventing constipation and fecal impaction.

A diet of approximately 1 gram of protein per kilogram of body weight and 1 gram of calcium per day seems to prevent osteoporosis and hypoproteinemia in the nonparalyzed individual. In cases of hypoproteinemia, the protein content should be approximately 1.5 grams per kilogram of body weight. Paralyzed patients who have experienced a severe loss of lean body mass develop a significant degree of osteoporosis that is impossible to prevent.[39, 40] These patients do not require a calcium supplement, since an excessive calcium intake would contribute to hypercalciuria and to renal lithiasis (assuming the presence of a concomitant urinary tract infection and renal stasis).

An adequate fluid intake is always necessary to prevent urinary complications unless the patient's cardiac condition is such that an increased fluid intake would create an unnecessary load to the heart muscle.

Sodium intake must be the usual one without the need to administer sodium supplements, since increased natriuresis is a transient occurrence and often inadvertent. Hypertensive patients should have a restricted sodium diet as required to maintain the blood pressure under control and to potentiate the effects of antihypertensive drugs, especially the thiazides.

Skin Hygiene. The immobilized patient must receive adequate skin hygiene. It is necessary to cleanse the skin thoroughly and to massage it adequately to maintain good turgor and avoid infections. This is particularly important in the skin of the dependent areas, since they are under constant pressure against the lying surface. Frequent trimming of all fingernails and toenails is a most important preventive measure.

In cases of immobilization due to paralysis, to heavy sedation, or to general debilitation, it is necessary to change the patient's position periodically in order to prevent prolonged, excessive pressure on the skin of the dependent areas. An accepted schedule is to change the body from one side to the back and from the back to the other side every two to four hours.

Summary

Rehabilitation physicians and allied health professionals who constitute the rehabilitation team must be aware of the pathophysiologic changes brought about by prolonged immobilization. These changes affect practically all systems of the body and may cause a greater degree of disability than the one produced by the illness or injury that caused the patient to remain in bed.

The most salient manifestations of the immobilization syndrome are (1) in the central nervous system, changes in sensation, decreased motor output, autonomic lability, emotional disturbances, and intellectual deficit; (2) in the muscular system, decreased strength and endurance, atrophy, and poor coordination; (3) in the skeletal system, osteoporosis, joint fibrosis, and ankylosis; (4) in the cardiovascular system, increased heart rate, decreased cardiac reserve, orthostatic hypotension, and phlebothrombosis; (5) in the respiratory apparatus, decreased vital capacity, decreased maximum voluntary ventilation, loss of respiratory endurance, regional changes in ventilation/perfusion, and impaired coughing; (6) in the digestive system, anorexia and constipation; (7) in the metabolic and renal systems, increased diuresis, hypernatriuresis, hypercalciuria, and renal lithiasis; and (8) in the integumentary system, atrophy of the skin and bed sores.

The prevention and treatment of the immobilization syndrome require (1) provision of environmental stimuli and intellectual challenges, (2) active isotonic or isometric exercises, (3) adequate position and passive mobilization of all joints, (4) gradual cardiovascular reconditioning through physical exercise and passive tilt, (5) respiratory and coughing exercises, (6) adequate nutrition and fluid intake with protein and calcium supplements when indicated, and (7) skin hygiene.

REFERENCES

1. Mendez, C.: Book of Bodily Exercise. English translation by Francisco Guerra. New Haven, Conn., E. Licht, 1960.
2. Cuthbertson, D. P.: The influence of prolonged muscular rest on metabolism. Biochem., 23:1328–1345, 1929.
3. Taylor, H. L., Erickson, L., Henschel, A., and Keys, A.: The effect of bed rest on the blood volume of normal young men. Am. J. Physiol., 144:227-232, 1945.
4. Dietrick, J. E., Whedon, G. D., and Shorr, E.: Effects of immobilization upon various metabolic and physiologic functions of normal man. Am. J. Med., 4:3-36, 1948.
5. Widdowson, E. M., and McCance, R. A.: Effect of rest in bed on plasma volume as indicated by haemoglobins and haematocrit. Lancet, 1:539-540, 1950.
6. Graybiel, A., and Clark, B.: Symptoms resulting from prolonged immersion in water. The problem of zero G asthenia. Aerospace Med., 32:181-196, 1961.
7. Miller, P. B., Johnson, R. L., and Lamb, L. E.: Effects of four weeks of absolute bed rest on circulatory functions in man. Aerospace Med. 35:1194-1200, 1964.
8. Space Medicine in Project Mercury. NASA SP-4003, 1965.
9. Gemini Summary Conference. NASA SP-138, 1967.
10. Biomedical Results of Apollo. NASA SP-368, 1975.
11. Biomedical Results from Skylab. NASA SP-377, 1977.
12. Browse, N. L.: The Physiology and Pathology of Bed Rest. Springfield, Ill., Charles C Thomas, Publisher, 1965.
13. Spencer, W. A., Vallbona, C., and Carter, R. E.: Physiologic concepts of immobilization. Arch. Phys. Med. Rehabil. 46:89-100, 1965.
14. Kottke, F. J.: The effects of limitation of activity upon the human body. JAMA, 196:117-122, 1966.
15. Long, C. L., and Bonilla, L. E.: Metabolic effects of inactivity and injury. In Downey, J. A., and Darling, R. C. (Eds.): Physiological Basis of Rehabilitation Medicine. Philadelphia, W. B. Saunders Company, 1971.
16. Millard, F. J. C., Nassim, J. R., and Woollen, J. W: Urinary calcium excretion after immobilization and spinal fusion in adolescents. Arch. Dis. Child., 45:399-403, 1970.
17. Rosen, F. J., Woolin, D. A., and Finberg, L.: Immobilization hypercalcemia after single limb fracture in children and adolescents. Am. J. Dis. Child., 132:560-564, 1978.
18. Grumbach, R., and Blanc, A.: The immobilization syndrome in the aged. Nouv. Presse Med., 2:1989-1991, 1973.
19. Gordon, D. L., and Reinstein, L.: Rehabilitation of the trauma patient. Am. Surg., 45:223-227, 1979.
20. Steinberg, F. U.: The immobilized patient. Functional pathology and management. New York, Plenum Publishing Co., 1980.
21. Downs, F.: Bed rest and sensory disturbances. Am. J. Nurs., 74:434-438, 1974.
22. Levy, R.: The immobilized patient and his psychologic well being. Postgrad. Med., 40:73-77, 1966.
23. Hammer, R. L., and Kenan, E. H.: The psychological aspects of immobilization. In Steinberg, F. U.: The immobilized patient. Functional pathology and management. New York, Plenum Publishing Co., 1980.
24. Hettinger, T., and Mueller, E. A.: Muskelleistung and Muskeltraining. Arbeitsphysiologie, 15:111-126, 1953.
25. Cardenas, D. D., Stolov, W. C., and Hardy, R: Muscle fiber numbers in immobilization atrophy. Arch. Phys. Med. Rehabil., 58:423-426, 1977.
26. Moore Ede, M. C., and Burr, R. G.: Circadian rhythm of urinary calcium excretion during immobilization. Aerospace Med., 44:495-498, 1973.
27. Claus-Walker, J., Spencer, W. A., Carter, R. E., Halstead, L. S., Meier, R. H., III, and Campos, R. J.: Bone metabolism in quadriplegia: Dissociation between calciuria and hydroxyprolinuria. Arch. Phys. Med. Rehabil., 56:327-332, 1975.
28. Raab, W., Silva, P. P., Marchet, H., Kiumra, E., and Starcheska, Y. K.: Cardiac adrenergic preponderance due to lack of physical exercise and its pathogenic implications. Am. J. Cardiol., 5:300-320, 1960.
29. Vallbona, C., Lipscomb, H. S., and Carter, R. E.: Endocrine responses to orthostatic hypotension in quadriplegia. Arch. Phys. Med. Rehabil. 47:412-421, 1966.
30. Wright, H. P., Osborn, S. B., and Hayden, M.: Venous velocity in bedridden medical patient. Lancet, 2:699-700, 1952.
31. Watson, N.: Venous thrombosis and pulmonary embolism in spinal cord injury. Paraplegia, 6:113-121, 1968.
32. Naso, F.: Pulmonary embolism in acute spinal cord injury. Arch. Phys. Med. Rehabil., 55:275-278, 1974.
33. Saltin, B., Blomqvist, G., Mitchell, J. H., Johnson, R. L., Wildenthal, K., and Chapman, C. B.: Response to exercise after bed rest and after training. Circulation, 38(Suppl. VII):1-78, 1968.
34. Greenleaf, J. E., Bernauer, E. M., Young H. L.,

Morse, J. T., Staley, R. W., Juhos, L. T., and Van Beaumont, W.: Fluid and electrolyte shifts during bed rest without isometric and isotonic exercises. J. Appl. Physiol., 42:59-66, 1977.

35. Claus-Walker, J., and Halstead, L.: Metabolic and endocrine changes in spinal cord injury: A review of the literature. Arch. Phys. Med. Rehabil. 62:595–601, 1981.

36. Kosiak, M.: Decubitus ulcers. *In* Kottke, F. J. (Ed.): Krusen's Handbook of Physical Medicine and Rehabilitation. Philadelphia, W. B. Saunders Company, 1982.

37. Lieberson, S., and Mendes, D. G.: Walking in bed. Phys. Ther., 59:1112, 1979.

38. Vallbona, C., Spencer, W. A., Cardus, D., and Dale, J. W.: Control of orthostatic hypotension in quadriplegic patients with the use of a pressure suit. Arch. Phys. Med. Rehabil, 44:7-18, 1963.

39. Hantman, D. A., Vogel, J. M., Donaldson, C. L., Friedman, R. J., Goldsmith, R. S., and Hulley, S. B.: Attempts to prevent disuse osteoporosis by treatment with calcitonin, longitudinal compression, and supplementary calcium and phosphorus. J. Clin. Endocrinol. Metab., 36:845-858, 1973.

40. Hulley, S. B., Vogel, J. M., Donaldson, C. L., Bayers, J. H., Friedman, R. J., and Rosen, S. N.: The effect of supplemental oral phosphate on the bone mineral changes during prolonged bed rest. J. Clin. Invest., 50:2506-2518, 1971.

Note: Page numbers in italics represent illustrations; *t* indicates tables.